KT-462-358

0912748

WITHDRAWN
FROM LIBRARY

BRITISH MEDICAL ASSOCIATION

ATLAS OF
IMAGING
IN SPORTS
MEDICINE

ATLAS OF
IMAGING
IN SPORTS
MEDICINE

SECOND EDITION

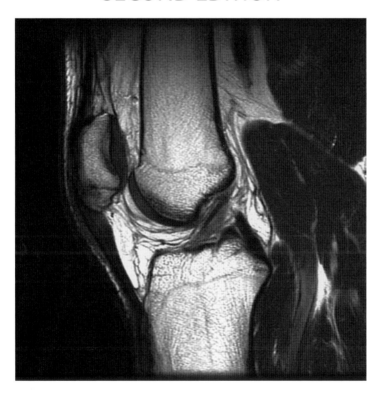

JOCK ANDERSON & JOHN W READ

BILL BREIDAHL, GUS FERGUSON, JAMES LINKLATER,
PHIL LUCAS, JENNIE NOAKES, TONY PEDUTO

The **McGraw·Hill** Companies

Sydney New York San Francisco Auckland
Bangkok Bogotá Caracas Hong Kong
Kuala Lumpur Lisbon London Madrid
Mexico City Milan New Delhi San Juan
Seoul Singapore Taipei Toronto

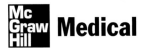

Notice

Medicine is an ever-changing science. As new research and clinical experience broaden our knowledge, changes in treatment and drug therapy are required. The editors and the publisher of this work have checked with sources believed to be reliable in their efforts to provide information that is complete and generally in accord with the standards accepted at the time of publication. However, in view of the possibility of human error or changes in medical sciences, neither the editors, nor the publisher, nor any other party who has been involved in the preparation or publication of this work warrants that the information contained herein is in every respect accurate or complete. Readers are encouraged to confirm the information contained herein with other sources. For example, and in particular, readers are advised to check the product information sheet included in the package of each drug they plan to administer to be certain that the information contained in this book is accurate and that changes have not been made in the recommended dose or in the contraindications for administration. This recommendation is of particular importance in connection with new or infrequently used drugs.

First edition 1998

Images and text © 2008 Dr I. F. Anderson and Dr J. Read
Illustrations and design © 2008 McGraw-Hill Australia Pty Ltd
Additional owners of copyright are acknowledged in on page credits, at the end of each chapter and on the general acknowledgments page.

Every effort has been made to trace and acknowledge copyrighted material. The authors and publishers tender their apologies should any infringement have occurred.

Reproduction and communication for educational purposes
The Australian *Copyright Act 1968* (the Act) allows a maximum of one chapter or 10% of the pages of this work, whichever is the greater, to be reproduced and/or communicated by any educational institution for its educational purposes provided that the institution (or the body that administers it) has sent a Statutory Educational notice to Copyright Agency Limited (CAL) and been granted a licence. For details of statutory educational and other copyright licences contact: Copyright Agency Limited, Level 15, 233 Castlereagh Street, Sydney NSW 2000. Telephone: (02) 9394 7600. Website: www.copyright.com.au

Reproduction and communication for other purposes
Apart from any fair dealing for the purposes of study, research, criticism or review, as permitted under the Act, no part of this publication may be reproduced, distributed or transmitted in any form or by any means, or stored in a database or retrieval system, without the written permission of McGraw-Hill Australia including, but not limited to, any network or other electronic storage.

Enquiries should be made to the publisher via www.mcgraw-hill.com.au or marked for the attention of rights and permissions at the address below.

National Library of Australia Cataloguing-in-Publication Data
Anderson, Ian F., 1941–.
Atlas of imaging in sports medicine.

2nd ed.
Bibliography.
Includes index.
ISBN 9780074715840 (pbk.).

1. Sports medicine – Atlases. 2. Sports injuries – Diagnosis. 3. Sports injuries – Imaging – Atlases. I. Read, John W., 1956–. II. Title.

617.1027

Published in Australia by
McGraw-Hill Australia Pty Ltd
Level 2, 82 Waterloo Road, North Ryde NSW 2113
Publisher: Nicole Meehan
Developmental Editor: Hollie Zondanos
Managing Editor: Kathryn Fairfax
Production Editor: Kim Ross
Copy Editor: Caroline Hunter, Burrumundi Pty Ltd
Illustrator: John Read, and Porcellato and Craig
Typesetter: Midland Typesetters
Proofreader: Pam Dunne
Indexer: Max McMaster
Printed in China on 105 gsm matt art by CTPS Limited

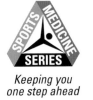

*Keeping you
one step ahead*

The **McGraw·Hill** Companies

Foreword

Associate Professor Jock Anderson and Dr John Read have, again, contributed to the science and advancement of imaging in sports medicine with the publication of this second edition of their book *Atlas of Imaging in Sports Medicine*. Jock and John have been assisted by a small group of fellow Australian musculoskeletal radiologists who have each contributed to an area of specific expertise.

The second edition of the Atlas summarises the current state of diagnostic imaging in sports medicine. The authors have preserved the feel of the initial Atlas and the previous emphasis on high-quality images has been taken to an even higher level. Both common and uncommon conditions are discussed and illustrated—embracing all commonly utilised imaging methods. This is important, as now, more than ever, the sports medicine practitioner requires a sound understanding of the appropriate roles, strengths and weaknesses of all imaging methods.

The book is well structured with a valuable introductory chapter discussing the basic principles of imaging and pathology in sports-related injuries. The following chapters provide a comprehensive overview of the conditions that occur in sport, by individual anatomical areas, with a final chapter discussing various diagnostic and therapeutic interventions.

Pictures are a powerful teaching tool; and, in the Atlas, more than 2200 well-selected, high-resolution images of sports injuries provide a unique learning resource and create lasting memories. A thorough understanding of sports injuries is aided by the use of numerous anatomical line drawings and a discussion that routinely includes both injury biomechanics and key clinical features. As with the first edition, this book is a tremendous adjunct to the clinical understanding and management of the injured athlete.

Mervyn J Cross
OAM, MB BS (Syd), MD (NSW), FRACS, FAOA, FASMF
Chairman, North Sydney Orthopaedic and Sports Medicine Centre
Director, Australian Institute of Musculo-Skeletal Research
Former chairman, Australian Society of Orthopaedic Surgeons
Member, International Hall of Fame of the American
    Orthopaedic Society of Sports Medicine

Brief contents

Contents

Preface

The authors are pleased to find copies of the first edition of the Atlas on the book-shelves of radiology reporting rooms, and in sports medicine and physiotherapy practices, throughout Australia and New Zealand. They hope that this new edition of *Atlas of Imaging in Sports Medicine* will be similarly embraced as it goes forward to reach an even wider international audience. When the first edition was written, the experiences of 15 years of sports medicine in Australia were beginning to trickle through the medical literature. The initial edition highlighted the potential of ultrasound and MRI, acknowledged the role of nuclear medicine and emphasised the pivotal role of a high standard of plain films in diagnosis. Sport, sports medicine and imaging technology have all altered significantly since that time and an update to the Atlas is well overdue.

A decade has passed since the first edition was written and the volume of sports medicine literature has undergone an extraordinary expansion as our understanding of injuries, tissue response and appropriate management have increased. This has occurred against a background of continuing change in sport at the community level. One major change has been the large amounts of money that are now poured into professional sport through contracts and sponsorships. Many of the previously traditional amateur activities have become full-time occupations. An injury is now viewed as dollars lost while the athlete is sidelined, placing pressure on all members of the medical team, including the radiologist. A quick, accurate diagnosis is essential for the implementation of appropriate management and early identification of complications. Working at the Sydney 2000 Olympics and the 2003 Rugby World Cup provided the authors with a valuable opportunity to personally experience the pressure that may be created by managers, trainers and athletes, themselves, following an injury. At the same time, the recreational athlete also continues to push for an early return to sport.

An additional chapter on intervention has been included in this second edition of the Atlas in response to an increasing demand for imaging-guided diagnostic and therapeutic procedures in the management of sports injuries. This chapter not only discusses the techniques of image-guided intervention, but it also reviews the ethical and legal considerations that accompany such procedures.

The authors have been extremely fortunate to work in the unique learning environment of the North Sydney Orthopaedic and Sports Medicine Centre and would like to acknowledge this association. The on-going close clinical interaction with the skilled sports physicians and surgeons of this institution over many years has provided the rich framework of experience and perspective on which much of the Atlas is based.

The authors

Associate Professor Jock Anderson MB BS, FRANZCR, FRACSP (Hon)

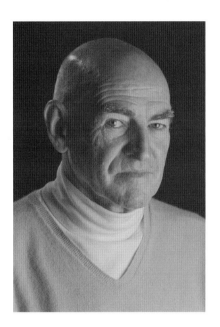

Jock Anderson has been involved in sports medicine imaging since 1985, with the development of Sports Imaging, a specialty musculoskeletal imaging practice. Since that time, sports medicine has enjoyed a remarkable growth through the creation of The Australian College of Sports Physicians and Jock has been intimately involved in the development and teaching of the imaging skills that are necessary for the management of sports injuries. Jock was awarded an honorary fellowship in this new college in 1993.

Jock is the Associate Professor in the sports medicine program at the University of NSW and a member of the International Skeletal Society and the Australasian Musculoskeletal Imaging Group.

Jock has been involved in many facets of sport and in 2000 he was awarded the Australian Sports Medal for his contribution to Australian swimming. He has also worked as a radiologist with the NSW and Australian Rugby Union.

In 1998, Jock was appointed director of medical imaging at the Sydney 2000 Olympic and Paralympic Games, attended the Winter Olympics as an observer in 2002 and was then appointed director of medical imaging for the Rugby World Cup in Australia, 2003.

Jock enjoys teaching, having lectured extensively both nationally and internationally, and has been author or coauthor of three previous texts on sports medicine, and now works as a radiologist with Castlereagh Imaging.

Dr John Read MB BS, FRANZCR, DDU

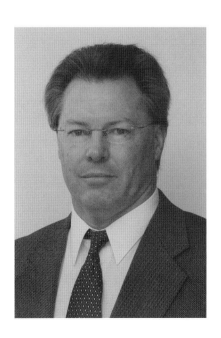

John Read is a skilled and dedicated musculoskeletal radiologist with a broad multi-modality imaging expertise, and a particular interest in the management of sports injuries. In the early years of the emergence of sports medicine, John recognised the specific challenges of making an early and precise diagnosis. Using his expertise in general ultrasound, knowledge of anatomy and interest in histopathology, John adapted and developed high-resolution musculoskeletal ultrasound.

Working with Jock Anderson and Jennie Noakes at Sports Imaging, John Read has played a pivotal role in the development of new ultrasound techniques that he has pioneered, refined and disseminated by extensive teaching—influencing clinical practice throughout Australia and New Zealand. His achievements include the development of an ultrasound methodology that has come to find an important role in the diagnosis and management of chronic athletic groin pain. Resulting from his influence, ultrasound is now commonly used to guide interventional procedures.

He participated in the imaging team at the Sydney 2000 Olympic and Paralympic Games, has previously served as both member and chairman of the RANZCR ultrasound committee, and currently holds an appointment as Conjoint Lecturer in the School of Medical Sciences at the University of NSW.

Chapter associate authors

Dr Bill Breidahl MB BS, FMGEMS, MRCP, FRANZCR

Bill Breidahl is a medical and radiological graduate, from Western Australia, who obtained an MRCP prior to radiology training. He is an outstanding musculoskeletal radiologist, with a special interest in musculoskeletal ultrasound and MRI. Bill currently works at the Royal Perth Hospital and as a partner in the Perth Radiological Clinic.

His career has been studded with awards, including the H. R. Sear prize in his final radiological exams, in recognition for the most outstanding performance in these Australia-wide exams. He subsequently received the Thomas Baker study fellowship to assist in his fellowship training overseas—also an Australia-wide competition. As a consequence of this award, Bill completed a musculoskeletal imaging fellowship at the University of Michigan.

Highlights of Bill's career so far include an appointment as the attending radiologist to all athletes at the Atlanta Olympic Games in 1996 and he was a radiologist at the Sydney 2000 Olympics. Bill supervised radiological services to the 2003 Rugby World Cup games held in Perth. He is currently president of the Australasian Musculoskeletal Imaging Group.

Dr Russell (Gus) Ferguson MB ChB, FRANZCR, FRCR

Gus Ferguson graduated from the Medical School at Otago University, New Zealand. He then completed his postgraduate radiological studies at the same university; and, on graduation, Gus was selected as the McKenzie Research Scholar to University College Hospital in London, allowing Gus to pursue further studies in the United Kingdom. He obtained a fellowship of the Royal College of Radiologists.

On returning to New Zealand, Gus was a consultant radiologist at the Dunedin Public Hospital. On moving to Brisbane in 1974, Gus has worked in private radiological practice, predominantly at St Andrew's War Memorial Hospital in Brisbane and Allamanda Private Hospital on the Gold Coast. He currently works at Nambour Selangor Private Hospital on the Sunshine Coast.

Gus has developed considerable skills and reputation as an interventionalist, with a particular interest in pain management. This subspecialty includes performing image-guided procedures, spinal intervention, spinal biopsy, percutaneous radiofrequency neurotomy (PRN) and other pain management procedures. A number of these procedures have been developed by Gus and his contribution to the book is greatly appreciated.

Dr James Linklater MB BS (Hons), B Med Sci, FRANZCR

James Linklater is a musculoskeletal radiologist at Sports Imaging in Sydney and St Vincent's Clinic. He trained in Sydney before undertaking a fellowship in musculoskeletal radiology at the Hospital for Special Surgery in New York, where, under the supervision of Dr Hollis Potter, he gained experience in musculoskeletal MRI. He is currently working for Castlereagh Imaging.

James is an enthusiastic presenter and has numerous papers to his credit. He acts as a reviewer for *Australasian Radiology* and *British Journal of Sports Medicine*, and is a Clinical Lecturer in the Sports Medicine Program at the University of NSW.

Being an habitual attendee of meetings, James belongs to the following radiological organisations:

- Australian Musculoskeletal Imaging Group
- International Cartilage Research Society
- Society of Skeletal Radiologists
- International Society of Arthroscopy, Knee Surgery and Orthopaedic Sports Medicine
- American Roentgen Ray Society
- Radiological Society of North America.

Dr Phil Lucas MB BS (Hons), FRANZCR

Phil Lucas is a talented musculoskeletal radiologist with a particular interest in sports medicine. Following undergraduate radiological training at The Royal North Shore Hospital in Sydney, Phil studied in the United States of America, obtaining a fellowship in musculoskeletal imaging at the University of Virginia, Charlottesville, under the supervision of Dr Phoebe Kaplan. Although Phil has a special interest in MRI, he is also extremely competent in all imaging methods.

He has a close involvement with sport, working as a radiologist with NSW Waratah Rugby and Manly Warringah Rugby League Club, and he was an important member of the medical imaging team for the Sydney 2000 Olympic and Paralympic Games.

Phil also has an involvement with education, and is a Clinical Lecturer at the University of NSW.

Jennie Noakes, B.Med, FRANZCR

Jennie Noakes is a musculoskeletal radiologist who has been working at Sports Imaging at the North Sydney Orthopaedic and Sports Medicine Centre since the early 1990s. At that time, Jennie enthusiastically applied her ultrasound skills to the diagnosis of sports injuries and this special interest has now evolved into a subspecialty. Jennie currently works for Castlereagh Imaging. Jennie is held in high regard for her competence with all imaging methods and has earned great respect for her musculoskeletal knowledge. Her contribution to the second edition of the Atlas has been greatly appreciated.

Jennie was a valuable member of the musculoskeletal imaging team at the Sydney 2000 Olympic and Paralympic Games.

Dr Tony Peduto MB BS, FRANZCR

Following his radiological training at The Children's Hospital and Westmead Hospital in Sydney, Tony Peduto expanded his interest in MRI with an MRI fellowship at Northwestern University, Chicago. He has subspecialised in both musculoskeletal and body MR imaging applications and has developed a particular interest in musculoskeletal anatomy as depicted by MRI.

Tony is director and supervising radiologist of the MRI unit at Westmead Hospital and head of the MRI Unit of Brain Dynamics Centre, Millennium Institute, Sydney University.

Tony is also involved in education at an undergraduate, postgraduate and fellowship level and is coordinator of medical student teaching, Western Clinical School, Sydney University and senior examiner in MSK, for the College of Radiology.

As the recipient of the 2005 Bill Hare Fellowship of the Royal Australian and New Zealand College of Radiology, Tony spent a year working as a research scholar at the University of California, San Diego. Tony is a radiologist with Castlereagh Imaging.

Acknowledgments

The production of a book such as this has required a contribution by many people. Jock Anderson and John Read are extremely grateful for the help that they received.

For Jock Anderson, the production of the Atlas was made difficult by illness; and a team of fellow musculoskeletal radiologists generously supplied images and time and provided a required momentum to the project during this difficult period. A brief biography of these radiologists has been provided. Jock would particularly like to give thanks to his neurologist, Dr Ron Joffe, and to acknowledge his role in permitting the book to be finished.

Peter Freeman of Freedom Graphics has worked tirelessly preparing images for publication and the extraordinary high standard of his work can be seen throughout the book. In addition, the artistic skills of John Read are in evidence in the many clear and informative illustrations, produced together with the publisher's illustrator. Special thanks goes to Dr Fiona Bonar, pathologist at Douglass-Hanly-Moir Pathology and a recognised authority with a particular interest in musculoskeletal disease. Fiona made an important contribution to the introductory chapter—Basic principles.

Many of the 2000, plus, images have been acquired from hospitals and private practices. The specific source of images has been acknowledged at the end of each chapter. In general, images have been supplied from The Royal North Shore Hospital by Dr David Brazier, Janeen Gibbs and Sandy Huggett. Many images have also originated from Gosford Hospital; and special thanks must be given to Raouli Risti, Barry Morgan, Bob Broug, Adam Loveday and Adam Hill. The authors are also grateful to Richard Moir at Hornsby Hospital for his help in digitising hard-copy images, and to the librarian at The Brisbane Private Hospital, Robyn Backholm, who was incredibly helpful in finding obscure references.

The majority of private practice images have been produced at Sports Imaging, a Castlereagh imaging practice, although others have come from other private practices owned by the I-med network and Symbion Health Ltd. The authors are grateful to these companies and acknowledge their role in this production.

Basic principles
Jock Anderson and John Read

1

The relentless pursuit of peak biological performance in sport requires the support of a skilled medical team to supply care and nurturing to our athletes. Within this team, the sports physician plays a pivotal role. When an injury occurs, the implications can be devastating for both professional and amateur athletes alike. As a consequence, sports medicine can often be a demanding discipline in which to work.

Characteristically, the athlete's hopes and expectations of management outcomes are high and the results of the medical support team's efforts are certain to be rapidly and severely tested. The successful management of sports injuries hinges upon many factors, the first of which is a fast and accurate diagnosis. Since medical imaging is an important member of this management team, it is vital that the sports physician and imaging specialty have a close working relationship and that the sports physician has a good understanding of the strengths, weaknesses and appropriate utilisation of the various imaging tools that are now available in clinical practice. Conversely, the radiologist requires a sound knowledge of the probable injury that results from particular biomechanics or an activity and how imaging can best help to reach a diagnosis.

The scope of sports medicine

Sports medicine is a diverse discipline that deals with conditions arising in individuals of all ages and abilities. At the extremes, the spectrum of injury can range from acute macro-trauma occurring in body contact and high-velocity sports to more subtle and chronic musculoskeletal problems of insidious onset. Sports medicine is becoming increasingly subspecialised as the volume of experience and knowledge increases. For example, paediatric sports medicine and sports medicine for athletes with disabilities are growing subspecialties. Not surprisingly, the same types of injuries that occur in sport can also be seen in other forms of repetitive physical activity and many aspects of sports medicine overflow into community medicine. Other expanding areas of subspecialised clinical practice include occupational medicine, military medicine and performing arts medicine.

Basic concepts

It must never be forgotten that imaging alone does not replace or reduce the need for a thorough clinical evaluation. It is the clinical assessment, coupled with a knowledge of the relevant anatomy and an understanding of the likely pathological process, which remains the cornerstone of accurate diagnosis. Only when a provisional clinical diagnosis has been reached can a rational decision be made about the need for additional tests and, when the results of such tests become available, can these be correctly interpreted.

Paradoxically, as imaging technology becomes more sophisticated and sensitive, the importance of clinical judgement in determining the relevance of any reported findings actually increases. For example, an incidental developmental variant may be demonstrated and asymptomatic age-related changes are commonly seen. With advancing age and a history of high-level sporting activity, incidental degenerative changes are increasingly prevalent. Studies have shown that subclinical pathology is present in a large proportion of asymptomatic or minimally symptomatic athletes (Sher et al. 1995; Orchard et al. 1998; Tempelhof et al. 1999; Haims et al. 2000; Cook et al. 2000; Beattie et al. 2005). There exists a natural temptation to overplay the significance of an abnormal test result. To add to the confusion, it has long been recognised that even gross pathological derangements, such as markedly osteo-arthritic joints, intervertebral disc protrusions and rotator cuff tears, can sometimes be completely asymptomatic. Consequently, the physician must always remember to 'treat the patient, not the scan'.

It is vitally important to provide a request form to the radiologist that offers a short guiding differential diagnosis or asks specific questions that the radiologist must attempt to answer. This significantly increases the likelihood of the detection of abnormalities by helping the radiologist to suggest an appropriate imaging protocol. Also, an informative request form focuses the radiologist's search pattern, which decreases the risk of overlooking subtle or equivocal findings. A relevant report depends upon a relevant request. In the language of computer science, 'garbage in = garbage out'.

When to image

Although imaging can be an extremely useful diagnostic tool, it should be employed only if the results can be used to guide management. In sports medicine, a specific anatomical diagnosis is not always required and does not necessarily constitute best practice (Orchard et al. 2005). For example, mild-to-moderate back pain in young adults without neurological signs can be safely and appropriately managed in the first instance with physiotherapy alone, irrespective of the actual anatomical diagnosis (Bigos and Davis 1996).

Imaging will play a role in any of the following circumstances:

- when the clinical diagnosis is uncertain and management may be affected
- when the clinical diagnosis is obvious but management decisions may change depending on the extent of injury or presence of complications
- when treatment has failed and the reasons for this are unclear
- when clinical 'red flags' (danger signals) are present, and sinister or systemic pathology must be excluded
- when objective documentation of disease existence, progression or resolution is required. This may occur in medicolegal situations
- when pre-operative localisation or planning information is needed.

Clinical red flags

It is not uncommon for sinister or systemic disease to first present as an apparent overuse or sports-related injury, and the sports physician must be on constant guard for this possibility (see Fig. 1.1). Therefore, before embarking on a trial of conservative management, imaging can play an important role in avoiding delayed or missed diagnoses if any of the following 'red flags' are present:

- if the patient's age is greater than 50
- if injury or disability is disproportionate to the mechanism
- if constitutional symptoms are present (e.g. generally unwell, fever, night sweats, weight loss)
- if there are unusually complex, bizarre or atypical symptoms
- if known risk factors are present (diabetes, osteoporosis, immune deficiency or steroid therapy)
- if symptoms are worse when supine or at night, or are associated with early morning stiffness
- if there is an unusually complex or sinister past history (e.g. various joints affected, previous malignancy)
- if there is a family history of inflammatory joint conditions
- if there are additional clues in other body systems (e.g. skin rash, progressive neurological deficit, urinary symptoms)
- if there is a poor response to therapy (see Fig. 1.2).

Which test?

In recent years, constantly improving imaging technology has significantly expanded our diagnostic capabilities. This has also made the choice of exactly which test to order, and when to use each one, increasingly difficult and somewhat challenging for the non-specialist. The medical literature offers few clear guidelines, but in everyday clinical practice a variety of factors can influence the final decision. These factors include:

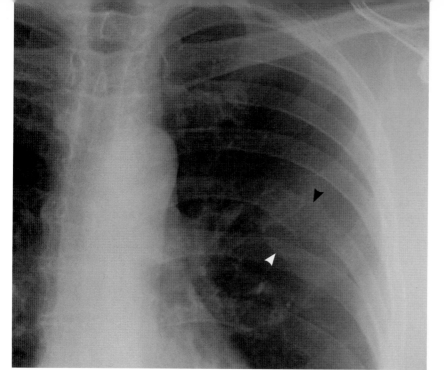

◄ Fig. 1.1(a) This case is an example of a clinical 'red flag'. A 60-year-old kayaker presented with localised left-sided rib pain. There was no history of acute injury and a stress fracture was provisionally diagnosed. A plain film showed mild expansion of the seventh rib (black arrowhead), with associated thickening of the extrapleural soft tissue (white arrowhead). This appearance was not consistent with a simple stress fracture and a computed tomography (CT) scan was performed.

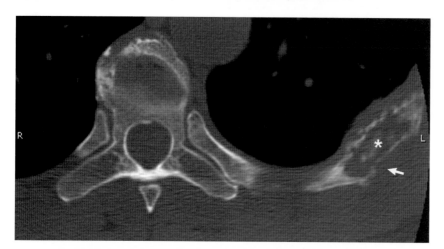

◄ (b) The CT scan demonstrated the presence of a destructive rib lesion (asterisk) with a complicating pathologic fracture (arrow). A biopsy revealed lymphoma.

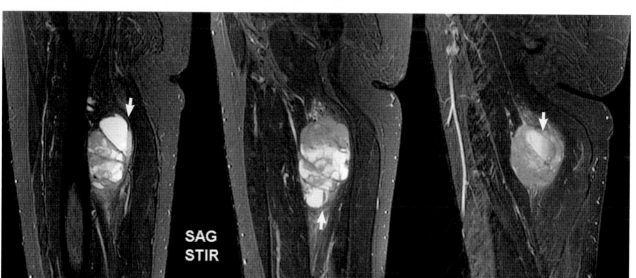

▲ Fig. 1.2 Poor response to therapy is another 'red flag'. A 35-year-old runner presented with acute thigh pain, and clinically the provisional diagnosis was a hamstring tear. An initial trial of conservative management did not produce the improvement that would normally be expected. Imaging was then requested. A plain film showed only vague and non-specific soft-tissue swelling. Magnetic resonance imaging (MRI) revealed a complex soft-tissue mass within the adductor magnus muscle, which proved to be a sarcoma. The mass contained haemorrhagic locules showing multiple red cell sedimentation levels (arrows).

- the provisional clinical diagnosis
- the local availability of appropriate imaging equipment and expertise
- patient considerations such as cost, convenience and compliance
- safety considerations such as patient age, radiation dose and contrast sensitivity
- costs such as those to the sporting body, tax payer or insurance company.

With few exceptions, whenever imaging is required, the work up should commence with plain radiographs (Lau 2001). Plain films provide a comprehensive anatomical overview in a user-friendly panoramic format at low cost and at an acceptable radiation dose. When combined with the clinical assessment, plain films alone will often allow a reasonable provisional diagnosis and management plan to be formulated without the need for more sophisticated tests. Even if the injury appears to involve soft tissue alone, plain films may still help to detect important background features that other tests may miss. These features may include soft-tissue calcifications, foreign bodies, bone spurs, accessory centres of ossification, clinically unsuspected fractures, old injuries and other predisposing conditions. Normal radiographs are not a waste of time, as they help to exclude or greatly reduce the likelihood of many conditions. Lastly, a failure to obtain plain films can lead to significant errors in the interpretation of other more complicated tests such as MRI, isotope bone scans and ultrasound. Consequently, it can be a mistake to bypass the traditional plain x-ray in favour of the more sophisticated tests.

Although plain x-ray may be the only imaging test required for the vast majority of sports injuries, some cases do require further imaging to reach a diagnosis and to help with the selection of management strategies. Every imaging method has particular strengths and weaknesses, and for the physician wondering which test to perform next, it is useful to think first of the individual anatomical structure and tissue type that may have been injured. It is only then, with additional consideration of cost, safety and convenience, that the most appropriate method can be chosen.

Bone

Nuclear bone scanning provides a 'functional' image of skeletal osteoblastic activity that is sensitive but non-specific. Bone scans are best used in sports medicine to identify and localise a bone or joint abnormality prior to targeted characterisation by another method. They may also be used to diagnose a few specific conditions, such as a long bone stress fracture, avascular necrosis, osteitis pubis and reflex sympathetic dystrophy (see Fig. 1.24 on page 19). A triple-phase study should be performed. After intravenous injection of the isotope, images are acquired immediately to show perfusion changes (the 'angiogram' phase). A few minutes later this is followed by the acquisition of images that depict the accumulation of isotope in vascular areas (the 'blood pool' phase). Finally, a few hours later, delayed images will show the distribution and metabolic activity of skeletal osteoblasts. About 80% of bone scans will be positive within the first 24 hours of bone injury, and 95% will be positive within 72 hours (Matin 1979).

The clinical context will heavily influence the interpretation of nuclear scans, since a number of pathologic processes such as degeneration, trauma, infection, tumour and osteonecrosis can produce similar appearances. Stress injuries of long bones are often characteristic, but similar pathology in small bones, especially those of the feet, may be less diagnostic and require further assessment. A combination of CT and MRI is usually necessary in this situation to differentiate bone stress reaction from a stress fracture or synovitis. It should also be remembered that soft-tissue disease may cause a localised increase in the metabolic activity of adjacent bone, producing bone scan findings that can be mistaken for primary bone pathology.

CT scanning is the ideal imaging method whenever cortical or trabecular architecture of bone or the bony anatomy of complex joints is to be examined. CT is better than MRI at showing fracture lines, small calcifications, loose bodies, subtle bone erosions and bone mineral loss or destruction. CT has the superior ability of resolving bony detail and is therefore the preferred method characterising a cortical fracture or an osteoid osteoma.

Although MRI resolves bone mineral poorly, it demonstrates the cellular marrow space superbly and is the best imaging method to characterise or determine the full extent of bone marrow pathology. This capability gives MRI a special place in the evaluation of osteochondral injury, avascular necrosis, bone bruising, bone stress, transient osteoporosis of the hip and bone tumours. MRI has a sensitivity equivalent to isotope bone scanning for the detection of bone stress, but provides considerably more anatomical information.

Joint

Articular cortical fractures and loose bodies are best resolved by CT. Injury to fibrocartilage such as a meniscal tear is generally best imaged by either standard non-contrast MRI or MR arthrography, which involves an intra-articular injection of gadolinium contrast agent. Conventional arthrography is now rarely performed. Multislice CT arthrography is another valid technique, but involves exposure to ionising radiation and provides only limited subsurface and parameniscal information. Ultrasound is effective in the demonstration of meniscal or parameniscal cysts.

Abnormalities of the surface of hyaline articular cartilage are most accurately resolved by CT arthrography or MR arthrography. However, these tests are invasive and do not reveal changes beneath the cartilage surface. In actual clinical practice, standard proton density-weighted fast spin-echo MRI sequences designed to optimise the signal contrast between cartilage and joint fluid provide both moderate sensitivity and the most practical routine approach to cartilage assessment. The MRI grading system for articular cartilage abnormalities is shown in Fig. 1.3.

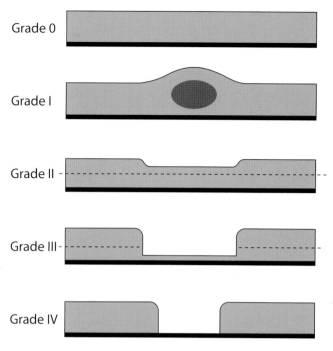

◀ **Fig. 1.3(a)** Schematic representation of the Modified Outerbridge classification used for MRI grading of chondral lesions.

Grade 0 = normal
Grade I = swelling or softening with signal increased or decreased
Grade II = superficial fibrillations or irregularities, loss of thickness less than 50%
Grade III = deep fibrillation or ulceration with loss of thickness greater than 50%
Grade IV = exposure of subchondral bone with associated marrow oedema

Source: Adapted from Drape et al. (1998).

▼ **(b)** This axial PD-weighted MR image of chondromalacia patellae illustrates the grading of chondral damage. There is focal chondral swelling and softening at the medial facet (Grade I change, arrowhead), and focal Grade II chondral surface fibrillation with underlying chondral softening at the lateral facet (arrow).

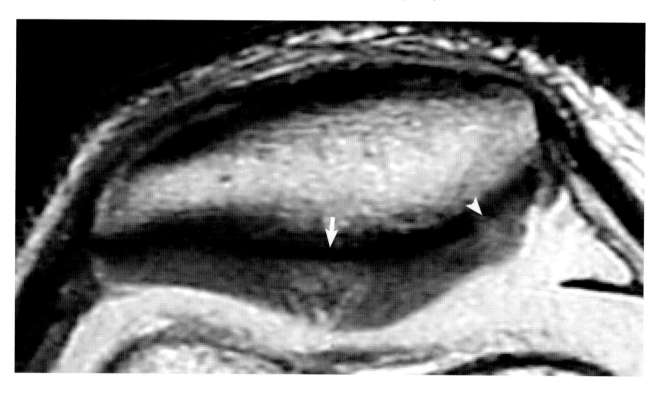

Capsular injuries are generally best imaged by either standard MRI or MR arthrography, particularly where deep joints such as the shoulder and hip are concerned. Standard MRI resolves the pericapsular structures and spaces in addition to the capsule itself very well, whereas MR arthrography provides an element of joint distension that can sometimes reveal the full extent of any capsular tear more sensitively. Minor capsuloligamentous injuries that produce symptomatic synovial cysts and mild localised post-traumatic synovitis are sometimes better appreciated by ultrasound than MRI. Small abnormalities tend to merge with the normal fluid signal of adjacent joint recesses on MRI and may not be seen. The loss of joint volume that occurs with shoulder capsulitis is best demonstrated by conventional arthrography, although the diagnostic value of this observation is negligible in clinical practice.

Ultrasound is an accurate and inexpensive solution for imaging conditions such as transient synovitis of the hip or septic arthritis where the aim of imaging is simply to detect a joint effusion or synovitis (see Fig. 1.4). Ultrasound also provides a simple method of accurately guiding a percutaneous needle aspiration procedure for fluid analysis.

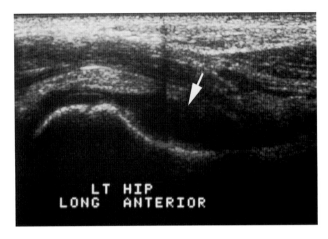

▲ **Fig. 1.4** Transient synovitis of the hip is shown by ultrasound. This is a fast, safe, painless and inexpensive method of detecting hip joint effusion. An arrow indicates fluid distending the inferior joint recess along the anterior aspect of the femoral neck.

When the role of further imaging is to assess non-weightbearing joint alignment, as with patellofemoral tracking or sternoclavicular joint dislocation, CT scanning is generally the preferred imaging method. This can include 3D image reconstructions if required.

Tendon

Provided adequate operator expertise is locally available, abnormalities of superficial tendons such as the Achilles and patellar tendons are generally best imaged with ultrasound. This imaging method is relatively inexpensive and can demonstrate the fine internal microarchitecture of a tendon. Compared to ultrasound, MRI has poorer spatial resolution but better diagnostic performance at depth and is therefore preferred for examining tendons that are deep or provide difficult acoustic access. Such tendons include the iliopsoas and thigh adductors. Importantly, the real-time imaging capabilities of ultrasound can also be used to assess the dynamics of tendon instability and tendon adhesion. The reliability of ultrasound is limited by operator dependence, a target depth from the skin surface of more than 3–4 cm, and poor acoustic or difficult transducer access. In these situations MRI may be a better alternative.

Tendon tears can be described on imaging according to a number of characteristics (see Fig. 1.5):

- age—acute, chronic, indeterminate
- size—partial thickness or full thickness, full width or partial width
- orientation—longitudinal or transverse
- visibility at operation—intrasubstance or surface breach
- position—insertional, juxta-insertional, mid-segment, proximal or musculotendinous junction
- degree of fibre retraction—retracted (with the gap measured), non-retracted
- other features—underlying tendinopathy, clean or ragged margin, complication

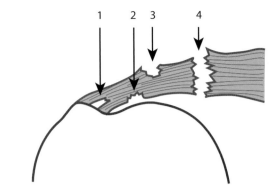

▲ **Fig. 1.5 (a)** Examples of tendon tear description.
1 = intrasubstance insertional tear
2 = articular-side, partial-thickness juxta-insertional tear
3 = bursal-side, partial-thickness mid-segment tear
4 = full-thickness tear

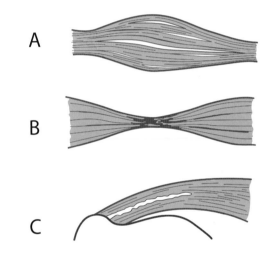

▲ **(b)**
A = degenerative longitudinal split tear
B = chronic tear with attenuation
C = intrasubstance lamination tear

Source: Adapted from Chhem and Cardinal (1999) and Rosenberg et al. (1988).

Ligament

Most ligament injuries are managed conservatively. Those that do require intervention are generally diagnosed clinically and graded on the basis of instability at physical examination. Therefore, in the acute or subacute setting, the primary role of imaging is usually to delineate other associated injuries that could alter management, such as meniscal tears or osteochondral fractures. MRI is the preferred imaging test in this situation, as it not only shows ligament well, but also demonstrates the related bony attachments, joint spaces and chondral surfaces. The MRI grading system for ligament tears is given in Table 1.1. Superficial ligaments that are not acoustically obscured by overlying bone can also be demonstrated by ultrasound and this imaging method is occasionally useful in the more chronic setting of persistent pain following a sprain (see Fig. 1.6).

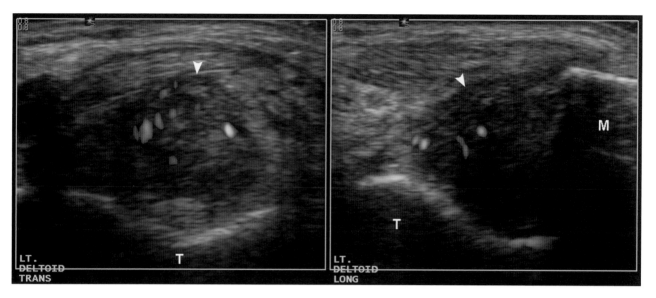

▲ **Fig. 1.6** An ultrasound examination of a chronically symptomatic deltoid ligament following impaction injury. The patient complained of persistent medial ankle pain and tenderness more than 10 months after an ankle inversion injury. The clinically suspected diagnosis was tibialis posterior tendinopathy, but transverse and long-axis Power Doppler ultrasound images instead demonstrated a thickened hypoechoic deltoid ligament (arrowheads) with convex bulge of the outer surface and intrasubstance hyperaemia. Talus = T. Medial malleolus = M.

Table 1.1 The grading system for ligament tears

Grade I	Pathology	= microscopic tearing (strain)
	Clinical	= tenderness but no ligament laxity
	MRI	= normal ligament thickness but increased periligamentous signal
Grade II	Pathology	= partial tear
	Clinical	= some ligamentous laxity but firm end-point
	MRI	= ligament thickening ± partial discontinuity, increased signal
Grade III	Pathology	= complete tear
	Clinical	= increased ligament laxity and no identifiable end-point
	MRI	= complete ligament discontinuity + oedema and haemorrhage

Muscle

Injuries that involve muscle bellies or musculotendinous junctions are best evaluated by MRI (note the grading system in Table 1.2). Ultrasound is also quite capable of demonstrating most Grade II–Grade III muscle tears. Ultrasound will accurately detect fluid collections, such as haematomata or post-traumatic muscle cysts (see Fig. 1.7). Any subsequent percutaneous needle aspiration procedure can also be guided by ultrasound imaging. However, the appreciation of low-grade muscle injuries by ultrasound can be difficult. MRI is clearly better at detecting oedema associated with low-grade muscle injuries (strains) and also gives an elegant panoramic demonstration of large-area muscles, allowing a more confident and precise determination of injury location and extent than ultrasound. Muscle ruptures due to direct compressive trauma occur at the site of applied force, whereas tears arising from distraction overload typically occur at the musculotendinous junction.

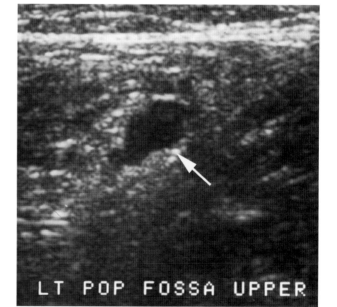

▲ **Fig. 1.7** A post-traumatic muscle cyst demonstrated by ultrasound. An ex-runner with a distant past history of a biceps femoris muscle tear complained of persisting posterior knee pain and was able to localise his pain precisely to one point at the upper end of the popliteal fossa. A small muscle cyst (arrowed) was evident when the ultrasound transducer was placed directly over this point.

Table 1.2 The grading system for muscle tears

Grade I	Pathology	=	microscopic tearing (strain), heals without defect
	Clinical	=	pain and tenderness, but no loss of function
	MRI	=	increased signal, no fibre discontinuity, perifascial hyperintensity
Grade II	Pathology	=	partial tear
	Clinical	=	often inseparable from Grade I tears, some loss of function
	MRI	=	increased signal, some fibres torn (irregular and slightly separated), haematoma at tear point, perifascial extension of fluid signal
Grade III	Pathology	=	complete tear
	Clinical	=	complete or near-complete loss of function, retraction, spasm
	MRI	=	complete muscle discontinuity, retracted tear margin, haematoma

Source: Blankenbaker and De Smet (2004).

Nerve

Nerve compressions arising at the spinal level are best imaged with CT scanning or MRI, although myelography still has a role in the demonstration of adhesive arachnoiditis. Nerve compression arising at a more peripheral level generally does not require imaging, but both MRI and ultrasound can image major nerve trunks and be used to exclude an intrinsic or extrinsic space-occupying lesion whenever this is clinically suspected. Occasionally, imaging can be helpful in the diagnosis of tunnel syndromes.

Vessel

Arteries and veins can be imaged using duplex ultrasound, contrast angiography or MR angiography. Post-traumatic false aneurysms (see Fig. 1.8) and deep vein thrombosis are both usually well detected with ultrasound. Thoracic outlet syndrome and vascular tumours may require angiography.

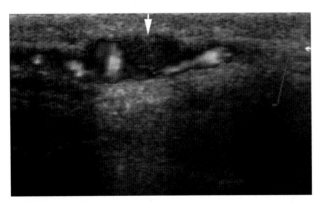

▲ **Fig. 1.8** A false aneurysm of the superficial temporal artery demonstrated by ultrasound. A rugby player sustained a direct blow to the head from the knee of an opponent. Colour Doppler ultrasound shows a flow void (arrow) due to thrombus within the focally dilated arterial segment.

Imaging standards

Effective radiographic diagnosis depends upon a number of factors, the first of which is image quality. The imaging findings that characterise both acute trauma and chronic overuse injury in sport can be quite subtle, sometimes involving anatomical structures of relatively small size. Consequently, the radiologist should take great care to optimise every link in the complex chain of factors that affect image quality. The radiologist must constantly endeavour to monitor and control the quality of each radiographic examination performed. The x-ray tube and x-ray generator combination must be able to produce short exposure times at 70 kV across a fine focal spot on large patients. A wide latitude single emulsion x-ray film and high-definition intensifying screen combination (or digital radiography system with equivalent characteristics) is required. The film processor should be configured to display an extended dynamic range without fogging. Any technically poor film should be repeated, unless the concern about irradiation outweighs the risk of missing a diagnosis. Other imaging methods can then be considered.

The following factors determine the quality of a plain film examination:

- *Exposure* A good musculoskeletal radiograph should clearly resolve the anatomy of both soft tissue and bone on the one film, under normal light-box viewing conditions (see Fig. 1.9). The correct exposure substantially eliminates the need for a bright light and is a key to the detection of subtle soft-tissue signs that are often vitally important clues to the diagnosis.

- *Fine detail* Good spatial resolution is critical to the demonstration of bone microarchitecture and is a key to fracture detection (see Fig. 1.10). Fine detail requires absence of motion blur, the use of an appropriate film–screen combination and a fine focal spot technique.

- *Positioning* Correct positioning is essential to the demonstration of important radiological anatomy. Incorrect positioning is one of the most common and serious errors made in musculoskeletal imaging. Some views are notorious for being poorly positioned and include the lateral wrist and lateral ankle (see Fig. 1.11). Whenever the relevant anatomy is not clearly demonstrated, the examination is technically inadequate and should be repeated.

- *Images series* A radiographic examination is inadequate if the film series does not demonstrate the relevant anatomy. An incomplete routine film series is a common mistake. For example, there is commonly a failure to include a skyline view of the patella in routine examinations of the knee and an axial view in an elbow series. The emergency departments of public hospitals are frequently responsible for limited views, claiming a policy that the exclusion of major trauma is a priority. What must be remembered is that patients will return to their local doctor, being told that they are radiologically normal. Mismanagement is a common outcome.

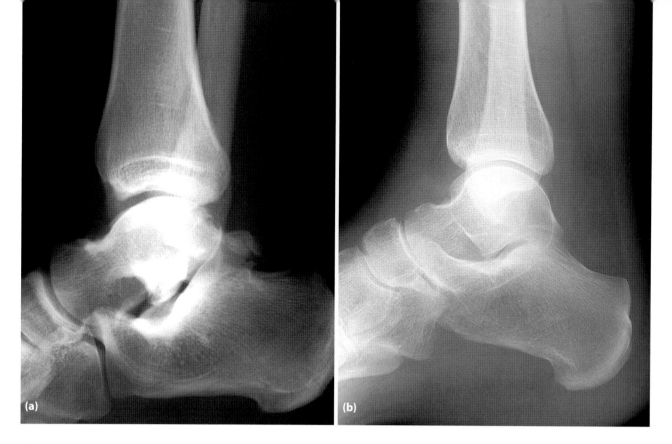

▲ **Fig. 1.9** A lateral view of the ankle is often substandard.
(a) This plain film of an ankle is technically poor. In a well-positioned lateral view, the malleoli will be superimposed and the articular margins and joint space will be well displayed. The film is also devoid of all soft-tissue detail due to the inappropriate exposure. **(b)** This examination is well positioned and the exposure is ideal. Note the calcaneonavicular coalition and soft-tissue swelling anteriorly.

▼ **Fig. 1.10** These images display the characteristics of a high-quality plain film. There is good definition of bony trabeculae together with soft-tissue detail. These films were obtained using single-emulsion film, high-definition screens and a fine focal spot. This standard of radiography is now easier to achieve due to the availability of computed radiography.

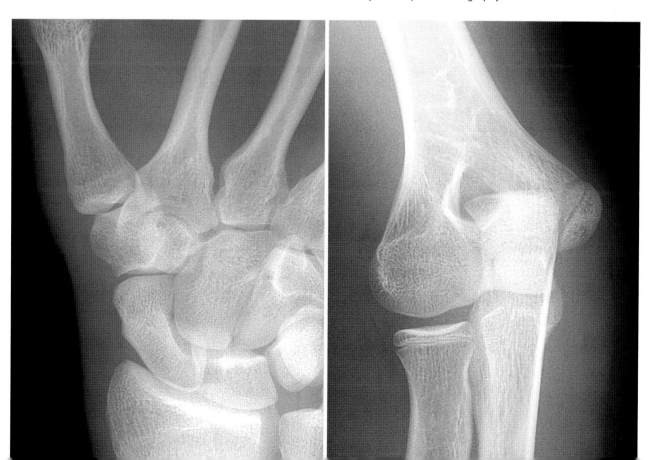

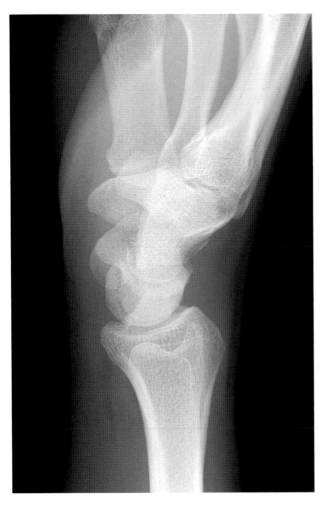

▲ **Fig. 1.11** This lateral wrist is poorly positioned. Assessment of carpal stability depends upon the third metacarpal being collinear with the long axis of the radius. Also, in a true lateral, the pisiform will be superimposed over the scaphoid tubercle.

An inadequate film series can also result from a poor clinical request that does not specify the site of interest or state a provisional clinical diagnosis. Whenever a limited film series has failed to show an abnormality despite high clinical suspicion, the use of additional views should be considered.

- *Additional views* The diagnosis of many sports injuries may require special views in addition to the standard views that are routinely performed. These are selected according to the specific clinical context.

Radiation dose

Ionising radiations such as x-rays and gamma rays are potentially harmful (Infante-Rivard et al. 2000; Morin Doody et al. 2000; Brenner et al. 2003; Brenner 2004; de Gonzalez and Darby 2004). It has been established that high radiation doses, such as those received by survivors of the atomic bomb at Hiroshima, can produce a variety of cancers. Low 'background' radiation levels, experienced to varying degrees by all human populations, have no detectable effect. Based chiefly

on data derived from Hiroshima, it is also known that adult reproductive tissues and children are particularly sensitive to radiation. Depending on their age, children can be up to ten times more sensitive to irradiation than adults, and imaging methods such as ultrasound and MRI (which are entirely free of ionising radiation) are therefore preferred in the paediatric age group whenever they offer diagnostic efficacy that is equivalent or superior to alternative methods.

It remains unknown whether radiation exposures generated by medical equipment:

- carry a risk that can be accurately calculated by simple linear regression from the doses and effects observed in atomic bomb survivors
- have a cumulative effect
- have an effect that varies with the rate of dose received.

Although it is doubtful whether standard doses associated with plain radiography cause problems, these unknowns have necessitated a cautious approach that is embodied in the ALARA principle. This states that an x-ray, a CT or nuclear medicine examination should be performed only if the potential clinical benefit clearly outweighs the theoretical radiation risk, and any exposure given should always be As Low As Reasonably Achievable (ALARA). In actual clinical practice, the radiation dose given should be titrated against the level of image noise that results. A complete absence of noise suggests an unnecessarily high dose, whereas too much noise risks a non-diagnostic examination. Consequently, it is good to have some level of noise in the image, as long as this does not compromise diagnostic efficacy!

Plain radiographs, nuclear scans and CT examinations all involve exposure to ionising radiation. In particular, the recent advent of multislice CT scanning has renewed concerns about the relatively large exposures that can be easily reached. The American Association of Physicists in Medicine (AAPM) has recently published a table of reference values (Gray et al. 2005) that indicate the 80th percentile of entrance skin exposures surveyed across the United States (see Table 1.3). This clearly shows that CT is a high-dose examination relative to plain x-ray.

Table 1.3 AAPM radiation exposure reference values

PA chest x-ray	0.25 mGy
AP cervical spine x-ray	1.25 mGy
AP abdominal x-ray	4.5 mGy
AP lumbar spine x-ray	5.0 mGy
CT head	60.0 mGy
CT abdomen	40.0 mGy

PA = posteroanterior. AP = anteroposterior.

However, the actual dose delivered in any given CT examination can vary greatly depending upon the type of scanner and the actual scan technique employed. It is therefore essential that radiologists and radiographic technologists understand and utilise best practice in tailoring exam protocols to minimise any radiation hazard. Bone offers high intrinsic image contrast and is therefore well suited to CT dose reduction measures—for example, adjusting factors for patient size, utilising high tube voltage (kVp) to reduce tube current (mAs), avoiding the use of overlapping slices, increasing pitch, increasing slice thickness if possible and adding beam filtration.

For plain x-ray examinations, there are many basic steps that can be taken to minimise radiation dose:

- Avoid repeats by taking due care with initial positioning, exposure and patient instructions.
- Collimate the beam to the region of interest.
- Use gonad shielding whenever possible. This is not possible if the area of critical interest may be obscured.
- Formulate technique charts and use these as established guidelines.
- Use dose-efficient film–screen combinations (or an equivalent digital radiography system).
- Set kVp at 70 rather than 65, which reduces the absorbed dose for only minor image contrast penalty.
- Use optimal beam filtration (2.5 mm or more of aluminium).
- Eliminate grids if possible, reducing the dose by 50%.
- Increase the focus-film distance from 100 cm to 120 cm, which reduces the dose by 8%.
- Use the fine focal spot if possible, producing greater image sharpness for no dose penalty.

Overuse injuries

The practice of sports medicine demands a comprehensive understanding of overuse injuries, as these disorders probably account for up to half of all sports-related conditions. In some sports the prevalence of overuse injury may be even higher. It has been reported that 50–75% of all running injuries relate to overuse (Van Mechelen 1992).

Overuse injuries may be acute or chronic, and may involve either 'hard' connective tissues such as bone or 'soft' connective tissues such as a tendon or bursa. Acute forms of overuse injury most frequently result from a frictional overload injuring a tendon sheath and causing acute tenosynovitis or injuring a bursa resulting in acute bursitis (bursopathy). Frictional overload is invariably due to some form of repetitive limb motion. A typical example is the development of de Quervain's disease following an unaccustomed weekend of tennis. Acute overuse syndromes rarely require imaging, as the diagnosis is obvious from the recent history and physical examination.

Characteristically, chronic overuse injuries have an insidious clinical onset and can therefore pose a greater diagnostic challenge. The following features are common to overuse syndromes:

- *The characteristic feature of the precipitating activity is its repetitive nature.* The causative loads involved are often small but invariably recurrent. Chronic repetitive trauma eventually overwhelms the normal process of tissue repair and symptoms then follow.

- *There has typically been a change in the type or degree of athletic activity.* Overuse injury will often manifest after a change of training routine. This may involve a change of sporting equipment as simple as new shoes, a change in training load or a subtle and often unintentional alteration in technique (see Fig. 1.12).

- *There is usually a delay in clinical presentation.* A time delay in presentation is a feature of chronic overuse injury. At first the athlete does not fully appreciate the significance of the symptom, as the onset is usually insidious and sport is normally accompanied by various aches and pains. In all sports, but particularly professional sports, there is pressure upon an athlete to be fit and to meet team commitments, so there is a tendency to ignore pain in order to extend tolerance (the 'no pain, no gain' philosophy).

▼ **Fig. 1.12(a)** Acute overuse injuries are often due to excessive unaccustomed activity. This young boy was extremely active, playing sport from dawn until dusk. Nevertheless, after receiving a scooter for Christmas, he developed a painful leg, which proved to be a stress fracture of the mid-tibial shaft. A plain film shows periosteal new bone on the lateral aspect of the tibial shaft.

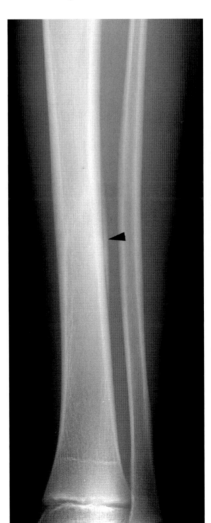

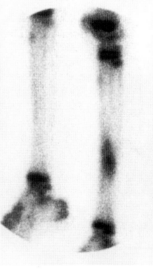

▼ **(b)** A bone scan shows an uptake of isotope, which is characteristic of a stress fracture.

Chronic bone stress

Chronic bone stress is a common problem in sports medicine (Flahive and Anderson 2004). Bone is a metabolically active tissue that normally undergoes continuous resorption and renewal. This activity is sensitive to stress, which accelerates the process. The response of bone to stress can be viewed as a dynamic continuum that ranges from normal remodelling to accelerated remodelling in response to increasing stress above the normal level, and finally to failure when the bone's ability to respond and lay down new bone is overwhelmed by the repetitive stress (Roub et al. 1979).

At the stage of accelerated remodelling, the athlete will usually develop symptoms but the plain film appearances may be normal. Only nuclear bone scanning or fat-suppressed MRI will detect changes at this level of stress. This stage of the continuum is known as 'bone stress'. However, with continuing stress, bone failure commences, reactive bony callus is laid down and eventually a fracture line will become evident.

So 'bone stress' is the result of accelerated remodelling and the plain films will become abnormal as periosteal or endosteal callus is laid down. Continued mechanical stress will then lead to a fracture line appearing on imaging and a 'stress fracture' is then present (see Fig. 1.13). A stress fracture can be diagnosed radiographically whenever there is a lucent line with surrounding callus. Initially the fracture line is partial, involving only one cortex, but with continuing insult it may become complete and then displace.

There are two types of stress fractures:

- A *fatigue fracture* occurs when abnormal stress is applied to bone that has normal elastic resistance. This is usually the case in the elite athlete.
- An *insufficiency fracture* occurs when normal stress is applied to bone with diminished elastic resistance. Stress

fractures of the calcaneum are often of the insufficiency type. In females, stress fractures should always be viewed with suspicion and osteodensitometry considered to exclude osteopaenia as a predisposing factor.

A rapid diagnosis is important, because early recognition will allow rapid recovery, since the reparative process, although overwhelmed, is already in place and active. Failure to investigate will result in continued injury, which may have devastating consequences for the athlete. Also, the underlying biomechanical cause for the bone stress should be investigated and the changes that have occurred in technique or training load should be identified and rectified.

Early diagnosis is aided by:

- educating the athlete to report unusual pain early
- investigating complaints of possible bone stress with early isotope scanning
- discussing problem cases directly with the radiologist.

Chronic tendon stress

In the course of normal life, tendons are exposed to a variety of stresses that can break their collagen fibril microlinkages. A constant process of microrepair is therefore required to maintain tendon integrity, and fibroblasts ('tenocytes') perform this function by manufacturing predominantly Type 1 collagen for tensile strength. Collagen is arranged in a hierarchical manner, with fibrils organised to form fibres, fibres organised to form bundles, and bundles organised to form fascicles. Tenocytes also produce an extracellular 'matrix' or 'ground substance' composed predominantly of complex hydrophilic high-viscosity gel-like proteoglycans macromolecules, which not only provide structural support for mature fibrils but also regulate the extracellular assembly of procollagen molecules into mature collagen. The rate of collagen manufacture and tendon repair is relatively slow.

A progressive breakdown of fibrils, so-called 'creeping tendon failure' (see Fig. 1.14), may occur if the normal rate of tendon repair is overwhelmed by the rate of repetitive tensile loading. This is seen in patellar tendonosis, which may result from the stress of constant jumping in activities such as basketball. Tendons may also be injured by exposure to persistent compressive or frictional forces such as a tendonosis developing due to impingement by an osteophyte. Whichever mechanism is involved, persistent or repetitive mechanical stress in sport is a common cause of tendon pain and swelling. The commonly occurring conditions of 'jumper's knee' and Achilles tendonosis show similar histopathological findings.

Connective tissue cells of all types are able to sense any alteration in loading ('mechanoreception') and can respond by changing their internal structure (Banes et al. 1995). As a consequence, chronic repetitive low-grade trauma causes connective tissue cells that are normally spindle-shaped and inconspicuous to become plump and spheroidal with contained mucoid vacuoles. There is also an increase in surrounding mucoid ground substance and fibrinoid degeneration

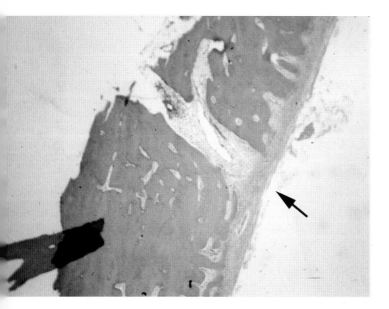

▲ **Fig. 1.13** Histopathology of a stress fracture shows a complete linear discontinuity of cortical bone (arrow), consistent with a fracture.

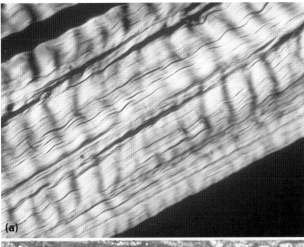

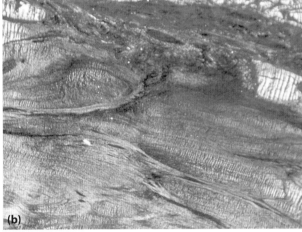

▲ **Fig. 1.14** The histopathological structure of normal tendon compared with tendonosis. Patellar tendon haemotoxylin and eosin (H&E) sections are viewed under polarised light.
(a) Normal tendon shows well-demarcated bundles of collagen closely apposed to one another and producing a dense homogeneous polarisation pattern.
(b) A low-power view of chronic tendonosis shows separation of collagen bundles, loss of the normal dense homogeneous pattern and an area of total disruption.

of collagen. This overall pattern of change is described as 'mucoid degeneration' or 'metaplasia' (Ledderhose 1893; King 1932). If the process continues, there is eventual diminution of collagen and a progressive accumulation of proteoglycans which culminate in advanced mucoid degeneration, fibrocartilagenous metaplasia, fibrinoid degeneration and fragmentation of collagen. Eventually, tendon macro-tear may result. These features are all characteristic of tendonosis (Fukuda et al. 1990; Kjellin et al. 1991; Regan et al. 1992; Potter et al. 1995; Jones et al. 1996). Associated microvascular ingrowth with capillary proliferation (see Fig. 1.15) and fibrinous exudate is common. If a recent tear is present, there may be organising granulation tissue with haemosiderin deposition. Attempted repair with fibroblastic and myofibroblastic proliferation may occur, the latter resulting in increased collagen production and scarring. Occasionally, dystrophic calcification and ossification may develop.

Tendonosis is particularly prone to occur at sites of relative tendon hypovascularity. There is often a sharp demarcation between the area of maximal degeneration and adjacent capillary, fibroblastic and myofibroblastic proliferation, further supporting the concept that local ischaemia plays a role. This is particularly evident at the patellar tendon (Khan et al. 1996). When the changes of

▼ **Fig. 1.15** The histopathology of microvascular ingrowth associated with patellar tendinopathy.
(a) Power Doppler ultrasound demonstrates increased tendon vascularity (white pixels) on a background of hypoechoic tendinopathy thickening. This is usually predictive of a symptomatic tendon. Despite the apparent large size of the vessels rendered by ultrasound, the flow depicted is actually microscopic and readily effaced by either excessive transducer pressure or tendon stretch. Note the paucity of vessels displayed when the tendon is scanned with the knee in a flexed position with the tendon on stretch.
Source: Read and Peduto (2000).
(b) The same tendon is floridly hyperaemic when the knee is extended and the fibres are relaxed.

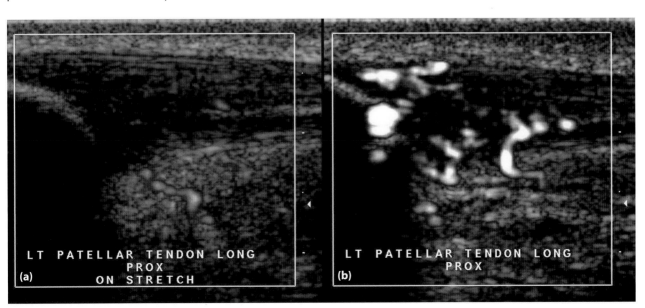

tendonosis are maximal at a bony insertion, there may be associated disruption of the tendon–bone interface with bony remodelling and sometimes small fragments of bony debris that suggest a 'tug' lesion. This is commonly seen in 'jumper's knee'. The progressive breakdown of collagen and accumulation of mucoid ground substance centrally within an area of advanced mucoid degeneration may result in a gel-like cyst or ganglion (see Fig. 1.16).

Tendonosis may or may not be symptomatic and has been shown to be the pathology that underlies up to 97%

of all spontaneous tendon ruptures (Kannus and Józsa 1991). Symptomatic tendonosis was previously known as tendonitis, but this term has now fallen out of favour as the underlying pathology is degenerative rather than inflammatory. The term tendinopathy is also used, although this is technically non-specific and could theoretically denote any type of tendon abnormality. Nevertheless, the sports medicine and radiological literature tends to use the term tendinopathy when referring to tendonosis.

The exact cause for the pain of symptomatic tendonosis remains unclear. Tendons contain stretch receptors but lack nociceptors, and the intratendinous imaging changes of tendonosis do not always correlate with symptoms. In fact, routine comparative ultrasound examinations of the 'normal' side in cases of symptomatic tendonosis attest to the high frequency of asymptomatic contralateral findings. A study of 200 elite athletes found sonographic changes of patellar tendonosis in up to 22% of individuals who had never experienced symptoms of anterior knee pain and about 40% of individuals who had previously suffered an episode of patellar tendonosis but were currently asymptomatic (Harcourt et al. 1995). Only sparse data is available concerning the reversibility of the imaging changes of tendonosis over time. A longitudinal study of 23 sonographically abnormal patellar tendons in 15 elite basketballers found that lesions may resolve, remain unchanged or progress. This study reached the conclusion that symptoms are not directly related to tendon morphology (Khan et al. 1997).

Of potential relevance to the source of pain in tendonosis is the imaging observation that symptomatic tendons almost always show accompanying changes in adjacent structures, such as within the paratenon, tenosynovium, adjacent fat pad, bursa or tendon enthesis (see Fig. 1.17). Corresponding histological changes have also been observed in the paratenon, including increased plumpness

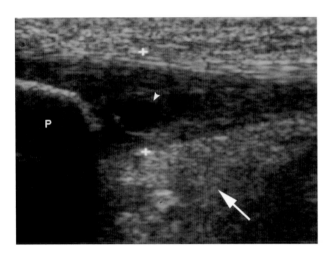

▲ **Fig. 1.16** A degenerative cyst associated with patellar tendinopathy. This long-axis ultrasound image of the proximal patellar tendon shows a central rounded anechoic focus of cystic degeneration (arrowhead) within a background of hypoechoic tendon thickening. The arrow indicates increased fat pad echogenicity adjacent to the involved segment of tendon. Callipers indicate superficial and deep tendon surfaces. Inferior pole of the patella = P.

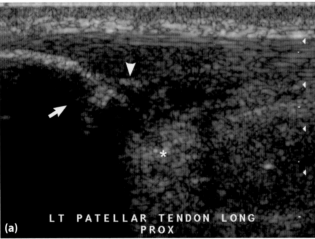

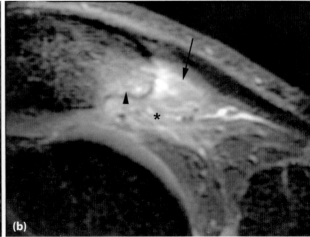

▲ **Fig. 1.17** Bone and fat pad changes associated with chronic patellar tendinopathy.
(a) Ultrasound shows irregularity at the patellar enthesis (white arrow) and increased fat pad echogenicity (white asterisk) on a background of proximal patellar tendinopathy. Also note the echogenic line of complicating intrasubstance tendon tear (white arrowhead).
(b) Fat-suppressed MRI shows abnormal marrow hyperintensity at the patellar apex (black arrowhead) and abnormal fat pad hyperintensity (black asterisk) in association with proximal patellar tendonosis (black arrow).

and roundness of connective tissue cells and increased mucoid ground substance on alcian blue and colloidal iron stains (see Fig. 1.18). Vascular channels in both tendon and peritendon appear more tortuous and prominent, and a moderately strong correlation between pain and increased tendon vascularity has been observed by Doppler ultrasound (Ohberg et al. 2001; Gisslen and Alfredson 2005). Associated fibrinoid degeneration of collagen is frequent, and in some instances frankly chondroid cells are seen within lacunae (Khan et al. 1996). Prolific CD 68 positivity (a histiocytic marker) can be demonstrated (personal observation, Dr Fiona Bonar, histopathologist, Douglas Hanley Moir Pathology, Sydney, 2005), and the degree of histiocytic differentiation could account for pain on the basis of increased lysosomal products.

Important imaging findings that suggest a symptomatic tendon include:

- localised tenderness to probing on real-time ultrasound scanning
- tendon hyperaemia on Doppler ultrasound scanning
- concurrent peritendon abnormality on ultrasound or MRI (e.g. within paratenon, tendon sheath, bursa, fat pad, enthesis).

Although most cases of tendon pain presenting to the sports physician will have a chronic mechanical aetiology, it is important to remember that other forms of *tendonitis* also occur. These include gout, pseudogout, seropositive and seronegative arthritides, and, rarely, infection (typical or atypical).

▼ **Fig. 1.18** Peritendon fat pad changes associated with tendonosis.
(a) In a normal knee, the infrapatellar fat pad shows normal fat cells, normal blood vessels and a clean, well-defined interface with the edge (arrowhead) of the normal patellar tendon.
(b) In a patient with symptomatic patellar tendonosis, the fat pad shows changes of mucoid degeneration. Fat cells can no longer be seen and are instead replaced by increased numbers of conspicuous plump connective tissue cells. There is a large amount of fuzzy background material that corresponds with mucinous ground substance on appropriate staining.

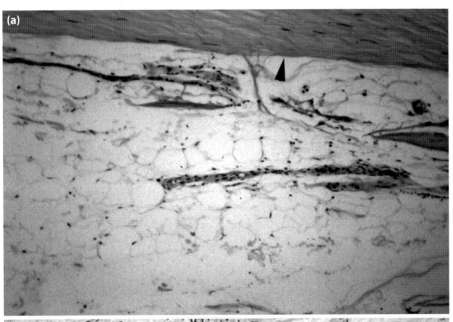
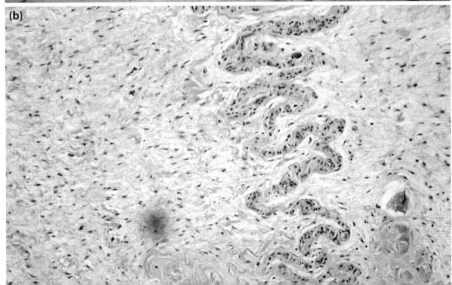

Chronic bursal stress

Synovial bursae are sacs that generally occur near synovial joints and may communicate with the joint cavity. They lie within fibroareolar tissue at sites of anatomical friction, such as tendon gliding against bone or skin gliding over a subcutaneous bony prominence. Most bursae develop in foetal life but some arise in later life as a response to local irritation ('adventitious' bursae). They are described according to their location with respect to surrounding structures, such as 'subtendinous', 'submuscular', 'subcutaneous', 'subacromial' and 'interligamentous'. A clinically swollen and painful bursa ('bursitis') may have a variety of causes including inflammatory arthritis (e.g. rheumatoid disease), gout, pseudogout, infection, acute trauma and chronic mechanical irritation. In clinical practice, the sports physician must be on constant guard for the possibility of a true inflammatory bursitis.

Bursitis in sport is most commonly due to either direct contusion or chronic repetitive low-grade trauma. Examples of chronic mechanical bursitis include shoulder impingement syndrome, pes anserinus bursitis and Haglund's syndrome. Histologically, the bursal wall is composed of a variably thick layer of fibrous tissue that is lined in part by organised granulation tissue and in part by a layer of synoviocytes. There is evidence of fibrinoid degeneration and often organising fibrinous exudate. Lymphocytes, plasma cells and neutrophils are not seen unless true inflammatory arthritis or infection is present (see Fig. 1.19).

In the absence of a true inflammatory infiltrate, terminology such as *overuse bursopathy* would therefore be technically more appropriate than bursitis. The surrounding tissues show features typical of chronic repetitive low-grade connective tissue trauma. There may be increased prominence and roundness of connective tissue cells, with increased mucoid ground substance and fibrinoid degeneration of collagen. Fibrocartilagenous metaplasia and lacuna formation are occasionally evident. Intraluminal protuberances composed of either subsynovial fat or granulation tissue are frequent, and these nodular foci often undergo necrosis attributable to trauma. Communicating bursae may simply reflect the pathology that is primarily present within the adjacent joint. For example, the bursae may contain fragments of hyaline cartilage and bone arising from a destructive arthropathy. Because bursae are lined by synovium, they may resorb debris from the lumen.

An acute episode of overuse may produce a transient bursal effusion, but the typical appearance of chronic bursal overuse is one of subtle hypoechoic soft-tissue thickening without effusion. A bursal thickness of more than 2 mm on ultrasound is nearly always abnormal (Van Holsbeeck and Introcaso 1991a), but measurements of less than 2 mm may also be abnormal and simple comparison with the contralateral asymptomatic side is therefore often a better yardstick. As a minimal finding on ultrasound, bursal thickening is easily overlooked by inexperienced operators and, as a source of high signal on MRI, it can be wrongly interpreted as a fluid effusion.

Mild bursal thickening and/or effusion is a frequent finding on imaging tests, but may be incidental and completely asymptomatic. Bursae thicken as a normal physiologic response to increased activity. Conversely, they become very thin and inconspicuous with chronic inactivity. Ultrasound in cases of chronic frozen shoulder, for example, will often show the subacromial-subdeltoid bursa to be thickened on the active asymptomatic side due to compensatory overuse, but thinned and inconspicuous on the painful inactive side. It is also common to see a mildly thickened and hyperintense pre-patellar bursa that is completely asymptomatic on MRI of the knee. Therefore, appropriate clinical correlation is the key to determining the significance of any apparent imaging abnormality.

Miscellaneous

Physiological changes

A variety of physiological changes are known to occur in musculoskeletal tissues with exercise. These changes should be taken into account when interpreting any imaging findings. Tendons show a variable increase in vascularity on Power Doppler imaging after exercise (Cook et al. 2005) and bones may show a transient asymptomatic marrow oedema pattern in response to altered weightbearing or biomechanics (Schweitzer and White 1996) (see Fig. 1.20). Muscles after exercise demonstrate a 10–15% increase in volume (van Holsbeeck and Introcaso 1991b), a subjective increase in vascularity on Power Doppler imaging (Newman et al. 1997) and a diffuse increase in MRI signal (Sjogaard et al. 1985) (see Fig. 1.21). Normal asymptomatic joints, bursae and tendon sleeves may all demonstrate effusions on MRI and ultrasound that are not statistically different in size or prevalence from those found in symptomatic cases (Schweitzer et al. 1994).

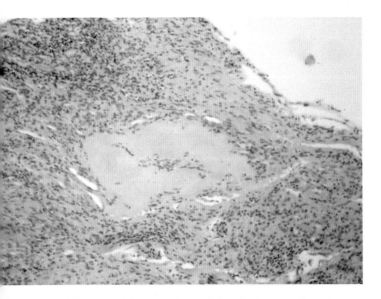

▲ **Fig. 1.19** Histopathology of chronic olecranon bursal reaction. Within the wall of the bursa there is organising granulation tissue and fibrosis. The bursa is lined by either inconspicuous or hyperplastic synoviocytes and shows areas of organising fibrinous exudates. There are no inflammatory cells.

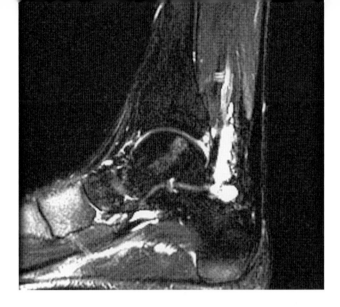

◀ **Fig. 1.20** Extreme physiological changes in the musculoskeletal system were constantly encountered in athletes at the Sydney 2000 Olympics. Fat-suppressed MRI of the feet and ankles of the majority of athletes competing at this level in track events were noted to show changes, including high signal in tarsal bones and muscle, joint space effusions and fluid around tendons, which normally would have been of concern. Clinical history was of great importance in helping to sort out which changes might indicate pathology. This athlete is a middle-distance runner with high signal in tarsal bones and scattered collections of fluid. Only the fluid associated with the flexor hallucis longus (FHL) tendon was clinically significant.

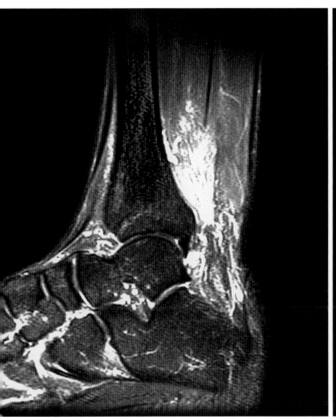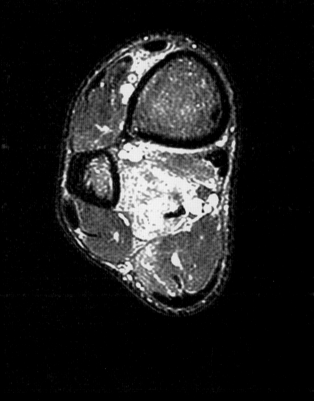

▲ **Fig. 1.21** An elite long-distance runner showed marked high signal in the distal FHL muscle in images obtained after a training run. Note the high signal in all the intertarsal regions. This athlete ran an exceptional race the following week, confirming that these physiological changes were clinically unimportant.

Spectrum of healing

Following injury, it is essential to consider the pattern of healing response that might be expected on imaging. Where does the process being imaged lie along the spectrum from acute to subacute to late subacute to chronic? Is there any discrepancy between the expected and the actual imaging appearances and, if so, what can be concluded? For example,

a healing late subacute stage tear of a ligament, tendon or fibrocartilage should appear as a bridging zone of intermediate signal scar (see Fig. 1.22) rather than a high signal line or gap, which would be more typical of an acute tear. Is the healing response inadequate or abnormal? Atrophy, non-union and remodelling together with hypertrophy and hyperplasia are all examples of abnormal healing responses that may have adverse consequences for the athlete (see Fig. 1.23).

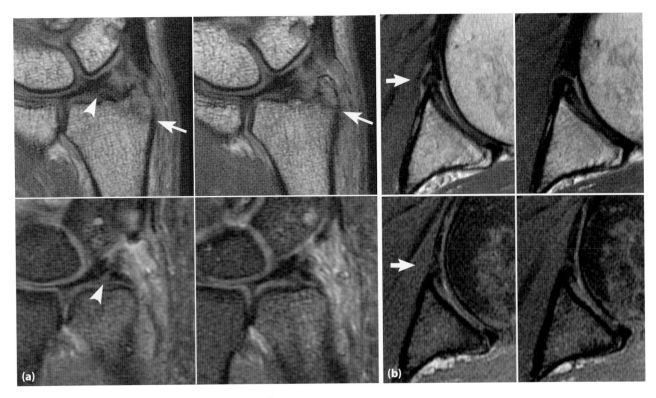

▲ **Fig. 1.22** MRI shows a healing subacute fibrocartilage tear.

(a) Images of the triangular fibrocartilage (TFC) obtained three months after injury show a peripheral proximal-side partial thickness tear. The tear demonstrates intermediate intensity on both proton density (PD) (top) and fat-suppressed PD (bottom) images (arrowhead), consistent with early subacute-stage scar (i.e. the tear brightness is lower than fluid but greater than mature fibrosis). Note the hypointense line of accompanying undisplaced fracture of the ulnar styloid process (arrow).

(b) Images of the anterior glenoid labrum obtained ten months after the injury show an undisplaced labral tear. The tear demonstrates intermediate PD intensity (top) and low fat-suppressed intensity (bottom), consistent with a late subacute stage scar with the tear brightness tending towards mature fibrosis.

▼ **Fig. 1.23** These images show the evolution of an anterior talofibular ligament (ATFL) tear. The ATFL is indicated by the arrows.

(a) A normal ATFL is demonstrated on a PD-weighted axial image (arrow).

(b) A PD-weighted MR image obtained three months after the injury shows a diffusely thickened ligament of intermediate-to-bright intensity with a linear partial thickness tear defect still visible (arrow).

(c) Eighteen months after the injury, the ligament remains thickened but now shows a uniform low signal in keeping with mature fibrosis. The tear defect is no longer evident (arrow).

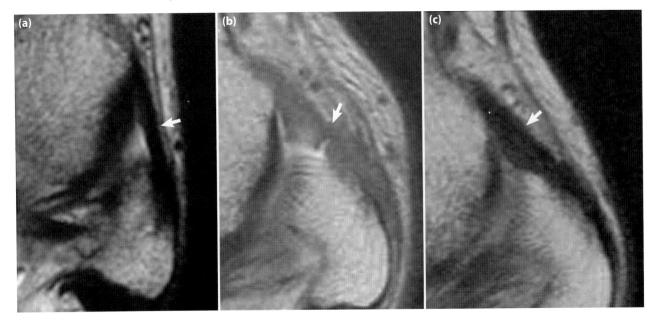

Reflex sympathetic dystrophy

Reflex sympathetic dystrophy (RSD) is a post-traumatic syndrome of pain, swelling, tenderness and stiffness that is thought to reflect a disturbance of sympathetic vasomotor control to the bone marrow. The symptoms involve the extremities and include local warmth in the early stages and cold sensitivity in the later stages. The clinical course may vary from months to years, and mild forms of this condition often go unrecognised. The usual plain film findings are those of non-specific osteopaenia and occasional chondromalacia. Severe RSD may produce an almost pathognomonic pattern of microcystic osteopaenia, which is most clearly resolved by CT scanning.

Nuclear bone scanning is the only sensitive, objective and specific method of diagnosis (see Fig. 1.24). MRI is not a reliable test for RSD because the appearances are variable and inconsistent. Nevertheless, 'warm-phase' RSD may show soft-tissue oedema, bone marrow oedema (see Fig. 1.25) and a joint effusion. The dystrophic phase of RSD may show muscle atrophy. Some patients have entirely normal MRI scans.

Arthrofibrosis

Arthrofibrosis is a condition of joint stiffness characterised by the hyperplastic proliferation of fibrous tissue in and around an affected joint after injury or surgical intervention (Eakin 2001). Excessive scar response involves both the intra-articular and extra-articular compartments as well as the joint capsule itself. Any joint may be affected, but the knee, elbow, shoulder, wrist, hand and ankle are the most frequently affected. In the authors' experience, arthrofibrosis occurs most frequently after total joint replacement and arthroscopic ACL reconstruction

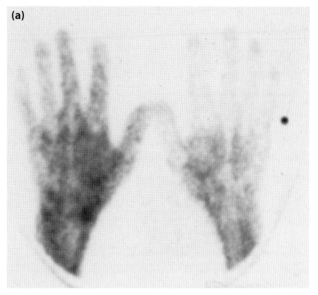
(a)

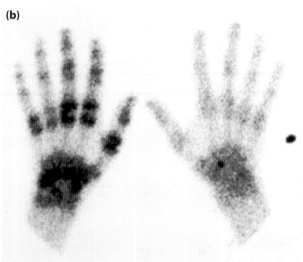
(b)

▲ **Fig. 1.24** RSD demonstrated by a nuclear bone scan.
(a) In the blood pool phase, images of the hands and wrists show a characteristic pattern of diffusely increased perfusion of the extremity on the affected left side.
(b) Delayed images also show a general increase in isotope uptake on the symptomatic side, with periarticular accentuation.

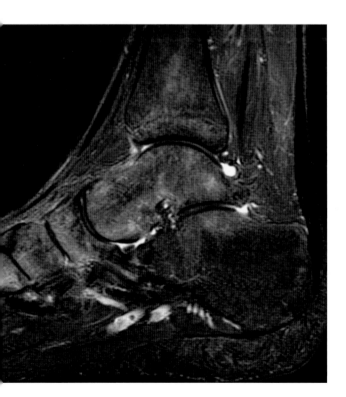

◀ **Fig. 1.25** A short tau inversion recovery MR image of warm-phase RSD demonstrates a coarse blotchy pattern of tarsal marrow oedema. There is also an area of soft-tissue oedema over the dorsal mid-foot region.

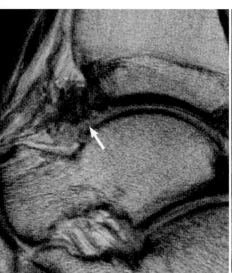
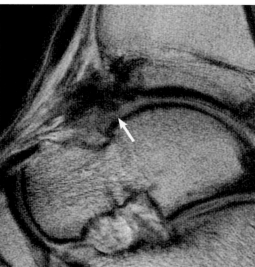
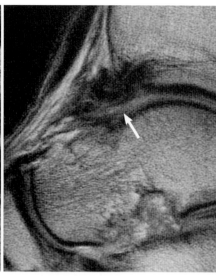

▲ **Fig. 1.26** Arthrofibrosis at the ankle is demonstrated by this PD-weighted MR image showing a localised irregular hyperplastic mass of hypointense fibrotic tissue at the anterior capsule of ankle joint (arrows). This had occurred following arthroscopy.

procedures. Relative post-surgical immobility is a known risk factor, and explains the importance of an immediate post-operative range of motion program. Fibrosis and associated capsular contracture can result in abnormal joint surface contact pressures and thereby predispose to osteoarthrosis. In the knee, fibrosis can lower the patella (patella baja or patella infera) and may cause a block to full joint extension secondary to impingement at the anterior intercondylar notch ('cyclops lesion'). MRI is the preferred imaging method (see Fig. 1.26), although examination quality may be suboptimal if a joint prosthesis is present.

Post-traumatic fat necrosis

Post-traumatic fat necrosis of the trunk or extremities is a condition of organising haemorrhage, fat necrosis and fibrosis (Tsai et al. 1997) that can result from direct trauma, crush or shear injury of the subcutaneous fat. Often there is a delay of weeks before a tender palpable lump is appreciated, and a majority of patients do not recall the inciting injury. In the early stages there may be an associated visible ecchymosis and high signal on MRI, which resolves. In the later stages, MRI may show only low signal and a loss of subcutaneous fat volume. On ultrasound there is a thickened, tender and indurated subcutaneous fat space containing poorly marginated areas of increased echogenicity with associated variable hyperaemia (see Fig. 1.27). Fat necrosis may occur at any age and is more common in women, occurring most often at sites that are prone to direct trauma, such as the breast, thigh and shin. The tender lump may take months to subside. Fat necrosis can cause residual subcutaneous contour deformity due to fibrosis, oil cysts (see Fig. 1.28) and radiographic calcifications.

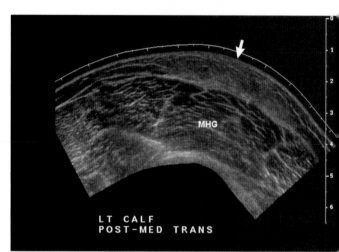
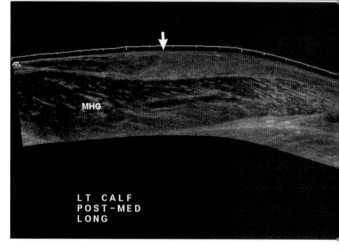

▲ **Fig. 1. 27** Post-traumatic fat necrosis presents as a tender swelling that had developed over the medial head gastrocnemius (MHG) calf muscle following overvigorous 'deep' massage treatment. Transverse and long-axis ultrasound images show a thickened subcutaneous fat space with increased echogenicity (arrows).

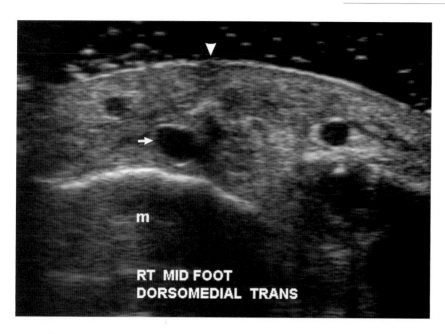

◀**Fig. 1.28** Fat necrosis demonstrated three weeks after a crush injury of the foot, imaged by ultrasound and MRI **(a)** Ultrasound shows a thickened echogenic subcutaneous space and a small oil cyst (arrow). An arrowhead indicates a cutaneous laceration that had been sutured. Metatarsal = M.

▼ **(b)** MRI confirms the oily nature of the cyst seen on ultrasound. The oil cyst shows high T1 signal (arrowhead), which completely suppresses with fat saturation (arrow). Also note the extensive bone bruising.

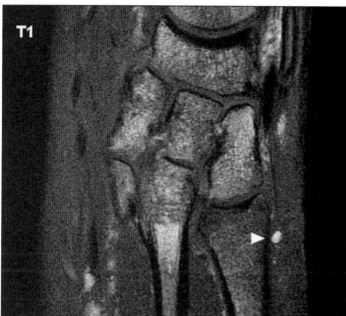
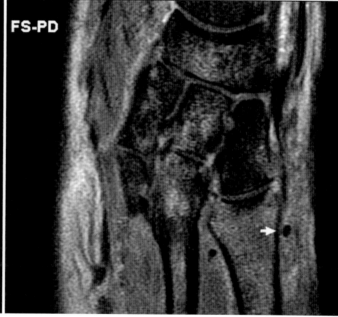

Paediatric injuries

Paediatric sports injuries often differ from those seen in adults. Some injuries are exclusive to the skeletally immature athlete, such as growth plate fractures and osteochondroses. Other injuries, although not unique to this particular age group, are nevertheless more likely to occur in the young. For example, 65% of all patellar subluxations and dislocations occur before the age of 18. Fractures that involve the growth plates of developing long bones can differ in both prognosis and management from adult fractures, and have been separately classified (see Fig. 1.29).

The paediatric population also presents diagnostic challenges that relate to the recognition of normal skeletal development and its many subtle variants. Some of these variants are clinically significant while others are unimportant. For example, the epiphysis at the base of first metatarsal, for

no apparent reason, is occasionally bifid and quite sclerotic. This finding is invariably asymptomatic and unimportant. However, particular developmental variants may eventually compromise the young athlete in later years. For example, an increased femoral neck angle may predispose to stress fracture. The recognition and differentiation of the normal from the possibly injured accessory ossicle or developing apophysis is clearly important yet not always easy, and radiographic comparison with the asymptomatic contralateral side is sometimes required.

Radiation dose is of particular concern, since susceptibility to leukaemia and other neoplastic conditions is higher in the paediatric age group. For all the above reasons, a close working relationship between the clinician and radiologist is even more important than in adult sports medicine, and can be vital in deciding upon an optimal pathway of investigation and any subsequent interpretation of the imaging findings.

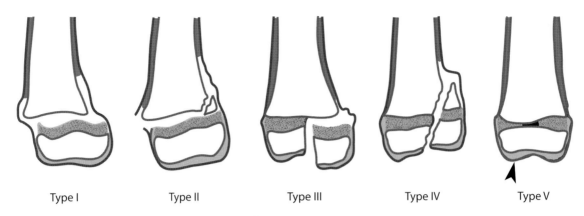

| Type I | Type II | Type III | Type IV | Type V |

▲ **Fig. 1.29** Salter–Harris classification of growth plate fractures.

Type I: The fracture involves the growth plate, sparing the metaphysis and epiphysis.
Type II: The fracture involves both the growth plate and metaphysis.
Type III: The fracture involves both the growth plate and epiphysis.
Type IV: The fracture line extends through the epiphysis, growth plate and metaphysis.
Type V: Crush injury to the growth plate (vector of force indicated by arrowhead).

Source: Adapted from Pitt and Speer (1982).

MRI concepts

MRI is a highly sophisticated and technically complex imaging modality in which a large number of variables may affect the type and quality of the image that is generated. Although a detailed description of the MRI techniques is well beyond the scope of this book, it is helpful to have a basic understanding of the method, terminology and image characteristics involved. The following brief discussion has been adapted from Read and Peduto (2000).

Routine MRI utilises the magnetic properties of unpaired hydrogen protons, and the chemical and magnetic environments in which they are found, to produce images of biological tissues. The spin of the positively charged hydrogen proton makes it behave like a tiny bar magnet. When placed in a strong external magnetic field these protons align themselves with that magnetic field. Electromagnetic energy is then pulsed at the natural or 'resonant' frequency of the proton (a radio frequency, or RF, pulse), temporarily exciting the protons to a higher energy state. When this external RF pulse is switched off, the protons 'relax' back into alignment with the external magnetic field (a lower energy state) and emit a corresponding amount of RF energy that can be detected and used to form an image.

Since the rate and nature of hydrogen proton relaxation are determined by the local chemical, structural and magnetic environments in which these protons are found (e.g. lipids, free water, proteins), there are significant differences in the resonant behaviour of different tissues. This different behaviour is the source of the superb image contrast provided by MRI. The rate at which excited protons realign with the main magnetic field is known as the T1 relaxation time. At the same time as T1 relaxation is taking place, protons are also precessing about the direction of the main magnetic field. The initial external RF pulse excites all hydrogen protons to precess in phase but, as time passes, these protons rapidly and

progressively de-phase due to inhomogeneities in their local molecular magnetic environments. This rate of de-phasing can be measured. It is known as the T2 relaxation time and is completely independent of the T1 relaxation time.

External RF energy is introduced in a series of pulses (known as a 'pulse sequence'), the timing of which determines which type of proton relaxation is emphasised in the resultant images—that is, whether an image is 'T1-weighted' or 'T2-weighted'. The chosen pulse sequence determines the number, strength and exact timing of the RF pulses delivered. The two most important pulse parameters are time to repetition (TR) and time to echo (TE). TR is the amount of time between consecutive groups of RF excitations, and TE is the time between the initial RF excitation and subsequent signal detection (see Fig. 1.30).

The wire coils or antennae that detect and measure the RF signal returning from the patient are critical determinants of image quality. These were initially incorporated into the wall of the magnet and the diagnostic role of MRI in the musculoskeletal system did not expand until the introduction of specialised extremity coils (known as 'surface' coils) in the late 1980s. These coils are positioned close to the structures of interest to improve the signal-to-noise ratio and allow images of high resolution. More recently, by combining multiple coils into a 'phased array' configuration, there have been further significant improvements in image quality.

The early years of clinical MRI were dominated by conventional spin-echo pulse sequences. These were prolonged acquisitions that were susceptible to patient movement, usually taking between 5 and 15 minutes each. Subsequently, the development of faster techniques has allowed higher resolution sequences to be performed in reasonable time frames of between 2 and 5 minutes each, and MRI examinations are now better tolerated with less risk of patient movement and additional imaging planes included. For musculoskeletal imaging, fast spin-echo (FSE) sequences have now become the general

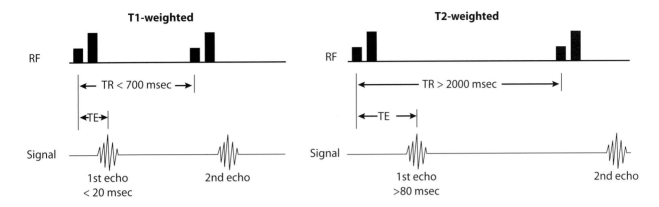

▲ **Fig. 1.30** Spin-echo pulse sequence, illustrating the concept of TR and TE.
Source: Adapted from Hesselink (2005).

workhorse. These sequences are usually used exclusively or in combination with other supplementary sequences such as short tau inversion recovery (STIR) or gradient-recalled echo (GRE). FSE techniques have also incorporated strategies to suppress the bright signal emanating from fat, which can obscure the high signal of pathology ('fat suppression').

Other techniques used to reduce artefacts arising from vascular pulsation, chemical shift and blurring are discussed below.

T1-weighted FSE sequences

T1-weighted FSE sequences utilise short parameters (TR < 700 msec, TE < 20 msec at 1.5 T field strength) and reflect the T1 characteristics of tissue within the image. They have a high signal-to-noise ratio and therefore provide good detail. However, they also make fluid appear grey and inconspicuous, fat very bright, 'magic angle' artefact (discussed below) most conspicuous and degenerative connective tissue signal more obvious. These factors can all cloud the delineation of anatomy or pathology and therefore limit the clinical value of T1-weighted images. T1-weighted sequences are most useful for the demonstration of fractures, meniscal tears and tumour characteristics.

T2-weighted FSE sequences

T2-weighted FSE sequences utilise long parameters (TR > 2000 msec, TE > 80 msec at 1.5 T field strength) and reflect the T2 characteristics of tissue within the image. They emphasise fluid and oedema. On FSE sequences, fat is shown at moderately bright intensity, whereas muscle appears hypointense. Tendons, ligaments and cartilage appear dark. 'Magic angle' artefact and degenerative signal in connective tissue is minimised. T2-weighted sequences can be helpful whenever 'magic angle' artefact or degenerative connective tissue signal may cloud the interpretation, such as suspected tendinopathy, because true pathology is usually brighter on T2 than on T1- or PD-weighted images. T2-weighted sequences are also useful in assessing tumour characteristics.

PD-weighted FSE sequences

PD-weighted FSE sequences utilise intermediate parameters (typically TR > 2000 msec, TE = 25–40 msec at 1.5 T field strength) and reflect the concentration of hydrogen protons (i.e. water) rather than the T1 or T2 characteristics of tissue within the image. PD-weighted sequences are the general workhorse of MRI in the musculoskeletal system because they are sensitive to oedema (a hallmark of pathology) and at the same time provide a high signal-to-noise ratio (i.e. good anatomical resolution) for reasonably fast scan times (see Fig. 1.31). At 1.5 T, optimal image contrast between articular cartilage and joint fluid is obtained using TE values of 25–35 msec. This provides an 'arthrographic effect', which is ideal for the assessment of joint surfaces. 'Magic angle' artefact remains moderately conspicuous.

STIR or 'Fat-Sat' sequences

STIR or 'Fat-Sat' sequences are used to achieve 'fat suppression' in order to overcome the problem of bright fat signal obscuring oedema. These images show relatively dark fat and bone marrow, but bright fluid signal and tissue oedema. STIR images achieve fat suppression by acquiring signal at a particular time in an 'Inversion Recovery' pulse sequence (inversion time or TI ~ 140 msec at 1.5 T field strength) when the signal from fat is almost 'nulled', while maintaining water and soft-tissue signal. Sub-total fat suppression allows a degree of anatomical information to be preserved, thus permitting the localisation of any detected abnormalities. STIR sequences are the most sensitive for oedema and are robust in the sense that uniform fat suppression can still be achieved even when the part being examined, such as a limb, may be off-centre within the bore of the magnet at a location where magnetic field homogeneity is suboptimal. However, they carry a penalty of longer acquisition times and consequently reduced spatial resolution. Frequency-selective fat-saturation ('Fat-Sat') sequences achieve fat suppression by applying an initial RF pulse that sets the magnetisation of fat to zero prior to the actual imaging pulses (see Fig. 1.31). These provide good spatial resolution and faster acquisition times, but are vulnerable to uneven fat suppression in cases requiring off-centre positioning within the magnet.

GRE sequences

GRE sequences (Gradient Echo sequences) are another distinct technique that utilises an additional parameter known as 'flip angle'. At large flip angles (45 to 90°) they give T1-weighted images, and at low flip angles (5 to 20°) they give a unique type of image described as having 'T2-star' (T2*) weighting rather than true T2-weighting (see Figs 1.31 and 1.32). GRE sequences provide high signal-to-noise ratio (i.e. high spatial resolution) images and can also be obtained as volumetric (3D) acquisitions, albeit with the penalty of long scan times. Unfortunately, GRE sequences greatly exaggerate degenerative signal within connective tissues and also markedly accentuate magnetic susceptibility artefacts arising in situations where there is an abrupt change in paramagnetic properties across a normal tissue interface, where residual micrometallic debris has occurred due to previous surgery, or where a prosthesis

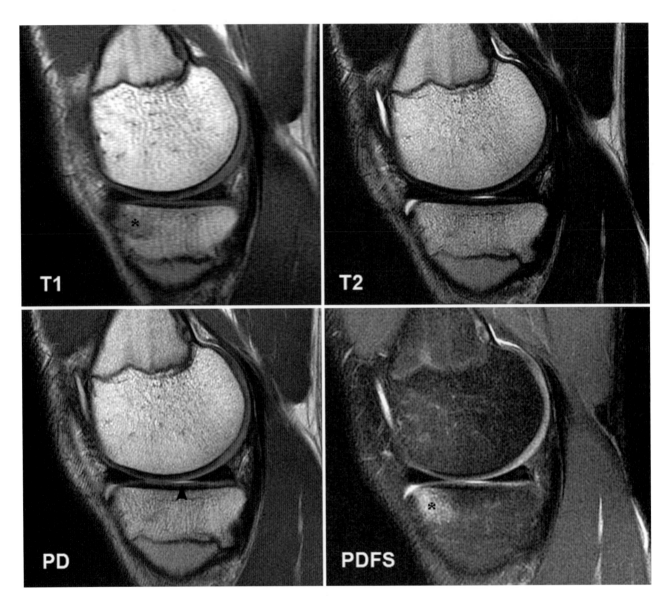

▲ **Fig. 1.31** These images illustrate the tissue signal characteristics for FSE and GRE pulse sequences.
Sagittal images obtained through the medial compartment of the knee joint show a localised bone bruise (asterisk) at the anterior tibial plateau, conspicuous on the T1 and fat-suppressed PD images but difficult to discern on the PD and T2 images. PD weighting provides a beautifully balanced overall rendering of musculoskeletal anatomy and also imparts a significant amount of T2 signal. This makes the differentiation of bright fat signal from bright water signal difficult, hence the importance of fat suppression as a component of any routine examination protocol. Also note the PD image shows good detail and contrast resolution (high signal-to-noise ratio) and produces an 'arthrographic' effect due to bright joint fluid clearly profiling the surface of intermediate signal articular cartilage (black arrowhead). Muscle and cartilage are darker on the T2 image. Joint fluid is grey and isointense with articular cartilage on the T1 image, greatly reducing clinical utility.

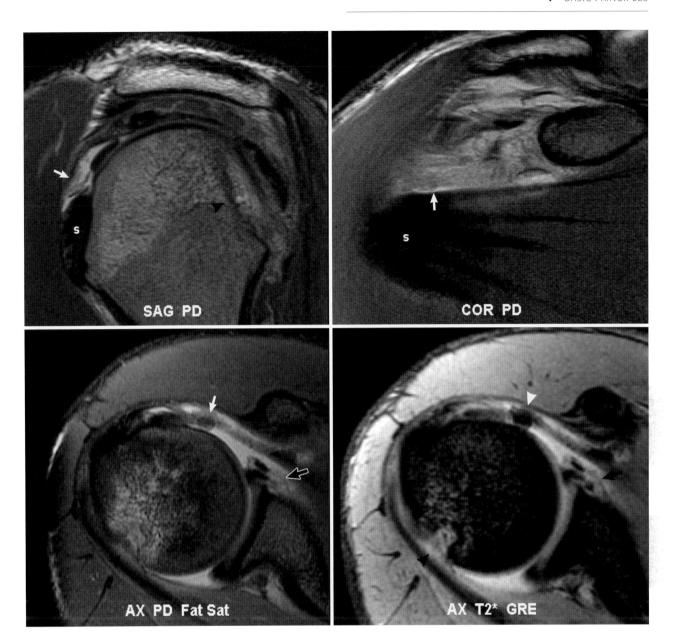

▲ **Fig. 1.32** Non-arthrographic multiplanar views of the shoulder have been obtained in a patient with anterior glenoid labral tear (black arrows), accompanying Hill-Sachs fracture (black arrowheads) and rotator interval synovitis (white arrows). An axial T2*-weighted GRE image has been included. Note the 'blooming' phenomenon associated with a frond of synovitis, which appears larger than on the corresponding PD image (white arrowhead). Bone marrow also appears relatively dark on the T2* image due to trabecular blooming, and articular cartilage is hyperintense. Supraspinatus = s.

or gas is present. Tissues with an increased concentration of paramagnetic compounds such as methaemoglobin, melanin, iron and manganese also have a 'blooming' effect on GRE images, making the affected areas appear larger than on corresponding FSE sequences. In practice, GRE sequences can sometimes be helpful in situations where the anatomical structures of interest are very small and/or orientated in awkward scan planes, or where extra tissue characterising information is sought, such as with haemosiderin, calcification or a loose body.

'Magic angle' phenomenon

'Magic angle' phenomenon (Erickson et al. 1991) describes spurious high signal that occurs along segments of structures in which there is highly organised collagen that is orientated at or near 55° to the main magnetic field of the scanner, such as may occur with a tendon (see Fig 1.33), articular cartilage or meniscus. This artefact arises only in short TE sequences (T1, PD and GRE) and the radiologist must be careful not to confuse the appearance with pathology.

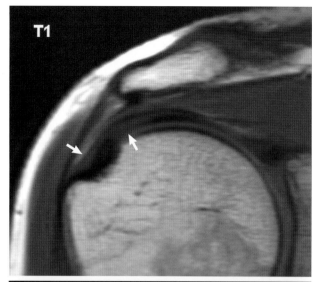

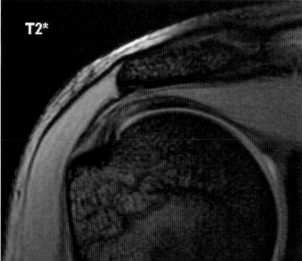

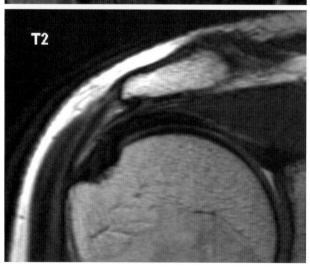

▲ **Fig. 1.33** MR images demonstrate the 'magic angle' artefact. Identically positioned coronal images obtained through a normal supraspinatus tendon show regions of spurious high signal (arrows) where fibre orientation is near 55° to the main magnetic field of the scanner. Note that short TE sequences (T1 and T2*) accentuate, and long TE sequences (T2) minimise, this artefact.

Contraindications to MRI

Contraindications to MRI include cardiac pacemakers (except in limited circumstances), ferromagnetic foreign bodies (particularly those near vital structures such as intraocular foreign bodies) and certain metallic and electronic implants, including ferromagnetic cerebral aneurysm clips. Most MRI units screen patients for the presence of these implants with extensive pre-scan questionnaires and interviews. Plain film radiographs of the orbits may be obtained if necessary.

References

Banes AJ, Tsuzaki M, Yamamoto J, Fischer T, Brigman B, Brown T, Miller L. 'Mechanoreception at the cellular level: the detection, interpretation, and diversity of responses to mechanical signals.' *Biochem Cell Biol* 1995, 73: 349–65.

Beattie K, Boulos P, Pui M, O'Neill J, Inglis D, Webber C et al. 'Abnormalities identified in the knees of asymptomatic volunteers using peripheral magnetic resonance imaging.' *Osteoarthritis Cartilage* 2005, 13: 181–6.

Bigos S, Davis G. 'Scientific application of sports medicine principles for acute low back problems.' *J Orthopaed Sports Phys Ther* 1996, 24: 192–207.

Blankenbaker DG, De Smet AA. 'MR imaging of muscle injuries.' *Appl Radiol* 2004, 33(4): 14–26.

Brenner D. 'Radiation risks potentially associated with low-dose CT screening of adult smokers for lung cancer.' *Radiology* 2004, 231: 440–5.

Brenner D, Doll R, Goodhead D, Hall E, Land C. 'Cancer risks attributable to low doses of ionizing radiation: assessing what we really know.' *Proc Natl Acad Sci USA* 2003, 100: 13761–6.

Chhem RK and Cardinal E (eds), *Guidelines and Gamuts in Musculoskeletal Ultrasound*. Wiley-Liss Publishers, New York, 1999.

Cook JL, Khan KM, Kiss ZS, Purdam CR, Griffiths L. 'Prospective imaging study of asymptomatic patellar tendinopathy in elite junior basketball players.' *J Ultrasound Med* 2000, 19(7): 473–9.

Cook JL, Kiss ZS, Ptasznik R, Malliaris P. 'Is vascularity more evident after exercise? Implications for tendon imaging.' *AJR* 2005, 185: 1138–40.

de Gonzalez A, Darby S. 'Risk of cancer from diagnostic x-rays: estimates for the UK and 14 other countries.' *Lancet* 2004, 363: 345–51.

Drape JL, Pessis E, Auleley GR, Chevrot A, Dougados M, Ayral X. 'Quantitative MR imaging evaluation of chondropathy in osteoarthritic knees.' *Radiology* 1998, 208: 49–55.

Eakin CL. 'Knee arthrofibrosis.' *The Physician and Sports Medicine* 2001, 29(3): 31–42.

Erickson SJ, Cox IH, Hyde JS, Carrera GF, Strandt JA, Estkowski LD. 'Effect of tendon orientation on MR signal intensity: a manifestation of the "magic angle" phenomenon.' *Radiology* 1991, 181: 389–92.

Flahive SR, Anderson IF. 'Bone stress in athletes at the Sydney 2000 Olympic Games.' *NZ J of Sports Med* 2004, 32: 2–12.

Fukuda H, Hamada K, Yamanaka K. 'Pathology and pathogenesis of bursal-side rotator cuff tears viewed from en bloc histologic sections.' *Clin Orthop* 1990, 254: 75–80.

Gisslen K, Alfredson H. 'Neovascularisation and pain in jumper's knee: a prospective clinical and sonographic study in elite junior volleyball players.' *Br J Sports Med* 2005, 39: 423–8.

Gray JE, Archer BR, Butler PF, Hobbs BB, Mettler FA, Pizzutiello RJ, Schueler BA, Strauss KJ, Suleiman OH, Yaffe MJ. 'Reference values for diagnostic radiology: application and impact.' *Radiology* 2005, 235: 354–8.

Haims AH, Schweitzer ME, Patel RS, Hecht P, Wapner KL. 'MR imaging of the Achilles tendon: overlap of findings in symptomatic and asymptomatic individuals.' *Skeletal Radiol* 2000, 29(11): 640–5.

Harcourt PR, Cook J, Khan K et al. 'Patellar tendon ultrasound of 200 active elite athletes: hypoechogenic lesions present in 40% of individuals.' In *Proceedings of the Australian conference of Science and Medicine in Sport, Hobart*, Sports Medicine Australia, Canberra, 1995.

Hesselink JR. 'Basic principles of MR imaging.' 2005 (http://spinwarp.ucsd.edu/NeuroWeb/Text/br-100.htm, accessed October 2005).

Infante-Rivard C, Mathonnet G, Sinnet D. 'Risk of childhood leukaemia associated with diagnostic irradiation and polymorphisms in DNA repair genes.' *Environ Health Perspect* 2000, 108: 495–8.

Jones AR, Lauder I, Finlay DB, Allen MJ. 'Chronic Achilles tendinitis: magnetic resonance imaging and histopathologic correlation.' *Sports Exercise and Injury* 1996, 2: 172–5.

Kannus P, Józsa L. 'Histopathological changes preceding spontaneous rupture of a tendon.' *J Bone Joint Surg* 1991, 73A: 1507–25.

Khan KM, Bonar F, Desmond PM et al. 'Patellar tendinosis (jumper's knee): findings at histopathological examination, US and MR imaging.' *Radiology* 1996, 200: 821–7.

Khan KM, Cook JL, Kiss ZS et al. 'Patellar tendon ultrasonography and jumper's knee in female basketball players: a longitudinal study.' *Clin J Sport Med* 1997, 96A: 374–85.

King ESJ. 'The pathology of ganglion.' *Aust NZ J Surg* 1932, 1: 367–81.

Kjellin I, Ho CP, Cervilla V et al. 'Alterations in the supraspinatus tendon at MR imaging: correlation with histopathological findings in cadavers.' *Radiology* 1991, 181: 837–41.

Lau L. *Imaging Guidelines*, 4th edn, RANZCR, Melbourne, 2001.

Ledderhose G. 'Die aetiologie der carpalen ganglion.' *Dtsch Zeit Chir* 1893, 37: 102.

Matin P. 'The appearance of bone scans following fractures, including immediate and long-term studies.' *J Nucl Med* 1979, 20: 1227–31.

Morin Doody M, Lonstein J, Stovall M, Hacker D, Luckyanov N, Land C. 'Breast cancer mortality after diagnostic radiography: findings from the US Scoliosis Cohort Study.' *Spine* 2000, 25: 2052–63.

Newman JS, Adler RS, Rubin JM. 'Power Doppler sonography: use in measuring alterations in muscle blood volume after exercise.' *AJR* 1997, 168: 1525–30.

Ohberg L, Lorentzon R, Alfredson H. 'Neovascularisation in Achilles tendons with painful tendinosis but not in normal tendons: an ultrasonographic investigation.' *Knee Surg Sports Traumatol Arthrosc* 2001, 9: 233–8.

Orchard J, Read J, Neophyton J, Garlick D. 'Ultrasound findings of inguinal canal posterior wall deficiency associated with groin pain in footballers.' *Br J Sports Med* 1998, 32(2): 134–9.

Orchard JW, Read JW, Anderson IF. 'The use of diagnostic imaging in sports medicine.' *MJA* 2005, 183(9): 482–6.

Pitt MJ, Speer DP. 'Radiologic reporting of orthopaedic trauma.' *Med Radiogr Photogr* 1982, 58: 14–18.

Potter HG, Hannafin JA, Morwessel RM et al. 'Lateral epicondylitis: correlation of MR imaging, surgical, and histopathologic findings.' *Radiology* 1995, 196: 43–6.

Read JW, Peduto AJ. 'Tendon imaging.' *Sport Med & Arthroscopy Rev* 2000, 8: 32–55.

Regan W, Wold LE, Coonrad R, Morrey BF. 'Microscopic histopathology of chronic refractory lateral epicondylitis.' *Am J Sports Med* 1992, 20: 746–9.

Rosenberg ZS, Cheung Y, Jahss MH, Noto AM, Norman A, Leeds NE. 'Rupture of posterior tibial tendon: CT and MR imaging with surgical correlation.' *Radiology* 1988, 169: 229–35.

Roub LW, Gumerman LW, Hanley EN Jr, Clark MW, Goodman M, Herbert DL. 'Bone stress: a radionuclide imaging perspective.' *Radiology* 1979, 132: 431–8.

Schweitzer ME, White LM. 'Does altered biomechanics cause marrow oedema?' *Radiology* 1996, 198: 851–3.

Schweitzer ME, van Leersum M, Ehrlich SS, Wapner K. 'Fluid in normal and abnormal ankle joints: amount and distribution as seen on MR images.' *AJR* 1994, 162: 111–14.

Sher JS, Uribe JW, Posada A, Murphy BJ, Zlatkin MB. 'Abnormal findings on magnetic resonance images of asymptomatic shoulders.' *J Bone Joint Surg [Am]* 1995, 77(1): 10–15.

Sjogaard G, Adams RP, Saltin B. 'Water and ion shifts in skeletal muscle of humans with intense dynamic knee extension.' *Am J Physiol* 1985, 248: 190–6.

Tempelhof S, Rupp S, Seil R. 'Age-related prevalence of rotator cuff tears in asymptomatic shoulders.' *J Shoulder Elbow Surg* 1999, 8(4): 296–9.

Tsai TS, Evans HA, Donnelly LF, Bissett GS, Emery KH. 'Fat necrosis after trauma: a benign cause of palpable lumps in children.' *AJR* 1997, 169: 1623–6.

Van Holsbeeck M, Introcaso JH. 'Sonography of bursae.' In 'Musculoskeletal ultrasound', *Mosby Year Book*, St Louis, 1991a.

Van Holsbeeck M, Introcaso JH. 'Sonography of muscle.' In 'Musculoskeletal ultrasound', *Mosby Year Book*, St Louis, 1991b.

Van Mechelen W. 'Running injuries. A review of the epidemiological literature.' *Sports Med* 1992, 14: 320–35.

Image acknowledgments

The authors wish to thank the following colleagues who kindly offered images for inclusion in this chapter:

- Dr James Linklater (Figures 1.3(b) and 1.23(a), (b) and (c))
- Dr Fiona Bonar (Figures 1.13, 1.14(a) and (b), 1.18(a) and (b) and 1.19)
- Dr Robert Cooper and Dr Stephen Allwright (Figure 1.24(a) and (b))
- Dr Karim Khan and Dr Steven Kiss (Figure 1.17(a) and (b)).

These images have significantly added to the quality of the chapter.

2

The hand and wrist
Jock Anderson and John Read

The 'hand' lies distal to the carpometacarpal (CMC) joints and provides fine control, with movement relying on a relatively simple arrangement of bones, tendons and ligaments. By contrast, the 'wrist', acting as a link between the hand and the forearm, is much more anatomically, functionally and radiographically complex.

Biomechanically, the wrist transfers forces from either the forearm to the hand (as in throwing) or the hand to the forearm (as occurs in swimming). To achieve efficient transfer of force, the wrist must be able to remain stable while under load during movement or in a fixed position.

The hand and wrist are particularly susceptible to injury due to their exposed position and their key role in many activities. Up to 9% of all sports injuries involve the hand and wrist (Lee and Montgomery 2002). Sports involving ball handling, gymnastics and fighting are the leading causes of injury. Sport is the most common cause of phalangeal fractures in 10- to 39-year-olds and produces 43% of all injuries in 10- to 19-year-olds (Snead and Rettig 2001).

In the past, sporting injuries of the hand and wrist were often casually and sometimes poorly managed. Injured fingers were frequently strapped to the neighbouring finger and painful wrists were supported with strapping to enable the athlete to continue playing or competing. It was not uncommon for strapping to be reapplied for months, with little attention paid to the nature of the underlying injury. An immediate or early return to sport was the clear priority.

However, experience has taught us that this relaxed approach to hand and wrist injuries can result in significant deformities and disabilities, many of which can be avoided with appropriate management at the time of the injury. The prompt restoration of stability and function is now recognised as essential to achieving an optimal treatment outcome. Imaging plays an important role in this process, contributing to a fast and accurate diagnosis.

A basic set of conventional radiographs is often all that is required to assess the hand. However, the wrist frequently needs further work up, with either special views or the use of additional imaging methods. Ultrasound has become an extremely valuable diagnostic tool used to assess foreign bodies (see Fig. 2.1), abnormalities of tendons and ligaments, soft-tissue masses such as ganglia, some vascular injuries, and synovitic processes affecting small joints (Read et al. 1996). Targeted high-resolution CT examination can further characterise bone lesions, including subtle or radiographically occult fractures and dislocations. MRI has an important role in the diagnosis of bone marrow changes, the triangular fibrocartilage complex (TFCC)

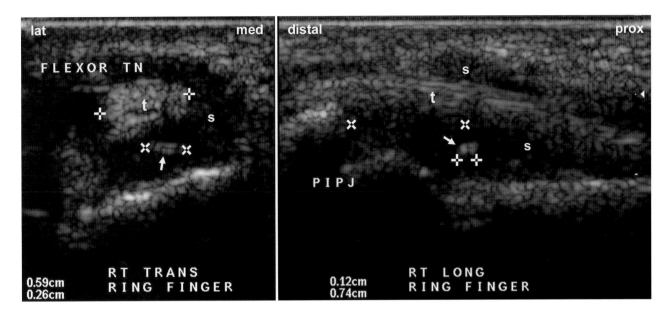

▲ **Fig. 2.1** Ultrasound has become an extremely valuable diagnostic tool. In this case, transverse and long-axis views of the ring finger flexor digitorum superficialis-flexor digitorum profundus (FDS-FDP) tendon complex (t) demonstrate a surrounding collar of hypoechoic flexor tenosynovitis (s) secondary to a wooden splinter (arrow) lying within the tendon sheath at the level of the proximal phalangeal neck.

and intrinsic ligament injuries, tendon pathology, synovitis, cartilage abnormalities, neural entrapment and impingement syndromes. Nuclear bone scans also provide a method of finding occult fractures and demonstrating marrow changes.

In determining which of these tests might be useful, the sports physician must, as always, be guided by a thorough history and physical examination. In particular, the history often holds the key to understanding the precise mechanism of the injury, and this information alone will usually suggest the probable diagnosis. It will also assist the radiologist in the selection of the most appropriate imaging protocol and direct the search for relevant imaging findings, which can sometimes be remarkably subtle and otherwise overlooked. Many bone and soft-tissue injuries occur in characteristic patterns. Consequently, an understanding of the mechanism of injury through an appropriate history is considered to be an essential component of radiological interpretation.

Imaging of the hand

As noted above, plain films play a major role in assessing injuries of the hand. A plain film series includes two standard radiographic views: a posteroanterior (PA) view and an oblique view. A PA view (see Fig. 2.2) should be obtained with the forearm resting prone on the table with the hand, elbow and shoulder in the same horizontal plane. This position is known as 'zero rotation' (see page 58). The fingers are slightly separated and the primary beam is centred on the head of the third metacarpal. It is possible to tell whether an examination has been obtained in the PA or anteroposterior (AP) position. When the image has been obtained in the PA position, the ulnar styloid process is positioned at the medial edge of the distal ulna, whereas if the examination is taken in the supine or AP position, the ulnar styloid process is projected more laterally or over the centre of

▼ **Fig. 2.2** A PA view of the hand provides a comprehensive overview of bone, joints and soft-tissue anatomy.

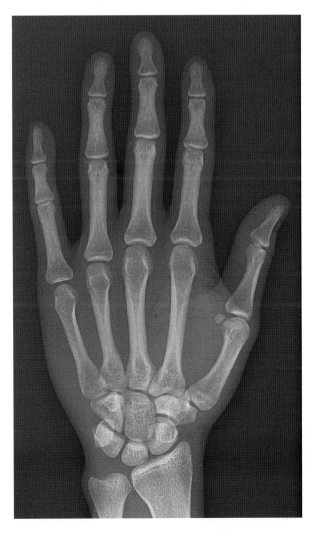

the distal ulna. An oblique view (see Fig. 2.3) is obtained by raising the radial side of the hand by resting the hand on a 45° sponge. As with the PA view, the fingers are slightly separated and the primary beam is centred on the head of the third metacarpal.

There are additional plain film views of the hand that may be helpful with certain particular clinical presentations (see Table 2.1). These views help to image specific anatomical structures that need to be examined given the injury that is clinically suspected.

Table 2.1 Additional plain film views of the hand

Additional plain film views of the hand are used in the following clinical situations:

- thumb injury
- possible ligamentous injury at the first metacarpophalangeal joint
- a suspected finger injury
- if a metacarpal fracture has been demonstrated on the routine films
- injury to the medial carpometacarpal joints
- a suspected intra-articular fracture of a metacarpal head.

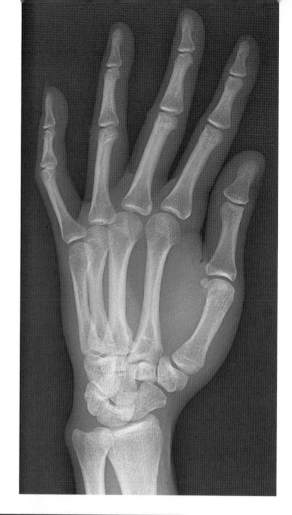

▶ **Fig. 2.3(a)** An oblique view adds a further dimension to radiographic assessment of the hand, without creating the confusion that would result from the superimposition of structures in a lateral projection.
▼ **(b)** This athlete has fractures of metacarpals three and four, which are difficult to see on the PA view. The fractures are well demonstrated when the hand is viewed obliquely. There is also evidence of old injury at the radial aspect of the bases of the second and third proximal phalanges.

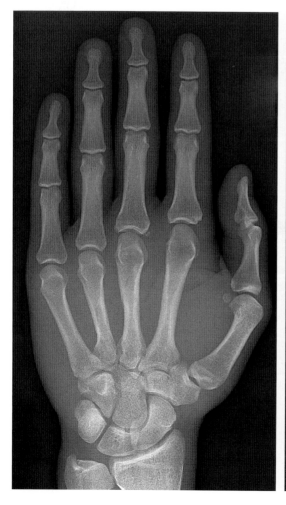

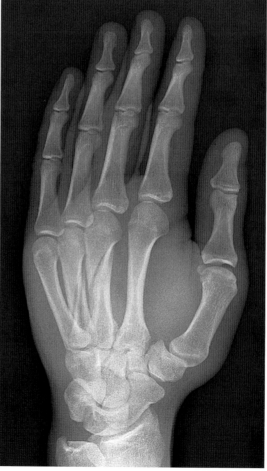

Specific views of the thumb (see Fig. 2.4) should be requested whenever there is clinical suspicion of a thumb injury. The anatomical plane of the thumb differs from that of the remainder of the hand and the thumb is therefore inadequately demonstrated on routine hand views.

A true lateral view is particularly important to allow adequate assessment of the first CMC joint, the first metacarpophalangeal (MCP) joint and the interphalangeal joint of the thumb. To obtain an AP view of the thumb, the hand is internally rotated until the dorsum of the thumb lies flat on the cassette. An oblique view is obtained by rotating the thumb to a position midway between an AP and a lateral view. All views are centred on the first MCP joint.

When a ligamentous injury at the first MCP joint is suspected, stress views may be helpful to assess the integrity of the ulnar and radial collateral ligaments. The radiographic technique, indications and contraindications for stress views are discussed on page 39.

All finger injuries require specific finger views (see Fig. 2.5(a)(i)–(iii)). A finger series includes a PA view (i), an oblique view (ii) and a true lateral view (iii). A technically good lateral projection is critical to the assessment of fracture-dislocation injuries. In acquiring the images, the finger should lie fully extended against the cassette with the primary beam centred on the proximal interphalangeal joint. Good collimation enhances detail. A lateral view of all fingers can be obtained by fanning and separating the fingers, as in Fig. 2.5(b).

When a metacarpal fracture has been demonstrated on the routine hand views, a slightly off-lateral view of the hand may be useful to help assess displacement, angulation or shortening at the metacarpal fracture site (see Fig. 2.6).

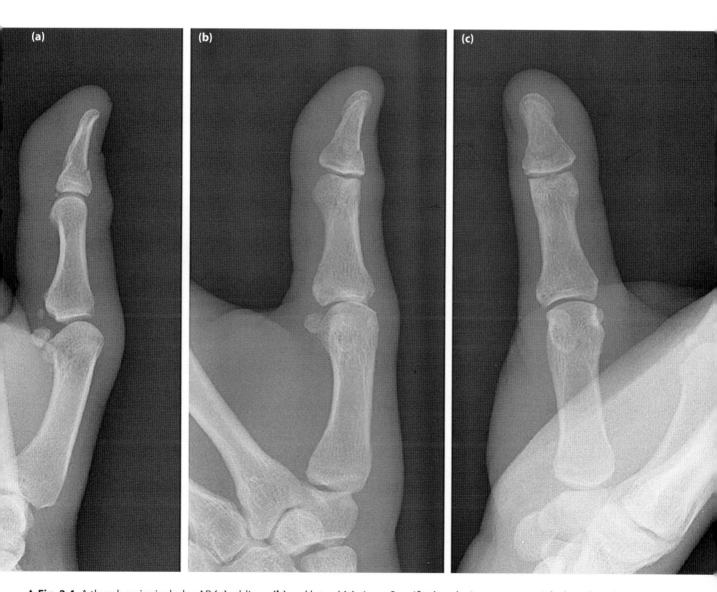

▲ **Fig. 2.4** A thumb series includes AP **(a)**, oblique **(b)** and lateral **(c)** views. Specific thumb views are essential when there has been a thumb injury, demonstrating the relevant anatomy in true AP, oblique and lateral projections. Note the recent fracture of the distal phalanx and an old injury to the anterior aspect of the base of the proximal phalanx, which has the appearance of an old volar plate avulsion.

▶ **Fig. 2.5(a)** A finger series includes a PA view **(i)**, an oblique view **(ii)** and a true lateral view **(iii)**. There is minor soft-tissue swelling centred on the proximal interphalangeal joint but no bone injury is seen.

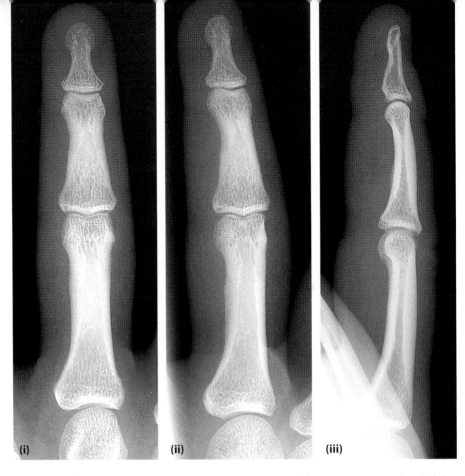

(i)   (ii)   (iii)

▼ **(b)** A lateral view of all fingers is possible using a single exposure, by fanning the fingers and resting them in the lateral position on a stepped foam wedge.

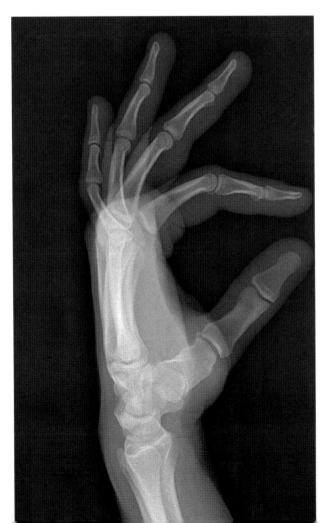

▼ **Fig. 2.6** When a metacarpal fracture is present, this slightly off-lateral view may be helpful to allow assessment of the angulation and shortening at the fracture site.

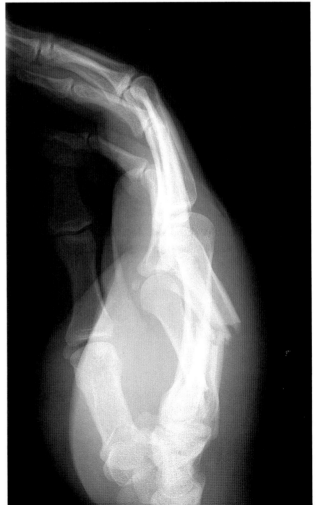

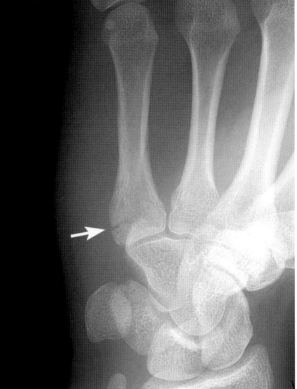

▶ **Fig. 2.7** This reversed oblique view shows an incomplete undisplaced fracture at the base of the fifth metacarpal (arrow) and enables examination of the hamate as well as the fourth and fifth CMC joints.

A reversed oblique view (see Fig. 2.7) is a useful additional view to demonstrate injury at the base of the fourth and fifth metacarpals and the adjacent carpals and medial CMC joints. The technique is discussed on page 45.

If an intra-articular fracture of a metacarpal head is suspected, Brewerton's view (Anderson 2000) is a valuable additional view (see Fig. 2.8). This view brings the majority of the articular surfaces of the MCP joints into profile and enables identification of small articular fractures. The radiographic technique to acquire this view is discussed on page 43.

Hand injuries

Hand injuries may involve bone, joints, tendons, ligaments and other soft tissues.

Bone and joint injuries

Finger injuries

Phalangeal fractures

Residual deformities following a phalangeal fracture may interfere with normal function. Consequently, all suspected phalangeal fractures require imaging, since particular fractures need orthopaedic assessment. If deviation (see Fig. 2.9) or rotation (see Fig. 2.10) of the distal fracture fragment has occurred and is left unreduced, fingers may cross when a fist is made. This would interfere with normal hand function. Other fractures, such as condylar fractures, are intrinsically unstable and usually require fixation (see Fig. 2.11).

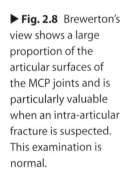

▶ **Fig. 2.8** Brewerton's view shows a large proportion of the articular surfaces of the MCP joints and is particularly valuable when an intra-articular fracture is suspected. This examination is normal.

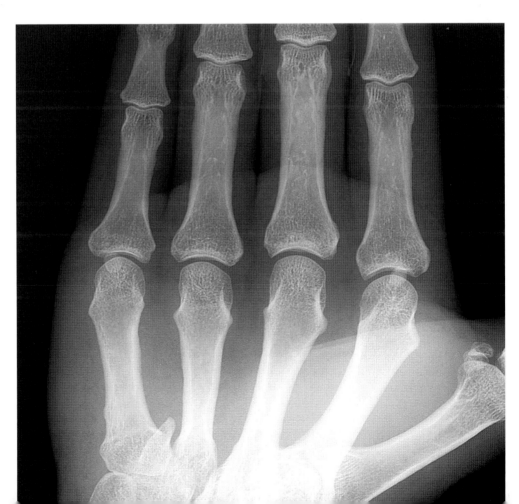

Interphalangeal joint injuries

Interphalangeal joints are hinge joints capable only of flexion and extension. The capsular ligament is reinforced on both sides by the collateral and accessory collateral ligaments (see Fig. 2.12). The volar plate protects the palmar aspect of the joint and acts as a constraint against hyperextension. The accessory collateral ligaments fuse with the lateral margins of the volar plate, increasing stability. The volar plate is membranous proximally and fibrocartilagenous distally. Joint injuries are often the result of an axial force, a so-called 'jamming' injury, forced hyperextension or violent deviation forces. Injury to the volar plates is a common injury and the radial collateral ligament is the ligament most injured. Direct trauma also occurs frequently, usually resulting from a fall, fighting or a stomping injury.

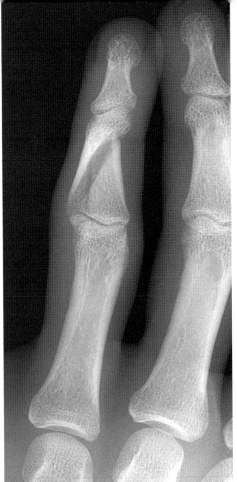

▼ **Fig. 2.9** If deviation such as this is uncorrected, overlapping of the fingers will result when the fingers are flexed.

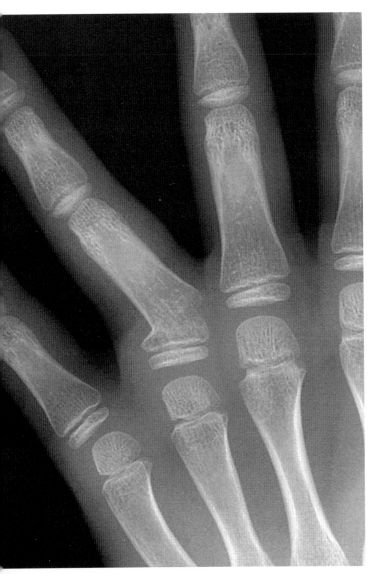

▲ **Fig. 2.10** There is a fracture of the middle phalanx with considerable rotation of the distal fragment. If this rotation is uncorrected, the fingers may overlap when a fist is formed.
▼ **Fig. 2.11** Uni- or bicondylar fractures **(a)** are usually unstable and require fixation **(b)**. Note that the distal screw has broken at surgery and the head of the screw has been removed.

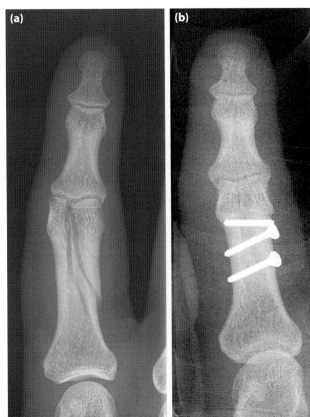

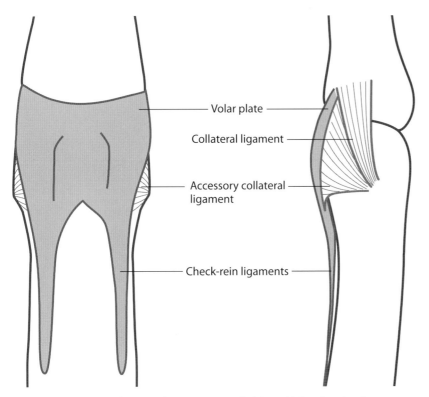

▲ Fig. 2.12 This line drawing depicts an interphalangeal joint showing ligaments and volar plate.

Volar plate
Collateral ligament
Accessory collateral ligament
Check-rein ligaments

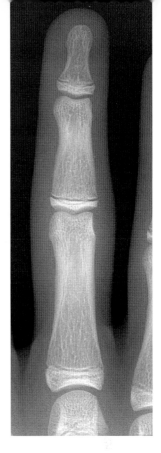

▲ Fig. 2.13 This is the typical appearance of a volar plate injury without a fracture. A fusiform soft-tissue swelling is seen, centred on the injured joint.

Volar plate injuries

Injury to the volar plate results from hyperextension and may occur with or without a characteristic associated phalangeal avulsion fracture. A volar plate injury without a fracture is an extraordinarily common occurrence in sports involving ball handling and is a source of discomfort every time the finger is 'jammed'. The athlete characteristically presents with soft-tissue swelling and tenderness centred on the injured joint (see Fig. 2.13). If an avulsion fracture is present, this will occur at the distal attachment of the plate, with proximal retraction of the bone fragment. The fragment avulsed is often tiny, and careful inspection of the anterior recess of the painful joint is warranted (see Fig. 2.14). When a large fragment is avulsed,

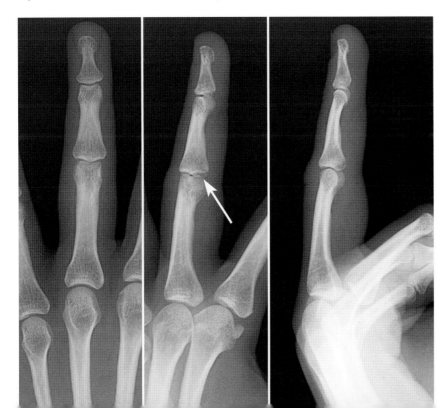

◄ Fig. 2.14 When traction by the volar plate separates a bony fragment, it is usually tiny and is often identified only after careful inspection of the anterior aspect of the injured interphalangeal joint. These tiny fragments are often best seen in the oblique view (arrow).

dorsal subluxation may occur (see Fig. 2.15). If 30–40% of the articular surface is separated, instability can be anticipated and fixation is usually considered (Palmer 1998). Occasionally a volar plate injury is suspected clinically but the plain films are normal. In such circumstances, the volar plate can be imaged by ultrasound (see Figs 2.16 and 2.17) or MRI (see Figs 2.18 and 2.19).

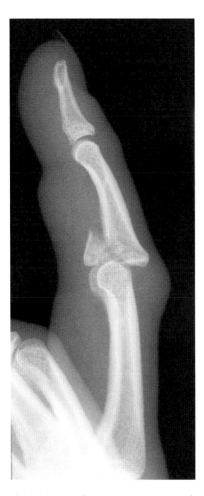

▲ **Fig. 2.15** A hyperextension injury has avulsed a large fragment from the volar aspect of the middle phalanx, which involves about 50% of the articular surface. This has resulted in instability and dorsal subluxation of the proximal interphalangeal (PIP) joint.

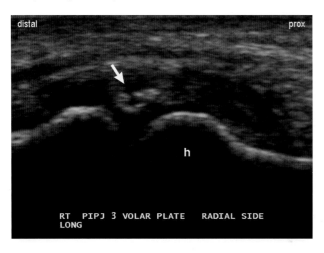

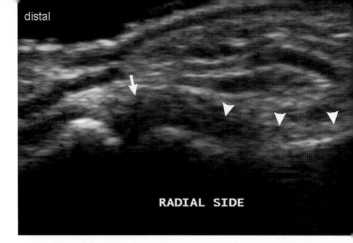

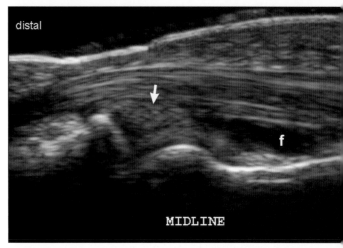

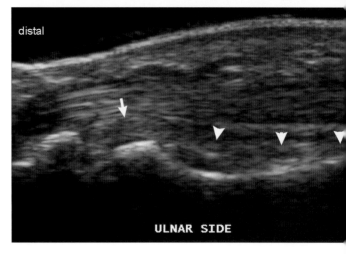

▲ **Fig. 2.16** A normal volar plate is demonstrated by ultrasound. Long-axis ultrasound images show the volar plate (arrows) of the PIP joint and its attachment to the proximal phalangeal neck via the check-rein ligaments (arrowheads). The check-rein ligaments are taut in finger extension but folded and lax in finger flexion. Note fluid (f) within the volar recess of the PIP joint between the check-rein ligaments.

◄ **Fig. 2.17** A subacute tear of the volar plate is demonstrated by ultrasound. This long-axis ultrasound image shows an irregular mixed hypo-hyperechoic cleft (arrow) indicative of a tear involving the volar plate of the middle finger PIP joint to the radial side of the midline. As the clinical management of volar plate tears is rarely altered, note that imaging beyond simple plain x-ray is *not* commonly performed. Proximal phalangeal head = h.

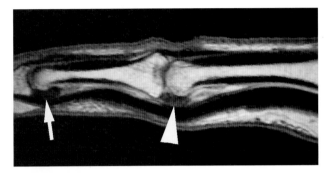

▲ **Fig. 2.18** This sagittal T1-weighted MR image shows normal volar plates at both the distal interphalangeal (DIP) joint (arrow) and PIP joint (arrowhead). Note that intact volar plates are continuous distally with the bases of the distal and middle phalanges, respectively.

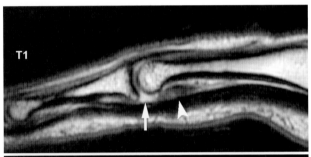

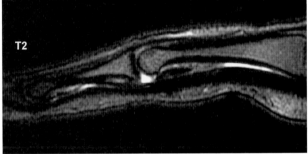

▲ **Fig. 2.19** A PIP joint volar plate tear is shown on T1-weighted and corresponding fat-suppressed sagittal T2-weighted MR images. A fluid-filled gap (arrow) indicates separation of the volar plate (arrowhead) from its normal attachment at the base of the middle phalanx.

Diagnostic imaging of phalangeal fractures and interphalangeal joints

Plain films are invariably the only imaging required for fractures of the phalanges and interphalangeal joints, although ultrasound and MRI may be used to image the volar plate. Interphalangeal joint dislocations are almost always dorsal (see Fig. 2.20). Rarely, volar dislocations can occur at the DIP joint when instability is produced by avulsion of a large dorsal fragment by the extensor tendon (see Fig. 2.21). Following a dislocation, post-reduction films are important and may reveal a previously unrecognised avulsed fragment. Occasionally, dislocations may be irreducible due to entrapment of either the joint capsule or the lateral band of the extensor tendon mechanism. Ultrasound or MRI can be valuable to confirm these complications.

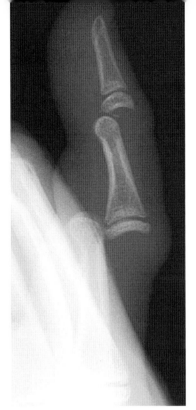

▲ **Fig. 2.20** A violent finger hyperextension injury occurred during a rugby game and produced dislocation of both the DIP and PIP joints. There is also a small fragment separated from the epiphysis at the base of the distal phalanx.

▼ **Fig. 2.21** Volar subluxation and dislocation are uncommon but occasionally may be seen at the DIP joint following avulsion of a large fragment by the extensor tendon. In this case, instability has resulted and there is slight volar subluxation. Also note the hyperextension of the PIP joint. This deformity is described as 'mallet deformity' due to the unopposed pull of the extensor mechanism on the middle phalanx (Lee and Montgomery 2002).

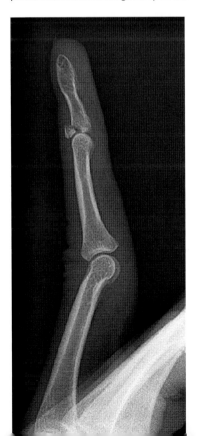

Metacarpal fractures and MCP joint injuries

Injury to the first MCP joint

Ligamentous injury occurs at the first MCP joint following a sudden and violent ulnar or radial deviation force applied to the thumb. A radial deviation injury may tear the ulnar collateral ligament (UCL) and produce a so-called 'skier's thumb' or 'gamekeeper's thumb' (Engkvist et al. 1982). An ulnar deviation force may tear the radial collateral ligament. The injury can result in a complete or incomplete tear of the collateral ligament, or in the avulsion of a bone fragment from the ligamentous attachment at the base of the first proximal phalanx. The diagnosis of a collateral ligament tear or an avulsion fracture is important, because instability may result if the injury is overlooked or inadequately managed. Most tears of the ulnar collateral ligament occur at the attachment to the proximal phalanx.

A stress view may be helpful to assess the integrity of the ulnar or radial collateral ligament when collateral ligament injury is suspected at the first MCP joint (see Fig. 2.22). To stress the UCL, a film of the MCP joint is obtained in the AP position with the joint in 30° of flexion (Lee and Montgomery 2002), while a valgus stress is applied to the MCP joint (see Fig. 2.23). Obviously, to stress the radial collateral ligament, a varus force is used (see Fig. 2.24). The view is abnormal when 30° or more of joint opening is produced on the symptomatic side compared to the normal side (see Fig. 2.25).

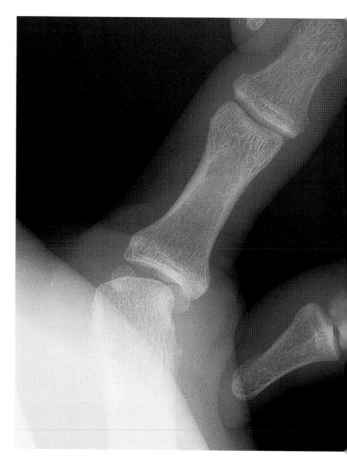

▼ **Fig. 2.22** There is loss of congruency at the first MCP joint suggesting that instability and ligamentous injury may be present. In this case, a stress view may be diagnostic.

▲ **Fig. 2.23** In the absence of an avulsed fragment, a view taken while applying a valgus stress to the UCL demonstrates abnormal opening of the medial side of the joint, indicative of a UCL injury.

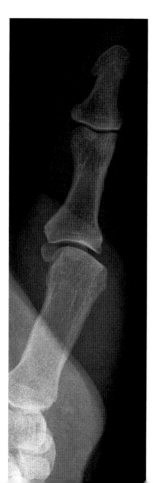

▼ **Fig. 2.24** Comparative views on stressing the ulnar collateral ligaments of both the symptomatic and asymptomatic sides show a diagnostic discrepancy. The symptomatic joint on the right opens abnormally, 30° more than the asymptomatic joint on the left, confirming rupture of the UCL of the thumb on the right.

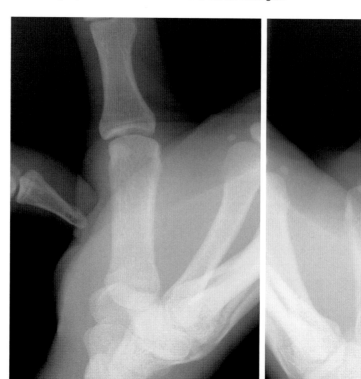

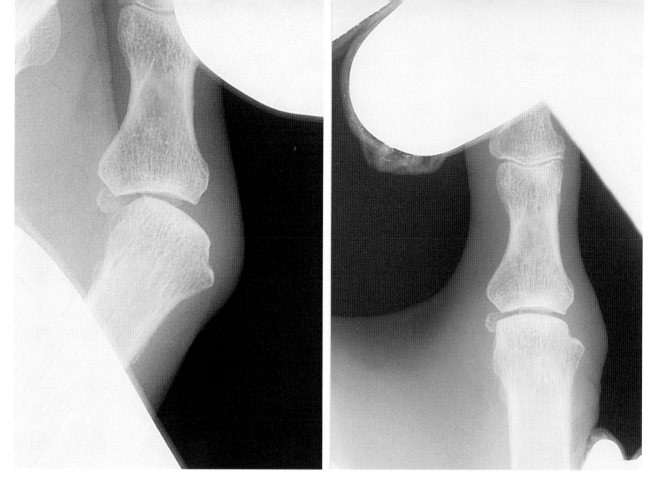

▲ **Fig. 2.25** Applying a varus stress to the radial collateral ligaments of both the asymptomatic thumb on the right and the symptomatic side on the left allows the diagnosis of a radial collateral ligament rupture on the symptomatic side.

An immediate surgical repair may be required to avoid instability. Conservative management is considered if there is a fracture that involves less than 30% of the articular surface of the base of the proximal phalanx and there is less than 1.5 mm of displacement. It is important to remember that a stress radiograph carries the risk of converting a non-displaced ligament tear or an in-situ avulsion fracture into a Stener lesion. A Stener lesion is present whenever the torn proximal stump of the UCL is displaced superficial to the adductor pollicis aponeurosis. Spontaneous ligament healing with restoration of MCP joint stability cannot then occur (see Fig. 2.26).

It is therefore inadvisable to perform a stress view if any of the following circumstances apply:

- an avulsion fracture has already been demonstrated on the routine film series (see Fig. 2.27)
- the local policy of surgical management is to explore these injuries regardless of the radiographic findings
- high-quality ultrasound (see Figs 2.28 and 2.29) or MRI (see Fig. 2.30) is available as an alternative method of imaging assessment (O'Callaghan et al. 1994).

▶ **Fig. 2.26** It is possible that an energetic stress view such as this may complicate a simple UCL avulsion by converting it into a Stener lesion.

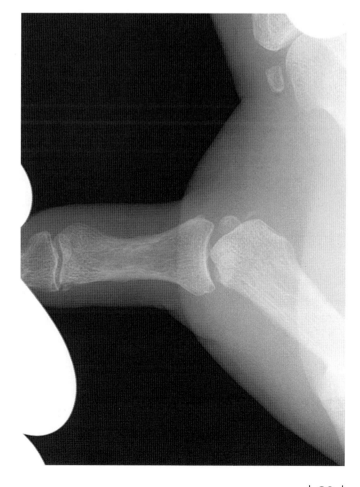

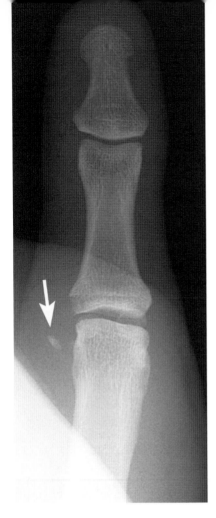

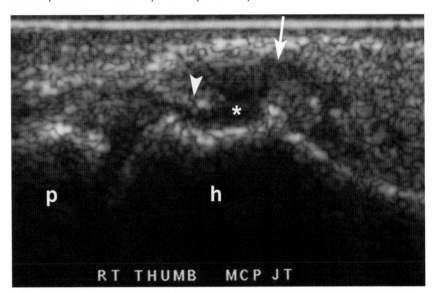

◀ **Fig. 2.27** A small bony fragment can be seen separated by the UCL (arrow). As the diagnosis of an avulsion with displacement is already available, a stress view should not be performed.

▼ **Fig. 2.28** A Stener lesion is demonstrated by ultrasound. A long-axis image of the UCL of the right thumb demonstrates a focal soft-tissue thickening adjacent to the metacarpal head, which represents the displaced proximal ligamentous stump. There is a hypoechoic gap at the usual site of the proximal segment (asterisk). Note the thin echogenic line of interposed adductor aponeurosis (arrowhead). Metacarpal head = h. Base of proximal phalanx = p.

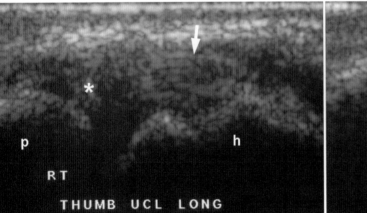

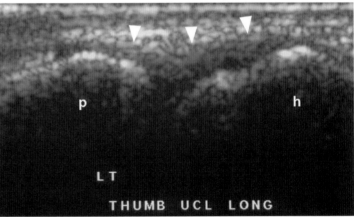

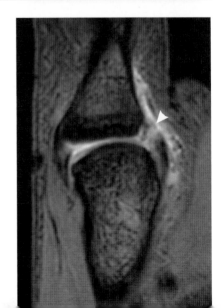

▲ **Fig. 2.29** A Stener lesion of the right thumb is demonstrated by ultrasound. The UCL of the *right* thumb MCP joint shows a hypoechoic zone distally that lacks discernible fibres (*), while the proximal portion of the ligament appears to have doubled in thickness (arrow) due to proximal folding and apposition of the torn and displaced distal portion. Arrowheads indicate a normal UCL of the *left* thumb MCP joint for comparison. Metacarpal head = h. Base of proximal phalanx = p.

▶ **Fig. 2.30** MRI demonstrates an undisplaced UCL tear at the thumb MCP joint. This fat-suppressed PD-weighted image shows a hyperintense defect in UCL fibre continuity (arrowhead) at the phalangeal attachment.

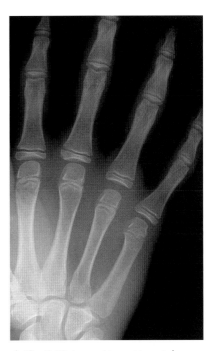

Dislocation and subluxation of the MCP joints

Dislocation and subluxation of the MCP joints are hyperextension injuries, with the proximal phalanx displaced dorsally (see Figs 2.31 and 2.32). The dislocations are characteristically difficult to reduce due to volar plate entrapment (see Fig. 2.33) or because occasionally the metacarpal head may be pushed through the volar plate or caught between the lumbrical and the long flexor tendon.

Metacarpal fractures

Metacarpal fractures are a common hand injury, usually resulting from punching (see Fig. 2.34) or direct trauma (see Fig. 2.35). A large percentage of metacarpal fractures

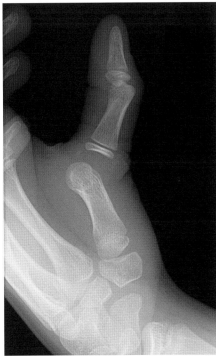

◀ **Fig. 2.31** During a game of rugby, a hyperextension force was applied to the thumb, resulting in dislocation of the first MCP joint.

▲ **Fig. 2.33** In an attempt to catch a cricket ball, this young cricketer has dislocated his fourth MCP joint. Joint space widening persists after reduction, suggesting volar plate entrapment within the joint space.

▼ **Fig. 2.32** An excessive hyperextension force to the hand has produced multiple dorsal dislocations of MCP joints two to five, with dorsal displacement of the proximal phalanges.

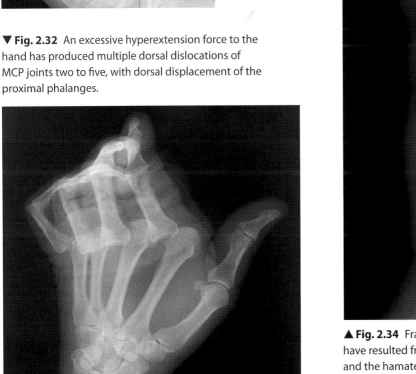

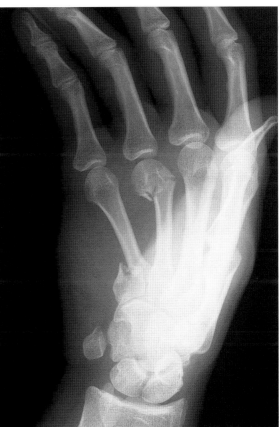

▲ **Fig. 2.34** Fractures of the fourth and fifth metacarpals have resulted from punching. The medial CMC joints and the hamate may also be injured as a result of this mechanism.

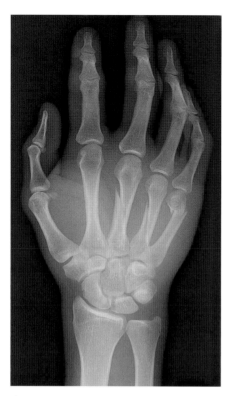

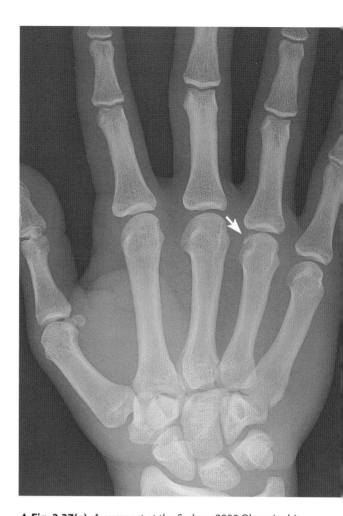

▲ **Fig. 2.35** Metacarpal fractures are also commonly caused by direct trauma. Fractures of the third, fourth and fifth metacarpals have resulted from a stomping injury suffered during a game of rugby.

▼ **Fig. 2.36** By far the most common metacarpal fracture is a fracture of the neck or distal shaft of the fifth metacarpal. Palmar angulation of the metacarpal heads will invariably occur. This is usually a punching injury, and on weekends casualty films always contain examples of this injury.

▲ **Fig. 2.37(a)** A gymnast at the Sydney 2000 Olympics hit his hand on the vaulting apparatus during a performance. An initial PA view shows possible bony density projected over the lateral margin of the head of the fourth metacarpal (arrow).
▼ **(b)** A Brewerton's view was obtained on the same athlete as in **(a)** and this view clearly shows an intra-articular fracture with displacement of the fragment.

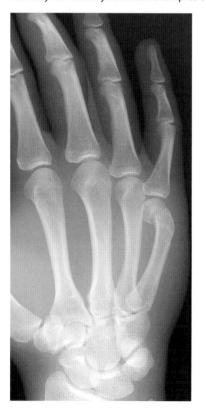

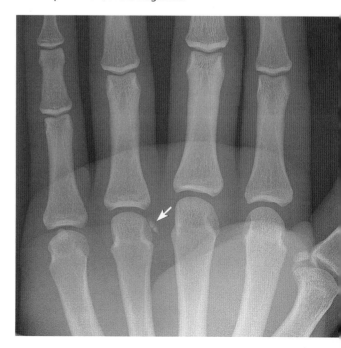

result from fighting and football. The most common type is a fracture of the fifth metacarpal neck (see Fig. 2.36): metacarpal fractures represent a third of all hand fractures, and fractures of the fifth metacarpal account for half of these (Lee and Jupiter 2000). Characteristically, palmar angulation of the metacarpal head occurs and this deformity is often accepted. However, it must be remembered that in some sports, such as cricket, golf and tennis where a comfortable bat, club or racquet grip is essential, reduction of the angulation may be necessary to avoid a bony lump in the palm of the hand. Rotational deformities are also functionally significant and it is important to appreciate this deformity on radiographs. For each 1° of malrotation at the metacarpal fracture site, there may be as much as a 5° malrotation at the finge tip (Opgrande and Westphal 1983). The acceptability of malrotation will vary with the manual activity required by the individual. There is a strong ligament that passes between metacarpal heads two to five. This ligament prevents separation of the metacarpals and adds stability to metacarpal shaft fractures. Fractures of the second and fifth metacarpals are consequently less supported as they have the ligament only on one side.

Metacarpal heads have a large articular surface at the palmar aspect of the neck, allowing increased metacarpophalangeal flexion. The size of the articular surface results in greater vulnerability to intra-articular fracture. A Brewerton's view is a valuable extra view that helps to examine a larger percentage of the articular surfaces when an intra-articular fracture is suspected (see Fig. 2.37(a)). The view is obtained with the hand AP and the dorsal surfaces of the fingers lying on the cassette. The MCP joints are flexed to 45° and the beam is centred on the third MCP joint using a straight tube (see Fig. 2.37(b)). If large enough, intra-articular fractures can often be identified by careful inspection of the routine plain film series (see Fig. 2.38).

Fractures and dislocations at the base of the first CMC joint

Fractures at the base of the first metacarpal require special attention and are classified as either stable or unstable, depending upon involvement of the first CMC joint. Bennett's fracture (see Fig. 2.39) and Rolando's fracture

▼ **Fig. 2.39(a)** A Bennett's fracture has resulted from axial loading of the first metacarpal. The volar ligament at the base of the first metacarpal has remained intact and a volar 'beak' fragment is separated from the volar aspect of the metacarpal base but remains undisplaced. **(b)** A Bennett's fracture. Muscular traction of the abductors and extensors has displaced the metacarpal shaft radially and dorsally, rotating the volar fragment away from the major fragment.

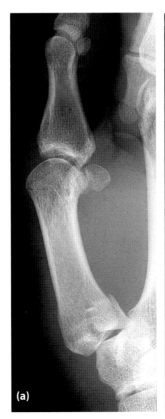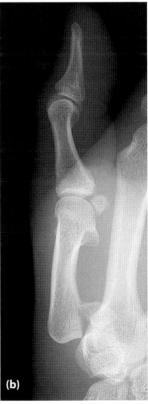

(a)　　(b)

▲ **Fig. 2.38** An intra-articular fracture of the head of the second metatarsal resulting from direct trauma is easily seen on routine hand views.

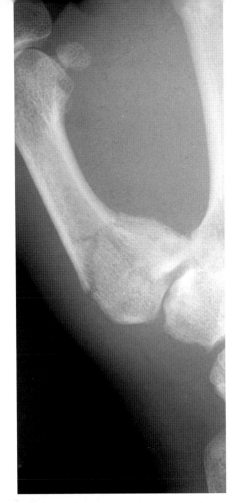

(see Fig. 2.40) are both unstable, as the pull of the abductors and extensors of the thumb will commonly produce displacement. Two stable fractures are also seen at the first CMC joint. These are fractures of the proximal metacarpal shaft (see Fig. 2.41(a)) and growth-plate fractures at the base of the first metacarpal in the skeletally immature (see Fig. 2.41(b)). Both fractures are extra-articular.

Subluxations and dislocations of the first CMC joint are uncommon and result from hyperextension injuries (see Fig. 2.42).

▲ **Fig. 2.40** A Rolando's fracture involves the first CMC joint. This is a comminuted T- or Y-shaped fracture involving the base of the first metacarpal, which commonly becomes displaced with dorsal displacement of the metacarpal shaft. This fracture also results from an axial force, with the ridge of the distal articular surface of the trapezium acting like a log splitter.

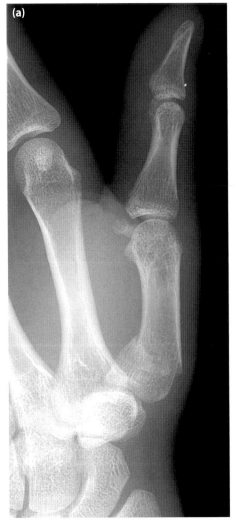
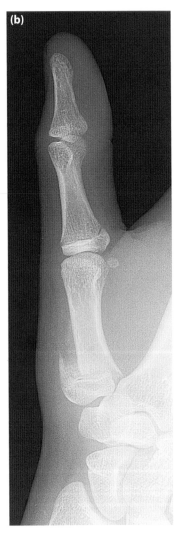

▲ **Fig. 2.41(a)** A fracture of the base of the first metacarpal. This is a stable fracture and does not involve the first CMC joint.
(b) A Salter-Harris II fracture involving the first metacarpal growth plate. This is also a stable fracture.

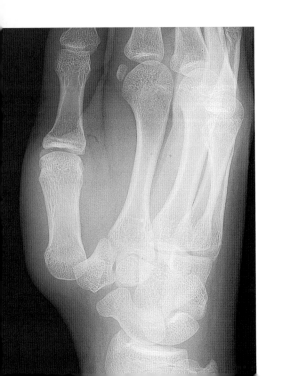

◄ **Fig. 2.42** Subluxation of the first MCP joint can result from hyperextension of the thumb. When subluxation of the first MCP joint has occurred, it is important to consider the possibility of an associated injury to the anterior ridge of the trapezium.

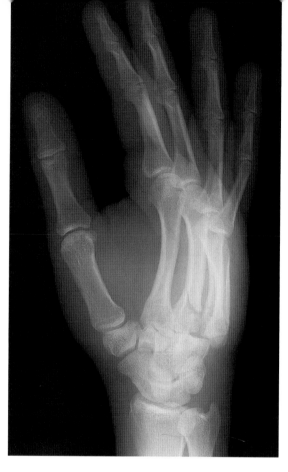

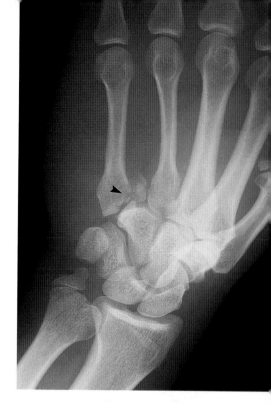

◀ **Fig. 2.43** A fracture of the third metacarpal and fracture/dislocations of the fourth and fifth CMC joints have resulted from a punching injury.

▶ **Fig. 2.44** A reversed oblique view shows a fracture of the base of the fifth metacarpal, which will be unstable and will act like a little Bennett's fracture.

Other CMC joint injuries

Apart from the first carpometacarpal joint, the CMC joints are relatively stable, being firmly restrained by ligaments. They are not required to move significantly with hand and wrist function. Consequently, the lesser CMC joints are rarely injured. Injury to the fourth and fifth carpometacarpal joints may occasionally result from punching trauma (see Fig. 2.43). When this injury is suspected, an additional reversed oblique view is worthwhile. This is a reversed oblique view. For this view, the hand is placed in an AP position with the radial side elevated 30° and the beam is centred on the fifth CMC joint. Fractures of the hamate are also shown well using this projection. If the fifth CMC joint is involved, these fractures may be the equivalent of Bennett's and Rolando's fractures, often requiring reduction and fixation to address instability (see Figs 2.44 and 2.45). Considerable force is required to dislocate other CMC joints (see Fig. 2.46).

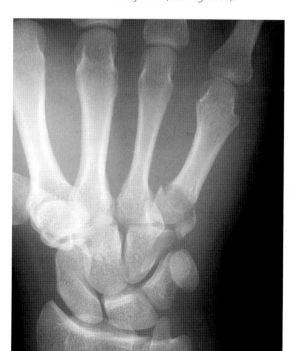

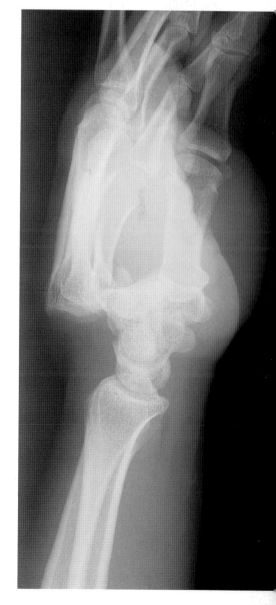

◀ **Fig. 2.45** A comminuted fracture involving the base of the fifth metacarpal, which is unstable and will behave in a similar manner to a Rolando's fracture of the first CMC joint.

▶ **Fig. 2.46** The CMC joints are intrinsically stable and an extremely forceful hyperextension injury would have been necessary to produce these dislocations of CMC joints two to five.

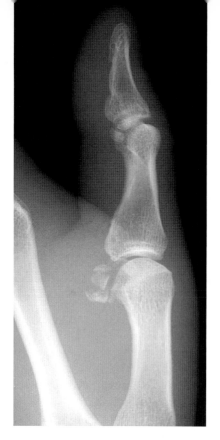

▲ Fig. 2.47 A cricketer fractured the thumb sesamoids by direct impact when attempting to catch a fast-travelling cricket ball.

Injury of the thumb sesamoids

The sesamoids lie within the volar plate of the first MCP joint and both the volar plate and sesamoids are susceptible to injury following a hyperextension injury or with direct trauma. Most direct injury occurs in sports involving the catching of a hard ball, such as in baseball and cricket (see Fig. 2.47).

Tendon injuries

Flexor tendon injuries

Knowledge of flexor tendon anatomy (see Fig. 2.48(a)) and the pulley system (see Fig. 2.48(b)) is important in the understanding of the flexor digitorum profundus (FDP) rupture 'climber's finger' and 'trigger finger' conditions. As the flexor tendons pass distally from the hand and along the finger, they pass through a fibro-osseous tunnel that extends from the mid-palm to the FDP insertion onto the distal phalanx. The FDP tendon has a broad insertion onto the anterior surface of the proximal third of the distal phalanx. A combination of annular and cruciate ligamentous fibres (pulleys) strap the FDS and FDP tendons down to the floor of the tunnel. Cruciate ligamentous fibres (pulleys) cross over the anterior aspect of the tendon at the interphalangeal joints, allowing a greater range of finger flexion. With flexion, these cruciate fibres become more transverse. The pulley system is essential for normal finger biomechanics and acts as a constraint against flexor tendon 'bowstringing'.

The pulleys are named in line with a standard classification produced by the American Society for Surgery of the Hand. The arcuate fibres are known as A1 to A5 depending on their position and the cruciate fibres are C1 to C3. The arcuate fibres can be demonstrated using ultrasound (see Fig. 2.49) and MRI (see Fig. 2.50) (Hauger et al. 2000).

▼ Fig. 2.48(a) Anatomy of the flexor tendon and the pulley system. **(b)** The pulley system of the finger.

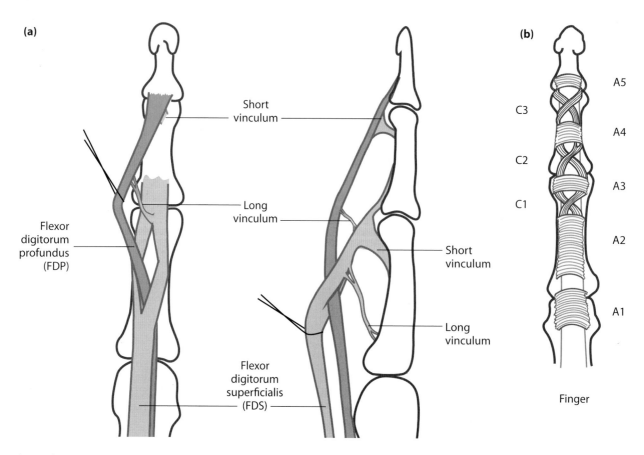

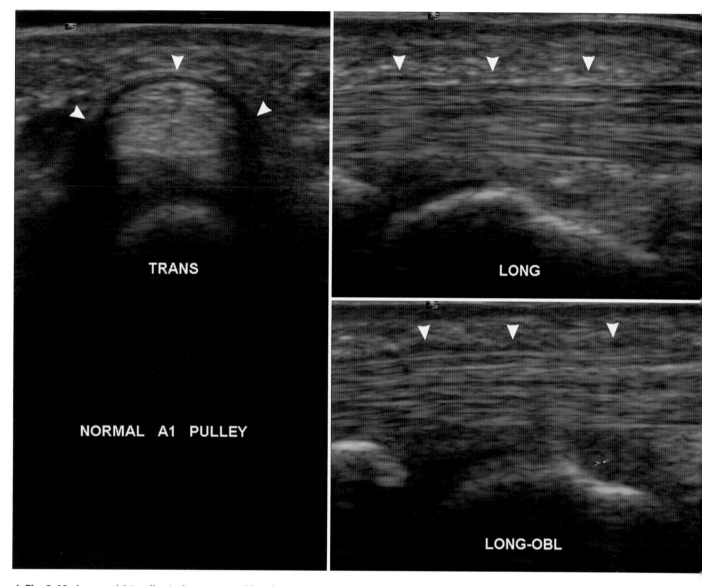

TRANS

LONG

NORMAL A1 PULLEY

LONG-OBL

▲ **Fig. 2.49** A normal A1 pulley is demonstrated by ultrasound. The A1 pulley is indicated by arrowheads. The transverse fibre orientation is best demonstrated on the transverse image (TRANS). On long-axis imaging (LONG), these fibres tend to blend with the adjacent tissues, but can be rendered conspicuous by angling the transducer slightly to render the fibres hypoechoic by anisotropy (long-oblique view, LONG-OBL).

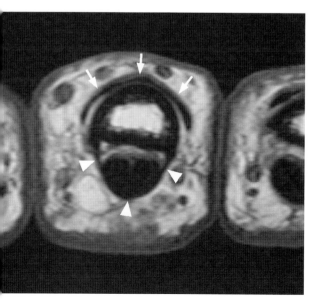

◀**Fig. 2.50(a)** A transverse T1-weighted MR image of a proximal phalanx shows a normal A2 pulley (arrowheads) and a normal extensor tendon complex (arrows). Note that normal tendons and ligaments appear uniformly hypointense on MRI.
▼ **(b)** A longitudinal MR image demonstrates a normal A2 (arrows) and A4 pulleys (arrowheads) profiled on the volar surface of the flexor tendon.

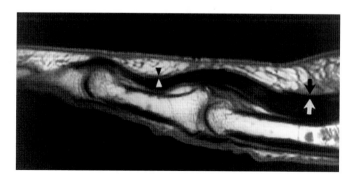

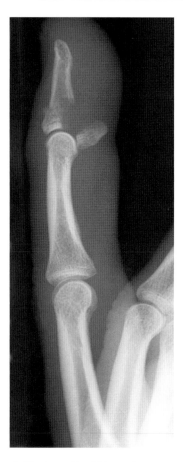 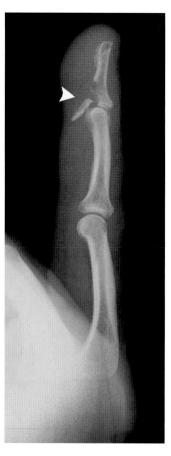

▲ **Fig. 2.51** The FDP tendon has avulsed a fragment from its insertion. The fragment has become rotated, hinged on the volar plate of the DIP joint.

▲ **Fig. 2.52** Following rupture of the FDP tendon, retraction of the tendon has been prevented by the avulsed fragment arrested on the A5 pulley (arrowhead).

▼ **Fig. 2.53** A fragment has been avulsed from the distal phalanx by the FDP tendon and retracted as far as the distal shaft of the middle phalanx. At this point the fragment is restrained by either an intact vinculum or the A4 pulley.

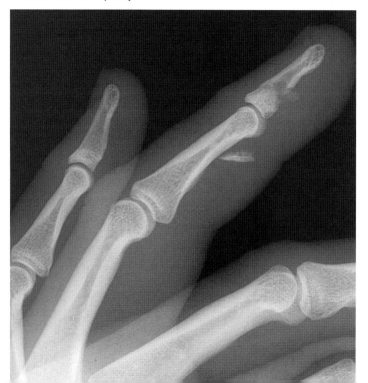

Injury to the FDP tendon

Injury to the FDP tendon occurs when there is sudden forced extension of a strongly flexed finger. This is classically encountered in rugby and is known as 'jersey finger'. A player attempts a tackle by grasping the jersey of an opponent who suddenly breaks loose, causing a violent extension of the tightly flexed fingers. The injury may involve any finger, including the thumb, but the ring finger is most commonly affected, representing 75% of all FDP injuries (Stamos and Leddy 2000). A bone fragment is usually avulsed from the tendon insertion at the distal phalanx, although the tendon itself may occasionally rupture.

In the heat of sport, a rupture of the FDP tendon may initially appear to be trivial and loss of flexion of the distal interphalangeal joint may not be appreciated. There is often a delay in the diagnosis being made. To further impede an early diagnosis, tenderness is most marked over the distal end of the retracted tendon and this may be some distance from the fracture bed in the distal phalanx.

Imaging of FDP injuries

In the vast majority of 'jersey finger' injuries, plain x-ray is the only imaging test required. Bony avulsion fragments tend to retract proximally with the tendon, but are invariably prevented from reaching the palm due to the fracture fragment being either held by its attachment to the volar plate at the DIP joint (see Fig. 2.51), held by an intact vinculum or caught on a flexor pulley (see Figs 2.52 and 2.53). It is obviously important to consider the diagnosis of FDP rupture whenever a bone fragment is seen at the anterior aspect of the finger on a lateral view. Other injuries such as volar plate avulsion fractures also produce small anterior bone fragments and are far more common than FDP avulsions. The differentiation relies on confirming that the size and shape of the displaced fragment corresponds to an equivalent bony defect at the phalangeal origin. Careful inspection of the insertion site of the flexor tendon may help exclude an FDP injury (see Fig. 2.54). Additionally, following an FDP avulsion fracture, it is important to determine whether the DIP joint is stable, remembering that instability is likely if 30–40% or more of the articular surface is separated. Instability is usually indicated by subluxation.

When the tendon ruptures and there is no bone fragment avulsed, the tendon may retract to any level and sometimes all the way into the palm of the hand. In this situation, ultrasound (see Fig. 2.55) or MRI (see Fig. 2.56) may be helpful for pre-operative localisation.

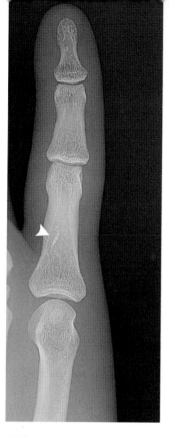
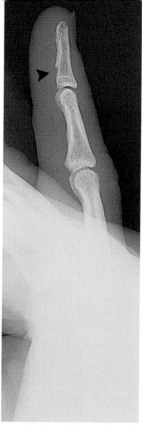

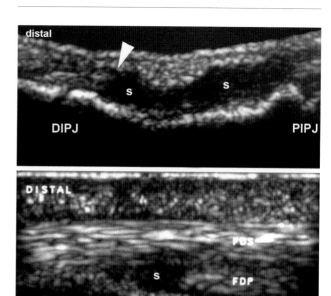

▲ **Fig. 2.54** The small bony fragment projected over the mid-shaft of the proximal phalanx (white arrowhead) is the same shape as the deficit at the FDP insertion (black arrowhead). The fragment is obscured in the lateral view. This fragment proved to be a fragment avulsed by the FDP tendon, which retracted until caught on the A2 pulley.

▲ **Fig. 2.55** Long-axis ultrasound images demonstrate a distal FDP tendon rupture and proximal retraction in a patient with underlying rheumatoid arthritis. The arrowhead indicates the tear margin of the distal tendon stump, which remains attached at the distal phalanx. The arrow indicates the retracted tear margin of the proximal tendon stump located at the level of metacarpal neck. There is intervening hypoechoic rheumatoid pannus (s), showing slightly lobulated contours. DIP joint = DIPJ. PIP joint = PIPJ. Metacarpal head = MC HEAD.

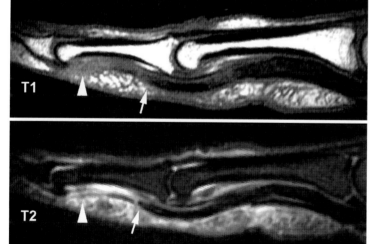

◄ **Fig. 2.56(a)** Sagittal T1- and corresponding fat-suppressed T2-weighted MR images demonstrate rupture of the distal FDP tendon. The arrowheads indicate the absent tendon and high signal within the tendon sheath at the middle phalanx level. The arrows indicate the tear margin of the proximal tendon stump retracted to C2 pulley level.

► **(b)** A sagittal T1-weighted MR image shows an avulsion of the FDP tendon with separation of a curvilinear cortical bone fragment (arrowhead). The tendon has retracted to the level of the proximal interphalangeal joint.

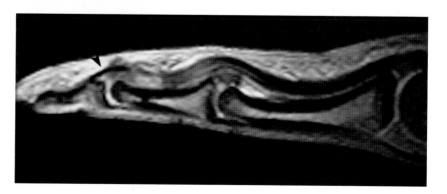

As a management guide, Leddy and Packer (1977) have classified 'jersey finger' into three types:

- *Type 1:* the tendon is retracted into the palm of the hand, implying rupture of the vincula and the absence of any significant bony fragment. Rupture of the vincula deprives the tendon of its blood supply, causing ischaemia, and the tendon becomes oedematous preventing rethreading. Surgical correction is a matter of urgency.

- *Type 2:* an avulsed bone fragment is retracted to the level of the PIP joint. This position would suggest that the fragment is snared on the A3 pulley and that the long vinculum remains intact with the blood supply maintained. Theoretically, the repair of this injury is less urgent. However, Trumble et al. (1992) found that six out of 12 of their series of patients with an FDP avulsion had pre-operative radiographs that underestimated the level of tendon retraction, suggesting that all FDP avulsions should be surgically repaired as soon as possible.

- *Type 3:* a large bone fragment is caught at the level of the A4 pulley. Although this scenario favours an intact blood supply, cases have been reported in which the tendon is no longer attached to the displaced fragment. This would support Trumble et al.'s belief that all FDP injuries should be referred for assessment as soon as possible.

Pulley injuries and 'bowstringing'

Flexor tendon pulley rupture most commonly occurs at either the A2 or A4 pulley. This injury usually occurs with a background of chronic repetitive overload and is typically seen in rock climbers and baseball pitchers. The ring and middle fingers are most often affected in climbers, whereas the middle finger is usually involved in baseball pitchers. Ultrasound (see Figs 2.57 and 2.58) and MRI (see Fig. 2.59) show thickening of the affected pulley and 'bowstringing' of the flexor tendons away from the underlying phalangeal bone surface at the level of rupture. Bowstringing is most dramatically demonstrated on real-time ultrasound examination as a dynamic phenomenon during resisted contraction. The changes become permanent, with scarring and soft-tissue thickening (see Fig. 2.60).

▶ **Fig. 2.58** Rupture of an A2 pulley is demonstrated by ultrasound. Long-axis views at the flexor aspect of the proximal and mid-segments of the proximal phalanx obtained in both flexion and extension show displacement of the FDS-FDP tendon complex (t) away from the underlying bone surface (callipers). 'Bowstringing' accentuates with finger flexion. Arrows indicate accompanying flexor sheath effusion.

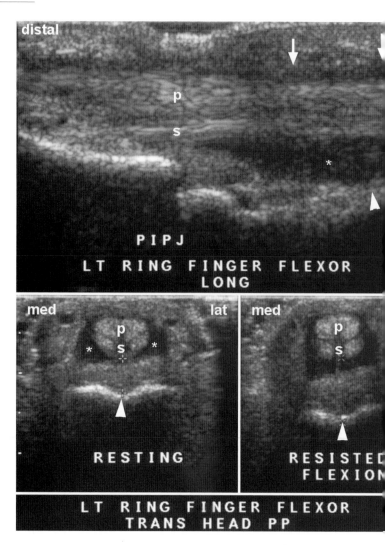

▲ **Fig. 2.57** Simultaneous rupture of both the A2 and A3 pulleys is demonstrated by ultrasound. Both transverse and long-axis images of the FDS-FDP tendon complex have been obtained at the level of the head and neck of the proximal phalanx. These show displacement of the tendons away from the underlying proximal phalangeal bone surface (arrowheads) indicative of pulley injury. This 'bowstringing' is further accentuated by resisted finger flexion (lower right image), as is apparent when compared with a resting view at the same level (lower left image). Note that there is accompanying flexor sheath effusion and/or synovitis (*). FDS tendon = s. FDP tendon = p. Arrows indicate thickened and abnormally hypoechoic A3 and A2 pulleys.

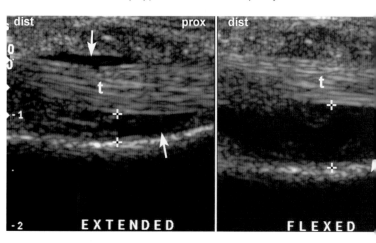

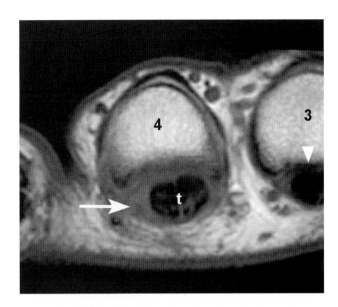

◀ **Fig. 2.59** A ring finger A2 pulley rupture is demonstrated by a transverse T1-weighted MR image. The arrow indicates the abnormally thickened ring finger A2 pulley showing increased signal intensity. The ring finger FDS-FDP tendon complex (t) is displaced away from the phalangeal bone surface when compared with the middle finger (arrowhead). Ring finger = 4. Middle finger = 3.
Source: Adapted from Stoller (2004).

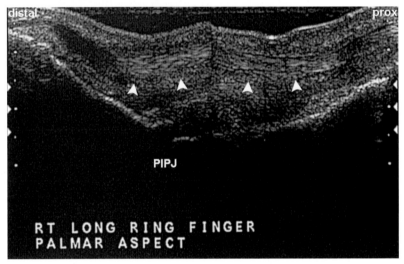

◀ **Fig. 2.60(a)** A long-axis ultrasound image demonstrates wide displacement of the flexor tendons (arrowheads) away from the phalangeal bone surfaces, consistent with multiple ruptured pulleys. Note the *absence* of accompanying tendon sheath effusion, indicative of chronic rather than recent injury. This occurred when the patient was thrown a lifeline after he was washed overboard during a sailing race in rough seas. The pulleys have failed under an extreme extension force similar to that which would operate during rock climbing. Note: Apparent abrupt angulation in the skin and tendon surface contours at the midpoint of this image is an artefact related to the split-screen juxtaposition of two separate images obtained with slightly different angles of insonation.
PIP joint = PIPJ.

▼ **(b)** A plain film of the injured finger shown in **(a)** shows a fixed flexion deformity and marked soft-tissue thickening due to scarring on the volar aspect of the PIP joint secondary to previous 'bowstringing'.

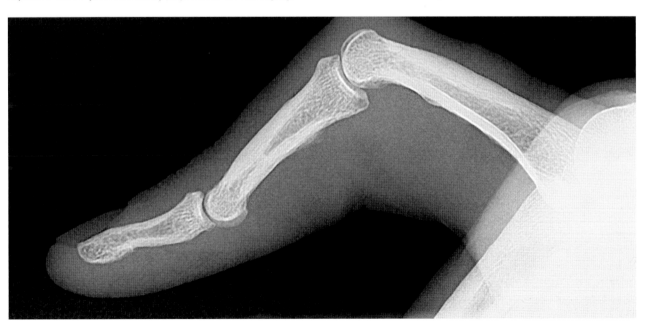

Injury to the FDS tendon

The FDS tendon passes through the flexor tunnel of each finger superficial to the FDP tendon. At the level of the mid-shaft of the proximal phalanx, the FDS tendon splits and passes on either side of the FDP tendon to insert into the shaft of the middle phalanx after becoming a single tendon. As with an FDP rupture, an FDS rupture occurs with sudden and violent finger extension against active flexion. Isolated rupture of the FDS tendon is an uncommon injury and the FDS and FDP tendons usually rupture together (Boyes et al. 1960). If they are ruptured, there is loss of ability to flex both the DIP and PIP joints together. Often the patient considers this a minor disability, and this commonly delays presentation and diagnosis. Plain films are required to exclude any associated bone injury, although it is rare to see an avulsion fracture. Pre-operative ultrasound or MRI can help to confirm the site of tendon rupture, assess underlying tendon quality and find the level of the retracted tendon stump. Usually, however, the end of the tendon is tender and can be felt as localised thickening.

Tendon adhesions

Tendon adhesions may follow trauma or an inflammatory process. The real-time imaging capability of ultrasound may be used to assess tendon glide and exclude tendon adhesion (see Fig. 2.61) differentiating it from tendon rupture.

Flexor tendon injury associated with a hook of hamate fracture

The base of the hook of hamate is closely related to both the FDP and FDS tendons (see Fig. 2.62(a)), which use the hook as a pulley (see Fig. 2.62(b)). Consequently, when there is a hook of hamate fracture, injury to the tendon and tendon sheath may occur due to bony irregularity, resulting in teno-synovitis, tendon attrition and tendon rupture. This process is aggravated by the common occurrence of non-union of a hook fracture. In a series reported by Bishop and Beckenbaugh (1988), 25% of patients with a hook of hamate fracture also had tenosynovitis, tendon fraying or rupture.

'Trigger finger'

Intermittent locking or catching of a finger (or thumb) during flexion and extension, with or without associated pain, can arise from a mismatch between the size of the flexor pulley and its enclosed tendon ('trigger finger' or 'stenosing tenosynovitis'). In most cases there is thickening of *both* the pulley and the FDS-FDP tendon complex. During finger flexion, the thickened tendon segment may produce a click as it passes proximally beneath the thickened pulley. On attempted finger extension, return glide of the thickened tendon segment through the abnormal pulley may then be difficult (i.e. the finger can become locked in the 'flexed trigger position'). Overuse is the most common cause, with activities that involve a powerful grip or repetitive forceful finger flexion predisposing to this condition. The diagnosis is obviously clinical, but dynamic ultrasound may provide details of the cause of the catch, as demonstrated in Figs 2.63 and 2.64.

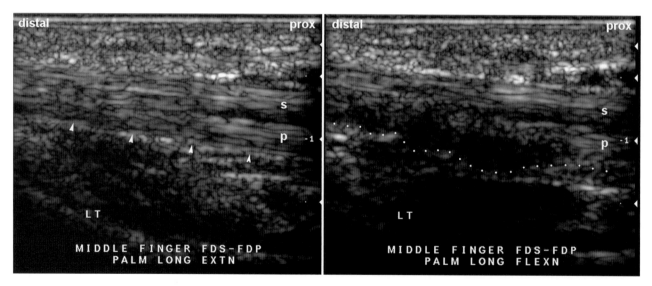

▲ **Fig. 2.61** An FDP tendon adhesion is demonstrated by ultrasound. Long-axis ultrasound images of the middle finger FDS (s) and FDP (p) tendons have been obtained at the same palm level with the finger alternately extended and flexed. On the finger extension view (EXTN), the FDP tendon shows normal straight contour (arrowheads) and normal fibrillar echotexture. On the finger flexion view (FLEXN), there is failure of normal FDP tendon glide due to adhesion, with consequent buckling of tendon surface contour (dotted line) and markedly hypoechoic tendon echotexture arising from poor tendon fibre reflectivity (fibre reflectivity being highly angle-dependent, a phenomenon known as anisotropy). Note that the FDS tendon shows normal glide with retention of normal contour and echotexture.

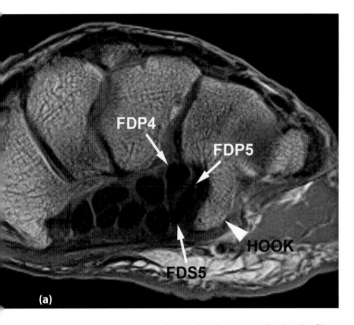
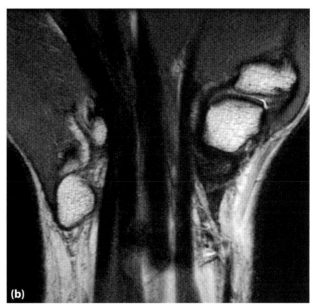

▲ **Fig. 2.62(a)** The close relationship between the hook of hamate and the flexor tendons of the ring and little fingers is demonstrated by this axial MR image. **(b)** The tendons of the ring and little fingers use the hook as a pulley, with alteration of their course shown in this coronal MR image. The tendons rub against the hook with finger flexion. Consequently, any bony irregularity caused by bone injury may produce tendon attrition.

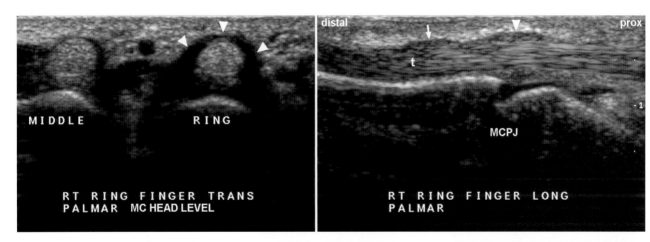

▲ **Fig. 2.63** An ultrasound examination shows the cause of 'trigger finger' in this case. Axial and longitudinal ultrasound images show thickening of the A1 (arrowheads) and A2 (arrow) pulleys of the ring finger. Note the transverse image of the middle finger shows a normal A1 pulley for comparison. FDS-FDP tendons = t.

▶ **Fig. 2.64** 'Trigger finger' syndrome is demonstrated by ultrasound. This long-axis ultrasound image of the flexor tendon apparatus at the level of the MCP joint shows focal hypoechoic nodular thickening of the FDS tendon (arrow). There is also hypoechoic thickening of the overlying distal fibres of the A1 pulley (arrowheads), and fusiform thickening of both the FDS and FDP tendons at the A2 pulley level (callipers).

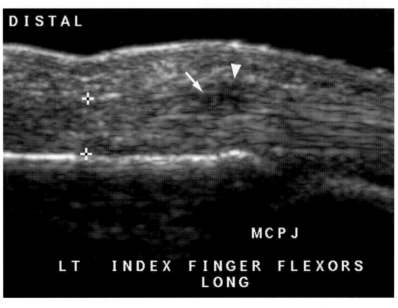

Extensor tendon injuries

'Mallet finger' deformity

The lateral bands of the extensor tendon join to form the distal conjoint extensor tendon, which inserts at the dorsal lip of the base of the distal phalanx. At this point the distal tendon is relatively thin, and an area of relative avascularity has been described 11–16 mm from its insertion (Scott 2000). This avascularity may contribute to spontaneous rupture of the tendon in this area. 'Mallet finger' deformity occurs following a flexion force to the DIP joint, usually due to an axial impact injury to the fingertip ('jamming'). This is most commonly seen in sports involving ball handling. This sudden and violent flexion can cause either rupture of the extensor digitorum tendon or an avulsion injury with separation of a bone fragment from the dorsal aspect of the base of the distal phalanx at the extensor insertion. Following injury, there is extensor lag at the DIP joint.

The DIP joint becomes slightly flexed due to the unopposed pull of the flexor digitorum profundus. Following a finger injury, it is important to consider the possibility of injury to the extensor tendon and testing for DIP movement will confirm loss of extension. Plain films are used to assess whether a bone fragment has been separated, the stability of the DIP joint and fragment displacement (see Figs 2.65, 2.66 and 2.67). A routine plain film series of finger views is required, taking particular care to obtain a high-quality lateral projection.

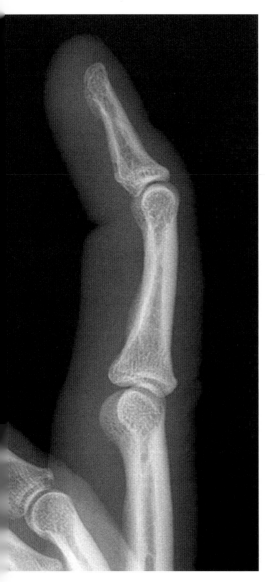

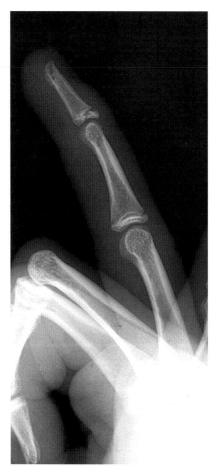

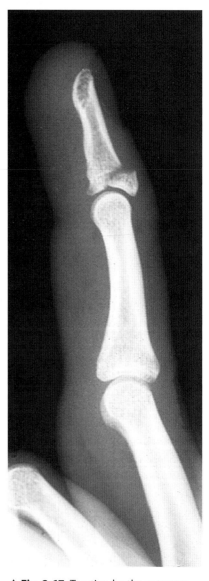

▲ **Fig. 2.65** A flexion deformity is present at the DIP joint. No bone injury can be seen. The appearance is of a 'mallet finger' deformity, consistent with a tear of the conjoint segment of the extensor tendon.

▲ **Fig. 2.66** In this immature athlete, there has been a 'mallet finger' injury with a small epiphyseal fragment avulsed. Slight fragment displacement has occurred.

▲ **Fig. 2.67** Traction by the extensor tendon has avulsed a large fragment. There is potential for instability as more than 40% of the articular surface of the distal phalanx is separated. At the time of the examination, no subluxation was apparent.

Boutonniere deformity

Knowledge of the anatomy of the extensor mechanism is essential for an understanding of boutonniere (buttonhole) deformity. The extrinsic and intrinsic extensor systems work together to enable simultaneous extension of the proximal and distal interphalangeal joints (see Fig. 2.68).

The long extensor digiti tendon (extrinsic) passes distally from the forearm along the dorsal aspect of the proximal phalanx and divides to form a middle slip and two lateral slips. The middle slip continues distally over the dorsal aspect of the PIP joint, replacing its dorsal ligament, and inserts into the base of the middle phalanx. The lateral slips form lateral bands, by fusing with contributions from the intrinsic extensor tendons (arising from the interossei and lumbricals). The lateral bands pass distally over the dorso-lateral aspect of the middle phalanx to join the midline dorsally and form a short terminal tendon that inserts on the dorsal aspect of the base of the distal phalanx. The lateral bands are maintained in their dorsolateral position by a triangular ligament. This ligament passes between the bands on the dorsal aspect of the middle phalanx and prevents palmar displacement of the bands in flexion. The dorsal bands are also prevented from dorsal movement in extension by retinacular ligaments.

Injury biomechanics

Boutonniere deformity may occur following injury to the central slip of the extensor tendon. This injury is usually the result of an actively straightened finger being forcibly flexed by a 'jamming' injury. Injury to the central slip may also result from a laceration or direct trauma.

Although there has been rupture of the central slip, the characteristic deformity does not appear immediately. Other progressive changes need to occur. Initially, extension of the PIP joint is still possible, employing the lateral bands that are maintained in a dorsal position by the triangular ligament. However, repetitive use of the lateral bands as extensors causes the triangular ligament to tear and eventually the lateral bands will be allowed to migrate anteriorly. At the same time, the head of the proximal phalanx will move dorsally due to absence of the central tendon (passing between the lateral bands like a buttonhole or 'boutonniere'). As a result of these changes, the lateral bands will eventually lie anterior to the axis of rotation of the proximal phalangeal head and, when this point is reached, the lateral bands will become flexors of the PIP joint. The lateral bands then become taut and cause extension of the DIP joint. This resultant flexion deformity of the PIP joint and extension of the DIP joint is known as boutonniere deformity.

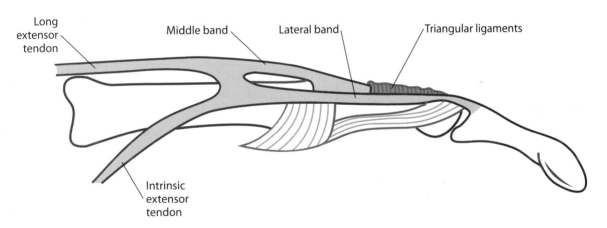

▲▼ Fig. 2.68
(a) A line drawing of the extensor mechanism shows important normal anatomy.
(b) Following rupture of the middle band of the extensor tendor there is dorsal migration of the head of the proximal phalanx, and tension of the lateral bands will produce DIP extension, creating a boutonniere deformity.

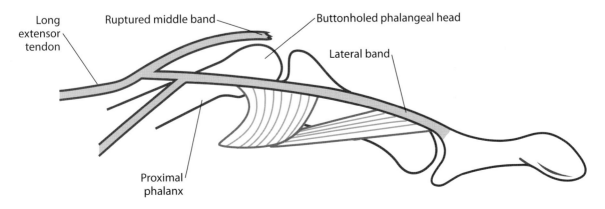

There are other causes of a flexion deformity of the PIP joint and these are known as pseudoboutonniere deformity. Confirming normal DIP movement will enable differentiation between pseudoboutonniere deformity and true boutonniere deformity.

Diagnostic imaging

A lateral view of the finger demonstrates the characteristic boutonniere deformity (see Fig. 2.69). An associated avulsion fracture is uncommon. Because the onset of deformity is often delayed, the inability to actively extend the PIP joint and flex the DIP joint is progressive. Dynamic ultrasound (see Fig. 2.70) can sometimes assist with early recognition, which is important, because the established deformity is difficult to treat.

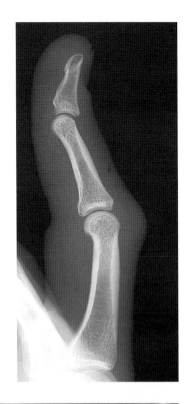

▶ **Fig. 2.69** A lateral view of the finger shows flexion at the PIP joint and extension at the DIP joint, typical of boutonniere deformity.

▼ **Fig. 2.70** Transverse and long-axis ultrasound images show a boutonniere deformity of the left ring finger. By comparison with the normal intact central extensor slip of the *right* ring finger (arrowheads), a rupture of the *left* ring finger central extensor slip is appreciated partly as a zone of fluid-filled attenuation or discontinuity (white arrows) and partly as a zone of frayed thickening (*). Also note the separation of the more lateral components of the extensor hood (black arrows) either side of the central tear on transverse imaging.

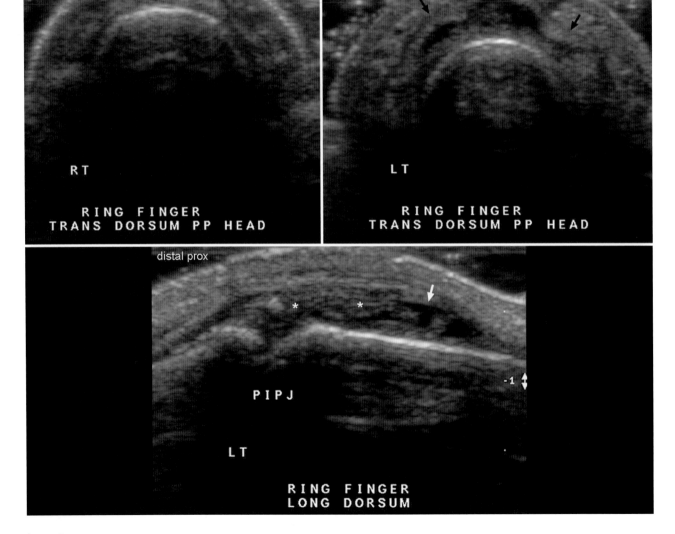

Extensor hood injury ('Boxer's knuckle')

The extensor hood is a structure that holds the common extensor tendon in the centre of the metacarpal head as it passes distally on the dorsal aspect of the MCP joints of the fingers. The hood is composed of fibres that anchor the tendon to the volar plate and the palmar transverse metacarpal ligament. The fibres are orientated transversely, obliquely and in the sagittal plane. The sagittal fibres originate from the sides of the extensor tendon and pass into the palm to attach to the volar plate, lying outside the joint capsule and collateral ligaments. Integrity of the extensor hood mechanism is essential for normal function and protects the underlying metacarpophalangeal joint.

The two most common mechanisms producing a tear in the hood are a forceful ulnar deviation of the fingers, tearing the radial sagittal fibres, or direct trauma, usually from a punch. The hood of the middle finger is the most frequently injured (Hame and Melone 2000), because the tendon is loosely held by the array of fibres. This is also the knuckle most traumatised in boxing. After injury to the hood, there will be tenderness and swelling over the knuckle and the swelling may obscure the subluxed tendon. There is pain every time the MCP joint is flexed and tendon subluxation is also painful. Subluxation of the tendon may occur in either a radial or an ulnar direction; ulnar dislocation is by far the most common.

Imaging with plain films simply shows soft-tissue swelling. Ultrasound is the examination of choice for establishing the diagnosis. With flexion of the MCP joint, the tear in the hood will open and become obvious (see Figs 2.71 and 2.72).

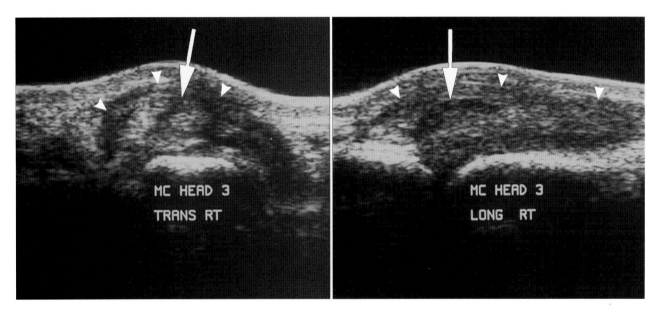

▲ **Fig. 2.71** 'Boxer's knuckle' is demonstrated by transverse and long-axis ultrasound images. There is a markedly thickened extensor hood over the third metacarpal head (arrowheads), with a superimposed subtle hypoechoic line of a complicating split tear (arrows).

▼ **Fig. 2.72** A boxer at the Sydney 2000 Olympics presented with a painful knuckle of the middle finger. This transverse ultrasound image obtained with flexion of the MCP joint demonstrates opening of a hypoechoic gap (indicated by callipers) at the site of the extensor hood tear. There is associated subluxation of the thickened lateral tendon component (arrow). The extensor hood more generally is thickened (t). There is a superficial zone of surrounding hypoechoic soft-tissue thickening, consistent with peritendonitis (arrowheads).

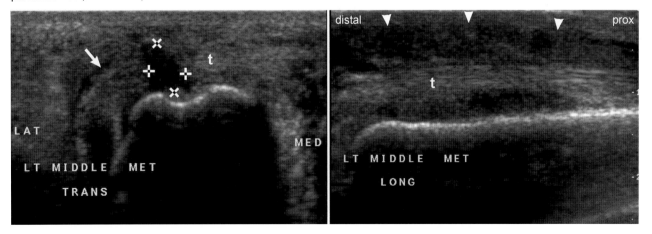

Imaging of the wrist

Management of a wrist injury commences with a thorough clinical history and physical examination. Because of the inherent complexity of the wrist, imaging is commonly used to confirm or exclude clinical suspicions. Considerable information can be obtained from good-quality plain films, although care must be taken to obtain an adequate series. These initial films can then be complemented by extra views to demonstrate particular structures. If there is continuing doubt about the diagnosis, the more sophisticated imaging methods such as ultrasound, nuclear medicine, CT scanning and MRI can all make a valuable contribution to the establishment of a diagnosis.

Plain films

There are three standard x-ray views:

(a) A *PA view* provides a good overview of the carpal bones and distal radioulnar joint (see Fig. 2.73). It is important that this view is obtained in a neutral position, with so-called 'zero rotation', eliminating both supination and pronation of the wrist. Zero rotation allows the relative lengths of the radius and ulna to be assessed for ulnar variance. Zero rotation is achieved by positioning the patient with their shoulder, elbow and wrist in the same horizontal plane (Hardy et al. 1987) (see Fig. 2.74).

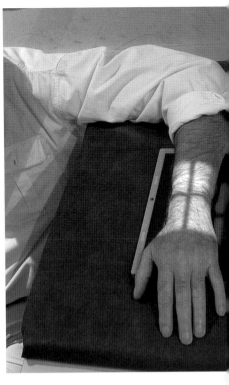

▲ **Fig. 2.74** This photo shows the correct positioning required to obtain a PA view in zero rotation. The key feature is having the shoulder, elbow and wrist at the same horizontal level, which prevents supination or pronation of the forearm.

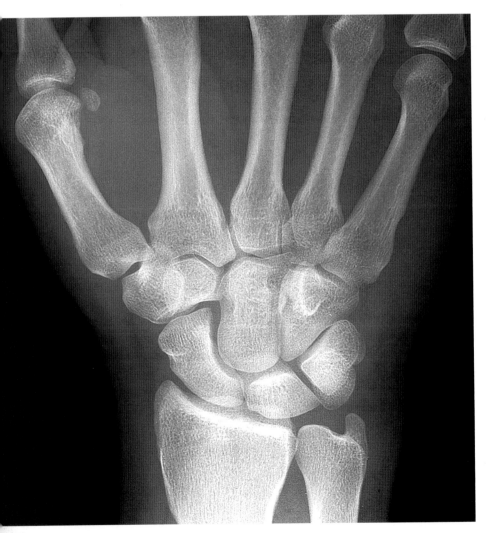

▲ **Fig. 2.73** A correctly positioned PA view will provide a good overview of the carpal bones, the radiocarpal and midcarpal arcs, the radiocarpal joint and the CMC joints.

(b) An *oblique view* adds a further dimension to the overall appreciation of the complex carpal anatomy and, more specifically, of important structures along the radial side of the wrist, including the radial styloid process, scaphoid, scaphotrapezial joints, trapezium, trapezoid and first carpometacarpal joint (see Fig. 2.75). The film is obtained in the PA position with the wrist resting on a 45° sponge, elevating the radial side.

(c) A *lateral view* holds the key to the diagnosis of many important conditions, and great care must be taken to ensure correct positioning. It is essential that the film is taken with the wrist in zero rotation and with the long axis of the radius colinear with the long axis of the third metacarpal. A true lateral view of the wrist in zero rotation is obtained with the patient leaning laterally, the humerus vertical and the elbow flexed to 90° (see Fig. 2.76). A correctly positioned lateral film will project the pisiform over the scaphoid tubercle and the radius superimposed upon and parallel with the ulna (see Fig. 2.77).

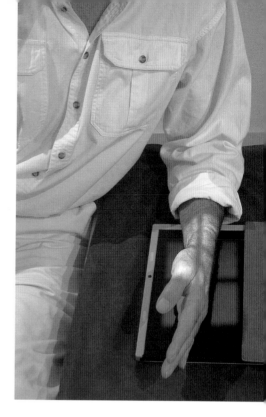

▲ **Fig. 2.76** To acquire a true lateral view of the wrist, the patient is required to lean across so that the humerus is vertical. The axis of the third metacarpal is colinear with the long axis of the radius. This photo shows correct positioning.

▼ **Fig. 2.75** An oblique view of the wrist may provide valuable information not evident on the PA view. The structures on the radial side of the wrist are particularly well demonstrated.

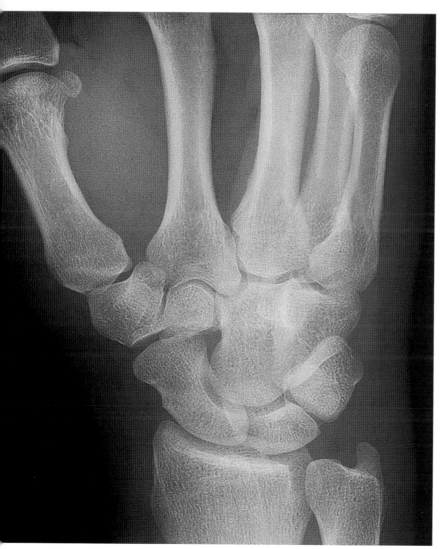

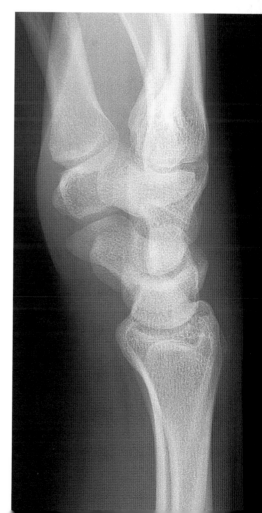

▶ **Fig. 2.77** A lateral view of the wrist obtained using the correct technique.

Tips on looking at plain films of the wrist

A large amount of information is available on the standard plain film series of the wrist and an organised search for abnormalities is important if the maximum amount of information is to be extracted. At first glance, the wrist appears to be a random collection of irregularly shaped bones. However, on further examination, order will be seen to be present and normal patterns will emerge. Armed with a clinical history of the injury biomechanics and physical findings, a search should begin for radiological clues of injury, the signs of which are often subtle. Significant changes can be found in bones, joints and soft tissue, so all structures have to be examined in turn and a search routine should be developed.

A normal PA view (see Fig. 2.78) will show smooth carpal arcs that are unbroken. The intercarpal joints should be uniform and congruent. If these criteria are not met, a dislocation or fracture may be present (see Fig. 2.79).

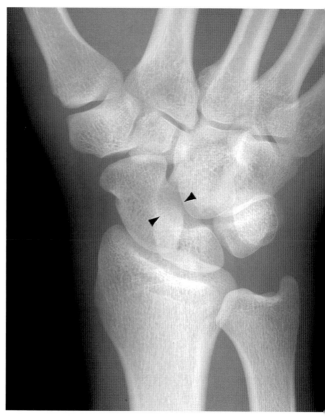

▲ **Fig. 2.79** There is disruption of the normal midcarpal arc with widening of the intercarpal joint between the scaphoid and the capitate (arrowheads), produced by a fracture of the capitate.

▼ **Fig. 2.80** A Type II lunate can be identified by noting a facet on the medial aspect of the distal surface of the lunate (arrowhead), a variant which disrupts the curvature of the midcarpal arc.

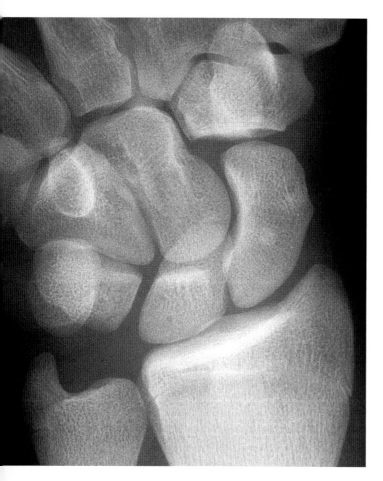

▲ **Fig. 2.78** A normal PA view shows smooth arcs between the proximal and distal carpal rows (the midcarpal arc) and between the distal radius and the proximal carpal row (the radiocarpal arc). If these arcs are disrupted, it is very likely that there is bony or ligamentous injury.

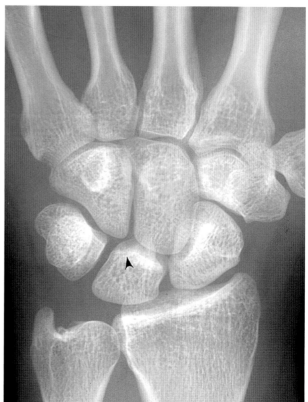

Another cause of disruption of the midcarpal arc is a fairly common anomaly called a 'Type II' lunate, which causes a step in the arc (see Fig. 2.80). This anomaly is present when the proximal pole of the hamate articulates with the lunate and can be readily identified by the presence of an articular facet on the medial aspect of the distal articular surface of the lunate (see Fig. 2.81). Noting this anomaly is more than an idle observation, because a Type II lunate may be symptomatic in up to 25% of cases due to the development of chondromalacia or more advanced degenerative changes at this anomalous articulation (Viegas, Wagner et al. 1990) (see Figs 2.82 and 2.83).

▼ **Fig. 2.81** The lunate variants are demonstrated by MRI. **(a)** This coronal PD-weighted image of a Type I lunate (*) obtained using a 9 cm field of view shows a *single* midcarpal articular facet. **(b)** This coronal PD-weighted image of a Type II lunate (*) obtained using a 7 cm field of view shows an *additional* midcarpal facet that articulates with the proximal pole of hamate (h) and produces a step in the contour of the midcarpal arc. In wrists with a Type II lunate, the proximal tip of hamate is a focal load-bearing structure with increased vulnerability to chondral wear. Note the improved spatial detail of image provided by using a smaller acquisition field of view (e.g. finer trabecular definition).

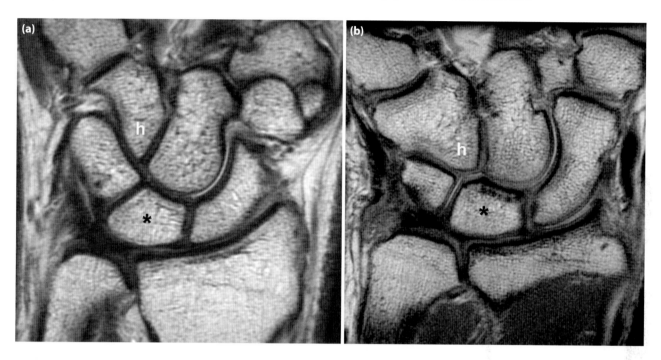

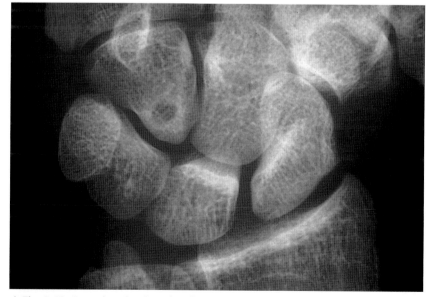

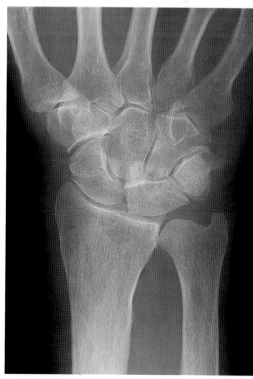

▲ **Fig. 2.82** A cyst has developed in the proximal hamate. This is an indirect indicator of overlying chondromalacia.

▶ **Fig. 2.83** The degenerative changes involving this anomalous articulation are more advanced, with joint space narrowing and subchondral cyst formation.

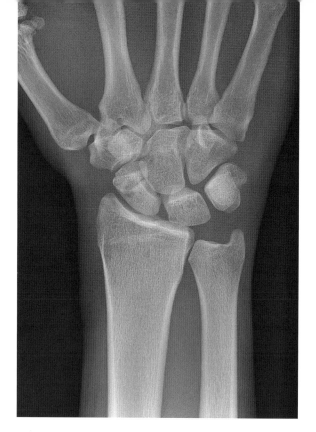

All intercarpal joint spaces should be of similar width. The scapholunate articulation is extremely important as widening ('Terry Thomas' sign) may be an indicator of ligamentous injury or instability and deserves careful inspection. However, it must be remembered that there are two causes of pseudo-widening of the scapholunate joint space. First, this space can appear widened in the presence of a scaphoid fracture due to shortening of the scaphoid (see Fig. 2.84). Second, the joint may also appear widened in children and adolescents (see Fig. 2.85). This 'pseudo Terry Thomas' sign was described by Light (2000) and arises because the developing scaphoid ossifies from the distal to the proximal pole (i.e. the apparent gap is due to unossified proximal pole cartilage). With advancing age and progressive ossification, the apparent joint space progressively decreases. The joint width averages 9 mm in 7-year-old children and 3 mm in 15-year-old adolescents (Light 2000).

Rotational displacement of the lunate and scaphoid occurs with various instabilities and is best assessed on the lateral view. With the wrist in the true lateral position, the capitolunate axis is normally within 10° of the metacarpal axis and the scapholunate angle is normally 30 to 60° (see Fig. 2.86). The scapholunate angle alters when there is ligamentous injury in the proximal carpal row, allowing the lunate to rotate independently of the scaphoid or triquetrum (see Fig. 2.87).

An examination of the soft tissues is often very rewarding. Soft-tissue changes include localised swelling, displacement or obliteration of fat planes and soft-tissue calcification. The scaphoid fat pad is a subtle space located between the radial collateral ligament of the wrist and the extensor pollicus longus (EPL) tendon

▲ **Fig. 2.84** There is an increase in the width of the scapholunate joint space associated with a scaphoid fracture, due to scaphoid shortening. This is a pseudo-widening and does not indicate injury to the SL ligaments. In fact, it is unusual for a scaphoid fracture and SL ligament injury to occur together.

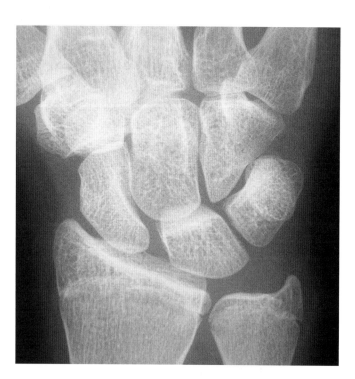

▲ **Fig. 2.85** Pseudo-widening of the scapholunate joint space is seen in the immature wrist due to developmental delay in ossification of the proximal pole of the scaphoid. A widened joint can be accepted as normal, although in the adolescent wrist, such as in this case, ligamentous injury cannot be absolutely excluded.

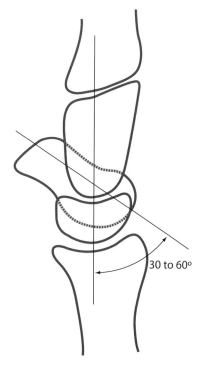

Normal scapholunate angle

▲ **Fig. 2.86** This line drawing demonstrates how to measure the scapholunate angle. Rotation of the lunate with respect to the scaphoid occurs in instabilities.

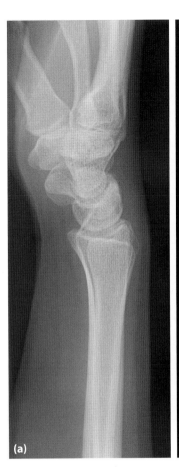
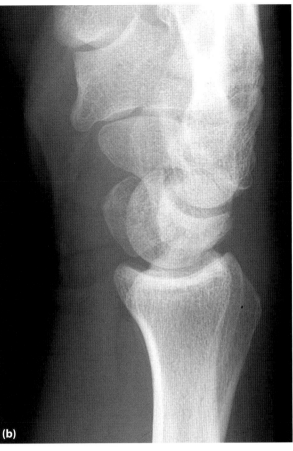

(a)

(b)

◀ **Fig. 2.87(a)** The scapholunate angle decreases when the lunate moves independently with respect to the triquetrum and rotates in a volar direction (volar intercalated segment instability (VISI) deformity). **(b)** When scapholunate dissociation is present, the lunate rotates in a dorsal direction, increasing the scapholunate angle (dorsal intercalated segment instability (DISI) deformity).

(see Fig. 2.88). It is consistently visualised in normal adults (see Fig. 2.89) but is inconsistently detected in children under the age of 12 (Rogers 1982). Lateral displacement or complete obliteration of the scaphoid fat pad often occurs with scaphoid fractures (see Fig. 2.90). Scaphoid fat pad changes are not entirely specific to scaphoid fractures and can occasionally be seen with injuries to the radial styloid, trapezium and first metacarpal base.

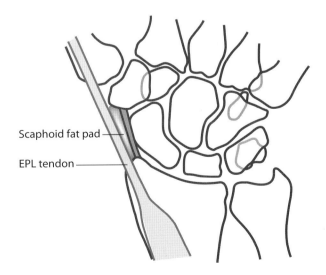

Scaphoid fat pad

EPL tendon

▲ **Fig. 2.88** Anatomy of a normal scaphoid fat pad. The scaphoid fat pad lies between the EPL tendon and the radial collateral ligament, and may be widened or obliterated when a scaphoid fracture is present.

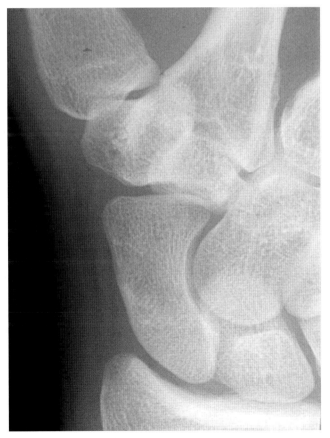

▲ **Fig. 2.89** The scaphoid fat pad is normal in this scaphoid view. An occult scaphoid fracture is unlikely.

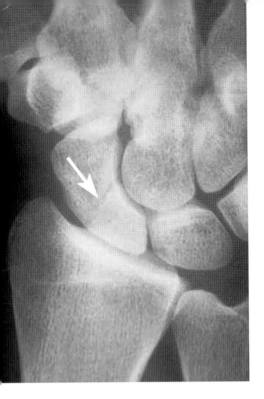

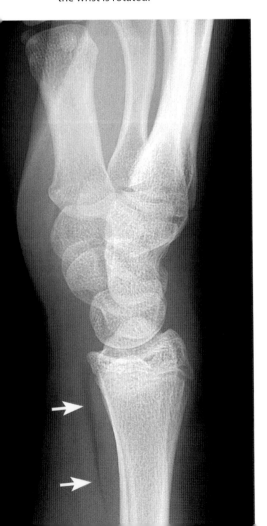

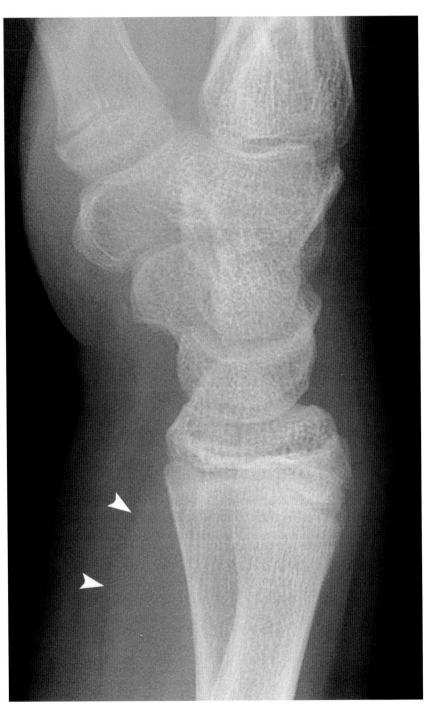

◀ **Fig. 2.90** The scaphoid fat pad is obliterated by a haematoma associated with a fracture of the scaphoid waist. Avascular changes are suspected in the proximal pole of the scaphoid.

In a true lateral view, a linear fat line is visible in the distal forearm overlying the pronator quadratus muscle (see Fig. 2.91). Fractures of the distal radius will displace or efface this pronator quadratus fat line. These changes are helpful in the detection of otherwise occult fractures of the distal radius and are especially valuable for detecting injury to the distal radial growth plate in children (see Figs 2.92 and 2.93). This fat line will be difficult or impossible to see on a poor-quality lateral view taken with obliquity.

▼ **Fig. 2.91** The pronator quadratus fat line is a thin straight fat line (arrows) that runs parallel to the long axis of the radius and should be identified in all well-positioned lateral views. This fat line may be difficult to see if the lateral view is technically poor, particularly if the wrist is rotated.

▲ **Fig. 2.92** Disruption of the distal radial growth plate has produced a haematoma, which displaces and bows the pronator quadratus fat line.

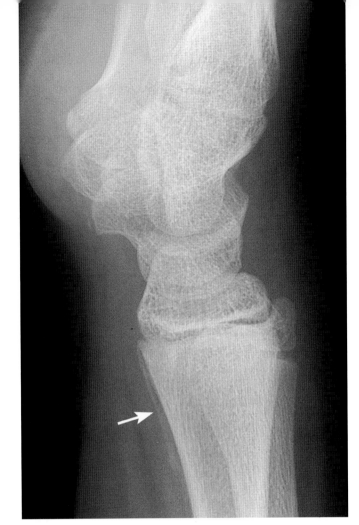

◀**Fig. 2.93** A progress examination of the same case as in Fig. 2.92 shows the fat line to have returned to a normal position. A periosteal reaction is now evident on the anterior aspect of the distal radius (arrow), due to periosteal injury at the time of the distal radial growth plate disruption.

Soft-tissue pathology may alternatively be suggested if localised swelling, calcification or bone reaction is present. De Quervain's tenosynovitis can usually be detected as soft-tissue swelling over the lateral aspect of the radial styloid process (see Fig. 2.94). Similarly, ECU tendinopathy can be detected by the presence of soft-tissue swelling medially (see Fig. 2.206 on page 112).

Additional radiographic views

Additional views are obtained when certain clinical situations are present. These views improve the visualisation of specific structures, contributing to the diagnosis and hopefully avoiding the necessity of using more expensive imaging methods. Extra views should be obtained when there is clinical suspicion of any of the following:

- a scaphoid fracture
- a fracture of the hook of hamate
- a fracture of the anterior ridge of the trapezium
- injury to the pisotriquetral articulation
- carpal instability
- distal radioulnar joint instability
- carpal boss syndrome.

The radiographic techniques used to obtain these extra views are described later in the chapter in the discussion of the relevant condition.

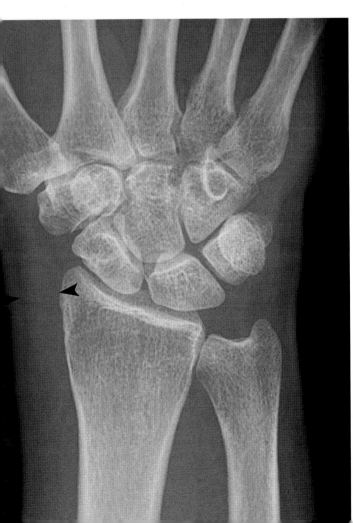

◀**Fig. 2.94** There is elongated soft-tissue swelling on the lateral aspect of the wrist (arrowheads). The position and shape of the swelling is typical of de Quervain's tenosynovitis.

Ulna variance

Ulna variance refers to an alteration in the normal relationship between the length of the radius and the ulna, due to a variation in the length of the ulna relative to that of the radius (see Fig. 2.95). When the ulna is relatively long, this is termed 'ulna plus variance' (see Fig. 2.96), while a short ulna is termed 'ulna minus variance' (see Fig. 2.97). This variation may be developmental or acquired and is often symptomatic.

Supination of the wrist significantly alters the relative length of the radius and the ulna, so ulna variance should be assessed only on a PA film taken in zero rotation (see page 58). Therefore, before making this diagnosis, it is important to be confident that the film has been obtained correctly.

Recently, there has been a change of thinking about the clinical importance of having a positive or negative variance.

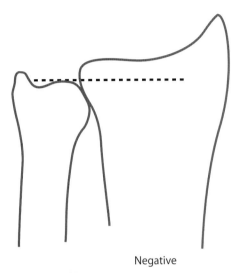
Negative

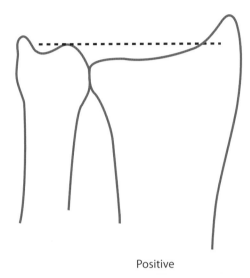
Positive

▲ **Fig. 2.95** Ulna variance. If the ulna is short, the condition is described as 'ulna negative (or minus) variance', whereas a relatively long ulna creates 'ulna positive (or plus) variance'.

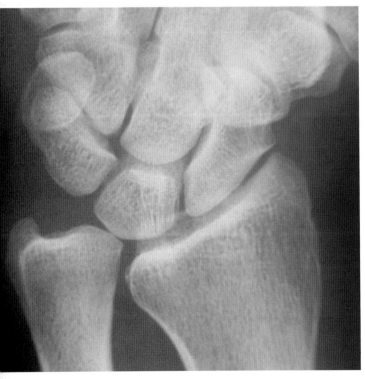

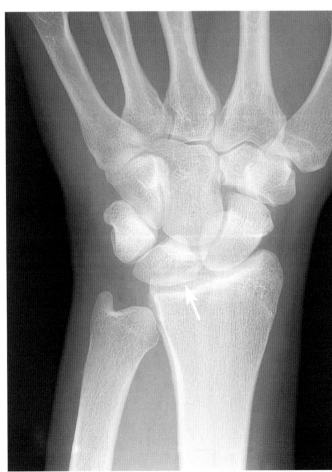

▲ **Fig. 2.96** Ulna plus variance (a positive variance) is present and ulnar abutment occurs even with radial deviation.

▶ **Fig. 2.97** The ulna is short with respect to the radius and is known as 'ulna minus variance' (a negative variance). An old compression fracture of the lunate is note (arrow).

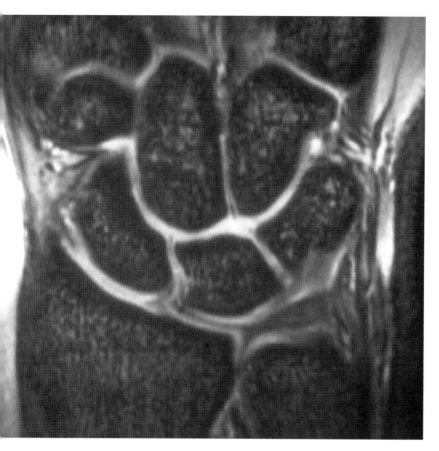

▲ **Fig. 2.98** Ulna minus variance is demonstrated on this coronal MR image. A thickened TFCC compensates for the short ulna.

▶ **Fig. 2.100** This T1-weighted MR image demonstrates evidence of ulnolunate abutment with focal subchondral sclerosis at the lunate (arrowhead) immediately adjacent to a tear of the triangular fibrocartilage (TFC) articular disc.

Previously, the significance of this anomaly was thought to be due to an alteration in the load distribution at the wrist. Loading at the wrist is normally shared between the radius and the ulna in an approximate 80:20 ratio. However, this ratio alters with a change in the length of the ulna relative to the radius. Werner et al. (1986) have noted that shortening of the ulna by as little as 2.5 mm reduces its share of the load to 4%, whereas lengthening of the ulna by 2.5 mm increases its share to 42%.

Recent literature suggests that ulna variance has less effect on variation in wrist loading than once thought. Previously, it was believed that both positive and negative variance caused injury to the TFCC. It is now recognised that when the ulna is relatively short, thickening of the articular disc compensates for the discrepancy (Dailey and Palmer 2000) and reduces the likelihood of injury (see Fig. 2.98). A far more important factor in injury to the TFCC is the variation in load across the disc produced by a dynamic positive variance, which occurs with a power grip and in sports requiring pronation and ulnar deviation of the wrist. If there is a pre-existing static positive or even neutral variance, the loading will be more marked than in an athlete with a negative variance. Transient positive variance is encountered in a number of sports (see the discussion on TFCC injury on page 100).

Complications associated with a long ulna include ulnar abutment syndrome (see Fig. 2.99) and TFCC injury (see Fig. 2.100). A short ulna has an association with avascular necrosis (AVN) of the lunate (Kristensen and Soballe 1987) (see Fig. 2.101).

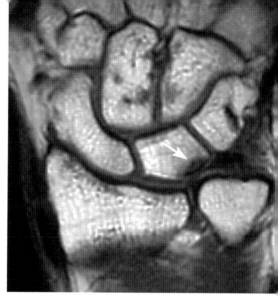

▲ **Fig. 2.99** This coronal T1-weighted MR image shows abutment due to an ulna plus variance. Subchondral changes are shown beneath the proximal articular surface of the lunate at the site of repetitive trauma (arrow). Attrition of the TFCC is also noted.

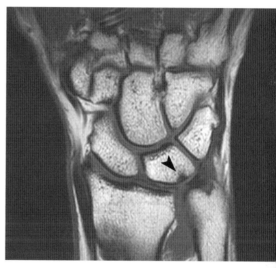

▼ **Fig. 2.101** There is an association between ulna minus variance and AVN of the lunate.

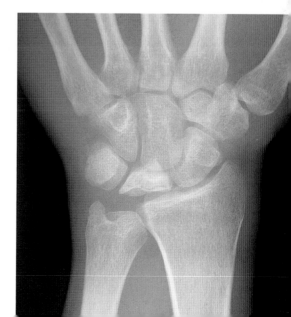

Specific wrist injuries

The biomechanics of wrist injuries

Understanding the biomechanics of a wrist injury goes a long way towards making a correct diagnosis. Particular wrist injuries will occur following the application of certain forces, and structures fail in characteristic sequences, producing diagnostic patterns. This enables imaging changes to be largely anticipated, allowing the most appropriate views to be obtained and the most appropriate imaging methods to be employed.

Whipple (1990), writing on the biomechanics of wrist injury in sport, has identified the principal actions of the wrist most likely to produce injury as throwing, weightbearing, twisting and impact.

The **throwing action** is common to sports such as cricket, baseball, racquet sports and golf. With this action, the wrist moves from extension and radial deviation to flexion and ulnar deviation and, in so doing, produces loading on the abductor pollicis longus (APL) and extensor pollicis brevis (EPB) tendons. This loading is accentuated by the weight of the racquet, club or bat. Tensile force is also applied to the flexor carpi ulnaris (FCU) tendon and, through this tendon, to the pisotriquetral complex. With overuse, the athlete may present with conditions such as de Quervain's tenosynovitis, FCU tendinopathy, injury to the pisotriquetral articulation resulting in degenerative joint disease, ganglion cyst formation or a stress fracture of the pisiform. If the throwing action also includes a component of wrist supination, such as 'undercutting' the forehand stroke in tennis and squash and off-spin bowling in cricket, additional stress occurs to the extensor carpi ulnaris (ECU) tendon. Excessive activity may then produce an ECU tendinopathy.

Weightbearing at the wrist occurs with activities such as weightlifting and gymnastics. In these sports, axial loading occurs with the wrist extended and radially deviated. The resulting volar stress may injure the FCU tendon, pisotriquetral complex and major volar carpal ligaments. If the degree of hyperextension force involved is extreme, a sequence of injuries may result, culminating in lunate dislocation. This mechanism is discussed on page 88.

Twisting injuries to the wrist are mainly seen in wrestling and gymnastics. Excessive pronation or supination characteristically causes injury to the triangular fibrocartilage and distal radioulnar ligaments, leading to instability of the distal radioulnar joint (DRUJ).

Impact injuries to the wrist are common and may result in a variety of injuries:

- A fall onto an outstretched hand commonly impacts the wrist in extension and may produce a fracture of the distal radius, the ulnar styloid process or the waist of scaphoid. Other potential injuries include rupture of the scapholunate (SL) or lunotriquetral (LT) ligaments, a tear of the triangular fibrocartilage, rupture of the volar radiocarpal ligaments or contusion of the dorsal radiocarpal ligaments.

- Impact with the wrist in flexion may avulse the dorsal joint capsule from the distal radius, rupture the SL ligament, fracture the waist of the scaphoid and fracture the distal radius.

- Punching may produce injury through axial loading of the wrist. The force is typically transmitted along the third metacarpal and the long axis of the capitate to the proximal pole of the scaphoid and lunate. If this is a repetitive force, chondromalacia commonly develops over the head of the capitate and on the convex articular surfaces of the lunate and scaphoid. Acute injury may present as a fracture of the proximal pole of the scaphoid or rupture of the dorsal band of the SL ligament. If the wrist is malpositioned in radial deviation during a punch, the impact force may injure the dorsal wrist capsule, fracture the neck of the fifth metacarpal (the most common punching injury) or cause injury to the fourth and fifth CMC joints.

- Direct impact injuries to the palmar side of the wrist may be acute or due to repetitive trauma, resulting from activities such as catching a baseball or cricket ball. Direct impact may result in a fracture of the pisiform, triquetrum, anterior ridge of the trapezium or hook of hamate.

Acute fractures

Individual carpal fractures

Fractures of the carpal bones may be extremely difficult to detect on routine views and specific additional views can often be helpful. Particular fractures that are commonly overlooked are listed in Table 2.2. Isotope bone scans, CT scanning and MRI scans can all help when clinical suspicion is high but the x-ray examination is equivocal or negative.

Table 2.2 Commonly missed fractures of the wrist

1.	Scaphoid fracture
2.	Fracture of the hook of hamate
3.	Fracture of the pisiform
4.	Fracture of the anterior ridge of the trapezium
5.	Fracture of the distal radial growth plate

Scaphoid fractures

Scaphoid fractures are common, representing 70% of all carpal fractures, and are often the result of sport. Approximately 70% of scaphoid fractures involve the waist of the scaphoid (see Fig. 2.102), 10–20% involve the proximal third (see Fig. 2.103) and the remainder involve the scaphoid tuberosity or distal articular surface (see Fig. 2.104(a)) (Kozin 2001). Distal fractures commonly occur in children. Because the distal pole of the scaphoid ossifies before the proximal pole, patterns of scaphoid fractures are different in children. The typical paediatric scaphoid fracture is an avulsion at the attachment of the scaphotrapezial ligament on the radial aspect of the scaphoid tuberosity. This fracture is often incomplete (see Fig. 2.104(b)).

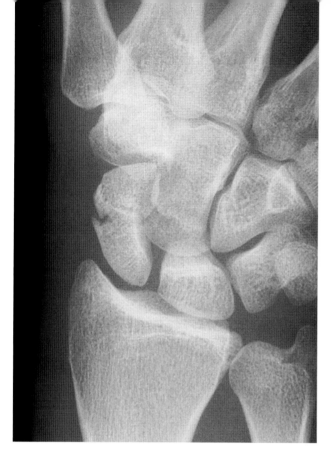

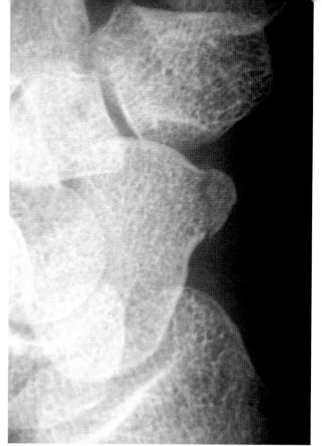

▲ **Fig. 2.102** This fracture involves the scaphoid waist. Displacement has occurred, producing a 'humpback' deformity. Note the increased scapholunate joint space associated with scaphoid shortening. There is also obliteration of the scaphoid fat pad.

▼ **Fig. 2.103** A fracture of the proximal pole of the scaphoid. AVN is almost inevitable with this type of fracture.

▲ **Fig. 2.104(a)** Fractures of the scaphoid tubercle are commonly seen in paediatric patients. This tubercle fracture extends to involve the distal articular surface of the scaphoid, predisposing to the development of degenerative changes in the scaphotrapezial joint in the future.

▼ **(b)** This fracture involves the radial aspect of the scaphoid tubercle. This is an avulsion fracture at the attachment of the radiotrapezial ligament.

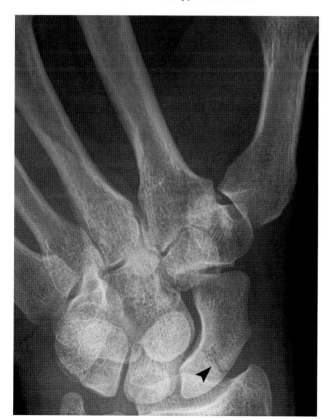

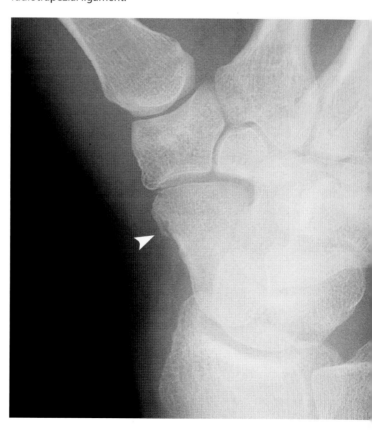

Injury biomechanics

Commonly, a scaphoid fracture is caused by a compressive force at the base of the thenar eminence during a fall on the outstretched hand, with the wrist extended and in radial deviation (Kozin 2001). Mayfield (1980) also produced scaphoid fractures in cadavers with hyperextension and ulnar deviation. In this position, the dorsal aspect of the scaphoid impinges on the dorsal rim of the radius, causing a fracture through the waist. A flexion injury may also produce a scaphoid fracture.

Dorsal subluxation and supination produce fractures of the proximal pole. This fracture may occur as a result of a punching injury when the punch is thrown with the wrist held in radial deviation.

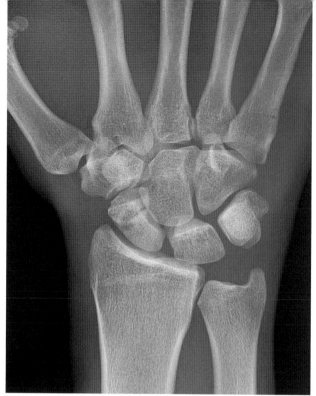

▲ **Fig. 2.105** Changes of delayed union of the scaphoid fracture are present, with clear demarcation of the fracture margins. Bony resorption is occurring laterally. Also note the increase in the scapholunate interval due to scaphoid shortening.

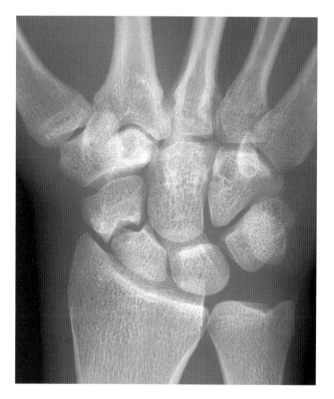

◀ **Fig. 2.106(a)** There is well-established non-union of the fracture of the waist of the scaphoid. The fracture margins are well defined and separated.

▼ **(b)** Non-union of a fracture of the waist of the scaphoid is well demonstrated by MRI. On the TI-weighted image **(i)**, the margins of the fracture site are seen to be sclerotic, and on the fat-suppressed T2-weighted image **(ii)** non-union is confirmed by the presence of fluid filling the fracture line (arrowhead). The proximal scaphoid fragment shows altered bony architecture with patchy sclerosis, but no oedema can be seen and there is maintenance of normal marrow signal. The appearances may be due to a previous ischaemic process.

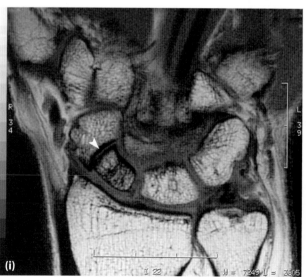

(i)

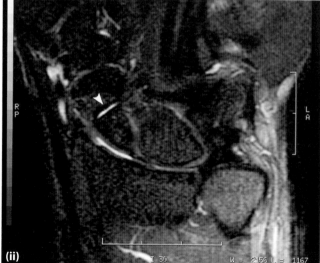

(ii)

Although the mechanism of injury is common to both a scaphoid fracture and SL ligament injury, it is rare for these injuries to occur together. Occasionally, an SL ligament injury may appear to be present with a scaphoid fracture. This is due to scaphoid shortening associated with a 'humpback' deformity, as shown in Fig. 2.102 on page 69. This shortening also pulls the lunate into extension, producing a pseudo-DISI deformity (Kozin 2001).

The following problems may be associated with a scaphoid fracture:

- Ligamentous traction on the fragments can result in scaphoid fracture instability. The proximal fragment is pulled into an extended position and is subjected to rotational forces. The distal fragment is flexed, causing a 'humpback' angulation deformity at the fracture site. The displacement of the fragments causes healing problems due to poor bony apposition and predisposes to delayed union (see Fig. 2.105) or non-union (see Fig. 2.106).

- The proximal pole of the scaphoid has a poor blood supply (see the section on carpal AVN on page 116). The site of the fracture is an important determinant of prognosis, because AVN is almost inevitable with proximal third fractures and occurs in 30% of all middle third fractures (Gelberman and Menon 1980).

- Even if fracture union occurs, there is still the possibility of decreased mobility, diminished grip strength and degenerative changes. Burgess (1987) showed that 5° of flexion deformity at the fracture site can produce a 24% loss of wrist extension. This is due to the altered relationship between the proximal and distal rows of the carpus.

- Following a scaphoid fracture, 5% of cases will develop degenerative change due to scaphoid shortening and altered biomechanics (Kozin 2001).

- When non-union occurs, degenerative changes seem inevitable and usually begin developing about five years after the trauma (Kozin 2001). The changes may be confined to the scaphoid, may involve the radioscaphoid articulation or may be generalised throughout the wrist (referred to as scaphoid non-union advanced collapse (SNAC) wrist).

Diagnostic imaging

Following trauma, a good-quality plain film series is essential. Precise positioning is important, and the exposure and resolution have to be adequate to define the scaphoid fat pad and scaphoid trabecular pattern. If a scaphoid fracture is suspected clinically, a specific scaphoid view should be included in the initial series. A specific scaphoid view provides a more detailed examination of the waist and tubercle of the scaphoid. The scaphoid fat pad is also well demonstrated. The view is obtained with the wrist in ulnar deviation and using a 20° cranial tube angle, with the beam centred on the scaphoid. Collimation is important and increases bony definition. This view slightly elongates the scaphoid waist (see Figs 2.107 and 2.108).

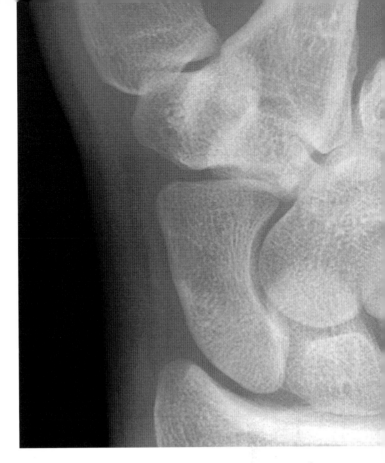

▲ **Fig. 2.107** A specific scaphoid view allows examination of the trabecular pattern of the scaphoid and the detection of subtle changes in the bone and adjacent soft tissues that may suggest a fracture. Here, the appearances are normal and the scaphoid fat pad is well demonstrated.

▼ **Fig. 2.108** A scaphoid view has been acquired. The scaphoid fat pad cannot be easily appreciated and there is the suggestion that it is displaced laterally. Although the bony structures appear normal, there is still a moderate chance that an occult fracture is present. Note that there is slight soft-tissue thickening lateral to the scaphoid when compared with Fig. 2.107. If clinical doubts persist, a nuclear bone scan or MRI would be advisable.

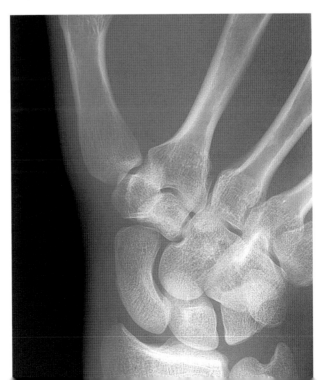

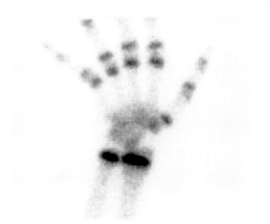

▲ **Fig. 2.109** A nuclear bone scan was performed in an acute wrist injury. The plain films were normal. The scan shows avascularity of the scaphoid initially, with increased vascularity appearing three days later.

It is a well-accepted fact that scaphoid fractures may be impossible to detect on the initial plain films. As a result, it has been traditional to immobilise the patient in a plaster cast and request a progress examination 10–14 days after the trauma. However, if this examination is taken in the cast, it is highly probable that the diagnosis will remain uncertain, as the cast will obscure detail. Even when a progress film is taken with the plaster removed, the diagnosis may still be uncertain. For the athlete, an isotope bone scan or MRI has the added advantage of providing a rapid diagnosis. A bone scan has a zero false negative rate in diagnosing a scaphoid fracture if obtained more than 48 hours after the injury (Gamel et al. 1979). Consequently, bone scans and MRI are useful in the diagnosis of scaphoid fractures (see Figs 2.109–2.115).

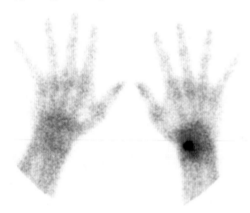

▲ **Fig. 2.110** An isotope bone scan demonstrates a scaphoid fracture. There is focal uptake of isotope across the waist of the scaphoid.

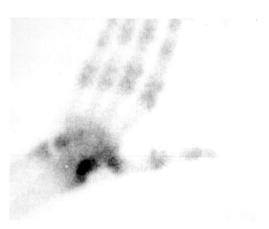

▲ **Fig. 2.111** A bone scan two months after an injury shows marked uptake of the isotope in the proximal pole of the scaphoid due to revascularisation following post-traumatic AVN.

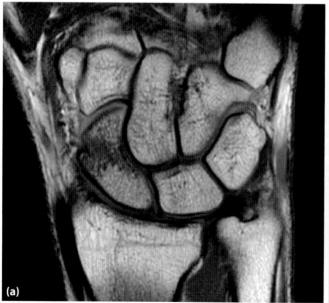

(a)

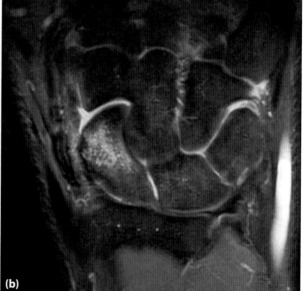

(b)

▲ **Fig. 2.112** A scaphoid bone bruise is demonstrated in the scaphoid following trauma.
(a) The T1-weighted image shows loss of the normal marrow signal extending from the medial aspect of the scaphoid waist to the lateral aspect of the tubercle. No fracture line can be seen.
(b) The fat-suppressed T2-weighted image shows high signal in the same distribution.

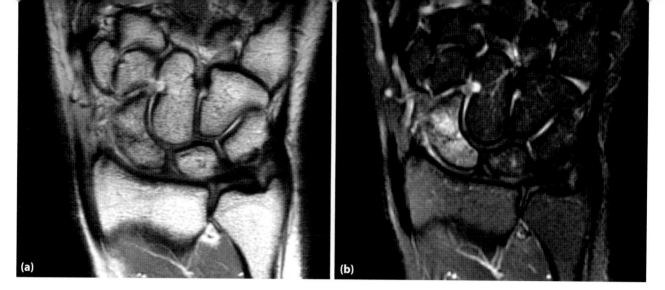

▲ **Fig. 2.113** An undisplaced scaphoid fracture is demonstrated by MRI.
(a) The TI-weighted image shows fracturing across the waist of the scaphoid.
(b) The T2-weighted image shows extensive hyperintense bone oedema throughout the entire scaphoid.

▼ **Fig. 2.114** MRI demonstrates an undisplaced fracture transversing the waist of the scaphoid. The hypointense fracture line is indicated by the arrows. An adjacent grey zone of intermediate signal on the coronal PD and sagittal T1 images, and the high signal on the fat-suppressed PD images, reflects associated bone marrow oedema. Note the prominent zone of accompanying oedematous and/or haemorrhagic peri-scaphoid soft-tissue swelling (arrowheads), which accounts for the indirect plain x-ray signs of scaphoid fracture that include obliteration or displacement of the scaphoid fat pad.

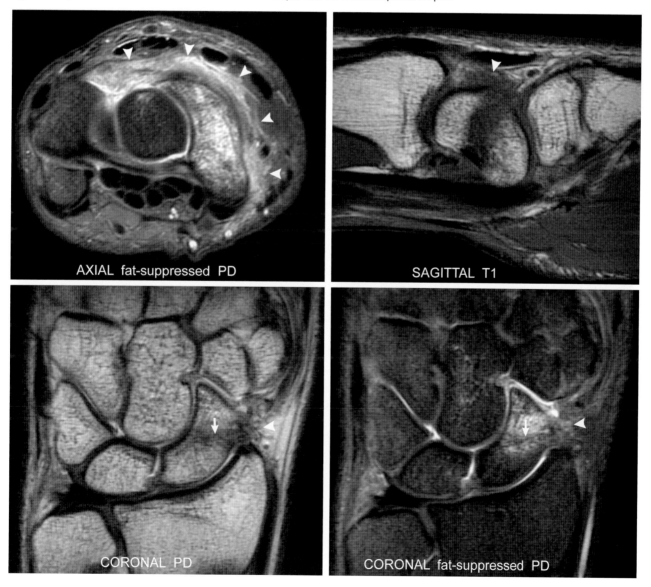

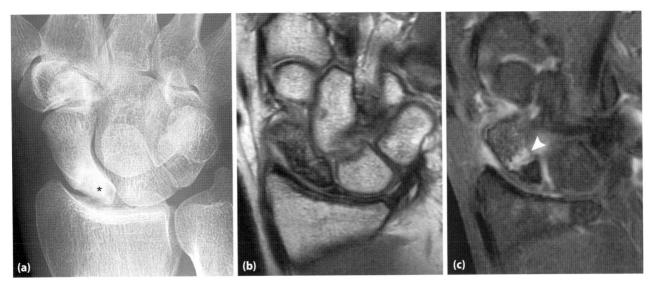

▲ **Fig. 2.115** Avascular bone changes may occur following a fracture at the waist and proximal pole of the scaphoid.
(a) The plain x-ray shows proximal pole scaphoid sclerosis and partial collapse (*), typical of osteonecrosis.
(b) The coronal T1-weighted MR image shows scaphoid marrow hypointensity at both the proximal and distal poles.
(c) The fat-suppressed coronal T2-weighted MR image indicates several different processes underlying and explaining the otherwise non-specific T1 imaging pattern of diffuse marrow hypointensity. The distal pole of the scaphoid shows diffuse low-grade marrow oedema compatible with any combination of hyperaemia, osteopaenia and increased stress loading. The waist of the scaphoid shows a broad band of marked hyperintensity (arrowhead) consistent with reparative granulation tissue that marginates the fracture line and indicates a vascularised zone of viability. Finally, the proximal pole of the scaphoid is diffusely and markedly hypointense, correlating with the sclerosis pattern noted on plain x-ray and also in keeping with dead bone in view of the complete absence of vascularised or viable (i.e. water-containing) marrow space (arrowhead).

Displacement with angulation at the scaphoid fracture site will invariably cause healing problems. CT is particularly useful in establishing the presence and degree of fracture deformity in the acute stage and later the degree of malunion. Amadio et al. (1989) established a protocol for this. The CT examination was performed with fine slices acquired along the long axis of the scaphoid and the images were assessed for carpal height and the radiocarpal, capitolunate, scapholunate and intrascaphoid angles. Malunion was assessed by measuring the 'lateral intrascaphoid' angle, which is the angulation of the scaphoid body seen in a sagittal plane of the scaphoid (see Fig. 2.116). Normal is

▼ **Fig. 2.116** A CT scan has been acquired through the long axis of the scaphoid and demonstrates volar displacement and angulation of the distal fragment at the scaphoid fracture site, a so-called 'humpback' deformity. In the image on the right, the lateral intrascaphoid angle exceeds 45°, suggesting that if the fracture is unreduced there may be malunion, ongoing pain, stiffness and degenerative changes.

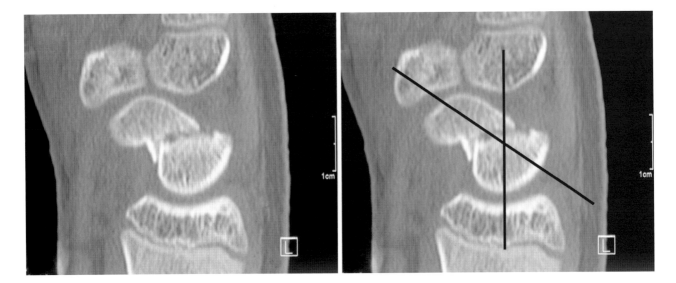

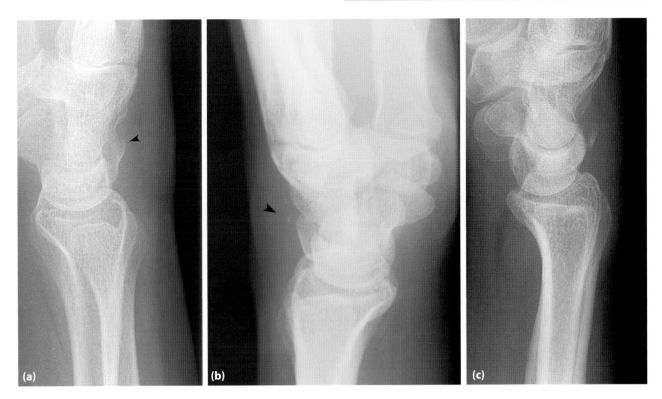

(a)   (b)   (c)

▲ **Fig. 2.117(a)** The fragment separated from the posterior tubercle of the triquetrum may be minimal or undisplaced (arrowhead). Marked soft-tissue swelling is invariably present and provides an important diagnostic marker.
(b) A small fragment is shown to be avulsed from the posterior tubercle of the triquetrum (arrowhead). The fragment is sometimes difficult to see and the dorsal margin of the carpus deserves careful inspection when dorsal pain and tenderness are present. Note the marked soft-tissue swelling, even though the fracture appears minimal.
(c) A violent traction by the dorsal radiocarpal ligament has separated the entire posterior tubercle.

less than 35° and malunion is present at an angle in excess of this figure. An angle greater than 45° is associated with ongoing pain, stiffness and degenerative change.

Triquetral fractures

After the scaphoid, the triquetrum is the second most common carpal bone fractured by sporting injury (Steinberg 2002). There are three different triquetral fractures: (1) fractures of the posterior tubercle of the triquetrum (see Fig. 2.117), the most common fracture; (2) fractures extending across the body of the triquetrum (see Fig. 2.118); and (3) fractures occurring with a pisotriquetral injury and involving the triquetral articular surface of this articulation.

Injury biomechanics

A dorsal triquetral avulsion fracture is usually the result of a fall on an outstretched hand with the wrist in ulnar deviation. The fracture is thought to be either due to an impingement of the posterior process of the triquetrum between the hamate and the ulnar styloid process (Lee and Montgomery 2002) or the result of traction by the dorsal radiocarpal and dorsal intercarpal ligaments.

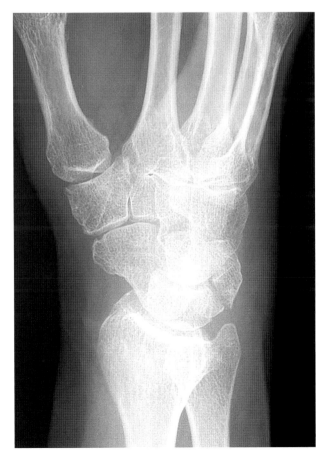

▶ **Fig. 2.118** A fracture of the body of triquetrum may occur in isolation or be a part of the 'greater arc' pattern of fractures. In this case, the fracture of the triquetral body is the only injury.

A second triquetral fracture is a fracture of the body of the triquetrum. This fracture occurs as a component of the 'greater arc' perilunate pattern of injury. Characteristically, this sequence of fractures starts on the radial side of the wrist, although it has been suggested that the pattern may commence on the ulnar side and the isolated triquetral fracture is presumably the beginning of the 'reverse' sequence. The biomechanics of perilunate injury is excessive hyperextension of the wrist in ulnar deviation (see page 88 for further discussion).

A fracture of the triquetrum may also occur at the pisotriquetral joint. The flexor carpi ulnaris inserts into the pisiform with the pisiform anchored by two ligaments, the pisohamate and pisometacarpal ligaments. A triquetral fracture as part of a pisotriquetral injury commonly results from direct trauma to the pisotriquetral joint, which occurs in sports involving ball catching, but may also result from a fall on the palm of the hand. Overuse injury to the pisotriquetral joint also occurs in throwing and racquet sports, rowing and golf due to repetitive loading during flexion and ulnar deviation of the wrist. Gymnastics, weightlifting, long-distance bike riding and the shot-put also stress the pisotriquetral articulation (see the discussion on page 68).

Diagnostic imaging

Triquetral fractures involving the posterior tubercle and body are usually diagnosed on plain films. Occasionally, a fracture of the posterior tubercle is incomplete or undisplaced, so the soft-tissue swelling on the dorsal aspect of the wrist in the lateral view becomes an important observation, as shown in Fig. 2.117. Often the exact origin of an isolated small bone fragment seen on the dorsal aspect of the carpus is uncertain. Experience would suggest that this is almost always a fragment separated from the posterior tubercle of the triquetrum.

Additional views and other imaging methods are often required to adequately assess the pisotriquetral joint. A pisotriquetral view, which is a steeply obliqued lateral view with slight dorsal rotation, demonstrates the pisotriquetral joint space (see Fig. 2.119). The joint is also well demonstrated in a carpal tunnel view (see Fig. 2.120). The pisotriquetral articulation is a common site of degeneration, sometimes occurring in surprisingly young athletes (see Fig. 2.121). Associated ganglia are well shown by ultrasound (see Fig. 2.122). CT will demonstrate small fractures of the articular surfaces of the pisotriquetral joint (see Fig. 2.123). A bone scan may be helpful in difficult cases (see Fig. 2.124), although if increased uptake is present, a CT scan is often additionally required to differentiate between bone injury and degenerative change and to show which bone is fractured.

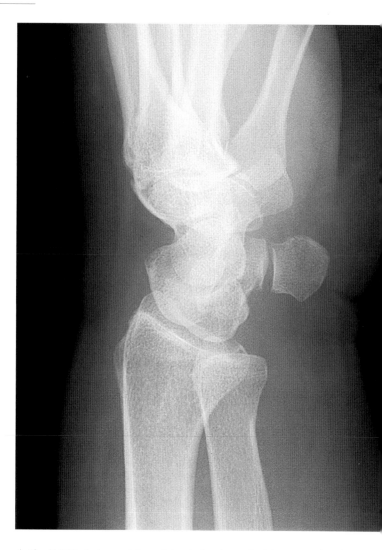

▲ **Fig. 2.119** A steep oblique lateral view is a valuable extra wrist view, enabling examination of the pisotriquetral joint space.

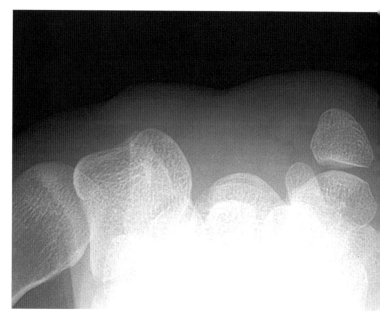

▲ **Fig. 2.120** Pisotriquetral articulation may also be examined by acquiring a carpal tunnel view.

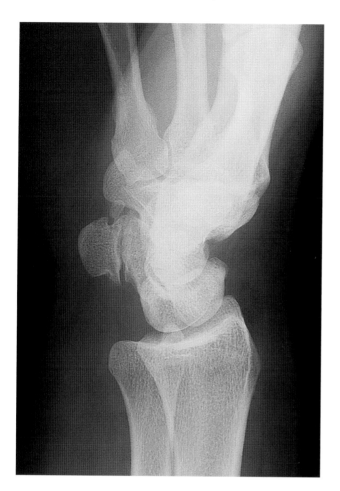

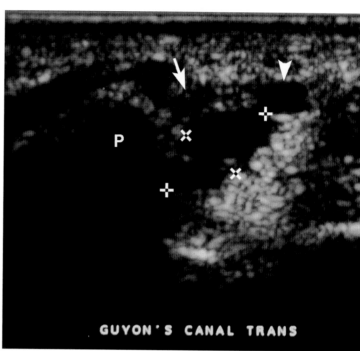

▲ **Fig. 2.121** Because of the important role played by the pisotriquetral joint in wrist extension and the repetitive direct trauma to the joint occurring with sport, degenerative changes in the pisotriquetral joint are common. Advanced changes are present in this relatively young athlete.

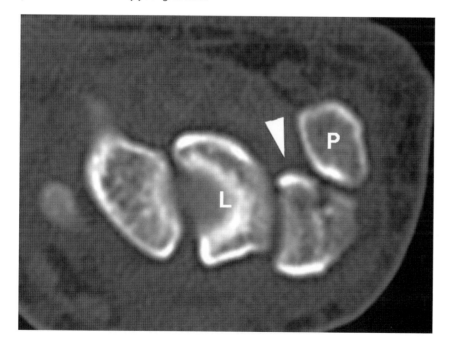

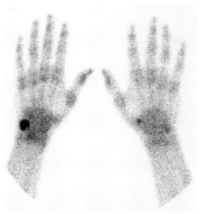

▲ **Fig. 2.124** Following a fall, a fracture of the pisotriquetral complex is demonstrated by nuclear scanning.

▲ **Fig. 2.123** This axial CT image shows a triquetral fracture (arrowhead) with involvement of the pisotriquetral joint. Lunate = L. Pisiform = P.

Pisiform fractures

Fractures of the pisiform (see Fig. 2.125) are usually the result of direct trauma and the most common cause is trauma from catching a speeding cricket ball or baseball. These fractures can be imaged using the same protocols as used for the pisotriquetral joint. Occasionally a PA view of the wrist with radial deviation will help reveal a pisiform fracture (see Fig. 2.126). A pisotriquetral joint view may also be useful for demonstrating a fracture of the articular surface of the pisiform (see Fig. 2.127).

Hook of hamate fractures

After the scaphoid and the triquetrum, a fracture of the hook of hamate is the third most common carpal bone fractured by sporting injury (Steinberg 2002). Diagnosis of this injury depends greatly on clinical awareness and competent imaging.

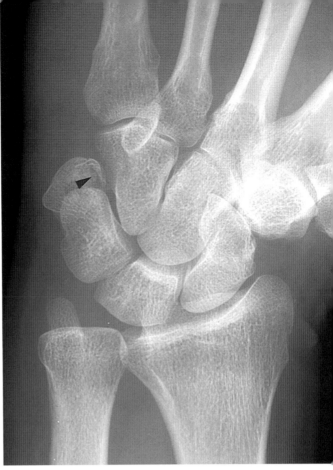

▲ **Fig. 2.126** A fall has resulted in a pisiform fracture (arrowhead). Radial deviation helps to demonstrate the fracture.

▼ **Fig. 2.127** A pisotriquetral view demonstrates a fracture of the articular surface of the pisiform (arrowhead). This extra view is well worth acquiring. The view is easy to obtain and can often provide important information.

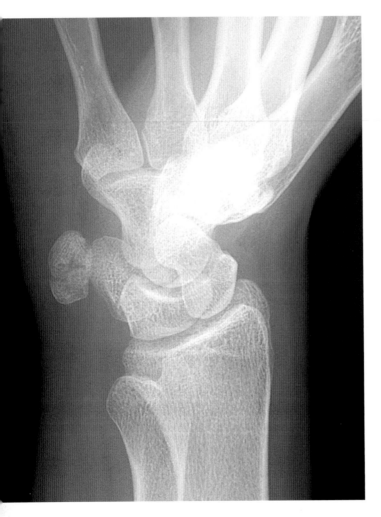

▲ **Fig. 2.125** A cricketer suffered a comminuted fracture of the pisiform from the impact of a cricket ball. This is well demonstrated in a steep lateral view.

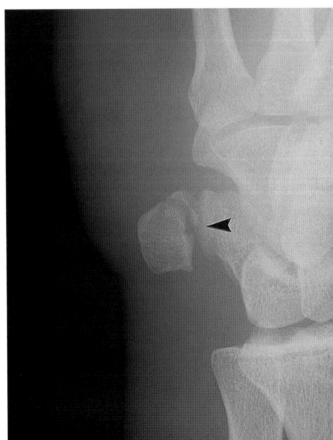

Injury biomechanics and presentation

The most common mechanism for this injury is direct force to the hook. This can be an acute injury or the result of repetitive trauma. There is often a history of repetitive stress preceding an acute episode. Stress can be applied to the hook by mechanisms other than repetitive direct trauma. Repetitive contraction of the flexor tendons of the ring and little fingers against the base of the hook has been suggested as a possible cause (Stark et al. 1977).

Repetitive impact to the hook also occurs in golf when the player takes a large divot or plays a shot from thick rough. This is particularly so when the golfer grips the club with the end of the grip resting against the hook. Similarly, the end of a baseball bat can also impinge on the hook, occurring particularly with 'bunting'. The body and hook of hamate may fracture in association with fourth and fifth CMC joint injuries.

Fractures of the hook of hamate cause ulnar-side wrist pain and there is usually tenderness on palpation over the hook. However, sometimes in a longstanding injury the tenderness may be absent or felt on the dorsum of the hand. The fracture is notorious for being undetected and the diagnosis delayed. This is largely due to the insidious clinical presentation and because the fracture is not readily seen on a routine series of plain films.

The hook projects anteriorly from the body of the hamate and develops from a separate ossification centre. The hook forms part of the ulnar border of the carpal tunnel and the radial border of Guyon's canal. It acts as an anchor for the transverse carpal and pisohamate ligaments and is the origin of the flexor and opponens digiti muscles. The contents of Guyon's canal are closely related to the hook, with the superficial sensory branch of the ulnar nerve passing close to the tip of the hook and the deep motor branch related to its base. As previously discussed, the flexor tendons of the ring and little fingers are closely related to the base of the hook, which acts as a pulley for these tendons in ulnar deviation and with a 'power grip', as shown in Fig. 2.62 (on page 53). There is poor vascularity in the mid-hook due to a poor anastomosis between vessels supplying the tip and the base (Walsh and Bishop 2000). A combination of fracture displacement and poor vascularity contributes to the high occurrence of non-union of hook fractures.

Diagnostic imaging

The hook of hamate can be seen in a well-positioned lateral view but usually superimposition makes the exclusion of a fracture impossible. A hook of hamate view will often demonstrate a hook fracture and is quick and cheap to obtain. The wrist is placed in the lateral position and a sponge under the fifth finger maintains radial deviation of the wrist. The wrist is then rolled slightly in a dorsal direction and the thumb extended anteriorly. Centring on the first web space with a straight tube will produce a lateral view of the hook (see Fig. 2.128). This view sufficiently demonstrates the hook (see Fig. 2.129) and fractures can be adequately shown (see Figs 2.130 and 2.131). The hook of hamate may also be examined in a carpal tunnel view (see Fig. 2.132).

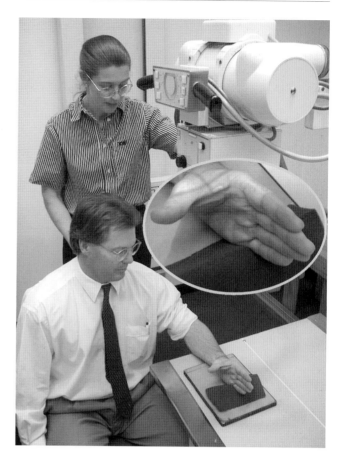

▲ **Fig. 2.128** This photograph shows the correct positioning of the wrist for a hook of hamate view.

▼ **Fig. 2.129** Using the plain film technique shown in Fig. 2.128, the hook of hamate can be well demonstrated. In this case, the hook appears normal.

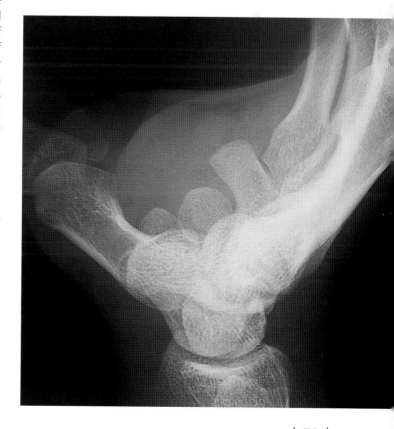

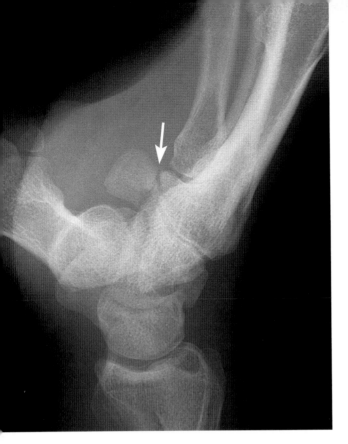

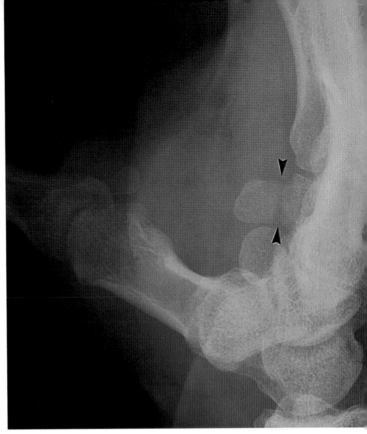

▲ **Fig. 2.130** Using the plain film technique shown in Fig. 2.128, a fracture of the hook of hamate is demonstrated involving the hook near its base (arrow).

▲ **Fig. 2.131** A fracture of the hook of hamate; slight displacement at the fracture site is noted (arrowheads). This displacement increases the chance of non-union and avascular change.

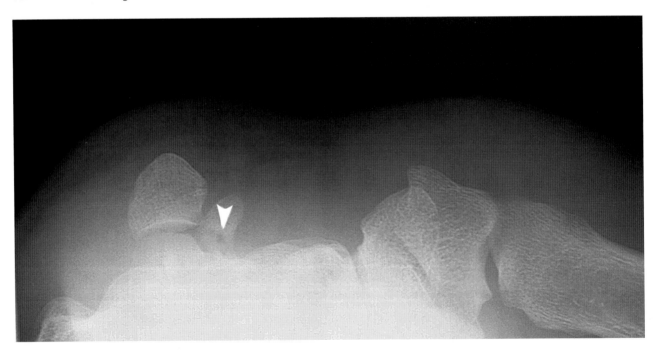

▲ **Fig. 2.132** A fracture of the hook of hamate shown in a carpal tunnel view (arrowhead). Further imaging with CT would be necessary to obtain fracture detail. Nevertheless, a carpal tunnel view is quick to obtain and can be extremely informative.

If the hook of hamate view is inconclusive, other imaging methods may be used. CT scanning (see Figs 2.133 and 2.134), nuclear medicine (see Fig. 2.135) and MRI (see Fig. 2.136) can all provide a diagnosis. Any displacement at the fracture site is likely to result in non-union and CT examination is particularly useful showing bony detail. Care must be taken to distinguish a fracture of the hook from an unfused secondary ossification centre for the hook, known as an os hamuli proprium (see Fig. 2.137).

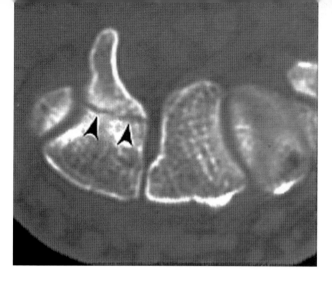

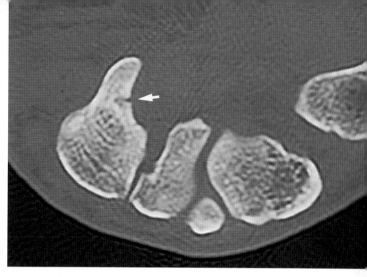

▲ **Fig. 2.133** A hook of hamate fracture (arrowheads) is well demonstrated by a CT scan (arrowheads). No displacement has occurred.

▲ **Fig. 2.134** A polo player presented with chronic pain in the medial aspect of the wrist. A stress fracture of the hook of hamate (arrow) is demonstrated by a CT scan. This has almost certainly been caused by the repetitive impact of the hook against the mallet.

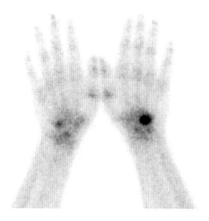

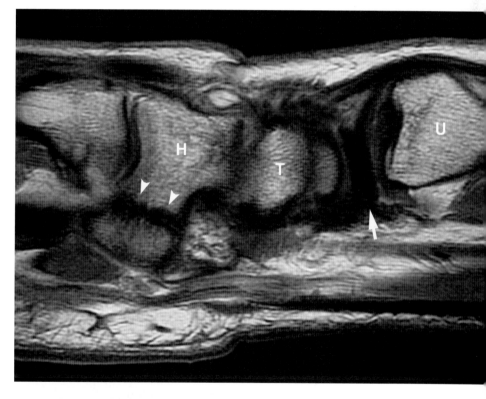

▲ **Fig. 2.135** An isotope bone scan is an efficient method of diagnosing a hook of hamate fracture and to exclude other medial side pathology. Other imaging methods would then be used to provide detail of the fracture.

▶ **Fig. 2.136** A hook of hamate fracture (arrowheads) is demonstrated by MRI. An arrow indicates the TFCC. Hamate = H. Triquetrum = T. Ulna = U.

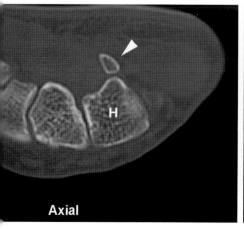

Axial

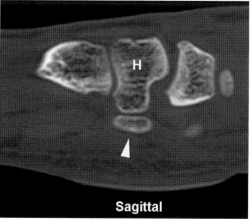

Sagittal

◀ **Fig. 2.137** An os hamuli proprium (arrowhead) is demonstrated on axial and reformatted sagittal CT images. Note the smooth corticated margins and normal trabecular architecture enabling differentiation between an accessory ossicle and a hamate fracture. Hamate = H.

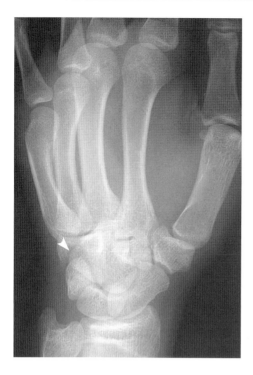

◀**Fig. 2.138** Punching has resulted in a fracture of the body of hamate (arrowhead). There is also evidence of an old punching fracture of the neck of the fifth metacarpal.

▼**Fig. 2.139** An axial CT shows a comminuted body of hamate fracture (arrows), also caused by punching.

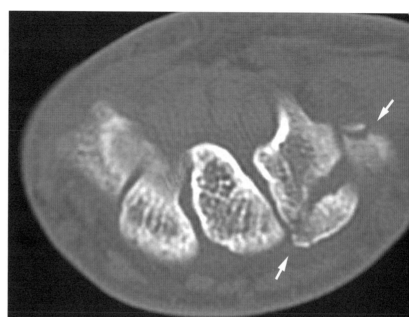

Fractures of the body of hamate

Injury to the fourth and fifth CMC joints may also extend to involve the body of hamate. These fractures are often the result of a punching injury (see Fig. 2.138). Plain films are usually sufficient to demonstrate a fracture but a CT examination is usually necessary to determine displacement (see Fig. 2.139). Occasionally, fractures of the body of hamate may occur as part of the 'greater arc' perilunate injury (see Fig. 2.158(a) on page 89).

Lunate fractures

The lunate fossa at the distal radial articular surface affords protection to the lunate and, as a result, lunate fractures are uncommon (see Fig. 2.140). When a fracture occurs, there is a high risk of subsequent AVN (Beckenbaugh et al. 1980). Small avulsion fractures may be associated with SL and LT ligament injuries. Ultrasound or a CT scan may be necessary to demonstrate these small avulsions (see Fig. 2.141).

▶**Fig. 2.140** In the absence of avascular changes, fractures of the lunate are uncommon. This impacted fracture was caused by a fall on the outstretched hand.

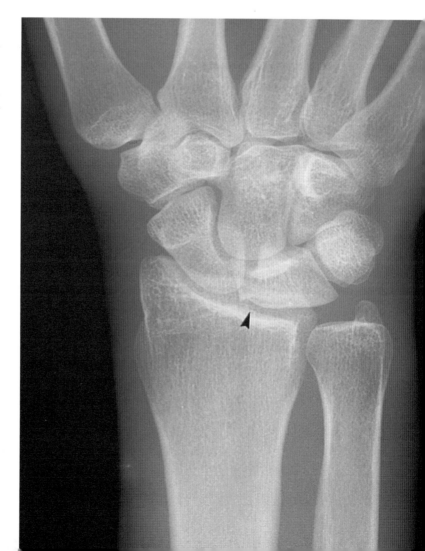

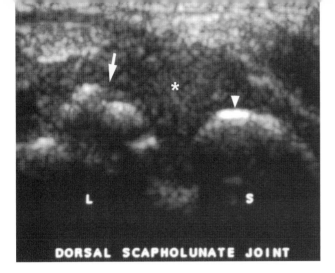

▲ Fig. 2.141 There is a comminuted avulsion fracture at the lunate attachment of the SL ligament. This transverse ultrasound image obtained over the dorsal aspect of the wrist shows an irregular fragmented lunate bone surface (arrow) compared with the smooth intact scaphoid surface (arrowhead). Note the hypoechoic soft-tissue swelling over the scapholunate interval (*) and the loss of normal dorsal band SL ligament fibre definition.

Fractures of the capitate

Fractures of the capitate may occur in isolation as a result of a hyperextension injury of the wrist (see Fig. 2.142). However, capitate fractures are more commonly associated with other carpal fractures or fracture-dislocations. A fracture through the waist of the capitate is commonly a part of the 'greater arc' pattern of carpal fractures (see Fig. 2.143). In the skeletally immature, fracture of the capitate is the second most common fracture after a scaphoid fracture (Le and Henz 2000). Plain films are usually the only imaging required for the diagnosis of a capitate fracture, and it is important to carefully examine the capitate in a patient with a scaphoid fracture.

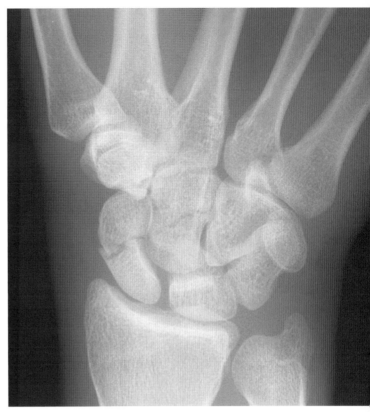

▲ Fig. 2.143 The capitate fracture is a part of a 'greater arc' pattern of injury. In this case the line of force has passed through the waist of the scaphoid and across the capitate. No hamate or triquetral fracture can be seen. The apparent widening of the scapholunate interval may be due to scaphoid shortening resulting from the scaphoid fracture.

▼ Fig. 2.142 An excessive hyperextension injury in a weightlifter has caused a fracture of the waist of the capitate. Considerable displacement has occurred, best seen in the lateral view.

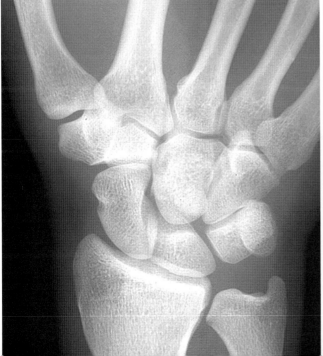

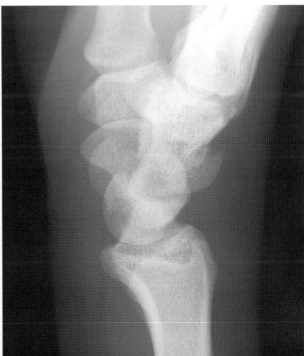

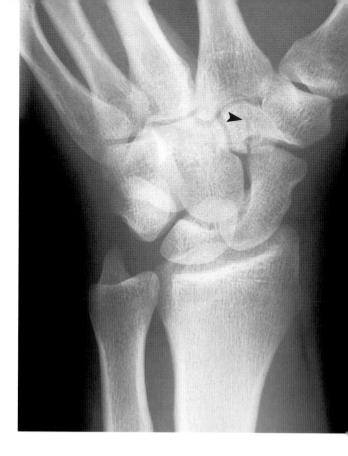

▶ **Fig. 2.144** A rare undisplaced fracture of the trapezoid (arrowhead).

Trapezoid fractures

The trapezoid lies in a well-protected position and undergoes little movement with wrist activity. As a result, fractures of the trapezoid are most unusual (see Fig. 2.144).

Fractures of the trapezium

The most common trapezial fracture seen as a result of sporting injury is a fracture of the anterior ridge, although fractures may also involve the body of the trapezium (see Fig. 2.145). The anterior ridge of the trapezium is in many ways similar to the hook of hamate and when the ridge is well developed it may be seen as a hooked structure on axial imaging (see Fig. 2.146). The flexor carpi radialis (FCR) tendon is closely related to the ridge and occupies a groove on its medial aspect. For this reason a fracture of the anterior ridge may produce important complications.

Fractures of the anterior ridge of the trapezium are uncommon, but when they occur they are often associated with a Bennett's fracture. Following an axial force to the first metacarpal, a vertical line of force separates the volar beak at the base of the first metacarpal and extends across the joint to separate the anterior ridge of the trapezium (see Fig. 2.147). The anterior ridge projects into the palm of the hand. A ridge fracture may also occur with direct trauma, usually caused by a fall on an outstretched hand. This fracture is also seen in association with subluxation or dislocation of the first CMC joint (see Fig. 2.148). As with hook of hamate fractures, fracture displacement occurs due to ligamentous and muscular attachments to the ridge. The flexor retinaculum attaches to the ridge, and the abductor pollicis brevis and opponens pollicis take origin from the ridge.

Fractures of the anterior ridge are prone to non-union, due to displacement. Irregularity at the fracture site may cause injury to the FCR tendon, resulting in tendon attrition with fraying of the tendon, tendinopathy and tendon rupture (see Figs 2.149 and 2.150). Swelling associated with this process may cause median neuropathy.

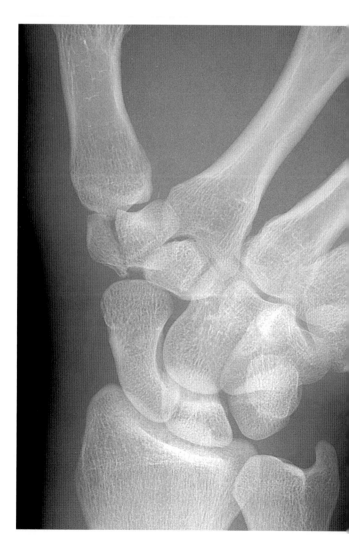

▶ **Fig. 2.145** A fracture involves the body of the trapezium, brought into prominence by ulnar deviation. Changes of nonunion are noted.

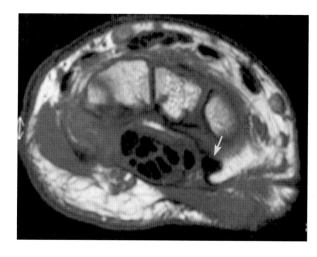

◀ **Fig. 2.146** The anterior ridge of the trapezium is seen on this axial MRI and shows its close association with the FCR tendon (arrow). The anterior ridge of the trapezium shows great similarity to the hook of hamate on the medial side of the wrist.

▼ **Fig. 2.147** A fracture of the anterior ridge of the trapezium has occurred in association with a Bennett's fracture (arrowhead). The line of force has presumably continued across the first CMC joint.

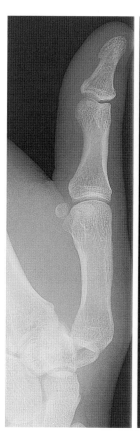

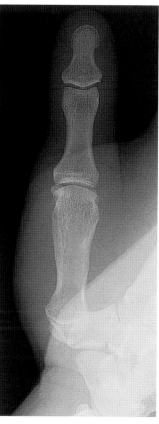

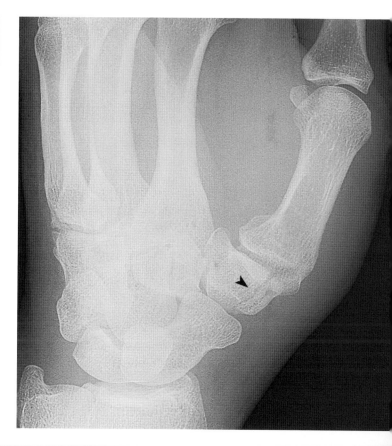

▲ **Fig. 2.148** An anterior ridge fracture has occurred in association with subluxation of the first CMC joint.

▶ **Fig. 2.149** An old fracture of the anterior ridge has healed with residual irregularity. This irregularity has caused FRC tendinopathy, due to the tendon rubbing against the irregularity. The bony irregularity is well shown in a carpal tunnel view (arrowhead).

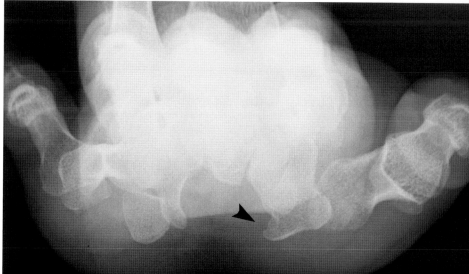

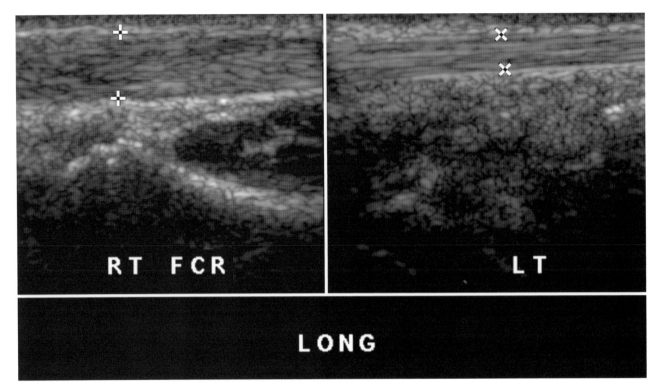

▲ Fig. 2.150 The bony irregularity resulting from the old fracture seen in Fig. 2.149 has produced a right FCR tendinopathy. This long-axis ultrasound image demonstrates a markedly thickened and mildly hypoechoic right FCR tendon compared with the normal left side.

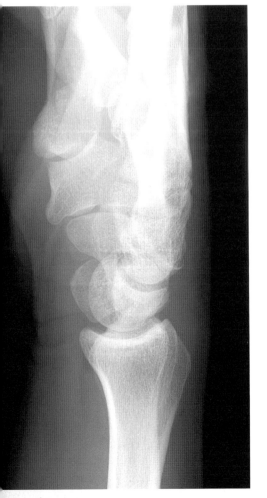

Diagnostic imaging

If an anterior ridge fracture is suspected clinically, additional plain film views should be obtained. The anterior ridge of the trapezium views can demonstrate the ridge both in the lateral projection and in profile. The anterior ridge can be well demonstrated with the wrist in a lateral position and then rolled forward slightly (see Fig. 2.151). The anterior ridge of the trapezium can also be examined in a carpal tunnel view, where it is seen in profile (see Fig. 2.149 on page 85). A bone scan may be helpful if plain films are normal or equivocal (see Fig. 2.152) and axial CT imaging can provide fracture definition. Ultrasound or MRI will detect associated tendinopathy, as shown in Fig. 2.150.

Stress fractures

Stress fractures occur at the wrist as a result of overuse and involve the hook of hamate, the pisiform and, most commonly, the distal radial growth plate (gymnast's wrist).

◄ Fig. 2.151 A slightly anteriorly rotated lateral view of the wrist shows the anterior ridge of the trapezium en face and is a valuable view for detecting fractures of the ridge. Note dorsal rotation of the lunate.

▶ Fig. 2.152 A fracture of the trapezium is detected by a nuclear scan. Note that the focal area of uptake is more distal than occurs with a scan of a scaphoid fracture.

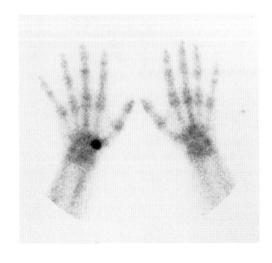

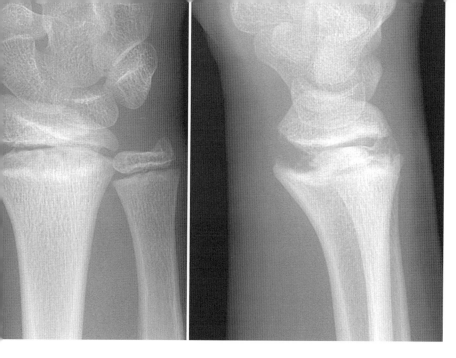

◀ **Fig. 2.153** Stress fractures of the distal radial growth plate occur in gymnasts. The condition is known as gymnast's wrist and this case is a typical example. The changes are shown in the PA and lateral projections. Bony resorption and irregularity mainly involve the metaphyseal side of the distal radial growth plate.

Stress fractures of the pisiform are uncommon. Israeli and Engel (1982) have reported stress fractures in volleyball players due to repetitive trauma. The pisiform is stressed in sports that require repetitive movement of the wrist from extension and radial deviation to flexion and ulnar deviation, or loading in an extended position, stressed through the action of the flexor carpi ulnaris. Degenerative changes in the pisotriquetral articulation are relatively common, resulting from the same mechanism.

All gymnastic events require extreme axial loading forces across the wrist with the wrist in hyperextension. Roy et al. (1985) described plain film changes occurring in the wrists of skeletally immature gymnasts. A stress reaction was described involving the distal radial growth plate producing widening of the growth plate and marginal irregularity (see Fig. 2.153). A common complication of this injury is radial shortening due to premature closure of the growth plate (see Fig. 2.154). This leads to an ulnar plus variance (see Fig. 2.155), ulnar impaction syndrome and TFCC injury (Caine et al. 1992; De Smet et al. 1994). Gymnastics is a major cause of wrist injury.

▼ **Fig. 2.154(a) and (b)** This gymnast was competing at the Sydney 2000 Olympics and presented to the Polyclinic with wrist pain. There are changes of gymnast's wrist bilaterally. The changes are producing retarded growth at the distal radial growth plate, and ulnar plus variance is already present on both sides.

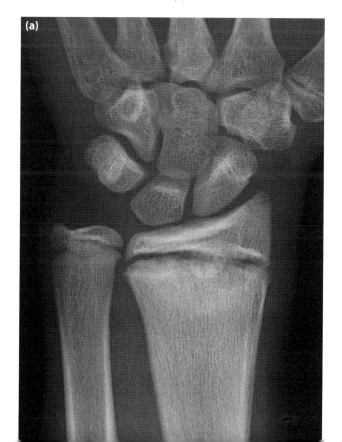

(a)

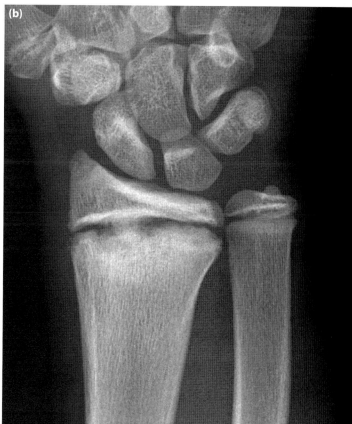

(b)

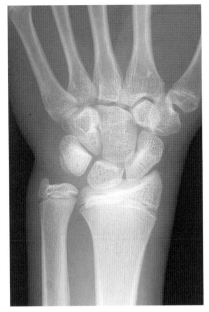

▲ Fig. 2.155 This is often the end result of gymnast's wrist. Premature closure of the distal radial growth plate is progressing, retarding radial growth. As a consequence, there is relative overgrowth of the ulna and ulnar plus variance is now present, with the associations of ulnar abutment syndrome and TFCC injury.

▼ Fig. 2.156 A lesser arc injury has progressed to liberate the lunate. The perilunate joints show incongruency indicating perilunate ligamentous injury.

Mandelbaum et al. (1989) reported a high incidence of wrist pain among competitive gymnasts. In their study, 75% of male gymnasts and 50% of female gymnasts complained of wrist pain. In male gymnasts, the symptoms were equally distributed between the radial and ulnar sides, whereas in females the pain was mainly ulnar-side. This was thought to be due to the different routines performed by each gender, with the majority of wrist problems in males produced by activity on the pommel horse. Clinically, it is important to remember that occasionally a gymnast with a stress fracture of the distal radial growth plate may present with a loss of dorsiflexion of the wrist rather than pain.

Patterns of fractures: perilunate injuries

Certain predictable patterns of injury occur in the wrist following trauma. They are centred on the lunate in two recognisable arcs (Melone et al. 2000). These types of injuries are due to severe trauma resulting in excessive wrist hyperextension and ulnar deviation. Intercarpal supination also plays a role.

Mayfield et al. (1980) described serial disruption of soft-tissue structures around the lunate that was termed the 'lesser arc' by Johnson (1980). This referred to a purely ligamentous injury. The sequence of failure commences on the radial side and progresses to the ulnar side. Although the lesser arc pattern usually commences with injury to radial-side ligaments including the scapholunate complex and volar ligaments, Mayfield et al. noted that, occasionally, fracture of the radial styloid commenced the lesser arc injuries.

Mayfield et al. described four stages of perilunar instability:

- *Stage I:* scapholunate dissociation caused by injury to the SL ligament complex and the volar extrinsic ligaments.
- *Stage II:* injury progresses with failure of the radial collateral ligament and midcarpal joint instability, disrupting the linkage between the lunate and the capitate and opening the space of Poirier.
- *Stage III:* continuing ligamentous injury involves the LT ligament and extrinsic stabilisers of the lunate, further liberating the lunate (see Fig. 2.156).
- *Stage IV:* with continuing force, the dorsal radiocarpal ligaments rupture and volar dislocation of the lunate occurs (see Fig. 2.157).

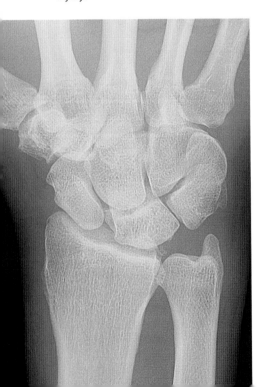

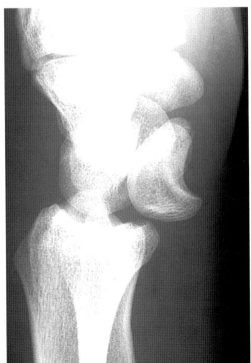

◀ Fig. 2.157 Further injury allows the lunate to dislocate, with the lunate rotating anteriorly through the space of Poirier. The other carpal bones remain in line with the radius.

Since this work by Mayfield et al., other researchers have shown that fractures of the scaphoid, capitate, hamate and triquetrum also occur in sequence, centred on the lunate but describing a more distal arc, called 'the greater arc'. These injuries are produced by a common mechanism that produces predictable patterns of fractures (see Fig. 2.158(a)) and fracture dislocations (see Fig. 2.158(b) and (c)).

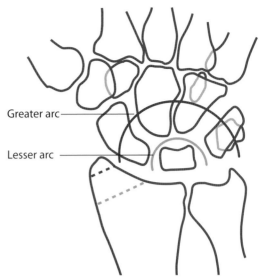

Greater arc

Lesser arc

▶ **Fig. 2.158(a)** The greater arc pattern (dark grey line) is an arc of fractures through the scaphoid, capitate, hamate and triquetrum, described by Mayfield (1980). The lesser arc pattern (light grey line) occurs when a force liberates the lunate by rupturing the ligaments that anchor the lunate and was first described by Johnson (1980). Cases have been encountered where both arcs commence with a fracture through the radial styloid process (dotted lines).

▼ **(b)** This is an example of a greater arc pattern of fractures. The line of force progresses across the wrist, causing fracturing through the waist of the scaphoid, and across the capitate, causing a comminuted fracture of the hamate. Unlike the classical greater arc injury, no triquetral fracture can be seen here.

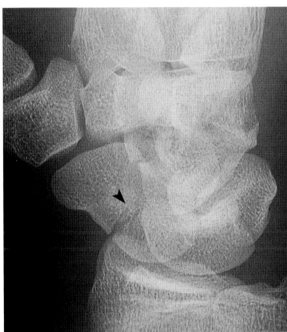
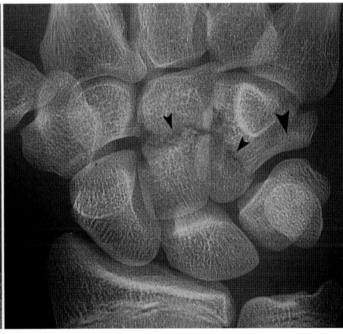

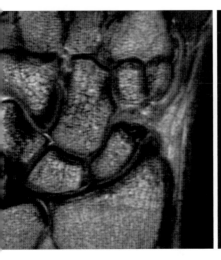
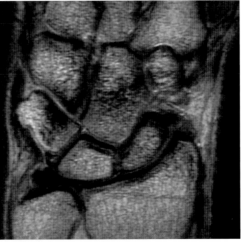

◀ **(c)** This interesting case provides further information regarding the greater arc pattern of injury. These coronal T1-weighted MR images were obtained from a female weightlifter with a painful wrist. Corresponding with the line of the greater arc, sclerotic changes pass through the triquetrum, through the proximal pole of the hamate, through the capitate and across the tubercle of the scaphoid. These changes almost certainly are in response to a repetitive line of force producing bone stress.

Other patterns of injury are also recognised (Herzberg et al. 1993). A fracture of the waist of the scaphoid may be associated with liberation of the lunate, with a trans-scaphoid perilunate fracture dislocation occurring (see Fig. 2.159). The greater arc sequence may commence with a fracture through the tip of the radial styloid process with the line of force continuing through the waist of the scaphoid (see Fig. 2.160). Also, a fracture involving the base of the radial styloid process may commence the lesser arc sequence and pass through the scapholunate interval (see Fig. 2.161).

However, these sequential patterns are not the entire answer. LT ligament injury can occur alone and ulnar-side injury is not necessarily preceded by scapholunate and lunocapitate injury. A reverse sequence from ulnar to radial side has been suggested to occur occasionally. The Mayo classification of fractures and fracture dislocations (Cooney et al. 1987) further widened the concept of predictable patterns of carpal injuries to include fracture dislocations.

Carpal ligament injuries and instabilities

To understand any type of instability, it is important first to recognise the stabilising structures and how they may fail. The scaphoid holds the key to carpal stability by providing a unique mechanical linkage between the radius and both carpus rows. Wrist function depends on normal and stable scaphoid movement.

The distal and proximal articular surfaces of the scaphoid are offset, with the distal articular surface lying anterior to the proximal surface. This means that reacting to axial loading of the wrist, the scaphoid will have an inherent tendency to volarflex. Intrinsic and extrinsic ligaments stabilise the scaphoid by providing a constraint against this flexion. As the wrist moves through flexion, extension and axial rotation, the scaphoid moves into different positions to accommodate available space. The scaphoid undergoes volar flexion when the lateral wrist is loaded by radial deviation or flexion and extends when there is an increase in the available space as a result of ulnar deviation and extension (Arkless 1966).

A number of papers in the 1940s and 1960s described scaphoid subluxation associated with rotation of the scaphoid (e.g. Russell 1949; Vaughan-Jackson 1949). It was noted that the pathological angulation of the scaphoid through its long axis and displacement of the proximal pole of the scaphoid dorsally were associated clinically with a painful click in the lateral wrist. The concept of scapholunate dissociation was first described by Linscheid et al. (1972) and this paper refocused attention on the loss of simultaneous movement of the scaphoid and the lunate, the abnormal rotation of the lunate, and the gap between the proximal pole of the scaphoid and the lunate. Scapholunate dissociation and DISI deformity were considered to be the primary instability. However, Blatt (1987) changed the approach to SL ligament injury again when he stated that 'the real clinical significance of SL dissociation is its role as a precursor to the much greater problem of rotary subluxation of the scaphoid'.

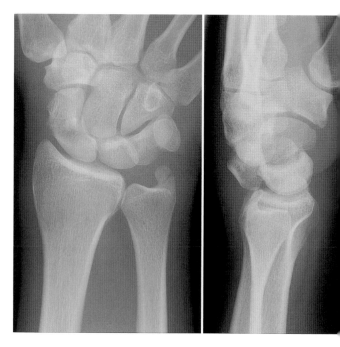

▲ **Fig. 2.159** A further pattern of injury following liberation of the lunate is a trans-scaphoid perilunate dislocation of the lunate, where the lunate and proximal pole of the scaphoid remain in line with the radius and the remaining carpus are displaced dorsally.

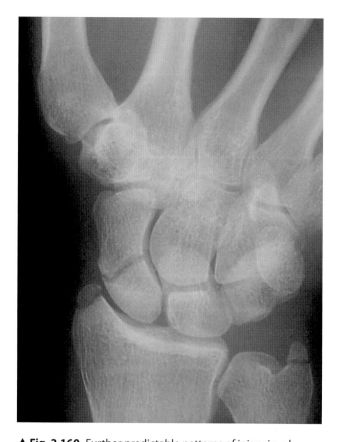

▲ **Fig. 2.160** Further predictable patterns of injury involve fractures of the radial styloid process. A line of force producing a fracture of the tip of the styloid process continues across the radiocarpal joint to involve the waist of the scaphoid. A fracture of the ulnar styloid is noted.

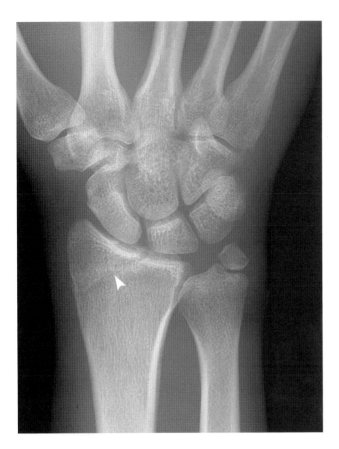

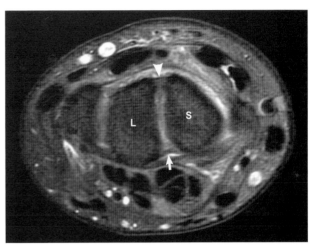

▲ Fig. 2.162 A normal SL ligament is demonstrated by MRI. The fat-suppressed axial PD-weighted MR image shows the normal volar band (arrow) and dorsal band (arrowhead) of the SL ligament. Lunate = L. Scaphoid = S.

▲ Fig. 2.161 A fracture of the base of the styloid process is shown to continue into the scapholunate interval with rupture of the SL ligaments.

Nathan and Blatt (2000) stressed that the significant clinical change is instability of the scaphoid at the radioscaphoid articulation rather than scapholunate dissociation that precedes the instability.

Patterns of instabilities

SL ligament injury

Anatomy of SL ligament injury and the concept of rotary subluxation of the scaphoid

Wrist stability depends on the integrity of both intrinsic and extrinsic ligaments. The primary stabilising intrinsic ligament is the SL ligament complex (Berger et al. 1982), which has three components: dorsal, volar and mid-substance. The dorsal component, the dorsal scapholunate ligament (DSLL), is the major stabiliser. The mid-substance or scapholunate interosseous ligament (SLIL) is fibrocartilaginous, similar to the proximal section of the LT ligament. If the SLIL is ruptured, there is no alteration to SL biomechanics or widening of the scapholunate joint space. The SL ligaments can be well demonstrated by MRI (see Fig. 2.162) and ultrasound (see Fig. 2.163). Rupture of both the DSLL and the SLIL is required to alter biomechanics and produces widening of the SL joint and the beginning of rotary deformity of the scaphoid (Berger et al. 1991) (see Fig. 2.164). The radioscaphocapitate extrinsic ligament prevents excessive scaphoid rotation

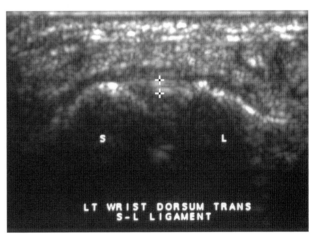

▲ Fig. 2.163 A normal dorsal band of SL ligament (callipers) is demonstrated on this transverse ultrasound section. Note the presence of continuous echogenic fibres extending between the scaphoid (S) and lunate (L) bones.

around its long axis (Linscheid et al. 1972) and stabilises the relationship between the lunate, the scaphoid and the distal radius. So, with continuing injury, the constraint against rotation is removed, dissociation between the scaphoid and the lunate will occur and there is instability of the radioscaphoid articulation. Excessive scaphoid flexion will then occur, and the proximal pole migrates laterally and dorsally towards the dorsal lip of the distal radial articular surface. The normal area of articulation between the scaphoid and the scaphoid fossa progressively decreases with increasing radioscaphoid instability. Consequently, rotary subluxation of the scaphoid is a progressive disability resulting from a continuum of ligamentous failure.

Degenerative changes will often occur in the radioscaphoid articulation due to radioscaphoid instability, producing joint space narrowing at the lateral aspect of the radioscaphoid

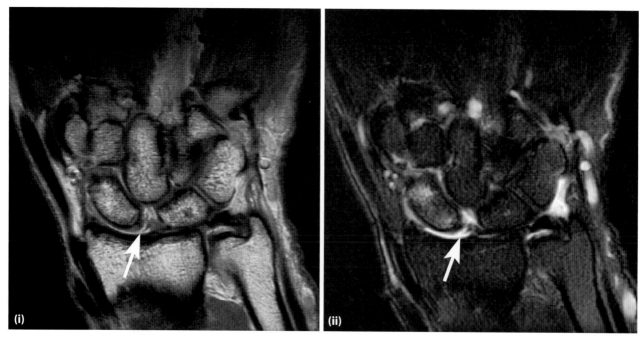

▲ **Fig. 2.164(a)** An SL ligament tear (arrow) is shown on **(i)** coronal T1- and **(ii)** fat-suppressed T2-weighted MR images. Note the high signal of marrow oedema within the scaphoid on the T2 image. Joint space widening has occurred indicating injury to both the DSLL and the fibrocartilaginous SLIL.

joint. Scapholunate advanced collapse (SLAC) wrist is a further late complication of this continuum of injury and occurs when the capitate migrates proximally through the widening space between the scaphoid and the lunate (see Fig. 2.165). The capitate may eventually articulate with the radius (Watson and Ballet 1984).

Clinical presentation

The majority of patients complain of radial-side wrist pain following trauma. There is often a delay in the appearance of the symptoms, with a painful click or clunk developing as rotary subluxation develops. The click or clunk characteristically occurs when the lateral side of the wrist is loaded by radial deviation and wrist flexion.

The clinical findings depend on the stage of the continuum of instability. Initially there is tenderness over the SL ligament and pain on movement of the scaphoid (Watson's Test). The pain is thought to be due to abnormal movement of the proximal pole against the dorsal rim of the radial fossa, and this manoeuvre will reproduce the patient's symptoms. With

▼ **(b)** This coronal PD MR image demonstrates rupture of the SLIL component of the SL ligament without significant joint space widening.

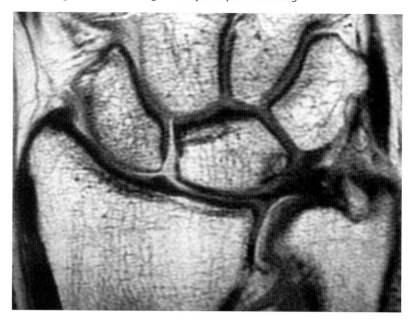

increasing instability, the proximal pole of the scaphoid can be made to sublux, producing a click or clunk. As the process progresses to a static stage, the scaphoid becomes dislocated from its articular fossa, fixed with the proximal pole palpable dorsally. As degenerative changes advance, pain, restricted wrist movement and crepitus may be felt.

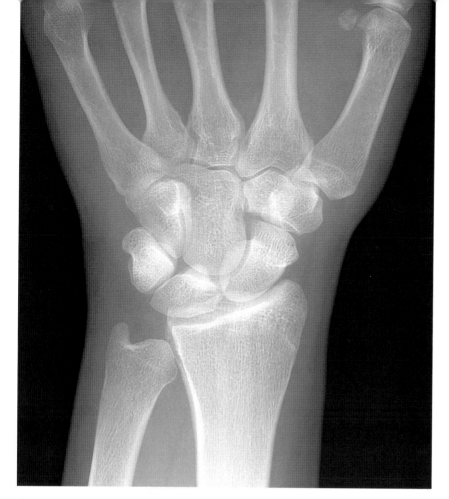

▲ **Fig. 2.165(a)** There is widening of the scapholunate joint space and the capitate has commenced the proximal migration of early SLAC wrist.

▼ **(b)** There is considerable widening of the scapholunate joint space and with an increased proximal migration of the capitate when compared with **(a)**, the capitate has now begun to interpose itself between the scaphoid and the lunate.

▼ **(c)** This plain film shows the advanced changes of SLAC wrist. The capitate has now almost reached the radius. Marked degenerative changes involve the radioscaphoid articulation.

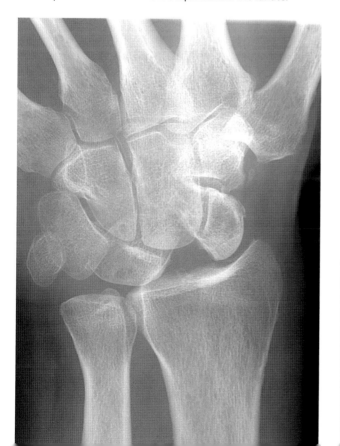

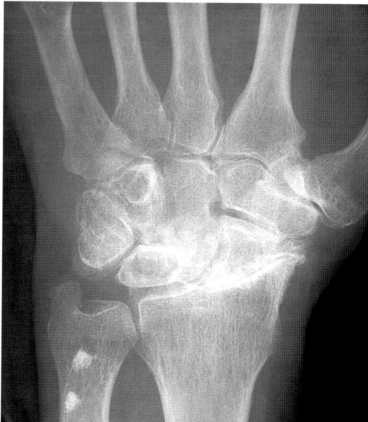

Diagnostic imaging

Initially, there may be a clinical suspicion of carpal instability but the plain film series is normal (Watson Type I). The SL ligament may be partially ruptured with an intact radiosca-phocapitate ligament preventing rotation of the scaphoid. At this stage, imaging of the scapholunate joint with ultrasound or MRI may demonstrate ligament injury (see Fig. 2.166). A bone scan may also provide evidence of SL ligament injury and help to exclude other traumatic changes (see Fig. 2.167).

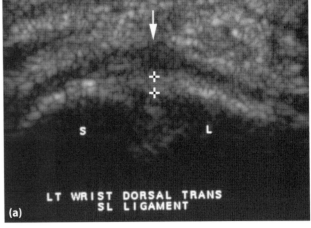

(a)

LT WRIST DORSAL TRANS
SL LIGAMENT

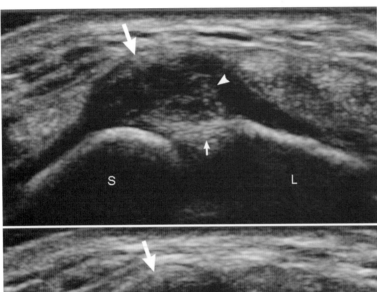

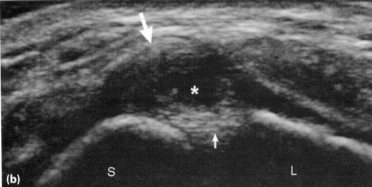

Fig. 2.166 Various patterns of SL ligament injury demonstrated by ultrasound

▲ **(a)** Localised post-traumatic dorsal synovitis (arrow) without cyst formation. Callipers indicate the dorsal SL ligament, which appears grossly intact.

(b)

▲ **(b)** Dorsal ganglion, indicated by asterisk, shown on two adjacent transverse images. Note the associated synovitis (arrowhead), underlying grossly intact SL ligament (small arrows), and displaced overlying dorsal radiocarpal ligament (large arrows).

▼ **(c)** Left SL ligament tear (arrow). Note the comparison view showing the intact right SL ligament (arrowhead). Scaphoid = S. Lunate = L.

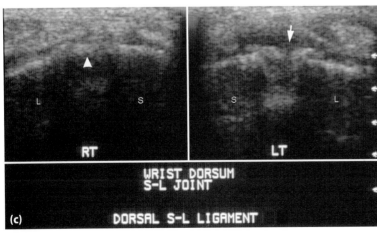

WRIST DORSUM
S-L JOINT

DORSAL S-L LIGAMENT

(c)

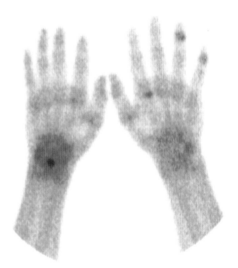

▲ **Fig. 2.167** A bone scan shows increased uptake of isotope over the SL ligament and is a useful tool for indicating injury in this region.

With progressive ligamentous failure, a clinical dynamic instability may develop. In the early stages, the plain film series is usually normal, but stress views will often provide a diagnosis. At the early stages of carpal instability minor widening of the scapholunate articulation may be present and stress views of the asymptomatic wrist as well as the symptomatic side can help to determine whether this widening is significant. Loss of congruency of the articular surfaces at the scapholunate interval is usually an indication of ligamentous injury and is an important observation to make (see Fig. 2.168).

Stress views are an attempt to load the scapholunate and lunotriquetral joints in a patient with a dynamic instability. The loading hopefully will reproduce the conditions that cause the intermittent instability. The series includes three films: radial and ulnar deviation views and a 'power grip' view. These can be obtained AP or PA. Movement into radial and ulnar deviation would normally produce ventral and dorsal rotation of the proximal carpal row. Widening of the scapholunate joint space with ulnar deviation is evidence of rupture or partial rupture of the SL ligament complex (see Fig. 2.169(a)). The third view in the series is a clenched fist or 'power grip' view, which drives the capitate into the scapholunate curve, stressing the ligamentous integrity between the lunate and both the scaphoid and the triquetrum (see Fig. 2.169(b)).

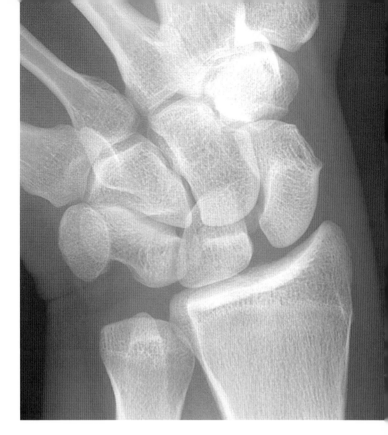

▲ **Fig. 2.169(a)** A stress view demonstrates rupture or partial rupture of the SL ligament. Ulnar deviation produces subtle but definite widening of the scapholunate joint space. A number of small bone fragments are projected over the distal end of the scapholunate joint space and these are almost certainly avulsed fragments.

▼ **(b)** A 'power grip' view shows widening of the scapholunate interval, which had not been evident on deviation views. With gripping, the capitate stresses the integrity of the ligaments in the proximal carpal row.

▼ **Fig. 2.168** Loss of congruity of the bony margins at the scapholunate interval indicates ligamentous injury.

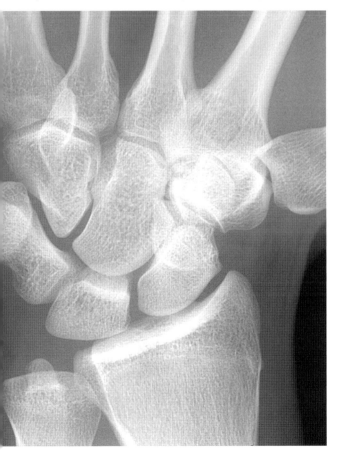

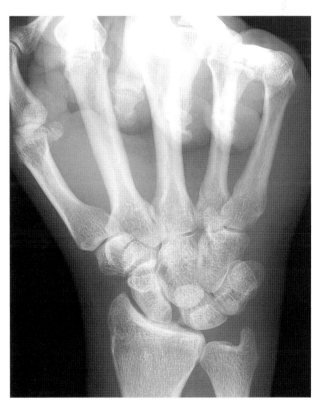

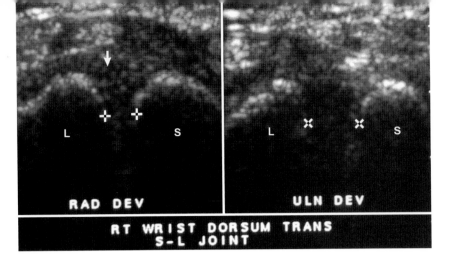

RAD DEV   ULN DEV

RT WRIST DORSUM TRANS
S-L JOINT

▲ **Fig. 2.170** Real-time ultrasound using either forced ulnar deviation or 'power grip' stress is an excellent dynamic method of assessing scapholunate joint stability. Transverse images have been obtained at the same location over the dorsal aspect of the scapholunate joint in forced radial deviation of the wrist (RAD DEV) and forced ulnar deviation of the wrist (ULN DEV). Significant widening (≥1.0 mm more than the normal side) of scapholunate joint space is demonstrated in ulnar deviation (callipers), indicative of SL joint instability. In cases of rotary subluxation of the scaphoid, the scapholunate joint space may not widen but abnormal rotary movement relative to the lunate can nevertheless be appreciated on real-time scanning by comparison with the normal side. Note the poor definition of dorsal SL ligament fibres in this case, particularly on the lunate side (arrow), suggestive of rupture. Scaphoid = S. Lunate = L.

▼ **Fig. 2.171** Rotary subluxation of the scaphoid is present with the scaphoid having become almost horizontal, and there is an increase in the scapholunate angle to about 90°. The proximal end of the scaphoid overhangs the dorsal rim of the distal radius. A fixed DISI deformity is present (Type III stage) and the changes are irreversible. Note the 'ring sign' in the PA view.

Dynamic ultrasound is another method of demonstrating widening of the scapholunate joint space (see Fig. 2.170). Radial deviation will stress the lunotriquetral joint.

If the instability becomes static, as occurs in the Type III stage, diagnostic changes will be evident on the plain film series and stress views will not add further information. At this stage, scapholunate dissociation is established, DISI deformity (see Fig. 2.171) is fixed and palmar flexion of the scaphoid is irreducible. In the lateral view there is an increased scapholunate angle. A 'ring' sign is described in the literature, produced by the scaphoid tubercle being seen end-on in the PA view (see Fig. 2.172) (Nathan and Blatt 2000).

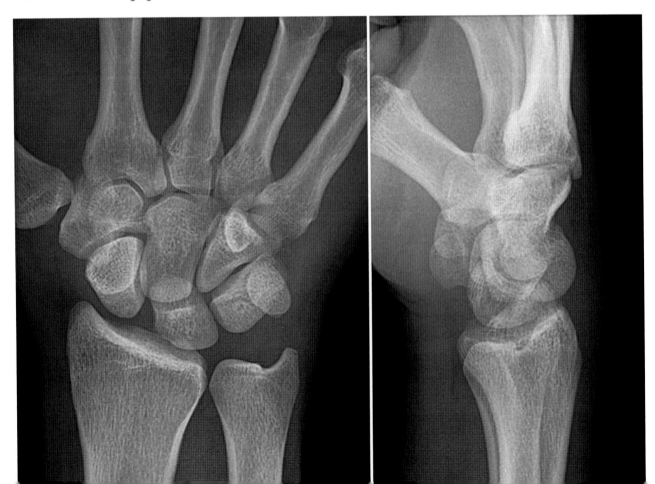

With altered wrist biomechanics, degenerative changes appear (Type IV). Degenerative changes are characteristically seen at the radioscaphoid joint laterally, the scaphotrapezial joints and at the lunocapitate articulation. A DISI deformity does not always indicate rupture of the SL ligament and other conditions can produce an identical deformity. When a pseudarthrosis develops following non-union of a scaphoid fracture, dissociation may occur at the pseudarthrosis site. The proximal pole fragment moves with the lunate, whereas the distal fragment is dissociated. A DISI deformity may develop (see Fig. 2.173(a)). Another condition that may mimic an SL ligament rupture is an avascular necrosis of the lunate, which can disrupt the stability of the proximal carpal row, resulting in a DISI deformity. AVN causing a DISI deformity is well demonstrated in Fig. 2.173(b).

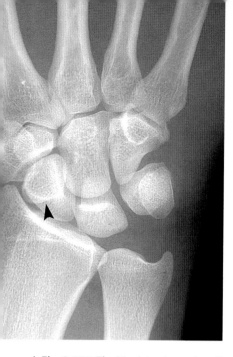

▲ **Fig. 2.172** The 'ring' sign (arrowhead) is created by volar rotation of the scaphoid, the ring being the tubercle viewed end-on.

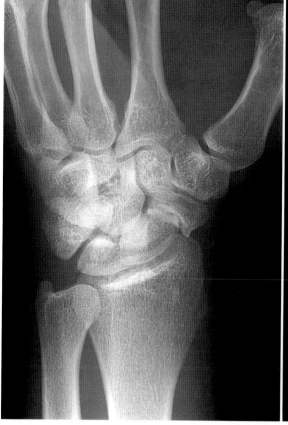
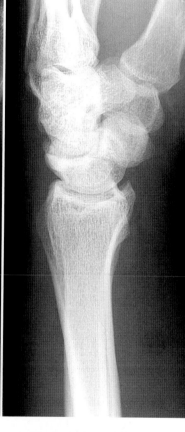

▶ **Fig. 2.173(a)** A DISI deformity is present, caused by non-union of the scaphoid with a pseudarthrosis. The dissociation occurs at the pseudarthrosis site rather than at the scapholunate joint.

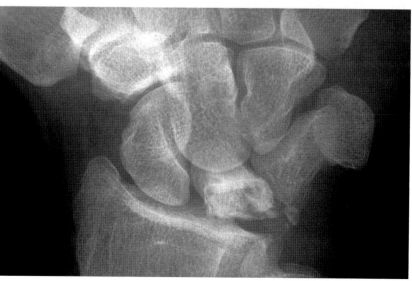

▶ **(b)** AVN of the scaphoid has produced a DISI deformity, with widening of the scapholunate joint space, and there is rotation of the proximal carpal row. There also appears to be a midtarsal instability present, with incongruity at the articulation between the hamate and the triquetrum. An ulna minus variance is noted.

LT ligament injury

Anatomy and injury biomechanics

Injury to the LT ligament is usually associated with other soft-tissue injury and rarely occurs in isolation. Tears of the LT ligament can be the result of trauma or degenerative change.

The LT ligament connects the lunate and triquetrum at the proximal half of the lunotriquetral joint and acts to stabilise the joint. Important extrinsic ligaments that attach to the posterior tubercle of the triquetrum afford further stability. These ligaments are the dorsal radiocarpal and dorsal inter-carpal ligaments.

The LT ligament consists of three distinct components: the dorsal and palmar segments of the LT ligament are joined across the proximal aspect of the joint by the third or proximal segment. The dorsal and palmar segments are true ligaments, whereas the proximal segment is fibrocartilaginous and is not a true ligament. The palmar segment is the most robust and the fibrocartilaginous proximal segment is the segment most injured (Ritter et al. 1999).

Tears of the LT ligament are relatively uncommon. The injury usually occurs in association with injury to the TFCC as a result of either acute trauma or ulnocarpal impaction syndrome. When LT ligament injury is the result of acute trauma, there has characteristically been a fall on the outstretched hand involving impaction and rotation (forced pronation). The wrist is usually in ulnar deviation and extension at impact (Werner and Plancher 1998). Lifting injuries may also tear the LT ligament.

The theory of progressive perilunar instability (Mayfield et al. 1980) would suggest that LT ligament injuries occur only after rupture of the scapholunate and lunocapitate structures in a continuum of liberating the lunate. However,

other researchers believe that there are patterns of injury that commence at the ulnar side of the wrist and that specific structures have to be injured to produce the characteristic VISI deformity. Ritt et al. (1998) demonstrated that division of the proximal or dorsal section of the LT ligament did not produce significant change in carpal kinematics, whereas division of the proximal and palmar sections produces VISI deformity. In addition, division of the dorsal radiocarpal (DRC) and dorsal intercarpal (DIC) ligaments increased the deformity. Viegas, Patterson et al. (1990) described a three-stage progressive instability pattern on the ulnar side of the wrist:

- *Stage I:* one component of the LT ligament ruptures (partial or complete) but the LT joint remains stable.
- *Stage II:* in addition, there is rupture of the palmar section, producing a dynamic instability.
- *Stage III:* additional injury to the DRC ligament will allow a static instability.

Diagnostic imaging

It is important to remember when investigating ulnar-side wrist pain that more than one cause may be present. For example, if a TFCC tear is found, other associated injuries should be excluded.

A routine plain film series will, as usual, contain PA and lateral views, taken in zero rotation to help access the true relative lengths of the radius and ulna. An oblique view completes the series. Additional stress views are necessary and will include PA views in ulnar and radial deviation and a 'power grip' AP view. In the authors' experience, widening of the lunotriquetral joint space is rare, and more often the clues to LT ligament rupture include a VISI deformity (see Fig. 2.174) and sometimes incongruency of the LT joint (see Fig. 2.175).

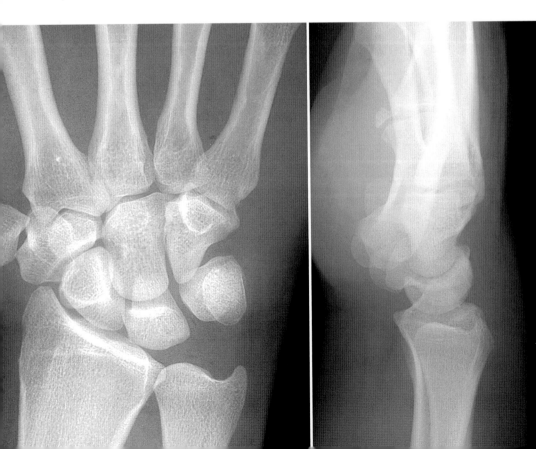

◀ **Fig. 2.174** There is moderate widening and congruency of the lunotriquetral joint space when stressed with radial deviation. In the lateral view, volar rotation of the lunate is present, typical of a VISI deformity.

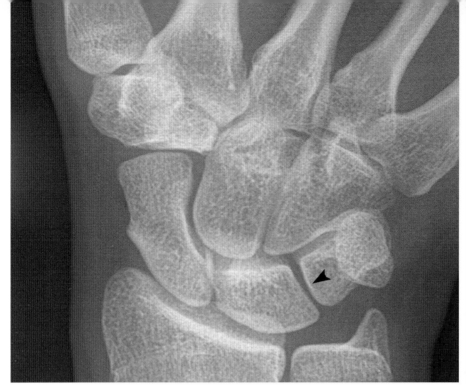

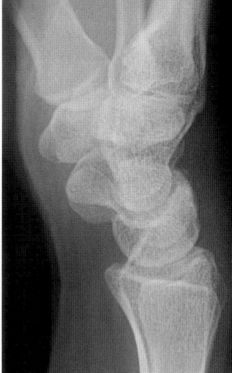

Arthrography may be helpful, although interpretation of a positive result should be viewed with some caution. Viegas, Patterson et al. (1990) showed that in a cadaveric study, 36% of that population had perforations of their LT ligament. Also, in a discussion on three-compartment injection arthrography, Palmer et al. (1991) reported a 14% false negative rate.

Although ultrasound (see Fig. 2.176) and MRI (see Fig. 2.177) can be performed with some confidence at the scapholunate joint, results at the LT joint have not been as reliable (Ritter et al. 1999). Arthroscopy at this stage would appear to be the most accurate method of assessment of LT injury.

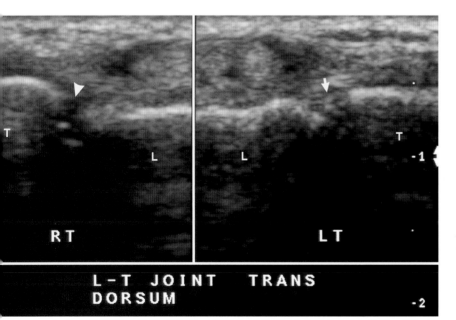

Fig. 2.176 Ultrasound demonstrates LT ligament rupture. A transverse image obtained over the dorsal aspect of the wrist with applied radial deviation stress shows a hypoechoic tear defect (arrowhead) interrupting the dorsal band of the *right* LT ligament. Compare this with the intact fibres of the normal *left* LT ligament (arrow). Also note the abnormal alignment on the right side when compared with the left, appreciated as a subtle asymmetric 'step-off' in the cortical contours of the lunate and triquetrum. Lunate = L. Triquetrum = T.

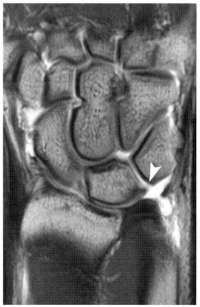

Fig. 2.177 A T1-weighted MRI arthrogram of a small full-thickness LT ligament rupture. High signal contrast injected at the radiocarpal joint spills through the tear defect (arrowhead) into the midcarpal joint. Note the Type II lunate.

Classification of carpal instabilities

Taleisnik (1988) introduced the concept of 'dynamic' and 'static' carpal instability. 'Dynamic' instability refers to the clinical situation where symptoms occur intermittently in certain wrist positions or with particular movements of the wrist. This deformity can be demonstrated only on radiographs taken with the wrist stressed. 'Static' deformity is constantly present and would consequently be seen on routine wrist views.

Watson et al. (1993) classified rotary subluxation of the scaphoid, combining clinical and radiological features at each stage of the continuum of injury:

- *Type I Predynamic:* when the radiographs are normal, but instability is demonstrated clinically.
- *Type II Dynamic:* changes are seen on stress radiographs.
- *Type III Static:* constant radiographic abnormality.
- *Type IV Degenerative:* rotary subluxation of the scaphoid is present and there are degenerative changes in the radioscaphoid joint or scaphotrapezial joint.
- *Type V Secondary:* rotary subluxation of the scaphoid due to other carpal lesions, such as AVN of the lunate or non-union of a scaphoid fracture.

Other carpal instabilities

Other carpal instabilities can occur but are uncommon. Mid-carpal instability (triquetro-hamate ligament injury) requires fluoroscopy for diagnosis and involves a sudden snap of the proximal carpal bones from minimal VISI to minimal DISI towards the end of movement from radial to ulnar deviation.

Proximal carpal instability due to extensive radiocarpal ligament injury results in ulnar translocation of the carpus. This is uncommon and is caused by forced pronation of the forearm on a fixed weightbearing hand. Injury occurs to both radiocarpal and ulnocarpal ligaments and requires extreme force (see Fig. 2.178).

TFCC injury and DRUJ instability

The triangular fibrocartilage complex is a composite structure on the ulnar side of the wrist created by the fusion of a triangular fibrocartilaginous articular disc within a ligamentous sling. The TFCC is important for normal function of the wrist and stability of the DRUJ. Injury of the complex commonly produces considerable pain and disability.

Anatomy of the TFCC and the DRUJ

The TFCC consists of a triangular fibrocartilagenous articular disc, dorsal and volar radioulnar ligaments, ulnocarpal ligaments (lunotriquetral and ulnolunate ligaments), the ulnar collateral ligament, the meniscal homologue and the sheath of the extensor carpi ulnaris tendon.

The TFC attaches to the sigmoid notch of the distal radius and creates a medial extension of the distal articular surface of the radius (see Fig. 2.179). Medially, the fibrocartilage is fixed to the base of the ulnar styloid process and, via the ulnocarpal

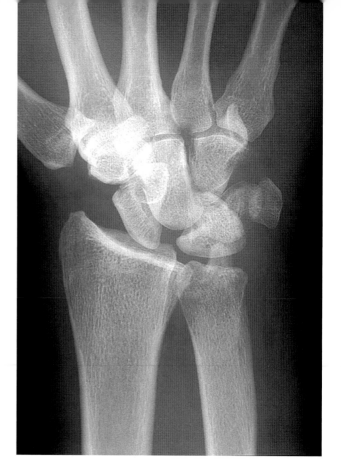

▲ **Fig. 2.178** An ulnar translocation of the carpus. This injury requires considerable rotational force causing radiocarpal and ulnocarpal ligament injury.

and the ulnar collateral ligaments, to the triquetrum, lunate, hamate and the base of the fifth metacarpal. The ulnolunate and ulnotriquetral ligaments are local thickenings in the capsule.

The dorsal and volar radioulnar ligaments merge with the borders of the articular disc and have superficial and deep layers (Dailey and Palmer 2000). The deep layer inserts into the fovea of the ulna and the base of the ulnar styloid process while the superficial layer extends to merge with the extensor carpi ulnaris sheath. The meniscal homologue is a shelf of ligamentous tissue originating from the ulnar collateral ligament (see Fig. 2.180). There is a variable opening adjacent to the meniscal homologue that communicates with the prestyloid recess. The opening is absent in about 10% of cases (Dailey and Palmer 2000). This variant is important to recognise as it can be mistaken for a TFCC tear on MR images.

The disc is largely avascular, with vessels reaching the peripheral 15% of the disc. Peripheral tears have been shown to heal.

TFCC injury

Injury biomechanics

The most common mechanism of TFCC injury is a fall on an outstretched hand producing axial loading with a rotational force. Traction forces on the ulnar side of the wrist may also cause acute injury to the TFCC.

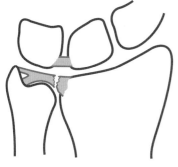 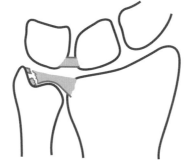 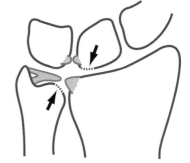

TYPE 1A
• traumatic 'central' tear

TYPE 1B
• traumatic 'peripheral' tear

TYPE 2
• degenerative 'central' wear or perforation
• chondromalacia lunate/ulnar head (arrows)
• LT and other ligament perforations
• DRUJ arthrosis

▲ **Fig. 2.179** Palmer classification of TFC tears (modified).

As discussed earlier in the section on ulnar variance, there is relative lengthening of the ulna when the wrist is pronated and shortening when the wrist is supinated (Epner et al. 1982). Chronic injury to the TFCC may occur in those sports where there is repetitive pronation, ulnar deviation and power grip activities, particularly if there is a pre-existing positive variance. It is important to remember that injury to the TFCC can occur when there is zero variance.

Dailey and Palmer (2000) describe the mechanisms of TFCC injury in sport as follows:

• Gymnasts subject their wrists to extreme axial loading and traction. The axial forces are transmitted through the TFCC and DRUJ, and ulnar-side problems are common. In addition, these forces acting on the immature wrist may produce a stress reaction at the radial growth plate, following which premature closure of this growth plate may occur, producing positive variance, abutment syndrome and a further cause of injury to the TFCC (De Smet 1994).

• Racquet sports employ pronation and ulnar deviation, producing a dynamic positive variance. A forehand hit with heavy topspin requires forearm pronation and both radial and ulnar deviation. In addition, at impact, axial loading will be present. In squash a flick shot is used, which, as well as impact loading, puts considerable strain on the ulnar side of the wrist.

• During a golf swing, there is also loading on the ulnar side of the wrist, with further loading occurring at impact. The right wrist, in a right-handed swing, pronates and moves from radial to ulnar deviation, producing dynamic positive variance. Impact loading is accentuated by taking a divot or by playing a shot from the heavy rough or sand, and a TFCC tear may result.

• Axial loading is produced across the TFCC in boxing, the shot-put and weightlifting.

• In waterskiing, traction forces are applied to the wrist and these forces may cause either an acute injury or a chronic injury to the TFCC.

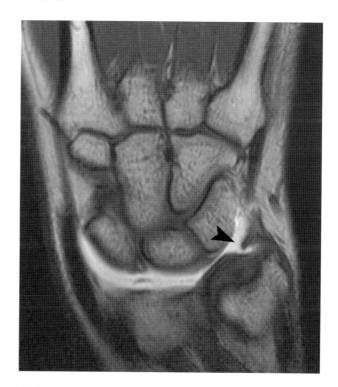

▲ **Fig. 2.180** The meniscal homologue is a shelf of ligamentous tissue (arrowhead) protruding laterally from and continuous with the ulnar collateral ligament. Adjacent to the meniscal homologue is an opening into the prestyloid recess. This opening is present in about 90% of the population.

Classification and presentation of TFCC injuries

Palmer (1989) developed a classification of TFCC injuries. Basically, there are two types:

- *Type I* is traumatic and includes perforations, ulnar and radial avulsions and distal tears on the volar aspect associated with the ulnolunate and ulnotriquetral ligaments.
- *Type II* is a degenerative injury, associated with ulnocarpal abutment syndrome.

An athlete can have either type or both types. Characteristically, the athlete will present with ulnar-side pain on activity, which is relieved by rest. This may be accompanied by a painful click or catch, and loss of power occurs in certain positions or with certain movements. On presentation, the biomechanics of the injury should be assessed and the position- and movement-producing symptoms identified.

DRUJ instability

The principal stabiliser of the DRUJ is the TFCC, through its thickened ligamentous margins forming the ventral and dorsal radioulnar ligaments. The interosseous ligament and the pronator quadratus also provide stability. Instability occurs only when the ventral or dorsal radioulnar ligaments, as well as the interosseous membrane, are ruptured (Kihara et al. 1995). The DRUJ has intrinsic instability. The joint surfaces are incongruent, with the radius of the sigmoid notch curve being greater than the curve of the head of the ulna head, allowing translation as well as rotation (Rozental et al. 2003).

Injury to the DRUJ may result from acute trauma (see Figs 2.181, 2.182 and 2.183), often involving hyperpronation or excessive supination. Injury may also be associated with a fracture of the ulna or the radial shaft, as occurs with a Galeazzi fracture. Occasionally, an injury to the distal radio-ulnar ligaments may produce an avulsion fracture, separating a fragment from the radial side of the DRUJ (see Fig. 2.184). Disruption of the DRUJ is also seen resulting from fractures of the distal radius that involve the DRUJ. A dislocation of the DRUJ may be difficult to reduce and the possibility of soft-tissue interposition should be considered. Occasionally, the extensor carpi ulnaris or extensor digiti minimi tendon may become caught in the joint (Rozental et al. 2003).

To demonstrate the presence of DRUJ instability on plain films, views of the distal radioulnar joint are acquired with pronation and supination. Instability is diagnosed when abnormal joint space widening occurs (see Figs 2.185 and 2.186). When the findings are marginal, stress pronation and supination may help to make the diagnosis with certainty. Subluxation at the DRUJ on wrist pronation implies rupture of the dorsal radioulnar ligament, whereas subluxation on wrist supination implies rupture of the volar radioulnar ligament. Subtle subluxation can be best imaged by CT examination in extreme supination and pronation. CT is also valuable in detecting occult fractures of the distal radius involving the sigmoid notch and the ulnar styloid process. MRI plays a role in demonstrating injury to the DRUJ stabilisers.

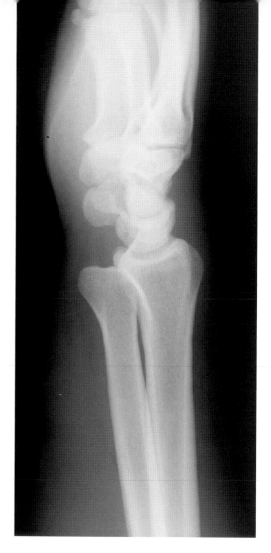

▲ **Fig. 2.181** Dislocation of the DRUJ demonstrated on a lateral view of the wrist. There is volar displacement of the ulna. This injury was caused by an attempted 'stiff-arm' tackle in a game of rugby.

▼ **Fig. 2.182** This fat-suppressed T2-weighted axial MR image shows an acute dislocation of the DRUJ. There is an impacted fracture of the ulnar head. A bone bruise on the volar rim of the distal radius suggests that there has been direct trauma. There is potential for the ECU tendon, which has subluxed, to become caught in the joint space, complicating reduction.

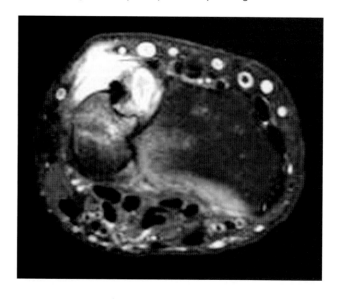

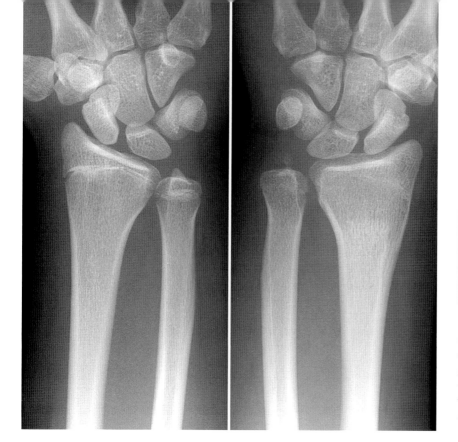

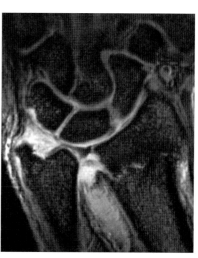

▲ **Fig. 2.185** This fat-suppressed coronal MR image demonstrates a distal radial fracture that involves the sigmoid notch of the radius, disrupting the DRUJ and producing a traumatic Type I peripheral detachment tear of the TFCC.

▲ **Fig. 2.183** AP views of both wrists of an adolescent ex-gymnast, showing a legacy from a sport that requires excessive pronation and supination of the wrist. There is instability of the right DRUJ with injury to the volar radioulnar ligament. Bilateral SL ligament rupture is present and a previous fracture of the distal radial shaft and ulnar styloid process on the right is noted, with premature closure of the distal radial growth plate on this side.

▼ **Fig. 2.184** The volar lip of the radial sigmoid notch has been avulsed by the ventral radioulnar ligament.

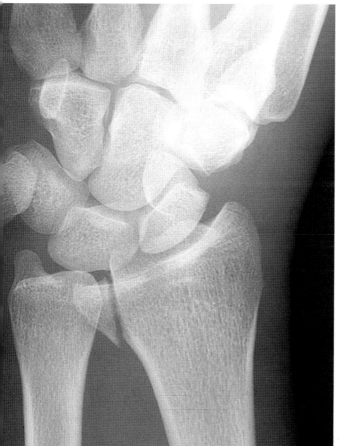

▼ **Fig. 2.186** This axial T1-weighted MR image demonstrates DRUJ instability. There is dorsal subluxation of the DRUJ due to injury to the ventral radioulnar ligament.

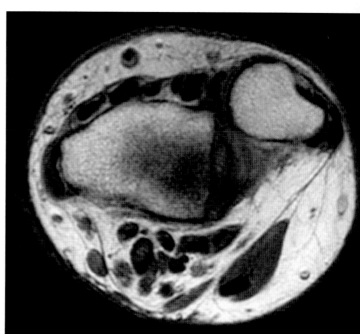

Diagnostic imaging

As usual, plain films are the initial examination. An assessment of ulnar variance is important in any wrist series, but is especially so when investigating possible TFCC injury. Consequently, care must be taken to acquire the PA and lateral views in zero rotation. Deviation views and a steep oblique view to examine the pisotriquetral joint may be extra views used in the investigation of ulnar-side symptoms. On plain films, a Type I injury can be suspected with the demonstration of fractures involving the sigmoid notch of the radius (see Fig. 2.187), a fracture of the ulnar styloid process or instability of the DRUJ (see Fig. 2.188).

Type II TFCC injury occurs as part of ulnar abutment syndrome, also known as ulnar impingement or impaction, and as previously discussed is usually associated with an ulnar plus variance or, less commonly, an unusually long ulnar styloid process (see Fig. 2.189). The head of the ulna or tip of the ulnar styloid process abuts the lunate when the wrist is in ulnar deviation and as a consequence DRUJ stress occurs. A plain film change of abutment provides indirect evidence suggesting that injury to the TFCC may be present.

Repetitive abutment produces changes of chondromalacia in the articular cartilage on the proximal surface of the lunate or triquetrum. The radiographic findings may include eburnation of the abutting surfaces (see Figs 2.190 and

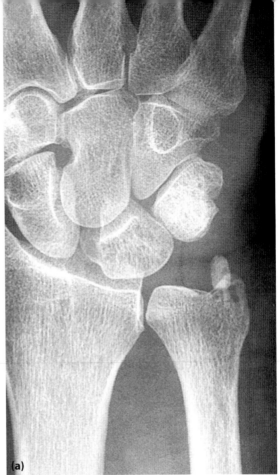

(a)

▲▼ **Fig. 2.188(a) and (b)** Instability of the DRUJ is demonstrated by widening of the DRUJ occurring with supination. This would indicate injury to the volar distal radioulnar ligament. There is also rupture of the SL ligaments, and a calcified density that moves with movement of the pisiform is almost certainly related to the FCU tendon.

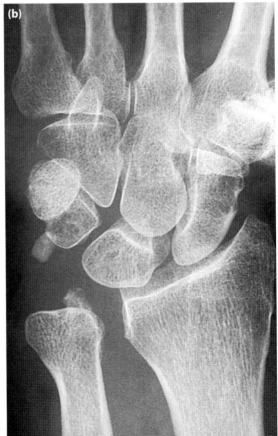

(b)

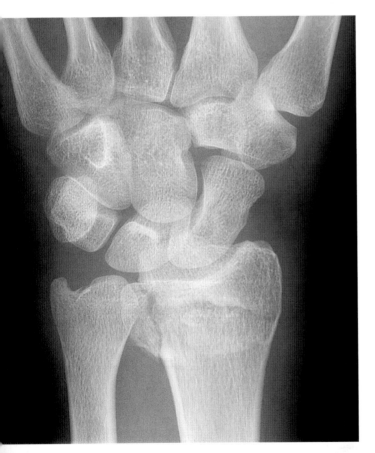

▲ **Fig. 2.187** A comminuted fracture of the distal radius is present with involvement of the sigmoid notch. There also appears to be a fracture in the region of the fovea at the distal ulna. There has almost certainly been injury to the TFCC.

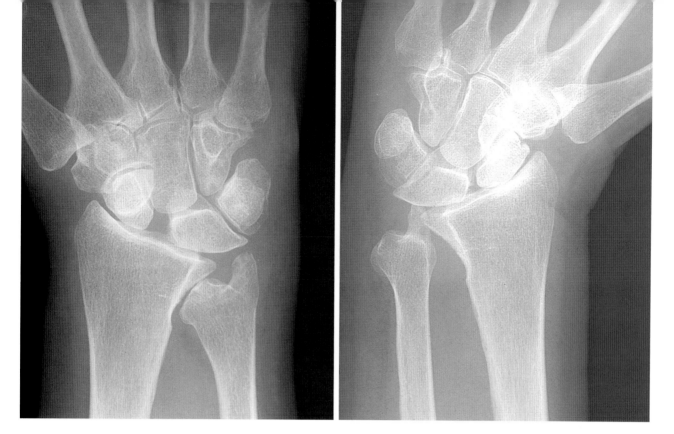

▲ **Fig. 2.189** Chronic impaction of an unusually long ulnar styloid process is present, with degenerative changes noted at the tip of the process. Ulna minus variance is present and there has been erosion of the radial sigmoid notch. Pronation and supination views show instability of the DRUJ, indicating injury to the TFCC. Note the coalition at the lunotriquetral articulation and the presence of rotary subluxation of the scaphoid.

▼ **Fig. 2.190(a) and (b)** Eburnation (polished thickened cortical bone) at the tip of the long ulnar styloid process and on the proximal articular surface of the lunate has resulted from repetitive impact and provides a plain film proof of abutment and TFCC injury. Repetitive abutment with supination has caused injury to the volar distal radioulnar joint, demonstrated on plain films by widening of the DRUJ in this position.

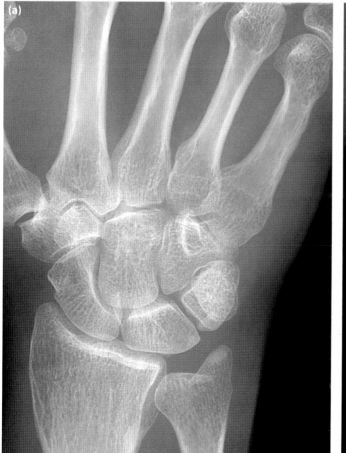

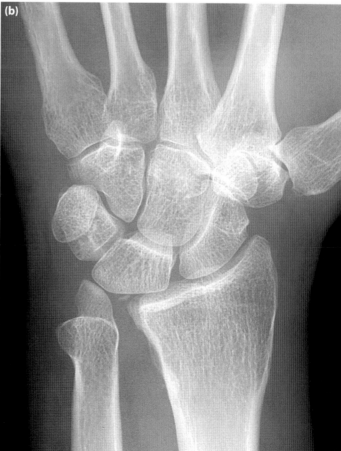

2.191) and subchondral cyst formation (see Fig. 2.192). A clenched fist view or a view in ulnar deviation may be used to demonstrate abutment. MRI and bone scans demonstrate early chondral or subchondral changes (Escobedo et al. 1995). Abutment produced by a long ulnar styloid process causes repetitive stress to the distal radioulnar joint when the wrist is supinated and eventually injury to the radioulnar ligaments occurs, manifest as instability of the distal radioulnar joint (see Fig 2.193).

MRI offers great potential in the imaging of injury to the TFCC. Using a dedicated wrist coil, perforation of the articular disc can usually be satisfactorily imaged (see Fig 2.194), and detection of partial tears is aided by the presence of fluid in the tear (see Figs 2.195 and 2.196). Injury to the distal radioulnar ligaments can also be well shown (see Fig. 2.197). Ultrasound can demonstrate some but not all TFC tears (see Fig. 2.198) and is better suited to tendon and ligamentous evaluation.

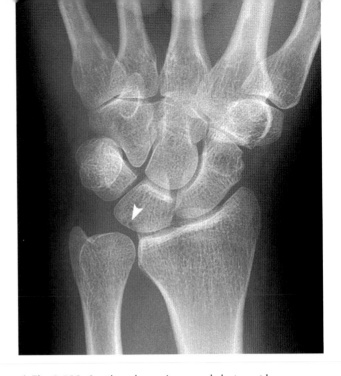

▼ **Fig. 2.191** Abutment occurs between the tip of the ulnar styloid process and the triquetrum. There is flattening of the tip of the ulnar styloid and at the area of impaction on the triquetrum.

▲ **Fig. 2.192** An ulna plus variance and abutment have produced subchondral cyst formation beneath the articular surface of the ulna in the area of contact (arrowhead).

▼ **Fig. 2.193** A nuclear bone scan shows increased uptake of isotope at the site of abutment on both the lunate and distal ulna.

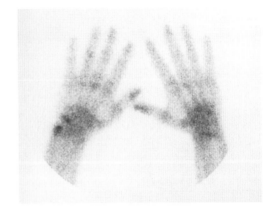

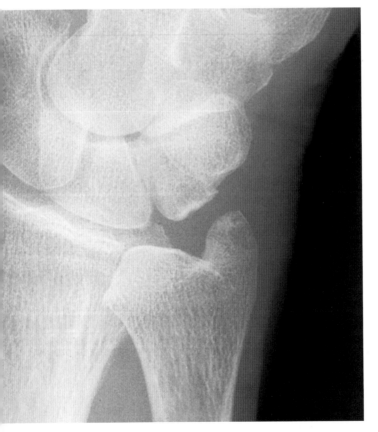

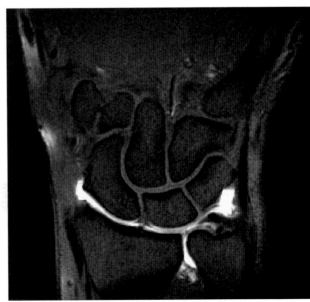

▶ **Fig. 2.194** A coronal fat-suppressed T1-weighted MR arthrogram shows ulna plus variance and a Type II perforation of the TFCC. Note that the contrast agent has spilled into the DRUJ from the injected radiocarpal joint compartment.

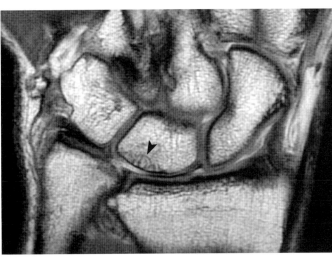
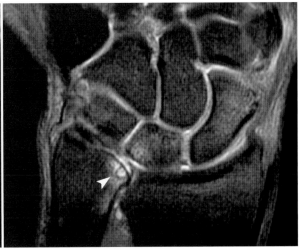

▲ **Fig. 2.195** A central tear of the TFC is demonstrated by coronal PD and fat-suppressed PD MRI sequences. Note the features of chronic ulnolunate abutment including ulna plus variance and subchondral cystic change with accompanying marrow oedema at the apposing surfaces of the lunate and ulna (arrowheads).

▼ **Fig. 2.196** Coronal T1- and fat-suppressed T2-weighted MR images demonstrate a partial Type I traumatic tear of the TFC involving the proximal surface of the disc (arrowhead). Fluid within the tear helps to identify the injury.

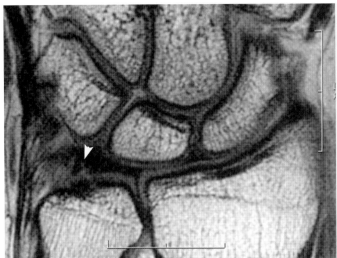
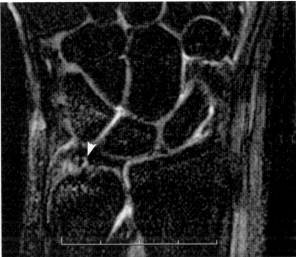

▼ **Fig. 2.197** An MR arthrogram shows a complete peripheral detachment of the TFC. Note the high signal contrast injected at the radiocarpal joint outlines an irregular tear defect at the styloid tip insertion (arrow), infiltrates the injured fibres of the foveal attachment (arrowhead) and spills into the DRUJ, indicative of a full-thickness communication.

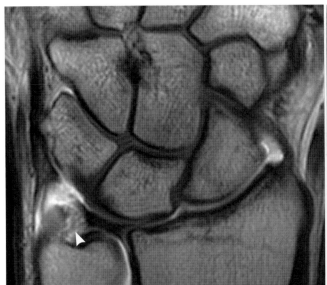
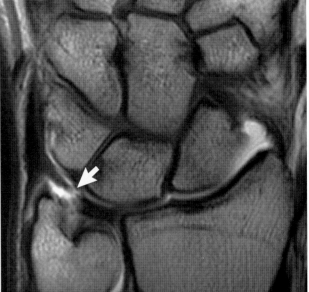

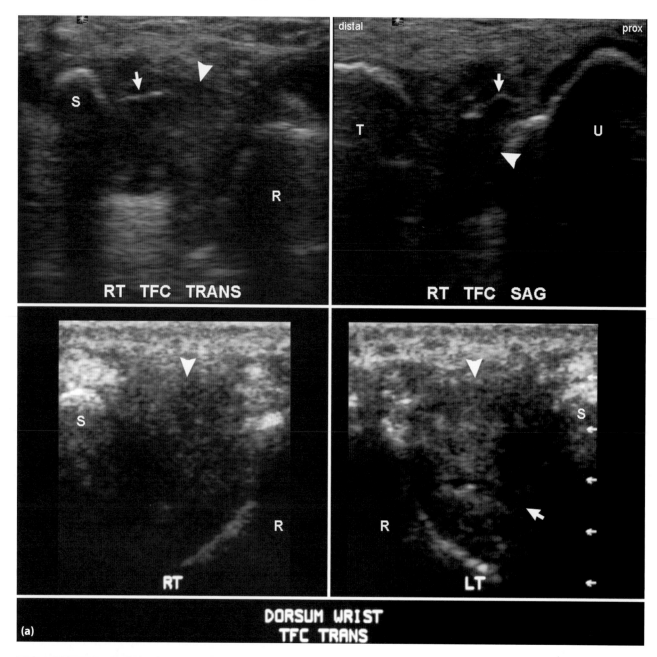

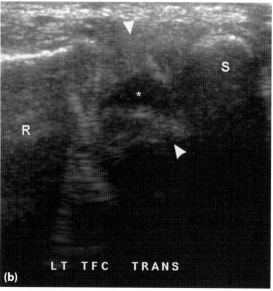

◀▲ Fig. 2.198 Separate cases illustrate the two different echotextural patterns of TFC tears that may be encountered on ultrasound examination.

(a) Upper images: a peripheral TFC tear is appreciated as a thin bright echogenic line (arrows) close to the ulnar styloid on the transverse view (TRANS) and traversing the full thickness of the articular disc immediately distal to the ulnar head on the sagittal view (SAG). Lower images: central TFC tear is appreciated as a linear anechoic space (arrow) traversing the otherwise normal and homogeneously grey triangular zone of the *left* TFC echotexture extending between the sigmoid notch attachment at the radius (R) and the ulnar styloid (S). Note the normal *right* side for comparison. Arrowheads in both cases indicate the TFCC margins.

(b) A transverse ultrasound image demonstrates a TFC perforation. The image is obtained over the dorsal aspect of the wrist and shows an ovoid anechoic fluid-filled central perforation defect (asterisk) in the otherwise normal and homogeneously grey triangular zone of the TFC echotexture (arrowhead), extending between the sigmoid notch attachment at the radius (R) and the ulnar styloid (S).

At the present time, arthroscopy has an accuracy rate for diagnosing TFCC injury approaching 100% (Dailey and Palmer 2000). Arthroscopy also has the advantage of being a therapeutic as well as a diagnostic procedure. However, with continuing technological development, ultrasound and MRI may provide a satisfactory level of diagnostic accuracy and may come to play a more routine role in diagnosis. A pre-arthroscopic diagnosis is considered to play an important role in an optimal outcome.

Tendinopathies

Tendon injuries from sporting activities usually result from repetitive overuse, sometimes accentuated by faulty technique. Initially the process is acute, although if the training habits or technique remain unchanged, chronic changes will develop. Tendon injury may also result from trauma produced by the tendon rubbing on a retinaculum or bony irregularity. The injury, whether a tenosynovitis or tendinopathy, will present with tenderness and swelling along the line of the tendon, together with pain on resisted movement. The clinical diagnosis can be confirmed by imaging with plain films (see Fig. 2.199), a nuclear bone scan (see Fig. 2.200), ultrasound (see Fig. 2.201) or MRI (see Fig. 2.202).

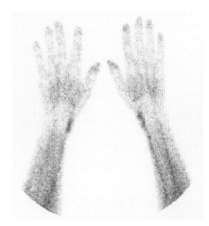

◀ **Fig. 2.200** This nuclear bone scan shows tendinopathy. In the blood pool phase, changes of bilateral de Quervain's tenosynovitis are demonstrated.

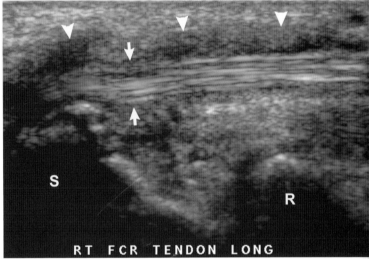

▲ **Fig. 2.201** FCR tendinopathy is demonstrated by ultrasound. A long-axis image obtained over the ventroradial aspect of the proximal carpal row shows subtle hypoechoic and fusiform FCR tendon thickening (arrows) and associated prominent surrounding tenosynovitis (arrowheads). Scaphoid with osteophytic irregularity at the distal pole as a source of tendon impingement = S. Distal end of radius = R.

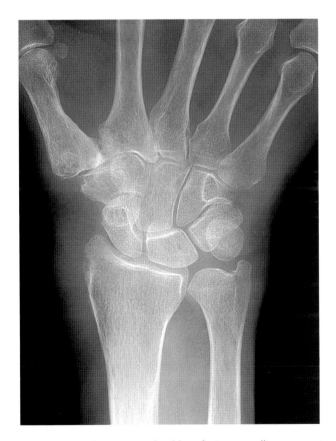

▲ **Fig. 2.199** There is considerable soft-tissue swelling over the lateral aspect of the radial styloid process typical of de Quervain's tenosynovitis. Erosion of the cortical margin along the lateral margin of the radial styloid process may be due to the increased vascularity associated with the soft-tissue changes and also indicates the chronicity of the process.

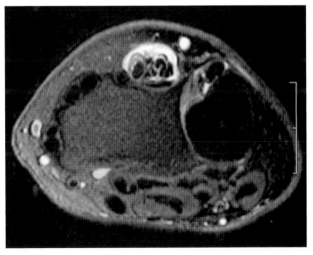

▲ **Fig. 2.202** This fat-suppressed axial T2-weighted MR image shows extensor tendinopathy, with a collar of high signal effusion distending the extensor digitorum tendon sheath.

Extensor tendinopathies

The first dorsal compartment is the most frequently involved, followed by the sixth and the third.

De Quervain's disease

The first compartment contains the APL and EPB tendons sharing a common sheath. Overuse injury will produce a tenosynovitis presenting with tenderness and swelling over the lateral aspect of the radial styloid process. Overuse may result from racquet and throwing sports or golf. If the activity is an unaccustomed one or the activity has been excessive, the tenosynovitis may be acute. The condition will become chronic with continued activity.

Plain films will show soft-tissue swelling over the radial styloid process (see Fig. 2.203) and, if the process is chronic, bony changes may be seen in the neighbouring styloid process. A bone scan is helpful to demonstrate the presence of tendinopathy and to exclude other radial side pathology (see Fig. 2.204).

Ultrasound will demonstrate a characteristic thickening of the extensor retinaculum, fusiform swelling of the tendons and occasional synovitis or effusion. When changes are subtle, comparison with the asymptomatic side will be helpful, although care must be taken, as it may be bilateral. Power Doppler is also useful, as retinacular and tenosynovial hyperaemia are frequent findings. Occasionally a septum separates the EPB and APL tendons, and, if present, the tendinopathy may predominantly affect the EPB tendon (see Fig. 2.205).

ECU tendinopathy

ECU tendinopathy is commonly associated with repetitive supination of the wrist, as may occur with undercutting a forehand at tennis or spin bowling. The tendon becomes traumatised against its restraining retinaculum and the retinaculum itself may be injured (either primarily or secondarily), allowing subluxation of the tendon from its groove along the medial aspect of the ulnar head. Subluxation usually produces a snapping sensation. This can be felt by palpating the sixth compartment as the wrist is supinated with ulnar deviation.

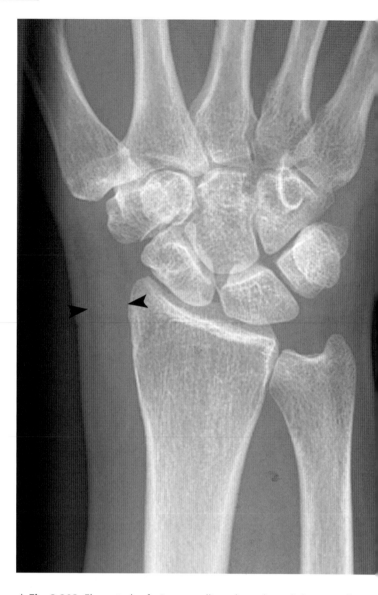

▲ **Fig. 2.203** Elongated soft-tissue swelling along the radial aspect of the radial styloid process is a characteristic appearance of de Quervain's tenosynovitis (arrowheads).

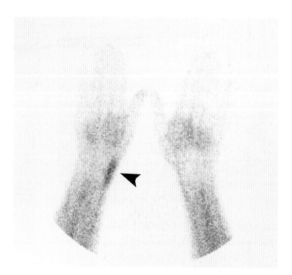

▲ **Fig. 2.204** A bone scan of de Quervain's shows a characteristic appearance in the blood pool phase (arrowhead).

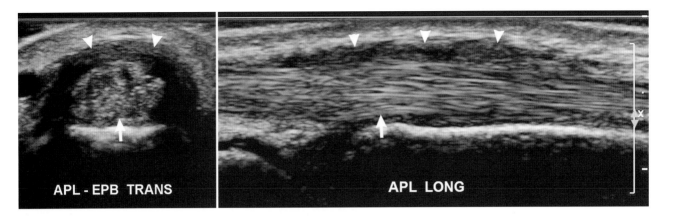

▲ **Fig. 2.205(a)** De Quervain's disease is demonstrated by ultrasound, predominantly involving the APL tendon. The APL–EPB tendon complex shows fusiform thickening most pronounced at the tip of the radial styloid level (arrowed on the long-axis image). In this case the first extensor compartment is a single undivided space, making it difficult to separate the APL tendon from the EPB tendon on the transverse image. The tendons demonstrate non-uniform echotexture typical of tendinopathy. Note the associated collar of hypoechoic peritendon soft-tissue thickening (arrowheads), which represents a combination of thickened extensor retinaculum (contained fibres being visible on the transverse image) and tenosynovitis.

▼ **(b)** Changes of de Quervain's disease are demonstrated by ultrasound, predominantly involving the EPB tendon. In this case the first extensor compartment of the *right* wrist is divided into separate APL and EPB spaces by a thickened hypoechoic septum (arrow). The presence of a dividing septum is an important finding, as it is a recognised cause for both failed corticosteroid injection therapy (if only one compartmental space is injected) and failed surgical release (if the septum is not removed). By comparison with the left, the right APL tendon shows subtle hypoechoic thickening, the right EPB tendon shows prominent thickening, and the overlying right extensor retinaculum shows marked thickening, particularly on the EPB side. Arrowheads indicate the extensor retinaculum. APL tendon = A. EPB tendon = E. Callipers on long-axis images indicate surfaces of EPB tendon. Superficial vein = V.

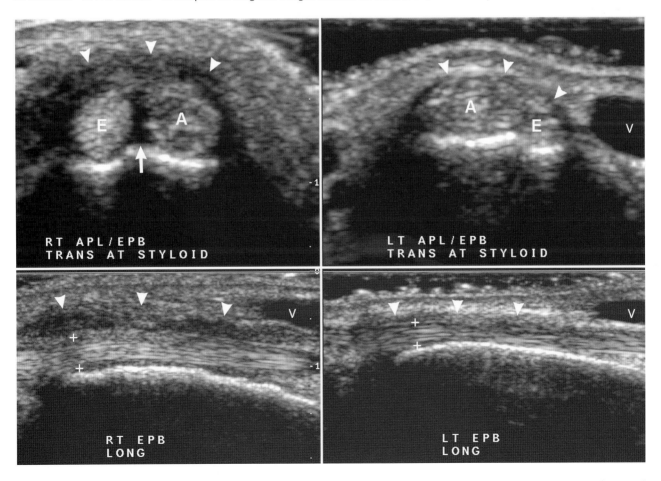

▶ **Fig. 2.206** Localised soft-tissue swelling and calcification on the medial aspect of the wrist overlying the distal ulna is due to ECU tendinopathy.

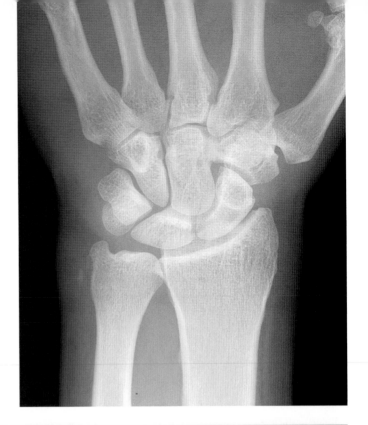

Soft-tissue swelling can be seen on the medial aspect of the wrist on plain films and, as the process becomes chronic, soft-tissue calcification can occur quite early in the process. Plain films (see Fig. 2.206), ultrasound (see Figs 2.207 and 2.208) and MRI (see Fig. 2.209) can be used to demonstrate the changes of ECU tendinopathy.

EPL tendinopathy

Tendinopathy may occur in the third dorsal compartment, resulting from attrition of the EPL tendon as it passes over Lister's tubercle. Irregularity of this tubercle may result from a previous wrist fracture, and history of a previous wrist fracture is significant.

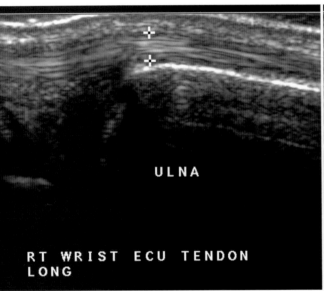

RT WRIST ECU TENDON LONG

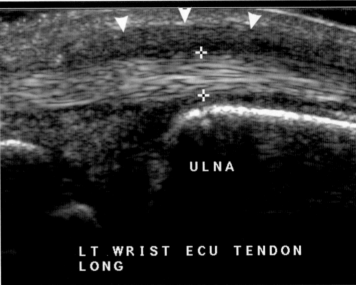

LT WRIST ECU TENDON LONG

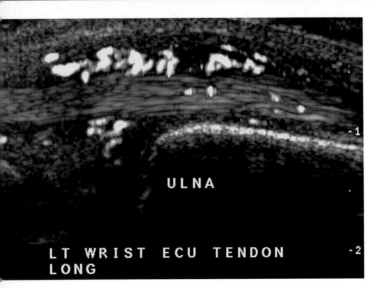

LT WRIST ECU TENDON LONG

▲ **Fig. 2.207(a)** Ultrasound demonstrates ECU tendinopathy. Comparative long-axis images show prominent fusiform thickening of the left ECU tendon and an associated collar of hypoechoic peritendon thickening comprised of both retinaculum and synovitis (arrowheads) at the level of ulnar head and styloid.
◀ **(b)** A Power Doppler image demonstrates accompanying florid tendon and peritendon hyperaemia.

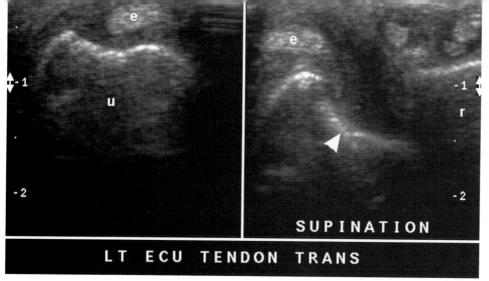

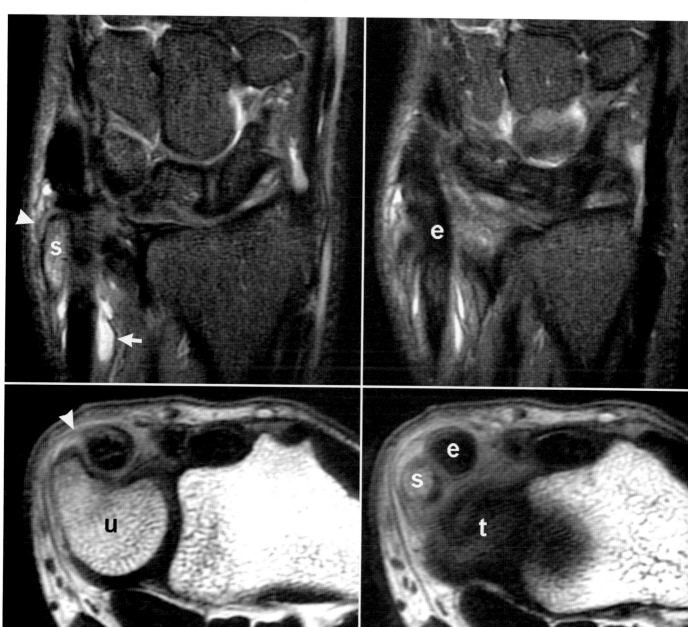

▲**Fig. 2.209** MRI demonstrates changes of ECU tendinopathy. Coronal fat-suppressed PD and axial T1-weighted images demonstrate marked fusiform ECU tendon thickening with low-grade intrasubstance hyperintensity. Also note the associated features of ECU tenosynovitis (arrow), reactive marrow oedema within the ulnar styloid and hyperintense thickening of the overlying extensor retinaculum (arrowheads). ECU tendon = e. Ulnar styloid = s. Ulnar head = u. TFC = t.

Intersection syndromes

Proximal intersection syndrome

Proximal intersection syndrome occurs due to tendinopathy and/or peritendonitis developing at the point where the APL and EPB tendons cross the radial wrist extensors (ECR tendons). The syndrome produces pain and a 'squeaky' sensation or crepitus on the dorsal aspect of the distal forearm on the radial side (Wood and Dobyns 1992). Intersection syndrome is most commonly seen in weightlifters and rowers. Changes can be demonstrated by ultrasound examination (see Fig. 2.210(a)) and MRI (see Fig. 2.210(b)).

Distal intersection syndrome

Distal intersection syndrome occurs at the point where the EPL tendon crosses the radial wrist extensors (ECR tendons). It usually presents as a lump due to focal tenosynovitis, and clinically mimics a ganglion (see Fig. 2.211).

Flexor tendinopathies

The FCU tendon is the flexor tendon most often injured due to overuse. The FCU tendon inserts into the pisiform and is commonly loaded in sporting activities requiring wrist hyperextension. These sports include throwing and racquet sports as well as weightbearing activities such as weightlifting and gymnastics.

As previously discussed, flexor tendons may also be injured in association with carpal fractures. The tendons of the fourth and fifth fingers may be injured in association with a hook of hamate fracture and the FCR tendon may be injured by a fracture of the anterior ridge of the trapezium. Because of their position within the carpal tunnel, when these finger flexors are injured, the associated swelling may cause a median neuropathy and may present as carpal tunnel syndrome.

The changes of tendinopathy are well demonstrated by ultrasound (see Fig. 2.212). Bone scan may provide a diagnosis and excludes other pathological processes in the area. The dynamics of tendon glide may be demonstrated by ultrasound scanning performed with finger and/or wrist flexion and extension.

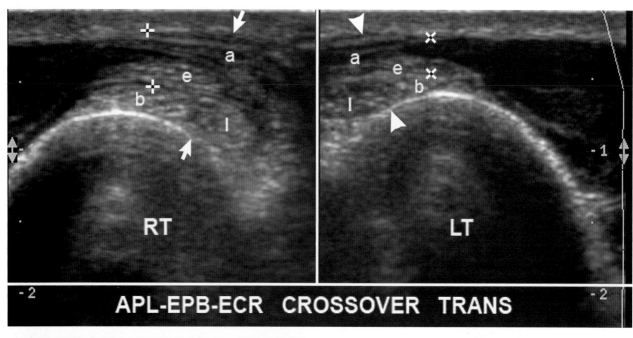

APL-EPB-ECR CROSSOVER TRANS

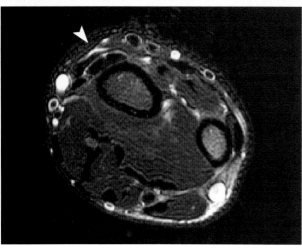

▲ **Fig. 2.210(a)** Proximal intersection syndrome is shown by ultrasound. The sonographic findings in this syndrome are typically subtle, with careful comparative transverse imaging being required. Pain, tenderness and occasionally crepitus are identified at the point of ECRL-ECRB (extensor carpi radialis longus-extensor carpi radialis brevis) crossover by the APL-EPB tendons. In this case, the abnormal right side shows overall tendon thickening (arrows) compared with the left (arrowheads) at the site of the symptoms. Also note the very thin line of hypoechoic peritendon thickening interposed between the right EPB and extensor carpi radialis brevis (ECRB) tendons. APL = a. EPB = e. ECRL = l. ECRB = b.
◀ **(b)** A companion MRI to (a). Note the high peritendon signal associated with the EPB tendon as it crosses the extensor carpi radialis (ECR) tendon (arrowhead).

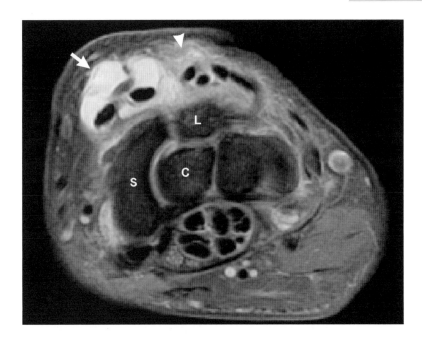

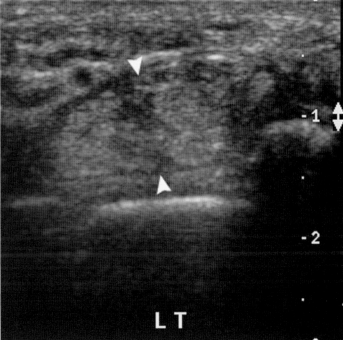

◀**Fig. 2.211** Distal intersection syndrome is demonstrated by MRI. This axial fat-suppressed T2-weighted image obtained at the level of scaphoid (S) shows prominent peritendon ganglionic change (arrow) encasing thickened ECRL, ECRB and EPL tendons. A broad zone of predominantly non-cystic hyperintense peritendon soft-tissue thickening (arrowhead) also encases the adjacent extensor digitorum tendon group, most pronounced on the radial side. Lunate = L. Head of capitate = C.

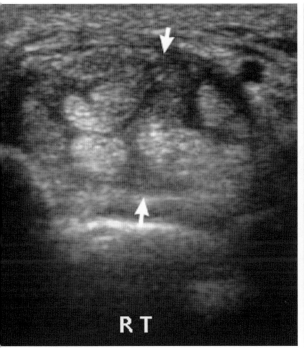

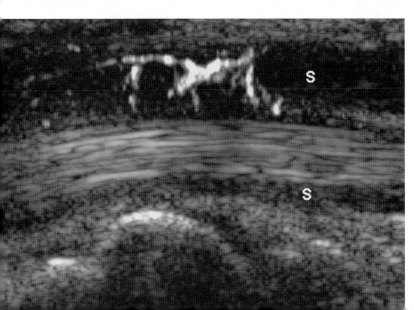

▲**Fig. 2.212(a)** Ultrasound shows changes of flexor tendinopathy. These views represent comparative transverse images of each carpal tunnel, demonstrating diffuse flexor tendon thickening and intervening zones of hypoechoic synovial thickening within the right flexor sheath. There is a corresponding increase in the AP diameter of the right carpal tunnel (arrows) when compared with the left (arrowheads).

◀**(b)** A Power Doppler image of the right carpal tunnel shows both hypoechoic synovial thickening (S) and colour fill of synovial hyperaemia within the flexor sheath.

Other sports-related conditions

AVN

The carpal bones most vulnerable to post-traumatic AVN are the scaphoid (see Fig. 2.213) and the lunate (see Figs 2.214, 2.215 and 2.216) and, less commonly, the trapezoid (see Fig. 2.213) and the capitate (see Fig. 2.217). AVN of the scaphoid was covered in the discussion on fractures of the scaphoid. Large areas of all these bones are supplied by a single extra-osseous blood vessel. The absence of an internal anastomosis also increases the risk of AVN in the hamate and trapezoid bones (Gelberman and Gross 1986).

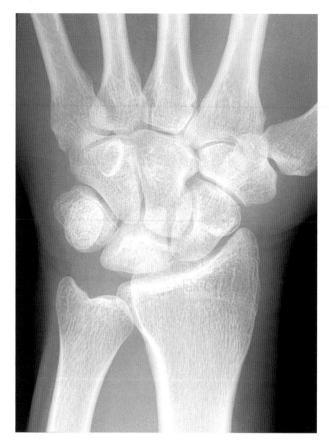

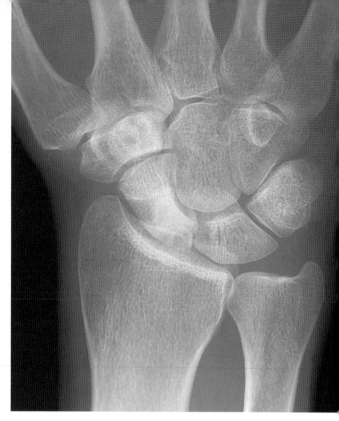

▲ **Fig. 2.213** AVN of the scaphoid, which appears on plain films to be revascularising. There is deformity of the proximal pole of the scaphoid due to previous trauma and a normal bone density is returning to this area. AVN of the trapezoid is also noted, with increased density present.

◀ **Fig. 2.214** Early avascular changes involve the lunate. There is a mild increase in the density of the lunate, with compression and fragmentation occurring laterally. There is rotation of the lunate with a 'ring' sign, suggesting rotary subluxation of the scaphoid.

▼ **Fig. 2.215** Coronal PD images with and without fat suppression show the changes of Stage II Kienbock's disease. Note the lunate marrow oedema and proximal subarticular hypointense line indicative of early trabecular collapse.

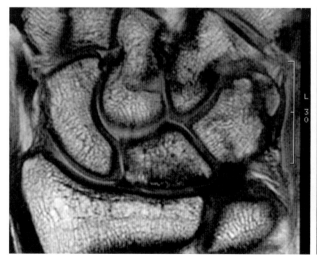

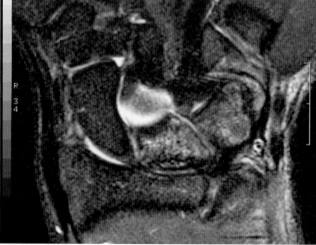

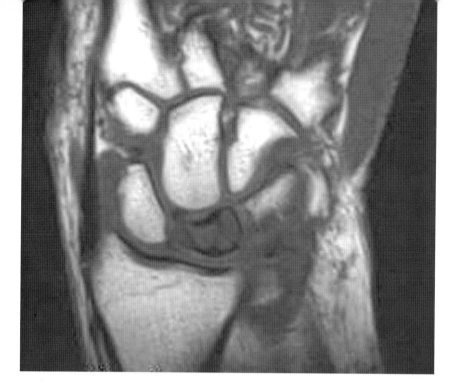

▲ **Fig. 2.216** This coronal T1-weighted MR image shows a complete absence of perfusion of the lunate due to AVN.

Carpal boss syndrome

Carpal bossing, also known as dorsal bossing or 'carpe bossu', describes a clinical syndrome of pain and tenderness localised in the region of a bony prominence normally found on the dorsal aspect of the base of the second metacarpal.

Diagnostic imaging begins with a plain film series that should include a dorsal boss view. This view is obtained with the wrist in a lateral position and then rotated slightly forward into a slightly supinated position. Ulnar deviation will profile the dorsal aspect of the second metacarpal base (see Fig. 2.218) to help differentiate a bone spur from an ossicle or a fracture (Conway et al. 1985).

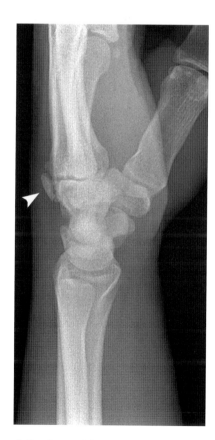

▲ **Fig. 2.218** A boss view is an easy extra plain view to obtain and may often prove to be an efficient way of demonstrating the cause of the patient's symptoms.

▲ **Fig. 2.217** Wrist pain in a gymnast proved to be due to AVN of the capitate. The capitate is sclerotic and there are suggestions of early fissuring and fragmentation.

In some individuals the bony prominence is an unfused apophysis, the os styloideum. There can be a separate ossicle (see Fig. 2.219), partial fusion of the apophysis (see Fig. 2.220) or degenerative changes that develop in the articulation between the metacarpal base and the apophysis (see Fig. 2.221). These changes are best demonstrated using CT scanning. In other cases, the prominence at the base of the second metacarpal may relate to osteophyte formation (see Fig. 2.222). Further possible causes of chronic pain related to a dorsal boss include ECRB insertional tendinopathy (see Fig. 2.223), arthritis, a ganglion cyst at the CMC joint, apophyseal separation or a fractured boss (Conway et al. 1985). A carpal boss may produce abnormal uptake on an isotope bone scan.

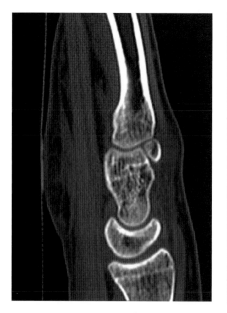

▲ **Fig. 2.219** A CT scan demonstrates an unfused secondary ossification centre, a separate ossicle called an os styloideum. The ossicle shows a smooth continuous cortical margin, helping to differentiate an ossicle from a fracture.

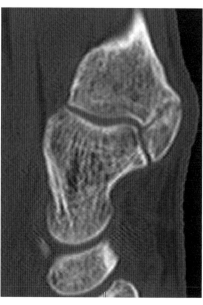

▲ **Fig. 2.220** Partial fusion of the apophysis is demonstrated by a CT scan.

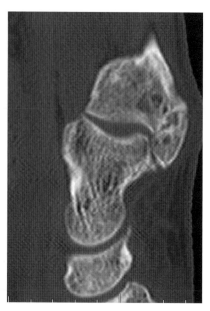

▲ **Fig. 2.221** Degenerative changes in the articulation between the apophysis and the base of the second metacarpal is demonstrated by a CT scan.

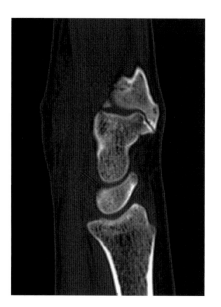

▲ **Fig. 2.222** Osteophyte formation on the dorsal aspect of the base of the second metacarpal causes a bony protrusion, which would presumably contribute to the patient's symptoms.

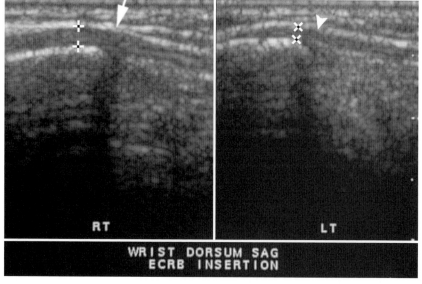

▲ **Fig. 2.223** ECRB insertional tendinopathy is shown by ultrasound. Corresponding with the indicated site of pain and localised tenderness to probing, long-axis ultrasound imaging demonstrates thickening of the right ECRB insertion (arrow) at the metacarpal base when compared with the opposite side (arrowhead).

Nerve entrapment syndromes

Entrapment neuropathies occurring in the hand and wrist as a result of sport are not uncommon and are seen in athletes involved in cycling, baseball, the martial arts and handball (Rettig 1990).

A routine role for imaging in the management of peripheral nerve entrapment syndromes such as carpal tunnel syndrome, ulnar nerve palsy and superficial radial nerve compression syndrome is difficult to justify. There already exists a well-established and validated work up algorithm involving clinical assessment and electrodiagnostic testing, and neuropathies due to clinically impalpable deep masses are uncommon. However, presentations that are atypical, have sudden onset, are rapidly progressive or have equivocal findings on electrodiagnostic testing can all benefit from careful imaging with either MRI or ultrasound. Imaging can show neural changes that help to confirm the presence and site of nerve compression. Imaging can also detect and characterise mass lesions and other space-occupying processes that my be responsible for nerve compression.

Median nerve entrapment occurs at the carpal tunnel level and presents as carpal tunnel syndrome. The athlete usually presents with pain in the wrist, radiating to the thumb, index, middle and the radial side of the ring finger. There may also be other sensory changes such as parathaesia in the same distribution. In sport this is most often seen in situations of repetitive wrist movements causing tendon swelling associated with flexor tendinopathy (see Fig. 2.224). A ganglion or functional hypertrophy of an anomalous or low-lying flexor muscle belly may compress the median nerve (see Fig. 2.225). Median nerve compression may also be caused by the pressure of the flexor retinaculum (see Fig. 2.226).

▼ **Fig. 2.224** Flexor tendinopathy is demonstrated as a cause of carpal tunnel syndrome. The top ultrasound image is a large field of view long-axis view of the carpal tunnel and palm showing flexor sheath effusion (e) and hypoechoic synovial thickening (arrowheads at palm level). The FDS and FDP tendons are indicated. The bottom view is a magnified long-axis image showing fusiform swelling of the median nerve (m) within the carpal tunnel level due to compression.

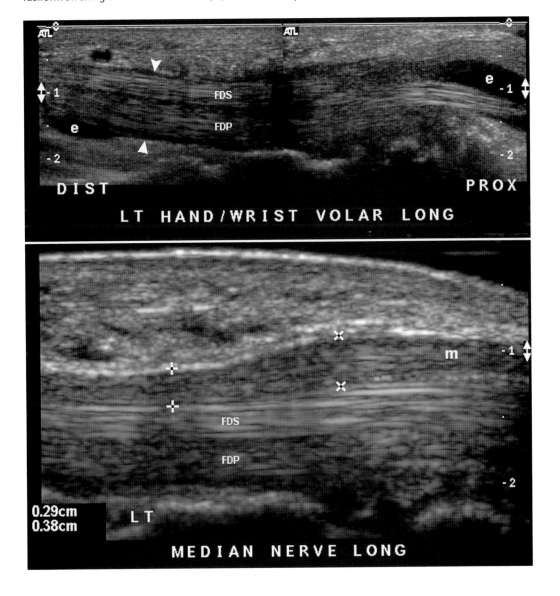

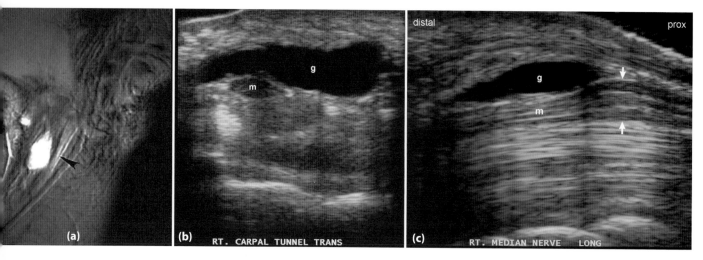

▲ **Fig. 2.225(a)** A coronal gradient-echo MRI obtained with T2-weighting and fat-suppression shows an ovoid hyperintense ganglion cyst immediately adjacent to an oedematous (high signal) median nerve (arrowhead). **(b)** and **(c)** Transverse **(b)** and long-axis **(c)** ultrasound images obtained at the carpal tunnel level show a well-defined anechoic space of ganglion cyst (g) compressing the subjacent median nerve (m). Note the prominent fusiform nerve swelling immediately proximal to the compression point (arrows). The ganglion shows a 'neck' that tapers gradually towards the radial side of the carpus (on real-time scanning the cyst appears to arise from the scaphotrapezial (STT) joint).

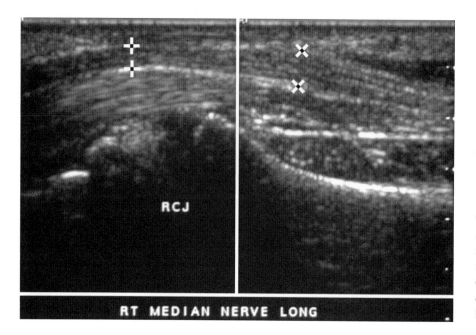

◄ **Fig. 2.226** Changes of carpal tunnel syndrome are demonstrated by ultrasound. This long-axis ultrasound image shows a fusiform segment of median nerve swelling immediately proximal to the flexor retinaculum, indicative of nerve compression within the carpal tunnel. This indirect imaging sign is often the only feature of raised pressure within the tunnel. However, it must be appreciated that imaging alone does not always predict carpal tunnel syndrome, because subclinical nerve compression is common. Consequently, appropriate clinical correlation is always required. Radiocarpal joint = RCJ.

Ulnar nerve entrapment at the wrist mostly occurs within the confined space of Guyon's canal. This condition is known as 'handlebar palsy', having been described in cyclists due to prolonged pressure from their grip on the handlebars.

Vascular injuries

Hypothenar hammer syndrome

Hypothenar hammer syndrome is generally seen in the dominant hand of male athletes and is due to ulnar artery occlusion in Guyon's canal. Repetitive trauma to the hypothenar

eminence may cause spasm, aneurysm and thrombosis of the ulnar artery (see Fig. 2.227), resulting in ischaemia of the hand and fingers. Repetitive trauma may cause intimal damage, resulting in thrombus formation and injury to the media can predispose to aneurysm formation (Le and Henz 2000). Because the ulnar nerve passes through the canal, injury to the artery may mimic or produce an ulnar nerve compression. This condition may occur in several sports including baseball (catcher's hand), cycling, handball, and stick and racquet sports (see Fig. 2.228). Rarely, direct trauma may cause false aneurysms at other locations (see Figs 2.229 and 2.230).

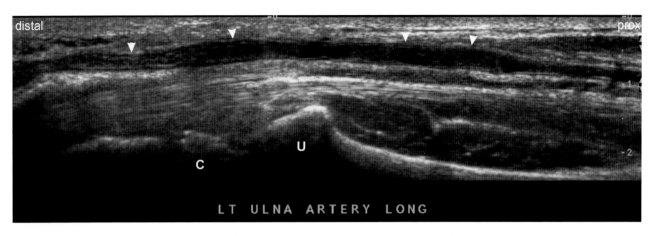

▲ **Fig. 2.227** A montage long-axis ultrasound image shows echogenic intraluminal thrombus (arrowheads) occluding an ulnar artery of variable calibre and producing a hypothenar hammer syndrome. Head of ulna = U. Proximal carpus = C.

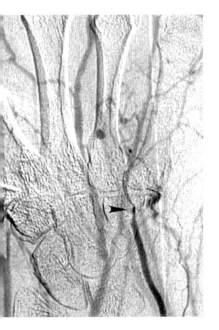

◄ **Fig. 2.228** A patient with hypothenar hammer syndrome is shown by arteriography to have intraluminal thrombus causing an abruptly tapering stenosis of the ulnar artery (arrowhead) adjacent to the hook of hamate.

► **Fig. 2.229** Ultrasound shows a false aneurysm (callipers) of the ulnar artery adjacent to the hook of hamate. The aneurysm has been caused by repetitive trauma against the hook and shows heterogeneous intraluminal echogenicity indicative of contained thrombus.

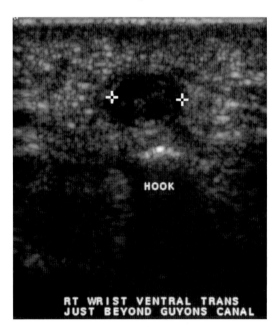

▼ **Fig. 2.230(a)** A false aneurysm is shown by arteriography in an athlete with hypothenar hammer syndrome arising from the ulnar side of the palmar arch and about 1.5 cm distal to the hook of hamate. Note the presence of a focal stenosis at the proximal margin of the aneurysm. **(b)** A large false aneurysm is demonstrated arising from the radial artery. The patient presented with a pulsating mass on the radial side of the wrist.

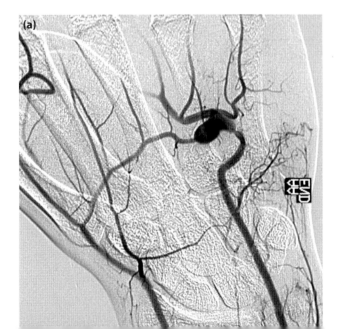

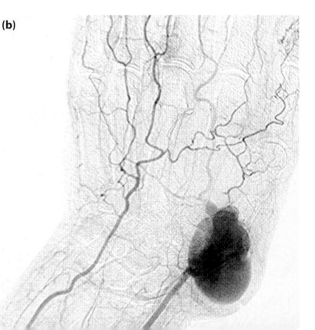

Axillary artery aneurysm

Repetitive trauma of the axillary artery related to repetitive compression or tension at the level of the pectoralis minor muscle in the throwing action of baseball pitchers may create a false aneurysm along the axillary artery or one of its branches (Kee et al. 1995). Intermittent episodes of embolic ischaemia occur in the hand or fingertips with pain, swelling and discolouration.

Effort thrombosis

Venous thrombosis of the upper extremity has been termed 'effort thrombosis' because of its common association with repetitive upper extremity activities. This usually involves hyperabduction of the arm, with consequent compression of the subclavian vein at the thoracic outlet. There are two subgroups of effort thrombosis: those with normal anatomy at the thoracic outlet; and those with an anatomical predisposition such as a fibrous cord or cervical rib. Symptoms include gradual onset of pain and swelling, often with a bluish discolouration to the affected limb. The diagnosis can be confirmed by colour Doppler sonography or contrast venography.

Wrist ganglia

Ganglia are the most common soft-tissue mass of the hand and wrist. The pathology of ganglia is discussed in detail in Chapter 10. Ganglia tend to occur at typical sites. Volar ganglia usually originate from the palmar capsule between the radioscaphocapitate ligament and the long radiolunate ligament, while dorsal ganglia typically arise from the dorsal band of the SL ligament. Imaging prevalence studies have shown ganglia to be common in asymptomatic wrists (Lowden et al. 2005). They usually present as either a lump or with pain. Pain arising from dorsal ganglia has been linked to compression of the posterior interosseous nerve. Ganglia may appear more complex if complicated by haemorrhage. Using ultrasound or MRI, ganglia typically appear as unilocular or multilocular anechoic masses (see Figs 2.231 and 2.232). Ganglia may also arise from tendon sheaths (see Fig. 2.233).

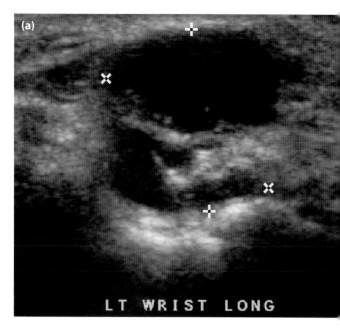

LT WRIST LONG

▲ **Fig. 2.231(a)** Ultrasound shows a large ganglion tracking via a complex pathway from the scapholunate articulation.
▼ **(b)** In contrast to **(a)**, ultrasound demonstrates a small ganglion (callipers) arising from the SL joint and communicating by a thread-like track.

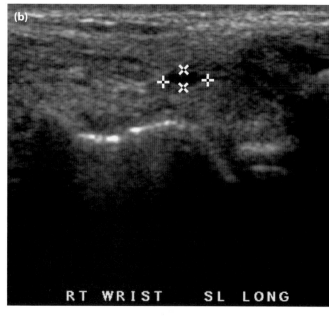

RT WRIST SL LONG

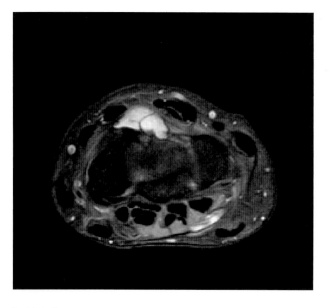

◀ **Fig. 2.232** This fat-suppressed axial MR image demonstrates a large septate dorsal ganglion overlying the scapholunate region.

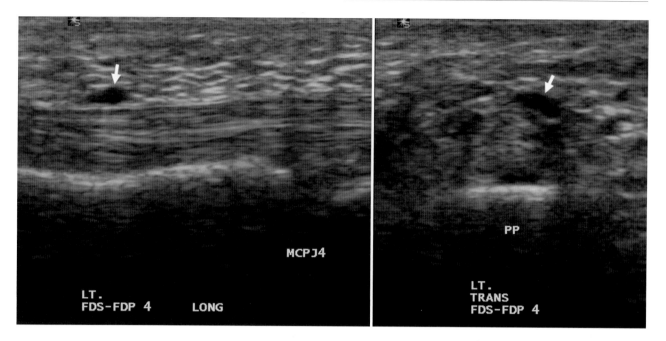

▲ **Fig. 2.233** Long-axis and transverse ultrasound demonstrate a small ganglion arising from a tendon sheath.

Muscle hypertrophy

Muscles in the hand may respond to increasing workload by physiological hypertrophy and then present clinically as a painful swelling or nerve entrapment syndrome. Included are the lumbricals (see Figs 2.234 and 2.235) and extensor digitorum manus brevis (see Fig. 2.236) (Anderson et al. 1995), flexor digitorum superficialis and abductor digiti minimi. Ultrasound will show an elongated structure with the normal echo-texture and functional contractility of muscle.

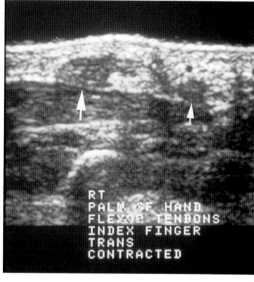

▲ **Fig. 2.234** Hypertrophy of the lumbricals on ultrasound. A transverse ultrasound image obtained at the site of soft-tissue swelling in the palm shows a prominent index finger lumbrical muscle (large arrow) compared with the adjacent middle finger lumbrical muscle (small arrow).

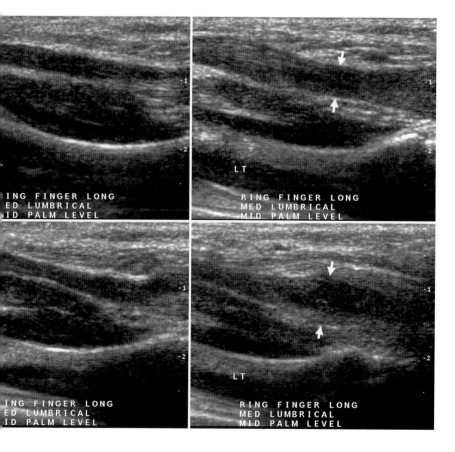

◄ **Fig. 2.235** Long-axis ultrasound demonstrates considerable hypertrophy of the ring finger lumbricals on the left side. The normal right lumbricals are shown for comparison. The athlete presented with a lump in the palm of the hand.

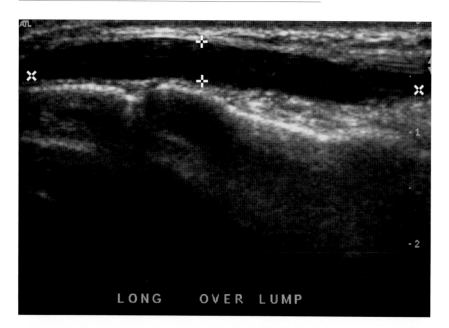

◀ **Fig. 2.236(a)** This long-axis ultrasound image demonstrates hypertrophy of the digitorum manus brevis, which clinically presented as a palpable lump on the dorsum of the hand.

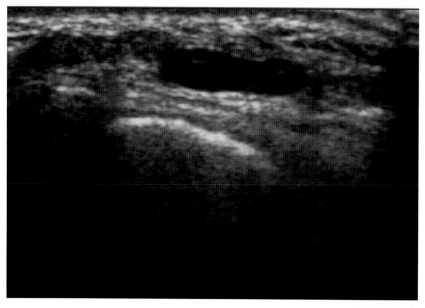

◀ **(b)** This ultrasound image is the companion transverse image to **(a)**.

Bowler's thumb

A traumatic ulnar digital neuroma of the thumb may occur in ten-pin bowlers (Howell and Leach 1970) due to repetitive friction caused by the grip hole of the bowling ball (see Fig. 2.237).

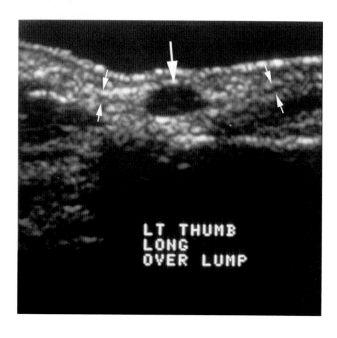

▶ **Fig. 2.237** This longitudinal ultrasound image shows a localised ovoid hypoechoic swelling (large arrow) along the path of the digital nerve (small arrows). This is a digital neuroma of the thumb, resulting from repetitive friction.

References

Amadio PC, Berquist TH, Smith DK et al. 'Scaphoid malunion.' *J Hand Surg (Am)* 1989, 14: 679–87.

Anderson IF. *An Atlas of Radiography for Sports Injuries.* McGraw-Hill Book Company, Sydney, 2000.

Anderson MW, Benedetti P, Walter J, Steinberg DR. 'MR appearance of the extensor digitorum manus brevis muscle: a pseudotumor of the hand.' *Am J Roentgenol* 1995, 164: 1477–9.

Arkless R. 'Cineradiography in normal and abnormal wrist.' *Am J Roentgenol* 1966, 96: 837–44.

Beckenbaugh RD, Shives TC, Dobyns JH, Linscheid RL. 'Kienbock's disease: the natural history of Kienbock's disease and consideration of lunate fractures.' *Clin Orthop* 1980, 149: 98–106.

Berger RA, Blair WF et al. 'The scapholunate ligament.' *J Hand Surg (Am)* 1982, 7: 87–91.

Berger RA, Kauer JMG et al. 'Radioscaphocapitate ligament: a gross anatomic and histological study of fetal and adult wrists.' *J Hand Surg (Am)* 1991, 16: 350–5.

Bishop AT, Beckenbaugh RD. 'Fracture of the hamate hook.' *J Hand Surg (Am)* 1988, 13: 135–9.

Blatt G. 'Capsulodesis in reconstructive hand surgery.' *Hand Clinics* 1987, 3: 81–102.

Boyes JH, Wilson JN, Smith JW. 'Flexor tendon ruptures in the forearm and hand.' *J Bone and Joint Surg (Am)* 1960, 42: 637.

Burgess RC. 'The effect of a simulated scaphoid malunion on wrist motion.' *J Hand Surg (Am)* 1987, 12: 774–6.

Caine D, Roy S, Singer KM, Broekhoff J. 'Stress changes of the distal radial growth plate. a radiographic survey and review of the literature.' *Am J Sports Med* 1992, 20: 290–8.

Conway WF, Destouet JM, Gilula LA, Bellinghausen HW, Weeks PM. 'The carpal boss: an overview of radiographic evaluation.' *Radiology* 1985, 156: 29–31.

Cooney WP, Bussey R et al. 'Difficult wrist fractures. Perilunate fracture-dislocations of the wrist.' *Clin Orthop* 1987, 214: 136–47.

Dailey SW, Palmer AK. 'The role of arthroscopy in the treatment of triangular fibrocartilage complex injuries in athletes.' *Hand Clinics* 2000, 16: 461–76.

De Smet L. 'Ulnar variance: facts and fiction review article.' *Acta Orthop Belg* 1994, 60: 1–9.

De Smet L, Claessens A, Lefevre J, Beunen G. 'Gymnast wrist: an epidemiological survey of ulnar variance and stress changes of the radial physis in elite female gymnasts.' *Am J Sports Med* 1994, 22: 846–50.

Engkvist O, Balkfors B, Lindsjö U. 'Thumb injuries in downhill skiing.' *Int J Sports Med* 1982, 3: 50–5.

Epner RA, Bowers WH, Guilford WB. 'Ulnar variance: the effect of wrist positioning and roentgen filming technique.' *J Hand Surg (Am)* 1982, 7: 298–305.

Escobedo EM, Bergman AG, Hunter JC. 'MR imaging of ulnar impaction.' *Skeletal Radiol* 1995, 24: 85–90.

Gamel A, Engel J, Oster Z et al. 'Bone scanning in the assessment of fractures of the scaphoid.' *J Hand Surg* 1979, 4: 540–3.

Gelberman RH, Gross MS. 'The vascularity of the wrist. Identification of arterial patterns at risk.' *Clin Orthop* 1986, 202: 40–9.

Gelberman RH, Menon J. 'The vascularity of the scaphoid bone.' *J Hand Surg (Am)* 1980, 5: 508–13.

Hame, SL and Melone, CP. 'Boxer's knuckle: traumatic disruption of the extensor hood', *Hand Clinic* 2000, 16: 375–80.

Hardy DC, Totty WG, Reinus WR, Gilula LA. 'Posteroanterior wrist radiography: importance of arm positioning.' *J Hand Surg (Am)* 1987, 12: 504–8.

Hauger O, Chung C et al. 'Pulley system in the fingers: normal anatomy and simulated lesions in cadavers at MRI, CT and US with and without contrast material distension of the tendon sheath.' *Radiology* 2000, 217: 201–12.

Herzberg G, Comtet JJ, Linscheild RL et al. 'Perilunate dislocations and fracture-dislocations.' *J Hand Surg (Am)* 1993, 18: 768–79.

Howell AE, Leach RE. 'Bowler's thumb. Perineural fibrosis of the digital nerve.' *J Bone Joint Surg (Am)* 1970, 52: 379–81.

Israeli A, Engel GA. 'Possible fatigue fracture of the pisiform bone in volleyball players.' *Int J Med* 1982, 3: 56–7.

Johnson RP. 'The acutely injured wrist and its residuals.' *Clin Orthop* 1980, 149: 33–44.

Kee ST, Dake MD, Wolfe-Johnson B, Semba CP, Zarins CK, Olcott C. 'Ischemia of the throwing hand in major league baseball pitchers: embolic occlusion from aneurysms of axillary artery branches.' *J Vasc Interv Radiol* 1995, 6: 979–82.

Kihara H, Short WH, Werner FW, Fortino MD, Palmer AK. 'The stabilising mechanism of the distal radioulnar joint during pronation and supination.' *J Hand Surg (Am)* 1995, 20: 930–6.

Kozin SH. 'Incidence, mechanism, and natural history of scaphoid fractures.' *Hand Clinics* 2001, 4: 515–24.

Kristensen SS, Soballe K. 'Kienbock's disease: the influence of arthrosis on ulnar variance measurements.' *J Hand Surg (Br)* 1987, 12: 301–5.

Le TB, Henz VR. 'Hand and wrist injuries in young athletes.' *Hand Clinics* 2000, 16: 597–607.

Leddy JP, Packer JW. 'Avulsion of the profundus tendon insertion in athletes.' *J Hand Surg (Am)* 1977, 2: 66–9.

Lee S-G, Jupiter JB. 'Phalangeal and metacarpal fractures of the hand.' *Hand Clinics* 2000, 16: 323–32.

Lee SJ, Montgomery K. 'Athletic hand injury.' *Orthop Clin N Am* 2002, 33: 547–54.

Light TR, 'Carpal injuries in children.' *Hand Clinics* 2000, 16: 513–22.

Linscheid RL, Dobyns JH et al. 'Traumatic instability of the wrist.' *J Bone Joint Surg (Am)* 1972, 54: 1612–72.

Lowden M, Attiah M, Garvin G et al. 'The prevalence of wrist ganglia in an asymptomatic population; magnetic resonance imaging evaluation.' *J Hand Surg* 2005, 30: 302–6.

Mandelbaum BR, Bartolozzi AR, Davis CA. 'Wrist pain syndrome in the gymnast: pathogenetic, diagnostic and therapeutic considerations.' *Am J Sports Med* 1989, 17: 305.

Mayfield JK. 'Mechanism of carpal injuries.' *Clin Orthop* 1980, 149: 45–54.

Mayfield JK, Johnson RP, Kilcoyne RF. 'Carpal dislocations: pathomechanics and progressive perilunar instability.' *J Hand Surg (Am)* 1980, 5: 226–41.

Melone CP, Murphy MS, Raskin KB. 'Perilunate injuries repair by dual dorsal and volar approaches.' *Hand Clinics* 2000, 16: 439–48.

Nathan R, Blatt G. 'Rotary subluxation of the scaphoid revisited.' *Hand Clinics* 2000, 16: 417–31.

O'Callaghan BI, Kohut G, Hoogewoud HM. 'Gamekeeper's thumb: identification of the Stener lesion with ultrasound.' *Radiology* 1994, 192: 477–80.

Opgrande JD, Westphal SA. 'Fractures of the hand.' *Orthop Clin North Am* 1983,14: 779–92.

Palmer AK. 'Triangular fibrocartilage complex lesions: a classification.' *J Hand Surg (Am)* 1989, 14: 594–606.

Palmer AK, Levinsohn EM, Rosen D et al. 'Wrist arthrography: the value of the three compartment injection method.' In *Proceedings of the American Society for Surgery of the Hand*, 46th Annual Meeting, Orlando, 1991.

Palmer RE. 'Joint injuries of the hand in athletes.' *Clin Sports Med* 1998, 17: 513–31.

Read JW, Conolly WB, Lanzetta M, Spielman S, Snodgrass D, Korber JS. 'Diagnostic ultrasound of the hand and wrist.' *J Hand Surg (Am)* 1996, 21A: 1004–10.

Rettig AC. 'Neurovascular injuries in the hand and wrist of athletes.' *Clin Sports Med* 1990, 9: 389.

Ritt MJPF, Bishop AT, Berger RA et al. 'Lunotriquetral ligament properties: a comparison of three anatomic subregions.' *J Hand Surg (Am)* 1998, 23: 425–31.

Ritter MR, Chang DS, Ruch DS. 'The role of arthroscopy in the treatment of lunotriquetral ligament injury.' *Hand Clinics* 1999, 14: 445.

Rogers LF. *Radiology of Skeletal Trauma*. Churchill-Livingstone, 1982.

Rozental TA, Beredjiklian PK, Bozentka DJ. 'Instability of the distal radioulnar joint: current diagnostic and treatment methods.' *Current Opinion in Orthopaedics* 2003, 14(4): 245–51.

Roy S, Caine D, Singer K. 'Stress changes of the distal radial epiphysis in young gymnasts: a report of 21 cases and a review of the literature.' *Am J Sports Med* 1985, 13: 301.

Russell TB. 'Inter-carpal dislocations and fractures-dislocations.' *J Bone Joint Surg Br* 1949, 31: 524–31.

Scott SC. 'Closed injuries to the extension mechanism of the digits.' *Hand Clinics* 2000, 16: 367–73.

Snead D, Rettig AC. 'Hand and wrist fractures in athletes.' *Current Opinion in Orthopaedics* 2001, 12: 160–6.

Stamos BD, Leddy JP. 'Closed flexor tendon disruption in athletes.' *Hand Clinics* 2000, 16: 359–65.

Stark HH, Jobe FW, Boyes JH et al. 'Fracture of the hook of hamate in athletes.' *J Bone Joint Surg (Am)* 1977, 59: 575–82.

Steinberg B. 'Acute wrist injuries in the athlete.' *Orthop Clin N Am* 2002, 33: 535–45.

Stoller, DW (ed.), *Diagnostic Imaging, Orthopaedics*, AMIRSYS, Salt Lake City, Utah, 2004.

Taleisnik J. 'Current concepts review: carpal instability.' *J Bone Joint Surg Am* 1988, 70: 1262–7.

Trumble TE, Vedder NB, Benirschke SK. 'Misleading fractures after profundus tendon avulsions: a report of six cases.' *J Hand Surg (Am)* 1992, 17: 902–6.

Vaughan-Jackson OJ. 'A case of recurrent subluxation of the carpal scaphoid.' *J Bone Joint Surg (Br)* 1949, 31: 532–3.

Viegas SF, Patterson RM, Peterson PD et al. 'Ulnar-sided perilunate instability: an anatomic and biomechanical study.' *J Hand Surg (Am)* 1990, 15: 268–78.

Viegas SF, Wagner K, Patterson R, Peterson P. 'Medial (hamate) facet of the lunate.' *J Hand Surg (Am)* 1990, 15: 564–71.

Walsh JJ, Bishop AT. 'Diagnosis and management of hook of hamate fractures.' *Hand Clinics* 2000, 16: 397–403.

Watson H et al. 'Rotary subluxation of the scaphoid: a spectrum of instability.' *J Hand Surg (Br)* 1993, 18: 62–4.

Watson HK, Ballet FL. 'The SLAC wrist: scapholunate advanced collapse pattern of degenerative arthritis.' *J Hand Surg (Am)* 1984, 9: 358–65.

Werner FW, Glisson RR, Murphy DJ, Palmer AK. 'Force transmission through the distal radioulnar carpal joint: effect of ulnar lengthening and shortening.' *Handchir Mikrochir Plast Chir* 1986, 18: 304–8.

Werner SL, Plancher KD. 'Biomechanics of wrist injuries in sport.' *Clin Sports Med* 1998, 17: 407–20.

Whipple TL. *The Upper Extremity in Sports Medicine*, Mosby, St. Louis, 1990.

Wood MB, Dobyns JH. 'Sports-related extraarticular wrist syndromes.' *Clin Ortho Nth Am* 1992, 23: 65–74.

Image acknowledgments

The authors wish to thank the following colleagues who kindly offered images for inclusion in this chapter:

- Dr James Linklater (Figures 2.106(b), 2.112(a) and (b), 2.114, 2.164(b), 2.209 and 2.215)
- Dr Phil Lucas (Figures 2.30, 2.50(a) and (b), 2.164(a), 2.177, 2.180, 2.194, 2.198 and 2.216)
- Dr Bill Breidahl (Figures 2.19, 2.115(a), (b) and (c), 2.137, 2.219, 2.220, 2.221, 2.222, 2.231(a) and (b), 2.233, 2.236(a) and (b))
- Dr Bruce Roberts (Figure 2.116)
- Dr Robert Cooper and Dr Stephen Allwright (Figures 2.109, 2.110, 2.111, 2.124, 2.152, 2.193, 2.200 and 2.204)

These images have significantly added to the quality of the chapter.

The elbow and forearm
Jock Anderson and John Read

The biomechanics of elbow injuries

The upper extremity operates as a linked system involving the shoulder, elbow, wrist and hand. A normally functioning elbow is an essential component of this system. The major function of the elbow is to position the hand in space, allowing the hand to move with precision, perform fine movements or operate with power. The elbow also serves as a pivot for forearm movement and anchors muscle groups that are responsible for wrist movements and for forearm pronation and supination.

The elbow joint is made up of precisely congruous articulations between the radius, ulna and humerus. The ulnohumeral joint is a hinge joint allowing flexion and extension, while the proximal radioulnar and radiohumeral joints are pivoting joints permitting rotation. These three joints are contained within the one joint capsule.

An understanding of the types of forces to which the elbow is subjected during sporting activities and the stabilising constraints of the elbow against these forces is fundamental to an understanding of how particular injuries and injury patterns occur. The major forces applied to the elbow during sporting activities are valgus and extension forces. Varus forces are rare in sport. The tremendous valgus force applied to the elbow in sports using the overhead throwing action is a common cause of elbow trauma in athletes. If the sporting activity requires this action to be repetitive, numerous overuse injuries can occur in all parts of the elbow joint.

Injury to the elbow may also be caused by direct trauma, such as falling on the out-stretched hand, and forces that cause rupture of the distal biceps or triceps tendon may be generated by a single violent muscular contraction. Elbow injuries in adult and immature athletes differ and are discussed separately.

Routine imaging of the elbow

Before discussing elbow injuries and how they might best be imaged, it is important to be familiar with the basic plain film series and additional views that may be helpful. The bony anatomy of the elbow is relatively simple and plain films are the mainstay of diagnostic imaging. A routine elbow examination consists of four views: anteroposterior, lateral-oblique, lateral and axial.

Anteroposterior (AP) view

An AP view is acquired with the shoulder, elbow and wrist all at the same level with supination of the elbow and hand. In this position the forearm bones are separated and parallel. The proximal radius and ulna and the distal humerus are well demonstrated and the joint spaces can be assessed (see Fig. 3.1). A straight tube is used, centred on the joint space.

Lateral-oblique view

A lateral-oblique view is a routine view obtained with the elbow extended in the AP position and then the hand and elbow turned with 40° of lateral rotation. This view shows the radial head and neck together with the anterior articular surface of the capitellum free of superimposition (see Fig. 3.2). A straight tube is used, centred on the joint space.

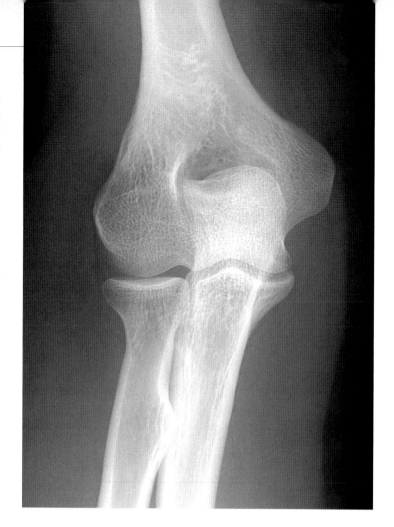

▶ **Fig. 3.1** A normal AP or supine view of the elbow. Correct positioning is important. Both the elbow and wrist must be fully supine, so that the forearm bones are parallel. In this view, the joint spaces and the bony structure of the proximal forearm and distal humerus can be assessed. The soft tissues adjacent to the medial and lateral epicondyles are also well displayed.

▼ **Fig. 3.2(a)** A lateral-oblique view is a particularly valuable projection for the examination of the lateral aspect of the elbow. Both the capitellum and the proximal radius are well displayed. **(b)** Changes in the subchondral bone of the capitellum are well demonstrated in a lateral-oblique view. In this case, areas of demineralisation in the subchondral region of the capitellum are typical of early osteochondritis dissecans (OCD) (arrow).

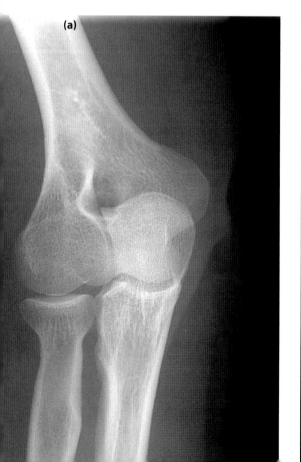

(a)

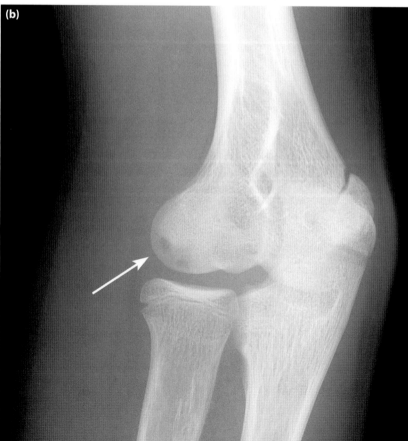

(b)

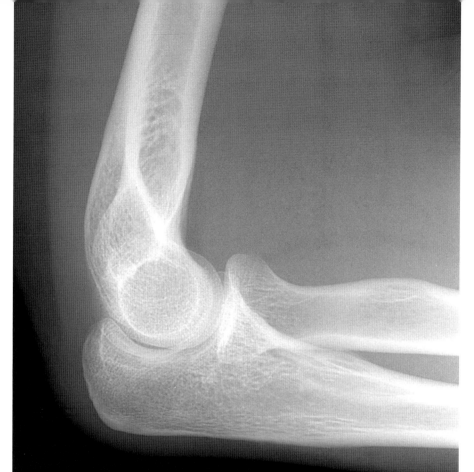

◀**Fig. 3.3** This well-positioned lateral view is a valuable component of the elbow series. If the view is not precisely lateral, the fat planes and fat pads will not be visible. In a well-positioned view, the forearm bones will be parallel and the condyles superimposed.

Lateral view

To obtain a lateral view, the wrist is placed in a lateral position and the elbow is flexed to 90°. The wrist, elbow and shoulder should lie in the same horizontal plane, bringing the condyles perpendicular to the film. Flexion of the elbow allows assessment of the fat planes and fat pads. This view also allows examination of the proximal radius and ulna and assessment of radiocapitellar alignment (see Fig. 3.3).

Axial view

To obtain an axial view, the elbow is flexed with the dorsal aspect of the upper arm lying flat on the cassette. The primary beam is at 90° to the humerus and is centred 5 cm from the tip of the olecranon. The olecranon and both epicondyles are profiled and the posterior aspect of the articular surfaces of the trochlea and trochlear notch are well displayed. Another advantage of this view is the demonstration of the posterior margin of the capitellum and the area between the lateral margin of the trochlear notch and the capitellum, which is a favoured site for loose bodies (see Fig. 3.4).

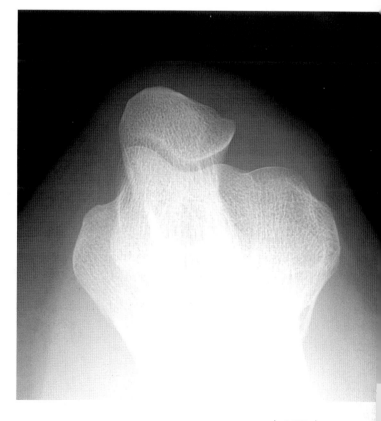

▶ **Fig. 3.4** When looking for injuries due to sporting activities, every elbow series should have an axial view. This view is a valuable projection for the assessment of the posterior aspect of the capitellum, the olecranon and the ulnohumeral joint space and its margins. Soft tissues adjacent to both epicondyles are also well demonstrated in this view.

▶ **Fig. 3.5** A stress view is acquired when a valgus stress is applied to the elbow to test the integrity of the MCL. It is an important inclusion in all series assessing the elbow for injuries produced by throwing. In this case, instability has been demonstrated as definite widening of the medial joint space (arrowheads). This may be the result of MCL attenuation from either chronic injury or acute MCL rupture.

Other helpful plain film views

Other helpful plain film views may be used in addition to the routine series.

A *stress view for medial collateral ligament (MCL) instability* is obtained as an AP view. The elbow is flexed between 30 and 40° to 'unlock' the olecranon from the olecranon fossa and then valgus stress is applied to the elbow joint. Abnormal opening of the medial joint space indicates injury to the MCL. Maloney et al. (1999) suggest that instability is present when there is 3 mm of medial joint space opening (see Fig. 3.5). However, other authors state that any degree of joint opening or reproduction of the patient's pain is an abnormal result (Cain et al. 2003).

An *epicondylar groove ('cubital tunnel') view* is used to determine whether there is bony encroachment on the cubital tunnel, causing or contributing to ulnar nerve entrapment. This view is an axial view, modified by 15° external rotation (see Fig. 3.6).

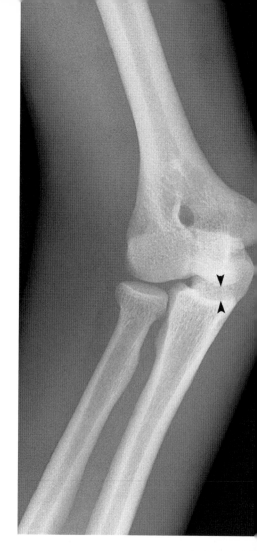

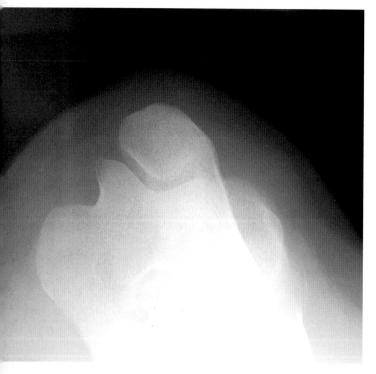

▲ **Fig. 3.6** Although this is known as a 'cubital tunnel view', it demonstrates the medial epicondylar groove, through which the ulnar nerve passes. This view will show any bony encroachment on the groove. An ossicle or bony spur may cause or contribute to ulnar nerve compression. Occasionally, if the groove is not well shown using a straight tube, 30 to 40° cranial angulation may help to demonstrate the tunnel more satisfactorily.

▶ **Fig. 3.7** When a fracture of the radial head or neck is clinically suspected, an angled radial head-capitellar view is extremely helpful. Fracture details are well displayed by eliminating any bony superimposition.

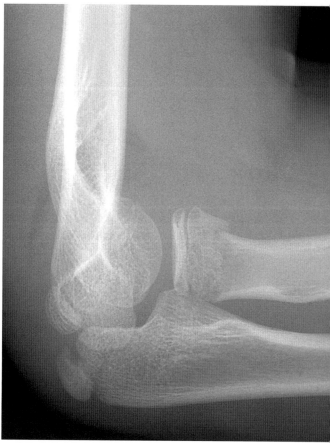

A *radial head-capitellar view* is useful when a fracture of the radial head or neck is suspected. It is indicated when the supinator fat plane is displaced, due to swelling in the region of the proximal radius. A radial head-capitellar view (see Figs 3.7 and 3.8) projects the radial head away from the ulna, and is obtained in the same position as a lateral view with the primary beam angled 45° towards the shoulder and centred on the radial head. This view also demonstrates the anterior aspect of the articular surface of the capitellum and may be helpful for demonstrating a subtle capitellar fracture or osteochondritis dissecans (OCD).

Other imaging methods

Other imaging methods play an important role in imaging sporting injuries to the elbow. Nuclear bone scans are useful for the identification of an occult fracture, bone stress, impingement and enthesopathy. CT scanning is important for imaging bone detail and is indispensable for the identification of loose bodies in the elbow joint. As sporting injury to soft tissues of the elbow is common, ultrasound and MRI are often helpful imaging methods. In addition to soft-tissue imaging, MRI can detect overuse or acute bone injury, impingement and enthesopathy.

The mature elbow

Tips on looking at plain films of mature athletes

Fortunately, the elbow does not have the anatomical complexity of some joints and often injury can be identified on a plain film series of high quality. The films must be examined mindful of the clinical presentation. There may be changes specific to the biomechanics of an injury or patterns of change resulting from a specific injury. For example, if a throwing athlete presents with medial elbow pain, the films should be painstakingly examined for changes of valgus instability, lateral-side compressive changes or evidence of extension overload, and a stress view will help assess the MCL (see Fig. 3.9).

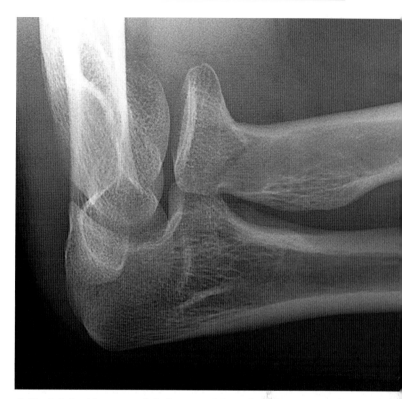

▲ **Fig. 3.8** In this case a subtle fracture of the radial neck could not be seen on the routine views but is well demonstrated with 45° tube angulation.

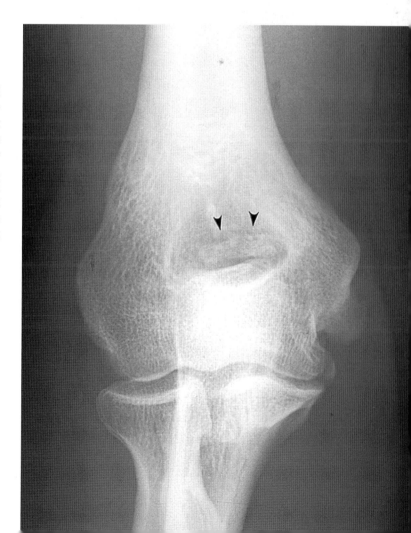

▶ **Fig. 3.9** An AP view of the elbow demonstrates a number of chronic throwing injuries. A loose body is projected over the olecranon fossa (arrowheads). There is also evidence of a previous healed avulsion from the medial epicondyle, and spur formation has developed at the distal end of the MCL on the medial corner of the coronoid. This spur appears to be detached, possibly due to recent trauma. Faced with considerable evidence of recurrent valgus stress, a careful search for other changes should be made. For example, a search for evidence of OCD would be advisable, as the origin of the loose body is not immediately evident. Further imaging may be considered.

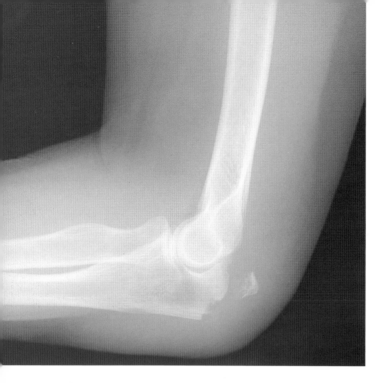

Fig. 3.10 There is considerable soft-tissue swelling associated with a triceps avulsion. A fragment of olecranon has been separated.

Fig. 3.11 In a normal lateral view of the elbow, the anterior fad pad is invariably identified as low density along the anterior border of the supracondylar region (arrowheads). The posterior fat pad is only occasionally seen in a normal elbow. In this case, it is not visible.

The soft tissues at the elbow are relatively easy to examine. Consequently, soft-tissue swelling can be detected due to displacement of fat planes. For example, it is usual for triceps rupture, fracture of the proximal radius and an acute rupture of the MCL to be suspected on plain films due to the associated swelling and obliteration of fat planes (see Fig. 3.10).

Fat pad displacement

The identification of particular fat pads and fat planes is important. A thin layer of fat is present between the fibrous and synovial layers of the elbow joint capsule, with pads of intra-capsular fat lying in both the coronoid and olecranon fossae. The fat pad in the coronoid fossa is usually visible on a lateral view of the elbow and occasionally the olecranon pad can also be seen. Because the capsule is not normally distended, the fat pads lie against the fossae and appear as elongated areas of low density against the anterior and posterior cortex of the distal humerus (see Fig. 3.11). Elbow joint effusions appear as rounded areas of water density that distend the capsule and displace these fat pads away from their respective humeral surfaces (see Fig. 3.12). The appearance has been likened to the billowing sails of a yacht. When this sign is present, an effusion can be diagnosed and there is increased probability of an occult intra-articular fracture. A progress examination or additional imaging may be considered.

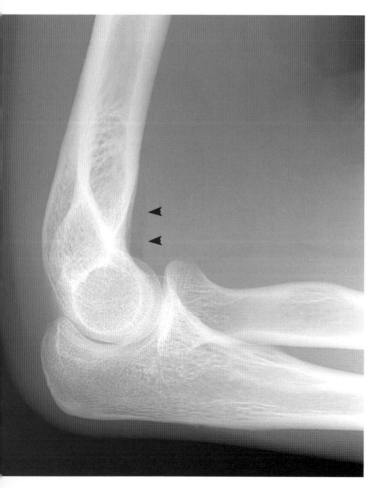

Fig. 3.12 When an effusion is present, the joint capsule is distended. As the fat pads lie within layers of the capsule, they are displaced away from the humerus and look like the sails of a yacht.

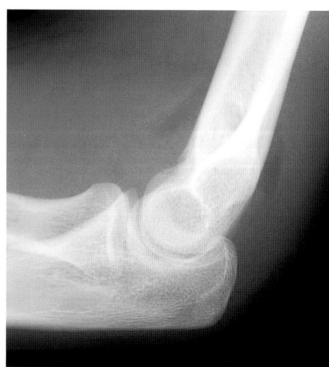

Supinator fat line

The surface of the supinator muscle is covered by a thin layer of fat that can be seen on a well-positioned lateral view of the elbow. The supinator fat line runs parallel to the anterior cortical margin of the proximal radius, and is separated from the radius by a distance of about 1 cm or so, depending on the patient's build (see Fig. 3.13). Following injury to the head or neck of the radius, the supinator fat line is displaced away from the radius by the associated haematoma (see Figs 3.14 and 3.15). This has proven to be a consistently accurate diagnostic marker of a fracture of the proximal radius and is particularly valuable when the fracture line is radiographically occult.

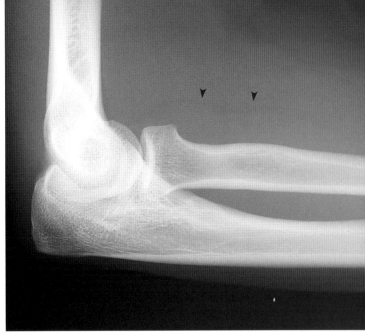

▲ **Fig. 3.13** The supinator fat line is seen in a normal lateral view as a line of low density running parallel to the proximal radius, separated about 1 cm or so from the anterior surface of the proximal radius (arrowheads).

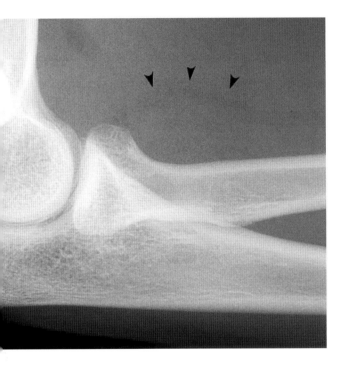

◄ **Fig. 3.14** When there has been injury to the radial head or neck, a haematoma will displace or bow the supinator fat line away from the radius. In this case, there is subtle displacement (arrowheads).

▼ **Fig. 3.15** In this case, there is a more marked displacement of the supinator fat line (arrowheads), again due to a fracture of the radial neck.

Soft-tissue calcification and ossification

Soft-tissue calcification and ossification are important to note, as they invariably denote a pathological process. About 20–25% of cases of medial and lateral epicondylitis will have associated calcification and there is often bony irregularity and ossification adjacent to the epicondyle. Although these changes can be seen on an AP view, the calcification or ossification is particularly well seen in an axial view (see Fig. 3.16). Areas of calcification or ossification may be seen in the line of the MCL and lateral collateral ligament (LCL), which indicate previous ligamentous injury (see Fig. 3.17). Calcific tendinopathy is another cause of soft-tissue calcification and is diagnosed when the calcification is projected in the line of a tendon. In Figure 3.72 on page 155, the calcification on the dorsal aspect of the olecranon is indicative of calcific triceps tendinopathy.

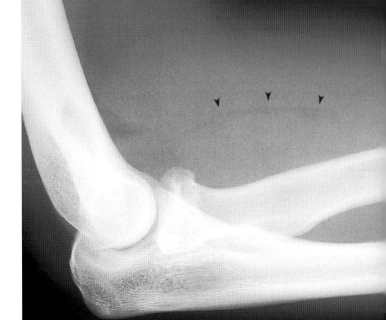

▶ **Fig. 3.16** An axial view shows calcification adjacent to the medial epicondyle (arrowhead). This calcification is almost certainly indicative of previous medial epicondylitis.

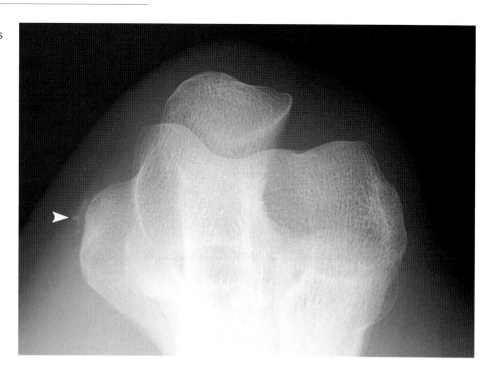

▼ **Fig. 3.17** There is ossification in the line of the lateral collateral ligament (arrowhead) indicating a previous ligamentous injury.

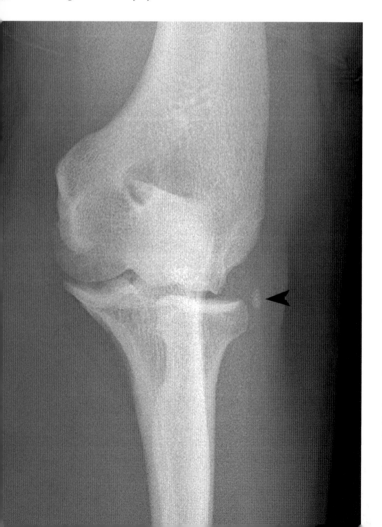

Loose bodies

Loose bodies are a common complication of a number of traumatic processes, and an ordered search for loose bodies requires examining those spaces in the joint where loose bodies often lie. Both the coronoid and olecranon fossae are favoured sites for loose bodies (see Figs 3.18, 3.19 and 3.20). Another site where loose bodies are often found is the sulcus between the capitellum and the trochlear and this space should be carefully examined (see Figs 3.21 and 3.22 on page 136). Loose bodies may be found in the trochlear notch and an axial view is required to demonstrate this area adequately (see Fig. 3.23 on page 137).

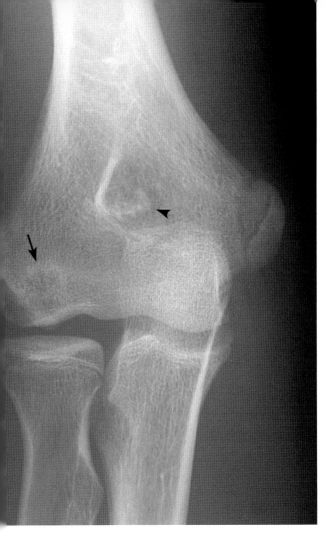

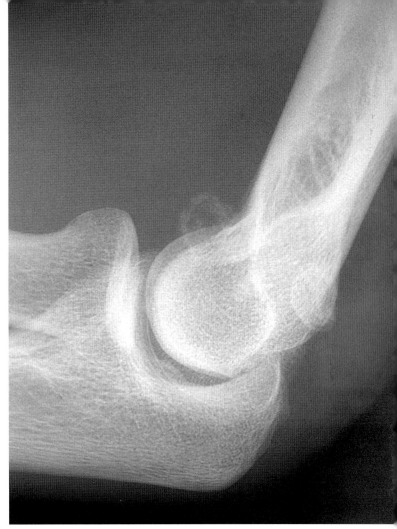

▲ **Fig. 3.18** A loose body originating from an area of OCD in the capitellum (arrow) lies in the olecranon fossa (arrowhead).

▲ **Fig. 3.19** Loose bodies are present in both the coronoid and olecranon fossae.

▼ **Fig. 3.20** Fragments of the articular surface of the capitellum have been separated and now lie in the coronoid fossa (arrowheads).

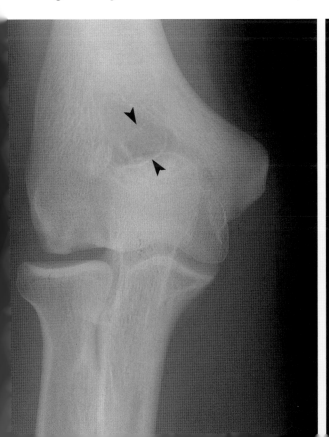

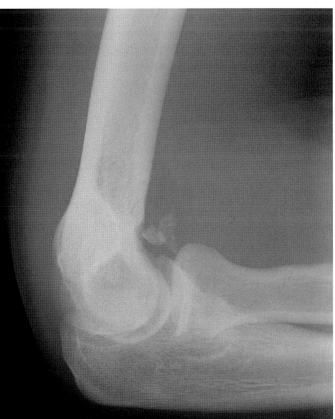

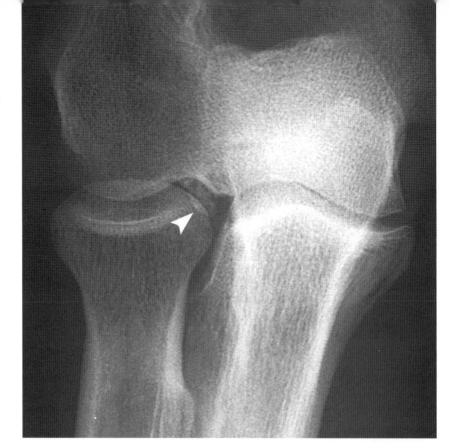

▶ **Fig. 3.21** When searching for loose bodies, it is important to remember that a favourite site for loose bodies is the sulcus between the capitellum and the trochlea. Loose bodies are present in this sulcus (arrowhead).

▼ **Fig. 3.22** Plain radiographs (top) show a loose body (arrowheads) lying in the sulcus between the trochlea and the capitellum (arrowheads). The origin of this fragment cannot be identified on the plain films. However, multiplanar CT reformations (bottom) not only demonstrate the exact location of the displaced osteochondral fragment (arrowheads) but also show that the fragment originated from the anterior aspect of the capitellum (arrow).

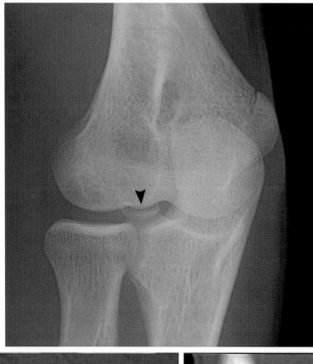
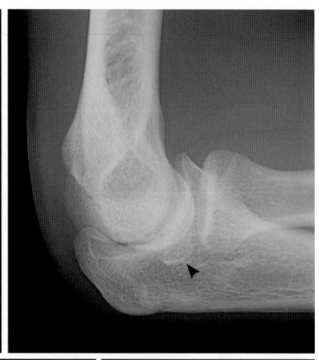

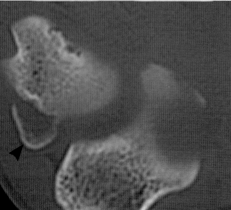
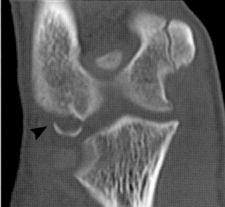
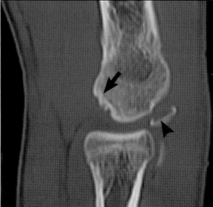

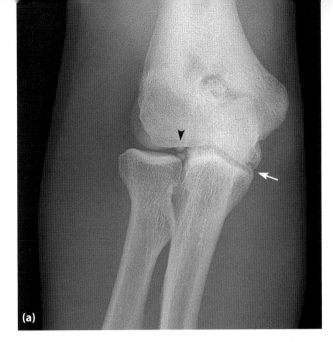

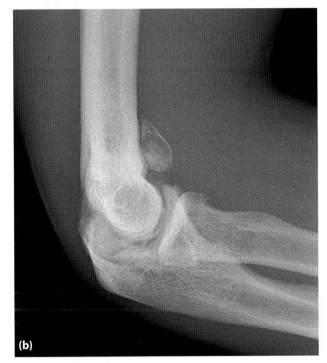

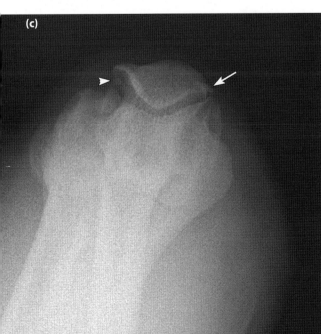

◀ **Fig. 3.23** This 24-year-old gymnast competed at the Sydney 2000 Olympics. Plain films display the ravages of gymnastics.
(a) In the AP view, a loose body is shown in the coronoid fossa and loose bodies are also present in the sulcus between the trochlea and the capitellum (arrowhead). Degenerative changes are demonstrated at the medial aspect of the ulnohumeral joint (arrow).
(b) The lateral view shows a large loose body within the coronoid fossa, enlargement of the tip of the coronoid process and degenerative changes involving the radiocapitellar articulation with osteophyte formation at the margins of the radial head.
(c) In the axial view, a loose body is shown in the trochlear notch (arrowhead) and an osteophyte on the medial aspect of the trochlear notch contributes to posterior impingement. OCD is demonstrated at the posterior aspect of the capitellum.

The mechanisms and patterns of elbow injuries

Trauma to the elbow may injure ligaments, tendons, bursae or bone together or in any combination. Certain patterns of injury emerge, the most prominent being injury produced in sports requiring the throwing mechanism. Because such sports cause so many injuries, a knowledge of the forces generated and the injuries produced enables the sports physician and radiologist to choose the most appropriate imaging method.

Valgus instability of the elbow is seen in athletes undertaking sports requiring throwing, such as cricket, baseball and the javelin, together with sports with similar biomechanics such as serving in tennis, volleyball, handball and water polo. A valgus stress on the elbow may occur in other sports such as gymnastics and weightlifting. In any of these sports, injury may be produced as a result of repetitive stress or occasionally as an acute injury. The majority of acute elbow injuries presenting to the Polyclinic at the Sydney 2000 Olympics were caused by weightlifting. All occurred when control of the weight was lost and the forearm was rotated laterally, producing a massive valgus force on the elbow and extensive injury.

To understand injury produced by a valgus force, the following need to be reviewed:

- the anatomy of the MCL
- the biomechanics of throwing
- valgus instability
- flexor-pronator injuries
- ulnar nerve entrapment
- radiocapitellar overload syndrome
- valgus extension overload
- olecranon stress fracture.

The anatomy of the MCL

The MCL is made up of three bands: the anterior-oblique band, the posterior-oblique band and the transverse ligament (see Fig. 3.24):

- The *anterior-oblique band* has parallel fibres running from the inferior aspect of the medial epicondyle to the medial corner of the tip of the coronoid process. Some fibres are taut throughout flexion and extension. The anterior-oblique band itself has three components: an anterior band, a posterior band and a central band. The anterior band functions as a constraint to valgus stress up to 90° of flexion, the posterior band contributes from 60° to full flexion and the central band functions as a constraint throughout the full range of motion (Armstrong et al. 2002).
- The *posterior-oblique band* is fan-shaped and fibres extend from the posterior aspect of the medial epicondyle to attach to the medial edge of the olecranon. This ligament is taut in flexion and lax in extension.
- The *transverse ligament* runs from the medial epicondyle to the inferomedial aspect of the coronoid process, is little more than capsular thickening and appears to be non-functional.

The biomechanics of throwing

The throwing action requires flexion and extension at the humeroulnar and humeroradial articulations with pronation and supination at the proximal radioulnar joint. The power of throwing commences in the lower extremities with coiling of the legs, trunk and upper extremities in sequence, followed by derotation of these segments (Maloney et al. 2002). Then, during the acceleration phase of throwing, the elbow pulls the arm forward, creating an extreme valgus stress and traction on the medial side structures, compressive forces on the lateral side of the joint and a shearing force posteriorly. As power is transferred to the forearm and subsequently to the object being thrown, the elbow is subjected to extension forces.

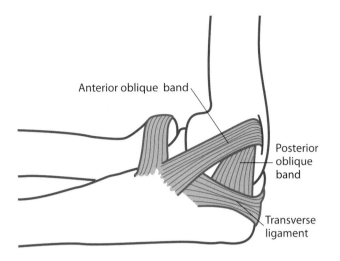

▲ **Fig. 3.24** A line drawing demonstrates the three separate components of the MCL.

There are both static and dynamic restraining forces helping to maintain elbow stability. The opposing articular surfaces at the elbow joints are tightly congruent and this, together with the MCL, the LCL and the anterior capsule, provides static stability. Dynamic stability is provided by the supporting muscles. O'Driscoll et al. (2000) demonstrated that compressive forces generated by dynamic muscle contraction protect the MCL against microscopic tears and rupture. The flexor carpi ulnaris and the flexor digitorum superficialis overlie the anterior band of the MCL and add a varus support to this static stabilising structure. The anterior capsule, biceps and brachialis absorb the forces of deceleration (Maloney et al. 2002).

Valgus instability

Repetitive valgus stress applied to the medial aspect of the elbow eventually causes injury to the MCL, producing micro-tears that may lead to attenuation of the ligament and eventually to rupture. MCL rupture may also occur as an acute injury. The normal MRI appearance of the MCL is shown in Fig. 3.25. MCL ruptures involve the epicondylar

▼ **Fig. 3.25** Coronal PD and fat-suppressed MRI show the appearance of a normal MCL (arrows). The normal ligament is characterised by homogeneous low signal with clearly defined proximal and distal attachments.

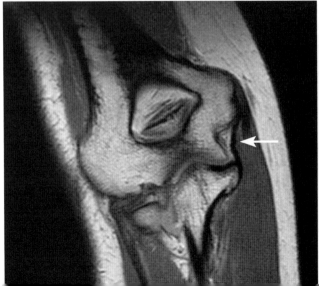
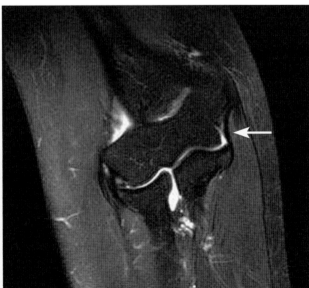

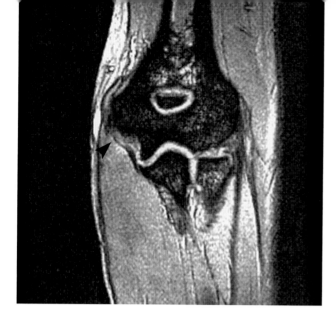

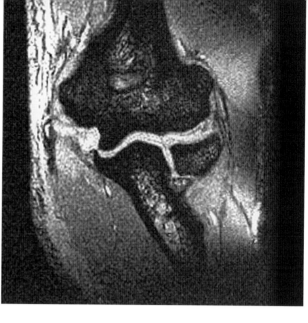

▲ **Fig. 3.26** Proximal MCL rupture demonstrated on a coronal T2*-weighted MR image. A female weightlifter at the Sydney 2000 Olympics lost control of the weight and a large valgus force was applied to her elbow, injuring the proximal end of the MCL. There is mild periligamentous oedema and high signal at the proximal end of the MCL.

▲ **Fig. 3.27** A more severe proximal MCL tear, also occurring in an Olympic weightlifter, shows considerable associated oedema and separation of the common flexor origin. These changes are demonstrated on a coronal T2*-weighted MR image.

end in 70% of cases (see Figs 3.26 and 3.27), the coronoid process end in 20% of cases (see Figs 3.28 and 3.29) and the mid-ligament in 10% of cases (see Figs 3.30 and 3.31) (Bennett and Tullos 1990). Ligamentous insufficiency may predispose to degenerative changes, and in particular spur formation develops at the bony attachment of the MCL at the coronoid process (see Fig. 3.32). Hypertrophy of the medial humeral condyle (see Fig. 3.33) and coronoid process has also been described (Chen et al. 2001). Enlargement of the coronoid process has been demonstrated in Fig. 3.23. Bone stress at the distal attachment of the MCL may be demonstrated by a nuclear bone scan (see Fig. 3.34). Nuclear bone scans can also be useful for demonstrating injury to the proximal MCL attachment (see Fig. 3.35) and increased uptake of isotope may indicate bone stress or bruising.

▶ **Fig. 3.28** A coronal PD-weighted MRI demonstrates injury to the distal MCL with stripping of the ligament from the coronoid process (arrowhead). There is also high signal in the adjacent flexor tendon.

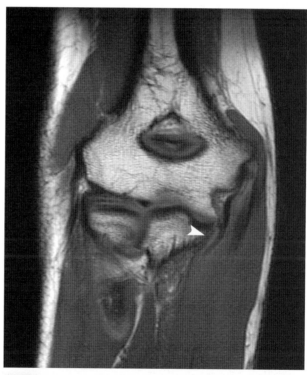

▶ **Fig. 3.29** MRI demonstrates a distal MCL tear. Coronal PD and corresponding fat-suppressed PD images together show a high-grade partial tear at the distal attachment of the MCL (arrow) and low-grade hyperintense signal indicative of strain at the proximal attachment of the MCL (arrowhead). There is oedema within the flexor muscle adjacent to the tear.

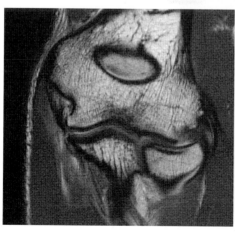

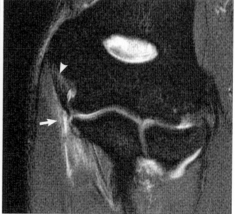

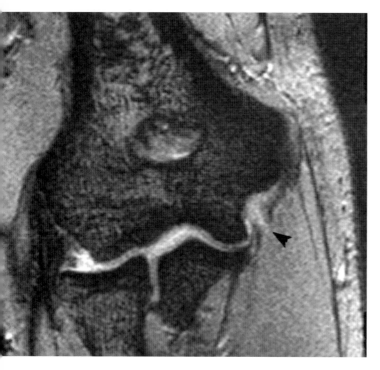

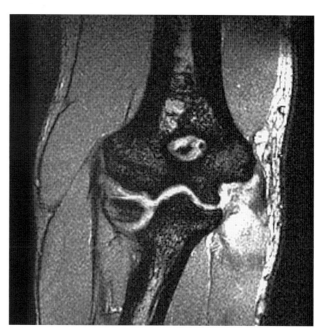

▲ **Fig. 3.31** A gross injury in a weight-lifter has caused diffuse interstitial rupture of the MCL and there is an accompanying tear of the common flexor origin. Considerable associated oedema is also shown. These changes are demonstrated on a coronal T2*-weighted MR image.

▲ **Fig. 3.30** A mid-segment MCL tear demonstrated on a coronal T2*-weighted MR image. There is minimal associated oedema, suggesting that the tear is a chronic injury.

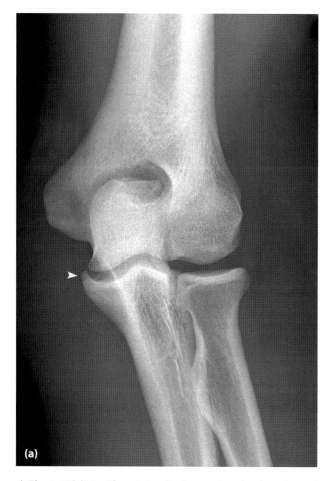

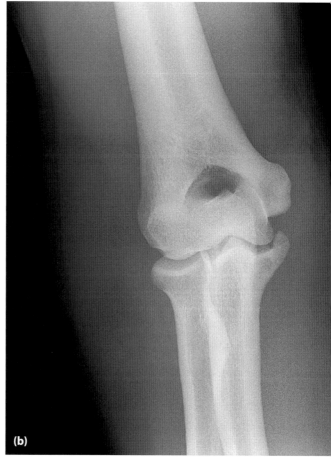

▲ **Fig. 3.32(a)** An Olympic javelin thrower has developed spur formation at the distal attachment of the MCL (arrowhead). **(b)** There is a large spur at the distal attachment of the MCL, indicating chronic stress in a weightlifter. This is the plain film of the injured weightlifter shown in Fig. 3.27.

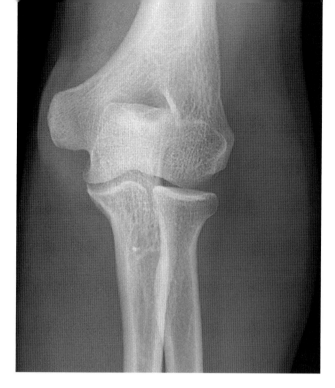

◄**Fig. 3.33** Chronic stress applied to the elbow by repetitive valgus forces in the developing skeleton may cause overgrowth and hypertrophy of structures at the elbow. In this athlete, there has been hypertrophy of the medial epicondyle.

▼**Fig. 3.34** Bilateral enthesopathy has developed at the medial epicondyles due to repetitive stress applied by the MCL. This change is demonstrated on a nuclear bone scan.

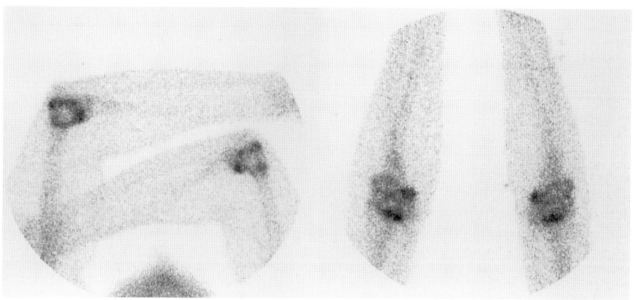

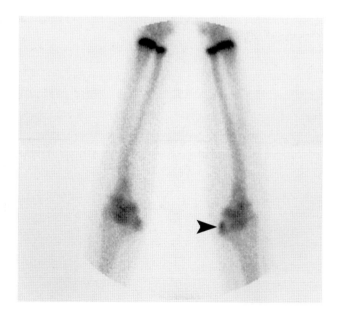

◄**Fig. 3.35** A nuclear bone scan demonstrates a traction injury to the medial epicondylar growth plate in an immature athlete (arrowhead).

Valgus instability is a clinical diagnosis, with the athlete usually presenting with medial elbow pain, a 'pop', on throwing and an inability to continue to throw. Nevertheless, imaging contributes valuable information to the management of this condition. Imaging begins with plain films. In addition to the routine series, a stress view is important and may be diagnostic of injury to the MCL if there is abnormal joint space opening (see Fig. 3.36) (Maloney et al. 1999). Plain films may demonstrate calcification associated with flexor tendinopathy (see Fig. 3.37) or ossification in the line of the MCL, providing evidence of a previous tear and haemorrhage (see Fig. 3.38). Plain films may also show spur formation, loose bodies or lateral compressive changes. These changes are discussed on the following pages.

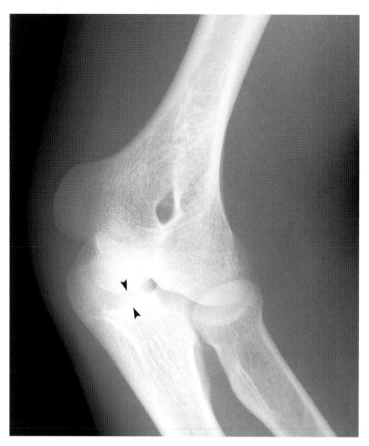

◀ **Fig. 3.36** This stress view demonstrates instability, with widening of the medial joint space (arrowheads) and the application of valgus stress to the elbow. The method of acquiring this image is described on page 130. This athlete is a javelin thrower, an activity with high risk of causing MCL injury.

▼ **Fig. 3.38** There is evidence of chronic MCL injury. Spur formation has developed at the distal attachment of the MCL to the coronoid process (arrowhead) and ossification within the MCL almost certainly indicates a previous tear and haemorrhage (arrow). Note the loose bodies in the sulcus between the trochlea and the capitellum. There is also deformity of the medial epicondyle suggesting an old avulsion.

▼ **Fig. 3.37** Calcification is present just below the medial epicondyle and its position suggests that this is associated with flexor-pronator tendinopathy.

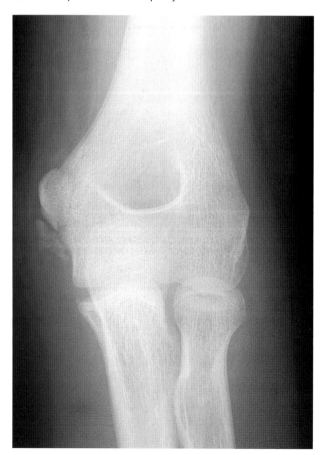

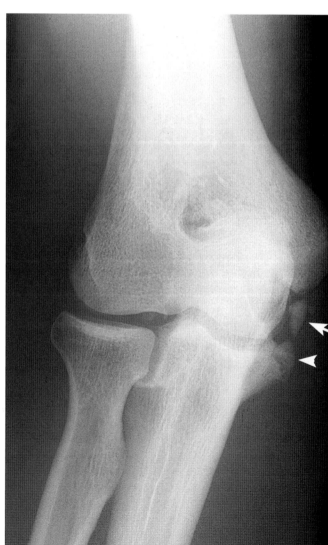

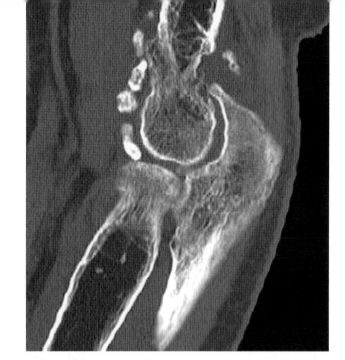

▶ **Fig. 3.39(a)** CT scanning demonstrates multiple loose bodies in this older elbow. Multiple loose bodies may indicate synovial osteochondromatosis.

▼ **(b)** A CT scan demonstrates the presence of loose bodies. Sagittal reformations through the trochlea (t) and radial head (r) have been generated from the axially acquired 'raw' image data. An OCD lesion of the capitellum shows an in-situ osteochondral fragment (arrowhead). A further displaced osteochondral fragment is seen within the olecranon fossa (arrow).

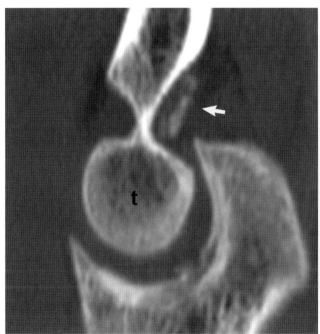

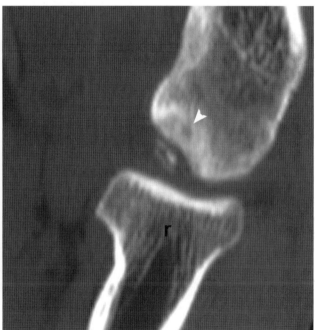

Due to bony superimposition at the elbow, computed tomography is extremely valuable for identifying loose bodies (see Fig. 3.39) and defining bone injury (see Fig. 3.40).

As the majority of changes occur in the soft tissues, ultrasound and MRI play major diagnostic roles. Figures 3.26–3.31 show MCL and flexor-pronator injuries demonstrated by MRI. Ultrasound offers a cheaper imaging option with the potential to obtain similar information (see Fig. 3.41). Both can image tendinopathy (see Fig. 3.42) and identify loose bodies (see Fig. 3.43). The ulnar nerve can also be imaged by either method. Ultrasound has the additional benefit of showing dynamic instability.

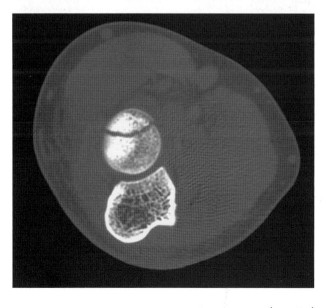

▶ **Fig. 3.40** A CT scan shows a fracture of the radial head that was not visible on plain films, although in retrospect the supinator fat line was displaced.

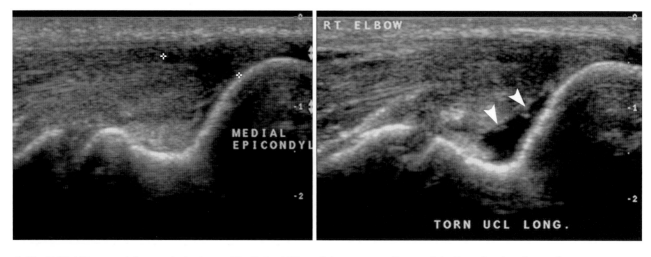

▲ **Fig. 3.41** Ultrasound demonstrates tears of both the MCL and the common flexor origin. Two closely adjacent long-axis ultrasound images obtained at the common flexor origin show a fluid-filled gap at the humeral attachment of the MCL (arrowheads) and a further small irregular intra-tendon fluid space indicative of an acute partial tear at the adjacent common flexor origin (callipers).

▶ **Fig. 3.42** Ultrasound imaging shows an uncomplicated flexor tendinopathy. A long-axis image of the common flexor tendon origin demonstrates a localised zone of hypoechoic tendon thickening (arrowhead) with preservation of underlying fibre continuity. Medial humeral epicondyle = h.

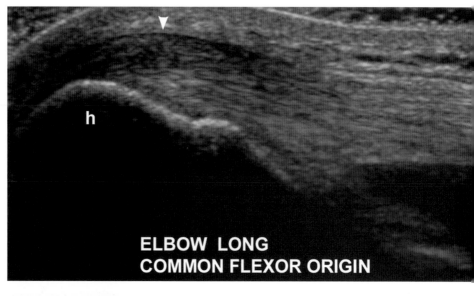

ELBOW LONG
COMMON FLEXOR ORIGIN

▼ **Fig. 3.43** A loose body is demonstrated on a sagittal T2-weighted MR image. The intra-articular body lies within the olecranon fossa of the elbow joint surrounded by fluid signal due to joint space effusion.

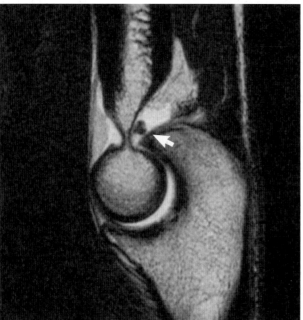

Flexor-pronator injuries

The flexor-pronator group of muscles plays an extremely important role in the throwing action. Not only does this muscle group act as an important dynamic restraint to valgus forces, but the FCR and FCU flex an extended wrist as part of ball release or tennis strokes and repetition of this activity may lead to enthesopathy or tendinopathy. In addition, as the flexor-pronator muscles become less effective with overuse, so the dynamic protection afforded the MCL is less effective, predisposing to MCL overload and injury.

The origin of the flexor-pronator muscle mass is from a number of sites on the medial epicondyle. Enthesopathy will develop from repetitive stress on these origins, mainly involving the pronator teres, the FCR and, less commonly, the FCU origins. The medial epicondyle becomes painful (see the discussion on medial epicondylitis on page 164).

Imaging of flexor-pronator injuries using plain films, nuclear bone scans, ultrasound and MRI has been discussed and demonstrated previously in the section on valgus instability.

Ulnar nerve entrapment

A more general discussion on cubital tunnel syndrome is found in the section on common tunnel syndromes at the elbow (see page 177). The following discussion relates to ulnar neuropathy associated with throwing injuries.

At the elbow joint, the ulnar nerve approaches the posterior aspect of the medial epicondyle by passing just medial to the posterior band of the MCL and medial joint capsule, giving off an articular branch at the joint level. The nerve then passes between the heads of the FCU muscle to enter the forearm. The nerve passes through the cubital tunnel, with the posterior band of the MCL and capsule lying on its lateral aspect, the medial epicondylar groove anteriorly and the arcuate ligament medially (Cain et al. 2003). The two most common sites of nerve compression are the epicondylar groove and where the nerve passes between the two heads of the FCU. There are other less common sites of compression. Wherever compression occurs, entrapment may be secondary to anatomical variants, synovitis, medial trochlear osteophytes (St John and Palmaz 1986), haemorrhage, ganglia, loose bodies, muscle hypertrophy or thickened retinaculum (Maloney et al. 2002).

An anomalous muscle, the anconeus epitrochlearis, may cause ulnar nerve compression. This muscle spans the cubital tunnel from its origin on the olecranon to its attachment on the medial epicondyle (see Fig. 3.44) (Cain et al. 2003).

The ulnar nerve may be injured by an isolated event, but injury is more often secondary to other processes at the medial aspect of the elbow. In particular, ulnar neuropathy occurs commonly in association with MCL injury, flexor-pronator strain and medial epicondylitis. About 40% of athletes with MCL insufficiency will present with ulnar nerve symptoms (Chen et al. 2001) and ulnar neuropathy has been reported to occur in 60% of patients with medial epicondylitis (Teitz et al. 1997). The neuropathy is thought to be due to compression, traction or local irritation. The nerve is surprisingly mobile and with full flexion and extension it will glide up to 9.8 mm (Rempel et al. 1999). Consequently, any process that tethers the nerve will produce traction.

The diagnosis of ulnar neuropathy is established clinically or by nerve conduction studies, but imaging with plain films (using the cubital tunnel view to exclude a bony cause of nerve compression), ultrasound (see Fig. 3.45) or MRI (see Figs 3.46 and 3.47) may assist in demonstrating the site and cause of the neuropathy.

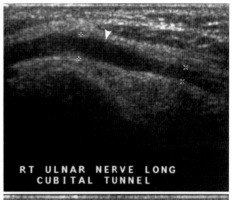
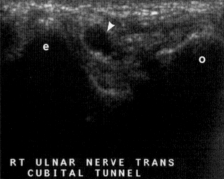

▲ **Fig. 3.45** Ultrasound demonstrates cubital tunnel syndrome. Transverse and long-axis images of the ulnar nerve at the cubital tunnel level show features of ulnar neuropathy. There is fusiform hypoechoic swelling of the ulnar nerve (arrowheads) and an associated zone of increased echogenicity in the perineural fat. Medial humeral epicondyle = e.

▼ **Fig. 3.44** MRI demonstrates an anconeus epitrochlearis muscle (asterisk) and its relationship to the ulnar nerve. The accessory anconeus muscle occurs in 4–34% of the population (O'Hara and Stone 1996). Muscle hypertrophy in response to weightlifting or overuse may cause ulnar nerve compression. Note ulnar nerve hyperintensity in this case (arrow).

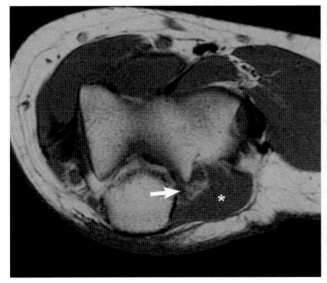
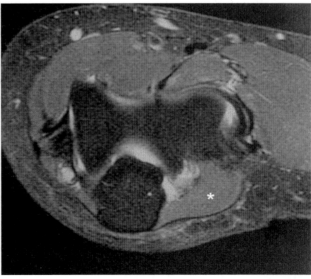

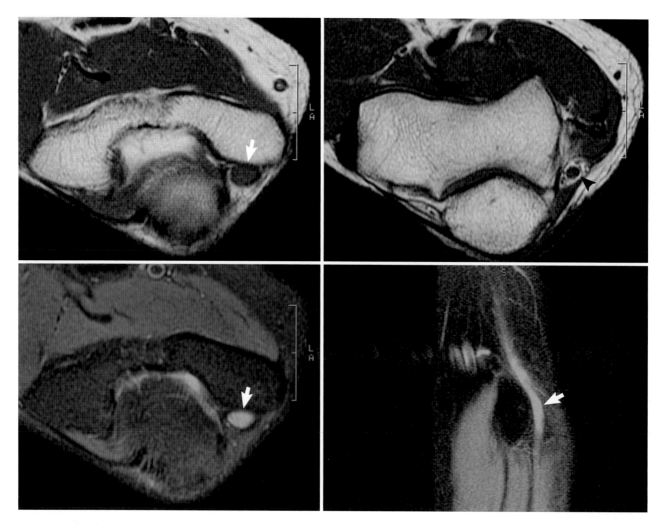

▲ **Fig. 3.46** MRI shows ulnar 'neuritis' in the cubital tunnel (cubital tunnel syndrome). Axial PD (top) and fat-suppressed axial and sagittal PD (bottom) images show the changes of ulnar neuropathy within the cubital tunnel. The ulnar nerve at the mid-to-upper cubital tunnel level is swollen and hyperintense (white arrows) when compared with the segment immediately distal to the cubital tunnel (black arrowhead).

▼ **Fig. 3.47** Direct trauma to the elbow joint during a game of wheelchair rugby ('murderball') in the Sydney 2000 Paralympics resulted in the development of ulnar neuropathy. This fat-suppressed axial MR image shows bone bruising of the olecranon and trochlea along the medial wall of the epicondylar groove. There is also high signal in the ulnar nerve and in the fat surrounding the ulnar nerve (arrowhead).

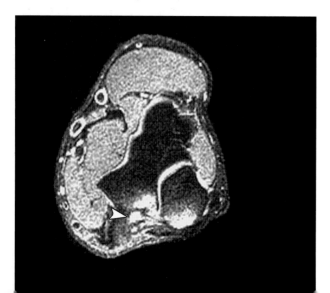

Radiocapitellar overload syndrome

Attenuation or rupture of the MCL leads to compressive forces laterally, with the radiocapitellar articulation acting as a static resistance to valgus instability (see Fig. 3.48). In the adult, changes in the lateral compartment are less common than those occurring medially and include the development of OCD and osteochondral fractures of both the capitellum and the radial head secondary to repetitive abutment of the radial head against the capitellum (see Fig. 3.49). Developing OCD may be demonstrated by a nuclear bone scan (see Fig. 3.50). OCD developing in the capitellum can be imaged by plain films (see Fig. 3.51) in a large number of cases. In doubtful cases, MRI is useful for demonstrating these changes (see Fig. 3.52). Lateral epicondylitis may also develop due to extensor-supinator muscle mass overuse from throwing (Fleisig at al. 1995) (see Fig. 3.53).

The repetitive impact of the radial head on the capitellum in the adult produces changes of chondromalacia (see Fig. 3.54) and bony degeneration leading to fracturing and loose body formation (see Fig. 3.55).

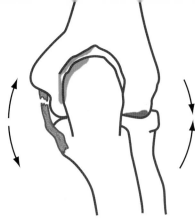

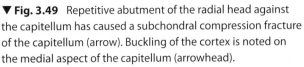

◀ **Fig. 3.48** The forces acting on the elbow that contribute to radiocapitellar overload syndrome.

▼ **Fig. 3.49** Repetitive abutment of the radial head against the capitellum has caused a subchondral compression fracture of the capitellum (arrow). Buckling of the cortex is noted on the medial aspect of the capitellum (arrowhead).

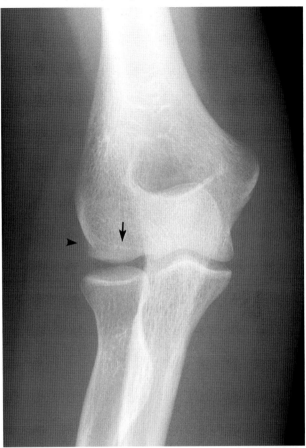

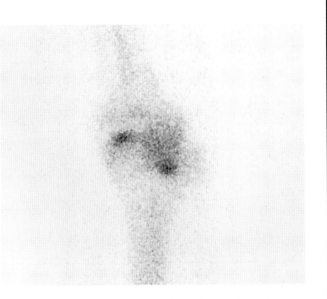

▲ **Fig. 3.50** A nuclear bone scan shows increased uptake of isotope in the right capitellum, typical of OCD. There is also evidence of olecranon abutment from valgus extension overload, with increased uptake of isotope in the olecranon.

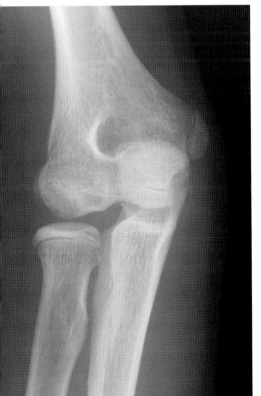

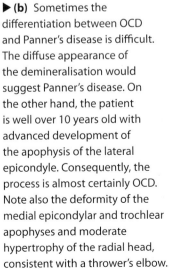

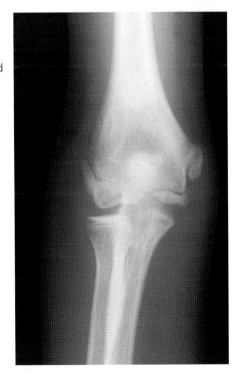

◀ **Fig. 3.51(a)** Plain film changes in the capitellum are typical of OCD. Considerable subchondral demineralisation has occurred and early fragmentation appears to be present. No loose body can be seen on this lateral-oblique view.

▶ **(b)** Sometimes the differentiation between OCD and Panner's disease is difficult. The diffuse appearance of the demineralisation would suggest Panner's disease. On the other hand, the patient is well over 10 years old with advanced development of the apophysis of the lateral epicondyle. Consequently, the process is almost certainly OCD. Note also the deformity of the medial epicondylar and trochlear apophyses and moderate hypertrophy of the radial head, consistent with a thrower's elbow.

▶ **Fig. 3.52** This coronal T2*-weighted MR image demonstrates an area of high signal in the subchondral region of the capitellum and there is subtle abnormal signal in the overlying articular cartilage (arrow). The appearances are those of OCD with chondromalacia in the overlying articular cartilage.

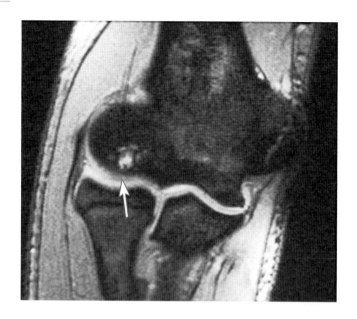

▼ **Fig. 3.53** Ultrasound demonstrates an LCL tear and extensor tendinopathy. Long-axis and transverse images of the common extensor tendon origin show an irregular fluid-filled gap in mid-segment LCL fibre continuity (arrows) and hypoechoic tendinopathy thickening of the adjacent common extensor tendon origin (arrowheads). Radial head = r. Lateral humeral epicondyle = h.

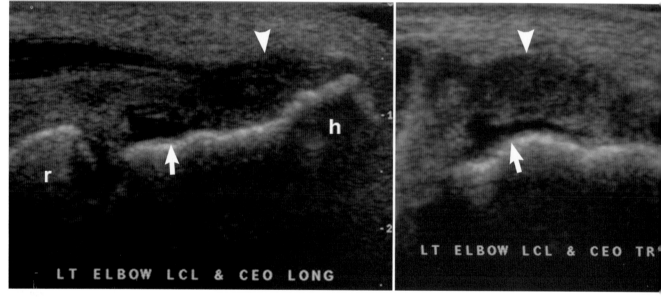

▼ **Fig. 3.54** MRI shows bone bruising in the capitellum resulting from abutment by the radial head. Coronal PD and corresponding fat-suppressed PD images together show bone marrow oedema indicating microtrabecular injury ('bone bruise') in the subchondral bone of the capitellum (arrowhead). There is also hypertrophy of the medial aspect of the tip of the olecranon with high signal present in this hypertrophied bone, indicating valgus extension overload (black arrow). A proximal tear of the MCL (white arrow) is noted.

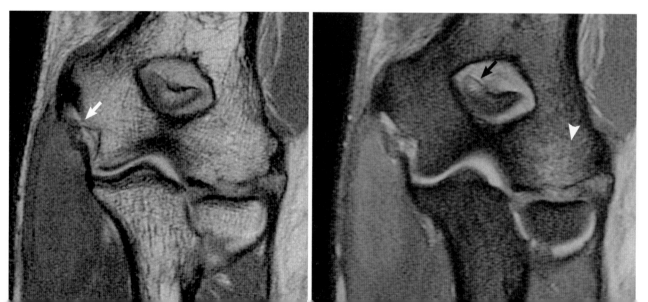

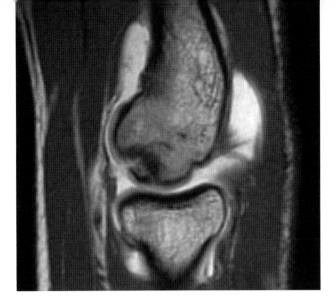

▲ **Fig. 3.55** This sagittal PD-weighted MR image shows OCD with a partly destabilised osteochondral fragment and joint space effusion.

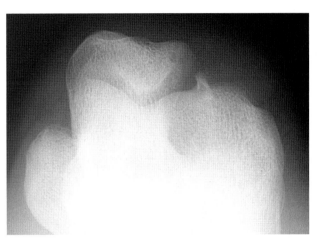

▲ **Fig. 3.57** Spur formation has developed at the lateral margin of the ulnohumeral articulation and is likely to cause posterior impingement. Subchondral cyst formation is noted in the apposing articular surface.

Valgus extension overload

The acceleration phase of throwing is largely resisted by the flexor-pronator muscles. The bony constraints are provided by the olecranon engaging the olecranon fossa and the radiocapitellar joint. So, if the deceleration phase is not controlled dynamically by the flexor muscles, the olecranon will repeatedly abut the olecranon fossa at full extension. In addition, King et al. (1969) noted that with MCL laxity there is a shearing force across the olecranon, which means that the posteromedial aspect of the olecranon will impinge on the medial wall of the olecranon fossa. This has been termed 'valgus extension overload'.

Repetitive bony impingement will cause pain with the development of chondromalacia on the articular surface of the abutting surfaces (see Fig. 3.56). Hypertrophy of the medial aspect of the olecranon may occur in response to the repetitive trauma. This change has been demonstrated in Figure 3.54. Osteophyte formation and loose bodies may develop, with loss of full extension caused by posterior impingement by osteophytes or locking due to loose bodies (see Figs 3.57, 3.58 and 3.59).

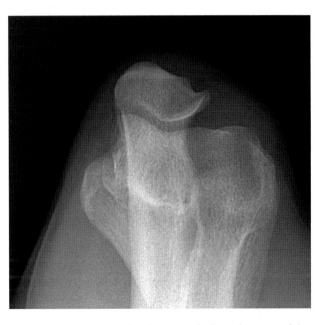

▲ **Fig. 3.58** Spurring is developing at the lateral margin of the trochlear notch. This is a degenerative change resulting from repetitive trauma.

▶ **Fig. 3.56** A nuclear bone scan demonstrates olecranon impingement on the right (dominant) side. There is a focus of uptake in the olecranon fossa.

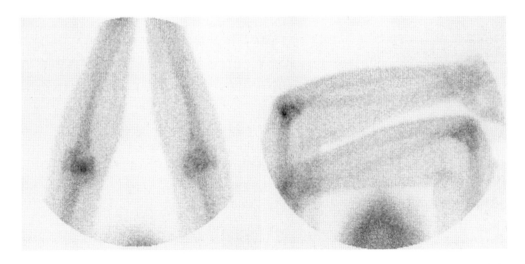

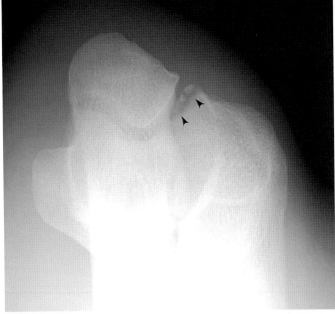

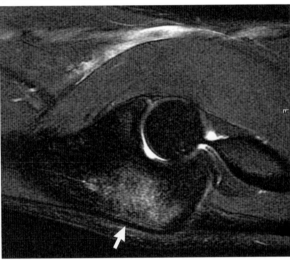

◀ **Fig. 3.59** Loose body formation is occurring at the posterolateral margin of the trochlea (arrowheads). The appearance suggests that this is an area of OCD resulting in the margin of the trochlea as a result of repetitive abutment.

▼ **Fig. 3.60(a)** MRI demonstrates an area of high signal in the olecranon (arrow). There is no history of acute trauma and the appearances are likely to represent bone stress associated with valgus extension overload. No fracture line can be seen.

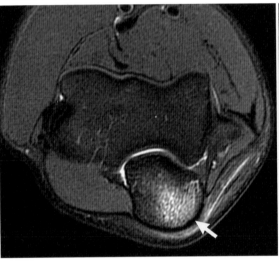

Olecranon stress fractures

Stress fractures of the olecranon have been described in gymnasts (Maffulli et al. 1992), javelin throwers (Hulkko et al. 1986) and baseball pitchers (Torg and Moyer 1977). These stress fractures are a result of valgus extension overload (Rao and Rao 2001) resulting from the repetitive abutment of the olecranon on the olecranon fossa (see Fig. 3.60). Gymnasts and wrestlers are at risk due to the requirement for repetitive explosive extension superimposed on weightbearing forces across the elbow. Transverse and oblique stress fractures have been described. It is thought that if the action of the triceps is the predominant force, the fracture line will be transverse, whereas oblique fractures are the result of the valgus shear across the olecranon with valgus extension overload (Suzuki et al. 1997). Maffulli et al. (1992) also noted that similar extension forces in the immature athlete may cause avulsion of the olecranon apophysis.

Elbow injuries

Injury to the LCL and posterolateral rotary instability of the elbow

The anatomy of the LCL

The LCL complex consists of four components (see Fig. 3.61):

- The *radial collateral ligament (RCL)*, the major component of the lateral ligament complex, originates from the lateral epicondyle and merges with the annular ligament.

- The *accessory lateral collateral ligament* is a separate band of annular ligament that attaches to a small prominence on the supinator crest, a ridge that extends distally from the inferior aspect of the radial notch.

- The *annular ligament* passes around the radial head and neck and attaches to the margins of the radial notch, holding the radial head firmly in the radial notch of the ulna. The annular ligament acts as a restraint against distal displacement of the radius. Injury to the annular ligament may be associated with a fracture of the radial head, producing incongruity of the proximal radioulnar joint and problems with supination and pronation.

- The *lateral ulnar collateral ligament (LUCL)* runs from the lateral epicondyle, its fibres blending with the remainder of the LCL. The ligament passes over the annular ligament and the posterior fibres fan out to insert on the posterior ulna behind the annular ligament. The anterior border attaches to the tubercle of the supinator crest. This ligament functions as an important static restraint against posterolateral subluxation of the radial head on the capitellum. This is a relatively recent concept (O'Driscoll et al. 1991).

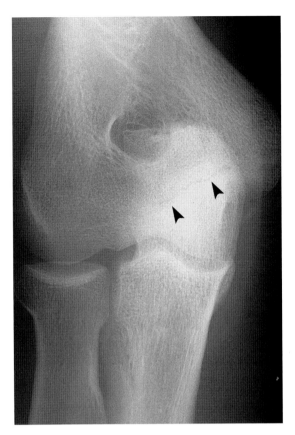

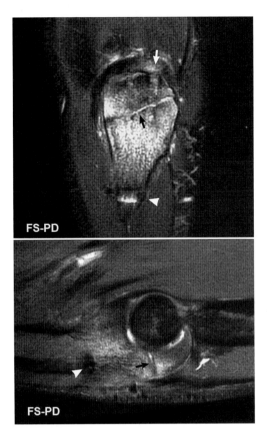

▲ **(b)** An olecranon stress fracture is demonstrated in a 19-year-old baseball pitcher who presented with recurrent gradual-onset elbow pain following a previous successful pin fixation and tension band wiring of a stress fracture. A subtle recurrent fracture line is evident on the AP film (arrowheads).

The four major static elbow-stabilising restraints are the articulations, the MCL, the LCL (particularly the LUCL) and the anterior capsule. It is suggested that on the lateral side, the lateral triceps, brachialis, extensor muscles and anconeus provide the dynamic restraint against varus stress (Conway and Singleton 2003).

The biomechanics of lateral elbow injury and elbow dislocation

Lateral instability is unusual. A continuum exists from mild laxity to recurrent dislocation. As varus elbow stress in sport is rare, LCL injury is uncommon, although forceful elbow flexion and supination may rupture the annular ligament component of the LCL and produce anterior dislocation of the radial head.

Posterolateral rotary instability of the elbow (PLRI), described by O'Driscoll et al. (1991), involves external rotation of the ulna in relation to the humerus together with pos-terolateral radial subluxation on the capitellum. The pattern of injury is described by Conway and Singleton (2003) as tissue disruption commencing on the lateral side of elbow, which progresses medially. Injury to the soft-tissue restraints begins initially with disruption of the LUCL and then injury occurs to the remaining components of the LCL. Failure of the anterior and posterior capsule is followed by injury to the posterior bundle of the MCL. Integrity medially is maintained

▲**(c)** Fat-suppressed PD-weighted images demonstrate the extent of the fracture as a thin hyperintense fluid line with sclerotic margins and surrounding marrow oedema. Note the magnetic susceptibility artefact within and around the olecranon due to micro-metallic debris from previous surgery. The fracture line is identified by black arrows, the tunnel associated with the previous tension wiring by white arrowheads and the bone tunnel associated with the previous pin by a white arrow.

by the anterior bundle of the MCL and this ligament provides a pivot around which dislocation occurs. Maintenance of an intact anterior bundle of the MCL also provides continuing valgus stability.

If this is not complex enough, the complete answer does not appear to be available. There is controversy regarding

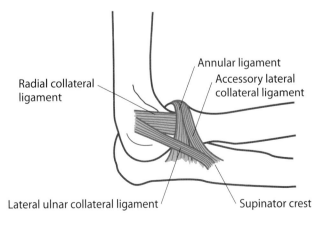

▲ **Fig. 3.61** The four components making up the lateral ligament complex are demonstrated.

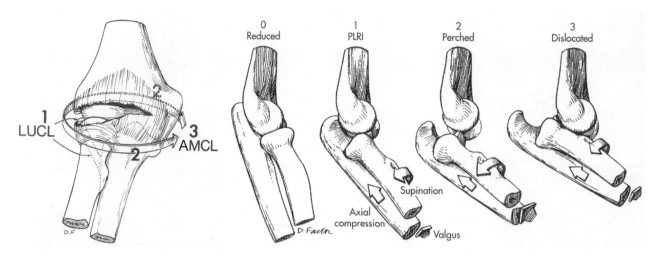

▲ **Fig. 3.62** A schematic of elbow instability. A 'circle of soft-tissue disruption' occurs from lateral to medial and is staged as follows:
Stage 0 Normal.
Stage 1 Disrupted LUCL: this causes posterolateral rotatory subluxation, which reduces spontaneously.
Stage 2 Further capsular disruption both anteriorly and posteriorly: this causes incomplete posterolateral dislocation ('perched elbow'), which can be reduced with minimal force.
Stage 3 All restraints are disrupted except the anterior band of the MCL: this causes complete posterior dislocation via the posterior rotatory mechanism, with the elbow pivoting about the intact anterior (band) medial collateral ligament (AMCL).
Stage 4 All restraints are torn: this causes gross varus and valgus instability (not shown).
Source: O'Driscoll SW, Morrey BF, Korineck S et al. 'Elbow subluxation and dislocation: a spectrum of instability.' *Clinical Orthopaedics & Related Research* July 1992, 280: 186–97.

the importance of the LUCL in PLRI. Dunning et al. (2001) demonstrated that dividing the LUCL does not produce PLRI if the annular ligament and RCL are intact. Research by Olsen et al. (1998) also found that division of the LUCL alone did not produce significant lateral joint laxity and that proximal disruption of both the RCL and LUCL is necessary to produce PLRI.

Dislocation of the elbow generally results from hyperextension, secondary to a fall on an extended arm. O'Driscoll et al. (1992) described stages of dislocation (see Fig. 3.62). As hyperextension progresses, the olecranon process is forced into the olecranon fossa and this acts as a lever to lift the trochlea over the coronoid process (see Fig. 3.63). Fractures/dislocations

are common with associated fractures occasionally involving the radial head, capitellum and coronoid process.

Imaging plays an important role in the management of the PLRI process. Plain films can be useful for demonstrating posterolateral subluxation of the radial head, the degree of dislocation, such as 'perched elbow' (see Fig. 3.64), and the presence of associated fractures. Fluoroscopy offers an imaging method of establishing the diagnosis of PLRI (see Fig. 3.65). MRI provides a valuable method of imaging the lateral ligament complex (see Figs 3.66, 3.67 and 3.68). In particular and of importance in the assessment of stability, MRI is able to image the LUCL (see Figs 3.69 and 3.70) and can also demonstrate PLRI (see Fig. 3.71).

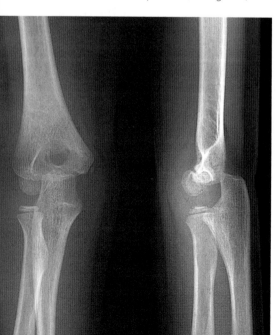

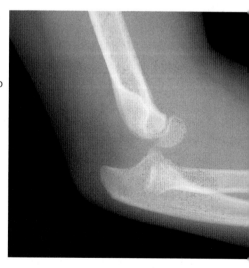

◀ **Fig. 3.63** The 'lever action' is occurring, demonstrated in the lateral view of this dislocated elbow. With continuing hyperextension, the olecranon process is used as a lever to lift the trochlea anteriorly.

▶ **Fig. 3.64** In O'Driscoll et al.'s Stage 2 of dislocation, the trochlea becomes perched on the coronoid process ('perched elbow').

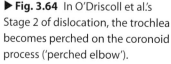

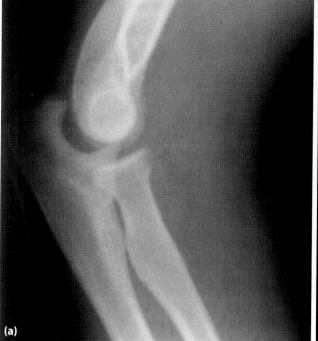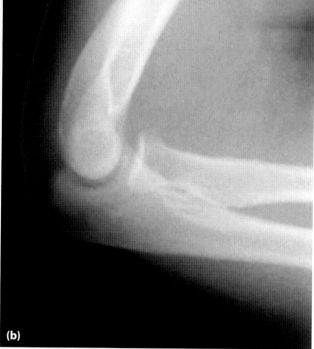

(a)　　(b)

▲ **Fig. 3.65** These fluoroscopic images demonstrate PLRI. The 'lateral pivot shift' of the proximal ulna on the humerus is the clinical test used to demonstrate PLRI secondary to LCL deficiency. This test is performed with the arm in an overhead position and is best done with the patient anaesthetised (an apprehension sign rather than a definite reduction clunk may otherwise result). Subluxation is first induced with the elbow held in extension by using a combination of axial compression, valgus and supination force **(a)**. With provocative force still applied, the elbow is then flexed and will at some point (typically at 30 to 60° of flexion) suddenly reduce with an accompanying palpable and visible clunk **(b)**.

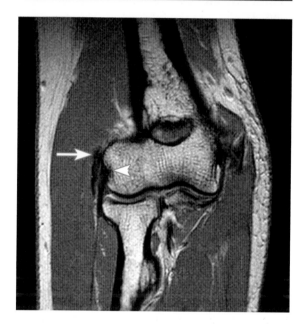

▶ **Fig. 3.66** This T1-weighted coronal MR image shows the normal appearance of the extensor tendon origin (arrow) and the LCL (arrowhead).

▼ **Fig. 3.67** Coronal PD and T2 fat-suppressed MR images demonstrate injury to the common extensor origin (arrow). High signal is present in the tendon substance consistent with oedema and a fluid gap is noted below the origin. The LCL appears normal.

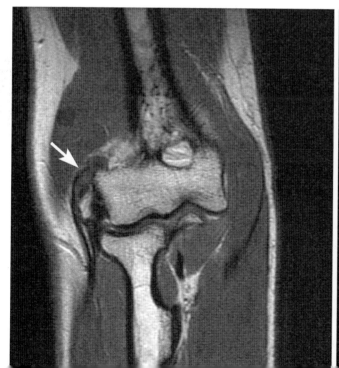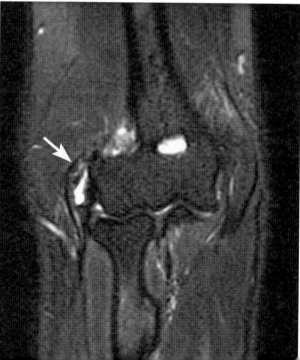

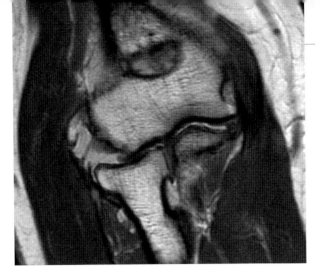

▲ **Fig. 3.68** Injury to both the LCL attachment and the common extensor origin is demonstrated on a coronal PD-weighted MR image. A large fluid gap is shown.

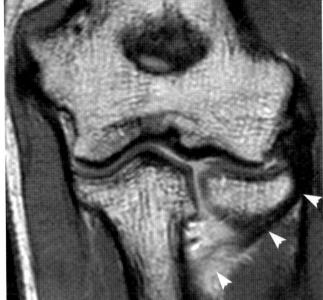

▲ **Fig. 3.69** An MR image of a normal LUCL. The ligament originates at the lateral epicondyle and passes over the annular ligament, and the posterior fibres fan out to insert on the posterior ulna behind the annular ligament (arrowheads).

◀ **Fig. 3.70** The LUCL is well demonstrated by this PD-weighted coronal MR image (arrowheads). There has been injury to the proximal segment of the LUCL with swelling and high signal present (arrow).

▼ **Fig. 3.71** These MR images demonstrate an LCL tear with associated PLRI. The fat-suppressed coronal PD-weighted image (COR) shows fluid signal traversing the normal interface between the epicondyle and the LCL (white arrow), consistent with a proximal avulsion of both the RCL proper and the LUCL. Arrowheads indicate intact distal fibres of the LUCL. Note the irregularity and haemorrhagic hyperintensity of the mid-segment fibres of the LCL and also an accompanying tear of the adjacent common extensor muscle. The sagittal image (SAG) demonstrates a joint space effusion, posterodistal displacement of the torn proximal segment LUCL (black arrow) and perching of the anterior rim of radial head against the capitellum.

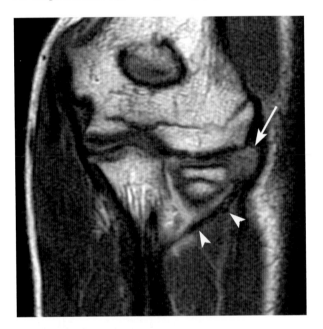

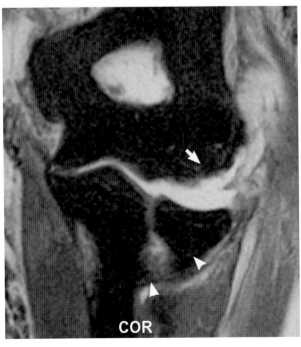

COR

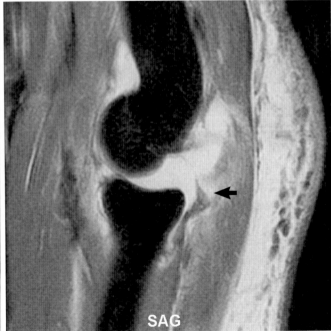

SAG

Tendon injuries at the elbow

Tendon injuries at the elbow include tendon rupture, enthesopathies and tendinopathies.

Rupture of the triceps tendon

Rupture of the triceps tendon is an unusual injury. Anzel et al. (1959) reviewed 1014 tendon injuries treated at the Mayo Clinic: only eight involved the triceps tendon, and four of these were lacerations (Vidal and Allen 2003).

The triceps tendon is usually avulsed from the olecranon and may separate a bony fragment or displace an olecranon apophysis when triceps tendon overload occurs as an acute injury due to powerful extension of the elbow. This is occasionally encountered in throwing, gymnastics, the shot-put, boxing and weightlifting. Intrasubstance ruptures also occur, and muscle tears and musculotendinous junction tears have been described as well (Boucher and Morton 1967). Rupture may also result from indirect trauma occurring due to a fall on the outstretched hand and is seen with chronic overuse as a complication of tendinopathy. The use of anabolic steroids and steroid injections has been implicated as a predisposing factor (Vidal and Allen 2003).

Diagnosis will usually be established by the history and physical examination, although imaging may be useful when the diagnosis is uncertain. Plain films may identify calcific tendinopathy (see Fig. 3.72), bony avulsion (see Fig. 3.73) or disruption of an olecranon apophysis (see Fig. 3.74). Soft-tissue swelling will invariably be present, as was shown in Figure 3.10. Nuclear bone scans are also helpful for diagnosing an enthesopathy at the triceps insertion (see Fig. 3.75).

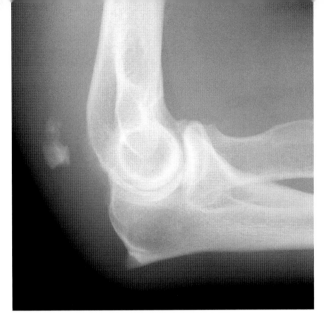

▲ **Fig. 3.73** A plain film shows an avulsion injury of the triceps with separation of a large bony fragment with retraction. Soft-tissue swelling is noted.

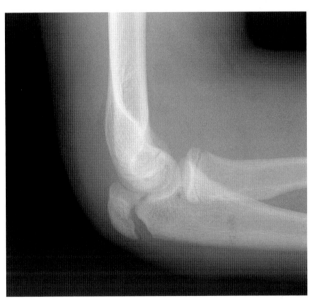

▲ **Fig. 3.74** A violent contraction of the triceps has disrupted the olecranon apophysis in an immature athlete. A fracture extends through the growth plate.

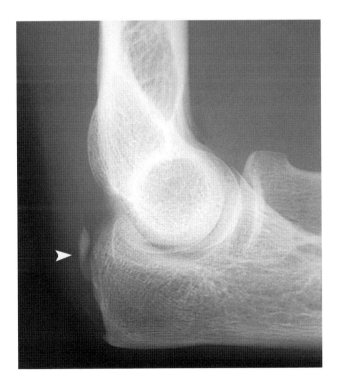

▲ **Fig. 3.72** A lateral plain film of the elbow demonstrates calcification (arrowhead) within the distal triceps tendon indicating calcific tendinopathy.

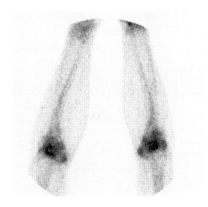

▲ **Fig. 3.75** A nuclear bone scan demonstrates an enthesopathy at the triceps insertion bilaterally, more marked on the left. Mild bilateral medial epicondylitis is also noted.

Triceps tendinopathy, a condition predisposing to a tendon tear, can be imaged using ultrasound (see Fig. 3.76) or MRI. Ultrasound and MRI can accurately identify the site of the injury (see Figs 3.77 and 3.78) and help determine whether the tear is partial or complete (see Fig. 3.79). There is usually tendon retraction if the rupture is complete, and details of the rupture and the degree of retraction can be demonstrated by MRI (see Figs 3.80, 3.81 and 3.82).

Biceps tendinopathy and rupture of the distal biceps tendon

Rupture of the distal biceps tendon is not common, although it is the most common acute tendinous injury around the elbow (Vidal and Allen 2003). The distal biceps tendon passes deep into the antecubital fossa and inserts onto the radial tuberosity. The biceps is the most powerful forearm supinator, increasing its role from 0 to 90° of elbow flexion. The biceps also acts to flex the forearm.

Injury at the biceps insertion characteristically results from hyperextension or repetitive pronation–supination activities. Violent extension or flexion against a heavy weight may also cause a distal triceps avulsion injury with a forceful concentric contraction of the biceps to a flexed supinated forearm. This injury typically occurs in males in their 50s or 60s (Morrey 2000). Seiler et al. (1995) described an area of hypovascularity within the distal tendon and suggested that attrition and rupture occur in this area. The use of anabolic steroids has been implicated as a predisposing factor leading to tendon rupture (Visuri and Lindholm 1994).

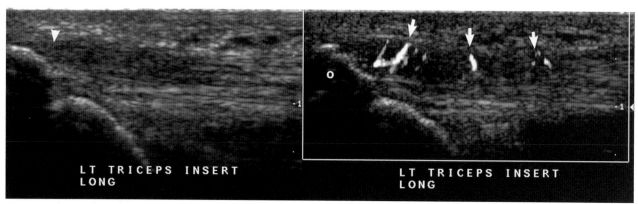

▲ **Fig. 3.76** Ultrasound demonstrates triceps tendinopathy. Long-axis greyscale and Power Doppler images show a strip of hypoechoic thickening and hyperaemia (arrows) along the distal triceps tendon segment (arrowhead). Note the preservation of the underlying fibrillar architecture. The olecranon = o.

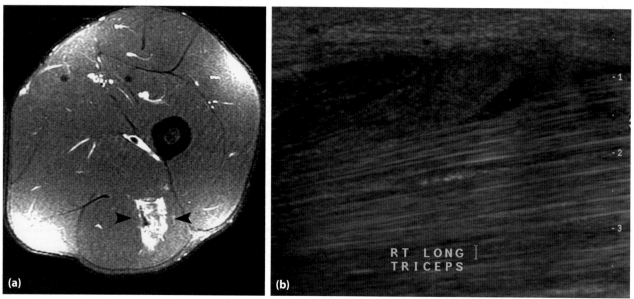

▲ **Fig. 3.77** During a high-bar routine at the Sydney 2000 Olympics, a gymnast suffered a tear in the triceps muscle at the musculotendinous junction. The injury was imaged by **(a)** axial MRI and **(b)** ultrasound.
(a) This axial fat-suppressed MRI image demonstrates a localised tear as an irregular area of high signal surrounding the central cord of the hypointense tendon (arrowheads).
(b) A longitudinal ultrasound image shows swelling and localised separation of the normal myofibrillar pattern by hypoechoic areas of haemorrhage.

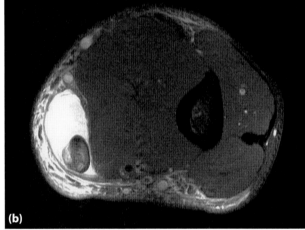

(a)

(b)

◀ **Fig. 3.78** An international rugby player suffered a tear at the musculotendinous junction of the triceps.
(a) This axial T2 fat-suppressed MR image obtained just proximal to the tear shows high signal haemorrhage infiltrating the retracted muscle in a typical feathery pattern and a lax hypointense central tendon.
(b) This axial image obtained immediately distal to the tear defect shows a large fluid space of haematoma with a contained 'bell-clapper' sign of the thickened stump of torn triceps tendon.

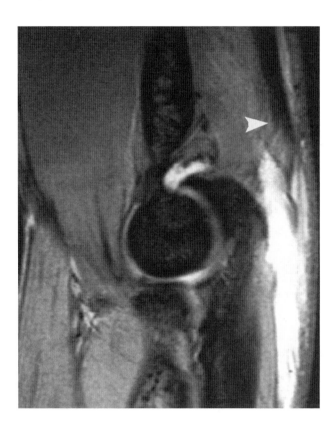

▶ **Fig. 3.79** This MR image shows avulsion of the triceps tendon from its insertion. Slight retraction has occurred (arrowhead). Associated haemorrhage is shown, tracking distally along the dorsal aspect of the elbow olecranon.

▼ **Fig. 3.80** These sagittal PD- and T2*-weighted GRE MR images of the elbow show triceps tendon avulsion and retraction. A component of muscle remains attached (arrowheads), which presumably has limited the degree of tendon retraction.

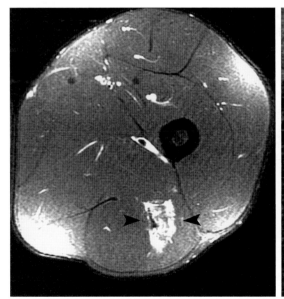

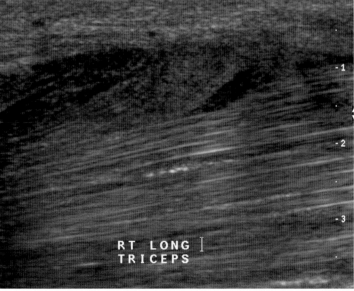

RT LONG
TRICEPS

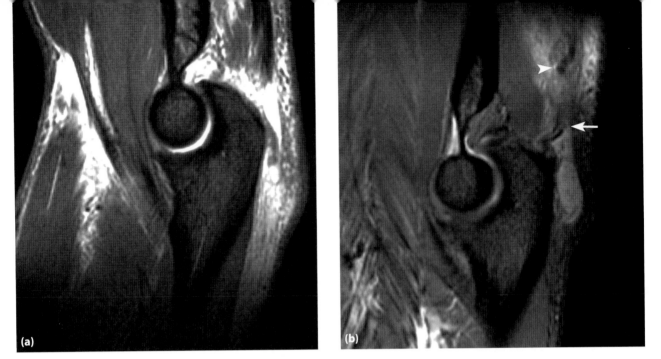

▲ **Fig. 3.81** Both these cases of complete triceps rupture occurred in judo players at the Sydney 2000 Olympics.
(a) This fat-suppressed MR image shows complete triceps avulsion from its insertion on the olecranon. There has been moderate retraction. Considerable bleeding has occurred throughout the surrounding soft tissues, profiling the distal biceps tendon.
(b) A mid-segment triceps tendon rupture is well demonstrated on this fat-suppressed PD-weighted MR image. There is separation of the torn ends. An arrow indicates the torn end of the distal fragment and an arrowhead shows the retracted proximal end.

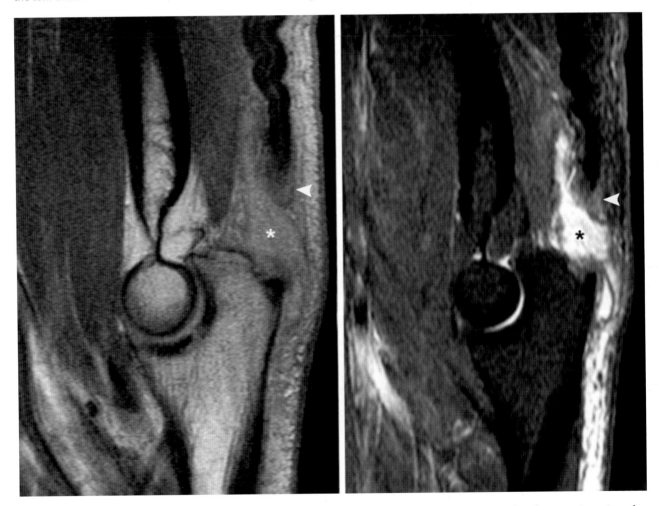

▲ **Fig. 3.82** These MR images demonstrate avulsion of the triceps tendon. Haemorrhage is present at the olecranon insertion of the triceps tendon (asterisk), interrupting tendon continuity. The proximal torn end of the triceps tendon has retracted proximally (arrowhead). The retracted tendon has a buckled appearance.

The diagnosis of distal biceps tendinopathy or partial tendon rupture is largely clinical, although when the findings are unclear, ultrasound (see Fig. 3.83) and MRI (see Fig. 3.84) may be helpful. A nuclear bone scan may be useful for demonstrating enthesopathy at the radial tuberosity (see Fig. 3.85). Sometimes the differentiation between tendinopathy and a partial tear may

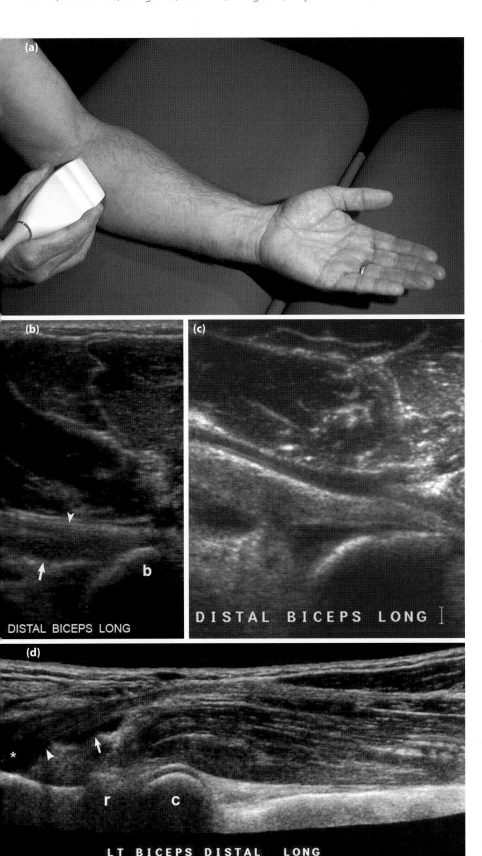

◀ Fig. 3.83(a) The scan technique and transducer position required for the demonstration of the distal biceps tendon is shown. The transducer is positioned at the medial aspect of the elbow to produce a coronal plane of tendon visualisation, while the biceps muscle is contracted, the elbow is flexed to straighten the distal biceps tendon and the forearm is fully supinated.
(b) A long-axis ultrasound image of the distal biceps tendon (arrowheads) has been obtained using the above scan technique, which is designed to straighten the tendon and visualise the radial tuberosity insertion. Note the focal fusiform hypoechoic tendon thickening, which indicates tendinopathy (arrow).
(c) A distal biceps insertional tear is demonstrated by ultrasound. The markedly hypoechoic space at the tendon/bone interface represents haemorrhage at the site of high-grade partial detachment. There is effusion in the bicipitoradial bursa, and the biceps tendon itself is diffusely tendinotic.
(d) Ultrasound demonstrates a partial tear of the distal biceps tendon. The deep fibre component of distal biceps tendon shows an abrupt linear pattern of fibre interruption (arrowhead) with an anechoic or markedly hypoechoic zone of haemorrhage just beyond (asterisk). There is an associated effusion within the bicipitoradial bursa (arrow). Capitellum = c. Radial head = r.

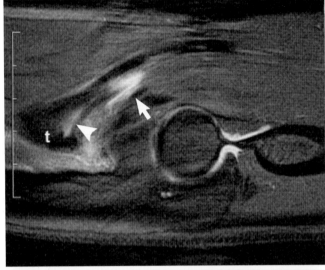

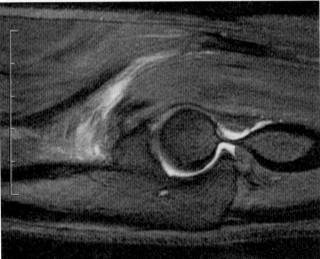

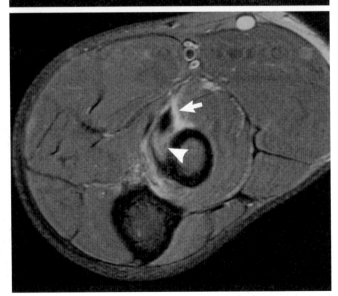

▲ **Fig. 3.84** MRI demonstrates a partial tear of the distal biceps tendon. Fat-suppressed axial and sagittal PD images of the distal biceps tendon show an incomplete pattern of interruption by high signal consistent with a partial tear. There is an associated effusion within the bicipitoradial bursa (arrows). Radial tuberosity attachment of biceps tendon = t.

be difficult. Plain films are of limited value. Spur formation may be present at the radial tuberosity as an indicator of the chronicity of stress, and in one case report (Meherin and Kilgore 1960) avulsion of the tuberosity had occurred. MRI may show high signal at the tuberosity indicative of bone injury (see Fig. 3.86).

A complete tear of the biceps tendon usually occurs at the tendon insertion and is well demonstrated by both ultrasound and MRI (see Fig. 3.87). Occasionally, a tear may occur at the musculotendinous junction.

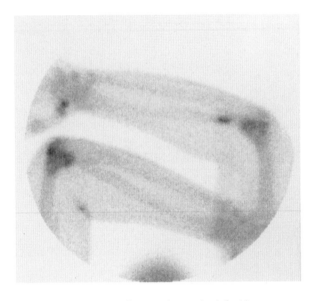

▲ **Fig. 3.85** Biceps enthesopathy on the left side demonstrated by a nuclear bone scan. There is also ulnar impingement on the left.

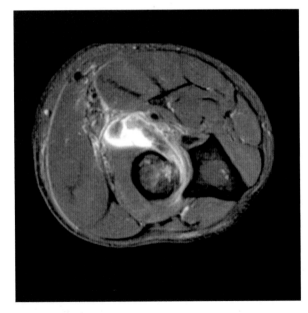

▲ **Fig. 3.86** This axial fat-suppressed MR image of the radial tuberosity shows high signal in the medulla and disruption of the cortex, consistent with a bony avulsion injury.

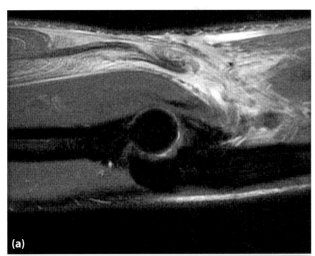

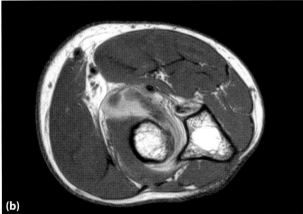

▲ Fig. 3.87 A complete insertional biceps avulsion with retraction is demonstrated by MRI. There is considerable tissue disruption and bleeding. The sagittal image **(a)** is a PD-weighted fat-suppressed image and the lower axial image **(b)** is PD-weighted.

Brachialis injury

Hyperextension forces may produce anterior elbow joint injuries. Hyperextension occurs in the throwing action, racquet sports, cricket (fast bowling), weightlifting and gymnastics. Hyperextension injuries can include tears of the brachialis muscle (see Fig. 3.88) and/or anterior joint capsule tears. Brachialis injury may cause a flexion contracture due to

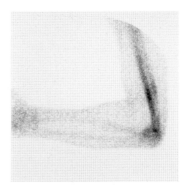

◄ Fig. 3.88 This nuclear bone scan shows considerable enthesopathy at the brachialis origin in an elite tennis player. This change indicates repetitive hyperextension overload.

subsequent fibrosis of the torn capsule. Other hyperextension injuries have been discussed above in the section on valgus extension overload.

Extensor and flexor origin rupture

Separation of the flexor origin may occur following elbow dislocation or violent valgus or force (see Fig. 3.89). Complete avulsion of the common extensor origin is rare because varus forces to the elbow are unusual in sport. Occasionally, a partial tear will occur (see Fig. 3.90).

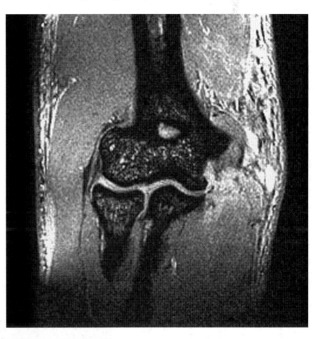

▲ Fig. 3.89 This coronal T2*-weighted MR image demonstrates a full-thickness tear of the common flexor tendon complex at the level of an associated mid-substance rupture of the MCL.

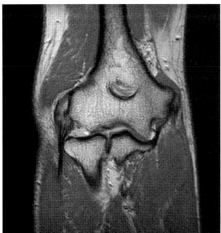 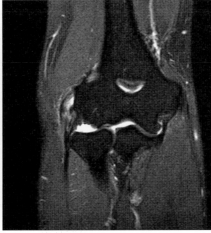

◄ Fig. 3.90 These PD and fat-suppressed coronal PD-weighted MR images demonstrate a high-grade partial tear of the common extensor origin.

Enthesopathies: lateral and medial epicondylitis

Lateral epicondylitis ('tennis elbow')

Clinically the term 'lateral epicondylitis' refers to pain at the common extensor origin on the lateral epicondyle. The pain is exacerbated by wrist extension. This condition is common in athletes besides tennis players and is quite often a work-related condition, where simple tasks may be painful. The process is a degenerative enthesopathy and there may be associated partial or complete tears of the extensor tendon. The ECRB is almost always involved (Kaminsky and Baker 2003). Diagnosis is usually made on clinical grounds, although imaging can play an important role.

Soft-tissue calcification is present in 25% of cases (Nirschl and Pettrone 1979). This calcification can often be seen in an AP view (see Figs 3.91 and 3.92), although it is particularly well shown in the axial view. Spur formation also occurs, indicating the chronic nature of the process (see Fig. 3.93).

Nuclear bone scans are sensitive to changes at the tendon/bone interface and demonstrate these changes best in delayed images (see Fig. 3.94). Ultrasound is also helpful for demonstrating calcification, tendinopathy and tendon tears (see Fig. 3.95). MRI is useful for defining the changes of lateral epicondylitis and tendinopathy in the neighbouring extensor tendon (see Figs 3.96 and 3.97).

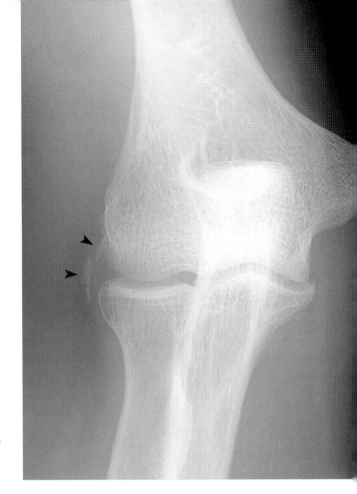

▲ **Fig. 3.91** There is extensive soft-tissue calcification adjacent to the lateral epicondyle (arrowheads). Its position and shape would suggest that this calcification lies in the extensor tendon, indicating calcific tendinopathy.

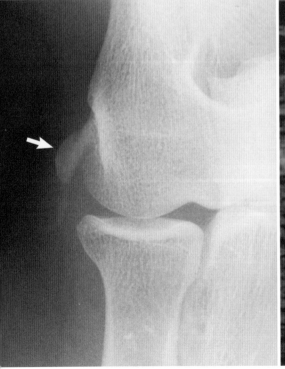

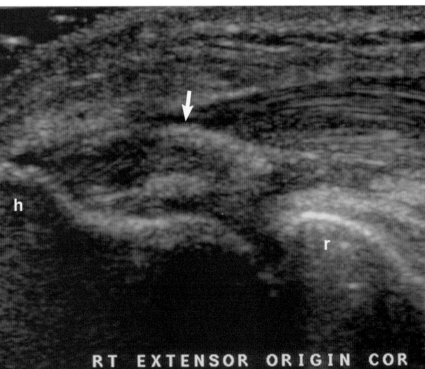

▲ **Fig. 3.92** Common extensor origin calcific tendinopathy imaged by ultrasound. Intrasubstance tendon calcification and ossification (arrows) is demonstrated on both plain x-ray and long-axis ultrasound imaging. Radial head = r. Lateral humeral epicondyle = h.

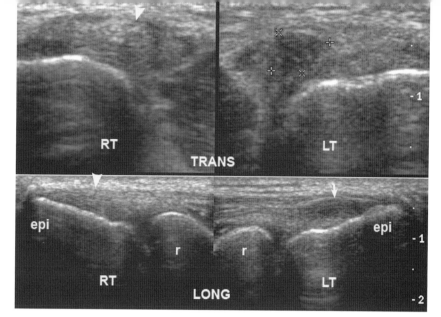

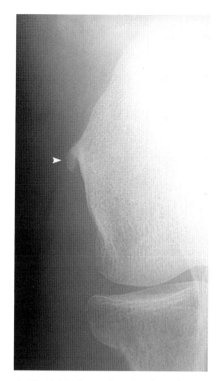

▲ Fig. 3.93 A spur has developed at the lateral humeral epicondyle in response to repetitive traction stress at the extensor origin.

▲ Fig. 3.95(a) Ultrasound demonstrates the changes of lateral humeral epicondylitis. Transverse (TRANS) and long-axis (LONG) views of both common extensor tendon origins demonstrate localised hypoechoic thickening typical of uncomplicated tendinopathy at the left ECRB origin (callipers on the transverse image and arrow on the long-axis image). Note that continuous fibres remain visible through the region of altered echotexture. The normal right ECRB tendon is indicated by the arrowheads. Lateral humeral epicondyle = epi. Radial head = r.

▼ (b) Ultrasound demonstrates lateral humeral epicondylitis with an underlying partial tear of the LCL. Comparative long-axis images of the common extensor tendon origins show a linear fluid gap consistent with a tear involving the proximal fibres of the right LCL (arrows). Note the thickened right common extensor tendon origin. Radial head = r. Lateral humeral epicondyle = h.

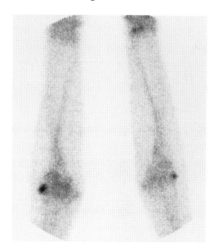

▲ Fig. 3.94 This nuclear bone scan demonstrates bilateral lateral epicondylitis, more marked on the right.

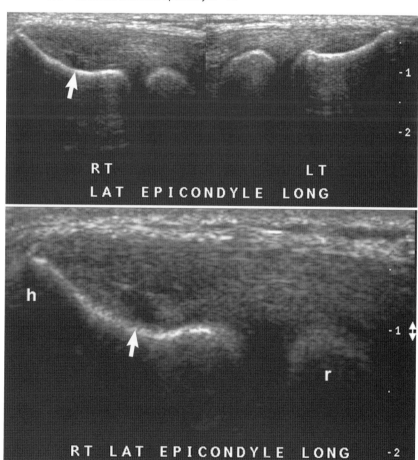

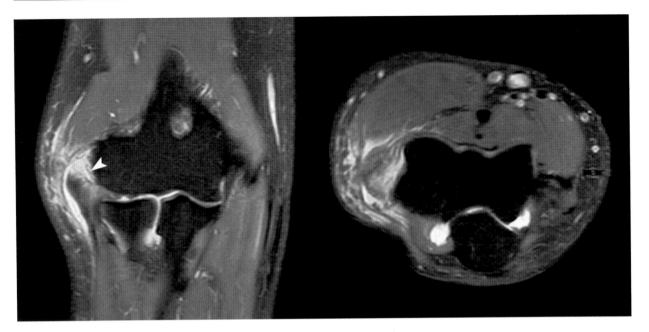

▲ **Fig. 3.96** Fat-suppressed axial and coronal MR images show changes of lateral extensor tendinopathy complicated by a tear. There is high signal at the lateral epicondyle at the bone/tendon interface, swelling of the tendon and a high-signal fluid line indicative of a tear at the extensor origin in the coronal image (arrowhead).

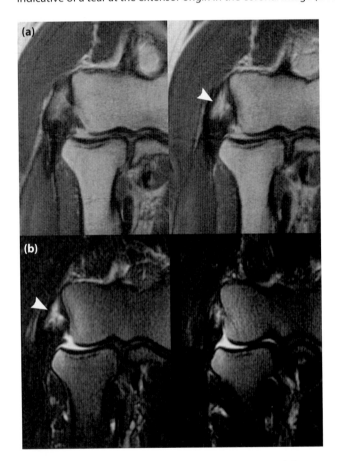

▲ **Fig. 3.97** MRI demonstrates lateral humeral epicondylitis with a complicating large partial tear. Coronal PD **(a)** and corresponding fat-suppressed PD **(b)** images show hyperintense thickening of marked tendinopathy at the common extensor origin with a superimposed high-grade partial tear appreciated as an irregular focus of much more pronounced hyperintensity equivalent to fluid (arrowheads).

Medial epicondylitis ('golfer's elbow')

Medial epicondylitis occurs at the bone/tendon interface at the origins of the flexor-pronator muscle group on the medial epicondyle, and is often associated with tendinopathy in the adjacent flexor tendons. The process is degenerative, with fibrillary degeneration of collagen, angiofibroblastic hyperplasia and fibrinoid necrosis seen pathologically (Teitz et al. 1997).

Clinically, there is increased pain with wrist flexion and forearm pronation. These findings differentiate medial epicondylitis from MCL injury. Medial epicondylitis is considered to be due to overuse, caused by repetitive stress. Although it is referred to as 'golfer's elbow', the condition can result from many sports and activities. In fact, any activity requiring repetitive wrist flexion and forearm pronation may cause medial epicondylitis. Medial epicondylitis may also occur after a single traumatic event (Leach and Miller 1987).

The tendons of the pronator teres and FCR arise from the anterior aspect of the medial epicondyle and are stretched during the acceleration phase of throwing (Ciccotti and Ramani 2003). In sport, the throwing action and the role played by the flexor-pronator muscle group as a secondary restraint against a valgus force is the principle cause of medial epicondylitis. In addition to throwing sports, medial epicondylitis has been reported in golf, tennis, bowling, archery, weightlifting, racquetball and American football. McCarroll (1990) attributed medial epicondylitis in golf to 'hitting from the top', which causes an excessive valgus stress on the dominant elbow. 'Hitting from the top' is a common fault among club golfers in which the club head is accelerated from the top of the backswing rather than through the hitting area.

As with lateral epicondylitis, diagnosis is usually established by the history and physical examination. Imaging may be useful to confirm or exclude the diagnosis in difficult cases and to examine the area for other causes of medial elbow pain.

Plain films have limited application but may demonstrate the presence of calcification and ossification. Calcification is present in 20–25 % of cases (Ciccotti and Ramani 2003). A nuclear bone scan is excellent for the demonstration of enthesopathy and can confirm the clinical suspicion of injury at the bone/tendon interface (see Fig. 3.98). Tendinopathy involving the flexor-pronator origin can be well demonstrated by ultrasound (see Fig. 3.99) and MRI (see Fig. 3.100).

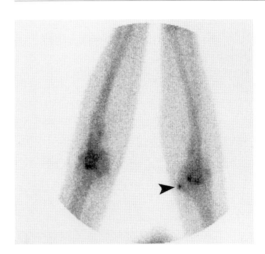

▶ **Fig. 3.98** This nuclear bone scan shows the changes of medial epicondylitis. There is a focal uptake of isotope at the left medial epicondyle (arrowhead).

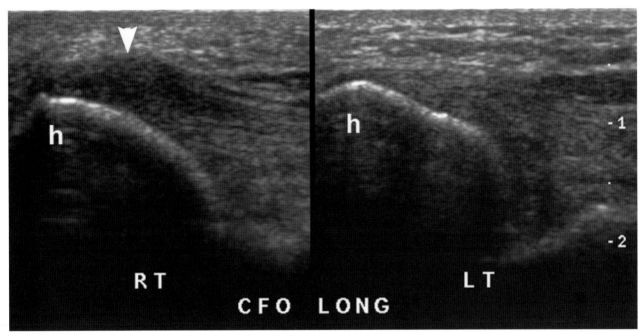

▲ **Fig. 3.99** Ultrasound shows the changes of uncomplicated flexor tendinopathy. Shown are comparative long-axis greyscale images of both common flexor tendon origins. On the abnormal right side there is localised hypoechoic tendon thickening with preservation of underlying fibre continuity (arrowhead). Medial humeral epicondyle = h.

▼ **Fig. 3.100** Coronal PD and fat-suppressed MR images demonstrate tendinopathy with a complicating partial tear at the common flexor origin (arrowhead).

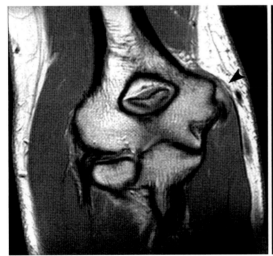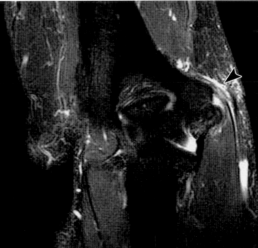

Bursae and ganglia

Olecranon bursopathy (see Fig. 3.101(a)) in a non-traumatic setting does not usually require imaging. The bursa separates the olecranon from the skin surface and may become enlarged with inflammation or infection. However, bursal distension also follows acute trauma and with this presentation a careful radiographic assessment of the olecranon process for fracture is advisable. An ultrasound examination may demonstrate fluid and synovitis within the bursa (see Fig. 3.101(b)). Bursae may be seen elsewhere in the elbow, developing anywhere where two adjacent surfaces move independently (see Fig. 3.102).

Ganglia are also seen around the elbow joint and may form in association with joints or tendon sheaths (see Fig. 3.103).

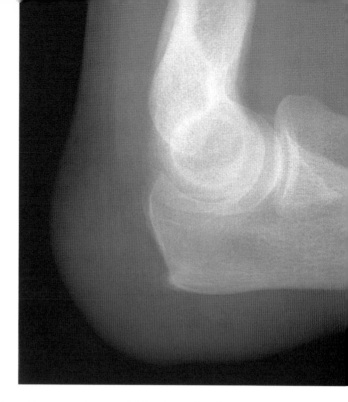

▶ **Fig. 3.101(a)** Olecranon bursopathy is demonstrated on a plain film. There is a large rounded mass at the tip of the elbow, surrounding the olecranon. The mass is not particularly dense and the appearance is typical of olecranon bursopathy.

▼ **(b)** Ultrasound demonstrates olecranon bursopathy. Long-axis and transverse images obtained over the olecranon process show fluid and synovial thickening in the overlying olecranon bursa (arrowheads).

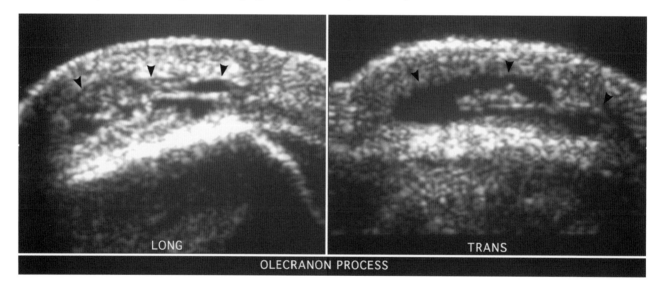

LONG

TRANS

OLECRANON PROCESS

▼ **Fig. 3.102(a)** A bursa adjacent to the distal biceps tendon (bicipitoradial bursa) demonstrated on fat-suppressed MR images. In the sagittal image **(i)**, the bursa appears lobulated and is closely related to the biceps tendon. In the axial image **(ii)**, the bursa partly envelops the tendon.

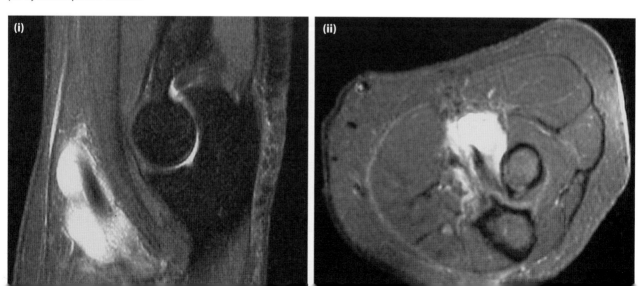

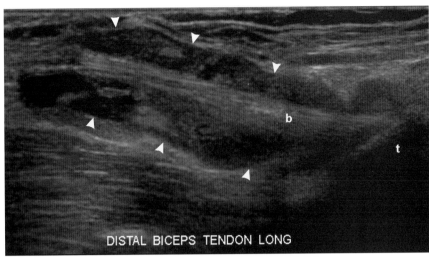
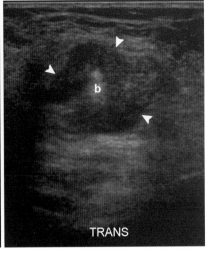

▲ Fig. 3.102(b) Ultrasound demonstrates changes of bursopathy adjacent to the distal biceps tendon. Transverse (TRANS) and long-axis (LONG) ultrasound images show a bicipitoradial bursa markedly distended by a combination of heterogeneously echogenic synovial thickening and effusion (arrowheads). Bursopathy may arise from either repetitive mechanical overload (with or without an underlying distal biceps tendon macro-tear) or an inflammatory arthritis such as rheumatoid arthritis (RA). In this case, the particularly marked degree of synovial proliferation would favour an inflammatory arthritis. Distal biceps tendon = b. Radial tuberosity = t.

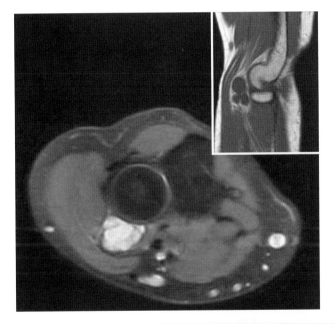

◄ Fig. 3.103 A loculated ganglion is demonstrated on sagittal T1 and axial fat-suppressed MRI images. The ganglion lies on the anterior aspect of the elbow (insert) and has a broad base against the annular ligament. It is possible that the ganglion has developed as a result of injury to the annular ligament.

Lateral synovial fringe syndrome

Lateral synovial fringe syndrome is due to the presence of a meniscus-like structure within the lateral aspect of the elbow (see Fig. 3.104). The presence of this synovial structure is often clinically silent but can occasionally produce symptoms of anterolateral elbow pain, stiffness, locking, popping or catching (Rosenberg et al. 1998).

► Fig. 3.104 PD-weighted coronal and sagittal MR images demonstrate a prominent or thickened lateral synovial fringe (arrowheads).

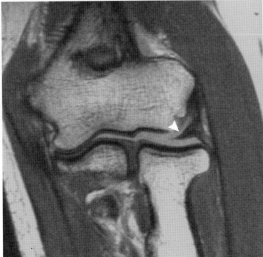
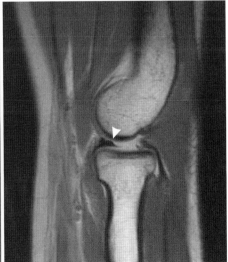

The immature elbow

Today, an increasing number of children are participating in organised sport, so elbow injuries in immature athletes are seen more commonly. Traditionally, children used to play all types of sports, but now there is a trend towards children being encouraged to participate in just one sport, resulting in an increasing number of injuries from overuse.

Although the biomechanics of injury are similar in immature and adult athletes, immature athletes have a different pattern of injury due to the presence of epiphyses, apophyses and growth plates. The changing strengths of the skeleton produce different patterns of injury from a particular force and alter with development.

Imaging immature elbow injuries

Imaging begins with plain films. The majority of changes are adequately demonstrated on a high-quality series, although it is conceded that it is not always possible to obtain technically perfect films of immature patients who are in pain.

Bone scans are sometimes difficult to interpret in children because the increased uptake in the numerous growth plates obscures the pathological details (Cooper et al. 2003). Nevertheless, bone scans play an important role in detecting injuries (some of which may be unexpected: see Fig. 3.105), especially considering that the history and physical examination are difficult and sometimes impossible. Bone scans are particularly helpful in the diagnosis of occult bone injury and OCD. With OCD, a 'cold' area in the capitellum is thought to be a poor prognostic sign.

Ultrasound has a role in examining soft tissues including cartilage and is particularly useful in examining the immature elbow. MRI is also useful in evaluating injuries, particularly if soft tissues are involved. MRI is a valuable method of assessing damage to articular cartilage and imaging bone stress and avascular changes in the capitellum.

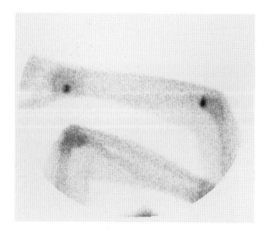

▲ **Fig. 3.105** A nuclear bone scan will show unexpected findings, especially in the paediatric population where the history and physical examination are difficult. An elbow scan will include the wrist and, in this case, the reason for this is well demonstrated. There is a fracture of the radial head and an unexpected fracture of the scaphoid.

Tips on looking at plain films of immature athletes

The developing elbow

Pappas (1982) suggested that elbow injury patterns relate to three stages of development:

- In childhood, prior to fusion of the secondary ossification centres, repetitive trauma can produce epiphyseal irregularity and fragmentation. This stage is completed with the appearance of all the secondary ossification centres.
- In adolescence, the increased physical strength of the young athlete can produce epiphyseal avulsions, particularly of the medial epicondyle, and AVN of the capitellum. This stage ends when the secondary ossification centres are fused.
- In adults, with completion of muscular development and epiphyseal fusion, musculotendinous injuries and avulsion fractures occur.

So, interpreting the plain films of an immature athlete begins with an assessment of the patient's age and stage of development. Ageing the elbow is not difficult. The most difficult decision involves working out whether there has been displacement of the secondary ossification centres, and comparison views of the non-injured elbow are often helpful if a slight epiphyseal or apophyseal displacement is suspected.

The condyles and epicondyles are cartilaginous at birth and the secondary ossification centres appear in a predictable sequence, as follows:

Centre	Age
Capitellum	1–2 years
Radial head	3 years
Medial epicondyle	5 years
Trochlea	7 years
Olecranon	9 years
Lateral epicondyle	10–11 years

Note that the centres appear roughly two years apart.

Important bony alignments that should be checked

There are two alignments that should be assessed in the immature elbow following trauma:

- A line drawn along the long axis of the radius must pass through the capitellar epiphysis irrespective of the projection (see Fig. 3.106). This is the *radiocapitellar alignment*. Anterior dislocation of the radial head may occur with forceful hyperextension and supination (Bonatus et al. 1995) or forceful flexion and supination of the elbow, and is diagnosed on plain films by loss of normal radiocapitellar alignment (see Fig. 3.107).

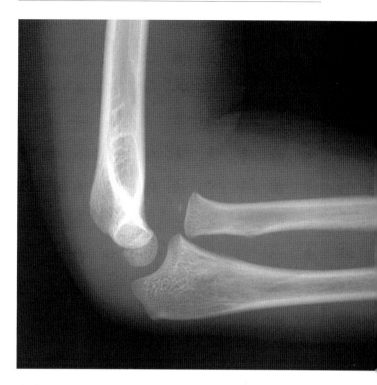

▲ **Fig. 3.107** The diagnosis of dislocation of the radial head depends on identifying loss of the normal radiocapitellar alignment.

▼ **Fig. 3.108** A line drawn along the anterior cortex of the humerus should pass through the middle third of the capitellar epiphysis.

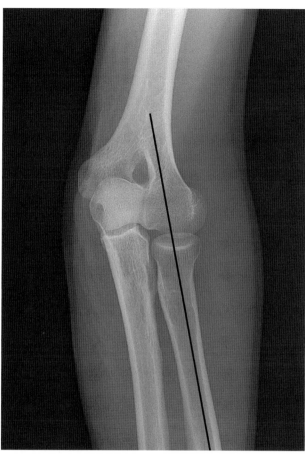

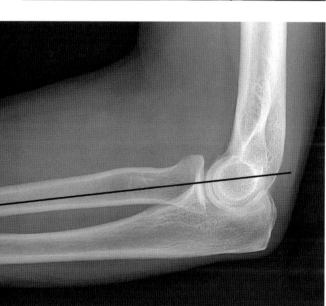

▲ **Fig. 3.106** In a normal elbow, a line drawn along the long axis of the radius in all views should pass through the capitellar epiphysis.

- A line drawn along the anterior cortex of the humerus must pass through the middle third of the capitellar epiphysis, remembering that there is a normal volar angulation of the capitellum of about 45° from the longitudinal axis of the humeral shaft (see Fig. 3.108). This is the *humero-capitellar alignment*.

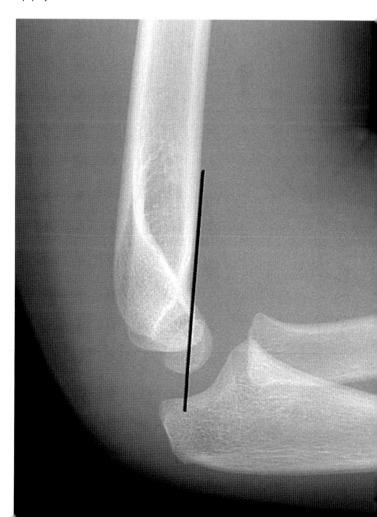

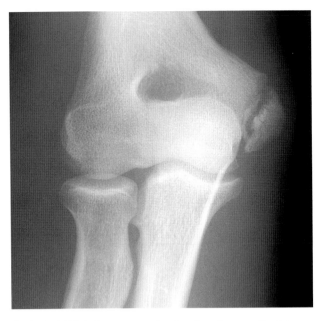

▲ **Fig. 3.109(a)** A stress reaction involves the growth plate of the medial epicondylar apophysis with minor apophyseal displacement. The reaction is characterised by the irregular widening of the growth plate.

▼ **(b)** Repetitive stress has caused a fragment to be separated from the medial epicondylar apophysis.

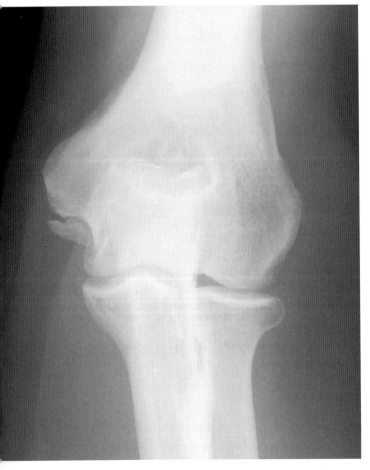

▶ **Fig. 3.110** Avulsion of the medial epicondylar apophysis has occurred as a result of violent traction by the MCL or the flexor-pronator muscle group.

Sporting injuries

Repetitive micro-trauma is now the most common cause of elbow injury in young athletes (Hughes and Paletta 2003). The major contributors to repetitive overuse injury are throwing sports (Larson et al. 1976), racquet sports (Hutchison et al. 1995) and gymnastics (Jackson et al. 1989). Injuries in these sports may also occur following a single trauma.

'Little leaguer's elbow' has become a generic term covering all throwing injuries in young athletes. The biomechanics of the throwing action is the same as in adults and consequently the injury pattern involves medial, lateral and posterior structures (Hughes and Paletta 2003).

On the medial side of the elbow, traction injury in immature athletes is most likely to produce injury to the epiphyses, apophyses and growth plates. MCL rupture is uncommon, with the likelihood of ligament injury increasing with muscular development. The occurrence of bone stress is also related to strength.

A number of different injuries are produced by repetitive stress to the medial epicondylar apophysis. A stress reaction may involve irregular widening of the growth plate with associated slight displacement of the apophysis. This reaction is related to delayed closure of the growth plate. In addition, repetitive stress may cause the apophysis itself to become fragmented and deformed (see Fig. 3.109). A secondary outcome of this trauma during development is hypertrophy of the medial condyle when the adult matures. This is presumably due to increased vascularity. An example of this has been seen in Figure 3.33. Avulsion of the medial epicondylar apophysis may occur as a result of a single violent valgus force superimposed on chronic changes or a powerful flexor-pronator contraction (see Fig. 3.110). Minor degrees of avulsion and rotation of the apophysis may be subtle and often require comparative views of the asymptomatic side for confirmation. Less commonly, a fracture of the apophysis may occur (see Fig. 3.111). MCL rupture is uncommon, although occasionally this occurs in adolescent athletes (see Fig. 3.112), and with increased strength bone stress may be demonstrated by a nuclear bone scan or MRI (see Fig. 3.113).

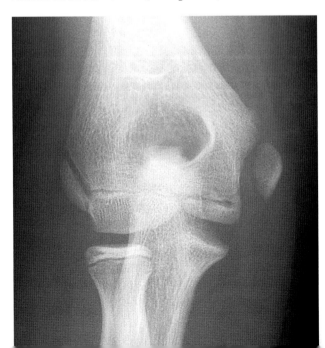

▶ Fig. 3.111 A violent valgus force on the medial epicondylar apophysis produced by the MCL or a flexor-pronator muscle contraction has caused avulsion of the apophysis and produced a fracture across the apophysis with moderate displacement of the fragments.

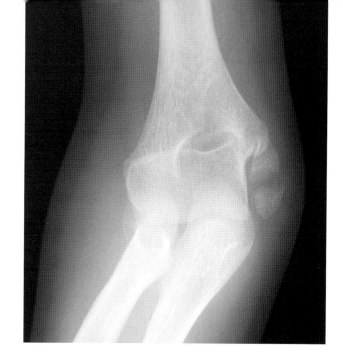

▼ Fig. 3.112 MR images demonstrate an acute MCL and flexor muscle tear in a 16-year-old athlete. Coronal PD (top) and corresponding fat-suppressed PD (bottom) images show complete detachment of the MCL from the medial epicondyle (displaced proximal end of ligament indicated by arrow). There has also been injury to the adjacent flexor muscle, which shows extensive high signal indicating oedema (asterisk). Note that the common flexor tendon appears intact (arrowhead).

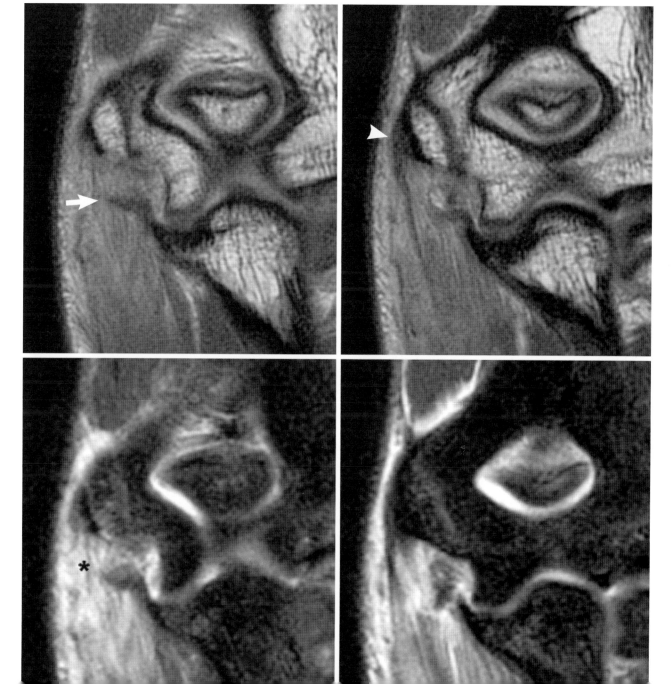

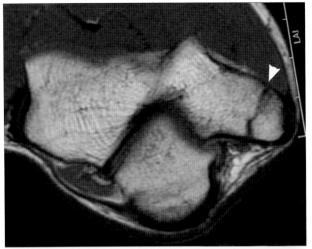

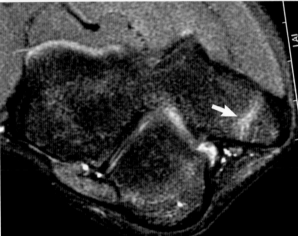

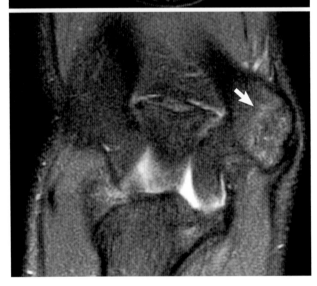

▲ **Fig. 3.113** A stress reaction at the growth plate of the epicondylar apophysis and bone stress involving the apophysis demonstrated by MRI. Coronal PD (top) and corresponding fat-suppressed axial PD (middle) and coronal (bottom) images of the medial humeral epicondyle show a band of bone marrow oedema (arrows) associated with a non-disrupted growth plate (arrowhead).

Lateral compressive forces produce injury more commonly in the immature elbow than in its adult counterpart. The most common changes occur in the capitellum as the result of repetitive compressive forces and include Panner's disease and OCD.

Panner's disease results from lateral compressive forces in children younger than 10 or 11 years old. Panner's disease is an osteochondrosis involving the capitellar epiphysis. The exact cause of the process is unknown. The athlete presents with lateral-side pain. Degeneration of the articular cartilage of the capitellum is followed by subchondral bony changes (see Fig. 3.114). In some cases, the bony changes may progress to involve the entire epiphysis, with disordered ossification and necrosis of the capitellum (see Fig. 3.115). This dramatic change is then followed by regeneration, which may take up to three years to become radiologically healed (Hughes and Paletta 2003).

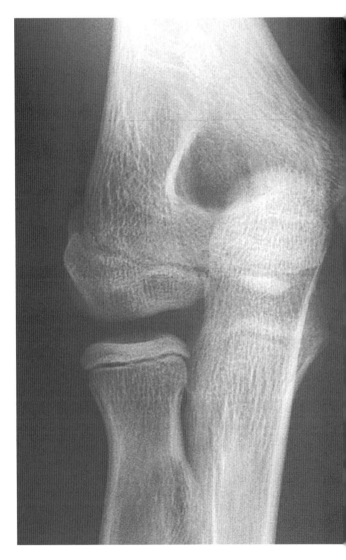

▲ **Fig. 3.114** This patient has extensive areas of demineralisation. The patient's age would suggest that this process is more likely to be OCD rather than Panner's disease, although it is possible that the appearance is that of resolving Panner's disease.

▶ **Fig. 3.115** This immature athlete is about 6 or 7 years old. The centres for the trochlea and olecranon have not yet appeared.
(a) An initial plain film study dated 25 July 2002 shows slight widening and irregularity of the growth plate of the capitellum, consistent with a stress reaction. The trabecular pattern of the capitellum appears normal. An effusion is noted.
(b) By 15 October 2002, the changes in the growth plate are less marked, but the normal trabecular pattern of the capitellum seen on 25 July has been replaced by a coarse pattern of patchy sclerosis and demineralisation, through which irregular linear clefts pass, indicating fragmentation. The entire epiphysis is involved and the appearance is that of Panner's disease. An effusion persists. These changes will almost certainly resolve and become normal without the production of loose bodies.

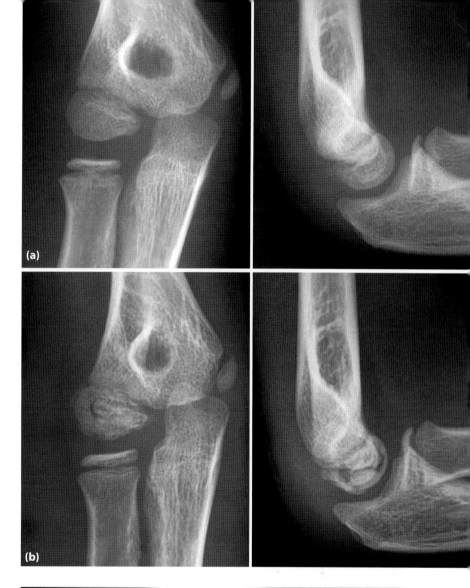

Throwing athletes and female gymnasts have the highest risk of developing OCD of the capitellum (Hughes and Paletta 2003), occurring in children over the age of ten and adolescents. In gymnastics, the weightbearing function of the elbow produces micro-trauma to the capitellum. Radiologically, the process behaves like an avascular process, beginning with subchondral demineralisation (see Fig. 3.116) and progressing to sclerosis and fragmentation (see Fig. 3.117) with the production of loose bodies (Woodward and Blanco 1975) (see Fig. 3.118). Research by Haraldsson (1959) has also suggested that OCD is the result of an avascular process, the most likely cause being repetitive micro-trauma produced by compression and impaction by the radial head. This repetitive trauma may cause overgrowth and deformity of the radial head (see Fig. 3.119(a)). Rarely, a stress fracture of the radial head or neck may develop (see Fig. 3.119(b)). A stress reaction may also develop in the capitellar growth plate (see Fig. 119(c)).

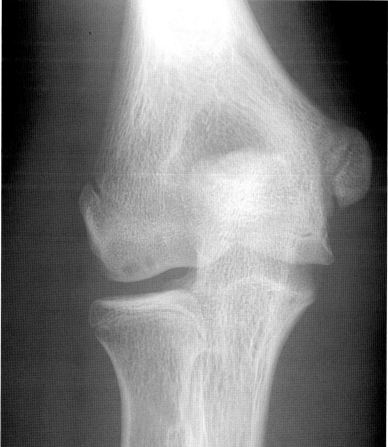

▶ **Fig. 3.116** A plain film shows the early subchondral changes of OCD. No sclerosis or fragmentation has occurred. The medial epicondylar apophysis is deformed and the head of the radius is prominent, consistent with thrower's elbow.

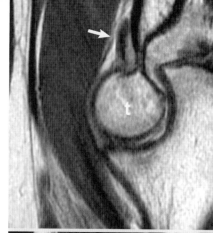

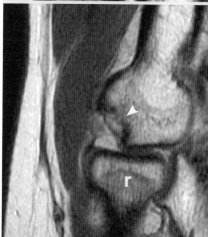

▶ **Fig. 3.117** MR images demonstrate capitellar OCD. Sagittal PD (top and middle) and fat-suppressed coronal PD (bottom) images demonstrate an osteochondral defect in the capitellum (arrowheads). A displaced osteochondral fragment lies within the coronoid fossa (arrow). Trochlea = t. Radial head = r.

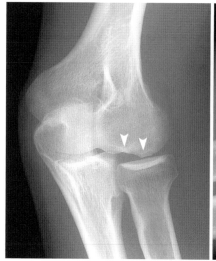

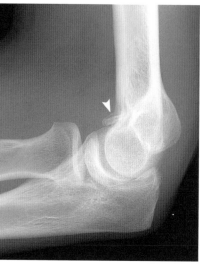

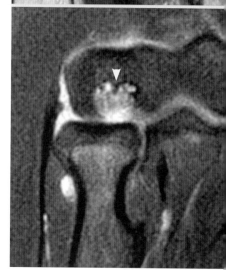

▲ **Fig. 3.118** Late-stage OCD shows a healed deformity of the capitellar articular surface and a loose body lying within the coronoid fossa.

▼ **Fig. 3.119(a)** In the developing skeleton, repetitive abutment of the radial head on the capitellum may produce overgrowth of the radial head, as shown here. Also note the deformity of the medial epicondylar apophysis.
(b) A stress fracture has developed in the radial neck as a result of repetitive radiocapitellar trauma in a junior elite tennis player.
(c) Repetitive impaction has caused a stress reaction in the growth plate of the capitellum. A bifid proximal radial epiphysis is also noted.

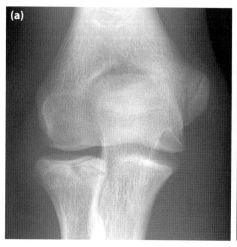

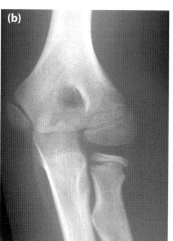

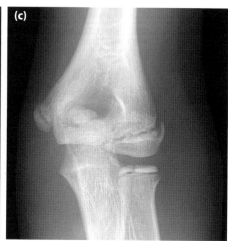

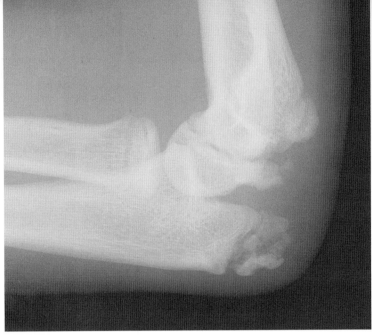
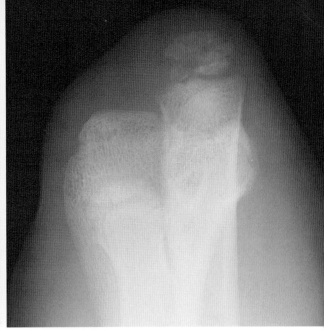

▲ **Fig. 3.120** Osteochondrosis of the olecranon apophysis with significant fragmentation. Deformity of the trochlear epiphysis is also noted. This will almost certainly lead to considerable hypertrophy of the olecranon process.

There are important differences between Panner's disease and OCD and recognition of these differences is important. In addition to different age groups being involved, in Panner's disease the entire ossification centre of the capitellum may be involved, although the anterior central area is most commonly affected. There is no associated loose body formation. However, the most important difference is that in Panner's disease the process is self-limited and the capitellar epiphysis will return to normal.

Posterior shear and traction injuries in immature athletes include osteochondrosis of the olecranon apophysis (see Fig. 3.120), which may result in hypertrophy of the olecranon. Fragmentation (see Fig. 3.121), delayed union and underdevelopment of the olecranon apophysis also occur (see Fig. 3.122).

▼ **Fig. 3.121** Underdevelopment and fragmentation of the olecranon apophysis, resulting from valgus extension overload.

▼ **Fig. 3.122** Occasionally, underdevelopment of the olecranon apophysis will be associated with delayed union.

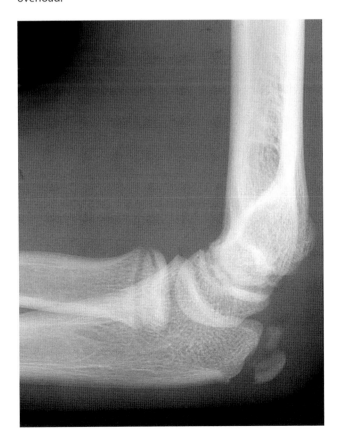
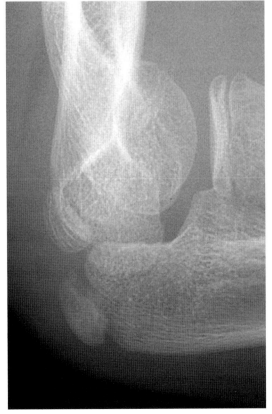

Paediatric elbow fractures

Fractures of the elbow occur more commonly in children than in adults. Elbow fractures vary in complexity from simple undisplaced low-energy fractures to complex high-energy injuries where the fracture is associated with injury to soft tissues, producing neurovascular and ligamentous problems. The most common elbow fracture is a supracondylar fracture of the humerus (see Fig. 3.123), which accounts for 60% of all paediatric elbow fractures and occurs most often between the ages of five and ten (Bartlett 2000). Complications are related to displacement at the fracture site. There is an increased likelihood of nerve injury if displacement of 90% or more of the shaft diameter has occurred (Kiyoshige 2000).

Radiologically, disruption of the distal humeral growth plate is difficult to identify. The key to making the diagnosis is that the capitellum maintains its relationship to the radial head but is displaced in its relationship to the humeral shaft (see Fig. 3.124).

Fractures of the lateral humeral condyle (see Fig. 3.125) account for 17% of paediatric elbow fractures, whereas fractures of the medial condyle account for only 2% and are difficult to diagnose because the trochlea is not visualised until 9 or 10 years of age (Bartlett 2000). Medial epicondylar fractures account for 17% of fractures in patients between the ages of five and 17.

Fractures of the radial neck and head usually result from a fall on the outstretched hand, make up 4–16% of elbow fractures and most commonly involve the proximal radial growth plate (Leung and Peterson 2000). These fractures rarely involve the articular surface of the radial head. Fractures of the olecranon are uncommon in children and are usually undisplaced. However, when they do occur, there is an associated elbow injury present in 77% of cases (Lins et al. 1999).

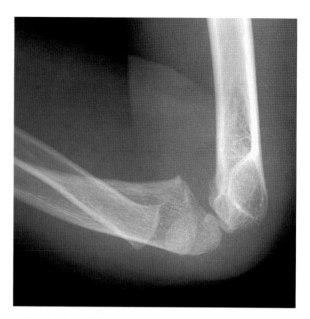

▲ **Fig. 3.124** With traumatic disruption of the distal humeral growth plate, the relationship of the radial head to the capitellum is maintained with displacement of the capitellum.

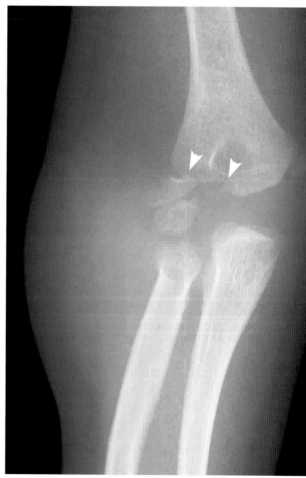

▲ **Fig. 3.125** A fracture involving the lateral condyle with displacement. This is a relatively common paediatric fracture.

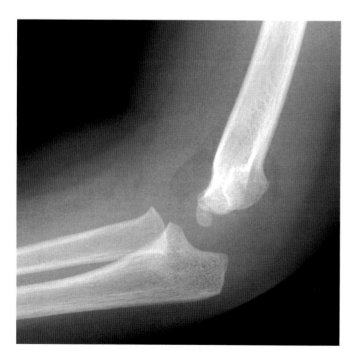

▲ **Fig. 3.123** A supracondylar fracture is the most common elbow fracture in children. In this case, the deformity is obvious. In more subtle cases an abnormality of the humerocapitellar alignment and an effusion provide valuable evidence of a supracondylar fracture.

Common tunnel syndromes at the elbow

The radial, median and ulnar nerves are each vulnerable to compression as they pass through their respective myofascial or fibro-osseous tunnels.

Supinator syndrome

The deep motor (posterior interosseous) branch of the radial nerve may be compressed as it passes beneath the tendinous arch of the superficial layer of the supinator muscle (arcade of Frohse) and between the two layers of the supinator muscle (see Fig. 3.126). This is known as supinator syndrome, posterior interosseous nerve entrapment or radial tunnel syndrome. It produces deep pain at the dorsal aspect of the forearm and localised tenderness to palpation just anterodistal to the lateral humeral epicondyle. There is then a gradual onset of weakness of extension of the fingers, thumb or wrist. There is no sensory disturbance. Consequently, this syndrome will initially have many similarities to lateral epicondylitis, which in some patients may coexist.

Supinator syndrome has a variety of causes, including supinator muscle hypertrophy following overuse in a number of sports, such as tennis (see Fig. 3.127), golf, rowing, swimming and weightlifting (Chumbley et al. 2000). Other causes include mass lesions such as a neuroma, ganglion cysts (see Fig. 3.128), lipomata (see Fig. 3.129) and general trauma with radial subluxation or a Monteggia fracture.

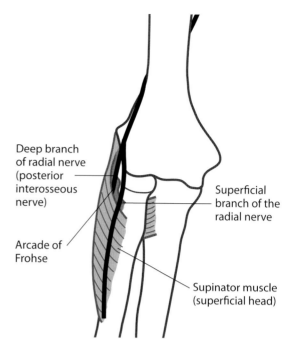

▲ Fig. 3.126 Radial nerve anatomy at the elbow is demonstrated by line drawing, showing the deep branch of the radial nerve entering the Arcade of Frohse.

▶ **Fig. 3.127** A right-handed tennis player presented with chronic right-sided lateral elbow pain and increasing finger weakness. Long-axis ultrasound images of both posterior interosseous nerves have been obtained at the radial neck level. The right posterior interosseous nerve shows subtle hypoechoic swelling at the entrance to the supinator tunnel (arrow) compared with the normal left side (arrowhead). On the right side, note that functional hypertrophy of the right supinator muscle has developed, causing supinator syndrome. Supinator muscle = s. Radial head = r. Callipers indicate posterior interosseous nerve.

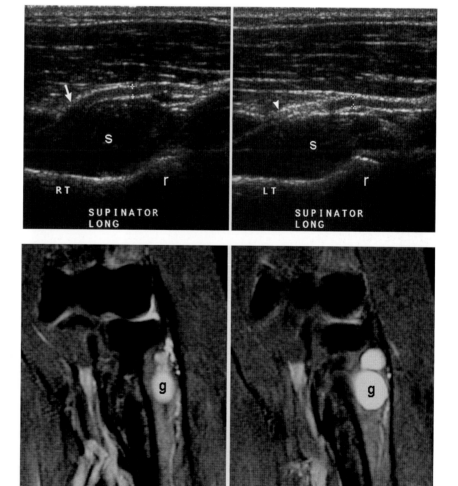

▶ **Fig. 3.128** These coronal PD fat-suppressed MR images show a deep ganglion cyst (g) over the anterior aspect of the supinator muscle. The ganglion was causing symptoms of supinator syndrome.

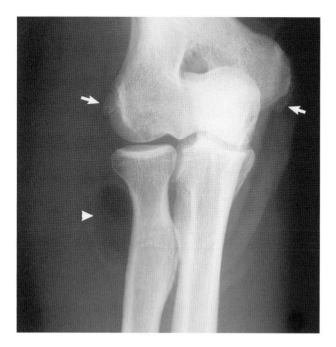

▲ Fig. 3.129 An intramuscular supinator lipoma responsible for supinator syndrome is demonstrated in a patient presenting with lateral elbow pain (arrowhead). Also note the presence of both medial and lateral humeral epicondylar soft-tissue ossifications (arrows), indicative of chronic epicondylitis. Lateral epicondylitis and supinator syndrome can sometimes coexist, a situation that may result in treatment failure if both problems are not recognised and addressed.

▶ Fig. 3.130 Median nerve anatomy at the elbow is demonstrated by line drawing. Note the median nerve passing between the humeral and ulnar heads of the pronator teres muscle.

Pronator syndrome

The median nerve may be compressed as it passes between the humeral and ulnar heads of pronator teres muscle, causing deep pain at the volar aspect of the forearm (see Fig. 3.130). This is known as pronator syndrome, anterior interosseous nerve entrapment or Kiloh-Nevin syndrome. A Tinel or Phalen sign is positive at the proximal forearm, and there are sensory disturbances in the thumb and radial-side two and a half digits and weakness of the thenar muscles. Importantly, sensory changes involve the palm (a useful differentiator from carpal tunnel syndrome). Causes include hypertrophy of the pronator teres muscle, a fibrous band of an accessory bicipital aponeurosis, a scarred lacertus fibrosis, a compressive tendinous arch of

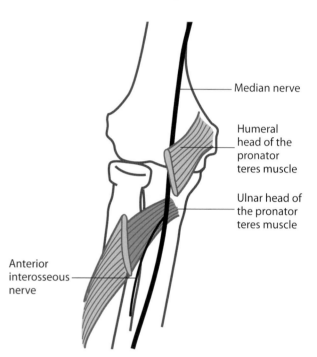

▼ Fig. 3.131 This long-axis ultrasound image shows fusiform hypoechoic thickening of the right median nerve (arrowhead) at the level of the pronator teres muscle (PT) compared with the normal left median nerve (arrow). Flexor digitorum profundus muscle = fdp.

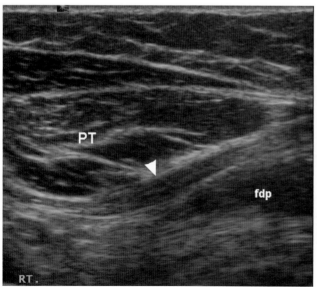
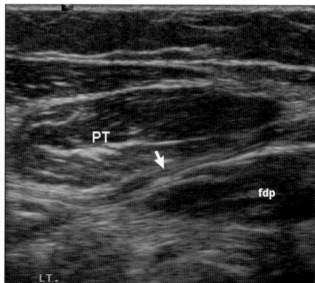

FDS and trauma leading to Volkmann's contracture (see Fig. 3.131). Overuse may occur in racquet and throwing sports (Chumbley et al. 2000). The differential diagnosis of median nerve entrapment secondary to a supracondylar process of the humerus and associated ligament of Struthers should also be remembered.

The anterior interosseous nerve branches from the median nerve trunk either within or just distal to the pronator teres tunnel. Compression of this purely motor nerve, often beneath the proximal tendinous arch of the FDS, produces a characteristic inability to pinch with the tips of the thumb and index finger. Pronator syndrome may occur together with median nerve entrapment within the pronator teres tunnel and some authors therefore regard it to be the same as pronator teres syndrome (Pecina et al. 1991).

Cubital tunnel syndrome

The ulnar nerve may be compressed beneath the tendinous arch (the arcuate ligament) connecting the humeral and ulnar heads of the FCU muscle as it leaves the cubital tunnel (see Fig. 3.132). This is known as cubital tunnel syndrome, flexor carpi ulnaris syndrome or sulcus ulnaris syndrome. Compression of the ulnar nerve at the elbow causes deep pain over the cubital tunnel region or forearm and sensory disturbance along the ulnar border of the hand and ulnar-side one and a half digits. Eventually, wasting or weakness of the intrinsic muscles of the hand will develop. There may be ulnar nerve tenderness and a positive Tinel's sign either within or just distal to the cubital tunnel.

Elbow flexion tenses the arcuate ligament and in turn compresses the ulnar nerve. Thus, individuals who work or sleep with their elbows flexed for many hours are at risk of cubital tunnel syndrome. Alternatively, the ulnar nerve may be compressed, or 'friction neuritis' may occur within the fibro-osseous cubital tunnel. Compression can be caused by a variety of factors including elbow joint osteophytes, loose bodies, proliferative synovitis and thickening of the cubital tunnel retinaculum, which dynamically compresses the nerve during elbow flexion. Other causes of nerve compression include thickening of the MCL, hypertrophy of an accessory anconeus muscle (see Fig. 3.133), ganglion cysts and other mass lesions.

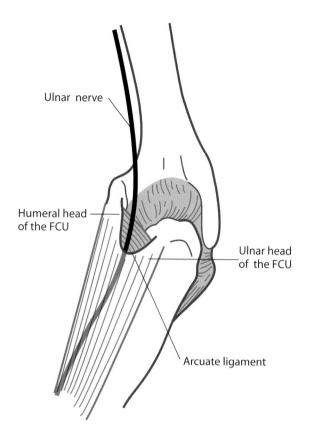

▲ **Fig. 3.132** A line drawing demonstrates ulnar nerve anatomy at the elbow. The ulnar nerve is shown to pass beneath the tendinous arch between the humeral and ulnar heads of the FCU muscle, as it leaves the cubital tunnel.

▼ **Fig. 3.133** These axial TI and fat-suppressed MR images demonstrate the presence of an anconeus epitrochlearis muscle (arrowheads). Although this accessory muscle is small, the relationship between this accessory muscle and the ulnar nerve (arrow) is well shown, with the nerve compressed against the medial humeral condyle. It is easy to imagine that hypertrophy of this accessory muscle would produce an ulnar neuropathy.

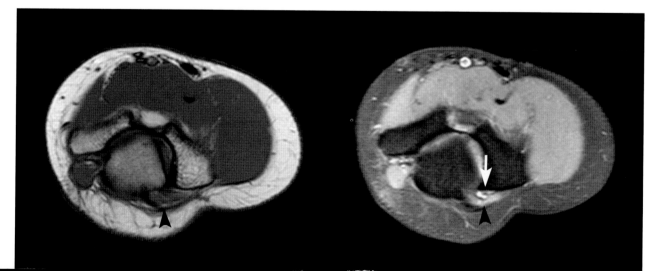

Congenital absence of the cubital tunnel retinaculum occurs in 10% of the population and is associated with anterior subluxation or dislocation of the ulnar nerve over the medial epicondyle during elbow flexion. With elbow flexion, as subluxation or dislocation of the ulnar nerve occurs, a 'snapping' sensation is experienced, often accompanied by an ulnar neuropathy (Fritz 1997).

Dislocation or subluxation of the ulnar nerve is sometimes associated with dislocation ('snapping') of the medial head of the triceps. This condition is associated with muscle hypertrophy, as occurs with body building and weightlifting. Snapping of the triceps occurs as the medial head of the triceps passes over the medial humeral epicondyle, producing a double-click. The diagnosis of dislocation of the medial head of the triceps can be made clinically and confirmed by ultrasound (Spinner and Golder 1998). The double-click distinguishes a snapping triceps from dislocation of the ulnar nerve occurring in isolation (which produces a single-click). Clinically, flexion greater than 100° against a resistance will reproduce medial elbow pain caused by the dislocation,

the double-click, and may produce ulnar neuropathy when the snapping triceps is associated with ulnar nerve dislocation. Dynamic ultrasound is performed with the elbow fully flexed and extended passively, actively and actively against a resistance (Jacobson et al. 2001).

Routine imaging of the forearm

The most common forearm injury in sport is an acute fracture caused by either a direct blow or an axial force resulting from a fall on the outstretched hand. Stress fractures have also been described involving the ulna in softball pitchers, tennis players and volleyball players. Repetitive torsion appears to be responsible for these stress fractures.

A routine series of films includes an AP view and a lateral view (see Fig. 3.134). Both views include the elbow and the wrist, and both views are centred on the mid-shaft of the forearm bones.

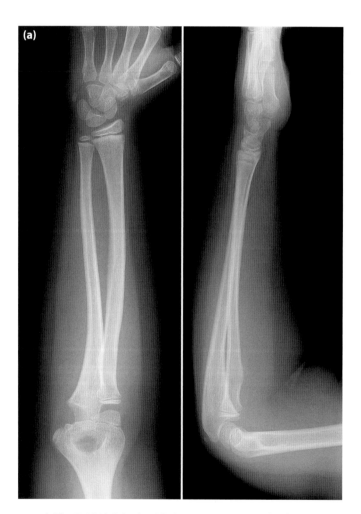

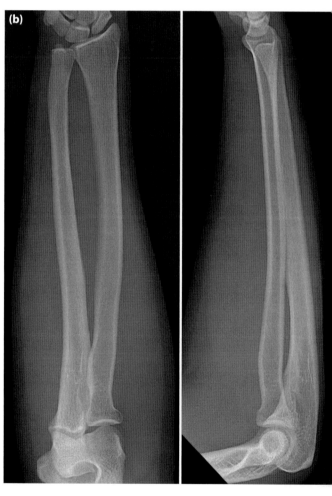

▲ **Fig. 3.134(a)** In the AP view, it is important that both the wrist and the elbow are in a true AP position. If this is achieved, the forearm bones will be parallel and not crossed. To produce a satisfactory lateral view of the forearm, it is important that both the wrist and the elbow are in a true lateral position, and both are included in each view. This is an immature athlete and the forearm and both joints can easily be included on a single film. **(b)** In the adult, the task of including the elbow and the wrist is more difficult and is best achieved by laying the forearm obliquely across the cassette for each view.

The biomechanics of pronation and supination

As previously discussed, the upper limb linkage allows 3D positioning of the hand, allowing infinite functions. The forearm's ability to execute the movements of supination and pronation add immensely to hand and wrist positioning. These movements are achieved by the two forearm bones rotating around themselves. The radius moves around the ulna, which has its position secured by its articulation with the humerus. The moving bone, the radius, takes the muscles and neurovascular bundles with it, preventing the twisting of these structures that would occur if there were a single forearm bone (Kapandji 2001).

In supination, the forearm bones are parallel. With pronation the radius moves around an oblique axis that passes through the proximal and distal radioulnar joints (see Fig. 3.135). The obliquity of the axis is compensated for by angulation of the elbow (physiological cubitus valgus). As a consequence, the hand remains collinear with the humerus.

The proximal radioulnar joint is very stable, with the radial head firmly secured in the radial notch by the annular ligament. As discussed in Chapter 2, the distal radioulnar joint is less firmly secured. The articular surfaces of the distal radioulnar joint are incongruent, and stability largely depends on the volar and dorsal radioulnar ligaments. The head of the ulnar moves distally and is translated laterally as the wrist is pronated, but the head of the ulna does not rotate. This has a practical implication. In all plain film views of the routine wrist series, the distal ulna is in the same position and fractures may be missed as the bone is examined in only one plane. Consequently, if a distal ulnar fracture is suspected, an AP view should also be acquired, to allow examination of the ulnar in two planes at right angles.

Forearm stability

The relationship between the forearm bones is stabilised as follows:

- The integrity of the proximal and distal radioulnar joints stabilises the forearm.
- The interosseous membrane has two layers, and the fibres of both layers are obliqued at 90° to each other, preventing proximal and distal translation of the radius.
- The pronator quadratus and flexors of the fingers also stabilise the forearm.

Problems with pronation and supination

Kapandji (2001) listed the following conditions that may interfere with normal supination and pronation:

- Deformity resulting from a poorly reduced fracture of either forearm bone may cause abutment and prevent normal supination and pronation. Obviously, cross-union following a fracture would also prevent normal movement.

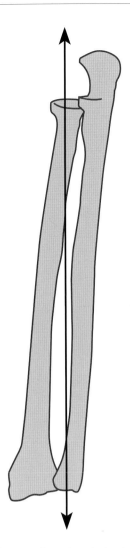

▲ **Fig. 3.135** The axis of rotation during forearm pronation is demonstrated by line drawing.

- There are two patterns of fracture/subluxations of the forearm that, if inadequately managed, may prevent normal supination and pronation. Monteggia's fracture/dislocation involves an ulnar fracture in combination with subluxation of the proximal radioulnar joint (see Fig. 3.136). Galeazzi's fracture/dislocation is a combination of a radial fracture and subluxation of the distal radioulnar joint.

An Essex-Lopresti lesion involves a fracture of the proximal radius, tearing of the interosseous membrane (IOM) and injury to the TFCC. Proximal migration of the radius may then occur (see Fig. 3.137). Axial forearm stability requires an intact radioulnar IOM and TFCC. Displaced or comminuted radial head fractures require additional assessment including testing of the integrity of the IOM and distal radioulnar joint to exclude longitudinal axial instability where the radial head fracture migrates proximally into the capitellum and the ulnar head impinges at the carpus. If both the IOM and the TFCC are sectioned, this may lead to 12–23 mm of proximal migration of the radius under axial loading. On axial stress x-ray, a change in ulnar variance greater than 10 mm is diagnostic of axial instability of the forearm (Bennett and Tullos 1990).

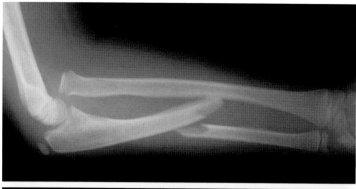

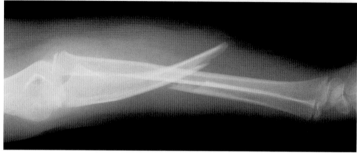

▲ **Fig. 3.136** Dislocation of the radial head and an ulnar fracture are the components of Monteggia's fracture/dislocation.

Stress fractures of the forearm

Bone stress injuries are relatively uncommon in the upper extremity. As previously discussed, stress reactions may involve growth plates, apophyses and epiphyses at the elbow joint, particularly in skeletally immature elite gymnasts. In the same group, stress reactions occur in the distal radial growth plate, producing so-called 'gymnast's wrist'.

Stress fractures of the shaft of the ulna are thought to result from torsion and have been reported in softball pitchers (Tanabe et al. 1991), elite tennis players (Bollen et al. 1993) and a female volleyball player (Mutoh et al. 1982). Interestingly, the bone stress reactions seen in elite tennis players involve the non-dominant forearm and most probably result from the forceful pronation that occurs during the double-handed backhand stroke (see Fig. 3.138). Although stress fractures of the radial shaft have not previously been described, the authors have encountered a single case of a stress fracture involving the proximal radial shaft of a female tennis player (see Fig. 3.139).

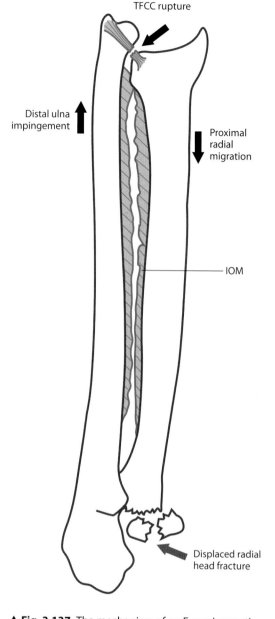

▲ **Fig. 3.137** The mechanism of an Essex-Lopresti lesion is demonstrated by line drawing.
Source: Modified from Nicholas and Hershman (1990).

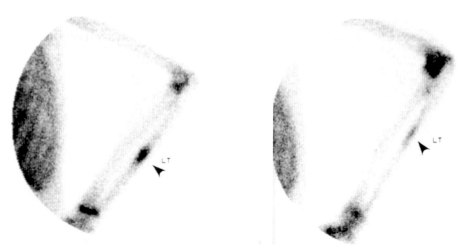

◀ **Fig. 3.138** These bone scans demonstrate a stress fracture in two separate elite tennis players. In each case, the increased isotope uptake involves a segment of the shaft of the ulna in the non-dominant forearm.

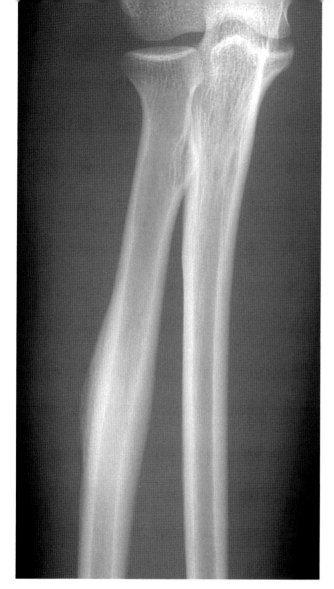

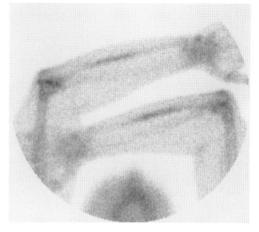

◀**Fig. 3.139** Typical plain film changes of a stress fracture are demonstrated in the proximal radial shaft of a female tennis player. This has probably resulted from stress at the supinator attachment caused by a repetitive backhand topspin action.

▲ **Fig. 3.140** A nuclear bone scan shows bilateral periosteal uptake along the ulnar shafts following overuse in the gym. This is the appearance of ulnar splints.

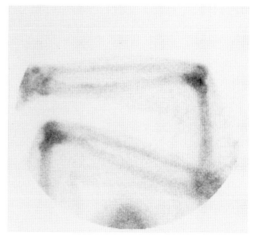

▲ **Fig. 3.141** Linear uptake along both the ulna and the radius bilaterally, indicating overuse and stress at muscle attachments.

Forearm splints

With overuse of the elbow and forearm musculature, forearm splints may develop. This is often associated with weight training, particularly following 'curls' (Cooper et al. 2003). This condition presents with forearm pain and changes may be demonstrated on nuclear bone scans (see Figs 3.140 and 3.141). Increased uptake of isotope may also be seen in muscle following heavy training (see Fig. 3.142).

▶**Fig. 3.142** Bilateral muscle uptake in the lower arms and proximal forearms following excessive 'workouts'.

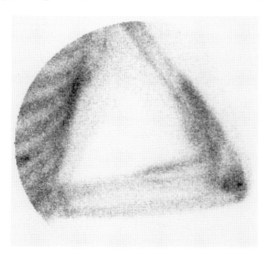
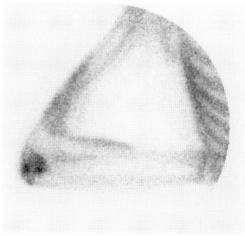

References

Anzel SH, Covey KW et al. 'Disruptions of muscles and tendons: an analysis of 1041 cases.' *Surgery* 1959, 45: 406–14.

Armstrong AD, Dunning CE, Faber KJ et al. 'Single-strand ligament reconstruction of the medial collateral ligament restores valgus elbow stability.' *J Shoulder Elbow Surg* 2002, 11: 65–71.

Bartlett CS. 'Elbow fractures.' *Curr Opinion in Orthop* 2000, 11: 290–304.

Bennett JB, Tullos HS. 'Acute injuries to the elbow.' In Nicholas JA, Hershman EB (eds), *The Upper Extremity in Sports Medicine*, Mosby, St Louis, 1990, pp. 326–7.

Bollen SR, Robinson DG, Crichton KJ, Cross MJ. 'Stress fractures of the ulna in tennis players using a double-handed backhand stroke.' *Am J Sports Med* 1993, 21: 751–2.

Bonatus T, Chapman MW, Felix N. 'Traumatic anterior dislocation of the radial head in an adult.' *J Orthop Trauma* 1995, 9: 441–4.

Boucher PR, Morton KS. 'Rupture of the distal biceps brachii tendon.' *J Trauma* 1967, 7: 626–52.

Cain EL, Dugas JR et al. 'Ulnar nerve injury in the throwing athlete.' *Sports Med and Arthroscopy Review* 2003, 11: 40–6.

Chen FS, Rokito AS, Jobe FW. 'Medial elbow problems in the overhead-throwing athlete.' *J Am Acad Orthop Surg* 2001, 9: 99–113.

Chumbley EM, O'Connor FG, Nirschl RP. 'Evaluation of overuse elbow injuries.' *Am Fam Physician* 2000, 61: 691–700.

Ciccotti MG, Ramani MN. 'Medial epicondylitis.' *Sports Med and Arthroscopy Review* 2003, 11: 57–62.

Conway JE, Singleton SB. 'Posterolateral instability of the elbow.' *Sports Med and Arthroscopy Review* 2003, 11: 71–8.

Cooper R, Allwright S, Anderson IF. *Atlas of Nuclear Imaging in Sports Medicine*. McGraw-Hill, Sydney, 2003.

Dunning CE, Zarbour ZDS, Patterson SD et al. 'Ligamentous stabilizers against posterolateral rotary instability of the elbow.' *J Bone and Joint Surg Am* 2001, 83: 1823–8.

Fleisig GS, Barrentine SW. 'Biomechanical aspects of the elbow in sports.' *Sports Med Arthrosc Rev* 1995, 3: 149–59.

Fritz RC. 'MR imaging in sports medicine: the elbow.' *Sem Musculoskel Rad* 1997, 1: 29–49.

Haraldsson S. 'On osteochondrosis deformans juvenilis capituli humeri including investigation of intra-osseous vasculature in distal humerus.' *Acta Orthop Scand* 1959, 38(suppl): 1–23.

Hughes PE, Paletta GA. 'Little leaguer's elbow, medial epicondyle injury, osteochondritis Dissecans.' *Sports Med and Arthroscopy Review* 2003, 11: 30–9.

Hulkko A, Orava S, Nikula P. 'Stress fractures of the olecranon in javelin throwers.' *Int J Sports Med* 1986, 7: 210–13.

Hutchison MR, Laprade RF, Burnett QM et al. 'Injury surveillance at the USTA Tennis Championships: a 6-yr study.' *Med Sci Sports Exerc* 1995, 27: 826–30.

Jackson D, Silvino N, Reimen P. 'Osteochondritis in the female gymnast's elbow.' *Arthroscopy* 1989, 5: 129–36.

Jacobson JA, Jebson PJL, Jeffers AW, Fessell DP, Hayes CW. 'Ulnar nerve dislocation and snapping triceps syndrome: diagnosis with dynamic sonography report of three cases.' *Radiology* 2001, 220: 601–5.

Kaminsky SB, Baker CL. 'Lateral epicondylitis of the elbow.' *Sports Med and Arthroscopy Review* 2003, 11: 63–70.

Kapandji A. 'Biomechanics of pronation and supination of the forearm.' *Hand Clinics* 2001, 17: 111–22.

King J, Brelsford HJ, Tullos HS. 'Analysis of the pitching arm of the professional baseball pitcher.' *Clin Orthop* 1969, 67: 116–23.

Kiyoshige Y. 'Critical displacement of neural injuries in supracondylar humeral fractures in children.' *J Pediatr Orthop* 2000, 20: 177–82.

Larson RL, Single KM, Bergstrom R et al. 'Little league survey.' *Am J Sports Med* 1976, 4: 201–9.

Leach RE, Miller JK. 'Lateral and medial epicondylitis of the elbow.' *Clin Sports Med* 1987, 6: 259–72.

Leung AG, Peterson HA. 'Fractures of the proximal radial head and neck in children with emphasis on those that involve the articular cartilage.' *J Pediatr Orthop* 2000, 20: 7–14.

Lins RE, Simovitch RW, Waters PM. 'Pediatric elbow trauma.' *Orthop Clin North Am* 1999, 119–32.

Maffulli N, Chan D, Aldridge MJ. 'Overuse injuries of the olecranon in young gymnasts.' *J Bone Joint Surg (Br)* 1992, 74: 305–8.

Maloney MD, Goldblatt J, Snibbe J. 'Elbow problems in the throwing athlete.' *Curr Op in Orthop* 2002, 13: 1–12.

Maloney MD, Mohr KJ, El Attrache NS. 'Elbow injury in the throwing athlete.' *Clin Sports Med* 1999, 16: 795–809.

McCarroll JR. 'Evaluation, treatment, and prevention of upper extremity injuries in golfers.' In Nicholas JA, Hershman EB (eds), *The Upper Extremity in Sports Medicine*, Mosby, St Louis, 1990, p. 883.

Meherin JM, Kilgore ES. 'The treatment of ruptures of distal biceps brachii tendon.' *Am J Surg* 1960, 99: 636–8.

Morrey BF. 'Injury of the flexors of the elbow: biceps in tendon injury.' In Morrey BF (ed.), *The Elbow and its Disorders*, WB Saunders, Philadelphia, 2000.

Mutoh Y, Mori T, Suzuki Y, Suzuira Y. 'Stress fractures of the ulna in athletes.' *Am J Sports Med* 1982, 10: 365–7.

Nicholas JA, Hershman EB (eds), *The Upper Extremity in Sports Medicine*, Mosby, St Louis, 1990.

Nirschl RP, Pettrone FA. 'Tennis elbow. The surgical treatment of lateral epicondylitis.' *J Bone Joint Surg (Am)* 1979, 61: 832–9.

O'Driscoll SW, Bell DF, Morrey BF. 'Posterolateral rotary instability of the elbow.' *J Joint Surg Am* 1991, 73: 440–6.

O'Driscoll SW, Jupiter JB, King GJ et al. 'The unstable elbow: instructional course lecture.' *J Bone Joint Surg (Am)* 2000, 82: 724–51.

O'Driscoll SW, Morrey BF, Korineck S et al. 'Elbow subluxation and dislocation: a spectrum of instability.' *Clin Orthop* 1992, 280: 186–97.

O'Hara JJ and Stone JH. 'Ulnar nerve compression caused by a prominent medial head of triceps and anconeus epitrochlearis muscle.' *J Hand Surg (Br)* 1996, 21: 133–5.

Olsen BS, Sojbjerg JO, Dalstra M et al. 'Posterolateral elbow joint instability: the basic kinematics.' *J Shoulder Elbow Surg* 1998, 7: 19–29.

Pappas AM. 'Elbow problems associated with baseball during childhood and adolescence.' *Clin Orthop* 1982, 164: 30–41.

Pecina MM, Krmpotic-Nemanic J, Markiewitz AD. *Tunnel Syndromes*, CRC Press, Boca Raton, 1991.

Rao PS, Rao SK. 'Olecranon stress fracture in a weight lifter: a case report.' *Br J Sports Med* 2001, 35: 72–3.

Rempel D, Dahlin L, Lundborg G. 'Pathophysiology of nerve compressive syndrome. Response of peripheral nerves to loading.' *J Bone Joint Surg* 1999, 81: 1600–10.

Rosenberg ZS, Bencardino J, Beltran J. 'MRI of normal variants and interpretation pitfalls of the elbow.' *Sem Musculoskel Rad* 1998, 2: 141–53.

Seiler III JG, Parker LM, Chamberland PD et al. 'The distal biceps tendon: two potential mechanisms involved in its rupture: arterial supply and mechanical impingement.' *J Shoulder Elbow Surg* 1995, 4: 149–56.

Spinner RJ, Golder R. 'Snapping of the medial head of the triceps and recurrent dislocation of the ulnar nerve.' *J Bone Joint Surg (Am)* 1998, 80: 239–47.

St John JN, Palmaz JC. 'The cubital tunnel in ulnar entrapment neuropathy.' *Radiology* 1986, 158: 119–23.

Suzuki K, Minami A, Suenaga N et al. 'Oblique stress fracture of the olecranon in baseball pitchers.' *J Shoulder Elbow Surg* 1997, 6: 491–4.

Tanabe S, Nakahira J, Bando E et al. 'Fatigue fractures of the ulna occurring in pitchers of fast-pitch softball.' *Am J Sports Med* 1991, 19: 317–21.

Teitz CC, Garrett WE, Miniaci A et al. 'Tendon problems in athletic individuals: instructional course lecture.' *J Bone Joint Surg (Am)* 1997, 79: 138–52.

Torg JS, Moyer RA. 'Non-union of a stress fracture through the olecranon epiphyseal plate observed in an adolescent baseball pitcher. A case report.' *J Bone Joint Surg (Am)* 1977, 59: 264–5.

Vidal AF, Allen A. 'Biceps tendon and triceps tendon injuries.' *Sports Med and Arthroscopy Review* 2003, 11: 47–56.

Visuri T, Lindholm H. 'Bilateral distal biceps tendon avulsions with use of anabolic steroids.' *Med Sci Sports Exer* 1994, 26: 941–4.

Woodward AH, Blanco AJ. 'Osteochondritis dissecans of the elbow.' *Clin Orthop* 1975, 110: 35–41.

Image acknowledgments

The authors wish to thank the following colleagues who kindly offered images for inclusion in this chapter:

- Dr James Linklater (Figures 3.41, 3.44, 3.46, 3.53, 3.54, 3.65, 3.84, 3.92, 3.97, 3.102(b), 3.112, 3.117 and 3.128)
- Dr Robert Cooper and Dr Stephen Allwright (Figures 3.34, 3.35, 3.50, 3.56, 3.75, 3.85, 3.88, 3.94, 3.98, 3.105, 3.138(a) and (b), 3.140, 3.141, and 3.142(a) and (b))
- Dr Phil Lucas (Figures 3.39, 3.78, 3.87, 3.102(a), 3.103, 3.128 and 3.133)
- Dr Bill Breidahl (3.25, 3.66, 3.67, 3.68, 3.69, 3.70, 3.90 and 3.104)
- Dr David Duckworth (Figure 3.60(b) and (c))

These images have significantly added to the quality of the chapter.

4

The shoulder, shoulder-girdle and thoracic cage

Jock Anderson and John Read with Phil Lucas

The shoulder (glenohumeral joint) is a component of the shoulder-girdle and acts as a pivot for the upper limb, allowing unlimited arm movements. Thousands of everyday functions and sporting activities rely on normal shoulder function. The glenohumeral joint has the greatest range of movement of any joint in the body, and to achieve this flexibility is traded for stability, making the shoulder inherently vulnerable. For the shoulder to function normally there has to be an important balance between strength, flexibility and stability, and this is particularly important for athletes who undertake repetitive overhead activity with the arm. When this balance is disrupted by injury, shoulder function is disturbed and pain and disability develop. Shoulder injuries resulting from sport usually present with symptoms produced by either instability or impingement. Although these injuries may be due to acute trauma, chronic overuse is the predominant cause.

Over recent years, our understanding of shoulder injury and injury biomechanics has improved, largely due to imaging and arthroscopy. Continuing technological upgrading of the imaging methods now enables greater precision in diagnosis and better characterisation of the pathological changes. An unexpected offshoot of this progress has been development of an entirely new shoulder language consisting of acronyms containing secret embedded codes which describe the injury, anatomy and sometimes even the injury management. We can now suffer with shoulder conditions known as SLAP, TUBS, AMBRI, GAGL, ALPSA, GLAD, GARD, HAGL, AIGHL and BHAGL and can even be placed in the ABER position.

Anatomy and biomechanics of the shoulder

The shoulder-girdle consists of four separate joints that must all work together if optimal upper limb function is to be achieved. The components of the shoulder-girdle comprise the glenohumeral or shoulder joint (GHJ), the acromioclavicular joint (ACJ), the sternoclavicular joint (SCJ) and the scapulothoracic articulation. The GHJ is an extremely versatile joint, capable of a wide range of complex movements under variable loads. The glenoid is small and shallow contacting only 25–30% of the humeral articular surface at any one time. This limited area of articulation allows great flexibility but means that bony structures do not contribute significantly to stability, which is instead provided by soft-tissue structures. Stabilising structures include the joint capsule, glenohumeral ligaments (see Fig. 4.1), glenoid labrum and rotator cuff.

The inferior glenohumeral ligament (IGHL) is believed to be the primary stabiliser, resisting anterior and posterior humeral displacement with the arm abducted (Turkel et al. 1981; O'Brien et al. 1995). Anterior displacement is also resisted by the middle glenohumeral ligament (MGHL), although this ligament plays a secondary role. The glenoid labrum contributes to stability by increasing the depth and surface area of the glenoid cavity, creating a 'suction cup' effect and acting to resist translation of the humeral head (Levine and Flatow 2000). The rotator cuff is a dynamic stabiliser that acts to maintain the humeral head centred on the glenoid. During abduction and external rotation, there is normal posterior movement of the head in relation to the glenoid (Howell et al. 1988). The rotators of the scapula (the trapezius, rhomboids and serratus anterior) position the glenoid to minimise the effect of destabilising forces.

Methods of imaging the shoulder

After obtaining a history and examining the shoulder, imaging is invariably the next step considered in the management of a shoulder injury. Plain films are an essential starting point for any imaging and the film series should be tailored to the clinical presentation (Anderson 2000). Significant errors in diagnosis may occur if basic radiographs are overlooked in favour of more sophisticated tests such as CT, MRI or ultrasound alone.

Following an initial series of films, additional plain film views or the use of other imaging methods may help to provide the diagnosis. A variety of imaging methods are available when additional imaging is required. These include conventional arthrography (single or double contrast), ultrasound, CT and CT arthrography, MRI and MR arthrography. At present there is wide variation in clinical practice and no general consensus exists regarding a single correct approach to shoulder imaging. Consequently, the choice of further test will vary, although the test chosen should obviously be that most likely to provide an accurate diagnosis. Even this will be subject to the

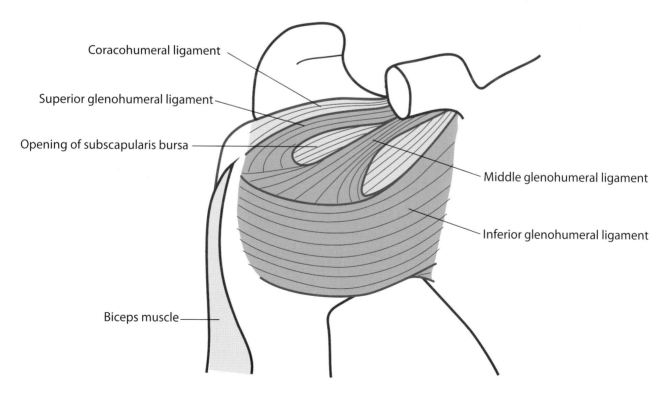

▲ **Fig. 4.1** A line drawing demonstrates the ligaments supporting the anterior GHJ. The anterior shoulder capsule shows a distinct 'Z' pattern formed by the superior glenohumeral, coracohumeral, middle glenohumeral and inferior glenohumeral ligaments.

constraints of the locally available radiological expertise and technology. Other factors for consideration include patient safety, comfort and cost.

Plain films

A plain film series will demonstrate bone and joint anatomy of the shoulder-girdle. A baseline series should include five views:

1 an AP view with external rotation
2 an AP view with internal rotation
3 a true AP view of the GHJ
4 an axial view
5 a lateral view.

These views are essential for all shoulder series. The limited trauma series consisting of AP and lateral views that is used in hospital emergency departments is inadequate for the exclusion of the many conditions resulting from sports injuries. Any plain film series must provide an effective screen for easily missed fractures (see Table 4.1).

Table 4.1 Easily missed fractures

- Avulsion of the greater tuberosity
- Direct trauma fracturing the greater tuberosity
- Bony Bankart lesion
- Hill-Sachs lesion
- Reverse Hill-Sachs lesion
- Fracture of the base of coracoid process
- Fractures of the acromion

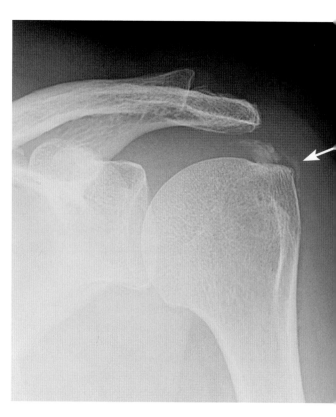

▲ **(b)** Calcific supraspinatus tendinopathy is well demonstrated by externally rotating the humeral head and using 10 to 15° of caudal tube angulation. In this case there is a large deposit of calcification present, with calcification leaking into the subdeltoid bursa (arrow).

▼ **Fig. 4.2(a)** An AP view of the shoulder in external rotation allows the greater tuberosity to be examined in profile. This is particularly important for demonstrating calcific supraspinatus tendinopathy or a fracture of the greater tuberosity.

▼ **(c)** A fracture of the greater tuberosity generally occurs from a fall onto the tip of the shoulder. The fracture is often subtle and may be easily missed without a well-positioned external rotation view.

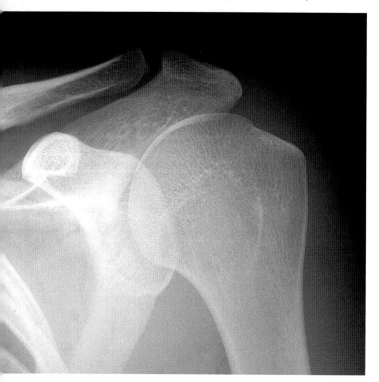

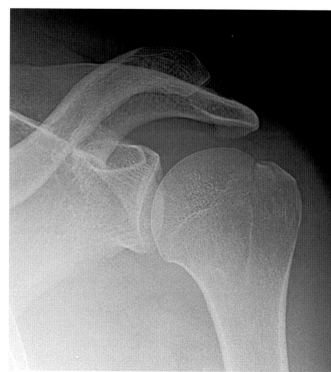

Details of routine plain film shoulder views

The scapula lies against the thoracic cage at a 40° angle to the coronal plane of the body. This places the axis of the articular surface of the glenoid at an angle, facing antero-laterally. Consequently, views taken with a straight tube (i.e. in the sagittal plane) will be oblique to the GHJ space and the articular surfaces of the GHJ will not be demonstrated on AP internal and external rotation views. For this reason a specific GHJ view must be included in all shoulder series.

AP view with external rotation

An AP view with external rotation is a standard view that demonstrates the greater tuberosity in profile (see Fig. 4.2(a)). The tube is centred on the GHJ space with 10 to 15° of caudal tube angulation to help display the subacromial soft-tissue space. The course of the supraspinatus can be examined to its insertion, allowing identification of calcific tendinopathy (see Fig. 4.2(b)). This view is also valuable for assessing bone injury at the greater tuberosity, the evidence of which is often subtle (see Fig. 4.2(c)). External rotation is best achieved by flexing the elbow to 90° and rotating the forearm laterally as far as possible, without abducting the arm. As usual, collimation is important and improves resolution.

AP view with internal rotation

An AP view with internal rotation displays the posterolateral aspect of the humeral head and neck in profile (see Fig. 4.3(a)) and is a particularly valuable view for the demonstration of a Hill-Sachs defect following glenohumeral dislocation (see Fig. 4.3(b)). This view also demonstrates the soft-tissue course of the infraspinatus tendon. As with the external rotation view, the primary beam is centred on the GHJ space with 10 to 15° of caudal tube angulation. Internal rotation is obtained by hyperpronation of the forearm and wrist.

True AP view of the GHJ

A true AP view is obtained with the patient rotated 40° away from the tube to bring the blade of the scapula perpendicular to the primary beam (see Fig. 4.4(a)). A straight tube is used, centred on the GHJ space. This demonstrates the articular surfaces of the GHJ in profile. The joint space can be assessed for evidence of degenerative joint disease, the articular surfaces can be displayed, and the relationship of the humeral head to the glenoid can be examined (see Fig. 4.4(b)).

Axial view

An axial view is a valuable component of the basic shoulder series. This view enables further assessment of the relationship of the humeral head to the glenoid in a plane 90° to that of the true AP view (see Fig. 4.5(a)). Examination of the coracoid process, the acromion, the scapular neck and the ACJ is also possible in this projection (see Fig. 4.5(b)). In particular, this view is essential for the diagnosis of a posterior subluxation or dislocation of the ACJ (see Fig. 4.5(c)). The axial view is obtained using a superoinferior projection. The patient sits at the end of

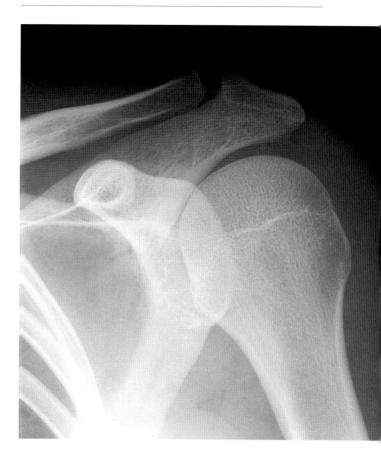

▲ **Fig. 4.3(a)** An AP view with internal rotation of the humeral head enables examination of the anterior and posterior surfaces of the humeral head and neck.

▼ **(b)** An internal rotation view enables even a small Hill-Sachs defect to be examined in profile (arrow).

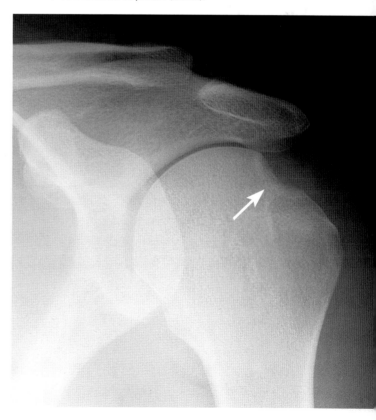

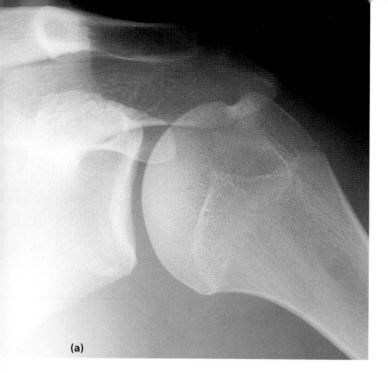

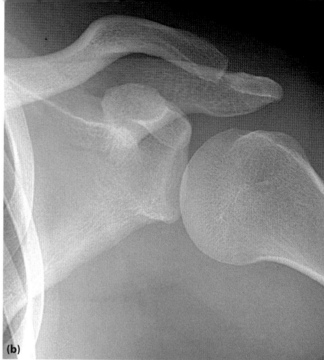

(a)

(b)

▲ **Fig. 4.4(a)** A true AP view is an important component of every shoulder series. This view enables the GHJ space and its articular surfaces to be assessed. The relationship between the humeral head and the glenoid is demonstrated in the superoinferior axis. **(b)** An AP view demonstrates a post-traumatic inferior subluxation of the humeral head in relation to the glenoid.

the table leaning across the cassette, which is elevated on a sponge to reduce the object–film distance. The arm is abducted to 90° on the side to be examined, with the elbow resting on the table. The elbow is flexed to 90°, with the hand resting palm down on the table. A straight tube is centred on the GHJ.

Lateral view

A lateral view is an essential view and is particularly important for the demonstration of a glenohumeral dislocation by assessing the relationship of the glenoid and the humeral head. The primary beam is directed along the plane of the body of the scapula, producing a 'Y' configuration of the coracoid and acromion processes and the body of the scapula. This is achieved with the patient standing facing the wall bucky and then obliqued with the affected side closest to the film. The exact degree of obliquity is assessed by palpating the plane of the scapula and rotating the patient until the scapula is perpendicular to the plane of the film. The patient's shoulder is extended with their forearm behind their back, or flexed slightly so that the humeral shaft is not projected over the body of the scapula (see Fig. 4.6(a) and (b)). A triangle is created by the tip of the coracoid process, the tip of the acromion process and the inferior angle of the scapula. Normally, the humeral head lies in the centre of this triangle. If an anterior dislocation is present, a large percentage of the humeral head will lie outside the anterior margin of the triangle (see Fig. 4.6(c)). In addition to demonstrating an anterior dislocation, this view is also used to confirm a satisfactory relocation of the humeral head following the reduction of a dislocated shoulder.

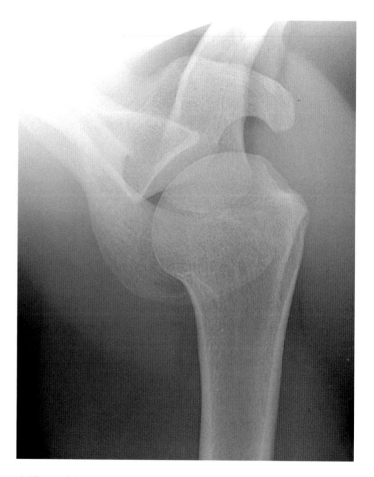

▲ **Fig. 4.5(a)** An axial view allows further assessment of the relationship of the humeral head to the glenoid and may demonstrate alteration in the anteroposterior axis. Viewed together with a true AP view, an axial view is important for the detection of subtle humeral head subluxation.

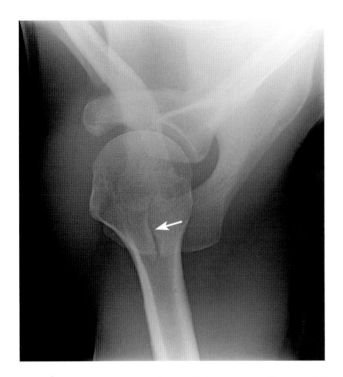

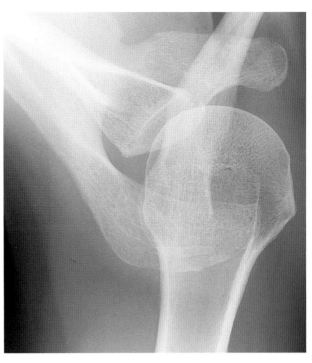

▲ **Fig. 4.5(b)** An os acromiale is well demonstrated by an axial view (arrow). This anomaly, produced by failure of fusion of the acromial apophysis, is a significant finding as a potential cause of impingement.

▲ **(c)** A posterior subluxation of the ACJ joint is demonstrated. This deformity cannot be appreciated on any other plain film view, so the axial view is an important component of plain film assessment of an ACJ injury.

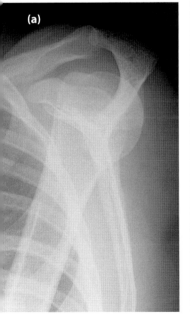

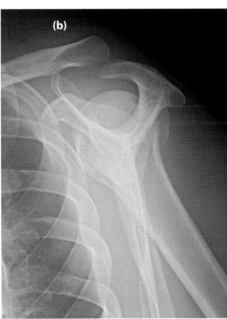

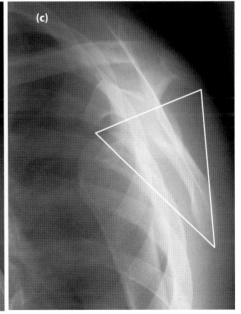

▲ **Fig. 4.6(a)** A lateral view demonstrates subluxation or dislocation of the humeral head. When the scapula is viewed side-on, a 'Y' is created by the tip of the coracoid process, the acromial process and the inferior angle of the scapula. Normally, the humeral head will lie in the centre of this triangle, overlying the glenoid. The shoulder should be extended or flexed, so that a scapular fracture is not missed by superimposition of the humeral shaft. In this case, the arm was in a sling and the shoulder was slightly flexed, so that the scapula was not obscured. **(b)** A lateral view has been obtained with the shoulder extended, with the patient's forearm behind their back. This is the preferred position. **(c)** The majority of the humeral head lies outside the triangle created by the tip of the coracoid and acromial processes and the inferior angle of the scapula, indicating that there is an anterior dislocation of the GHJ.

Details of additional shoulder views

Additional plain film views of the shoulder may contribute valuable information, often replacing the need for the use of more sophisticated and expensive imaging methods. As previously noted, athletes tend to present with a clinical picture suggestive of either an instability or an impingement problem. Views are added to the baseline series of five images to produce a different series for each symptomatic group, displaying specific structures that are important to examine. These series are listed in Tables 4.2 and 4.3.

Table 4.2 Routine instability series

View	Role
AP with external rotation	Detects fractures of the greater humeral tuberosity
	Shows a reverse Hill-Sachs lesion
AP with internal rotation	Demonstrates a Hill-Sachs lesion
True AP view	Shows abnormal GHJ alignment
	Detects loss of congruity of the GHJ
Axial view	Shows GHJ alignment
	Detects hypoplasia of glenoid
	Detects posterior glenoid rim fracture
	Assesses voluntary subluxation
Westpoint view (alternatively Garth or modified Garth view)	Shows anteroinferior glenoid rim fracture (Bankart lesion)

Table 4.3 Routine impingement series

View	Role
True AP view	Shows superior subluxation of the humeral head
	Demonstrates GHJ osteoarthrosis
AP with external rotation	Detects calcific deposits within supraspinatus tendon
	Shows degenerative changes at the greater tuberosity
AP with internal rotation	Localises calcification (especially if multiple deposits)
Axial view	Assesses glenohumeral alignment
	Detects os acromiale
	Helps localise calcification
	Checks ACJ alignment
Outlet view	Detects acromial spurring
	Detects ACJ osteophytes
	Assesses acromial shape
AP view with 30° of caudal tilt	Detects an anterior acromial spur

Outlet view

The patient is positioned as for a true lateral view and a caudal tube angulation of 25 to 30° is used. A correctly acquired view will demonstrate the sweep of the acromioclavicular arch and profiles the acromion in a true lateral position (see Fig. 4.7(a)). An outlet view demonstrates the tunnel through which the supraspinatus passes and will show bony encroachment on the

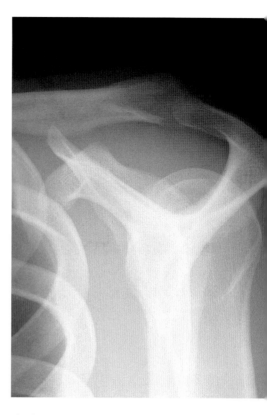

▲ **Fig. 4.7(a)** An outlet view is an extremely valuable impingement view, demonstrating the soft-tissue pathway of the supraspinatus beneath the bony coracoacromial arch and enabling detection of bony encroachment on this outlet tunnel. Bony encroachment is usually caused by a subacromial spur, osteophytes projecting inferiorly from the ACJ or an os acromiale.

▼ **(b)** A large bony spur is demonstrated by an outlet view (arrowhead). The spur is similar to that shown in Fig. 4.8(b), being imaged in profile using this view.

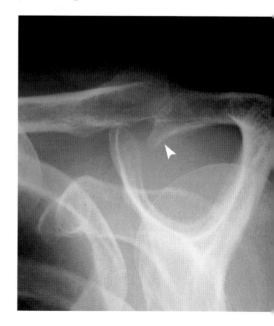

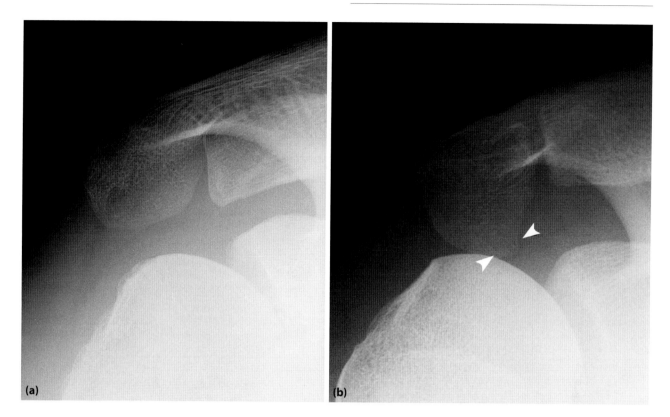

▲ **Fig. 4.8(a)** An AP view with 30° of caudal angulation, centred on the anterior margin of the acromion, is a useful view to acquire in a patient presenting with impingement. Bony spurs commonly arise from the anterior margin of the acromion. This case is normal, with the anterior margin of the acromion well defined. **(b)** A spur arises from the anterior border of the acromion (arrowheads) and would almost certainly contribute to the patient's impingement. Using this view, the spur is imaged 'en face'. Note the shallow Hill-Sachs defect in the humeral head.

tunnel (see Fig. 4.7(b)). This view is also valuable for displaying the shape of the acromion and definition of the coracoid. The outlet view has been found to be so valuable that the authors (who work in a specialty sports medicine centre) include this view in all shoulder series (a sixth routine view).

AP view with 30° of caudal tilt

This angled AP view is used to profile the anterior margin of the acromion, a common site for spur formation (see Fig. 4.8(a)). Spurs tend to form along the line of the coracoacromial ligament (Kilcoyne et al. 1989). An AP view with 30° of caudal tube angulation is centred on the anterior margin of the acromion. The outlet view shows the spur in profile, whereas the angled AP view adds further information by showing the spur 'en face', which is important if surgery is being contemplated (see Fig. 4.8(b)).

Stryker's notch view

A Stryker's view is an additional view that may occasionally be used to demonstrate a Hill-Sachs defect or the bony spur of a Bennett lesion (see Fig. 4.9). It is unwise to use this view in the immediate post-reduction period when elevation of the arm should be avoided. A Stryker's view is obtained with the patient supine and the cassette placed under the shoulder. The palm of the hand of the affected shoulder is placed on top of the head, with the fingers directed towards the back

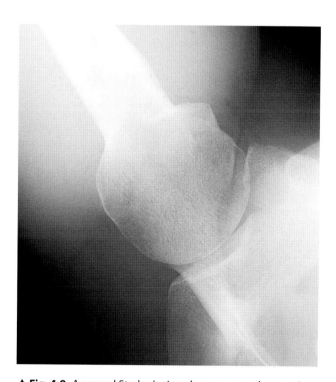

▲ **Fig. 4.9** A normal Stryker's view demonstrates the anterior and posterior margins of both the humeral head and the glenoid. This has been a favoured view for the demonstration of a Hill-Sachs defect, but an internal rotation view is now the most widely accepted view for this purpose.

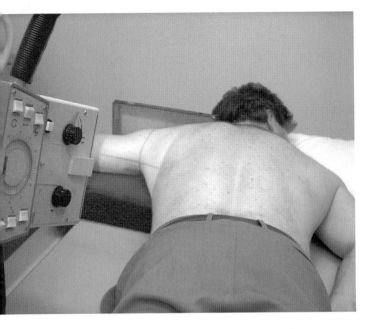

▲ Fig. 4.10(a) A Westpoint view is acquired with elevation of the shoulder to be examined using a pad and the patient's arm abducted and hanging over the side of the table, palm facing towards the feet. There is 30° of caudal tube angulation to the horizontal and also 30° of medial angulation. The beam is centred on the shoulder joint through the axilla.

▼ (b) A Westpoint view is an essential additional view for any patient with recurrent instability. The detection of a fracture at the anteroinferior aspect of the glenoid is an important finding and will affect management decisions. When the view has been taken correctly, the fracture is projected between the GHJ and the coracoid process (arrow).

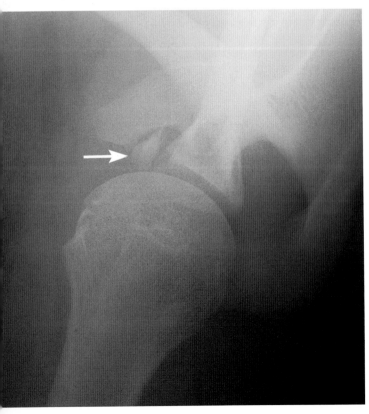

of the head and the elbow pointing straight upwards, so that the arm and forearm lie in the sagittal plane. The x-ray beam is angled 10° towards the head and centred over the coracoid process. This view has previously enjoyed popularity, but an internal rotation view is generally considered the easiest way of examining the shoulder for a Hill-Sachs defect.

Westpoint view

During glenohumeral dislocation, a Bankart fracture of the anteroinferior aspect of the glenoid rim may result from impaction by the humeral head. This fracture may predispose to recurrent instability (Richards et al. 1994) and is discussed in more detail later in the chapter. A Westpoint view specifically profiles the anteroinferior section of the glenoid rim. The patient is prone, lying with a 6 cm pad elevating the symptomatic shoulder from the tabletop. The arm is abducted and hangs freely over the side of the table with the hand pronated. There is cranial tube angulation, with 30° of angulation medially and a 30° tilt to the horizontal plane. The beam is centred on the GHJ through the axilla. In some x-ray rooms medial rotation of the tube housing is not possible, and this is overcome by the patient being angled 30° to the long axis of the table (see Fig. 4.10(a)). If the view has been acquired correctly, the anteroinferior margin of the glenoid is projected through the gap between the humeral head and the coracoid process (see Fig. 4.10(b)).

Garth and modified Garth views

Garth and modified Garth views (Garth et al. 1984) are preferred to the Westpoint view by some radiologists to demonstrate a fracture of the anteroinferior rim of the glenoid. Each method has its supporters. The authors prefer the Westpoint view.

A Garth view (see Fig. 4.11(a)) is obtained with the patient seated with their arm by their side. The patient is rotated 40° to bring the spine of the scapula parallel to the cassette. The tube is then centred on the coracoid process with 45° of caudal angulation. A Garth view has the advantage of being able to be obtained with the patient's arm immobilised.

A modified Garth view (see Fig. 4.11(b) and (c)) is obtained with the same centring and tube angulation, but with the arm held in a mild ABER (ABducted and Externally Rotated or 'stop sign') position. This position has the advantage of rotating the anteroinferior glenoid rim into profile. This view cannot be used following acute trauma, as the ABER position runs the risk of redislocating a recently reduced glenohumeral dislocation. A modified Garth view can be used for the routine investigation of instability when there has been no recent acute trauma.

Other shoulder-girdle views

A number of other plain film views may be acquired when there are symptoms localised to other bones and joints of the shoulder-girdle. If there has been trauma to the scapula, an AP view and a lateral view of the scapula should be added to the routine shoulder series. In addition, there are specific views to demonstrate the scapular neck, the scapular spine, the suprascapular notch, the acromion and coracoid processes, the bicipital groove and the scapulothoracic articulation.

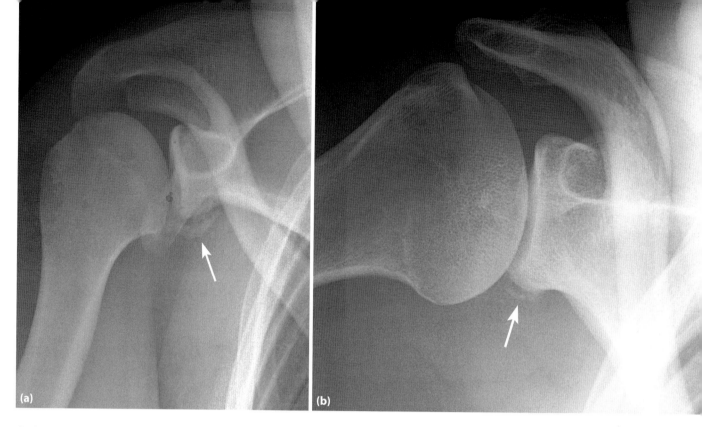

(a)

(b)

▲ **Fig. 4.11(a)** A Garth view will demonstrate a fracture of the anteroinferior aspect of the glenoid rim. This view is obtained with the patient sitting, their arm by their side. A cassette is placed behind the shoulder, parallel to the plane of the scapula. The primary beam is centred on the glenohumeral joint at 45° to the coronal plane of the thorax and 45° caudally. In this case a bony Bankart fragment is shown separated from the glenoid (arrow). **(b)** A modified Garth view demonstrates a bony Bankart fracture (arrow). Note that this view requires abduction of the arm into the ABER position, which is unwise following a recent reduction of a shoulder dislocation.

▼ **(c)** These images show the similarity of the Westpoint and modified Garth views. The Westpoint view **(i)** and the modified Garth view **(ii)** both adequately demonstrate a fracture of the anteroinferior glenoid rim in the same patient (arrows).

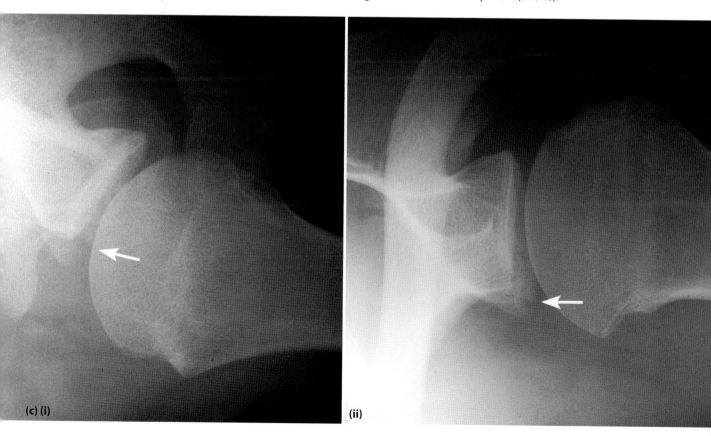

(c) (i)

(ii)

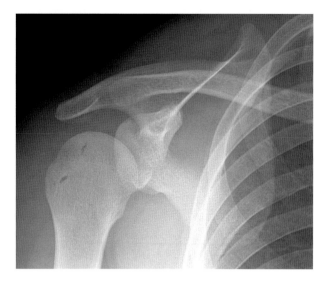

▲ **Fig. 4.12** In this true AP view of the scapula, the entire scapula is shown 'en face'. Positioning and angulation is similar to a true AP view of the GHJ, with centring on the centre of the body of the scapula. However, less than 40° is often necessary to prevent superimposition of the sternum over the medial border of the scapula. Less than 40° has been used in this case.

▼ **Fig. 4.13** A lateral projection of the body of the scapula is obtained with the patient's hand resting on their head to prevent superimposition of the humeral shaft over the scapula. The body of the scapula can be palpated and positioned at 90° to the film.

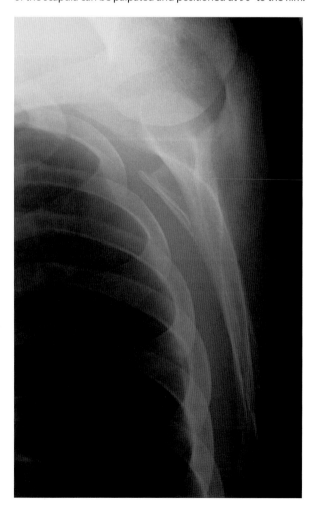

There are also specific views of the ACJs, the clavicle and the SCJs.

True AP view of the scapula

For a true AP view of the scapula, the scapula is required to be at 90° to the primary beam. This is achieved by rotating the patient 35 to 40° to the symptomatic side, as for a GHJ view. Often, when the patient is rotated to 40°, the sternum is projected over the medial border of the scapula, so less rotation is usually used (as is the case in Fig. 4.12). The view is centred on the centre of the body of the scapula.

Lateral view of the scapula

A lateral view is obtained with the body of the scapula parallel to the primary beam. The patient stands with their affected side closest to the cassette. The plane of the scapula can be palpated, enabling correct positioning. The patient rests their forearm on top of their head to prevent the humerus overlying the scapula (see Fig. 4.13). This view is usually obtained with the patient standing against the wall bucky, but it can also be obtained prone oblique.

Scapular neck view

A scapular neck view is useful when there is a suspicion of injury in this region. This is not the ideal view for demonstrating a Bankart fracture, but it is valuable for the detection of a scapular neck fracture or a Bennett lesion, which is ossification of the inferoposterior aspect of the GHJ capsule producing a traction spur in athletes who frequently undertake overhead activity with the arm. This lesion is also well demonstrated using a Stryker's notch view or by CT scanning. This view is an AP view with the patient's arm abducted and elbow flexed as though the patient is making a 'stop sign' (the ABER position) (see Fig. 4.14).

▼ **Fig. 4.14** Abducting the arm causes the scapula to rotate in a clockwise direction, displaying the scapular neck. This is a valuable extra view when an abnormality of the neck is suspected clinically or on the routine views.

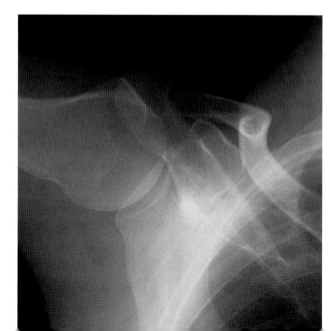

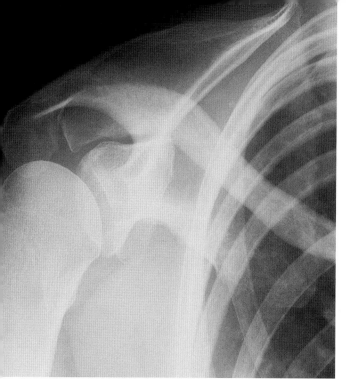

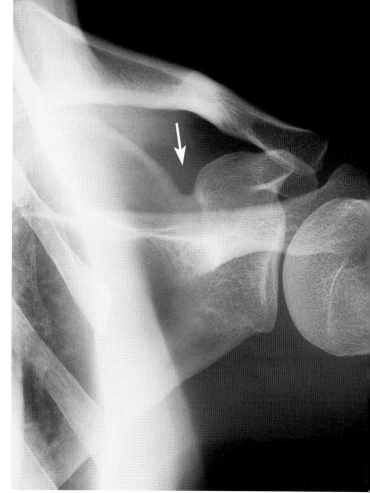

▲ **Fig. 4.15** Imaging of the scapular spine may be important if there is tenderness localised to the spine following trauma. With the patient lying supine, the spine can be projected away from the body of the scapula by using 45° of caudal angulation with the beam centred on the spine.

Scapular spine view

When there has been direct trauma to the spine of the scapula, a view of the spine is often useful to exclude a fracture. This is obtained in the supine position using 45° of caudal tube angulation, with the primary beam centred on the scapular spine (see Fig. 4.15).

Suprascapular notch view

The suprascapular notch is an important anatomical structure to display if there has been injury to the suprascapular nerve. The nerve may be injured by a fracture involving the notch or if there is bony or soft-tissue encroachment on the notch. A true AP view with 40° obliquity and 20° of cranial tube angulation (see Fig. 4.16) will demonstrate the notch (arrow).

Acromion and coracoid processes view

These processes are usually adequately shown in the routine axial and outlet views, but if further definition of the coracoid process is required, an AP view with 30° of cranial tube angulation will demonstrate the tip of the coracoid (see Fig. 4.17).

▲ **Fig. 4.16** An important step in investigating a post-traumatic supraspinatus nerve injury is to examine the suprascapular notch for evidence of bone injury. This is a simple view. The patient is turned 40° as for a GHJ view and 20° of cranial tube angulation is used. In this case the notch appears normal.

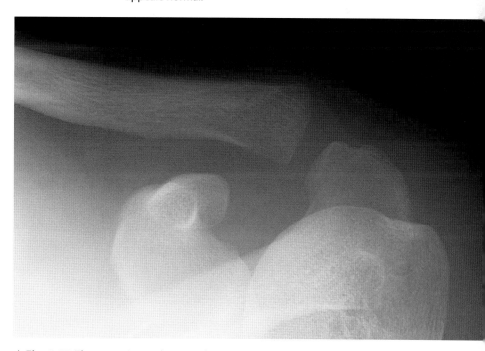

▲ **Fig. 4.17** The acromion and coracoid processes are well seen on outlet and axial views. If a further view of the tips of the processes is required, an AP view with 30° of cranial tube angulation is an excellent view for demonstrating the tips in profile.

Scapulothoracic articulation view

A scapulothoracic articulation view is obtained with the patient facing the bucky and turned with the symptomatic side closest to the film. The patient can have their hand either on their head or behind their back to move the humerus so that it is not superimposed over the scapulothoracic space. The plane of the body of the scapula can be palpated and placed at 90° to the film. The scapulothoracic joint can be widened by asking the patient to place their hand behind their back and push their shoulder forwards with their humerus angled backwards (see Fig. 4.18).

Bicipital groove view

A bicipital groove view is obtained with the patient in the supine position, arm by their side and hand supinated. A cassette stands resting against the superior surface of the shoulder. A 10° caudal tube angulation to the horizontal plane is used, with centring on the superior aspect of the femoral head (see Fig. 4.19). For many x-ray tables the humerus has to lie in the middle of the table, making the view difficult to obtain in larger patients using this method. For larger patients, the examination can be performed with the patient sitting at the side of the table, holding a cassette on their forearm in the horizontal plane and with their shoulder extended 10 to 15°. The humerus has to lie in the sagittal plane. Obliquity in this plane is the most common cause of failure. As before, the beam is centred on the anterior margin of the humeral head.

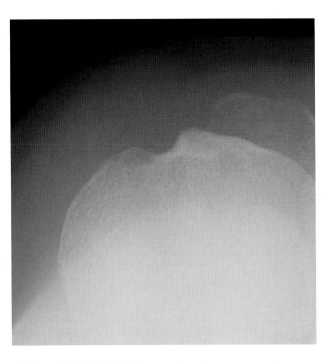

▲ **Fig. 4.19** This bicipital groove view shows a normal groove. Biceps tendinopathy may be due to encroachment by an osteophyte on the groove or to a steep bicipital groove wall. A shallow groove may predispose to tendon subluxation.

ACJ views

When there has been injury to the ACJ, plain films may demonstrate a fracture, dislocation or subluxation. Comparative views of both sides are obtained to help in the assessment of subtle alignment abnormalities or joint space widening. The joints can be examined on one film, although the authors' preference is to examine the joints separately as this will improve definition with the use of individual collimation. An AP view is obtained with 15° of cranial tube angulation to project the joint away from the shoulder. Views are obtained both with and without weightbearing. The patient's arms hang by their sides and internal rotation of the shoulders is important to allow muscle relaxation (see Fig. 4.20). When weightbearing is used, weights should hang from the patient's wrists by straps, as gripping the weights may increase muscle tension around the shoulder. There is further discussion on the shoulder-girdle and ACJ imaging later in the chapter.

Clavicular views

Two views are used to examine the clavicle. Ideally, these views should be obtained in the prone or erect PA position, although with recent trauma to the clavicle, these positions may be too uncomfortable and AP projections will suffice. A PA view or an AP oblique view must always be obtained in combination with a straight PA or AP view, to project the clavicle away from the ribs (see Fig. 4.21 on page 200). About 30° of obliquity is used, but this angle will vary depending on the patient's build. This angulation will be caudal in a PA projection and cranial in an AP view. Clavicular fractures are discussed later in the section on the shoulder-girdle.

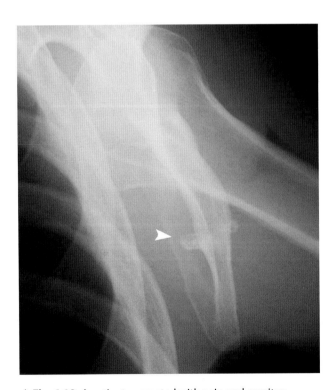

▲ **Fig. 4.18** A patient presented with pain and crepitus related to movement of the scapulothoracic articulation. A scapulothoracic view opens the space between the scapula and the rib cage and demonstrates a small exostosis on the undersurface of the scapula.

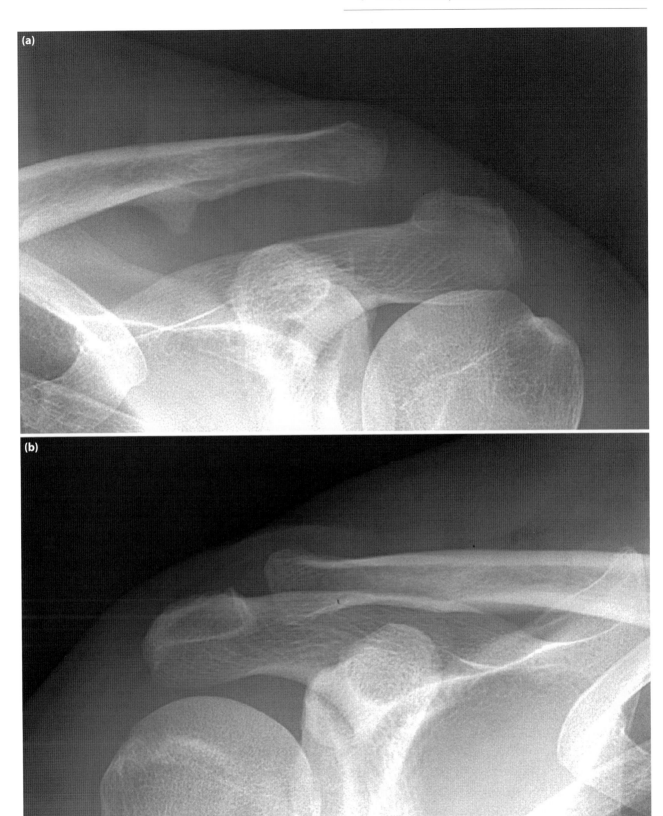

▲ **Fig. 4.20** Following trauma to the left shoulder, images of both the ACJs were obtained for comparison. Images are obtained with and without weightbearing with the shoulders in internal rotation to reduce muscle tension around the shoulders. These are the weightbearing images, obtained with weights hanging from the patient's wrists.

(a) There is widening and superior subluxation of the left ACJ. Widening of the coracoclavicular space indicates rupture of the coracoclavicular ligament. A bony spur is present just medial to the conoid tubercle suggesting previous injury to the coracoclavicular ligament at the conoid ligament attachment.

(b) The right ACJ appears normal.

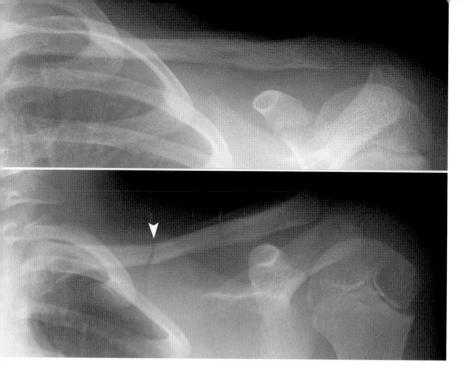

▲ **Fig. 4.21** Clavicular fractures in the immature athlete may be subtle, and in this case the fracture would have been missed if an angled AP view had not been obtained. This view shows a greenstick-type fracture (arrowhead).

SCJ views

Plain film examination of the SCJs includes a PA view and PA oblique views, to help exclude a fracture or disruption of the joints. In practice, even after obtaining these views, a CT examination is invariably required to display detail of the joints, and so it makes sense to obtain CT or, if available, MDCT images in the first instance instead of plain films (see the following discussion on the shoulder-girdle).

If CT is unavailable, a PA view is obtained with the patient prone, their arms by their sides and their palms facing upwards (see Fig. 4.22(a)). In this position, the shoulders roll forward, reducing angulation of the clavicles. A straight tube is centred on T3 and tight collimation is paramount if a high-quality image is to be produced.

Oblique views are obtained by rolling the patient 20 to 30° one way and then the other to project the sternoclavicular joints away from the spine (see Fig. 4.22(b)). Both joints are imaged to allow a comparative assessment.

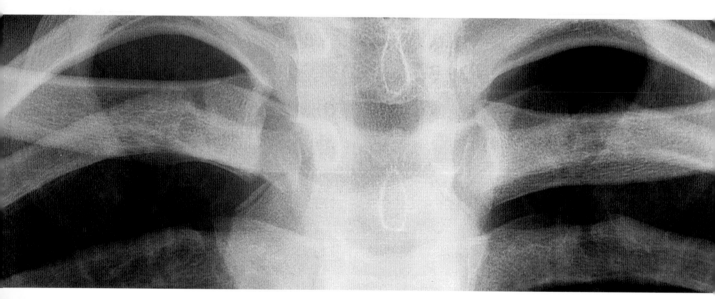

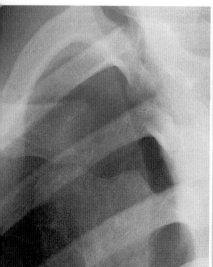
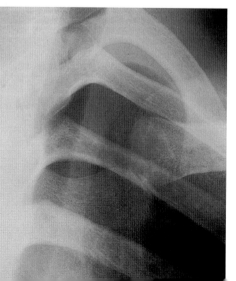

▲ **Fig. 4.22(a)** Plain films of SCJs have largely become superfluous, and a CT examination should be performed if a sternoclavicular injury is clinically suspected. If CT is unavailable or difficult to access, plain films including a PA and PA oblique views may provide valuable information. In this case, a PA view of the SCJs shows asymmetry of the joints, consistent with subluxation of the right SCJ.
◀ **(b)** Oblique views in the same case confirm the right SCJ subluxation seen on the PA view. A CT examination is still required to provide information concerning displacement and injury to the surrounding soft tissues.

Tips on looking at plain films of the shoulder

The extraordinary flexibility of the shoulder allows the complex bony anatomy to be relatively easily demonstrated and examined by plain films. The range of clinical presentations of sports-related shoulder problems is limited, and the plain film examination and interpretation is considerably influenced by the clinical history. As always, a request form containing a full history and results of a thorough physical examination greatly help in the assessment of plain films and make the report more meaningful. An understanding of the biomechanics of a particular injury assists in the identification of plain film abnormalities and helps in the selection of the subsequent diagnostic pathway to follow if plain films are normal.

The examination of shoulder joint images usually involves an initial overall assessment, followed by a careful search for specific changes that may be responsible for a particular symptomatology. An important part of the initial assessment is confirming that the examination is of adequate radiographic standard and contains the views appropriate for investigation of the patient's symptoms. Satisfied that the films are adequate, a careful and orderly search pattern commences, looking for pathological changes in bony structures, joint spaces and soft tissues.

The examination of the bony structures of the GHJ is made difficult by the spherical shape of the humeral head and the complex angulations and superimpositions of the acromion and coracoid processes. Each view in the series and the use of additional views will help to unravel these anatomical complexities and, by using each view in turn, every structure can be examined in different planes. In examining the bony structures, it is important to inspect the bony architecture, noting sclerosis, demineralisation and cystic areas. Processes such as degenerative joint disease (see Fig. 4.23) and avascular necrosis will be identified (see Fig. 4.24). Generalised demineralisation of the humeral head and neck commonly occurs with a frozen shoulder (see Fig. 4.25).

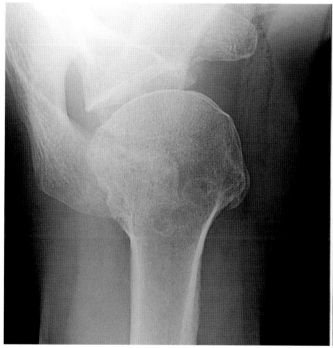

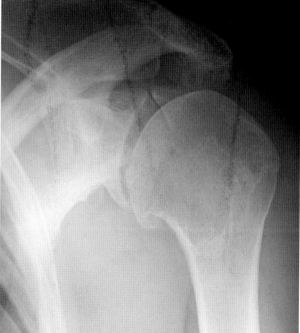

▲ **Fig. 4.23** Advanced degenerative joint disease is present. There is loss of the normal bony architecture with sclerosis and cyst formation. Osteophytes have developed at the margins of the humeral articular surface. Although the joint space appears well maintained in the axial view on the left, inferior subluxation and incongruity of the articular surfaces occurs in the erect position, due to the weight of the arm demonstrating joint laxity (right image). Gross spur formation originates from the undersurface of the acromion.

▶ **Fig. 4.24** There is destruction of the cortex and subchondral bone of the articular surface of the humeral head. A band of sclerosis surrounds this area and the appearance is that of the advanced stages of AVN. A small Hill-Sachs defect is also noted.

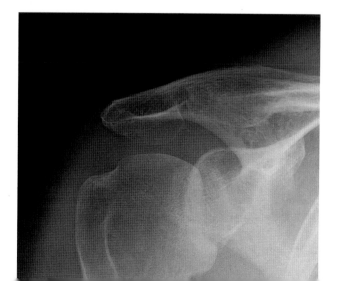

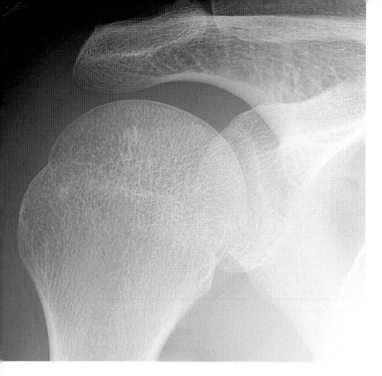

▲ **Fig. 4.25** There is generalised demineralisation of the humeral head and neck, typical of a frozen shoulder (adhesive capsulitis).

Fracture identification is greatly assisted by an understanding of the biomechanics of the injury. The age of the athlete also affects the search pattern. If the patient is adult and the history suggests a fracture, sites most often involved are carefully examined for evidence of a cortical break. The most common shoulder fractures occur as the result of glenohumeral dislocation (see Fig. 4.26). Fractures of the greater tuberosity are also common in mature athletes, usually caused by a fall on the tip of the shoulder. These fractures may be extremely subtle (see Fig. 4.27). Also, if the head of the humerus has been driven superiorly by a fall on the outstretched hand or elbow, unexpected and difficult-to-see fractures of the coracoid and acromion are occasionally present and it is important to remember to look for these fractures (see Figs 4.28 and 4.29). Disruption of the ACJ may be difficult to identify on a shoulder series and specific acromioclavicular views should be acquired if symptoms are localised to the ACJ. These specific views are discussed later in the chapter. Plain films have limitations in the diagnosis of glenoid fractures, although Westpoint and Garth views may demonstrate fractures of the all-important anteroinferior aspect of the glenoid rim. CT scanning is indicated if there is a suspicion of a fracture of the articular surface of the glenoid.

Fractures occurring in the immature athlete are likely to involve the clavicle, the humeral neck or the proximal humeral shaft. Consequently, the clavicle needs to be examined in its entirety and, as previously shown in Fig. 4.21, it is important to remember that a clavicular fracture in children can be extraordinarily subtle and easily missed. There must also be special focus on the proximal humeral shaft, growth plate and metaphysis.

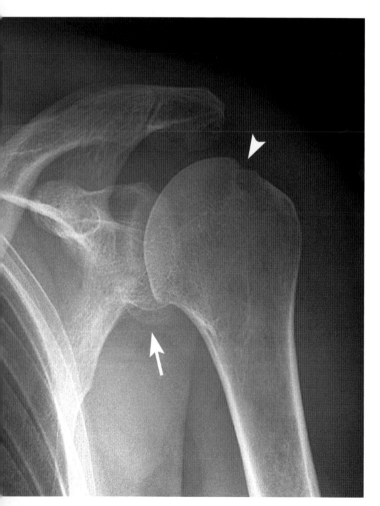

▲ **Fig. 4.26** The most frequently seen fractures of the shoulder occur following a GHJ dislocation. In this case there is a small Hill-Sachs defect (arrowhead) and a bony Bankart lesion (arrow).

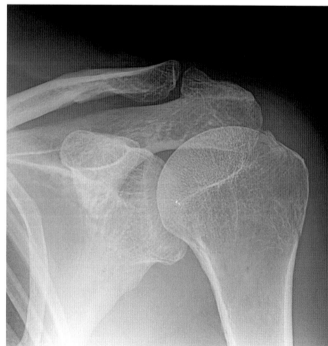

▲ **Fig. 4.27** The greater tuberosity requires a careful examination in patients who have fallen on their shoulder. This is a typical example of a greater tuberosity fracture. The fracture is not easily seen, in spite of its considerable size.

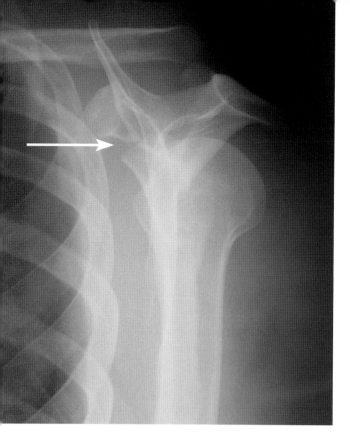

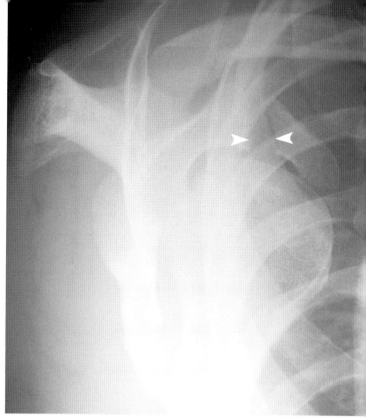

▲ **Fig. 4.28** If the head of the humerus is driven upwards, fractures of the coracoid process may occur and these fractures may be difficult to see. This case shows a fracture through the base of the coracoid process (arrow).

▲ **Fig. 4.29** There is an anterior dislocation of the shoulder and a fracture of the coracoid process has occurred due to the impact of the humeral head as it was driven upwards by a fall. This fracture is difficult to see due to superimposition of the ribs (arrowheads).

The GHJ space and its articular surfaces can be assessed in two planes at 90°, displayed on the 40° AP and axial views in combination. These views make the relationship of the humeral head to the glenoid easily assessed. Normally, the centre of the curvature of the humeral head apposes the centre of the concavity of the glenoid articular surface and the articular surfaces are parallel (congruous). This relationship may be disrupted if there is instability or a developmental anomaly (see Fig. 4.30). Nerve injury or a large joint effusion may cause inferior subluxation of the humeral head, also disrupting congruity (see Fig. 4.31). Superior migration of the humeral head occurs with rotator cuff degeneration (see Fig. 4.32).

The articular surfaces will also become incongruent when a dislocation is present. It is important to remember that the articular surfaces may appear to be congruent on an AP view when a posterior dislocation is present, and for this reason this condition is often overlooked on plain films (see Fig. 4.33). When a posterior dislocation is present, the humeral head is locked in internal rotation and, as will be discussed later, this is a crucial diagnostic sign to recognise. Injury to the other shoulder-girdle joints (ACJ and SCJ) will be discussed in detail later.

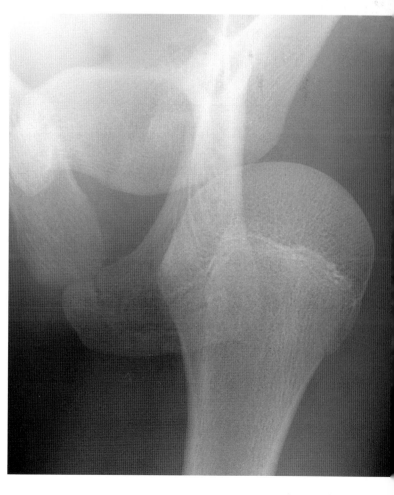

▶ **Fig. 4.30** A developmental anomaly is present with hypoplasia of the glenoid and acromion. There is an abnormal relationship between the abnormal glenoid and the humeral head with a slight posterior subluxation. This anomaly produces laxity and allows excessive movements.

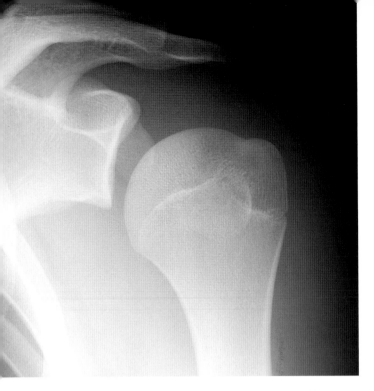

▲ **Fig. 4.31** Inferior subluxation of the humeral head has occurred following blunt trauma to the shoulder and injury of the circumflex nerve.

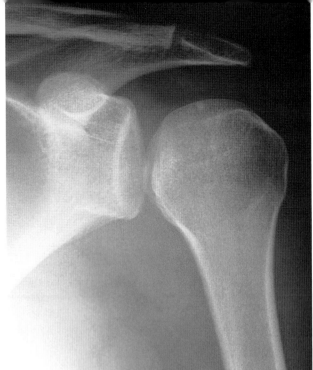

▲ **Fig. 4.33** A posterior dislocation is present. Note that the articular surfaces of the humeral head and the glenoid are roughly parallel, suggesting congruity. A large percentage of posterior dislocations are missed because of this appearance. The humerus is internally rotated and this is a sign that should raise the possibility of a posterior dislocation, a diagnosis confirmed on a lateral view.

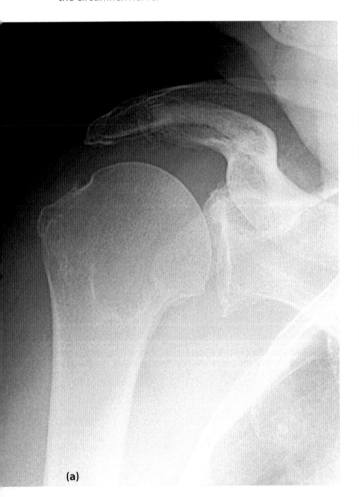

(a)

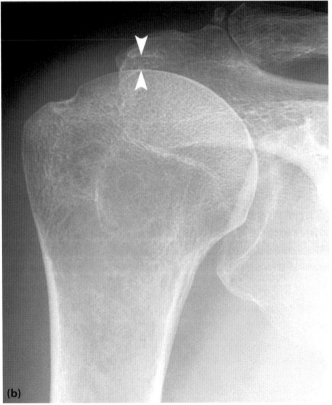

(b)

▲ **Fig. 4.32(a)** Early superior migration of the humeral head and narrowing of the subacromial space indicates failure of the rotator cuff to maintain humeral head depression. **(b)** An advanced stage of the process seen in **(a)** is almost complete obliteration of the subacromial space (arrowheads). When the space is completely narrowed, excavation of the undersurface of the acromion may occur (as shown in Fig. 4.123).

Having generally examined the shoulder plain film series, those structures of special significance with regard to the patient's symptoms should be reassessed. When the presentation involves instability, structures such as the glenoid rim and the posterolateral aspect of the humeral head and neck deserve a second look (see Fig. 4.34). Also, a check on developmental changes such as the shape of the humeral head and the size, orientation and degree of concavity of the glenoid articular surface is well worthwhile (see Fig. 4.35).

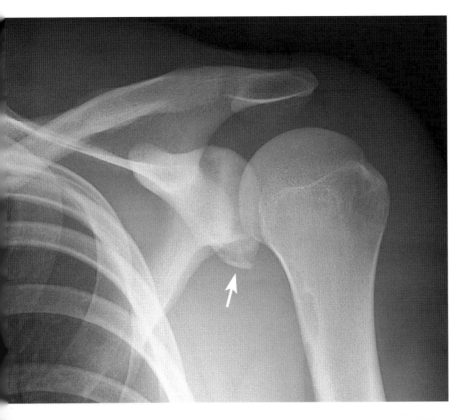

◀**Fig. 4.34** An AP view in internal rotation demonstrates a bony Bankart fracture (arrow) and a shallow Hill-Sachs defect in profile. These changes indicate a previous dislocation and possibly predispose to continuing instability.

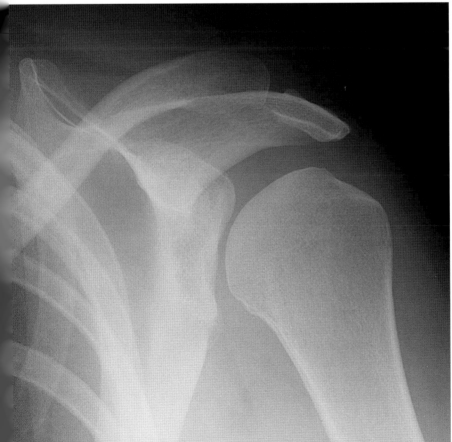

◀**Fig. 4.35** The glenoid is abnormally shallow and elongated in the superoinferior axis. The humeral head is flattened posterolaterally due to a shallow Hill-Sachs defect, suggesting that chronic instability is present.

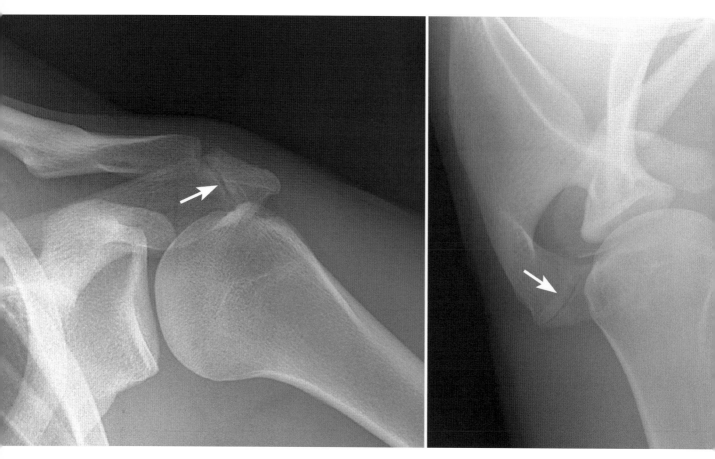

▲ **Fig. 4.36** Changes of an os acromiale are seen in angled AP and axial views.

▼ **Fig. 4.37(a)** An outlet view shows a spur in profile. Impingement on the soft-tissue outline of the supraspinatus is well shown (arrow).

▼ **(b)** An AP view with 30° of caudal tube angulation demonstrates the spur seen in the outlet view in **(a)** (arrow). This spur is likely to contribute to impingement.

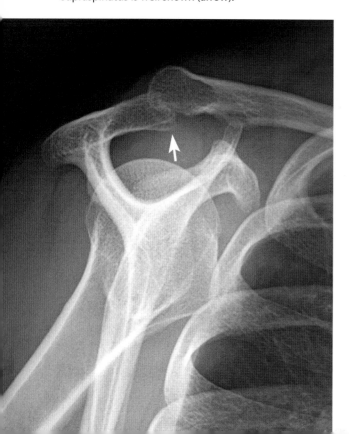

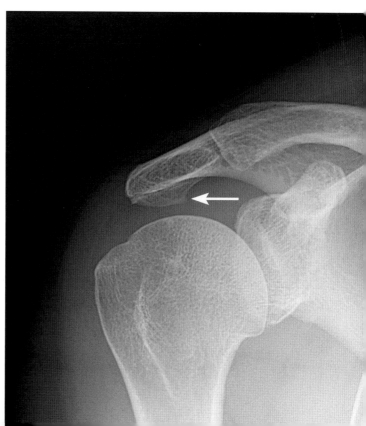

▶ **Fig. 4.38** A large deposit of supraspinatus calcification is present. Areas of both soft and dense calcification can be seen, the significance of which will be discussed later. The deposit increases the bulk of the tendon, producing subacromial impingement.

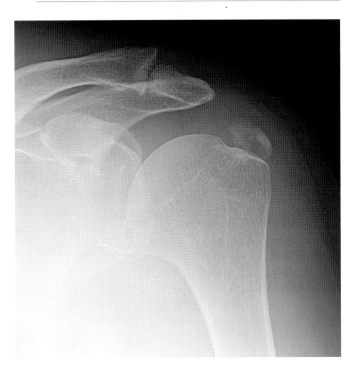

If the patient presents with impingement, a double-check of the shape of the acromion, evidence of an os acromiale on the axial view (see Fig. 4.36) and reassessment of the undersurface of the acromioclavicular arch in the outlet view often pay dividend. Subacromial new bone, spur formation and inferior protrusion of osteophytes from the ACJ are all significant findings (see Fig. 4.37).

In addition, sclerosis and cystic changes seen on the posterosuperior aspect of the humeral head in athletes who throw frequently may be indicative of an internal impingement. Calcific tendinopathy may also be present with impingement due to tendon swelling, and calcification is an important finding in this group of patients (see Fig. 4.38).

Soft-tissue changes around the shoulder are generally limited to the identification of a loose body in the GHJ and searching for evidence of rotator cuff calcific tendinopathy. Calcification is most commonly seen in the supraspinatus tendon 1–2 cm from its insertion, although any of the cuff tendons may be involved and accurately placing the calcification is not always easy (see Fig. 4.39). The calcification may leak into the subacromial-subdeltoid (SA-SD) bursa and this is also an important observation (see Figs 4.40 and 4.41). Calcific tendinopathy of the rotator cuff tendons is discussed in detail later. Although loose bodies are occasionally seen around the humeral head, the vast majority lie in the infraglenoid recess of the shoulder joint, which acts as a sump (see Fig. 4.42). When scattered ossifications are present, osteochondromatosis may be present (see Fig. 4.43).

▼ **Fig. 4.39** Sometimes it is difficult to accurately localise calcification. In this case there is faint calcification that lies in the supraspinatus tendon (arrowhead). The exact position of the denser and larger collection is more difficult to determine and this may lie in the SD bursa (arrow).

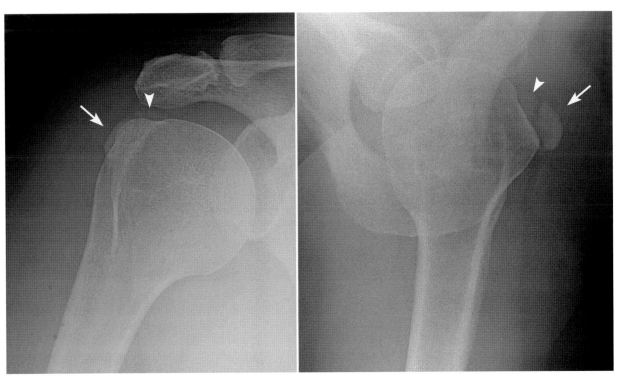

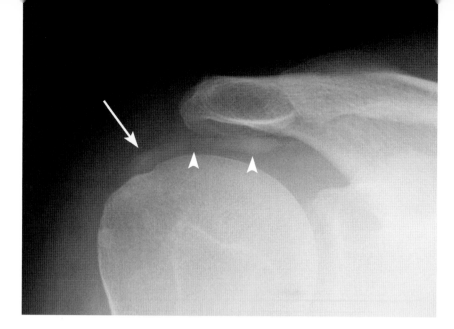

▶ **Fig. 4.40** There is calcific tendinopathy involving the supraspinatus (arrow), and a considerable percentage of the calcification has leaked into the subacromial bursa (arrowheads).

▼ **Fig. 4.41** Calcification has leaked from the infraspinatus tendon into the SD bursa (arrow).

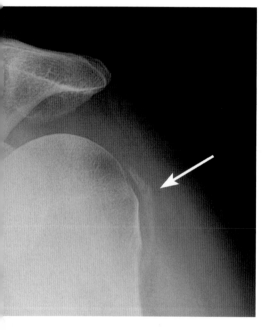

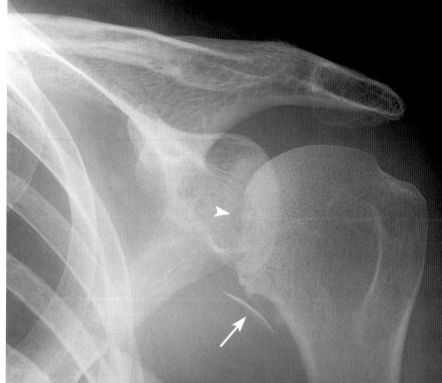

▶ **Fig. 4.42** AVN involves the humeral head. The cortical surface of the involved area has become separated following extensive subchondral bony resorption (arrowhead). This cortical fragment is a loose body and lies in the infraglenoid recess (arrow).

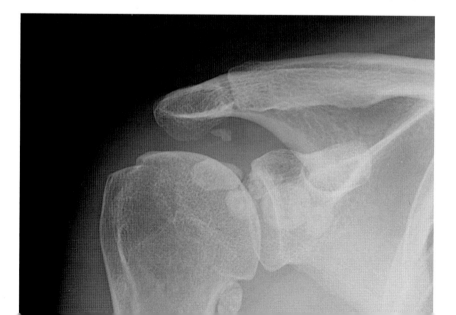

▶ **Fig. 4.43** Multiple ossicles are present and the appearance is that of osteochondromatosis.

Ultrasound

High-resolution ultrasound is a relatively inexpensive and entirely safe test for shoulder imaging. This method is often seen as an attractive alternative to MRI. Ultrasound has become established as a major method of assessing rotator cuff tears (see Fig. 4.44) and abnormalities of the long head of the biceps (LHB) tendon, and occasionally as a method of detecting occult fractures (see Figs 4.45 and 4.46). Ultrasound can also detect posterior and superior perilabral cysts (see Fig. 4.47). However, labral tears are not reliably imaged using ultrasound. Achieving consistently accurate results with ultrasound depends on having a skilled operator using high-quality equipment. Therefore, if adequate sonographic expertise is not available locally, MRI or some form of shoulder arthrography may be a better choice for additional imaging.

A clinical diagnosis of subacromial impingement can be confirmed using the dynamic capabilities of real-time ultrasound, although a normal examination does not totally exclude impingement (Farin et al. 1990; Read and Perko 1998). Additional applications of dynamic ultrasound include the assessment of frozen shoulder, stability of the biceps tendon and ACJ stability (see Fig. 4.48).

Ultrasound also plays a significant interventional role and can be used for the percutaneous aspiration of calcific tendinopathy or perilabral cysts. In addition, accurate therapeutic injections can be performed using ultrasound imaging control. These interventional procedures are discussed at length in Chapter 10. The most commonly performed interventional procedures are the injection of the SA-SD bursa (see Fig. 4.49), the GHJ, the biceps sheath and the ACJ.

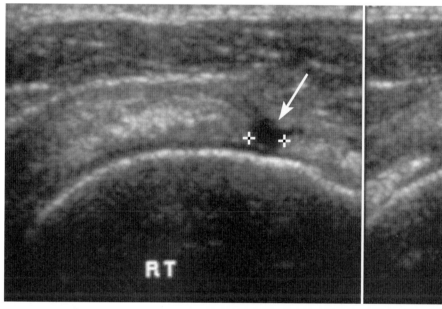
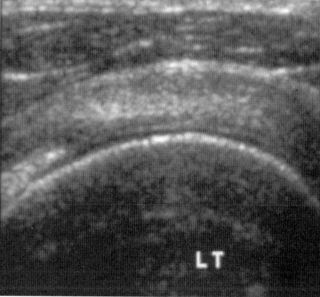

▲ **Fig. 4.44** Comparison transverse ultrasound images of the rotator cuff show a small fluid-filled gap (arrow), indicative of a full-thickness tear (callipers) at the anterior aspect of the right supraspinatus tendon.

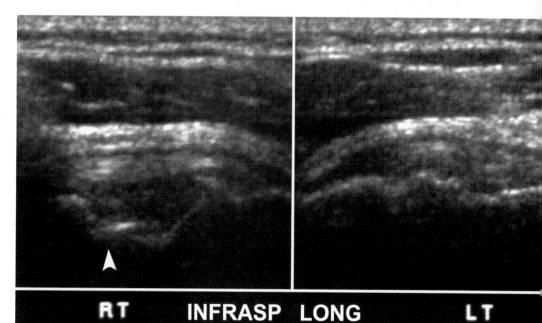

▶ **Fig. 4.45** A transverse ultrasound image obtained over the posterior aspect of the right humeral head shows depression of cortical bone, typical of a Hill-Sachs fracture (arrowhead). A comparison image of the left side has also been obtained.

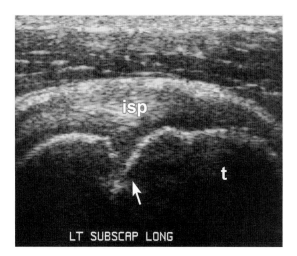

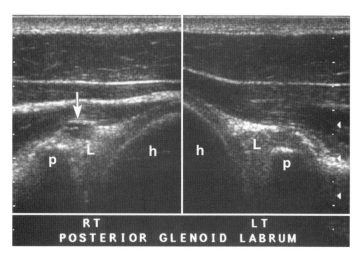

▲ **Fig. 4.46** A reverse Hill-Sachs lesion is shown by ultrasound. A transverse image obtained over the anterior aspect of the humeral head shows an abruptly angulated impaction fracture (arrow). Note the overlying infraspinatus tendon (isp) inserting at the lesser humeral tuberosity (t).

▲ **Fig. 4.47** Ultrasound demonstrates a glenoid perilabral cyst. Transverse images obtained over the posterior glenoid labrum (L) of both shoulders show a small, rounded perilabral cyst (arrow) on the right. This finding is a reliable indicator of an underlying glenoid labral tear. Bony posterior glenoid rim = p. Humeral head = h.

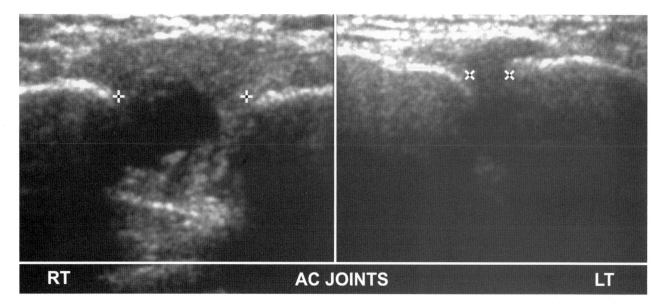

▲ **Fig. 4.48** Ultrasound demonstrates an ACJ subluxation injury. Comparative images of the right and left ACJs show an abnormal appearance on the right side, which includes widening (+ callipers), superior capsular thickening and heterogeneous intra-articular echotexture with effusion. Dynamic assessment performed during shoulder flexion and extension manoeuvres will demonstrate relative hypermobility on the symptomatic side. The normal left ACJ space is indicated by × callipers.

▶ **Fig. 4.49** An injection of the SA-SD bursa has been guided by ultrasound. A long-axis view of the supraspinatus tendon (ssp) shows the injecting needle (arrowheads) with the tip located in the bursal space (b) immediately deep to the peribursal fat stripe (f). Acromion = a. Humeral head = h.

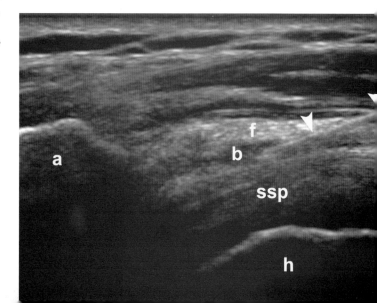

CT scanning

Non-contrast CT scanning is helpful in the detection and evaluation of fractures (see Fig. 4.50) and has an important role in the pre-operative assessment of comminuted fractures of the humeral head or fractures of the glenoid being considered for internal fixation (see Figs 4.51 and 4.52). The recent development of MDCT technology has significantly improved the resolution of reformatted images, making CT arthrography a valid alternative to MRI for the assessment of internal joint derangements (see Fig. 4.53) and rotator cuff tears. Nevertheless, as CT arthrography is invasive and involves exposure to ionising radiation, this imaging method is generally best reserved for situations in which MRI is unavailable, contra-indicated or of limited sensitivity due to previous surgery. High-quality 3D image reconstructions can also be helpful when complex anatomical relationships cannot be readily understood or demonstrated with individual 2D sections alone (see Fig. 4.54 on page 213).

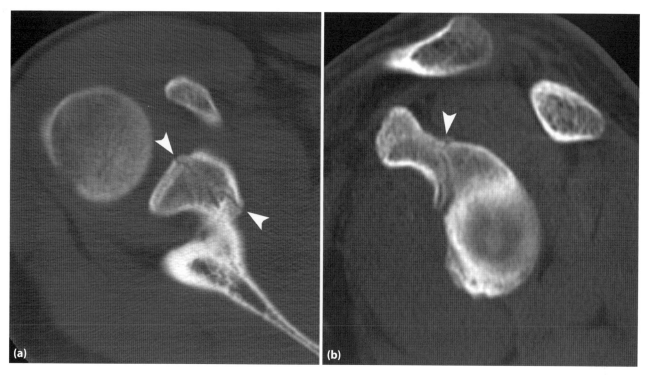

(a)   (b)

▲ **Fig. 4.50** Axial **(a)** and reformatted sagittal **(b)** images from an MDCT examination show an undisplaced fracture at the base of the coracoid process which was occult on plain x-ray (arrowheads).

▼ **Fig. 4.51** A comminuted fracture of the greater humeral tuberosity is demonstrated by CT, giving an appreciation of fragment position and displacement which was unavailable on plain films.

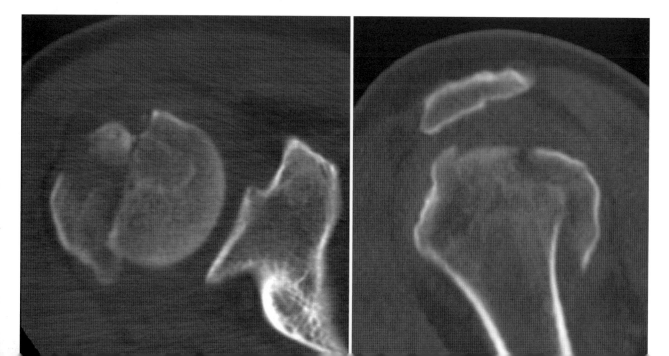

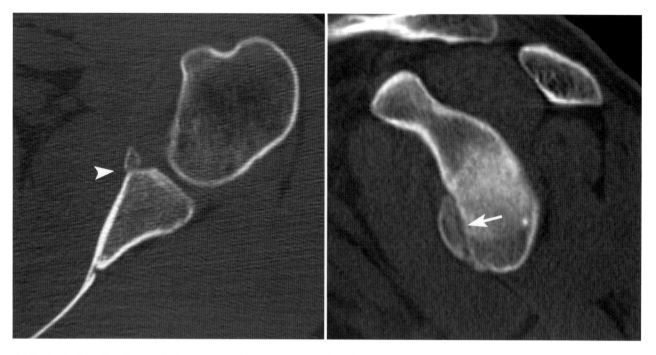

▲ **Fig. 4.52** A Bankart fracture is demonstrated by CT scanning. The left image is an axial image demonstrating the Bankart fracture (arrowhead). A reformatted sagittal image, shown on the right, allows an accurate assessment of fracture size, position and degree of comminution prior to surgical fixation (arrow).

▼▶ **Fig. 4.53** These images are examples of MDCT arthrography.

(a) A reformatted coronal image shows a laterally directed line of contrast within the superior glenoid labrum (arrow), indicative of a SLAP tear.

(b) An axial image shows a tear at the base of the anterior glenoid labrum (arrow) and periosteal reaction indicative of capsuloperiosteal stripping at the anterior aspect of the scapular neck (arrowhead) due to a Perthes lesion.

(c) A reformatted ABER image shows an undetached tear at the base of the anteroinferior glenoid labrum (arrow).

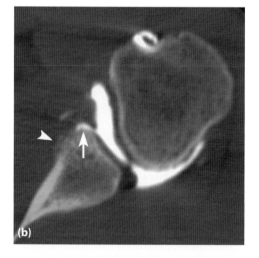

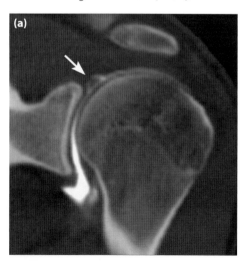

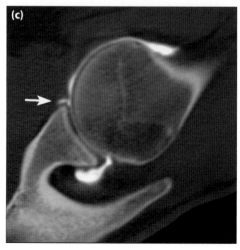

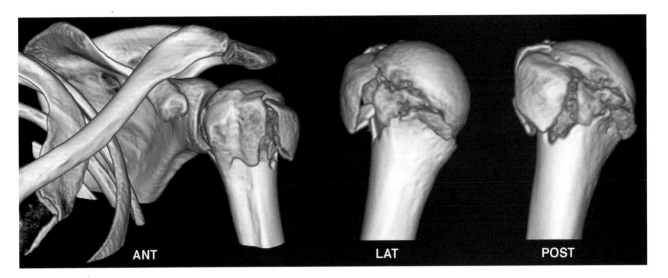

▲ **Fig. 4.54** 3D bone reconstructions obtained from an MDCT examination demonstrate overall alignment at a comminuted fracture of the proximal humerus. Note the ability to perform a virtual disarticulation of the shoulder joint to better evaluate the articular surfaces.

Nuclear medicine

Nuclear bone scans have a valuable imaging role to play around the shoulder-girdle and thoracic cage following a sports-related injury. They remain an excellent method of identifying occult fractures (see Figs 4.55 and 4.56). Enthesopathies (see Figs 4.57, 4.58 and 4.59) are well shown, and muscle tears may also be well demonstrated (see Fig. 4.60). Examples of overuse injuries demonstrated by nuclear bone scans are shown later in the chapter.

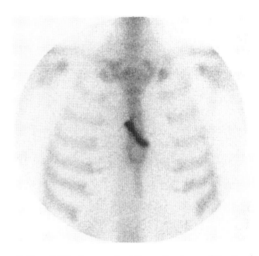

▲ **Fig. 4.56** An occult oblique fracture of the body of the sternum is demonstrated.

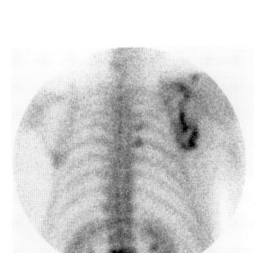

▲ **Fig. 4.55** Nuclear bone scans play a valuable role in the identification of occult fractures around the shoulder-girdle. There has been extensive fracturing of the scapula, which was not appreciated on plain films. There is also abnormal uptake of isotope in left ribs 5 and 6 adjacent to the tubercle of the ribs. In addition, an unexpected fracture of the superior endplate of L1 is shown.

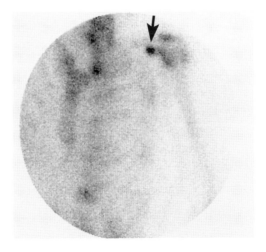

▲ **Fig. 4.57** A left coracoid enthesopathy is shown by a nuclear bone scan (arrow).

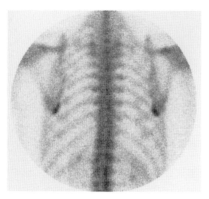

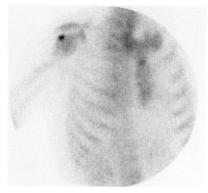

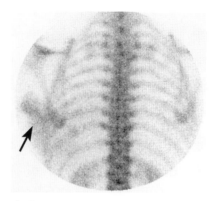

▲ **Fig. 4.58** A weight-lifter has developed symptoms of serratus anterior enthesopathy, and a nuclear bone scan showing increased uptake of isotope at the inferior angle of the scapular bilaterally.

▲ **Fig. 4.59** There is right supraspinatus enthesopathy, with localised uptake of isotope at its insertion.

▲ **Fig. 4.60** An acute muscle tear of the left latissimus dorsi is demonstrated by bone scan. The abnormal uptake is confined to the soft tissues.

MRI

MRI is a well-established imaging method for a wide range of conditions around the shoulder (see Fig. 4.61). The ability to obtain panoramic images in a variety of planes has enabled comprehensive assessment of the complex bone and soft-tissue anatomy of the shoulder. MRI enjoys a special place in both diagnosis and surgical planning. Advances in surface coil design and imaging sequences have created imaging techniques that are useful in the detection and characterisation of rotator cuff pathology, occult fractures, bone bruising, labral tears, chondral lesions and capsuloligamentous injuries. Using fat-suppressed FSE sequences, the accuracy of MRI is high, with sensitivities of 84–100% and specificities of 77–97% reported for full-thickness tears and slightly lower accuracy for partial-thickness tears (Tuite 2004).

▼ **Fig. 4.61** MRI provides a panoramic demonstration of both bone and soft-tissue anatomy at the shoulder. Non-arthrographic axial and coronal images obtained with PD weighting illustrate the detail provided by this imaging method. Acromion = A. Anterior = ANT. Coracoid process = C. Coracohumeral ligament = CHL. Inferior glenohumeral ligament = IGHL. Infraspinatus tendon = ISP. Long head of the biceps tendon = LHB. Middle glenohumeral ligament = MGHL. Posterior = POST. Subacromial-subdeltoid bursa = SA-SD (thickened in this example). Subscapularis tendon = SCP. Supraspinatus tendon = SSP. Superior = SUP.

There is continuing debate as to the additional diagnostic sensitivity and place of MR arthrography. Nevertheless, some authorities have adopted a policy of selectively using intra-articular gadolinium to increase the sensitivity of the MRI examination for both labral and rotator cuff tears in patients less than 30 years old and in professional athletes with chronic shoulder problems. The rationale for such an approach is to minimise the chance of missing subtle healed tears that have developed a synovial cover. Whether or not intra-articular gadolinium is given,

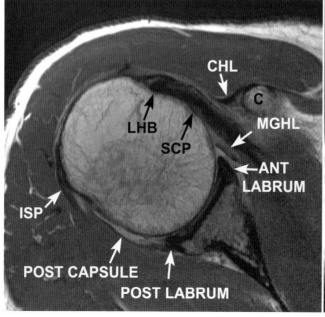

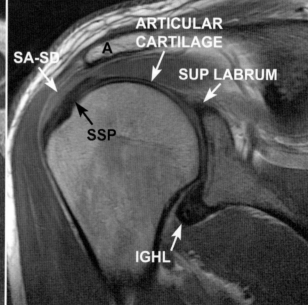

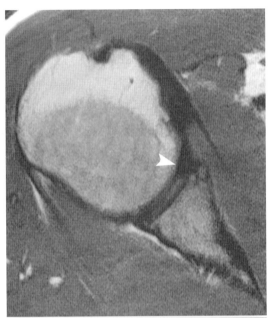

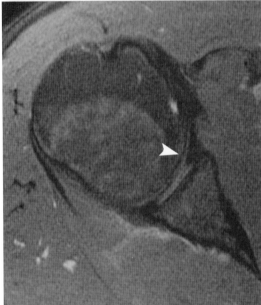

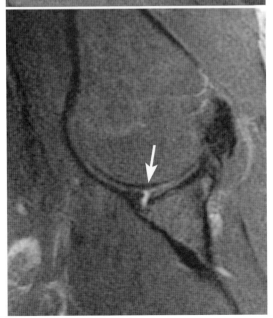

◀**Fig. 4.62** The value of the ABER position is demonstrated on relevant images from a non-arthrographic MRI series. The standard axial PD sequence (top image) and fat-suppressed PD-weighted sequence (middle image) show no discernible labral tear (arrowheads). However, a fat-suppressed ABER sequence (bottom image) applying traction to the anteroinferior GHJ capsule reveals a tear at the base of the anteroinferior labrum (arrow). Note the absence of any associated tear or stripping of the scapular periosteum in this case.

the sensitivity of MRI can be significantly improved by including an imaging sequence in which the arm is placed in the ABER position (Tirman, Bost et al. 1994; Cvitanic et al. 1997) (see Fig. 4.62). In the ABER position, the arm is abducted and the elbow flexed. The forearm rests on the table with the hand behind the neck, placing traction on inferior structures of the shoulder joint.

Arthrography

Arthrography involves the injection of an intra-articular contrast agent followed by imaging. A variety of imaging methods can be used to detect rotator cuff and glenoid labral tears. Conventional arthrography with plain films is able to demonstrate the reduction in joint volume that occurs with GHJ capsulitis, but is rarely used as far more information is available using CT or MR arthrographic techniques. MR arthrography and MDCT arthrography both provide high-quality coronal oblique images that will profile the superior glenoid labrum and demonstrate SLAP tears, which are superior labrum anterior to posterior tears (see Fig. 4.63). However, MRI is better at demonstrating any associated perilabral cyst. CT and MR arthrography are of equal value in detecting Bankart lesions, although if the bony fragment is small or a periosteal reaction with a labral detachment is to be imaged, CT will provide better resolution. MRI provides a superior overall assessment of associated ligamentous injuries, bone bruising and rotator cuff injuries.

▼**Fig. 4.63** An MR arthrogram demonstrates a SLAP tear. A fat-suppressed coronal T1-weighted MR image shows a laterally directed line of high signal representing gadolinium contrast agent extending into a tear of the superior glenoid labrum (arrow).

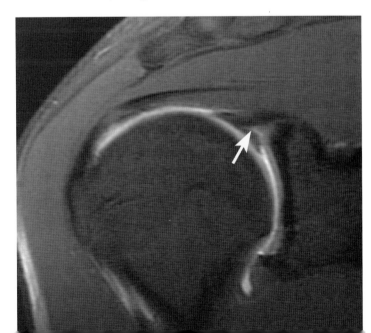

There are many normal anatomical variations in the pattern of the glenoid labral and capsular attachment that are potential traps for the novice in the interpretation of shoulder arthrograms (Mosely and Overgaard 1962; Neumann et al. 1991). The most common variations include the sublabral foramen or hole at the anterosuperior labrum (see Figs 4.64 and 4.65) and the Buford complex, which is a deficient anterosuperior labrum and cord-like middle glenohumeral ligament (MGHL) (Williams et al. 1994) (see Fig. 4.66). The anteroinferior labrum has a consistent firm attachment to the glenoid and any cleft seen at the base of the labrum in this quadrant can be safely regarded as pathological. Variations in the normal pattern of anterior capsular attachment at the scapula have the potential of being mistaken for periosteal stripping. Type I attachments occur on or near the labrum; Type II attachments occur at the scapular neck, within 1 cm of the labrum; and Type III attachments occur medial to the scapular neck, more than 1 cm from the labrum (see Fig. 4.67). Types II and III have an increased incidence of anterior instability.

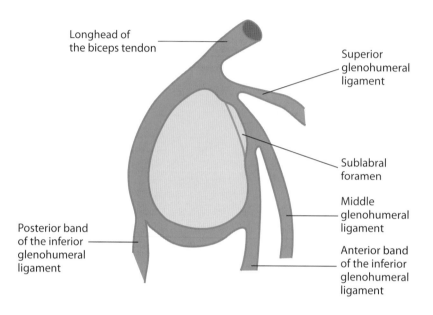

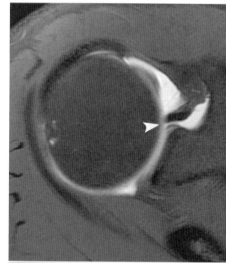

▲ Fig. 4.64 A line drawing of a sublabral foramen.

▶ Fig. 4.65 A sublabral foramen is demonstrated by MR arthrogram. A thin smoothly marginated line of contrast extends beneath the anterosuperior glenoid labrum (white arrowheads). This diminishes at the glenoid equator (white arrow). The MGHL is indicated by black arrows.

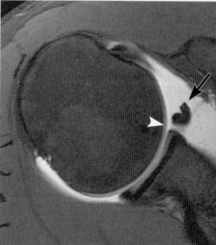

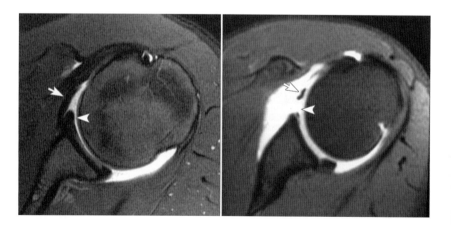

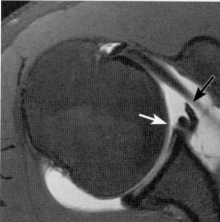

▲ Fig. 4.66 The MR arthrogram on the left shows a well-formed anterior labrum (arrowhead) and normal MGHL (arrow) with a capsular insertion that occurs closely adjacent to the labrum, which is Type I. The MR arthrogram on the right shows a Buford complex consisting of an absent anterior glenoid labrum (arrowhead) and a small but nevertheless cord-like MGHL (arrow). Note the far medial (Type III) attachment of the anterior joint capsule in this case.

Type I

Type II

Type III

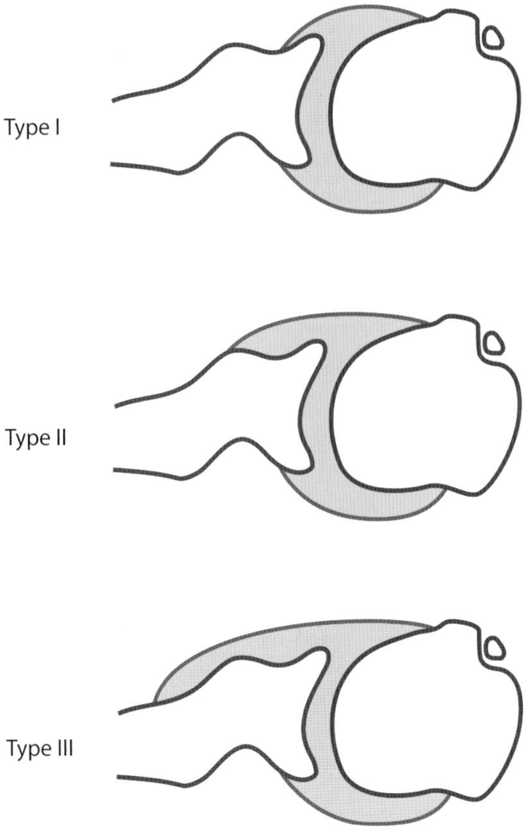

▲ **Fig. 4.67** A line drawing showing the three types of capsular attachment.

Glenohumeral instability

Glenohumeral instability describes an inability to keep the humeral head centred within the glenoid fossa. This condition has a variety of types, and may have numerous causes and appearances, with two broad groups recognised. 'Microinstability' describes a group of instabilities that encompass injury to any of the stabilisers at the superior aspect of the shoulder. Displacement of the unstable humeral head is limited by the adjacent coracoid, acromion and intervening rotator cuff. This group is discussed in more detail below. 'Macroinstability' describes injury to any of the stabilisers at the anterior or posterior aspects of the shoulder, producing a variety of clinical presentations that can range from mild apprehension to frank glenohumeral dislocation. Dislocations can be isolated or recurrent, unidirectional or multidirectional, voluntary or involuntary.

Categories of instability with respect to the age of the athlete

Injury patterns in younger patients

In younger patients (aged less than 35 years), two main dislocation categories have been described: TUBS (traumatic, unidirectional, Bankart, surgical) and AMBRI (atraumatic, multidirectional, bilateral, rehabilitation, inferior capsular shift) (Matsen et al. 1990).

TUBS

TUBS injuries usually result from a fall onto an outstretched, externally rotated and abducted arm. TUBS injuries account for 96% of dislocations (Rowe 1956) and are typically unidirectional (see Fig. 4.68). An

▼ **Fig. 4.68** An acute anterior shoulder dislocation is demonstrated by AP and lateral plain film images. Note that the majority of the humeral head lies anterior to a triangle formed by the tip of the coracoid and acromial processes and the inferior angle of the scapula. The humeral head lies in a subcoracoid position.

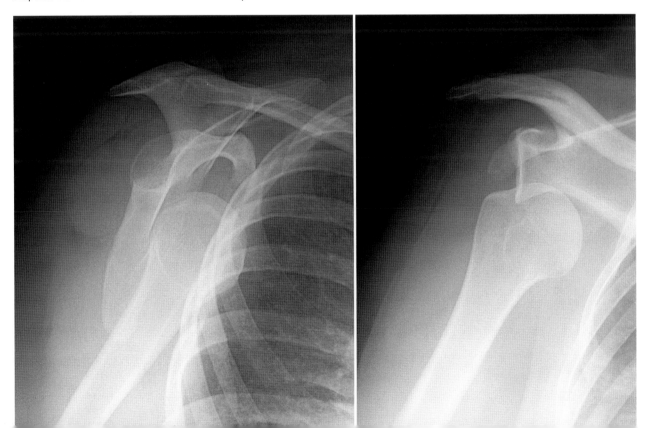

▶ **Fig. 4.69** The mechanism of a Hill-Sachs injury is demonstrated with impaction of the humeral head against the anteroinferior glenoid rim, producing a large depression fracture. Such fractures are diagnostic of anterior instability and occur in about 50% of dislocations.

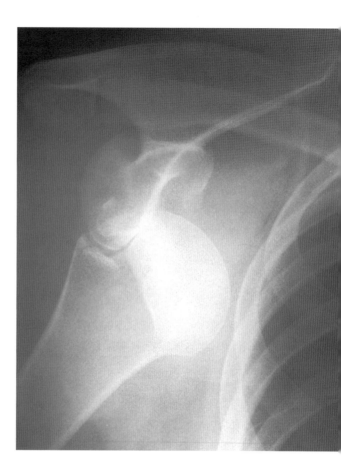

anatomical defect such as a capsulolabral tear, a Hill-Sachs fracture (see Fig. 4.69) or a Bankart lesion (see Fig. 4.70) may result, predisposing the athlete to recurrent dislocation. These changes may be demonstrated by imaging and, if dislocation is recurrent, surgical intervention may be required.

AMBRI

Patients with AMBRI injuries have laxity of the inferior gleno-humeral ligament, which is either congenital or acquired from overuse activities such as weightlifting, swimming and pitching in baseball. Congenital causes include glenoid dysplasia or hypoplasia, glenoid retroversion (see Fig. 4.71), far medial anterior capsular attachment at the scapula, small or absent glenohumeral ligaments, and systemic conditions such as Ehlers-Danlos syndrome. The condition is often multidirectional and bilateral, presenting as subacromial impingement secondary to rotator cuff overload. Imaging tests are often negative, although plain films may demonstrate glenoid hypoplasia. Capsular redundancy, glenoid or labral hypoplasia may be demonstrated by MR or CT arthrography.

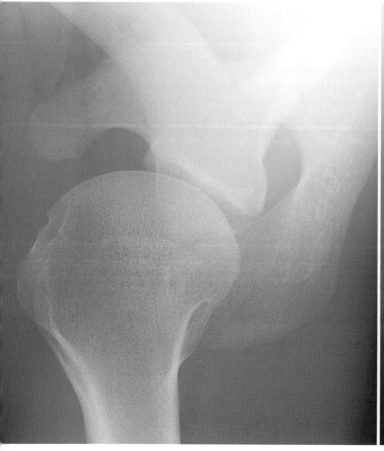

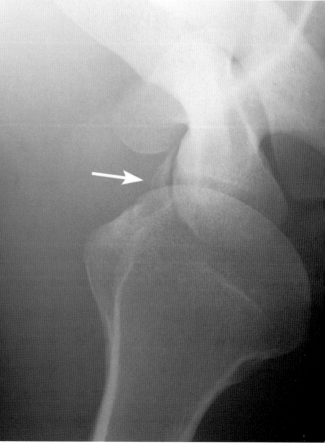

▲ **Fig. 4.70** Following shoulder trauma, a routine axial view (left image) appears normal. A Westpoint view of the same shoulder shows a bony Bankart lesion with a moderate-sized fragment separated from the anteroinferior glenoid rim (right image).

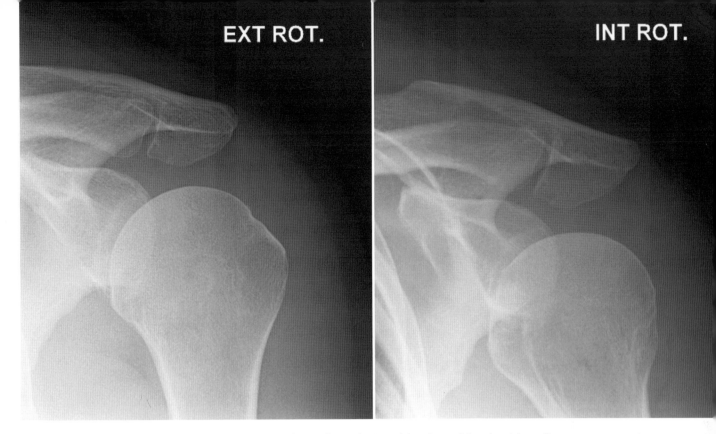

EXT ROT.

INT ROT.

▲ **Fig. 4.71** Glenoid retroversion is present. This anomaly, involving sloping of the plane of the glenoid, predisposes to recurrent instability.

Injury patterns in older patients

In older patients (aged over 35 years), injury patterns associated with first-time anterior shoulder dislocations may be quite different from those of the TUBS group (Neviaser et al. 1988, 1993). Humeral head dislocations in this group have a tendency to occur over an intact labroligamentous hinge and manifest as supraspinatus or subscapularis tears or avulsions, or as an avulsion fracture of the greater tuberosity. There may also be tears of the anterior band of inferior glenohumeral ligament (AIGHL).

Categories of instability with respect to the patterns of glenohumeral dislocation

Although glenohumeral dislocations are separated into the two categories TUBS and AMBRI with respect to direction, it must be appreciated that there are many cases with features of multidirectional instability which will have components of both anterior and posterior instability.

Anterior instability

By far the most common form of shoulder instability is anterior glenohumeral dislocation. Acute trauma is the main aetiological factor, but other causes can include overuse, particularly in throwing sports as well as general ligamentous laxity. In fact, the dividing line between normal laxity and pathological instability is not always clear. Some individuals with particularly lax joints are able to produce voluntary atraumatic shoulder

dislocations, although in time these may eventually become involuntary. Anterior shoulder dislocations are almost always caused by forceful abduction, external rotation and extension of the arm. Disruption of the anterior capsulolabral restraints allows the humeral head to dislocate, most commonly into a subcoracoid position. Impaction of the humeral head against the anterior glenoid margin during this process frequently produces a tear of the anteroinferior glenoid labrum and scapular periosteal attachment producing a soft-tissue Bankart lesion, an injury that has been reported in up to 85% of anterior dislocations (Singson et al. 1987).

Imaging of anterior instability

Ideally, following acute trauma producing a GHJ dislocation, an initial plain film is advisable to exclude a fracture before reduction is attempted. This is often not possible. A plain film is certainly mandatory if reduction is difficult, since a large interposed fracture fragment may be preventing relocation. Immediately following reduction, a plain film should be obtained to confirm reduction and exclude a fracture. The examination is limited to AP and lateral views if the shoulder is immobilised by strapping or a sling, which should not be removed for imaging.

In the non-acute setting, a full plain film instability series of films should be obtained, including a Westpoint or Garth view (see Table 4.2 on page 192). A number of fractures may be associated with anterior instability and dislocation. In addition to a Hill-Sachs lesion and a Bankart fracture (see Fig. 4.72), a BHAGL lesion (bony humeral avulsion of the glenohumeral ligament) may be demonstrated (see Figs 4.73 and 4.74). Other fractures that are uncommonly seen include a coracoid

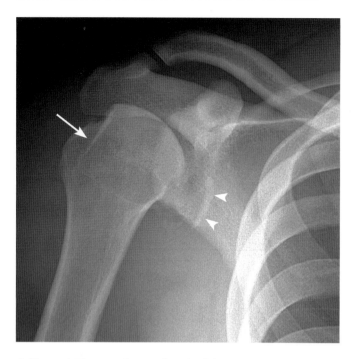

▲ **Fig. 4.72** There is a large Hill-Sachs defect (arrow) and a comminuted fracture of the anteroinferior glenoid rim (arrowheads). Continuing anterior instability would be anticipated.

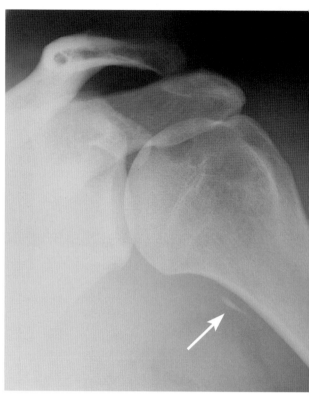

▲ **Fig. 4.74** A BHAGL fragment is present, lying in the infraglenoid fossa (arrow).

▼ **Fig. 4.73** An avulsion of a small bony fragment from the humeral attachment of the inferior glenohumeral ligament is a BHAGL lesion (arrow).

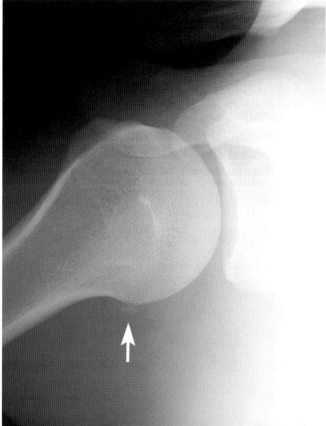

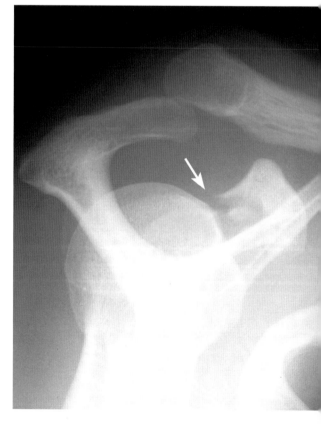

▲ **Fig. 4.75** Fracture of the coracoid process occurs due to an impact by the humeral head during an anterior shoulder dislocation. In this case, a fracture has occurred through the base of the coracoid process (arrow).

process fracture caused by direct impact by the humeral head (see Fig. 4.75) and a fracture of the greater tuberosity due to rotator cuff avulsion. Even when no fracture has occurred, plain films obtained several weeks after the injury may show periosteal reaction at the anteroinferior glenoid rim or scapular neck due to either a periosteal tear associated with a labral Bankart lesion or periosteal stripping associated with a Bankart variant such as a Perthes lesion (see Fig. 4.76). Careful inspection of the scapular neck and glenoid rim is important in all views (see Fig. 4.77). Incongruity of the articular surfaces of the GHJ may also indicate instability (see Fig. 4.78).

Imaging recurrent anterior instability

Following an initial traumatic dislocation, the athlete may subsequently develop recurrent GHJ subluxation or dislocation as shown in Fig. 4.78. The younger the athlete, the greater is the likelihood of recurrent instability, with a reported incidence of more than 90% in the under-20 age group (Rowe and Sakellarides 1961).

MRI plays a major role in detecting abnormalities associated with an initial traumatic dislocation and assists in surgical planning. The following may all predispose to recurrent instability: a Hill-Sachs lesion (see Fig. 4.79), a BHAGL lesion (see Fig. 4.80), a Bankart fracture (see Fig. 4.81), a labral Bankart lesion (see Fig. 4.82), a Perthes lesion (see Fig. 4.83), an ALPSA (anterior labroligamentous periosteal sleeve avulsion) lesion (see Figs 4.84 and 4.85) and a HAGL (humeral-side avulsion of the inferior glenohumeral ligament) lesion (see Fig. 4.86).

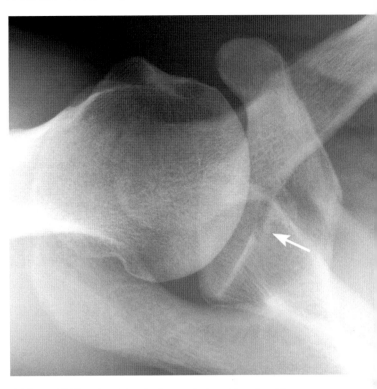

▲ **Fig. 4.77** The glenoid articular cortical contour should be examined carefully on all views. In this case, a displaced fracture of the glenoid rim is seen on an axial view, with the fracture extending to involve the articular surface of the glenoid (arrow). A CT scan would further define this fracture and define the articular deformity.

▼ **Fig. 4.76** Periosteal new bone is present on the anteroinferior aspect of the scapular neck (arrow). The appearance is almost certainly indicative of periosteal stripping (Perthes lesion). No fracture is evident.

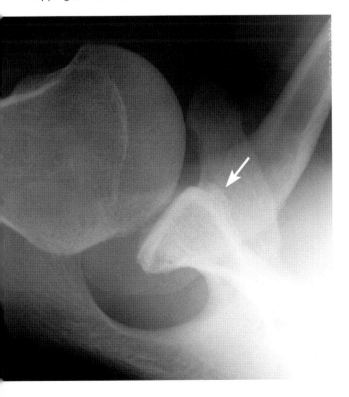

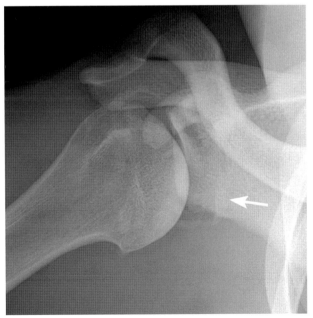

▲ **Fig. 4.78** There has been a previous comminuted fracture of the anteroinferior aspect of the glenoid rim in this 28-year-old athlete (arrow). Anteroinferior subluxation of the humeral head has resulted and secondary degenerative changes are developing. Apparent joint space narrowing is likely to be due to a combination of the subluxation and injury to the articular cartilage.

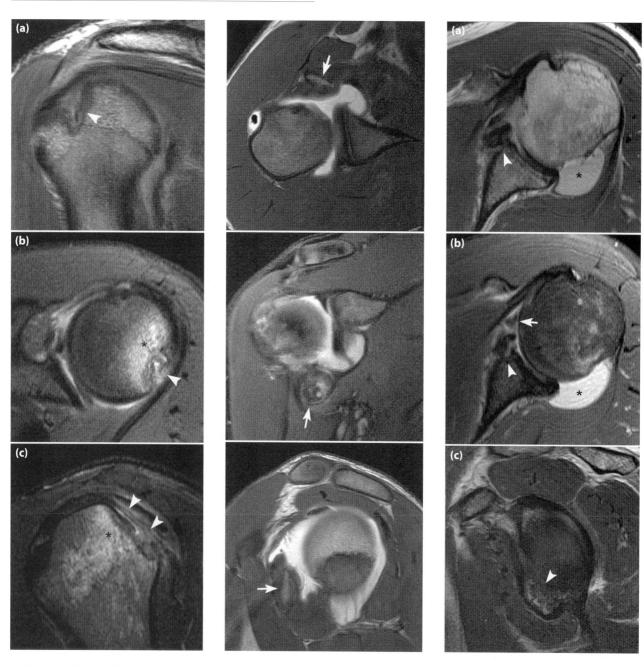

▲ **Fig. 4.79** Recent Hill-Sachs lesions are shown by MRI. Coronal PD (**a**), fat-suppressed axial PD (**b**) and sagittal STIR (**c**) sequences all demonstrate localised cortical impaction at the posterior convexity of the humeral head (arrowheads). Note the associated bone marrow oedema (asterisk).

▲ **Fig. 4.80** An MR arthrogram demonstrates a BHAGL lesion. Axial, coronal and sagittal PD-weighted images are shown. The anterior band of the IGHL has avulsed a bone fragment (arrows) from the humeral insertion.

▲ **Fig. 4.81** A Bankart fracture is demonstrated by MRI. Axial PD (**a**), axial fat-suppressed PD (**b**) and sagittal PD (**c**) images show a separated and slightly displaced fracture of the anteroinferior glenoid rim (arrowheads). These fractures can sometimes be surprisingly difficult to appreciate on axial MRI sequences, and careful scrutiny of the sagittal images is often necessary. Note the associated haemarthroses (asterisk) and in (**b**) the injured MGHL (arrow).

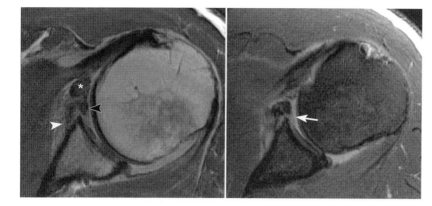

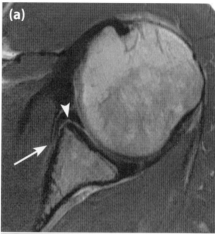

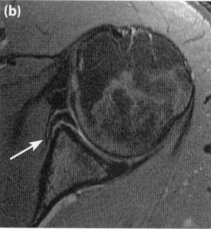

▲ **Fig. 4.82** A labral Bankart lesion consists of an anterior labral tear with associated IGHL destabilisation due to an accompanying tear of the scapular periosteum. An example of a recent Bankart lesion is demonstrated by axial PD (left image) and fat-suppressed PD (right image) sequences from a non-arthrographic MRI exam. Note the linear high signal indicative of a tear at the base of the anteroinferior glenoid labrum (white arrow) and hyperintense marked thickening with overlying haemorrhage indicative of torn periosteal attachment of the anteroinferior capsulolabral complex (white arrowhead). In this case, there is accompanying injury to the MGHL (asterisk) and glenoid articular cartilage. The anterior glenoid labrum is indicated by the black arrowhead.

▶ **Fig. 4.83** A non-arthrographic MRI demonstrates a Perthes lesion. Axial PD **(a)**, fat-suppressed axial PD **(b)** and fat-suppressed ABER **(c)** images are shown. This injury is a labroligamentous avulsion, which is differentiated from a labral Bankart lesion by the presence of a stripped but still intact scapular periosteum (arrow). Note the intact fat plane overlying the stripped periosteum, with an absence of haemorrhage. An arrowhead indicates the point of labral separation.

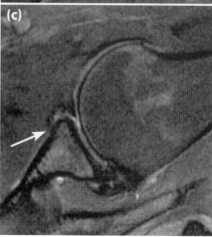

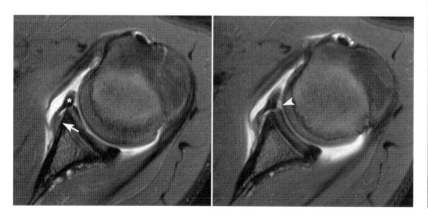

▲ **Fig. 4.84** MRI demonstrates an acute ALPSA lesion. Haemarthrosis produces an arthrographic effect on these fat-suppressed axial PD images. The injury is a labroligamentous avulsion, which is differentiated from a labral Bankart lesion by the presence of an intact scapular periosteum (arrow) and is differentiated from a Perthes lesion by medial displacement and rotation of the labrum (asterisk). The rotated labrum can completely displace onto the scapular neck, but in the case shown here the degree of displacement is only mild. The arrowhead indicates the point of labral separation. A chronic healed and resynovialised ALPSA lesion can be difficult to recognise at arthroscopy.

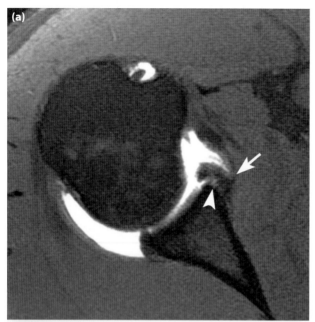

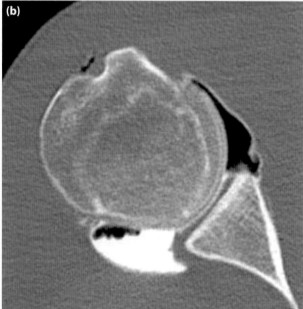

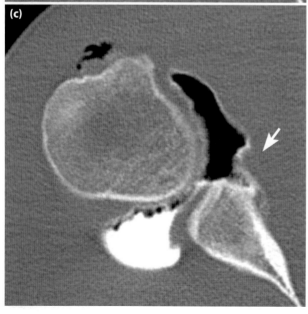

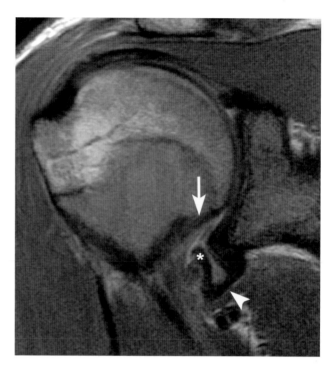

◀ **Fig. 4.85** A chronic ALPSA lesion demonstrated by MR arthrogram **(a)** and CT arthrogram (**(b)** and **(c)**) in two different cases. Both examples show the rounded soft-tissue prominence of a 'medialised' anterior labroligamentous complex at the anterior glenoid rim (arrows). The MR arthrogram also shows a localised zone of mixed high and low signal consistent with reparative granulation tissue and fibrosis filling the interval between the displaced labrum and glenoid rim (arrowhead). Smooth contrast coating at the point of the labral detachment is indicative of healing and chronicity.

▲ **Fig. 4.86** A HAGL lesion. A coronal PD-weighted image from a non-arthrographic MRI examination shows a detached stump (asterisk) of the inferior glenohumeral ligament separated by a high signal line of joint fluid from the normal site of humeral attachment (arrow). An arrowhead indicates the intact IGHL mid-segment.

Although the abovementioned injury patterns are common, many variations are also encountered. These can include purely ligamentous disruptions such as a glenoid-side avulsion of the IGHL from the labral attachment (a GAGL lesion), non-detached labral tears which incorporate an avulsed fragment of adjacent articular cartilage (a glenolabral articular disruption or GLAD lesion) (see Fig. 4.87) and other chondral or osteochondral defects of the glenoid cavity and glenoid rim (Yu et al. 1998) with or without loose bodies (see Fig. 4.88). As a consequence, it is important to recognise that complex injury patterns cannot always be placed into neat diagnostic pigeonholes (see Fig. 4.89).

Posterior instability

Only 2–4% of all shoulder instabilities are purely posterior in direction (Boyd and Sisk 1972). These occur either as the result of a single acute trauma event or due to repetitive micro-trauma.

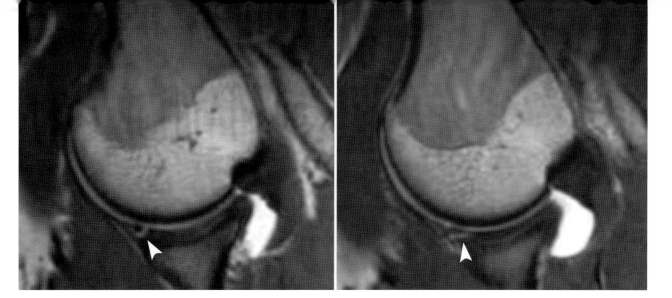

▲ **Fig. 4.87** A GLAD lesion is demonstrated by PD-weighted MR arthrogram images obtained in the ABER position. These images show a partial-thickness tear of the glenoid labrum (arrowheads), with an associated glenoid articular cartilage avulsion. The involved labral segment is not completely detached and there is no capsular stripping. Consequently, this lesion is clinically stable but may produce pain.

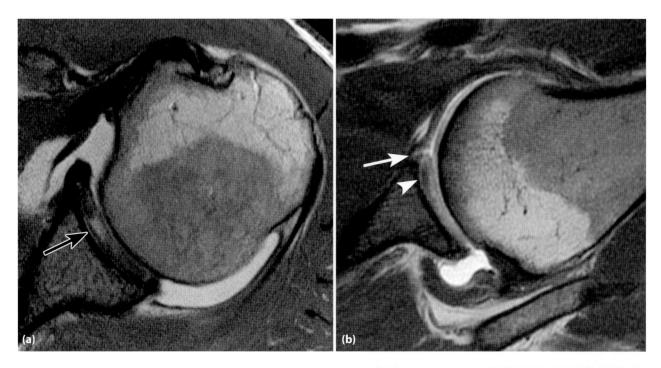

(a)

(b)

▲ **Fig. 4.88** MR images show chondral injury associated with anterior instability. PD-weighted axial **(a)** and ABER **(b)** images show an incomplete and non-displaced tear of the anteroinferior glenoid labrum (white arrow) with an accompanying glenoid chondral fracture (black arrow). Note that there is a subtle high signal line extending beneath the anterior glenoid articular cartilage on the ABER sequence, consistent with chondral flap (arrowhead).

▶ **Fig. 4.89** Injury patterns associated with GHJ instability cannot always be confidently or neatly categorised by a specific acronym! Consequently, the most practical and helpful radiology reports are generally those that simply describe the morphologic features of the injury and avoid the use of questionable and confusing acronyms. The MRI example shown here is a variant pattern that combines an unstable labral Bankart lesion (a capsuloperiosteal tear is indicated by the black arrow) with an avulsed fragment of articular cartilage (white arrowhead).

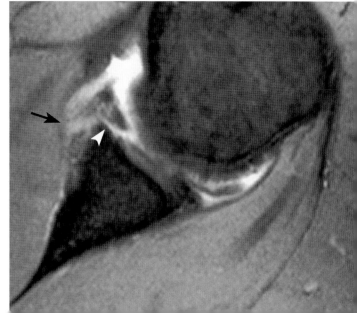

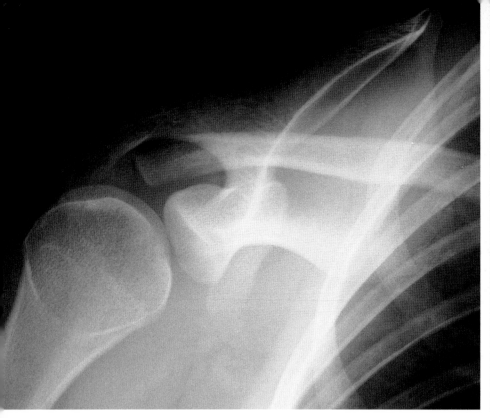

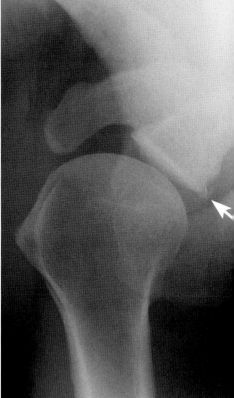

▲ **Fig. 4.90** This injury to the right shoulder resulted from karate. The scapula is rotated and locked in this position with widening of the scaphothoracic joint space. An AP view of the shoulder shows a posterior dislocation at the GHJ, demonstrating the two characteristic features: the articular surfaces of the humeral head and glenoid are roughly parallel and may be mistaken for congruity; and the humeral head is locked in internal rotation.

▲ **Fig. 4.92** An axial view of the shoulder shows a fracture of the posterior glenoid rim (arrow). This is a reverse Bankart lesion resulting from a posterior dislocation.

▼ **Fig. 4.91** Plain films show the mechanism of a reversed Hill-Sachs lesion produced by posterior glenohumeral dislocation. On the left image, the humeral head is locked by a reverse Hill-Sachs defect. On the post-reduction film (right image), an axial view of the shoulder demonstrates a reverse Hill-Sachs defect (arrow).

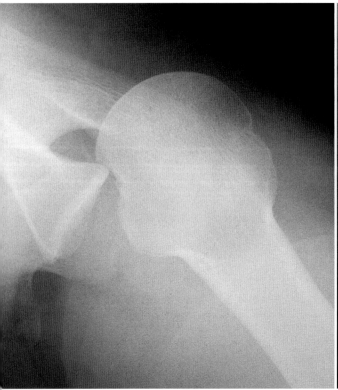

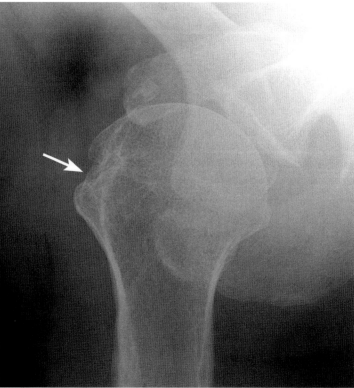

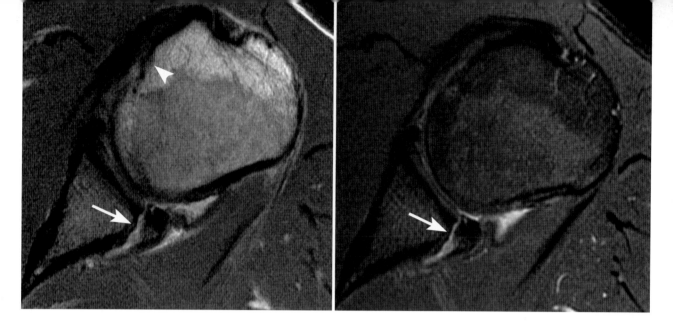

▲ **Fig. 4.93** Non-arthrographic axial PD and fat-suppressed PD MR images demonstrate a reverse Bankart fracture (arrow) and a shallow reverse Hill-Sachs lesion (arrowhead). Note the relative absence of bone marrow oedema, consistent with the subacute-on-chronic clinical presentation of this 20-year-old rugby player with no specific recalled injury.

Other causes include capsuloligamentous laxity, glenoid retroversion or hypoplasia, muscle imbalance and violent muscle contractions (Bergfeld 1990). Acute traumatic posterior dislocations usually result from a direct anterior blow to the shoulder, or a forceful flexion, adduction and internal rotation of the arm. Occasionally a posterior dislocation will be seen as the result of a convulsion (including those associated with electrocution) and a fall onto the outstretched hand.

If possible, a full plain film instability series should be obtained and carefully assessed, remembering to look for additional features of anterior instability that may be simultaneously present in cases of multidirectional instability. It has been estimated that 60–80% of all posterior dislocations are missed at their initial presentation (Rockwood 1984). Disturbance of normal GHJ alignment may be subtle on AP radiographs obtained prior to reduction. As previously noted, the major clue to the diagnosis of posterior dislocation is that the humerus is locked in internal rotation (see Fig. 4.90). Following reduction, plain films may show an impaction fracture at the anteromedial aspect of the humeral head. This is a reverse Hill-Sachs lesion (see Fig. 4.91). There may also be a reverse Bankart fracture of the posterior glenoid rim (see Fig. 4.92).

Recurrent posterior subluxations may develop following the initial injury. In sport, recurrent posterior subluxations due to acquired capsular laxity are reported in butterfly swimmers, rowers and archers. Repetitive impact micro-trauma in which the humeral head is driven posteriorly against the glenoid rim occurs in punching, blocking in football, and weightlifting. Voluntary subluxation can be produced by some individuals with particularly lax joints, as has been shown in Fig. 4.30 on page 203. As with anterior shoulder instability, the clinical presentation may actually be that of a subacromial impingement syndrome due to increased dynamic loading of the rotator cuff producing a secondary tendinopathy.

Imaging is used to demonstrate changes that might contribute to recurrent posterior instability. Plain films,

CT and MRI can all be used to identify those significant injuries and anatomical variants, which include a reverse Bankart fracture, a reverse Hill-Sachs lesion (see Fig. 4.93), a Bennett lesion (periosteal ossification related to posterior capsuloligamentous avulsion) (Ferrari et al. 1994) (see Fig. 4.94), glenoid hypoplasia and glenoid retroversion. CT arthrography and MRI can demonstrate tears of the posterior glenoid labrum (see Figs. 4.95, 4.96 and 4.97). Rarely, a GARD (glenoid articular rim divot) lesion may occur (see Fig. 4.98). This is a post-traumatic osteochondral lesion producing cystic change in the central posterior glenoid rim with an accompanying posterior labral tear (Sanders et al. 2000).

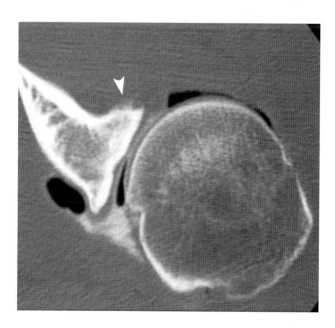

▲ **Fig. 4.94** An axial CT arthrogram image demonstrates bony irregularity and a periosteal reaction at the attachment of the posterior GHJ capsule to the glenoid (a Bennett lesion).

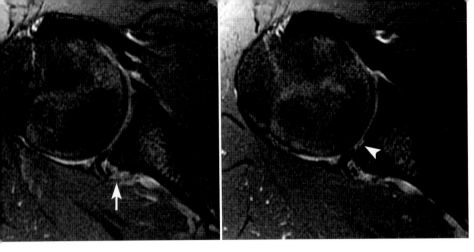

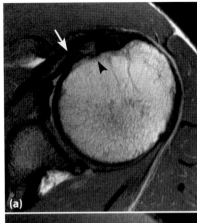

(a)

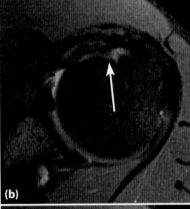

(b)

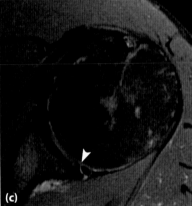

(c)

▲ **Fig. 4.95** Non-arthrographic MRI demonstrates posterior glenohumeral instability. Axial fat-suppressed PD-weighted images show a combination of a reverse Perthes lesion (stripped scapular periosteum indicated by an arrow) and a posterior glenoid rim chondral fracture (arrowhead).

▶ **Fig. 4.96** Posterior glenohumeral instability is demonstrated by non-arthrographic MRI. Axial PD **(a)** and fat-suppressed PD (**(b)** and **(c)**) images show a tear of the posterior glenoid labrum (white arrowhead) without a periosteal tear or stripping. A small reverse Hill-Sachs lesion is indicated by a black arrowhead with accompanying marrow oedema (long white arrow). An associated articular-side partial-thickness tear of the subscapularis tendon with proximal laminar intrasubstance extension is indicated by the short white arrow.

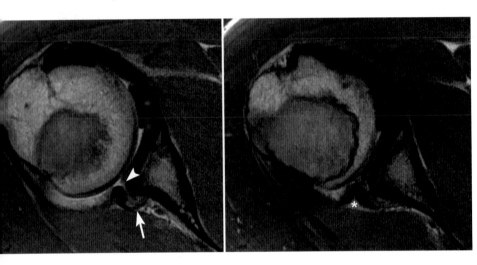

▲ **Fig. 4.97** A reverse Perthes lesion is demonstrated by non-arthrographic axial PD images. A labral tear is indicated by an arrowhead and an arrow indicates the stripped and injured but still grossly intact scapular periosteum. Note the clean overlying fat plane (asterisk). Glenoid retroversion is present, predisposing to posterior instability.

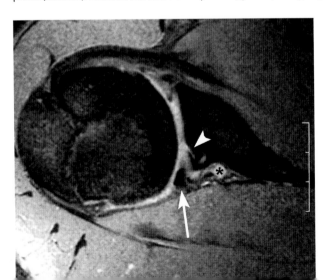

◀ **Fig. 4.98** An axial GRE image in a 22-year-old man after an impact injury to his shoulder demonstrates a displaced posterior labral tear (large arrow) in conjunction with an osseous defect in the posterior aspect of the glenoid rim (arrowhead). This is a GARD lesion. An asterisk indicates a small associated labral cyst.
Source: With permission from Sanders et al. (2000).

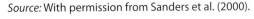

Inferior instability

Inferior dislocation (luxatio erecta) (see Fig. 4.99) is a rare condition associated with martial arts and wrestling. In acute traumatic inferior dislocation, the inferior GHJ capsule is usually torn and there may be injury to the brachial plexus and axillary artery. There may also be an associated avulsion fracture of the greater humeral tuberosity.

Transient inferior subluxation (or 'pseudosubluxation') is not a true dislocation and describes inferior displacement of the humeral head following a post-traumatic haemarthrosis, which may be associated with poor rotator cuff muscle tone due to a neurapraxia (Laskin and Schreiber 1971; Connolly 1982). An example of transient neurapraxia was shown in Fig. 4.31.

Superior instability (microinstability)

As previously discussed, 'microinstability' is a general term that includes a variety of injuries to the stabilisers along the upper half of the GHJ which can result in superior displacement of the humeral head, limited by the coracoid and acromion processes and the rotator cuff. Injuries to the rotator interval ligaments, the coracohumeral ligament (CHL), the superior glenohumeral ligament (SGHL), the superior glenoid labrum (SLAP tears) and the rotator cuff may produce microinstability. These injuries either can occur as acute traumatic events or are the result of chronic overuse, associated with repetitive overhead activities. The clinical and imaging diagnosis can be challenging, with supplementary arthroscopy often being the final arbiter. Symptoms can include a subjective sensation of instability or weakness, thrower's 'dead arm', non-specific shoulder pain with overhead or cross-body activities and subacromial impingement. The athlete may report a sensation of 'popping', 'catching', 'grinding' or 'clunking'. MRI or MR arthrography is the imaging method of choice, but multislice CT arthrography is a valid alternative when MRI is either unavailable or contraindicated.

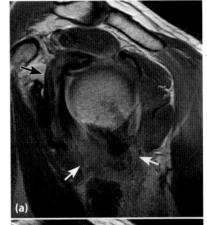

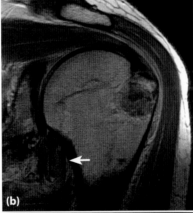

Major patterns of SLAP tears

A SLAP tear occurs at the glenolabral attachment of the long head of the biceps tendon. The classification of these tears has expanded, although four main types of SLAP tear were originally described (Andrews et al. 1985; Snyder et al. 1990):

- *Type I:* there is marked fraying of the superior glenoid labrum with the biceps still attached.
- *Type II:* a tear is present at the base of the superior labrum and associated biceps 'anchor'.
- *Type III:* a bucket-handle tear of the superior labrum occurs with the biceps still attached.
- *Type IV:* a bucket-handle tear of the superior labrum extends distally along the biceps tendon.

The reliable detection and differentiation of SLAP tears into these four types by MRI may be difficult, largely due to variations in the anatomy of the superior labrum and difficulty in consistently demonstrating biceps tendon destabilisation at the supraglenoid tubercle (see Figs 4.100, 4.101 and 4.102).

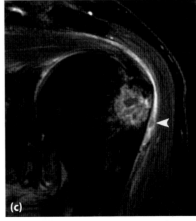

▶**Fig. 4.99** MRI of recent luxatio erecta. Sagittal PD **(a)**, coronal PD **(b)** and coronal fat-suppressed T2 **(c)** images from a non-arthrographic examination show an undisplaced avulsion fracture of the greater humeral tuberosity with accompanying marrow oedema. The capsular injury is diffuse, with haemorrhagic thickening of both the inferior GHJ capsule (white arrows) and anterosuperior GHJ capsule (black arrow). A haemorrhagic effusion is also present within the SA-SD bursa (white arrowhead).

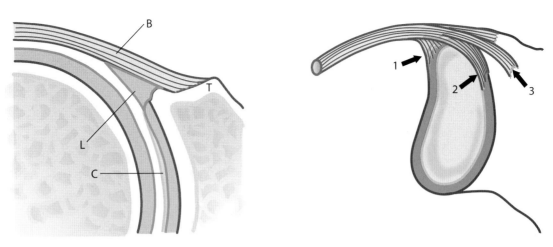

▲ **Fig. 4.100** Line drawings depict the anatomy of the biceps tendon attachment. The diagram on the left is a coronal section through the biceps 'anchor': note the tendon (B) primarily attaches to the supraglenoid tubercle (T) and secondarily attaches to the superior labrum (L), while the labrum attaches to both the glenoid articular cartilage (C) and the bony glenoid rim. A common variation, not shown here but observed in 73% of MR arthrograms, is the presence of a sublabral recess extending beneath the labral attachment (Smith et al. 1996). The diagram on the right illustrates the additional anterior and posterior extent of attachment of the biceps 'expansion': (1) posterosuperior labrum, (2) anterosuperior labrum and (3) base of coracoid process. *Source:* Modified with permission from De Maeseneer et al. (2000).

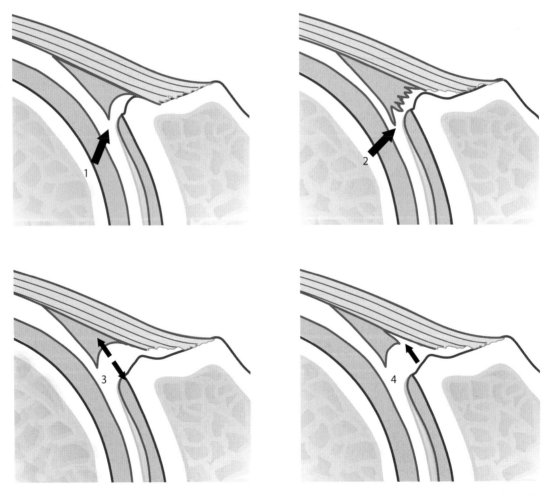

▲ **Fig. 4.101** Type II SLAP tear versus normal superior sublabral recess. Coronal schematics of the labral-bicipital attachment are shown: (1) normal recess with a sharp free edge of the labrum (arrow); (2) Type II SLAP tear with an irregular free edge of the labrum (arrow); (3) Type II SLAP tear with wide separation between the superior labrum and the glenoid (arrows); and (4) Type II SLAP tear with lateral extension of the labral tear (arrow). *Source:* Modified with permission from De Maeseneer et al. (2000).

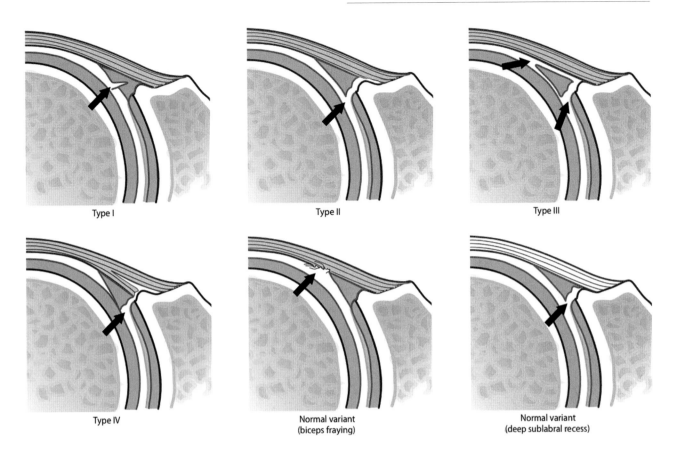

▲ **Fig. 4.102** Coronal schematic drawings of SLAP tear types and normal anatomical variants. Note the potential difficulty in differentiating a Type II SLAP tear from a normal superior sublabral recess on MRI or CT arthrography. Imaging features that can help to confirm a SLAP tear in this circumstance include an abnormally wide separation between the labrum and glenoid, an irregular labral base, and lateral extension of high signal from the sublabral recess (see Fig. 4.101).
Source: Adapted with permission from De Maeseneer et al. (2000).

In addition, some patients have combined or 'complex' SLAP tears, in which features of both Types II and III or II and IV are simultaneously present (Nam and Snyder 2003). If non-arthrographic MRI is used, careful attention to high-resolution scan technique is important (Connell et al. 1999). The inclusion of at least one sequence with LHB traction can be helpful. MR arthrography can theoretically improve the detection of a tear, but a prospective study performed to determine its accuracy in the pre-operative diagnosis of SLAP tears yielded an overall sensitivity of 0.89, specificity of 0.91 and accuracy of 0.9, showing that this technique is effective but does not entirely eliminate error (Bencardino et al. 2000).

Many athletes with a SLAP tear cannot recall a previous injury. In others, the mechanism of injury may be either traction to the LHB tendon, occurring in activities such as water-skiing, throwing or involving sudden weight loads, or as a component of a GHJ dislocation. The mechanism may also involve compression of the superior labrum by the humeral head caused by injuries such as a fall onto an outstretched hand or direct trauma. In the latter case, if the compressive forces are large enough, an additional chondral or osteochondral fracture of the humeral head ('SLAP fracture') may result (Nam and Snyder 2003). This fracture is similar to a Hill-Sachs lesion but the location is more anterior and superior. In about one-third of cases chronic superior instability also leads to secondary rotator cuff tears that begin as partial-thickness tears on the articular side (Morgan et al. 1998).

Type I SLAP tears

This grading of SLAP tear describes labral fraying that is believed to be degenerative and usually affects middle-aged to older patients. Underlying rotator cuff degeneration and dysfunction with consequent superior migration of the humeral head may be a contributing factor (see Fig. 4.103).

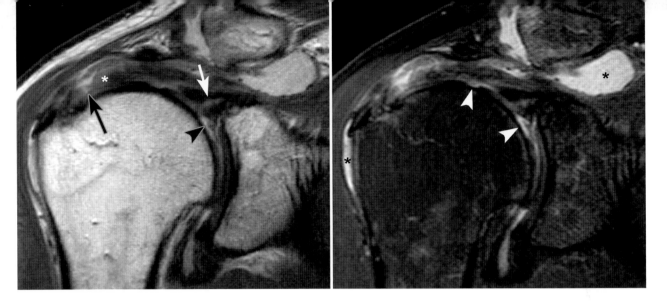

▲ **Fig. 4.103** A Type I SLAP tear is demonstrated by MRI. Coronal PD and fat-suppressed PD MR images show fraying of the superior glenoid labrum (black arrowhead) on a background of labral degeneration (white arrow). There are other degenerative findings present including supraspinatus tendinopathy (white asterisk), with a complicating small full-thickness tear (black arrow). An accompanying SA-SD bursal effusion is indicated by black asterisks and areas of Grade III chondral wear at the humeral head are indicated by white arrowheads. There is also a small GHJ effusion and marked ACJ degeneration with an associated effusion.

▼ **Fig. 4.104** A Type II SLAP tear is an avulsion of the superior labrum and an incomplete avulsion of the LHB tendon at the supraglenoid tubercle attachment. A coronal MR arthrogram demonstrates a line of high signal contrast extending along the tendon/bone junction at the supraglenoid tubercle, indicating partial destabilisation of the bony attachment of the LHB tendon (arrow). Note the absence of irregularity at the labral base and the non-widened superior sublabral sulcus, making the MRI finding of partial supraglenoid tubercle detachment the only means of differentiating a Type II SLAP tear from the normal variant of a deep sublabral sulcus. This case would probably be difficult to diagnose with standard non-arthrographic MRI, with intra-articular gadolinium providing high signal contrast.

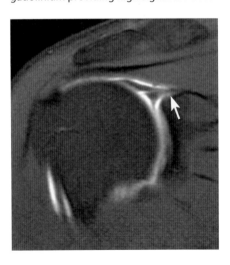

Type II SLAP tears

Type II SLAP tears are the most common subtype. Although labral edge fraying is usually present, Snyder et al. (1990) noted that the key features include an avulsion of the superior labrum from the glenoid rim and partial detachment of the biceps 'anchor' due to an incomplete tear at the supraglenoid tubercle insertion of the biceps tendon (Nam and Snyder 2003). As a consequence, the primary attachment of the biceps tendon is unstable (see Figs 4.104, 4.105 and 4.106).

Sub-classification of Type II SLAP tears

Morgan et al. (1998) and Burkhart et al. (2000) have suggested that Type II SLAP tears can be sub-classified into the following types: anterior (SLAC), posterior ('posterior peel-back') and combined anterior and posterior (or 'classic').

- A SLAC (superior labral anterior cuff) tear is characterised by a tear of the anterosuperior labrum and articular-side fraying or a partial-thickness tear at the anterior 'non-crescentic' aspect of the supraspinatus tendon (Savoie et al. 2001). Overhead activities are the most common cause. There may be an accompanying injury of the rotator interval producing changes that can include an SGHL tear or laxity, a CHL tear, subcoracoid bursopathy and interval synovitis. The SLAC tear causes anterosuperior instability, but a component of straight anterior instability can also be present if the labral tear extends to involve a high MGHL attachment.

- A 'posterior peel-back' SLAP tear is a tear of the posterosuperior labrum that occurs in athletes who throw overhead. The suggested mechanism is a torsional 'dish-rag' shortening of the LHB tendon due to the wind-up phase of throwing, which causes the biceps anchor to peel off the bone. Although this tear produces posterosuperior instability as the primary abnormality, throwers also commonly acquire posterior capsular tightness (PIGHL contracture) that leads to an anterior translational force on the humeral head and compensatory laxity of the anteroinferior capsule. In about one-third of cases there is articular-side fraying or a partial-thickness tear at the posterior insertion of the supraspinatus tendon due to 'internal impingement' (internal impingement is discussed in detail later in the chapter).

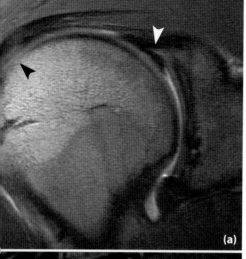
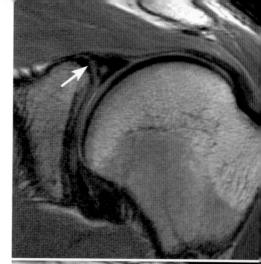

(a)

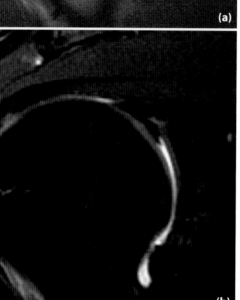

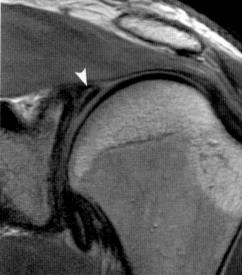

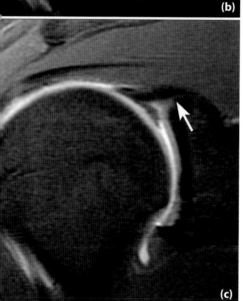

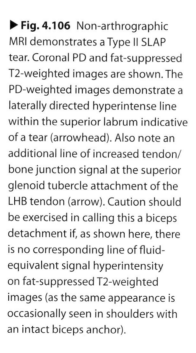

(b)

◀Fig. 4.105 An MR arthrogram demonstrates a Type II SLAP tear. There is a hyperintense line (arrowhead) indicative of a tear extending laterally into the superior labrum on coronal PD **(a)**, fat-suppressed T2 **(b)** and fat-suppressed T1-weighted sequences **(c)** images. Abnormal signal at the supraglenoid tubercle attachment is indicative of biceps tendon destabilisation and this can best be appreciated on the fat-suppressed T1-weighted image (arrow), with contrast provided by injected intra-articular gadolinium. Note the associated shallow articular-side partial-thickness tear of the supraspinatus tendon (black arrowhead).

▶Fig. 4.106 Non-arthrographic MRI demonstrates a Type II SLAP tear. Coronal PD and fat-suppressed T2-weighted images are shown. The PD-weighted images demonstrate a laterally directed hyperintense line within the superior labrum indicative of a tear (arrowhead). Also note an additional line of increased tendon/bone junction signal at the superior glenoid tubercle attachment of the LHB tendon (arrow). Caution should be exercised in calling this a biceps detachment if, as shown here, there is no corresponding line of fluid-equivalent signal hyperintensity on fat-suppressed T2-weighted images (as the same appearance is occasionally seen in shoulders with an intact biceps anchor).

(c)

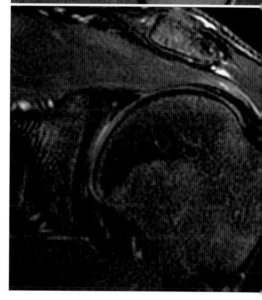

- A 'classic' Type II SLAP tear is a tear that involves both the anterior and posterior portions of the superior labrum, including the 'anchor' of the biceps tendon to the labrum and supraglenoid tubercle. The most common mechanism is a fall onto an outstretched arm, with the shoulder positioned in abduction and slight forward flexion at the time of impact. However, athletes who throw overhead are also affected. Articular-side partial-thickness rotator cuff tears are frequently associated with 'classic' SLAP tears. These tears typically occur at the posterior insertion of the supraspinatus tendon.

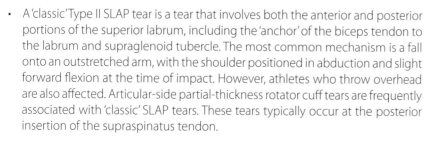

Glenoid labral tears, including Type II SLAP tears, are often associated with perilabral cysts, which are analogous to parameniscal cysts at the knee (Tirman, Feller et al. 1994). The detection of a perilabral cyst by MRI or ultrasound is a strong indicator of an underlying labral tear irrespective of whether the tear itself can be directly visualised (see Figs 4.107 and 4.108). Superior perilabral cysts can be up to 3–4 cm in diameter and may cause compression of the suprascapular nerve at the suprascapular or spinoglenoid notch (see Fig. 4.109), producing a nerve entrapment syndrome in which there is infraspinatus weakness with or without supraspinatus weakness and pain. MRI can detect corresponding changes of muscle denervation with wasting and increased signal intensity on T2-weighted images, shown later in Figs 4.146 and 4.147 on page 255. At times there are signs and symptoms of denervation of the infraspinatus and supraspinatus muscles without any visualised compressive nerve lesion. This painful condition has been called brachial neuritis or Parsonage-Turner syndrome and is diagnosed on MRI by the presence of denervation muscle oedema with no evidence of an underlying ganglion cyst (Helms et al. 1998) (see Fig. 4.110).

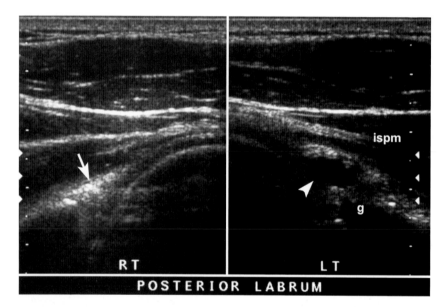

▲ Fig. 4.107 A posterosuperior glenoid perilabral cyst (arrowhead) is associated with a SLAP tear, demonstrated by an MR arthrogram.

◀ Fig. 4.108 Ultrasound demonstrates a small posterior glenoid perilabral cyst. Comparison transverse images obtained over the posterior glenoid rim show a normal echogenic triangle of intact posterior labrum on the right (arrow) and a small, rounded anechoic ganglion cyst obscuring the posterior labrum on the left (arrowhead). An underlying tear of the posterior glenoid labrum is almost certainly present. Infraspinatus muscle = ispm. Posterior glenoid rim = g.

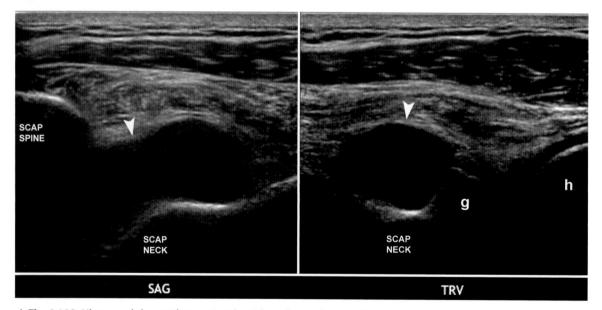

▲ Fig. 4.109 Ultrasound shows a large spinoglenoid notch ganglion. Sagittal and transverse images obtained over the posterior glenoid neck demonstrate a large well-circumscribed anechoic mass lesion typical of a ganglion cyst (arrowheads). Glenoid rim = g. Humeral head = h.

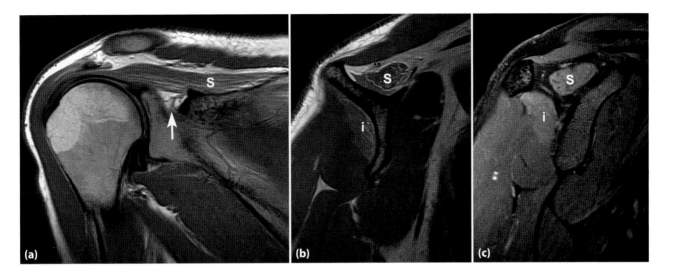

▲ **Fig. 4.110** MRI demonstrates Parsonage-Turner syndrome. A subacute brachial neuritis pattern is shown on coronal PD **(a)** and sagittal PD **(b)** images, which demonstrate atrophy and fatty infiltration of the supraspinatus (s) and infraspinatus (i) muscles. A fat-suppressed sagittal PD image **(c)** shows diffuse muscle hyperintensity due to denervation oedema. Note the absence of any space-occupying lesion at the scapular notch (arrow).

Type III SLAP tears

A Type III SLAP tear is present when there is a bucket-handle tear of a meniscoid superior labrum with the biceps anchor remaining intact (see Fig. 4.111).

Type IV SLAP tears

This grading is similar to Type III, except that the bucket-handle tear extends into the biceps tendon (see Fig. 4.112).

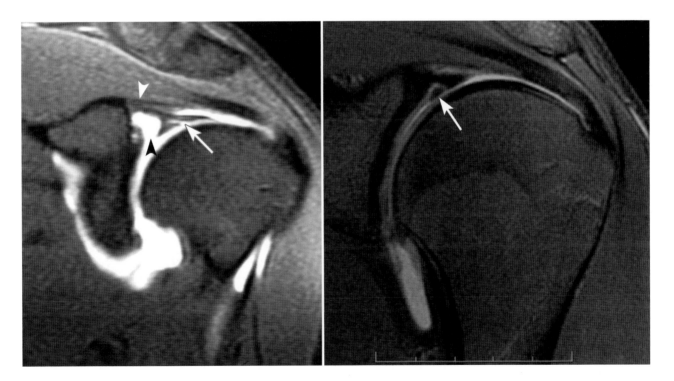

▲ **Fig. 4.111** A Type III SLAP tear is demonstrated by MRI. This tear is a bucket-handle tear of the superior glenoid labrum with an intact supraglenoid tubercle insertion of the LHB tendon. **(a)** A coronal MR arthrogram image shows a bucket-handle tear with complete detachment of the labrum from both the glenoid rim (black arrowhead) and the LHB tendon (arrow). Note the intact biceps tendon insertion (white arrowhead). **(b)** A coronal MR arthrogram image shows a bucket-handle fragment of superior labrum (arrow). Note the large ('meniscoid') superior labrum.

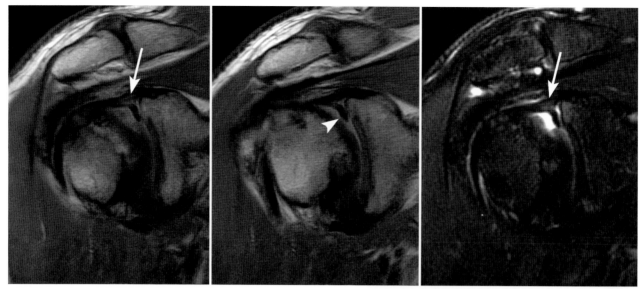

▲ **Fig. 4.112** A Type IV SLAP tear is a bucket-handle tear of a meniscoid superior labrum which extends into the biceps tendon. Non-arthrographic coronal PD and fat-suppressed T2-weighted MR images demonstrate linear signal hyperintensity of the tear extending distally along the proximal biceps tendon segment (arrow) and mild inferior prolapse of the bucket-handle fragment of superior labrum (arrowhead).

▶ **Fig. 4.113 (a)** A normal acromioclavicular arch is well demonstrated by an outlet view. The supraspinatus passes through a rigid tunnel, the roof of which is created by the undersurface of the acromion and ACJ. Bony encroachment on the tunnel invariably occurs from the roof, and the outlet view is a valuable component of a shoulder series.

▼ **(b)** In the left image, soft-tissue calcification is demonstrated in the supraspinatus tendon adjacent to its insertion (arrow). Degenerative changes are also noted, with narrowing of the GHJ space, and there is osteophyte formation at the margins of the humeral articular surface. An acromioclavicular arch view (right image) shows the calcification in the tendon seen end-on (arrow).

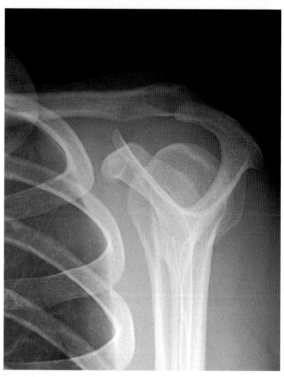

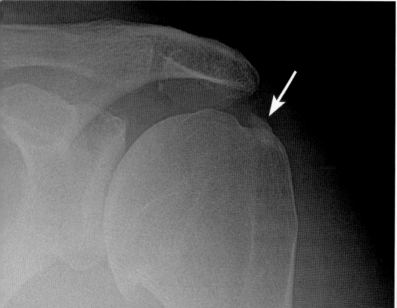

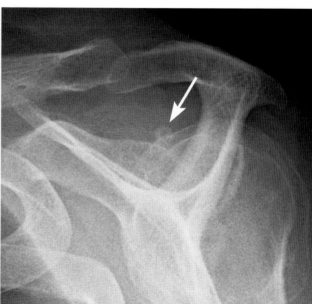

Shoulder impingement and rotator cuff tendinopathy

Several types of impingement syndrome are recognised at the shoulder.

Subacromial impingement syndrome

Subacromial impingement syndrome, or painful arc syndrome, describes a common condition of shoulder pain that characteristically occurs during mid-range abduction. The early and late stages of abduction are usually pain-free. For a variety of reasons, rather than moving freely, the greater tuberosity with its related soft-tissue structures such as the supraspinatus tendon may impinge upon the acromioclavicular arch (see Table 4.4 and Fig. 4.113). There is debate as to whether subacromial impingement syndrome follows the classical pathological and clinical paths described by Neer (1983) (see Table 4.5). Neer (1983) proposed that an acromial osteophyte and/or a thickened tight coracoacromial ligament contribute to impingement, leading to a progressive bursal-side cuff wearing and eventual tearing of the tendon. A more recent theory is that the primary pathology is degeneration of the rotator cuff tendons due to chronic overload and micro-trauma, leading to cuff weakness and secondary impingement. Whatever the case, the process may be greatly accelerated in athletes who frequently undertake overhead activity with the arm due to the excessive overuse that may be associated with training and competition.

As some degree of friction must always occur between the rotator cuff and the coracoacromial arch during shoulder abduction (hence the intervening bursa), subacromial impingement could theoretically be said to be present in all normal shoulders. Subclinical impingement is remarkably common, with imaging features of impingement frequently seen in shoulders that have few or no symptoms. The term 'subacromial impingement syndrome' should be used to describe a clinical presentation of pain in individuals with appropriate symptoms and signs. It is important to remember that the diagnosis of subacromial impingement syndrome is clinical and not radiographic. Consequently, the MRI radiologist who may be reporting findings without having personally examined the patient must adopt a guarded approach to the interpretation of features that indirectly suggest impingement. On the other hand, the ultrasound specialist who has personally examined the patient and has had an opportunity to directly correlate the imaging with the clinical findings is much more appropriately placed to make a firm diagnosis.

Subacromial impingement syndrome is most often due to overuse, arising from any form of repetitive overhead activity with the arm, such as in swimming, tennis and throwing. Acute overuse produces acute rotator cuff tendinopathy and an acute SA-SD bursopathy with an accompanying effusion. Chronic overuse leads to rotator cuff tendinopathy and chronic SA-SD bursopathy. With tendinopathy there are collagen micro-tears, which cause a loss of tensile tendon strength (Kjellin et al. 1991). These collagen micro-tears may

Table 4.4 Causes of subacromial impingement syndrome

• Subacromial soft-tissue swelling
Thickening of the SA-SD bursa resulting from overuse Calcific tendinopathy of the rotator cuff Non-calcific rotator cuff tendinopathy (GHJ instability) Avulsion fracture of the greater tuberosity Rotator cuff contusion
• Supraspinatus outlet encroachment
Anterior acromial bone spur Acromial undersurface hyperostosis Type II (curved) or Type III (hooked) acromion AC joint osteophyte or capsular hypertrophy (OA) An os acromiale
• Humeral depressors overpowered by the deltoid
Supraspinatus tendon rupture LHB tendon rupture Suprascapular nerve palsy

Table 4.5 Neer's stages of subacromial impingement

Stage I	Acute tendinopathy/bursopathy
Stage II	Chronic tendinopathy/bursopathy ± partial-thickness cuff tear
Stage III	Full-thickness rotator cuff tear
Stage IV	Cuff tear arthropathy

Source: Neer (1983).

gradually coalesce to form a 'degenerative' macro-tear. A sudden high-energy stress to an already weakened tendon may also produce an acute macro-tear, which is visible on imaging. It has been demonstrated that extrinsic compression of the cuff due to subacromial impingement generates concentrations of stress sufficient to cause tearing not only at the bursal surface but also at the articular surface and within the tendon (Matava et al. 2005).

Degenerative tears initially tend to delaminate the tendon, forming longitudinal intrasubstance defects that eventually extend to either the bursal or articular surfaces of the cuff as partial-thickness lesions (Seibold et al. 1999) (see Fig. 1.6 on page 7). Delamination tears may be up to 2–3 cm in length and can produce marked weakness. With continuing insult, partial-thickness cuff tears may progress to full-thickness lesions, which slowly increase in size or extend suddenly to further exacerbate the symptoms of impingement.

It is highly unlikely that a normal rotator cuff without predisposing attritional degeneration will tear due to a single episode of acute trauma. This is reflected in the age distribution of cuff tears, which are strongly skewed towards the older population (50+ years). Degenerative rotator cuff tears have a common distribution, usually starting at the anterior supraspinatus insertion within the critical zone of hypovascularity (Codman 1934) and from this point extending backwards along the rotator 'crescent'. The rotator 'crescent' is a thinner and relatively avascular zone of cuff tissue that is prone to degenerative tearing. Initially these tears are intrasubstance lesions, not visible at arthroscopy, but seen with ultrasound and MRI.

In addition to partial-thickness cuff tears associated with the more common mechanisms of subacromial impingement and cuff degeneration, it is also important to recognise that other mechanisms of cuff tear also exist. These include internal impingement and the spectrum of GHJ micro-instability, both of which produce articular-side tears that are typically more posterior in location. These entities are discussed below.

Unfortunately, location alone is not a reliable means of differentiating the aetiology, as some degenerative tears may also start posteriorly.

A brief review of rotator cuff structure at the sub-tendon level can provide a better understanding of partial-thickness tears and their imaging characteristics. The supraspinatus and infraspinatus tendons both comprise five distinct histological layers and are intimately connected to the CHL and biceps pulley (Clark and Harryman 1992):

▶ **Fig. 4.114** Transverse ultrasound images of a normal supraspinatus tendon illustrate the sonographic artefact that may be produced by the histological layering of the tendon. Images have been obtained at the same level but with slightly differing transducer angulation. **(a)** Layer 2 is artefactually hypoechoic (arrows). **(b)** Transducer angulation has been optimised to provide maximal reflectivity from layer 2 as well as the other components of the tendon. Note that the differing composition of the layers together with the presence of transition zones between layers results in a heterogeneous echo-pattern.

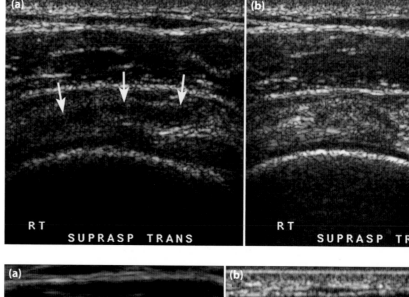

▶ **Fig. 4.115** Normal sonographic rotator cuff tendon anatomy is demonstrated. The orientation of the tendon fibres in layer 2 differs from that of the deeper fibres in layer 3. The longitudinal curvature of superficial and deep tendon fibres also differs at the humeral insertion. This can lead to artefactual alterations in tendon echogenicity that must not be mistaken for partial-thickness tears. Simply changing the angulation of the transducer will typically reveal normal fibrillar echotexture or render the connective tissue transition zones between the cuff layers much less conspicuous. An important diagnostic tip is that the background tendon shows normal sonographic architecture and echotexture without evidence of thickening, tendinopathy or peritendon abnormality. **(a)** Arrowheads indicate a hypoechoic line of transition between layers 2 and 3; **(b)** an arrowhead indicates a mixed hypo-hyperechoic line of transition between layers 2 and 3; **(c)** an arrowhead indicates a subtle hyperechoic line of transition between layers 2 and 3; and **(d)** an arrow indicates a hypoechoic zone typically present at the humeral insertion of the deep fibres of the rotator cuff due to anisotropy arising from steep longitudinal curvature.

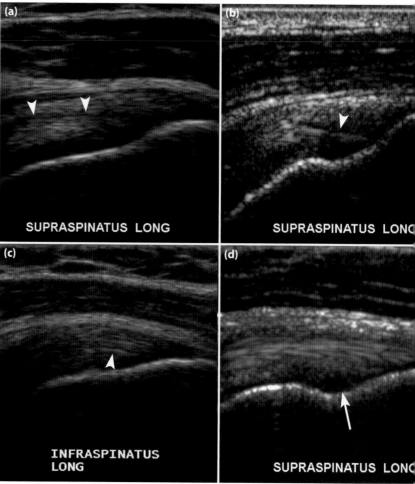

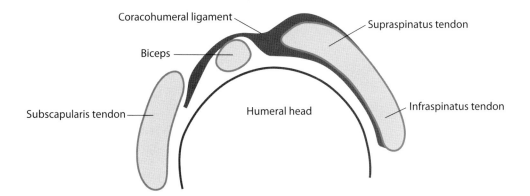

▲ **Fig. 4.116** A line drawing demonstrates CHL anatomy. The CHL is a thick, tent-like band of fibrous tissue extending from the base of the coracoid process over the rotator interval surface of the GHJ capsule to the greater and lesser humeral tuberosities between the supraspinatus and subscapularis tendons. The CHL blends with the rotator interval segment of the GHJ capsule and anterior leading edge of the supraspinatus tendon to form the roof of the rotator interval, and also sends a 1 cm wide band of posterior extension along both the superficial and deep surfaces of the supraspinatus tendon to the posterior margin of the infraspinatus tendon. *Source:* Clark and Harryman (1992) with permission.

- Layer 1 measures up to 1 mm thick and contains obliquely oriented fibres of the CHL.
- Layer 2 measures 3–5 mm thick and contains large (1–2 mm in diameter) longitudinally oriented fibre bundles.
- Layer 3 measures about 3 mm thick and is a criss-crossing meshwork of fibres that contribute to cuff fusion.
- Layer 4 comprises loose connective tissue and thick collagen bands that merge with the deep extension fibres of the CHL.
- Layer 5 is the GHJ capsule.

The fibre orientation differences between the cuff layers result in variable appearances on imaging tests that are a potential pitfall to interpretation.

This complex arrangement of layers helps to explain why articular-side partial-thickness tears are more frequent. The articular-side fibres of the cuff are both less vascular and only half as strong as the bursal-side fibres due to thinner and less uniformly arranged bundles (Matava et al. 2005). In addition, the presence of connective tissue transition zones between adjacent fibre bundles or layers can produce intrasubstance lines of variable echogenicity (see Figs 4.114 and 4.115). An understanding of CHL (see Fig. 4.116) and 'biceps pulley' anatomy at the rotator interval can also aid in image interpretation, as cuff tears can cross the interval and lead to biceps tendon dysfunction.

It is likely that the main pain generator in subacromial impingement syndrome is the SA-SD bursa, which develops a frictional bursopathy with accompanying effusion and hyperaemia in acute or acute-on-chronic impingement settings. There may be superior recess thickening without an effusion in chronic impingement. The cardinal imaging feature of an early (Neer Stage I) subacromial impingement syndrome is superior recess SA-SD bursopathy (see Fig. 4.117). Imaging changes of supraspinatus tendinopathy may also be demonstrated on both ultrasound and MRI, and cases in which the sole imaging feature is insertional tendinopathy are also occasionally seen (see Fig. 4.118). Dynamic assessment with real-time ultrasound will usually, but not invariably, show bunching of the SA-SD bursa against the coracoacromial arch during shoulder abduction (see Fig. 4.119). Irrespective of this finding, the essential diagnostic observation during

▶ **Fig. 4.117** Neer Stage 1 chronic shoulder impingement syndrome is demonstrated by ultrasound. A long-axis ultrasound image of the supraspinatus tendon (s) shows SA-SD bursal thickening (callipers) confined to the superior bursal recess. Note the absence of bursal effusion. Greater humeral tuberosity = gt.

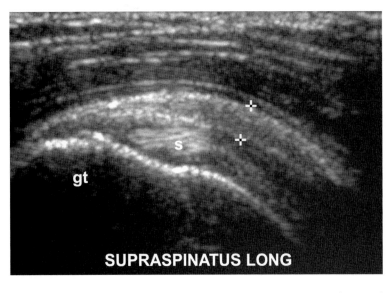

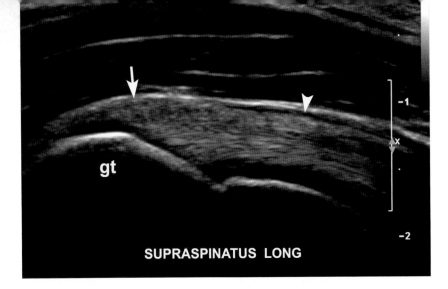

SUPRASPINATUS LONG

gt

◀Fig. 4.118 Subacromial impingement associated with an insertional tendinopathy without the imaging features of active SA-SD bursopathy. A long-axis ultrasound image of the supraspinatus tendon shows focal swelling and an echotexture of tendinopathy, predominantly involving the superficial fibres at the humeral insertion (arrow). This area was focally tender to probing. Note the normal appearance of the SA-SD bursa (arrowhead). Greater humeral tuberosity = gt.

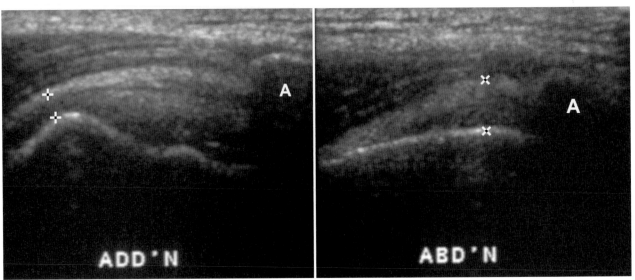

ADD'N   ABD'N

▲ Fig. 4.119 Dynamic ultrasound assessment of subacromial impingement is demonstrated. Long-axis images of the supraspinatus tendon have been obtained in both adduction and abduction. Thickening of the SA-SD bursa is observed dynamically throughout the abduction arc at a fixed visual reference point located over the tip of greater humeral tuberosity (indicated by callipers). Note the 'bunching' of the bursa against the acromial margin in the abducted position. However, before making an ultrasound diagnosis of subacromial impingement syndrome, it is essential to know whether these changes were accompanied by a simultaneous arc of pain (with or without a palpable click), as the supraspinatus tendon insertion passes beneath the acromial margin. It is also important to recognise that cases of symptomatic subacromial impingement are occasionally encountered in which these changes of bursal thickening and dynamic bursal bunching are not present. Acromion process = A.

this manoeuvre is the production of pain through an arc that coincides with the passage of the supraspinatus insertion beneath the acromial margin. The painful arc occurs on elevation of the arm or return of the arm from the fully abducted position, is absent at end-range abduction and is occasionally associated with a palpable click. Injection of local anaesthetic and steroid into the subacromial, often performed under ultrasound guidance for improved accuracy (see Fig. 4.49 on page 210), offers good diagnostic confirmation of the pain source and is a useful therapeutic procedure.

Plain films may reveal an anatomical factor that predisposes to frictional overload of either the bursa or cuff by narrowing the subacromial space. These factors include an os acromiale (see Fig. 4.120) and an adverse acromial shape (see Figs 4.121 and 4.122). MacGillivray et al. (1998) described a method of MRI assessment to assess lateral acromial downslope in the coronal plane relative to the distal end of the clavicle. They classified the

Type A acromion as having a lateral downslope of 0 to 10° and the Type B acromion as having a lateral downslope of >10°, and found that 83% of Type B acromions were associated with Neer Stage II or III subacromial impingement. Osteophytes projecting from the inferior margin of the AC joint and GHJ instability may also produce a reduction in the subacromial space.

Plain films may show superior subluxation of the humeral head if there is a large full-thickness supraspinatus or LHB tendon tear. These structures normally act as depressors of the humeral head. Superior migration of the humeral head may also result from muscle imbalance, when neglected external rotators are effectively overpowered by well-trained and overdeveloped internal rotators, producing subacromial impingement (Richardson 1990). Superior subluxation is best assessed on a true AP view of the shoulder, which profiles the GHJ (see Fig. 4.123).

Other causes of subacromial impingement syndrome include conditions such as acute or non-acute calcific rotator

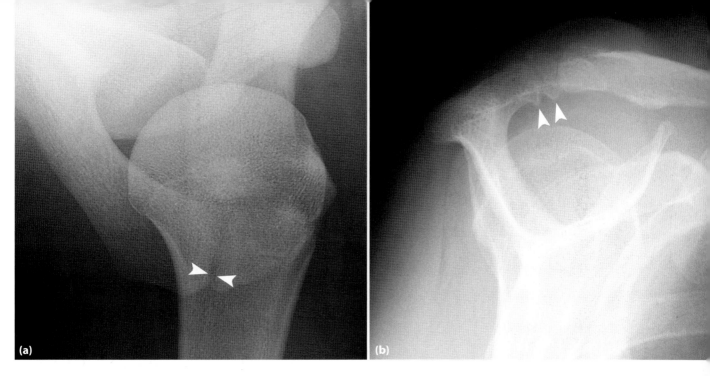

▲ **Fig. 4.120** An os acromiale is demonstrated in **(a)** an axial view and **(b)** an outlet view. Note the small bone spurs protruding inferiorly from the margins of the synchondrosis.

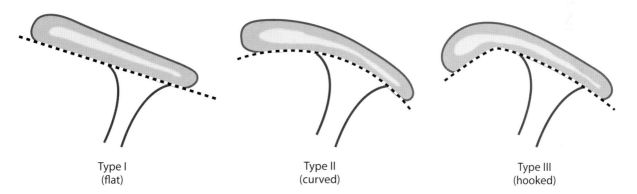

| Type I (flat) | Type II (curved) | Type III (hooked) |

▲ **Fig. 4.121** A line illustration showing Bigliani classification of acromial morphology assessed on an outlet view. There is a higher incidence of rotator cuff tears in shoulders with Type II and Type III acromions. An analysis of age distribution indicates a consistent and gradual transition from a flat acromion in early life towards an increasingly hooked acromion in later life. *Source:* Bigliani et al. (1991) and MacGillivray et al. (1998).

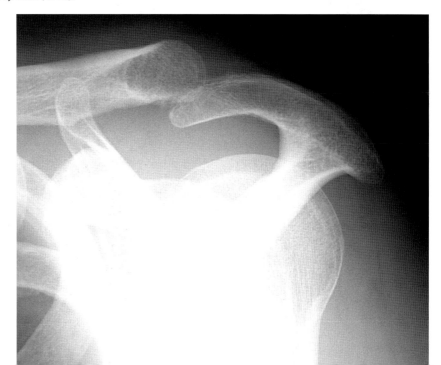

▶ **Fig. 4.122** An outlet view demonstrates a Type III hooked acromion.

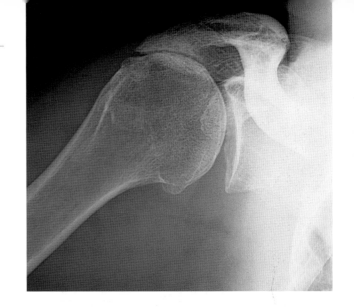

▶ **Fig. 4.123** A true AP view of the shoulder shows advanced degenerative changes with absence of the rotator cuff. Superior subluxation of the humeral head has obliterated the subacromial space. There is excavation of the undersurface of the acromion. Incongruity of the joint space suggests joint laxity, and advanced loss of articular cartilage is almost certainly present.

▶ **Fig. 4.124** MR images show subacromial impingement secondary to rotator cuff calcification. Coronal PD and fat-suppressed PD images show a hypointense calcific deposit within the distal supraspinatus tendon. Note the resultant tendon swelling and superior recess SA-SD bursopathy (arrowheads).

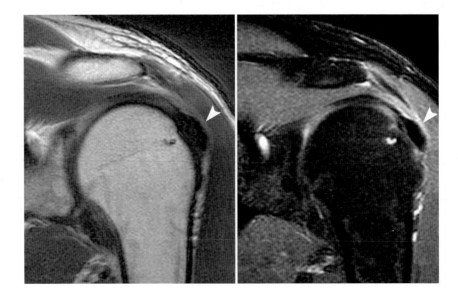

▼ **Fig. 4.125** MRI demonstrates degenerative ACJ hypertrophy causing narrowing of the supraspinatus outlet. A coronal PD-weighted image shows degenerative bony and capsular hypertrophy of the ACJ (white arrowhead). There is associated supraspinatus impingement appreciated as a corresponding localised distortion of the subjacent muscle contour. Also note supraspinatus tendon thickening due to marked tendinopathy (arrow) with a complicating full-thickness insertional tear (black arrowheads).

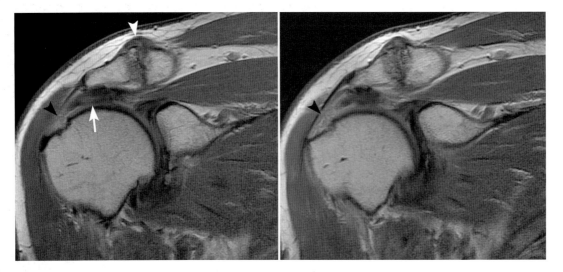

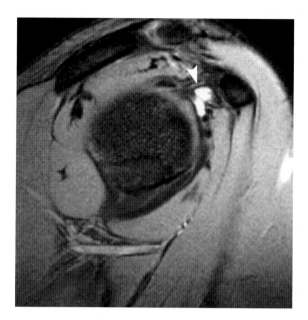

▲ **Fig. 4.126** A fat-suppressed PD-weighted sagittal MRI shows a superior glenoid labral cyst (arrowhead).

cuff tendinopathy (see Figs 4.124 and 4.125), rotator cuff contusion, spontaneous rupture of the LHB tendon and a fracture of the greater tuberosity. ACJ osteoarthrosis (see Fig. 4.126) and suprascapular nerve palsy due to either acute injury or a superior labral cyst (see Fig. 4.127) may also produce an impingement syndrome.

Plain films also play an important role in demonstrating new bone formation on the undersurface of the acromion and in showing the presence of spurs that commonly occur at the anterior margin of the undersurface of the acromion, following the direction of the coracoacromial ligament. Two views in the impingement series will demonstrate a spur in two planes at 90° to each other. Occasionally unusually long spurs are present suggesting ligamentous ossification (see Fig. 4.127). The new bone formation and subacromial spurs reduce the volume of the rigid canal through which the supraspinatus passes (see Fig. 4.128) and characteristically predispose to bursal-side abrasions and partial or full-thickness tendon tears. These can be imaged with either ultrasound or MRI (see Figs 4.129–4.133).

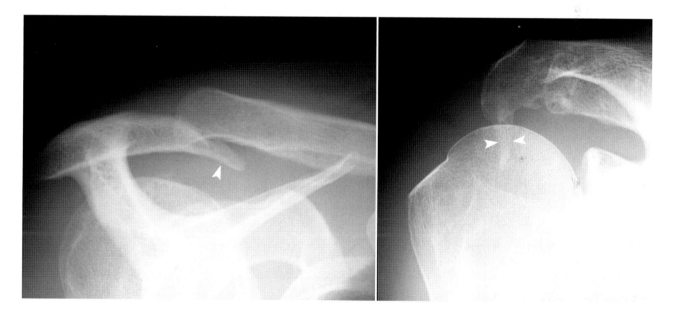

▲ **Fig. 4.127** An unusually long anterior acromial spur is shown on an outlet view and an angled-down AP view.

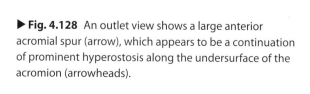

▶ **Fig. 4.128** An outlet view shows a large anterior acromial spur (arrow), which appears to be a continuation of prominent hyperostosis along the undersurface of the acromion (arrowheads).

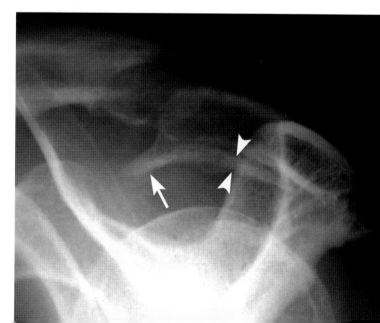

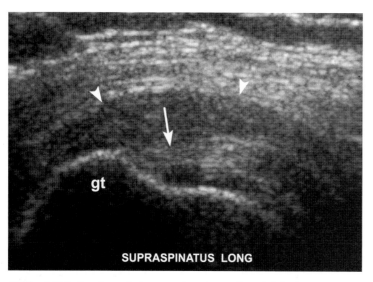

SUPRASPINATUS LONG

◀**Fig. 4.129** A bursal-side abrasion or a partial-thickness tear of the supraspinatus tendon is demonstrated by ultrasound. This long-axis ultrasound image of the supraspinatus tendon shows a localised shallow distal tendon surface concavity consistent with bursal-side abrasion or a tear (arrow). Subacromial impingement is inferred from the grossly thickened overlying superior recess of the SA-SD bursa (arrowheads). Note the absence of an effusion, which indicates a chronic bursopathy. Bursal echotexture tends to merge with that of the underlying tendon, making the tendon surface contour abnormality inconspicuous. Greater humeral tuberosity = gt.

▼**Fig. 4.130** A gallery of ultrasound patterns of partial-thickness rotator cuff tears is shown. In each example the tear is indicated by an arrow or arrowhead. Greater humeral tuberosity = gt. Lesser humeral tuberosity = t.

(a) A small articular-side hypoechoic defect is present. It is important that a finding of this kind is carefully interrogated to confirm reproducibility, visibility in both transverse and long-axis planes of section, and freedom from anisotropy.

(b) A small linear hypoechoic defect of an intrasubstance type is demonstrated. With subtle changes of this kind, similar comments to those in **(a)** apply with regard to lesion reproducibility.

(c) A linear anechoic fluid-filled cleft of intrasubstance lamination tear is shown. Note that chronic lamination tears may be echogenic or mixed hypo-hyperechoic.

(d) Ultrasound demonstrates a degenerative deep fibre intrasubstance or articular-side tear of curvilinear and mixed hypo-hyperechoic echotexture. Note the irregular enthesial bone pitting at the adjacent greater tuberosity.

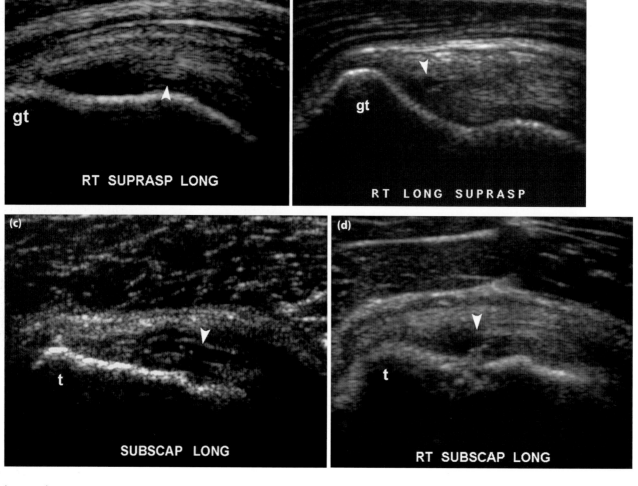

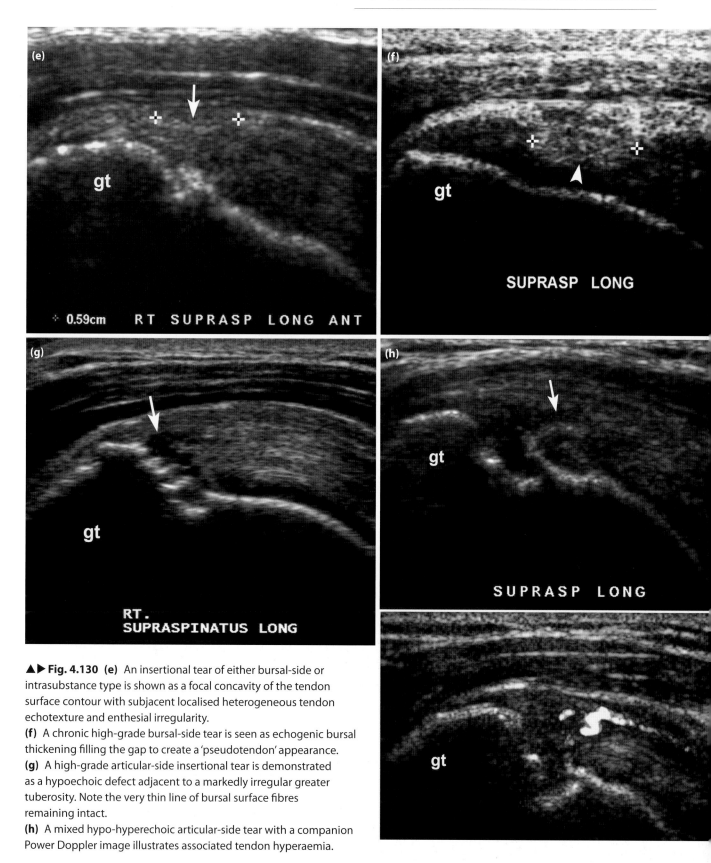

▲▶ **Fig. 4.130** **(e)** An insertional tear of either bursal-side or intrasubstance type is shown as a focal concavity of the tendon surface contour with subjacent localised heterogeneous tendon echotexture and enthesial irregularity.

(f) A chronic high-grade bursal-side tear is seen as echogenic bursal thickening filling the gap to create a 'pseudotendon' appearance.

(g) A high-grade articular-side insertional tear is demonstrated as a hypoechoic defect adjacent to a markedly irregular greater tuberosity. Note the very thin line of bursal surface fibres remaining intact.

(h) A mixed hypo-hyperechoic articular-side tear with a companion Power Doppler image illustrates associated tendon hyperaemia.

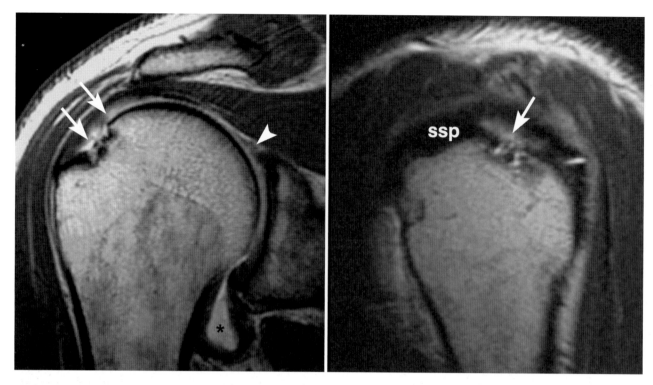

▲ **Fig. 4.131** Non-arthrographic MRI demonstrates an articular-side partial thickness rotator cuff tear. Coronal and sagittal PD-weighted images show a high-signal interruption of normal deep fibre tendon hypointensity consistent with a tear extending proximally from a localised area of enthesial irregularity at the greater tuberosity (white arrows). The tear involves the posterior supraspinatus and superior infraspinatus insertions. Note the slightly irregular superior glenoid labrum of intermediate signal suggestive of degeneration and fraying (arrowhead). Internal impingement would therefore have to be considered as a possible explanation for the posterosuperiorly located cuff tear identified in this case. There is a small GHJ effusion (asterisk). Supraspinatus tendon = ssp.

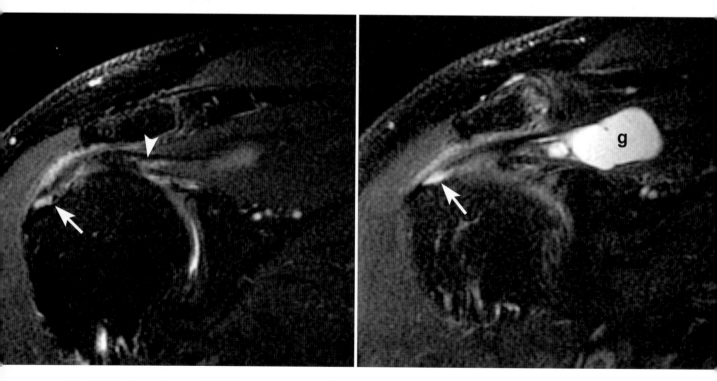

▲ **Fig. 4.132** Non-arthrographic MRI shows a partial-thickness supraspinatus tendon tear. Fat-suppressed coronal T2-weighted images demonstrate signal hyperintensity of a high-grade articular-side tear at the supraspinatus insertion (arrows). There is a proximal intrasubstance laminar extension (arrowhead) into an intra-muscular ganglion cyst (g).

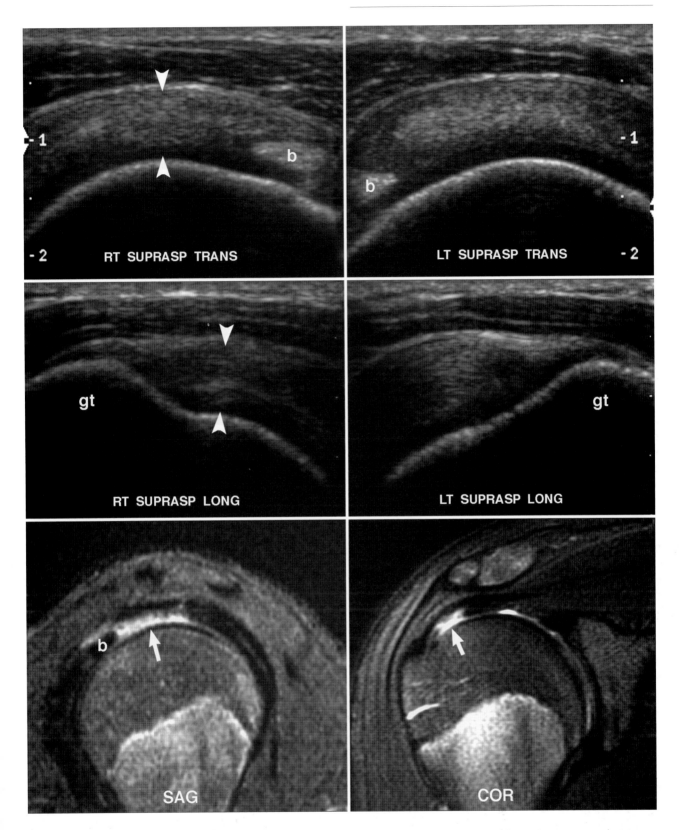

▲ **Fig. 4.133** An articular-side partial-thickness supraspinatus tendon tear is demonstrated by ultrasound and MRI. A 12-year-old softball player experienced sudden right shoulder pain as she contacted the ball and subsequently complained of a painful click. An ultrasound examination was requested to exclude a rotator cuff tear. Asymmetric supraspinatus tendon thickness was noted (white arrowheads), but this appeared diffuse and no focal echotextural defect was identified. In view of the unexplained symptoms, an MRI was advised and this non-arthrographic study showed a high-grade articular-side partial-thickness tear with retraction of the torn deep fibres and corresponding fluid-filled gap (arrows). This illustrates the difficulty that ultrasound sometimes has in perceiving the presence of an articular-side tear. It also shows that, although uncommon, rotator cuff tears can occur in surprisingly young patients. LHB tendon = b. Greater humeral tuberosity = gt.

▼ **Fig. 4.134** A full-thickness rotator cuff tear is demonstrated indirectly. Comparative transverse images have been obtained through the bicipital groove at both the upper level (top images) and lower level (bottom images). On the symptomatic right side there is effusion simultaneously present within the SA-SD bursa (arrowheads) and LHB tendon sleeve (arrow). This finding is an indirect but strong predictor of an intervening full-thickness cuff tear, having a positive predictive value of 95%. LHB tendon = b.

In late-stage impingement (Neer Stage III) and rotator cuff tendinopathy, a progressive full-thickness rotator cuff tear may develop (see Figs 4.134, 4.135 and 4.136). This can be large, often involving the full width of the supraspinatus tendon and occasionally extending into the infraspinatus and subscapularis tendons (see Fig. 4.137). Accompanying LHB tendon ruptures are common (see Fig. 4.138) and secondary GHJ osteoarthrosis will eventually result. Large full-thickness tears of the supraspinatus tendon that are longstanding will have associated wasting and fatty replacement of the supraspinatus muscle, making them unsuitable for surgical repair. These muscle changes are best demonstrated and assessed with MRI (see Fig. 4.139), but can also be appreciated with ultrasound (see Fig. 4.140). A system of grading the degree of fatty atrophy of the rotator cuff muscles has been devised for CT and MRI (Goutallier et al. 1994) (see Table 4.6 on page 251). The cuff is surgically unrepairable if the muscle shows greater than 50% fatty infiltration. Occasionally, disruption of the inferior capsule of the ACJ may lead to the development of a ganglion at the upper joint surface. Arthrographic opacification of this has been described as the 'geyser sign' (Craig 1984).

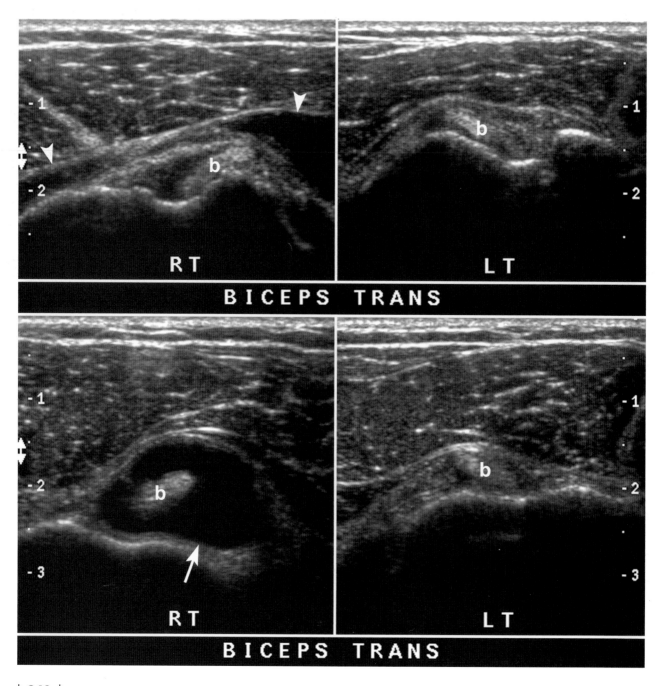

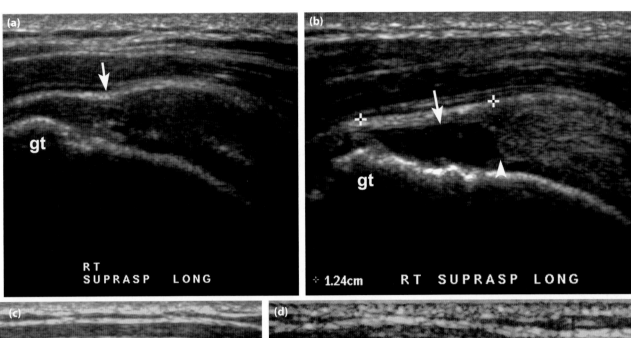

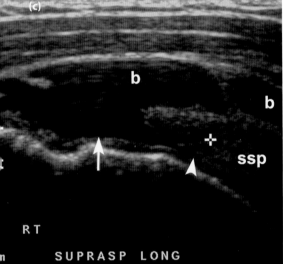

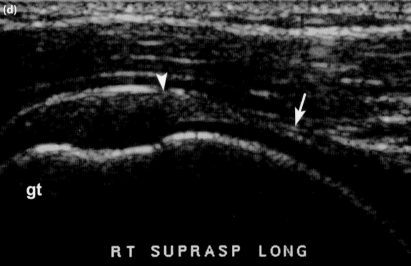

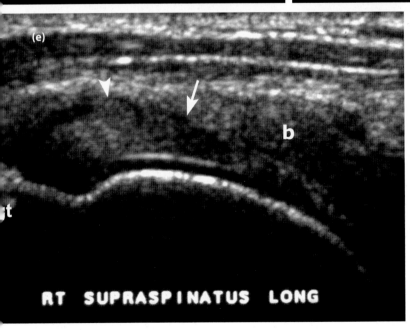

◄▲ Fig. 4.135 A gallery of ultrasound patterns of full-thickness rotator cuff tears. In each example the tear is indicated by an arrow and, if visible, the torn tendon edge is indicated by an arrowhead. Greater humeral tuberosity = gt.

(a) A small tear is seen as a focus of full-thickness heterogeneous echotexture with overlying surface contour concavity.

(b) A moderate-sized tear is appreciated as a full-thickness anechoic fluid-filled gap.

(c) A large tear is demonstrated as a full-thickness fluid-filled gap with a retracted supraspinatus tendon (ssp) and an associated prominent SA-SD bursal effusion (b).

(d) A large tear is seen as a complete tendon absence (arrow) apart from a small residual stump of tissue at the greater tuberosity (the proximal margin of the stump is indicated by an arrow).

(e) A large tear of similar geometry to that in **(d)** is seen but with the tendon gap filled by an area of echogenic SA-SD bursal thickening (b).

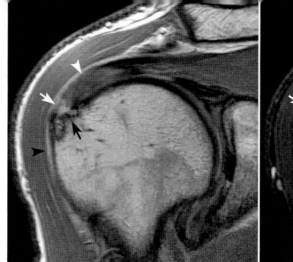
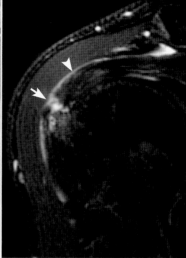

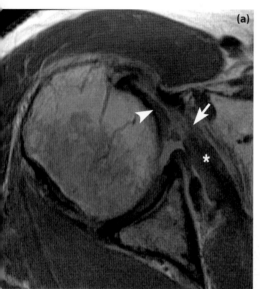

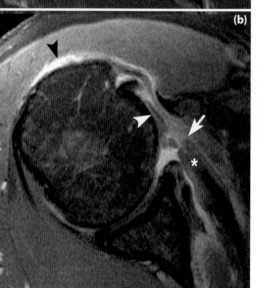

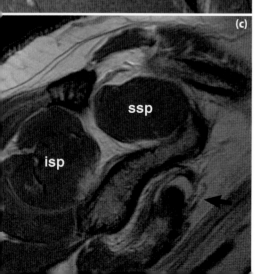

▲ **Fig. 4.136** Non-arthrographic MRI demonstrates a small full-thickness insertional tear of the supraspinatus tendon. Coronal PD and fat-suppressed T2-weighted images show the high signal defect of a tendon tear (white arrows) with degenerative enthesial bone pitting at the adjacent greater tuberosity (black arrow). There are background changes of tendon swelling with intermediate signal indicative of marked supraspinatus tendinopathy (white arrowheads). Note the associated SA-SD bursopathy (black arrowhead).

◄ **Fig. 4.137** Non-arthrographic MRI shows a large full-thickness insertional tear of the subscapularis tendon. Axial PD **(a)** and axial fat-suppressed PD-weighted **(b)** images show the proximal stump of the subscapularis tendon (asterisk), which has retracted to the level of the glenoid rim. White arrows indicate the level of the end of the tendon, and only irregular capsulosynovial thickening plus scant effusion is present in the tendon 'gap' (white arrowheads). The black arrow indicates fluid in the SA-SD bursa. A sagittal PD image **(c)** obtained through the rotator cuff muscles shows associated marked fatty atrophy of the mid and upper subscapularis belly (black arrow) indicative of a chronic cuff tear. Supraspinatus muscle = ssp. Infraspinatus muscle = isp.

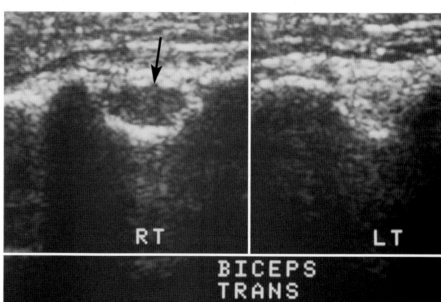

▲ **Fig. 4.138** Full-thickness proximal rupture and retraction of the right LHB tendon is shown by ultrasound. After a real-time search has first ruled out medial dislocation of the biceps tendon, a complete absence of any echogenic tendon within the humeral groove and rotator interval on comparison transverse ultrasound images (arrow) is diagnostic of proximal rupture and retraction.

Table 4.6 CT and MRI grading of rotator cuff muscle fatty atrophy

Mild	Some fatty streaks within the muscle
Moderate	More muscle than fat
Severe	As much or more fat than muscle (surgically unrepairable)

Source: Goutallier et al. (1994).

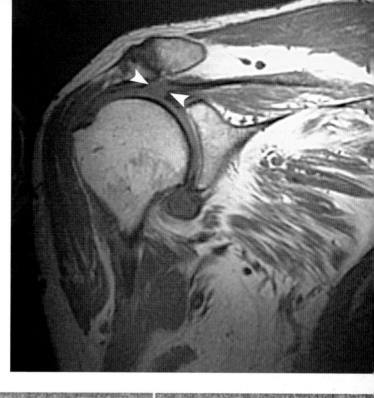

▶ **Fig. 4.139** A large chronic full-thickness rotator cuff tear is demonstrated by MRI. A coronal T1-weighted image shows diffuse marked fatty atrophy of the supraspinatus and subscapularis muscles secondary to a cuff tear. Arrowheads indicate the tendon defect produced by the tear.

▶ **Fig. 4.140(a)** Comparative long-axis ultrasound images of the supraspinatus muscles within the suprascapular fossae allow evaluation of supraspinatus muscle quality following a full-thickness rotator cuff tear. The images show the normal symmetrical appearance of muscle echotexture with an echogenic central tendon and only mild overall size difference in a right-side dominant patient (arrowheads).

▼ **(b)** Similar ultrasound images obtained in a patient with a large chronic left-sided rotator cuff tear show diffuse fatty atrophy of the left supraspinatus muscle appreciated as increased echogenicity and reduced muscle size (arrows).

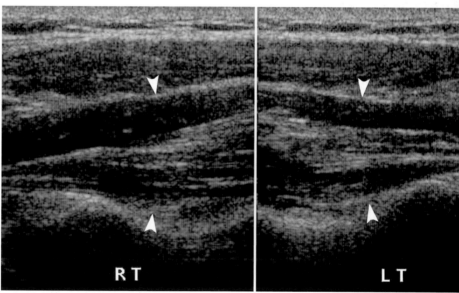

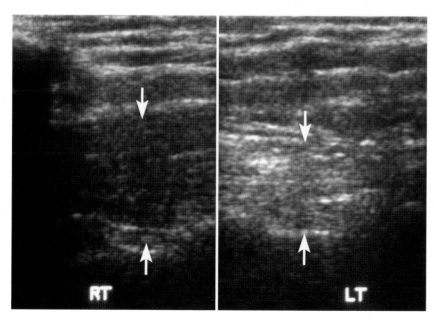

Internal impingement syndrome

Internal impingement, also called posterosuperior gleno-humeral impingement, is a syndrome of posterior shoulder pain that occurs predominantly in athletes who use an over-head throwing motion, with repeated movement of the GHJ into an extreme ABER position during the late cocking and early acceleration phases of throwing. This action results in exaggerated impact of the posterosuperior cuff insertion and humeral head against the posterosuperior glenoid rim (see Fig. 4.141). A range of injuries can be produced, including scuff-ing and eventual articular-side partial-thickness tears of the posterosuperior cuff insertion (Walch et al. 1991). Tears of the posterosuperior glenoid labrum may develop together with subcortical cystic and chondral changes at the posterosuperior margin of the humeral head (see Fig. 4.142). Additional factors may contribute to this impingement mechanism in throwers. There may be acquired anterior capsular laxity and posterior capsular tightness, which lead to increased anterior translation and external rotation of the humeral head. Posterosuperior GHJ instability secondary to a 'posterior peel-back' SLAP tear, decreased humeral head retroversion, poor throwing mechanics and scapular muscle imbalance may also occur (Matava et al. 2005). MRI or MDCT arthrography performed with the shoulder in the ABER impingement position is the imaging test of choice.

▶ **Fig. 4.141(a)** A line drawing depicts the mechanism of internal impingement syndrome. The posterosuperior rotator cuff insertion impacts against the posterosuperior glenoid rim (arrow). This type of glenohumeral contact can occur in the normal stable shoulder, but repetitive or excessive impact is required to produce the injury pattern and symptoms associated with internal impingement syndrome.
▼ **(b)** Corresponding PD-weighted MR arthrogram images obtained in the ABER position show an articular-side partial-thickness cuff tear (arrow) and cystic change at the point of the greater humeral tuberosity abutment (arrowhead).

Coracoid impingement syndrome

The soft-tissue structures over the lesser humeral tuberosity (the subscapularis tendon and SA-SD bursa) may impinge on the coracoid process, producing a dull anterior shoulder pain associated especially with forward elevation, internal rotation and cross-arm adduction manoeuvres (Bigliani and Levine 1997). This syndrome has been called coracoid, subcoracoid or coracohumeral impingement and, although uncommon, should be considered in the differential diagnosis of anterior shoulder pain. The aetiology can be idiopathic, traumatic or iatrogenic (Gerber et al. 1985). Reported causes have included chronic overuse, mal-union of a coracoid process or gle-noid fracture, iatrogenic alteration in anatomic relationships associated with glenoid osteotomy or other anterior shoulder surgery, and an intra-tendon subscapularis ganglion (Ferrick 2000). Anterior GHJ instability is another potential predisposing factor (Patte 1990). In the authors' experience, the condition is often encountered in weight-lifters and body builders.

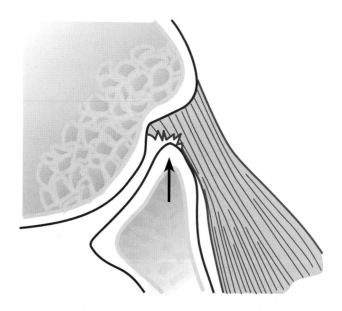

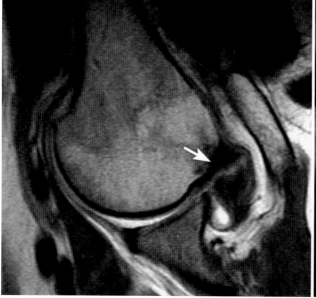

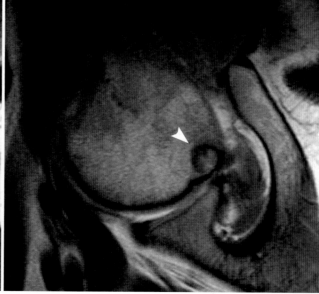

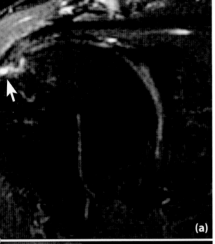

(a)

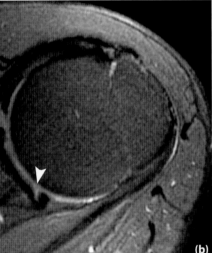

(b)

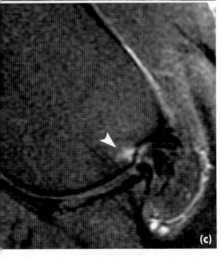

(c)

◀ **Fig. 4.142** MRI demonstrates internal impingement. Fat-suppressed coronal T2 **(a)**, fat-suppressed axial PD **(b)** and fat-suppressed ABER PD-weighted **(c)** images demonstrate features of a posterosuperior articular-side partial-thickness cuff tear (arrow), non-detached posterosuperior glenoid labral tear (arrowhead on **(b)**) and focal hyperintensity of either bone bruising or early cystic change at the posterosuperior corner of the humeral head (arrowhead on **(c)**). Note the direct juxtaposition of all these findings on the ABER image, which replicates the impingement position.

Compression of the SD bursa may be seen on dynamic ultrasound assessment as a 'bunching' phenomenon adjacent to the coracoid tip during internal shoulder rotation (see Fig. 4.143) and cross-arm adduction manoeuvres. As with subacromial impingement, this appearance can be regarded as clinically significant only when presenting as a distinct syndrome with correlating pain. The potential for subcoracoid impingement may also be suggested on axial imaging with CT or MRI, when the interval between the maximally internally rotated lesser tuberosity and the coracoid process measures less than 11 mm and there is buckling of the subscapularis against the coracoid process (Bonutti et al. 1993; Friedman et al. 1998) (see Fig. 4.144).

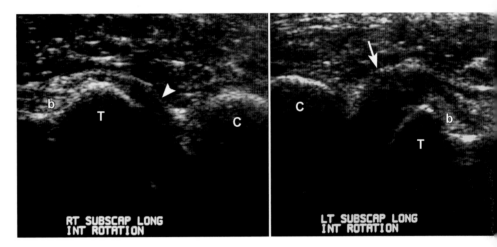

▲ **Fig. 4.143** Ultrasound demonstrates coracoid impingement. Comparative images have been obtained at the level of the coracoid tip, transverse to the bicipital groove, and hence in the long axis of the subscapularis tendon. On dynamic real-time assessment, the patient complained of anterior pain at the left shoulder, which coincided with bunching of the subscapularis tendon and overlying SA-SD bursa (arrow) adjacent to the tip of the coracoid process (C) during internal shoulder rotation. Note the normal soft-tissue contour on the right (arrowhead). Lesser humeral tuberosity = T. LHB tendon = b.

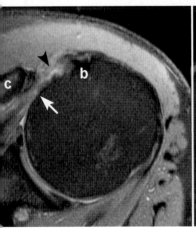

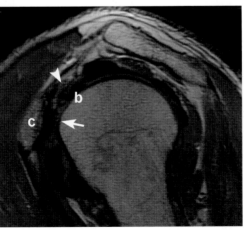

◀ **Fig. 4.144** Coracoid impingement is demonstrated by MRI. Non-arthrographic axial fat-suppressed PD and sagittal PD images show an elongated coracoid process (C), a narrow coracohumeral interval (arrows), a subscapularis tendon tear (black arrowhead) and adjacent rotator interval synovitis (white arrowhead). Inferior to the coracoid level on the sagittal image, changes of diffuse subscapularis tendinopathy with a superimposed laminar tear component are also demonstrated. LHB tendon = b.

▼ **Fig. 4.145(a)** Ultrasound demonstrates an acute full-thickness rupture and retraction of the left LHB tendon. Comparison transverse images obtained at the lower bicipital groove level show a normal echogenic LHB tendon on the right (arrowhead) but a markedly distended biceps sheath filled with heterogeneous low-to-medium level echo on the left. This appearance is indicative of haemorrhage and/or horsetail fraying of torn tendon fibres (arrow).

Abnormalities of the LHB tendon
LHB tendon rupture

Tears of the LHB tendon usually occur either at the glenolabral attachment or along the extra-articular tendon segment in the bicipital groove between the greater and lesser tuberosities. As the LHB tendon normally functions in part as a depressor of the humeral head, ruptures may present clinically as secondary subacromial impingement syndrome. Ultrasound or MRI can identify the tendon rupture (see Figs 4.145, 4.146 and 4.147). It is not uncommon to discover longstanding glenolabral detachments of the biceps tendon that have remained clinically silent. There may not be total loss of function, as the retracted tendon often spontaneously reattaches to the bicipital groove or lesser humeral tuberosity.

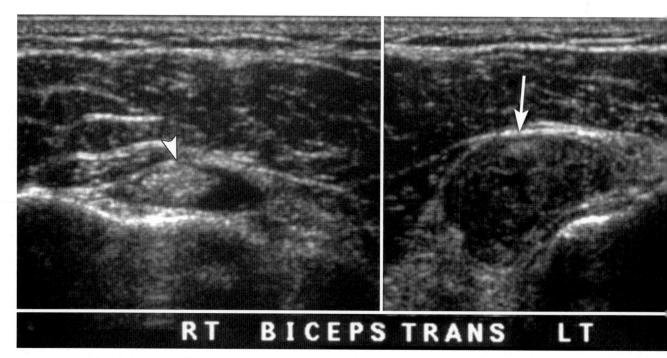

▼ **(b)** A long-axis image of the bicipital groove shows a distended biceps sheath (arrows) with markedly hypoechoic echotexture indicative of effusion and no contained tendon (note that the cranial aspect of the image is to the left).

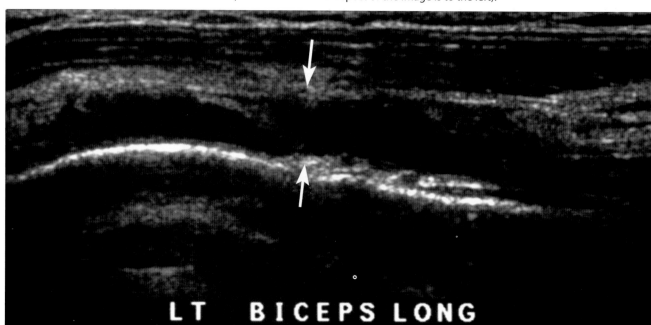

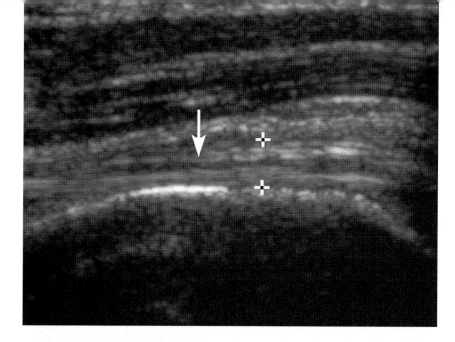

◄ Fig. 4.146 A long-axis ultrasound image shows the extra-articular segment of the LHB tendon (callipers) at the humeral groove level. This case illustrates a dilemma that occasionally confronts the radiologist. A hypoechoic cleft (arrow) is demonstrated extending along the length of the biceps, representing either a longitudinal tear or synovitis interposed between the limbs of a bifid (normal variant) tendon. The lack of apparent underlying tendinopathy in this case would favour the latter possibility.

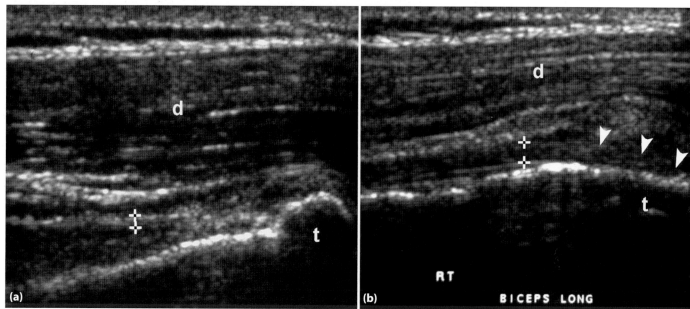

▲ Fig. 4.147 Two ultrasound examples demonstrate chronic LHB tendon rupture without marked retraction.
(a) A long-axis image at the bicipital groove level shows a thin atrophic LHB tendon (callipers) attaching at a well-developed bony shelf (t) arising from the floor or lesser tuberosity margin of the upper humeral groove.
(b) A similar view obtained in another patient shows a more subtle variation of the same phenomenon. The LHB tendon (callipers and arrowheads) inserts into a shallow bony shelf (t) at the upper end of the bicipital groove.

Attritional ruptures of the intra-articular segment of the LHB tendon may be gradual and clinically silent. If the vinculum at the bicipital groove remains intact, the LHB tendon will not completely retract to the mid-shaft humerus level and, as demonstrated in these two cases, may spontaneously reattach at the humeral groove and induce bony remodelling. Deltoid = d.

LHB tendinopathy

Bicipital tendinopathy (see Figs 4.148 and 4.149) can result from overuse with activities such as weightlifting and may occur secondary to subacromial impingement. This is especially so with a Neer Stage III impingement, where the presence of a full-thickness rotator cuff tear exposes the biceps tendon to even greater attrition. Bicipital groove stenosis secondary to osteophytes can also contribute to tendinopathy and may be demonstrated by plain films using a bicipital groove view (see Fig. 4.150), or by ultrasound or CT scanning. Bicipital grooves with unusually steep medial wall angles (approaching 90°) have also been associated with tendon constriction and bicipital tenosynovitis (Cone et al. 1983).

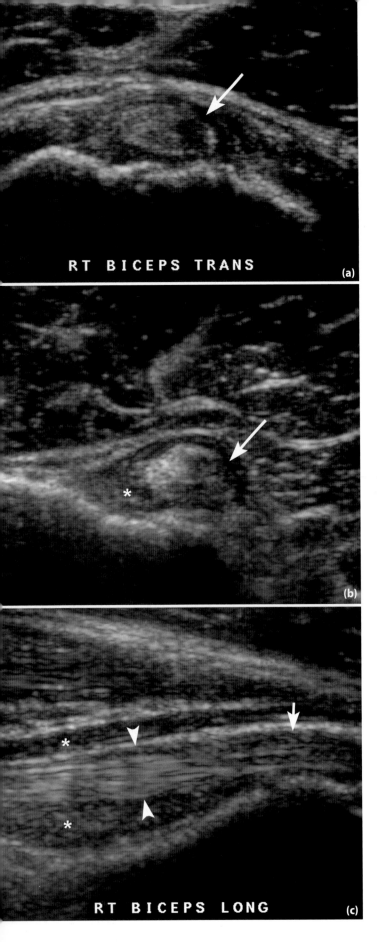

RT BICEPS TRANS **(a)**

* **(b)**

RT BICEPS LONG **(c)**

▶ **Fig. 4.150** A normal bicipital groove view has been acquired by the method described on page 194 in the section 'Other shoulder-girdle views'.

◀ **Fig. 4.148** Ultrasound demonstrates LHB tendinopathy and tenosynovitis. Transverse images have been obtained at the rotator interval **(a)** and lower bicipital groove **(b)** levels, and a long-axis view **(c)** of the LHB tendon has been obtained at the bicipital groove level. The LHB tendon is swollen (arrowheads) and shows areas of mildly hypoechoic tendinopathic echotexture (arrows). A normal biceps tendon should not exceed 4 mm in thickness. Extensive tenosynovial thickening (asterisk) is present within the biceps sheath.

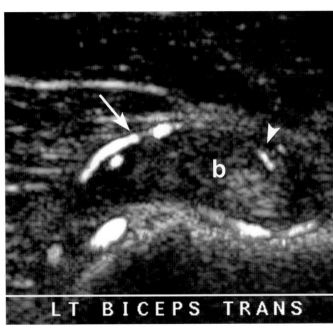

LT BICEPS TRANS

▲ **Fig. 4.149** Doppler ultrasound shows the appearance of bicipital tendinopathy and tenosynovitis. A transverse Power Doppler image obtained at the lower bicipital groove level shows a thickened LHB tendon (b) with tendinopathic echotexture and intrasubstance hyperaemia (arrowhead). An associated collar of hyperaemic tenosynovial thickening (arrow) is also present.

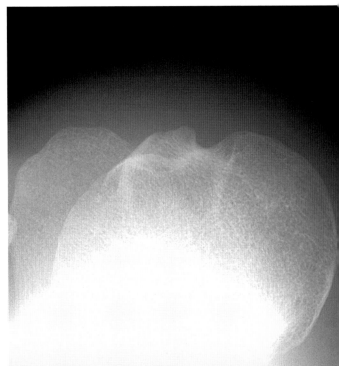

LHB tendon instability

An unstable tendon of the LHB may be a source of shoulder pain and produce a click. Tendon subluxation occurs in a medial direction and may be intermittent, occurring with external shoulder rotation. Biceps tendon subluxation or dislocation from the intertubercular sulcus is commonly associated with rotator cuff tears, and may lead to displacement of the tendon into the anterior recess of the GHJ. This indicates that there is a full-thickness subscapularis tear (see Fig. 4.151). Extra-articular dislocation reflects a partial-thickness tear of the subscapularis tendon or the transverse humeral ligament, which is essentially a lateral extension of the superficial fibres of the subscapularis (see Fig. 4.152). A hypoplastic bicipital groove predisposes to subluxation. Cone et al. (1983) determined the average medial wall angle to be 48° and found that angles of less than 30° were associated with tendon instability. Ultrasound and MRI can both demonstrate biceps tendon subluxation, but ultrasound has the special advantage of providing a dynamic assessment, helping to determine reducibility.

Another more subtle form of biceps tendon instability is the 'pulley lesion', also called the 'hidden lesion' due to the difficulty in seeing this lesion at arthroscopy. The biceps pulley stabilises the LHB tendon at the lateral aspect of the rotator interval and the upper end of the bicipital groove, and is formed by the reflection of insertional fibres of the CHL, SGHL and superior border of the subscapularis tendon. Consequently, a partial tear of the subscapularis tendon may extend into the medial portion of the biceps pulley and produce a medial subluxation of the LHB tendon at the superior aspect of the

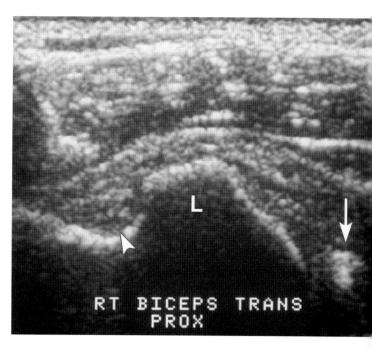

▲ **Fig. 4.151** Medial dislocation of the LHB tendon is demonstrated by ultrasound. A transverse ultrasound shows the echogenic displaced biceps tendon (arrow), lying deep to the apparent path of the subscapularis tendon. In fact, a full-thickness rupture of the distal subscapularis tendon was also present in this case, and the echogenic space immediately anterior to the displaced biceps tendon is haematoma. Note the 'empty' bicipital groove (arrowhead). Lesser humeral tuberosity = L.

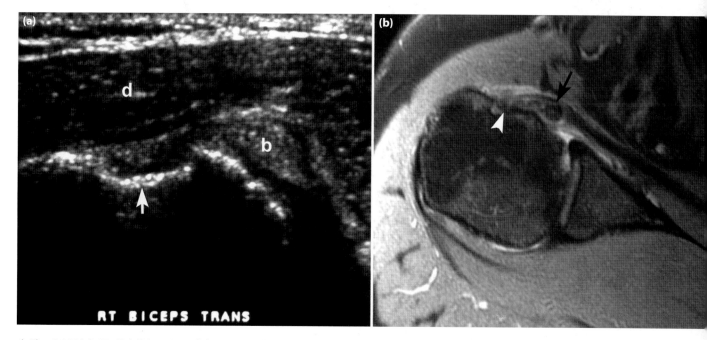

▲ **Fig. 4.152(a)** Medial dislocation of the LHB tendon is demonstrated by ultrasound. A transverse ultrasound image at the mid-bicipital groove level shows medial dislocation of the LHB tendon (b) from an 'empty' and relatively shallow humeral groove (arrow). In this case, only the superficial fibres of the subscapularis have been split and the displaced tendon does not reach the GHJ space. Deltoid muscle = d. **(b)** In another case of dislocation of the LHB tendon, a fat-suppressed axial PD-weighted MR image at the mid-bicipital groove level shows medial dislocation of the LHB tendon (black arrow) from an 'empty' and shallow humeral groove (arrowhead). In this example, the LHB tendon lies at the deep surface of the subscapularis and has therefore reached the GHJ space.

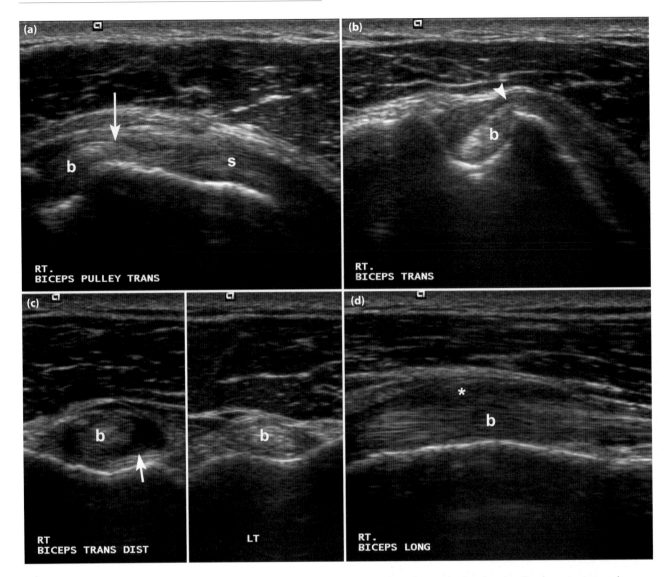

▲ **Fig. 4.153** Ultrasound demonstrates a 'hidden lesion'. Transverse images have been obtained at the distal rotator interval through the most distal portion of the rotator interval **(a)**, at the upper bicipital groove level **(b)** and at the lower bicipital groove level **(c)**, respectively. A single long-axis image of the LHB tendon (b) at the bicipital groove level has also been included **(d)**. The biceps tendon shows early medial subluxation (long arrow) with associated splitting of the superficial fibres of the subscapularis tendon (s). The biceps tendon shows subtle patchy hypoechoic echotexture indicative of tendinopathy and is also swollen, as evidenced by the single comparison view of the left biceps tendon as well as the early 'spill' of the tendon edge over the medial corner of the humeral groove (arrowhead). Note biceps sheath effusion (short arrow) and synovial thickening (asterisk) due to associated tenosynovitis.

bicipital groove and lateral aspect of the rotator interval. It has been shown that 47% of all subscapularis tears involve the SGHL/CHL complex (Bennett 2001). This can lead to refractory anterior shoulder pain and accompanying impingement symptoms arising from secondary LHB attrition and tendinopathy (see Figs 4.153 and 4.154).

Other conditions of the shoulder

Shoulder capsulitis

Shoulder capsulitis describes a generally self-limiting clinical syndrome of shoulder pain associated with a global pattern of passive GHJ restriction. The condition has a slight female preponderance and is most common in the 40–60 year age group. The initial or 'freezing' phase involves shoulder pain without motion restriction and usually lasts 10–36 weeks. Next comes the 'frozen' phase characterised by pain and

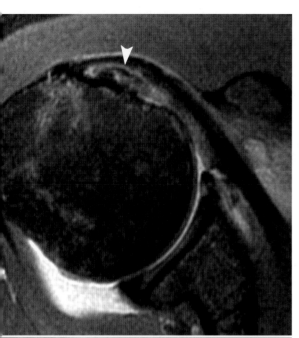

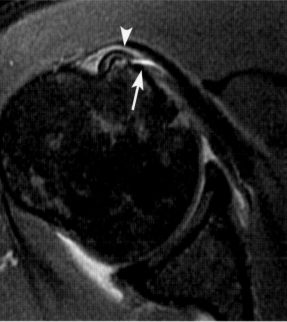

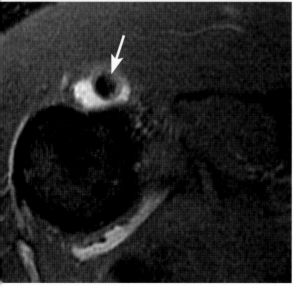

◄ **Fig. 4.154** Non-arthrographic MRI demonstrates a 'hidden lesion'. Fat-suppressed axial PD-weighted images (top and middle images) show medial subluxation of an irregular, attenuated and tendinotic biceps tendon at the pulley level (arrowheads). There is also a high signal line of a partial tear at the superior humeral insertion of the subscapularis tendon (arrow). In the lower image, a swollen biceps tendon is demonstrated at the lower bicipital groove level (arrow). Note the accompanying GHJ effusion.

progressive end-range multidirectional GHJ passive motion restriction, which usually lasts 4–12 months. External shoulder rotation is usually most severely affected, but the overall pattern and severity of motion restriction can vary from case to case. The final or 'thawing' phase is one of gradual recovery that takes place over the next 1–2 years (Miller et al. 1996), although a small proportion of cases can smoulder for many years.

Arthroscopy shows synovial hypertrophy and hyperaemia in the 'freezing' phase of the condition (Hannafin 1999), but the dominant histologic changes are those of fibroplasia involving the subsynovial capsule and pericapsular structures such as the coracohumeral ligament (Ozaki et al. 1989; Bunker and Anthony 1995; Dahan et al. 2005). Some authors use the term 'adhesive capsulitis' for this condition, but there are no structural intracapsular or extracapsular adhesions.

The aetiology of frozen shoulder remains unclear. Suggested causes have included upper limb trauma, calcific tendinopathy, viral infection, nerve root irritation due to cervical spondylosis, suprascapular nerve entrapment, sympathetic dysfunction and ischaemic heart disease. Diabetes mellitus appears to be a predisposing factor. In the authors' clinical practice, shoulder impingement syndrome, shoulder trauma and surgery appear to be the most frequent recognisable precursors.

The diagnosis of established frozen shoulder is usually clinical and straightforward. However, in the early stages of the condition, before the characteristic pattern of GHJ motion restriction has manifested, the clinical diagnosis can be more difficult, and confusion with subacromial impingement syndrome is common. In cases where impingement has been the trigger for capsulitis, the clinical features of both conditions may be present.

Plain films usually demonstrate demineralisation of the humeral head and neck (see Fig. 4.155). Depending on the clinical stage, conventional arthrography can show a reduced GHJ capacity with effacement of the normal joint recesses. However, the diagnostic value of this finding is limited when the clinical features are already established. There is no single sonographic finding that is either diagnostic or consistently present in all cases. Ultrasound which includes both dynamic and Doppler components is nevertheless the most helpful imaging test for early capsulitis and will generally allow a confident diagnosis when the findings are taken together with the clinical context.

In the active synovitic phase of the condition there is usually diffuse low-grade tenderness to probing over the GHJ capsule. Dynamic ultrasound interrogation will commonly demonstrate a typical pattern of multidirectional passive end-range GHJ motion restriction (or 'blocking'), with an absence of compressive bursal bunching on shoulder abduction, except when impingement is concurrently present (see Fig. 4.156). Doppler ultrasound will often show localised capsulosynovial hyperaemia at the rotator interval most marked in the line of the SGHL-CHL complex (see Fig. 4.157).

▶ **Fig. 4.155** Demineralisation of the humeral head is commonly evident on plain films in a patient with a frozen shoulder.

▼ **Fig. 4.156** Ultrasound of the left shoulder shows changes of capsulitis. A comparative dynamic ultrasound examination, performed in the long axis of the supraspinatus tendon during active shoulder abduction, shows the typical pattern of 'blocking' without bursal bunching on the left. On the right side, where the range of abduction is normal, the tip of the greater humeral tuberosity has passed beneath the acromion process and out of view. On the symptomatic left side, the key observation is that there is an abrupt mechanical block to normal end-range abduction and that pain occurs at this premature end-point. In the example shown here, where the block to abduction has occurred at only 60° elevation of the left arm, the tip of the greater humeral tuberosity could not pass beneath the acromion. Note the absence of SA-SD bursal bunching (arrows), which differs from subacromial impingement. It is nevertheless important to recognise that, in some cases, elements of both capsulitis and impingement may coexist in the same patient and produce mixed sonographic features.

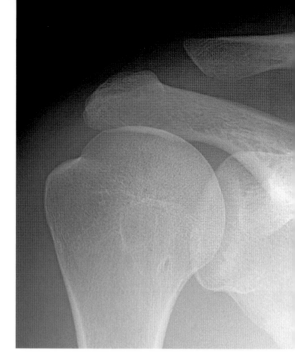

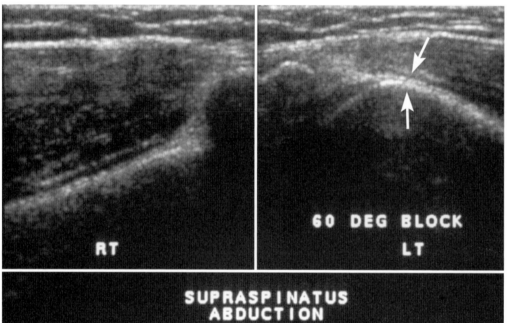

▼ **Fig. 4.157** Glenohumeral capsulitis is demonstrated by ultrasound. Greyscale and Colour Doppler images are oriented transverse to the LHB tendon (b) within the mid-to-distal rotator interval. These images show the most commonly observed distribution of capsulosynovial hyperaemia (arrow) along the line of the SGHL-CHL complex (arrowheads). Successful elicitation of this sign requires equipment with good Doppler sensitivity, and an appropriate scan technique including optimised Doppler settings, a very light transducer pressure, the cuff tissues taken off stretch and the muscles relaxed. Supraspinatus tendon = ssp. Subscapularis tendon = scp.

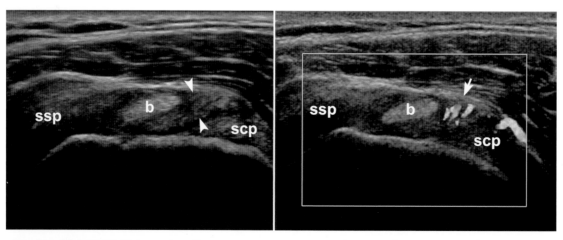

Frequently, both ultrasound and MRI reveal an associated scant GHJ effusion (see Fig. 4.158). A GHJ capsule thickness of more than 4 mm at the level of the axillary recess has been reported as an MRI finding (Emig et al. 1995). In the authors' experience, capsular hyperintensity, which is most objectively assessed at the posterior glenohumeral recess, and capsulosynovial thickening within the rotator interval are the most useful MRI signs of capsulitis (Mengiardi et al. 2004) (see Figs 4.159 and 4.160). Imaging with ultrasound or fluoroscopy can be used to accurately guide the therapeutic injection of the GHJ in patients with capsulitis (discussed in Chapter 10). We believe this to be of greatest value early in the course of the disease.

Calcific tendinopathy

Calcific tendinopathy is an idiopathic self-limiting condition of calcium hydroxyapatite crystal deposition that occurs in adults of any age and produces pain. Acute symptoms may be severe and usually subside spontaneously over several weeks. Some patients experience chronic symptoms that tend to take months or years to resolve. Small age-related rotator cuff calcifications of presumed degenerative aetiology are common, especially in the subscapularis tendon. These calcifications can be found in 3–20% of patients with painless shoulders (Woodward 2004) and tend not to resolve with time. Consequently, a finding of calcification on plain films does not necessarily indicate a symptomatic tendinopathy. Symptomatic calcifications are non-dystrophic, occurring

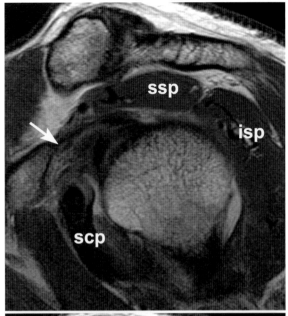

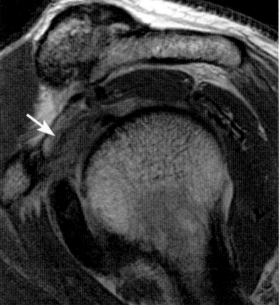

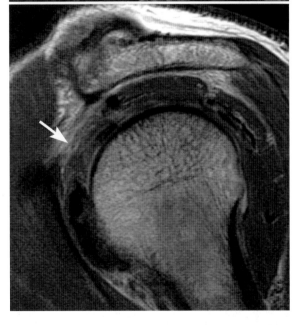

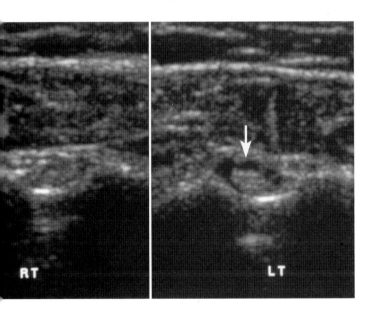

▲ **Fig. 4.158** Transverse ultrasound images of a patient with left shoulder capsulitis show an associated small biceps tendon sheath effusion (arrow) by comparison with the normal right side.

▶ **Fig. 4.159** Glenohumeral capsulitis is demonstrated by non-arthrographic MRI. Sequential PD-weighted sagittal images demonstrate a localised zone of intermediate signal within the proximal rotator interval (arrows) indicative of capsulosynovial thickening. Note the effacement of normal subcoracoid fat signal. Supraspinatus tendon = ssp. Subscapularis tendon = scp. Infraspinatus tendon = isp.

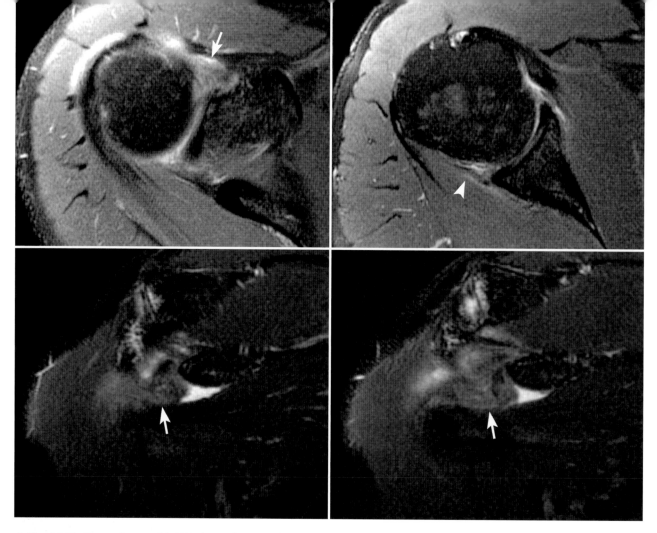

▲ **Fig. 4.160** Non-arthrographic MRI shows changes of glenohumeral capsulitis. Fat-suppressed coronal T2 and fat-suppressed axial PD-weighted images show capsulosynovial thickening within the rotator interval (arrows). There is also thickening and hyperintensity in the line of the posterior GHJ capsule (arrowhead) and a small GHJ effusion. Changes of ACJ degeneration, supraspinatus tendinopathy and SA-SD bursopathy are also incidentally present.

in viable rather than necrotic tissue. These most commonly involve the supraspinatus tendon about 1–2 cm proximal to its insertion, although any of the rotator cuff tendons can be involved and there may be painful leakage of the calcified material into the SA-SD bursa (see Figs 4.161 and 4.162).

The peak incidence of symptomatic calcifications occurs in a younger population than the degenerative type occurs in. Deposits are most commonly chalky but can occasionally have a semi-liquid consistency similar to toothpaste. A 'soft' radiographic appearance or non-shadowing sonographic appearance favours acute over chronic crystal deposition (see Fig. 4.163). Dense and well-circumscribed calcifications of more chronic appearance with posterior acoustic shadowing can also be associated with acute symptoms (see Fig. 4.164). Calcific deposits may be difficult to detect on MRI. They appear as 'black' signal voids within the tendon, perhaps distorting the tendon contour and are usually associated with a peri-tendinitis or bursopathy (see Fig. 4.124 on page 242). Both acute and chronic deposits of soft-tissue calcification can produce tendon and bursal swelling, which may contribute to shoulder impingement (see Fig. 4.162). Ultrasound is useful for the real-time guidance of therapeutic percutaneous needle aspiration and injection, as described in Chapter 10.

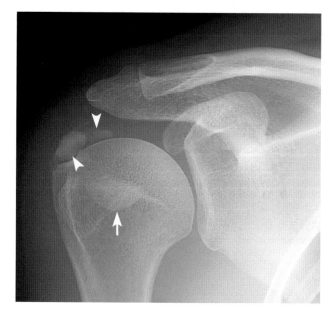

▲ **Fig. 4.161** Calcific rotator cuff tendinopathy is demonstrated by plain film. Calcific deposits are illustrated within both the subscapularis (arrow) and supraspinatus tendons (arrowheads). Both dense and soft deposits are present and there is rupture into the SA-SD bursa.

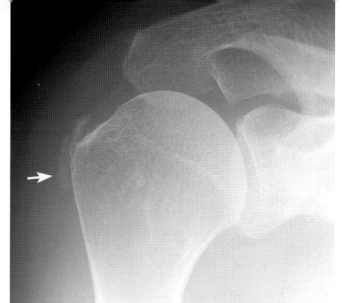

▶ **Fig. 4.162** Calcific supraspinatus tendinopathy is present, with rupture of soft calcification into the SA-SD bursa (arrow).

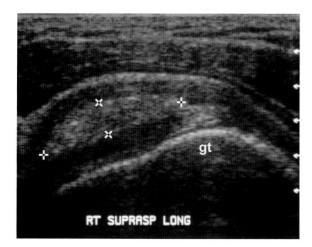

▲ **Fig. 4.163** A long-axis ultrasound image of the distal supraspinatus tendon shows a large echogenic focus of contained non-shadowing calcification. Greater tuberosity = gt.

Lateral acromial apophysitis

Repeated traction on the lateral acromion by the deltoid can produce a painful apophysitis in the skeletally immature athlete. This is most common between the ages of 16 and 17, when the developing athlete's power is starting to increase. Plain films show typical changes of osteochondritis in the acromial apophysis with fragmentation, compression and demineralisation (see Fig. 4.165). The process resolves without complication.

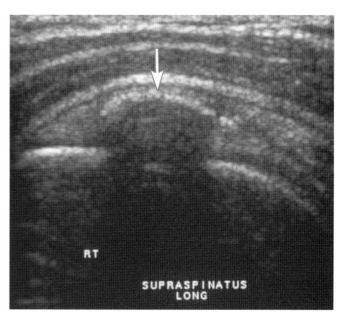

▲ **Fig. 4.164** Chronic calcific supraspinatus tendinopathy is shown on a long-axis ultrasound image. Only the superficial surface of the calcific deposit can be appreciated as an echogenic line (arrow). Detail posterior to this is obscured by acoustic shadowing.

▼ **Fig. 4.165** Changes of apophysitis are demonstrated involving the unfused acromial apophysis. There is patchy demineralisation and early fragmentation.

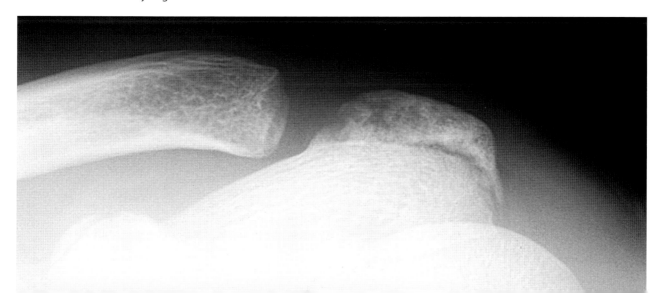

▶ **Fig. 4.166** Following an avulsion injury, dense myositis ossificans has developed at the pectoralis major insertion.

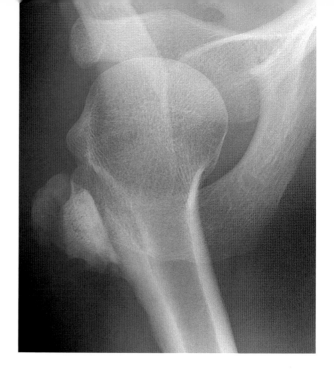

Avulsion of the pectoralis major

Pectoralis major ruptures most commonly occur at the humeral attachment (see Fig. 4.166) but may occasionally involve the musculotendinous junction. A frequent mechanism of pectoralis major injury is body building with bench presses in the gymnasium. Anabolic steroid use is an obvious factor that may increase the chance of muscle or tendon rupture. The diagnosis is usually clinically obvious. Imaging may help in determining management options. If the tear is full-thickness at the humeral attachment, early repair may be indicated, whereas a partial-thickness tear at the musculotendinous junction may be treated conservatively. MRI is the modality of choice in assessing these injuries (see Fig. 4.167), although ultrasound can also detect tears (Zvijac et al. 2006) (see Fig. 4.168).

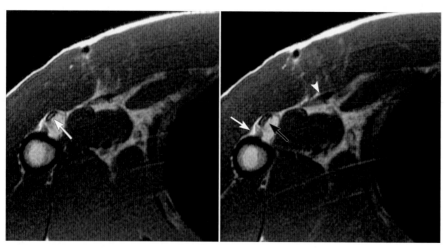

◀ **Fig. 4.167** Avulsion of the pectoralis major tendon from its humeral insertion is demonstrated by MRI. A professional basketball player was injured when he was transiently caught by the arm in a basketball hoop during a slam-dunk competition. Contiguous axial PD-weighted MR images show a complete avulsion of the pectoralis major tendon at or very close to its humeral insertion (white arrow) with retraction of the proximal tendon stump (white arrowhead). Note the consequent mild anterior prolapse of the LHB tendon (black arrow).

▼ **Fig. 4.168** A tear at the pectoralis major musculotendinous junction is demonstrated by ultrasound. Long-axis ultrasound images have been obtained along the length of the pectoralis major tendon and muscle. Humerus = h.

(a) This panoramic view of the muscle shows a broad zone of mixed echotexture due to haemorrhage at the musculotendinous junction (asterisks). Note that the distal tendon can be followed to the humeral insertion and appears intact (arrowhead), while the proximal stump of pectoral muscle has retracted and bunched (arrow). **(b)** This detailed view of the distal tendon and humeral attachment confirms the presence of a normal fibrillar echopattern and continuity.

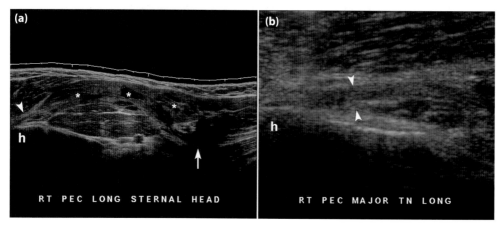

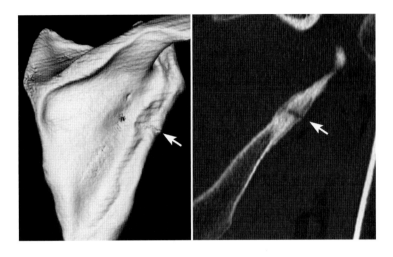

▶ **Fig. 4.169** A stress fracture of the lateral border of the scapula is demonstrated by CT. There is a fracture line with adjacent sclerosis and periosteal reaction, demonstrated on both 3D reconstruction (left image) and coronal plane reformation (right image).

▼ **Fig. 4.170** A nuclear bone scan shows increased uptake of isotope on the lateral border of the scapula in a thrower (arrow). This most probably represents an enthesopathy, possibly due to overuse of the serratus anterior.

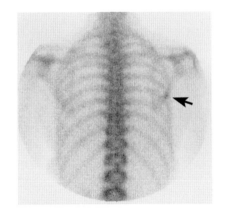

Stress fractures of the shoulder

Stress fractures of the shoulder occur with pitching (Branch et al. 1992), weight-lifting (Horwitz and DiStefano 1995) and tennis. The literature also reports stress fractures involving the inferior glenoid rim in pitchers (Bennett 1941), the clavicle in a diver (Waninger 1997), the acromion (Schils et al. 1990; Ward et al. 1994; Hall and Calvert 1995), the coracoid process of the scapula in a trap shooter (Sandrock 1975), the lateral border of the scapula (Brower et al. 1977) (see Figs 4.169 and 4.170) and the superomedial portion of the scapula in a jogger who ran with weights in both hands (Veluvolu et al. 1988).

Scapulothoracic bursopathy

A syndrome of snapping pain or crepitus described as scapulothoracic bursopathy or 'snapping scapula' usually occurs in athletes who throw frequently. Symptoms are most often experienced at the inferior angle of the scapula in the late cocking and acceleration phases of the throwing action. The cause is usually obscure, but possible mechanisms include bony changes that alter congruence between the scapula and chest wall, such as a malunited rib fracture or an osteochondroma (see Fig. 4.171). Also, there are several bursae described about the scapula, and an overuse-induced chronic bursopathy may affect one or more of these. Plain films or CT are indicated to exclude a bony cause. Ultrasound can be used to guide an injection of the scapulo-thoracic space in the region of the symptoms (see Fig. 4.172).

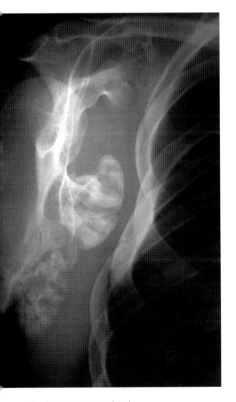

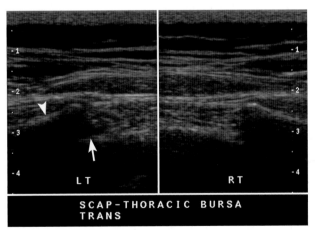

▲ **Fig. 4.171** Multiple osteochondromata arise from the scapular fossa and encroach on the scapulothoracic joint. Note the associated rib deformity.

▲ **Fig. 4.172** Scapulothoracic bursopathy is demonstrated by ultrasound. Corresponding with an area of pain and localised tenderness, comparison transverse ultrasound images demonstrate subtle hypoechoic bursal thickening beneath the medial edge of the left scapula (arrow). An ultrasound-guided therapeutic injection is possible. The arrowhead indicates the scapula.

Paediatric shoulder injuries

Sports-related injuries to the shoulder-girdle in children and adolescents are becoming common as their participation in organised competitive sports increases. As discussed in Chapter 1, paediatric injuries differ from those seen in adult athletes, although adult patterns emerge in the adolescent years as strength develops. Both acute and overuse injuries occur in this age group.

Acute paediatric shoulder injuries

Acute injuries that occur commonly in children and adolescent athletes include fractures of the clavicle and proximal humerus and glenohumeral dislocation.

A fracture of the clavicle is the most common childhood fracture and usually follows a fall on the tip of the shoulder or, less commonly, a fall on the outstretched hand (see Fig. 4.173). As the clavicle is subcutaneous, little soft-tissue protection is available and a direct trauma across the clavicle may also produce a clavicular fracture. Nearly 50% of all clavicular fractures occur in children under seven years of age.

A fracture of the proximal humerus results from direct trauma or a fall backwards with the arm behind the body. Most of these fractures occur in children between the ages of 10 and 14 (Kohler and Trilland 1983). Two-thirds involve the metaphysis (see Fig. 4.174) and one-third involve the growth plate (Salter–Harris Type I or II) (see Fig. 4.175). Imaging with plain films is invariably the only imaging required.

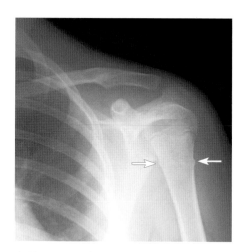

▲ **Fig. 4.174** There is a greenstick-type fracture of the metaphysis/proximal shaft of the humerus (arrow). These fractures are often subtle and may result from a fall on the outstretched hand or elbow.

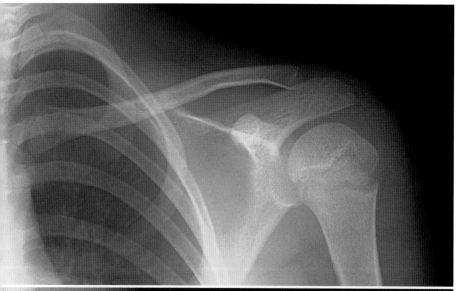

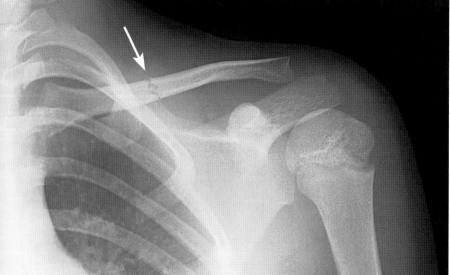

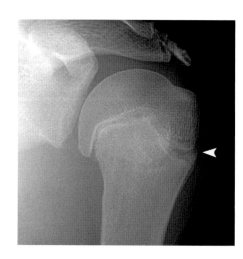

▲ **Fig. 4.173** There is a fracture of the middle third of the clavicle, without displacement (arrow). This fracture would have been missed without the AP view with cranial tube angulation.

▲ **Fig. 4.175** There is a Salter–Harris fracture of the proximal humeral growth plate, following direct trauma.

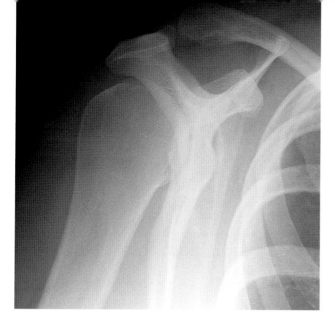

▲ **Fig. 4.176** Dysplastic changes involve the scapula, with a dysplastic, retroverted glenoid predisposing to multidirectional instability.

Overuse paediatric shoulder injuries

Young athletes may also develop chronic overuse injuries resulting in glenohumeral instability, a stress reaction in the proximal humeral growth plate, tendinopathy and bone stress at the outer end of the clavicle. Rib fractures rarely occur in children.

- Recurrent shoulder instability in children raises the possibility of developmental laxity of the glenohumeral ligaments or glenohumeral dysplasia allowing multidirectional instability. An instability series may demonstrate dysplastic changes (see Fig. 4.176), a Hill-Sachs defect (see Fig. 4.177), a Bankart fracture or other cause of recurrent instability.

- A stress reaction involving the proximal humeral growth plate has been reported to occur exclusively in throwing sports and is known as 'Little League' shoulder. This develops most commonly between the ages of 11 and 16 (Ireland and Andrews 1988). Plain films may show widening of the proximal humeral growth plate with associated resorption and sclerosis developing on the metaphyseal side of the growth plate (see Fig. 4.178).

- Sports that involve overhead action such as throwing, swimming or tennis commonly cause rotator cuff tendinopathy in young athletes. This may be combined with glenohumeral instability. Multidirectional instability is commonly associated with impingement due to translation of the humeral head superiorly.

- Osteolysis of the outer end of the clavicle has been reported in adolescents, usually associated with weight-lifting (Cahill 1992).

- Rib fractures in the paediatric age group require consideration. Rib fractures are uncommon because children younger than 14 have a compliant rib cage and may absorb considerable force without a fracture occurring. So if rib fractures are present, it is likely that there has been significant trauma. The costovertebral and costochondral

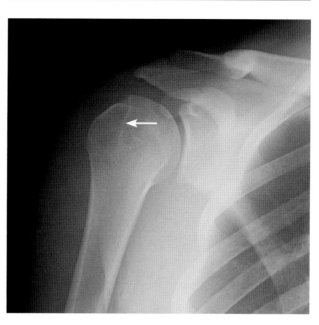

▲ **Fig. 4.177** A large Hill-Sachs defect is present, predisposing the immature athlete to continuing instability.

▼ **Fig. 4.178** There has been disruption of the proximal humeral growth plate with slight displacement of the humeral head epiphysis (arrow) in a young athlete involved in sports requiring repetitive overhead activity. In the absence of recent acute trauma, this change was considered to be an overuse injury ('Little League' shoulder).

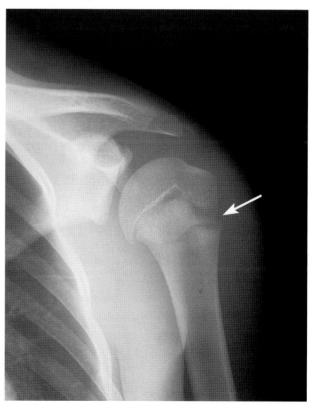

junctions are usually involved and are difficult to identify on a chest x-ray and rib views (Westcott et al. 2000). Child abuse must be considered when fractures are found (rib fractures account for 5–27% of all fractures in abused children).

Sporting injuries of the ACJ, clavicle and SCJ

The ACJ, clavicle and SCJ provide a mobile strut connecting the axial skeleton to each upper limb. The clavicle articulates with the acromion at the ACJ and the sternum through the SCJ. Many ligamentous structures stabilise these joints, and muscles insert and originate from the clavicle providing both stability and mobility. ACJ injuries are more prevalent than SCJ injuries and occur frequently in contact sports due to direct or indirect trauma. SCJ disruptions occur infrequently during sporting activities. Less than 1% of SCJ dislocations are sports-related (Rodosky and Jari 2001).

The ACJ

The ACJ is located between the distal end of the clavicle and the medial margin of the acromion process of the scapula. The articular surfaces of hyaline cartilage are separated by a fibrocartilagenous disc, which invariably degenerates with age and is usually non-functional beyond the age of 40. There is a considerable normal variation in the inclination of the joint in the coronal plane (Galatz et al. 2001). The plane of the joint is usually vertical (see Fig. 4.179), but may also be inclined downwards and medially as much as 50° as a normal variant, with the clavicle overriding the acromion. This oblique inclination is present in approximately 50% of normal cases (see Fig. 4.180).

Approximately 75% of ACJ injuries are due to trauma occurring during contact sports (Rodosky and Jari 2001). Injury to the ACJ often follows a fall on the tip of the shoulder or onto the outstretched hand, commonly occurring in contact sports such as rugby and ice hockey and in high-velocity activities such as skiing and equestrian sports. If the clavicle does not fracture, the ACJ and the coracoclavicular ligament may be injured. ACJ joint problems also have an association with weightlifting as a part of an upper-body conditioning program (Cook and Tibone 1988). ACJ injury is a problem in sports involving throwing, but this usually relates to the weight training associated with the sport.

Stability of the ACJ is maintained by the coracoclavicular ligaments, the acromioclavicular capsular ligaments and the deltopectoral fascia. There are superior, inferior, anterior and posterior acromioclavicular ligaments, which insert on the clavicle about 1.5 cm from the ACJ. The acromioclavicular ligaments mainly act as a constraint against anteroposterior displacement and the coracoclavicular ligaments prevent superior displacement of the distal clavicle. The deltoid and trapezius muscles also contribute to the stability of the ACJ by blending with the superior acromioclavicular ligament, which is the strongest of the acromioclavicular ligaments.

The coracoclavicular ligament consists of two parts—the conoid ligament and the trapezoid ligament—which act to anchor the clavicle over the coracoid process of the scapula. The conoid ligament passes superiorly and slightly posteriorly from the coracoid process and inserts on the conoid tubercle on the undersurface of the clavicle. The trapezoid ligament passes anterolaterally to the conoid ligament and attaches

to a ridge on the undersurface or outer end of the clavicle (see Fig. 4.181). These ligaments prevent the acromion from passing under the outer end of the clavicle when a force is applied to the lateral aspect of the shoulder. The coracoclavicular ligament is the prime suspensory ligament of the upper limb.

Rockwood (1984) described six types of ACJ injury with varying degrees of disruption and subluxation. This classification can be found in orthopaedic texts. In practice, plain films are usually the only imaging required.

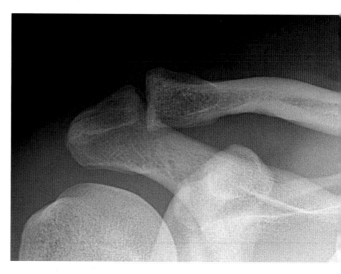

▲ **Fig. 4.179** The orientation of the ACJ is usually vertical.

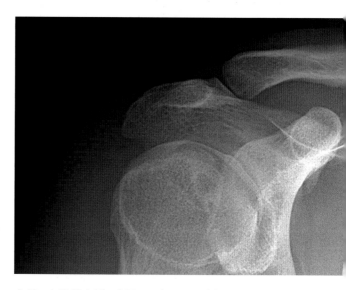

▲ **Fig. 4.180(a)** The ACJ may have an oblique orientation. Up to 50° is accepted as normal and some obliquity is seen in up to 50% of the population.
▼ **(b)** Chronic subluxation is demonstrated in an oblique joint.

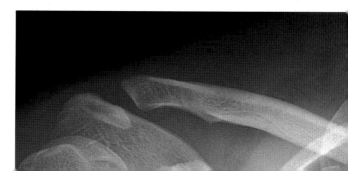

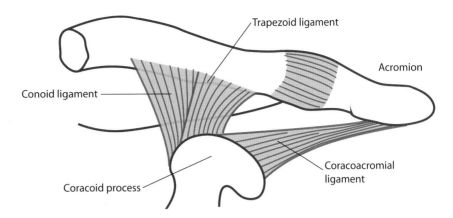

▶ **Fig. 4.181** A line drawing shows the configuration of the conoid and trapezoid components of the coracoclavicular ligament (see text).

Imaging the ACJ

As previously discussed in the section 'Other shoulder-girdle views', there are two standard plain film views: an AP view with 15° of cranial tube angulation and an axial shoulder view.

AP view with 15° of cranial tube angulation

There are some important points to remember about imaging the ACJ using an AP view with 15° of cranial tube angulation.

• Comparison with the asymptomatic side will help determine subtle joint space widening or an increased coracoclavicular space on the injured side. This can often be obtained on one film (see Fig. 4.182(a)), but definition is improved by obtaining separate collimated images (see Fig. 4.182(b)).

• This view is obtained with and without weightbearing to stress the joints, which helps assess subtle instability (see

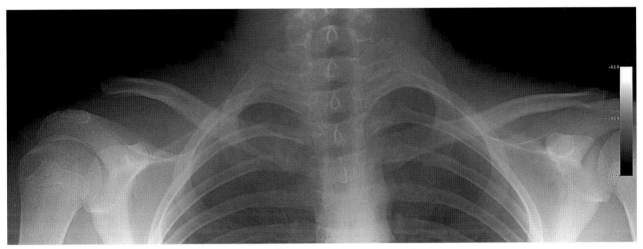

▲ **Fig. 4.182(a)** The two ACJs can be compared on one film. In this case, there is obvious dislocation of the right ACJ and the left joint appears normal. Note that the two joints barely fit on the one film, which is a deficiency of this technique. No bone injury can be seen.

▶ **(b)** The authors prefer the ACJs to be imaged separately, as collimation increases resolution. These four views and an axial view of the symptomatic side make up the routine series used by the authors. The upper two images are obtained with weightbearing and the lower images are taken at rest. The sides are compared, the shoulders are internally rotated and the weights hang from the hands, rather than being gripped for the weightbearing views (as discussed in the text).

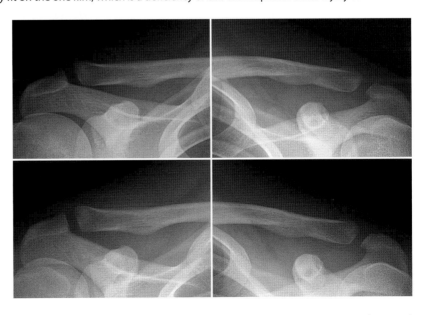

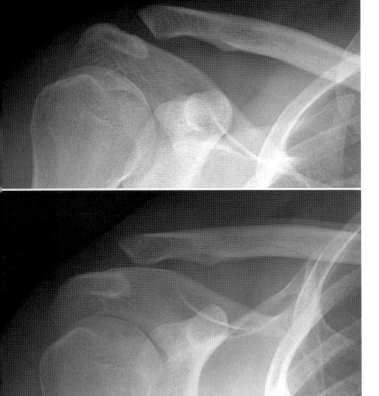

Fig. 4.183). It is important that the weights hang from the wrists, as gripping a weight will commonly tense the shoulder musculature, which may mask minor instability. Sandbags with straps attached are ideal.

- For the same reason, it is essential that the shoulder is internally rotated while ACJ integrity is being tested. Internal rotation relaxes the surrounding muscles and, not uncommonly, simply internally rotating the shoulder alone will cause ACJ widening and increase subluxation if there has been ligamentous injury (see Fig. 4.184).

In the immature athlete there is an apophysis on the upper surface of the coracoid at the attachment of the coracoclavicular ligament. This apophysis may be avulsed by the coracoclavicular ligament and the position of this apophysis should be examined and compared with the asymptomatic side (see Fig. 4.185). There is also an apophysis on the undersurface of the outer end of the clavicle which will fuse to form the trapezoid ridge. This is demonstrated in Figs 4.185 and 4.192 (on page 274).

▲ **Fig. 4.183** Weightbearing views should be obtained with the weights hanging by straps from the patient's wrists. Gripping weights causes tension in the shoulder musculature, which may prevent joint widening or subluxation. The upper image was obtained without weights, and an increased widening of the coracoclavicular and acromioclavicular joint spaces is seen in the lower image with weightbearing.

▼ **Fig. 4.184** Simple internal rotation of the shoulder alone will produce an increased widening of the coracoclavicular and acromioclavicular joints. There is external rotation of the humeral head in the upper image and internal rotation in the lower image.

▼ **Fig. 4.185** In an immature athlete there is a normally occurring apophysis at the point of attachment of the coracoclavicular ligament to the coracoid (black arrows). There has been avulsion of this coracoid apophysis on the left, resulting in minor subluxation of the left ACJ. There also appears to be avulsion of an apophysis on the undersurface of the outer end of the clavicle at the attachment of the trapezoid ligament.

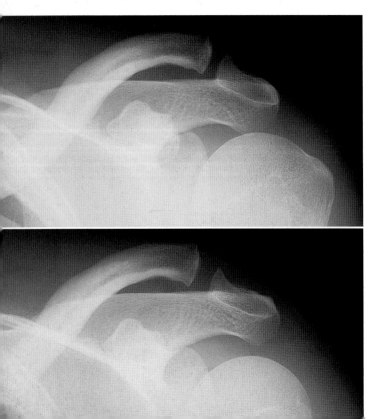

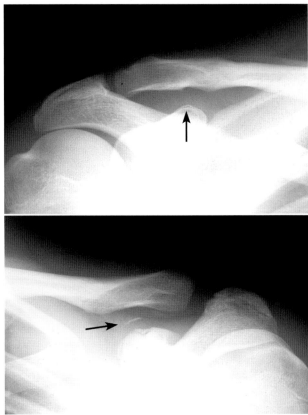

Axial view

The method of obtaining this view is described in the section on routine GHJ views. This is an extremely important view when there is a clinical suspicion of posterior dislocation of the ACJ. It is not possible to appreciate posterior displacement on a frontal projection, although often the joint space appears widened (see Fig. 4.186).

If doubt remains after reviewing the plain films, further imaging may be helpful. MRI can detect ligamentous injury (see Fig. 4.187) and dynamic ultrasound can further assess ACJ stability if required.

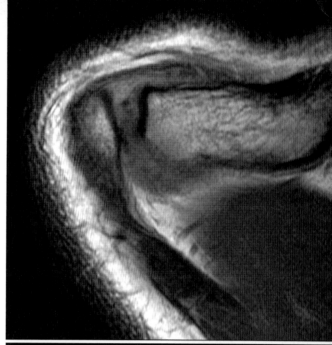

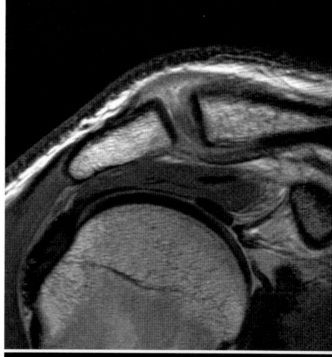

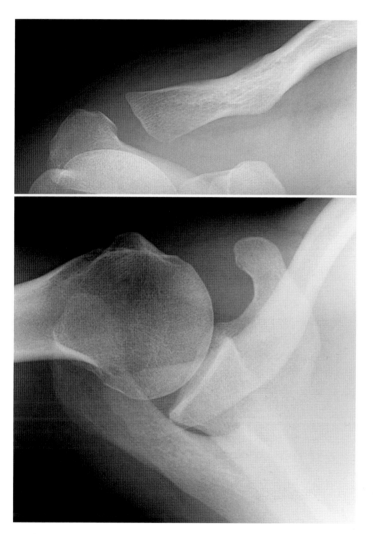

▲ **Fig. 4.186** Posterior dislocation of the AC joint is well demonstrated using an axial view. An AP view shows only mild widening of ACJ space, and the 15° angled-up view does not allow appreciation of a posterior displacement. However, the axial view clearly demonstrates posterior ACJ dislocation. This is an uncommon injury that implies complete rupture of the acromioclavicular and coracoclavicular ligaments as well as buttonholing of the outer end of the clavicle through the trapezius muscle.

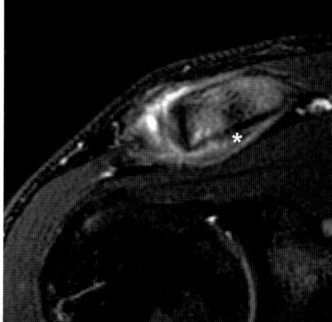

▶ **Fig. 4.187** MRI demonstrates ACJ injury. Axial PD, coronal PD and fat-suppressed coronal T2-weighted images show diffuse capsular thickening and hyperintensity, disruption of the anterosuperior attachment of the articular disc, and capsuloperiosteal stripping along the undersurface of the outer end of the clavicle (asterisk). Accompanying bone marrow oedema is present.

Injury to the clavicle

The clavicle is an S-shaped bone that functions as a strut between the sternum and the GHJ. Many ligaments attach to the clavicle, stabilising its attachment to the acromion and sternum (as discussed in the sections on the ACJ and SCJ). Three muscles originate from the clavicle—the sternohyoid, the pectoralis major and the deltoid—and three muscles insert onto the clavicle—the sternomastoid, the subclavius and the trapezius. These muscles apply deforming forces when a fracture occurs, and an understanding of these forces helps to explain displacement of clavicular fractures. The clavicle rotates 40 to 50° about its longitudinal axis with full abduction of the arm. As the outer end of the clavicle rotates upwards, scapulothoracic rotation occurs through the clavicular attachments to the scapula via the conoid and trapezoid ligaments. Its subcutaneous position exposes the clavicle to injury and, as a consequence, fractures of the clavicle are common, representing about 5–10% of all adult fractures. Previously, the most common mechanism of a fractured clavicle was thought to be due to a fall on the outstretched hand. However, Nordqvist and Petersson (1994) found that only 6% of clavicular fractures were caused by this mechanism and a direct fall on the shoulder is a much more common cause.

There are important structures closely related to the clavicle and complications of a clavicular fracture are often related to these surrounding structures. Consequently, a search for other fractures of the shoulder-girdle and ribs is important and the possibility of pulmonary contusion, pneumothorax and haemothorax should be considered. In addition, vascular trauma may occur due to laceration of the subclavian vessels (see Fig. 4.188(a)). Thoracic outlet syndrome may occur as a complication of a comminuted clavicular fracture (see Fig. 4.188(b)).

The classification of clavicular fractures is complex, with the most commonly used classification containing a modification of middle third fractures introduced by Nordqvist and Petersson (1994). The management significance of the classification of clavicular fractures is found in orthopaedic texts.

▼ **Fig. 4.188(a)** A tragic fracture of the clavicle occurred during a rugby match resulting from a tackle onto the point of the shoulder. This post-mortem chest film shows a comminuted fracture of the outer third of the clavicle (arrow). During impact, a sliver of bone tore the left subclavian artery resulting in exsanguination into the left side of the chest. The left hemithorax is opacified by blood and there is a marked shift of mediastinal structures to the right.

▼ **(b)** This image is borrowed from Chapter 8. Coronal and sagittal T1-weighted images show a displaced bone fragment (arrowhead) originating from a comminuted mid-sharft clavicular fracture pressing on the brachial plexus of an athlete and causing a C6 neuropathy.

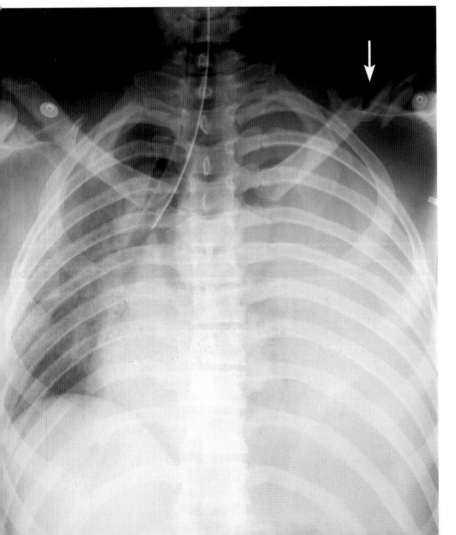

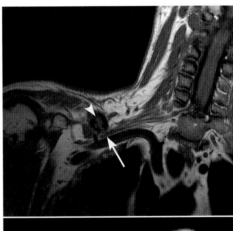

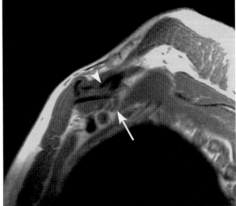

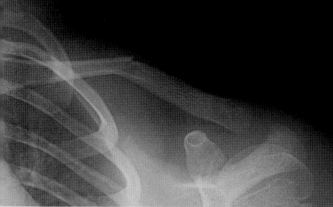

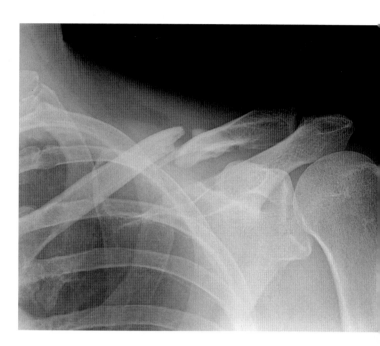

Group I: middle third fractures

Approximately 80% of all clavicular fractures occur in its middle third and are classified as Group I (see Figs 4.189 and 4.190). Shortening of the middle third fracture is important to demonstrate and note. There is a 15% incidence of non-union in a middle third fracture when shortening greater than 2 cm is demonstrated on the initial examination (Wick et al. 2001) (see Fig. 4.191).

▲ **Fig. 4.189** A fracture involves the middle third of the clavicle with upward angulation resulting at the fracture site. This deformity is common and may result in a subcutaneous bony lump if not reduced.

▼ **Fig. 4.190** Commonly, clavicular shortening will result at a middle third clavicular fracture site, due to overriding of the medial fragment. There is a 15% chance of non-union if shortening greater than 2 cm is demonstrated initially.

▲ **Fig. 4.191** A fracture involves the junction of the middle and outer thirds of the clavicle. There is overriding of the medial fragment and comminution is present. Non-union has occurred.

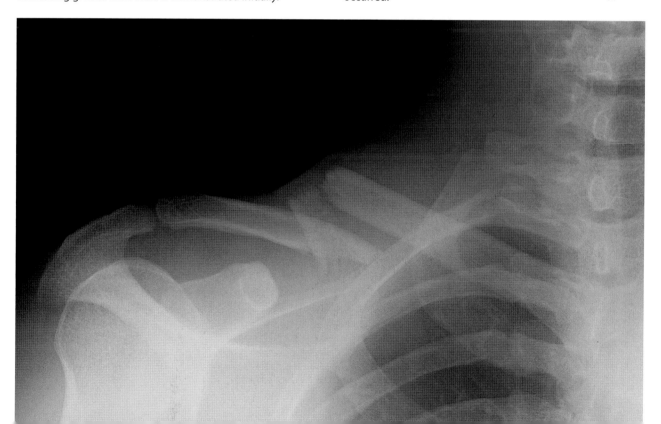

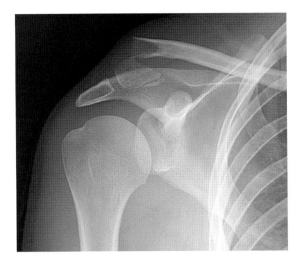

▲ **Fig. 4.192** A fracture involves the distal third of the clavicle and demonstrates the role played by the ligaments and tendons in displacement of outer third fractures. With rupture of the conoid ligament, there is loss of restraint to the elevation of the medial fragment and superior displacement occurs. The trapezoid ligament remains intact and there is no disruption of the ACJ. Possible minor displacement of the apophysis on the undersurface of the outer end of the clavicle has occurred (also noted in Fig. 4.185 on page 270).

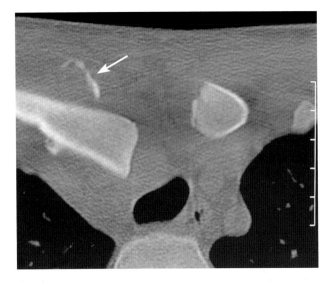

▲ **Fig. 4.193** CT demonstrates a fracture involving the growth plate at the proximal end of the clavicle with considerable displacement. There is anterior displacement of the epiphysis (arrow) and considerable posterior displacement of the medial end of the clavicle. Considerable soft-tissue injury is present, with tracheal compression demonstrated.

▶ **Fig. 4.194** An early resorptive stage of osteolysis is demonstrated by a plain film. There is subchondral demineralisation and irregular bony resorption (arrowheads). A band of sclerosis is noted deep to the demineralisation.

Group II: fractures of the outer third

Approximately 15% of all clavicular fractures involve the outer end and are classified as Group II. Group II fractures are further divided into three types depending on the displacement, which is related to whether the coracoclavicular ligament is intact. When injury to the coracoclavicular ligament has occurred, there is widening of the space between the coracoid process and the clavicle (see Fig. 4.192).

Group III: proximal third fractures

Proximal third fractures are rare and represent only 2% of all clavicular fractures. There are five types of Group III fractures related to displacement and depending on whether the SCJ is involved, and epiphyseal separation may occur in athletes up to 25 years of age. This growth plate is late in closing, and dislocated sternoclavicular dislocations are often growth plate fractures in younger athletes (see Fig. 4.193).

Post-traumatic osteolysis of the clavicle

This painful condition follows recurrent ACJ trauma and is mostly seen in footballers and weight-lifters. Bench presses and military presses have been strongly implicated (Scavenius et al. 1987). Onset may occur several weeks to several years following trauma, and the lytic phase can last 12–18 months if left untreated. Plain films show resorption of the outer end of the clavicle (see Figs 4.194 and 4.195). Ultrasound demonstrates local tenderness, capsulosynovial thickening, hyperaemia and a variable degree of articular cortical irregularity. MRI will show hyperintensity of the joint capsule, marrow oedema at the outer end of the clavicle on T2-weighted sequences, and bony irregularity of osteolysis.

Stabilising occurs and then resolution will progress over four to six months with the outer end of the clavicle often remaining smoothly tapered and the ACJ permanently widened (Levine et al. 1976). It has been postulated that the condition represents either a bone stress reaction or slowly progressive post-traumatic synovitis.

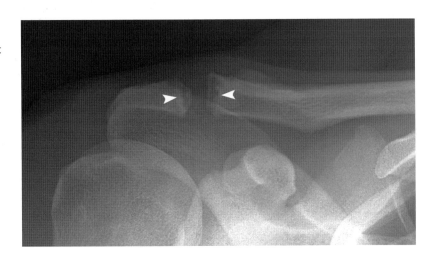

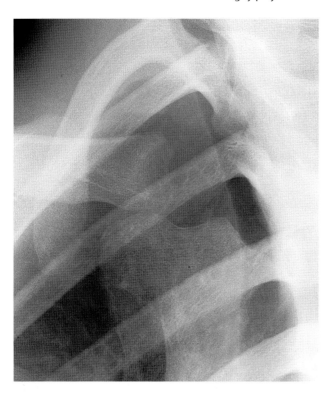

▲ **Fig. 4.195** Well-established post-traumatic osteolysis of the clavicle is demonstrated in an international rugby player.

▲ **Fig. 4.196** An anterior dislocation is demonstrated on an oblique plain film view. CT should now be performed to better define the displacement and to help assess soft-tissue injuries. It seems sensible to perform CT in the first instance, if this imaging method is available.

▶ **Fig. 4.197** A CT scan shows a posterior dislocation of the right SCJ. No significant haematoma or tracheal compression can be seen. The medial end of the right clavicle is indicated by an arrow.

The SCJ

The clavicular articular surface of the SCJ is saddle-shaped and articulates with a simple notch in the sternum. The clavicular articular surface is larger than the sternal articular surface and the joint surfaces are not congruous. The incongruity of the articular surfaces is accommodated by the presence of an articular disc.

Injury to the SCJ is unusual, accounting for 1–4% of shoulder injuries (Wettstein et al. 2004), and is most commonly seen following a direct or indirect trauma during contact sport (Carmichael et al. 2006). Anterior subluxation is the more common displacement, occurring three times more frequently than posterior dislocation (see Fig. 4.196). Rare posterior dislocations may create a medical emergency due to tracheal compression and other complications similar to the case shown in Fig. 4.193. Carmichael et al. (2006) noted that as many as 30% of posterior-directed medial clavicular injuries had concomitant injuries to the trachea, oesophagus or great vessels.

Plain films play a limited role in the examination of the SCJ, mainly due to the difficulty in obtaining a diagnostic series of films, and a CT examination is usually performed regardless of the care and attention paid in obtaining good plain films. Carmichael et al. also noted the frequency of delayed and missed diagnoses reported in the literature when plain films have been relied on as the imaging method.

A plain film series of the SCJ consists of an AP view, both oblique plain film views and a lateral view, and the method of obtaining these views has been described earlier in the chapter, in the section 'Other shoulder-girdle views'. When assessing the plain films, careful comparison of the joint spaces is necessary to detect or suspect displacements. The incongruity of the articular margins makes the interpretation of the plain films difficult, and minor displacement is virtually impossible to detect.

As a consequence, CT becomes a valuable imaging method. CT scanning provides better definition, enables small bone fragments to be detected and demonstrates injuries in the adjacent soft-tissue structures (see Fig. 4.197). The use of MDCT provides easy-to-interpret images (see Fig. 4.198).

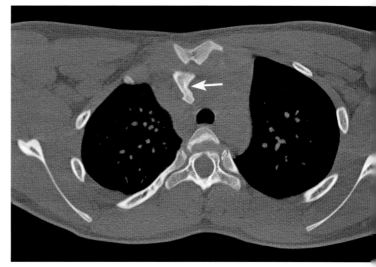

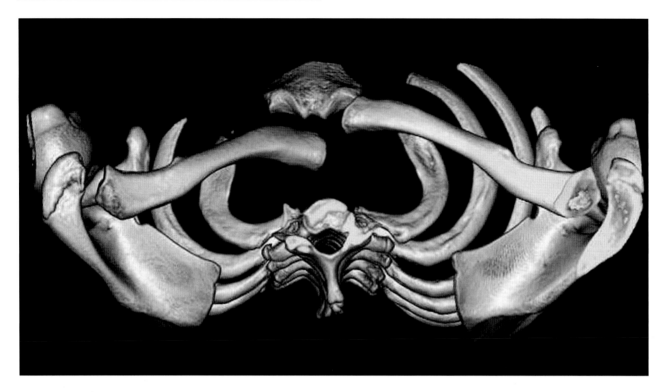

▲ **Fig. 4.198** An improved understanding of the dislocation and displacement is provided by a volume-rendered (3D) reconstruction of the data from the case demonstrated in Fig. 4.197.

Rib injuries in sport

Rib fractures may be the result of acute trauma or repetitive stress, and both acute and stress fractures regularly result from sporting activities.

Imaging guidelines for acute rib fractures

Rib fractures most commonly involve ribs five to nine. This is thought to be due to the protection provided to the upper ribs by the shoulder-girdle and the fact that the lower ribs resist fracture due to their inherent mobility and pliability.

Acute rib fractures are a common sporting injury and are particularly prevalent in contact sports. A fractured rib is a painful injury and whether imaging is worthwhile has been the subject of much discussion. This subject has been investigated by the American College of Radiology and guidelines were issued in 2000. In drawing up guidelines for imaging rib fractures, Westcott et al. (2000) noted that studies had found that neither plain films nor ultrasound were efficient at identifying rib fractures. One study compared ultrasound and plain films (chest x-ray and one oblique rib view) in a group of 50 patients with fractured ribs, and found that plain films detected 8 of 83 fractures and ultrasound diagnosed 6 of 39 fractures. However, ultrasound was able to show fractures of the costochondral junction and rib cartilage (see Fig. 4.199). Westcott et al. stated that a further study of 37 patients using ultrasound had found rib fractures in 40% of patients, all of whom had normal plain film examinations.

MDCT is being used more frequently for trauma assessment, having the added advantage of being able to identify chondral fractures and demonstrate complications such as visceral injury. Nuclear bone scans are especially helpful in the diagnosis of occult rib fractures in athletes (see Fig. 4.200) and are also valuable for the diagnosis of costochondral and chondral fractures (see Figs 4.201 and 4.202).

The imaging guidelines suggest that it is usually unnecessary to perform rib radiography in addition to a chest film, unless the clinical picture suggests that a complication exists. It was noted that certain fractures carry an increased risk of specific complications. Fractures involving the first and second ribs carry a risk of injury to the subclavian and innominate vessels and may constitute a medical emergency. Lower ribs are more likely to be associated with injury to abdominal viscera. The twelfth rib in particular has an association with renal contusion and lacerations. Westcott et al. noted that when three or more ribs were fractured, there was an increased incidence of pneumothorax, haemothorax, abdominal injury and mortality.

Stress fractures of the ribs

Stress fractures of the ribs are uncommon but occasionally present in a specialised sports medicine imaging practice. As elsewhere in the skeleton, bone stress is the result of repetitive muscular activity, and because this occurs in a variety of different sports, an eclectic collection of cases is presented (see Figs 4.203–4.209).

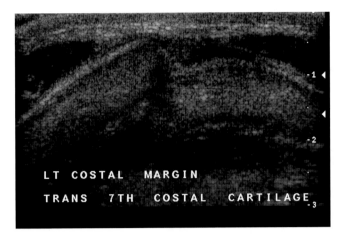

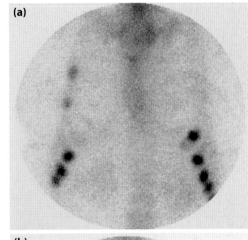

(a)

▲ Fig. 4.199 A fracture of rib cartilage is clearly demonstrated by ultrasound. The fracture occurred in a wrestler at the Sydney 2000 Olympics. The fracture was the result of a bear hug.

▶ Fig. 4.200(a), (b) and (c) Occult rib fractures are extremely common because plain radiography is an inefficient method of imaging fractured ribs. Each of these three cases had normal plain films consisting of a chest x-ray and an oblique rib view and these were considered to be normal. Nuclear bone scans are an excellent method of identifying rib fractures, although often a positive result does not significantly change the patient's management. Even in body contact sports, rib fractures tend to be treated symptomatically, but it may be important to identify the fractures if complications are thought to be likely.

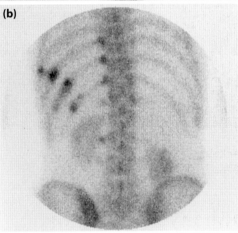

(b)

▶ Fig. 4.201 An injury to a costochondral junction is shown by a nuclear bone scan (arrow) and is best seen in the lateral projection.

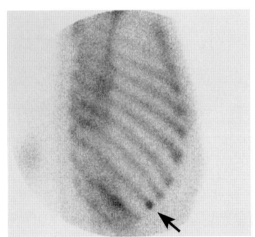

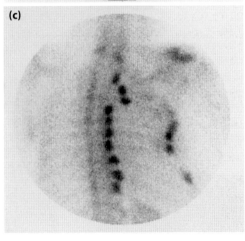

(c)

▶ Fig. 4.202 A tear in a left lower costal cartilage is clearly defined by a nuclear bone scan. Increased uptake of isotope has occurred at the site of the costal cartilage injury (arrow), and the changes can be well localised to the sixth costal cartilage.

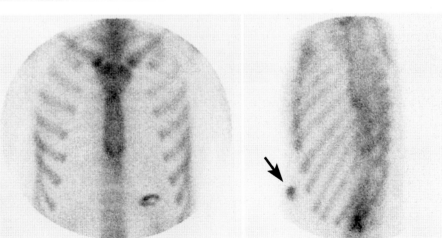

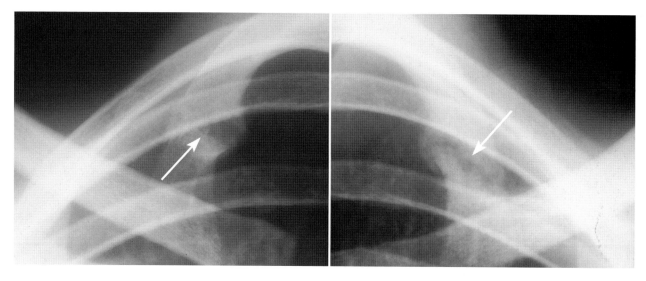

▲ **Fig. 4.203** A principal male dancer complained of pain in both first ribs aggravated by lifting and holding female dancers above his head. Plain films show bilateral stress fractures (arrows). The majority of first rib stress fractures occur across the groove for the subclavian artery, between the attachments of the scalenus anterior and scalenus medius muscles. This is the thinnest segment of the rib and research suggests that stress occurs across the groove with the scalenus anterior and scalene medius producing forces pulling the rib upwards, while the intercostals and serratus anterior pull downwards (Curran and Kelly 1966; Gurtler et al. 1985).

▶ **Fig. 4.204** A nuclear bone scan shows linear uptake of isotope in the left eleventh rib of a cricket fast bowler (arrows). This change is almost certainly indicative of traction stress.

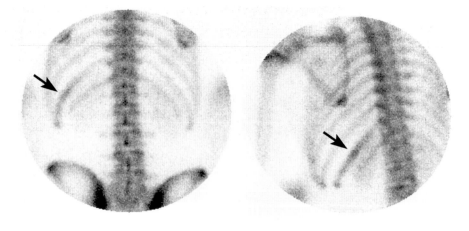

▼ **Fig. 4.205** There is a stress fracture involving the posterior half of the right first rib in a baseball pitcher. This particular type of stress fracture characteristically occurs in baseball pitchers and has been described in the segment of rib posterior to the scalenus medius (Takeshi et al. 2005).

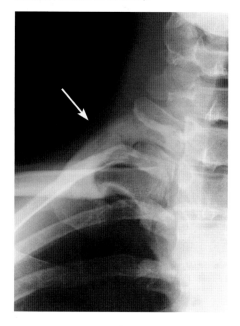

▼ **Fig. 4.206** Bilateral stress fractures of the first ribs have developed in a scuba diver (arrow). These fractures have presumably resulted from the stress of swimming with tanks.

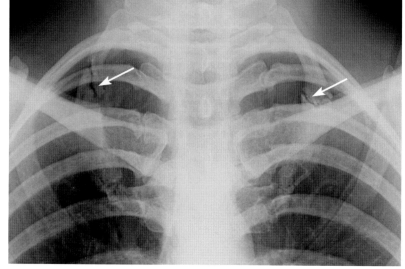

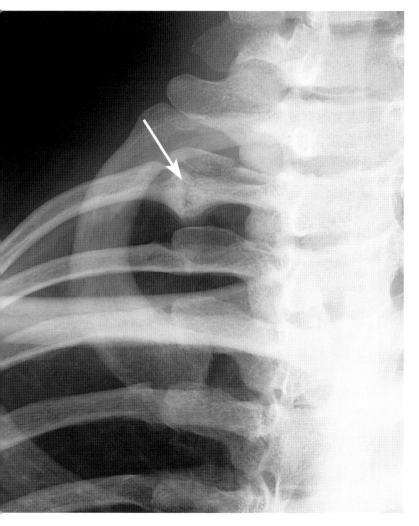

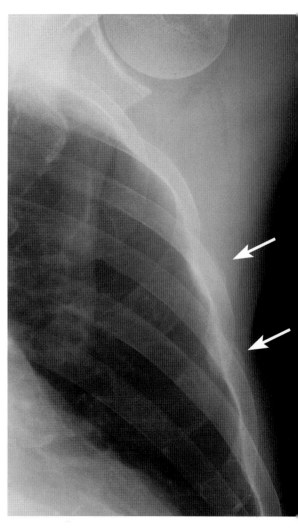

▲ **Fig. 4.207** A stress fracture of the tubercle of the second right rib has developed in a ballerina.

▲ **Fig. 4.209** Stress fractures of the left fourth and fifth ribs have developed in a golfer. This golfer was an overenthusiastic beginner who spent considerable time hitting balls at a golf driving range. Golf produces localised stress: ribs four to six are generally involved posterolaterally or posteriorly and the golfer is usually a beginner. The contralateral side is affected—that is, in a right-handed golfer, the stress fracture is likely to be on the left. Fatigue of the serratus anterior is thought to contribute to the bone stress. Progress plain films commonly confirm the diagnosis when the easily recognised changes of healing appear.

▼ **Fig. 4.208** There is a stress fracture of the anterolateral aspect of the right seventh rib in an elite rower. Stress fractures of the ribs are common in rowers. Approximately 6–12% of rowers develop stress fractures of the ribs (Warden et al. 2002). With rowing, there is a general stress loading of the entire rib cage as a unit, so no specific muscle loading at any particular level is identified.

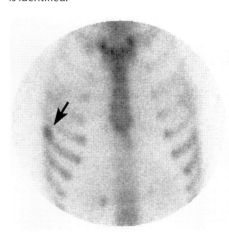

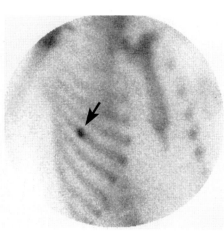

Neural abnormalities

Suprascapular neuropathy

Entrapment of the suprascapular nerve most commonly occurs at either the suprascapular notch or the spinoglenoid notch, due to a space-occupying lesion such as perilabral ganglion cyst (see Fig. 4.210) or to repetitive micro-trauma (Safran 2004). The suprascapular nerve can also be acutely injured by an adjacent scapular fracture, traction associated with an acute GHJ dislocation, a penetrating injury or surgical procedure. Suprascapular nerve palsies have been reported in a range of sports that require repetitive overhead shoulder action, such as baseball, tennis, weightlifting, swimming and volleyball. Entrapment at the suprascapular notch produces weakness, a variable degree of posterolateral shoulder pain, and wasting of both the supraspinatus and infraspinatus muscles. Entrapment at the suprascapular notch is prone to affect athletes who frequently use a throwing action and most often produces painless wasting and weakness of the infraspinatus muscle alone. The imaging test of choice is MRI, which can demonstrate the suprascapular nerve, exclude space-occupying lesions and evaluate muscle wasting.

Axillary nerve injury

Injury to the axillary nerve is usually due to direct contusion secondary to acute blunt trauma, traction associated with an acute GHJ dislocation or quadrilateral space syndrome (Safran 2004). Acute injuries can often be asymptomatic but may produce weakness ranging from early fatigue with heavy lifting and overhead activity through to obvious loss of abduction strength or inability to raise the arm. Quadrilateral space syndrome produces poorly localised posterolateral shoulder pain of dull aching or burning quality. The symptoms are of insidious onset and are usually exacerbated by activity and may have associated overhead weakness. This syndrome is most commonly seen in athletes who throw overhead due to repetitive micro-trauma, but can also relate to space-occupying lesions such as ganglion cysts (see Fig. 4.211) or follow direct trauma such as a fall onto the outstretched hand. The most frequently identified predisposing factor is the presence of fibrous bands in the quadrilateral space. On MRI, the deltoid and teres minor muscles may show acute or subacute denervation changes (see Fig. 4.212) and subsequent denervation atrophy (see Fig. 4.213).

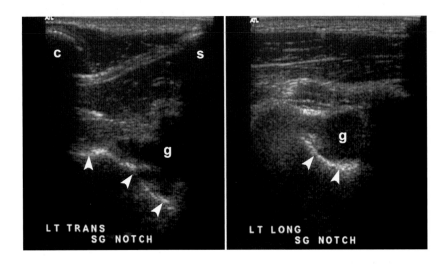

◀**Fig. 4.210(a)** A spinoglenoid notch ganglion is demonstrated by ultrasound. Transverse and longitudinal ultrasound images have been obtained with the transducer placed superiorly over the region of the spinoglenoid notch. These images demonstrate a lobulated anechoic ganglion cyst (g) abutting the posterosuperior surface of the scapular neck (arrowheads). This finding indirectly implies the presence of an adjacent glenoid labral tear. Secondary entrapment of the suprascapular nerve is likely, and decompression of the cyst is feasible using needle aspiration under real-time ultrasound control. Clavicle = c. Scapular spine = s.

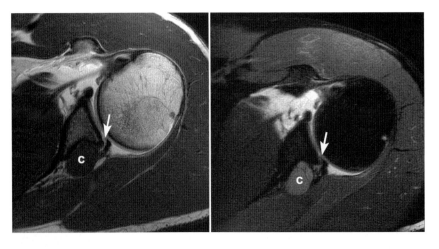

◀**(b)** A posterior glenoid labral tear is demonstrated together with an associated perilabral cyst. Axial T1 and fat-suppressed T1-weighted MR arthrogram images show a full-thickness tear traversing the posterior glenolabral junction (arrow) and extending into a septate perilabral cyst (c) abutting the posterior surface of the scapular neck. Gadolinium has not entered the cyst. The location of the cyst would potentially cause suprascapular nerve entrapment. However, the infraspinatus muscle in this case shows no apparent denervation effect.

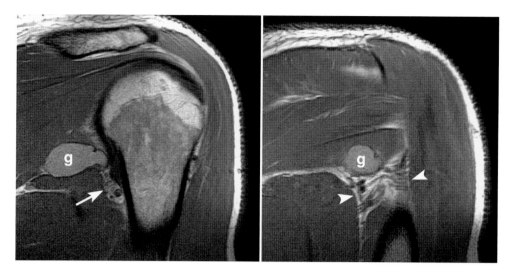

▲ **Fig. 4.211** MRI shows a quadrilateral space ganglion. Coronal and sagittal PD-weighted images demonstrate a lobulated ganglion cyst (g) at the superior margin of the quadrilateral space (arrowheads) adjacent to the contained axillary nerve and posterior circumflex humeral vessels (arrow). In this case the teres minor muscle shows no evidence of denervation effect to suggest axillary nerve entrapment.

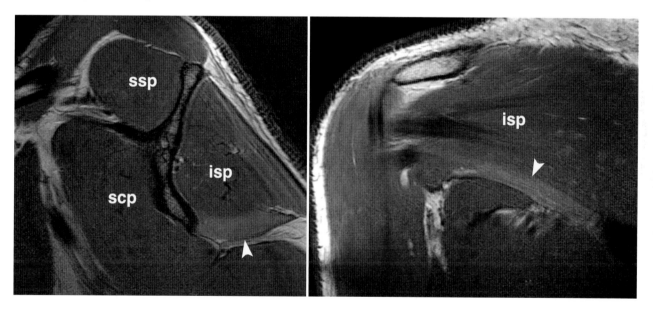

▲ **Fig. 4.212** A case of subacute quadrilateral space syndrome is demonstrated by MRI. Sagittal and coronal PD-weighted MR images show diffuse teres minor muscle hyperintensity (arrowheads), without underlying structural defect or surrounding oedema. This appearance is consistent with subacute denervation secondary to axillary nerve injury. Supraspinatus muscle = ssp. Infraspinatus muscle = isp. Subscapularis muscle = scp.

▼ **Fig. 4.213** Chronic axillary nerve injury. Sagittal and coronal PD-weighted MR images demonstrate selective fatty infiltration of the teres minor muscle (arrowheads) indicative of chronic denervation atrophy. Infraspinatus muscle = isp.

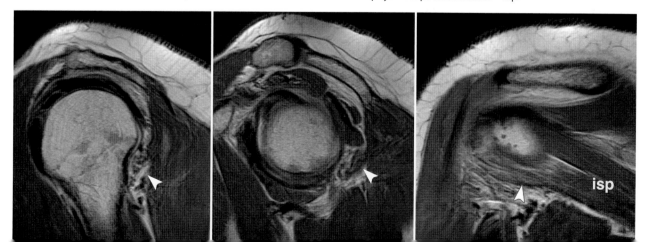

Vascular abnormalities

'Effort' thrombosis is a form of axillary and subclavian vein thrombosis due to thoracic outlet compression. It occurs infrequently but has been reported in sports such as swimming (Vogel and Jensen 1985) and wrestling (Medler and McQueen 1993).

A false aneurysm of the axillary artery, or one of its branches, may occur due to repetitive trauma of the humeral head against the axillary artery in the throwing action of baseball pitchers (Kee et al. 1995). Intermittent episodes of embolic ischaemia can then affect the hand or fingertips with pain, swelling and discolouration.

References

Anderson IF. *An Atlas of Radiography for Sports Injury*, McGraw-Hill, Sydney, 2000.

Andrews JR, Carson WG Jr, McLeod WD. 'Glenoid labrum tears related to the long head of the biceps.' *Am J Sports Med* 1985, 13(5): 337–41.

Bencardino JT, Beltran J, Rosenberg ZS, Rokito A, Schmahmann S, Mota J, Mellado JM, Zuckerman J, Cuomo F, Rose D. 'Superior labrum anterior-posterior lesions: diagnosis with MR arthrography of the shoulder.' *Radiology* 2000, 214(1): 267–71.

Bennett GE. 'Shoulder and elbow lesions of the professional baseball pitcher.' *JAMA* 1941, 117: 510–14.

Bennett WF. 'Subscapularis, medial and lateral head coracohumeral ligament insertion anatomy. Arthroscopic appearance and incidence of "hidden" rotator interval lesions.' *Arthroscopy* 2001, 17(2): 173–80.

Bergfeld JA. *Acromioclavicular Complex*, Mosby, St Louis, 1990.

Bigliani LU, Levine WN. 'Subacromial impingement syndrome.' *J Bone Joint Surg (Am)* 1997, 79(12): 1854–68.

Bigliani L, Morrison D, April E. 'The morphology of the acromion and its relationship to rotator cuff tears.' *Orthopaedic Transactions* 1991, 10: 228.

Bonutti PM, Norfray JF, Friedman RJ, Genez BM. 'Kinematic MRI of the shoulder.' *J Comput Assist Tomogr* 1993, 17(4): 666–9.

Boyd HB, Sisk TD. 'Recurrent posterior dislocation of the shoulder.' *J Bone Joint Surg (Am)* 1972, 54(4): 779–86.

Branch T, Partin C, Chamberland P, Emeterio E, Sabetelle M. 'Spontaneous fractures of the humerus during pitching. A series of 12 cases.' *Am J Sports Med* 1992, 20(4): 468–70.

Brower AC, Neff JR, Tillema DA. 'An unusual scapular stress fracture.' *Am J Roentgenol* 1977, 129(3): 519–20.

Bunker TD, Anthony PP. 'The pathology of frozen shoulder. A Dupuytren-like disease.' *J Bone Joint Surg (Br)* 1995, 77(5): 677–83.

Burkhart SS, Morgan CD, Kibler WB. 'Shoulder injuries in overhead athletes. The "dead arm" revisited.' *Clin Sports Med* 2000, 19(1): 125–58.

Cahill BR. 'Osteolysis of the distal clavicle, a review.' *Sports Med* 1992, 13: 214–22.

Carmichael KD, Longo A, Lick S, Swischuk L et al. 'Posterior sternoclavicular epiphyseal fracture-dislocation with delayed diagnosis.' *Skeletal Radiol* 2006, 35: 608–12.

Clark JM, Harryman DT II. 'Tendons, ligaments, and capsule of the rotator cuff. Gross and microscopic anatomy.' *J Bone Joint Surg (Am)* 1992, 74(5): 713–25.

Codman EA. *The Shoulder. Rupture of the Supraspinatus Tendon and Other Lesions in or About the Subacromial Bursa*, Thomas Todd Company, Boston, 1934.

Cone RO, Danzig L, Resnick D, Goldman AB. 'The bicipital groove: radiographic, anatomic, and pathologic study.' *Am J Roentgenol* 1983, 141(4): 781–8.

Connell DA, Potter HG, Wickiewicz TL, Altchek DW, Warren RF. 'Noncontrast magnetic resonance imaging of superior labral lesions. 102 cases confirmed at arthroscopic surgery.' *Am J Sports Med* 1999, 27(2): 208–13.

Connolly JF. 'Inferior shoulder subluxation associated with a surgical neck fracture of the humerus.' *Nebr Med J* 1982, 67(1): 11–12.

Cook FF, Tibone RA. 'The Mumford procedure in athletes.' *Am J Sports Med* 1988, 16: 97–100.

Craig EV. 'The geyser sign and torn rotator cuff: clinical significance and pathomechanics.' *Clin Orthop Relat Res* 1984, 191: 213–15.

Curran JP, Kelly DA. 'Stress fracture of the first rib.' *Am J Orthop* 1966, 8: 16–18.

Cvitanic O, Tirman PF, Feller JF, Bost FW, Minter J, Carroll KW. 'Using abduction and external rotation of the shoulder to increase the sensitivity of MR arthrography in revealing tears of the anterior glenoid labrum.' *Am J Roentgenol* 1997, 169(3): 837–44.

Dahan TH, Roy A, Fortin L, Dahan B. 'Adhesive capsulitis.' *eMedicine*, 2005 (www.emedicine.com/pmr/topic8.htm).

De Maeseneer M, Van Roy F, Lenchik L, Shahabpour M, et al. 'CT and MR arthrography of the normal and pathological anterosuperior labrum and labral-bicipital complex.' *Radiographics* 2000, 20: S67–S81.

Emig EW, Schweitzer ME, Karasick D, Lubowitz J. 'Adhesive capsulitis of the shoulder: MR diagnosis.' *Am J Roentgenol* 1995, 164(6): 1457–9.

Farin PU, Jaroma H, Harju A, Soimakallio S. 'Shoulder impingement syndrome: sonographic evaluation.' *Radiology* 1990, 176(3): 845–9.

Ferrari JD, Ferrari DA, Coumas J, Pappas AM. 'Posterior ossification of the shoulder: the Bennett lesion. Etiology, diagnosis, and treatment.' *Am J Sports Med* 1994, 22(2): 171–5, discussion pp. 175–6.

Ferrick MR. 'Coracoid impingement. A case report and review of the literature.' *Am J Sports Med* 2000, 28(1): 117–19.

Friedman RJ, Bonutti PM, Genez B. 'Cine magnetic resonance imaging of the subcoracoid region.' *Orthopedics* 1998, 21(5): 545–8.

Galatz LM, Barrett S, Williams GR et al. 'Rehabilitation in throwing and overhead sports.' *Sports Med and Arthro Rev* 2001, 9: 44–51.

Garth WP Jr, Slappey CE, Ochs CW. 'Roentgenographic demonstration of instability of the shoulder: the apical oblique projection. A technical note.' *J Bone Joint Surg (Am)* 1984, 66(9): 1450–3.

Gerber C, Terrier F, Ganz R. 'The role of the coracoid process in the chronic impingement syndrome.' *J Bone Joint Surg (Br)* 1985, 67(5): 703–8.

Goutallier D, Postel JM, Bernageau J, Lavau L, Voisin MC. 'Fatty muscle degeneration in cuff ruptures. Pre- and postoperative evaluation by CT scan.' *Clin Orthop Relat Res* 1994, 304: 78–83.

Gurtler R, Pavlov H, Torg JS. 'Stress fracture of the ipsilateral first rib in a pitcher.' *Am J Sports Med* 1985, 13: 277–9.

Hall RJ, Calvert PT. 'Stress fracture of the acromion: an unusual mechanism and review of the literature.' *J Bone Joint Surg (Br)* 1995, 77(1): 153–4.

Hannafin JA. 'Arthroscopic findings and treatment of the frozen shoulder.' San Diego Shoulder Arthroscopy Library, 1999 (www.shoulder.com/hannafin_frozenshoulder.pdf).

Helms CA, Martinez S, Speer KP. 'Acute brachial neuritis (Parsonage-Turner syndrome): MR imaging appearance—report of three cases.' *Radiology* 1998, 207(1): 255–9.

Horwitz BR, DiStefano V. 'Stress fracture of the humerus in a weight lifter.' *Orthopedics* 1995, 18(2): 185–7.

Howell SM, Galinat BJ, Renzi AJ, Marone PJ. 'Normal and abnormal mechanics of the glenohumeral joint in the horizontal plane.' *J Bone Joint Surg (Am)* 1988, 70(2): 227–32.

Ireland ML, Andrews JR. 'Shoulder and elbow injuries in the young athlete.' *Clin Sports Med* 1988, 8: 473–94.

Kee ST, Dake MD, Wolfe-Johnson B, Semba CP, Zarins CK, Olcott CT. 'Ischemia of the throwing hand in major league baseball pitchers: embolic occlusion from aneurysms of axillary artery branches.' *J Vasc Interv Radiol* 1995, 6(6): 979–82.

Kilcoyne RF, Reddy PK, Lyons F, Rockwood CA Jr. 'Optimal plain film imaging of the shoulder impingement syndrome.' *Am J Roentgenol* 1989, 153(4): 795–7.

Kjellin I, Ho CP, Cervilla V, Haghighi P, Kerr R, Vangness CT, Friedman RJ, Trudell D, Resnick D. 'Alterations in the supraspinatus tendon at MR imaging: correlation with histopathologic findings in cadavers.' *Radiology* 1991, 181(3): 837–41.

Kohler R, Trilland JM. 'Fracture and fracture separation of the proximal humerus in children: report of 136 cases.' *J Pedriatr Orthop* 1983, 3: 326–32.

Laskin RS, Schreiber S. 'Inferior subluxation of the humeral head: the drooping shoulder.' *Radiology* 1971, 98(3): 585–6.

Levine AH, Pais MJ, Schwartz EE. 'Posttraumatic osteolysis of the distal clavicle with emphasis on early radiologic changes.' *Am J Roentgenol* 1976, 127(5): 781–4.

Levine WN, Flatow EL. 'The pathophysiology of shoulder instability.' *Am J Sports Med* 2000, 28(6): 910–17.

MacGillivray JD, Fealy S, Potter HG, O'Brien SJ. 'Multiplanar analysis of acromion morphology.' *Am J Sports Med* 1998, 836–40.

Matava MJ, Purcell DB, Rudzki JR. 'Partial-thickness rotator cuff tears.' *Am J Sports Med* 2005, 33(9): 1405–17.

Matsen F, Thomas S, Rockwood C Jr. *Anterior Glenohumeral Instability*, WB Saunders, Philadelphia, 1990.

Medler RG, McQueen DA. 'Effort thrombosis in a young wrestler. A case report.' *J Bone Joint Surg (Am)* 1993, 75(7): 1071–3.

Mengiardi B, Pfirrmann CW, Gerber C, Hodler J, Zanetti M. 'Frozen shoulder: MR arthrographic findings.' *Radiology* 2004, 233(2): 486–92.

Miller MD, Wirth MA, Rockwood CA Jr. 'Thawing the frozen shoulder: the "patient" patient.' *Orthopedics* 1996, 19(10): 849–53.

Morgan CD, Burkhart SS, Palmeri M, Gillespie M. 'Type II SLAP lesions: three subtypes and their relationships to superior instability and rotator cuff tears.' *Arthroscopy* 1998, 14(6): 553–65.

Mosely H, Overgaard B. 'The anterior capsular mechanism in recurrent anterior dislocation of the shoulder.' *J Bone Joint Surg (Br)* 1962, 44(B): 913–27.

Nam EK, Snyder SJ. 'The diagnosis and treatment of superior labrum, anterior and posterior (SLAP) lesions.' *Am J Sports Med* 2003, 31(5): 798–810.

Neer CS II. 'Impingement lesions.' *Clin Orthop Relat Res* 1983, 173: 70–7.

Neumann CH, Petersen SA, Jahnke AH. 'MR imaging of the labral-capsular complex: normal variations.' *Am J Roentgenol* 1991, 157(5): 1015–21.

Neviaser RJ, Neviaser TJ, Neviaser JS. 'Concurrent rupture of the rotator cuff and anterior dislocation of the shoulder in the older patient.' *J Bone Joint Surg (Am)* 1988, 70(9): 1308–11.

Neviaser RJ, Neviaser TJ, Neviaser JS. 'Anterior dislocation of the shoulder and rotator cuff rupture.' *Clin Orthop Relat Res* 1993, 291: 103–6.

Nordqvist A, Petersson C. 'The incidence of fractures of the clavicle.' *Clin Orthop* 1994, 300: 127–32.

O'Brien SJ, Schwartz RS, Warren RF, Torzilli PA. 'Capsular restraints to anterior-posterior motion of the abducted shoulder: a biomechanical study.' *J Shoulder Elbow Surg* 1995, 4(4): 298–308.

Ozaki J, Nakagawa Y, Sakurai G, Tamai S. 'Recalcitrant chronic adhesive capsulitis of the shoulder. Role of contracture of the coracohumeral ligament and rotator interval in pathogenesis and treatment.' *J Bone Joint Surg (Am)* 1989, 71(10): 1511–5.

Patte D. 'The subcoracoid impingement.' *Clin Orthop Relat Res* 1990, 254: 55–9.

Read JW, Perko M. 'Shoulder ultrasound: diagnostic accuracy for impingement syndrome, rotator cuff tear, and biceps tendon pathology.' *J Shoulder Elbow Surg* 1998, 7(3): 264–71.

Richards R, Sartoris D, Pathria M, Resnick D. 'Hill-Sachs lesion and normal humeral groove: MR imaging features allowing their differentiation.' *Radiology* 1994, 190: 665–8.

Richardson A. *Overview of Soft Tissue Injuries of the Shoulder*, Mosby, St Louis, 1990.

Rockwood C. *Subluxations and Dislocations About the Shoulder*. J.B. Lippincott, Philadelphia, 1984.

Rodosky M, Jari R. 'Acromioclavicular and sternoclavicular injuries in athletes.' *Curr Opinion in Orthop* 2001, 12(4): 325–30.

Rowe CR. 'Prognosis in dislocations of the shoulder.' *J Bone Joint Surg (Am)* 1956, 38A(5): 957–77.

Rowe CR, Sakellarides HT. 'Factors related to recurrences of anterior dislocations of the shoulder.' *Clin Orthop* 1961, 20: 40–8.

Safran MR. 'Nerve injury about the shoulder in athletes, Part 1.' *Am J Sports Med* 2004, 32(3): 803–19.

Sanders TG, Morrison WB, Miller MD. 'Imaging techniques for the evaluation of glenohumeral instability.' *Am J Sports Med* 2000, 28(3): 414–34.

Sandrock AR. 'Another sports fatigue fracture. Stress fracture of the coracoid process of the scapula.' *Radiology* 1975, 117(2): 274.

Savoie FH III, Field LD, Atchinson S. 'Anterior superior instability with rotator cuff tearing: SLAC lesion.' *Orthop Clin North Am* 2001, 32(3): 457–61.

Scavenius M, Iversen BF, Sturup J. 'Resection of the lateral end of the clavicle following osteolysis, with emphasis on non-traumatic osteolysis of the acromial end of the clavicle in athletes.' *Injury* 1987, 18(4): 261–3.

Schils JP, Freed HA, Richmond BJ, Piraino DW, Bergfeld JA, Belhobek GH. 'Stress fracture of the acromion.' *Am J Roentgenol* 1990, 155(5): 1140–1.

Seibold CJ, Mallisee TA, Erickson SJ, Boynton MD, Raasch WG, Timins ME. 'Rotator cuff: evaluation with US and MR imaging.' *Radiographics* 1999, 19(3): 685–705.

Singson RD, Feldman F, Bigliani L. 'CT arthrographic patterns in recurrent glenohumeral instability.' *Am J Roentgenol* 1987, 149(4): 749–53.

Smith DK, Chopp TM, Aufdemorte TB et al. 'Sublabral recess of the superior glenoid labrum: study of cadavers with conventional nonenhanced MR imaging, MR arthrography, anatomic dissection, and limited histologic examination.' *Radiology* 1996, 201: 251–6.

Snyder SJ, Karzel RP, Del Pizzo W, Ferkel RD, Friedman MJ. 'SLAP lesions of the shoulder.' *Arthroscopy* 1990, 6(4): 274–9.

Takeshi S, Yasunobu K et al. 'First rib fracture in a sidearm baseball pitcher: a case report.' *J Sports Science and Med* 2005, 4: 201–7.

Tirman PF, Bost FW, Steinbach LS, Mall JC, Peterfy CG, Sampson TG, Sheehan WE, Forbes JR, Genant HK. 'MR arthrographic depiction of tears of the rotator cuff: benefit of abduction and external rotation of the arm.' *Radiology* 1994, 192(3): 851–6.

Tirman PF, Feller JF, Janzen DL, Peterfy CG, Bergman AG. 'Association of glenoid labral cysts with labral tears and glenohumeral instability: radiologic findings and clinical significance.' *Radiology* 1994, 190(3): 653–8.

Tuite M. 'Shoulder, rotator cuff injury (MRI).' *eMedicine*, 2004 (www.emedicine.com/radio/topic894.htm).

Turkel SJ, Panio MW, Marshall JL, Girgis FG. 'Stabilizing mechanisms preventing anterior dislocation of the glenohumeral joint.' *J Bone Joint Surg (Am)* 1981, 63(8): 1208–17.

Veluvolu P, Kohn HS, Guten GN, Donahue PM, Isitman AT, Whalen JP, Collier BD. 'Unusual stress fracture of the scapula in a jogger.' *Clin Nucl Med* 1988, 13(7): 531–2.

Vogel CM, Jensen JE. '"Effort" thrombosis of the subclavian vein in a competitive swimmer.' *Am J Sports Med* 1985, 13(4): 269–72.

Walch G, Liotard JP, Boileau P, Noel E. 'Postero-superior glenoid impingement. Another shoulder impingement.' *Rev Chir Orthop Reparatrice Appar Mot* 1991, 77(8): 571–4.

Waninger KN. 'Stress fracture of the clavicle in a collegiate diver.' *Clin J Sport Med* 1997, 7(1): 66–8.

Ward WG, Bergfeld JA, Carson WG Jr. 'Stress fracture of the base of the acromial process.' *Am J Sports Med* 1994, 22(1): 146–7.

Warden SJ, Gutschlag FR et al. 'Aetiology of rib stress fractures in rowers.' *Sports Med* 2002, 32: 819–36.

Westcott J et al. 'Rib fractures. American College of Radiology. ACR Appropriateness Criteria.' *Radiology* 2000, 215(Suppl): 637–9.

Wettstein M, Borens O, Garofalo R et al. 'Anterior subluxation after reduction of a posterior traumatic sterno–clavicular dislocation: a case report and review of the literature.' *Knee Surg Sports Traumatol Arthrosc* 2004, 12: 453–6.

Wick M, Muller EJ et al. 'Midshaft fractures of the clavicle, with a shortening greater than 2 cms predispose to non-union.' *Arch Orthop Trauma Surg* 2001, 121(4) 207–11.

Williams MM, Snyder SJ, Buford D Jr. 'The Buford complex—the "cord-like" middle glenohumeral ligament and absent anterosuperior labrum complex: a normal anatomic capsulolabral variant.' *Arthroscopy* 1994, 10(3): 241–7.

Woodward AH. 'Calcifying tendonitis.' *eMedicine* Specialties (Orthopaedic Surgery) 2004 (www.emedicine.com/orthoped/topic379.htm).

Yu JS, Greenway G, Resnick D. 'Osteochondral defect of the glenoid fossa: cross-sectional imaging features.' *Radiology* 1998, 206(1): 35–40.

Zvijac JE, Schurhoff MR, Hechtman KS, Uribe JW. 'Pectoralis major tears: correlation of magnetic resonance imaging and treatment strategies.' *Am J Sports Med* 2006, 34(2): 289–94.

Image acknowledgments

The authors wish to thank the following colleagues who kindly offered images for inclusion in this chapter:

- Dr Bill Breidahl (Figures 4.63, 4.65, 4.66, 4.85(a), 4.87, 4.104, 4.05, 4.144 and 4.152(b))
- Dr Phil Lucas (Figures 4.85(b) and (c), 4.107, 4.124, 4.126, 4.132, 4.169 and 4.210)
- Dr James Linklater (Figures 4.79, 4.80, 4.81, 4.84, 4.99, 4.103, 4.110, 4.131, 4,136, 4.137, 4.139, 4.141(b), 4.159, 4.187, 4,188(b) and 4.213)
- Dr Peter Briscoe (Figure 4.188(a))
- Raouli Risti at Gosford Hospital CT (Figures 4.54, 4.193, 4.197 and 4.198)
- Dr Richard de Villiers (Figure 4.169)
- Dr Robert Cooper and Dr Stephen Allwright (Figures 4.55, 4.56, 4.57, 4.58, 4.59, 4.60, 4.170, 4.201, 4.202, 4.204 and 4.209).

These images have significantly added to the quality of the chapter.

5

The pelvis, hip and thigh
Jock Anderson and John Read

Every sporting activity depends upon normal function of the pelvis and hips. Whether the athlete is walking, throwing, high jumping, rowing or running, transfer of power is required through the pelvis and hips from the spine to the legs or from the legs to the spine. In addition, as the site of attachment of many large muscles, the pelvis and hips combine to function as the body's powerhouse and as such are subjected to considerable endurance stresses and explosive forces. Sporting injuries involving the pelvis and hips are commonly due to overuse and may involve either bone or soft tissues, or both.

Management of these injuries must begin with an accurate diagnosis. This is dependent upon an understanding of injury biomechanics, correct interpretation of clinical findings and the appropriate use of the currently available diagnostic imaging techniques. It is wise to remember that more than one injury is often present, either occurring at the same time or developing due to a change in stresses and biomechanics resulting from an initial injury. As a consequence, if the presentation is complex or the response to management is unexpectedly poor, a search for other injuries is worthwhile (see Fig. 5.1).

Radiographic anatomy of the hip

Due to its anatomical structure, the hip joint offers both stability and mobility. This classic ball-and-socket joint comprises the acetabulum (providing the socket) and the spherical femoral head (the ball). The normal joint has perfectly congruent surfaces which, together with the acetabular labrum, contribute to stability and mobility. Radiological examination of the hip requires systematic identification and assessment of a number of structures (see Fig. 5.2).

The acetabulum is directed anterolaterally and inferiorly, requiring the femoral neck and head to be angled in an anteromedial and cranial direction. The degree of inferior tilt of the acetabulum is an important factor when considering whether there is adequate acetabular coverage of the femoral head in the weightbearing area. The method of determining whether this tilt is adequate is discussed later in the section on hip dysplasia. The acetabular labrum is a rim of fibrocartilage that is triangular in

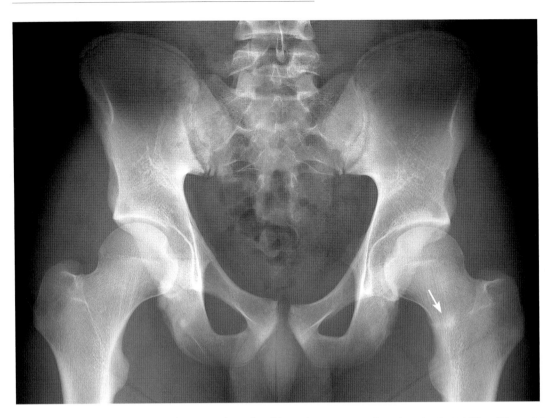

▲ **Fig. 5.1** This young footballer has a number of problems that appear to be related to instability of the pelvis:
- There is evidence of an old injury, with rotation of the right hemi-pelvis, disrupting the pubic symphysis and the right sacroiliac joint. This had resulted from a high-level impact.
- There is also subtle lateral sloping of the acetabular roof on both sides, more marked on the right. These changes may indicate mild hip dysplasia (discussed later).
- A stress fracture of the left femoral neck (arrow) has almost certainly developed from the repetitive stress of training together with the altered biomechanics from either or both of the above two conditions.
- Demineralisation at the left hamstring origin indicates a stress reaction, with developing ischial apophysitis.

▶ **Fig. 5.2** For assessment of the hip, various structures should be examined.
- On the acetabular side of the joint, these structures include (a) the acetabular roof ('eyebrow'), (b) the medial wall of the acetabulum, (c) the 'teardrop', (d) the acetabular notch and (e) the acetabular fossa.
- The relationship between the femoral head and neck also requires examination. A line drawn along the centre of the femoral neck should pass through the centre of the femoral head (f). The radius of the head from the centre to the superior border should be equal to the inferior radius. As will be discussed later, any change in the normal head/neck relationship may predispose to the development of degenerative changes and impingement. The femoral head should be a perfect sphere, apart from a small indentation, the fovea centralis (g), which is the site of attachment of the ligamentum teres.
- Finally, if an AP pelvis image is available, the joint spaces of both hips should be examined and compared for evidence of articular cartilage wear. If only the symptomatic hip has been imaged, the joint space is examined for uniformity (h).

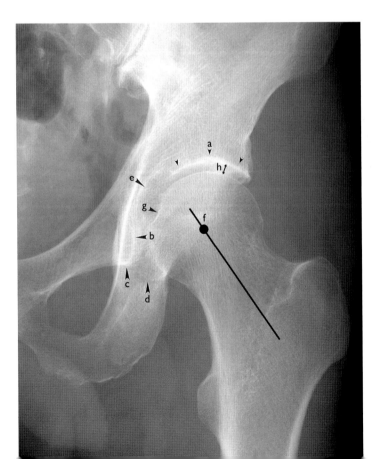

cross-section and attaches adjacent to the peripheral margin of the acetabulum. The labrum increases hip joint stability by increasing the surface area of the acetabulum by 22% and the acetabular volume by 33% (Seldes et al. 2001). Evidence suggests that an intact labrum may also enhance stability by providing a negative intra-articular pressure within the hip joint (Takechi et al. 1986).

The acetabular notch is a deficiency in the bony rim of the acetabulum inferiorly. The transverse acetabular ligament blends with the inferior continuation of the labrum and traverses this notch. The acetabular fossa is a nonarticular depression at the base of the acetabulum that contains a fat pad known as the 'pulvinar'. This fibrofatty tissue contains vessels and nerves from the posterior branch of the obturator nerve. The acetabular articular cartilage surrounds the acetabular fossa in a horseshoe configuration, with the opening of the horseshoe spanning the acetabular notch.

The weightbearing area of the acetabular roof can be identified on plain films as a dense, thickened cortical line known as the 'eyebrow'. It is important to note the length, shape and orientation of this weightbearing area, as these features may provide evidence of hip joint dysplasia (see Fig. 5.3). The medial and lateral ends of the eyebrow should be at the same horizontal level. This is discussed in more detail at a later stage.

▼ **Fig. 5.3** The weightbearing area of the acetabular roof is sclerotic and can be readily identified. This linear sclerosis is known as the 'eyebrow'. To be normal, the 'eyebrow' should curve upwards with both of its ends at the same horizontal level. Departure from this may indicate hip dysplasia. The shape and length of the weightbearing area should be noted.

(a) This is the appearance of a normal 'eyebrow'.

(b) A short roof should be noted, as this may be associated with insufficient coverage of the femoral head, (Type II hip dysplasia). The method for measuring this anomaly is discussed on page 368.

(c) Minor to moderate dysplastic changes are present, with sloping of the acetabular roof.

(d) Marked sloping of the acetabular roof is present, indicating prominent hip dysplasia. There is also reduced coverage of the femoral head.

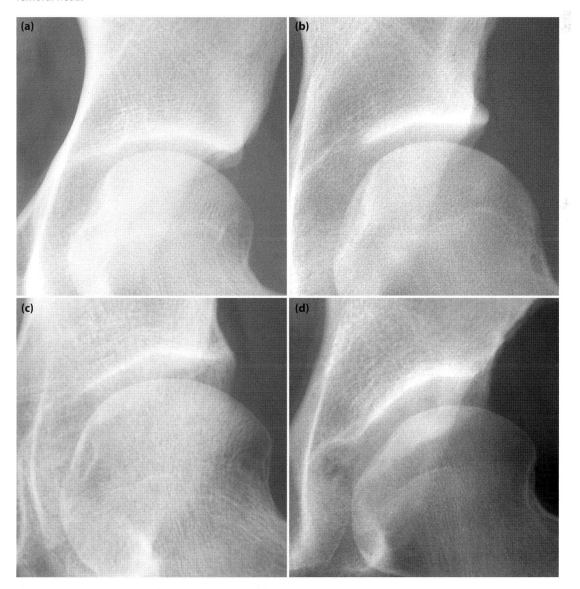

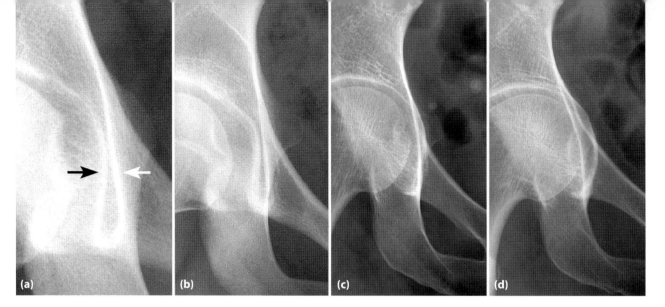

▲ **Fig. 5.4** The 'teardrop' is formed by the junction of the medial wall of the acetabulum and the quadrilateral plate of the ilium. A rounded configuration results and this structure is used as a constant landmark to help assess changes in position of the femoral head. These examples of 'teardrops' demonstrate varying appearances.

(a) The 'teardrop' is formed by the junction of the medial wall of the acetabulum (black arrow) and the quadrilateral plate (white arrow).

(b) This is an example of a normal 'teardrop'. The medial wall of the acetabulum lies on the lateral side of the quadrilateral plate.

(c) If the medial wall of the acetabulum crosses the quadrilateral plate of the ilium by more than 2 mm, there is abnormal protrusion of the acetabulum centrally into the pelvis. This condition is called protrusio acetabulae deformity. In this case, there is a minor degree of protrusio acetabular deformity.

(d) This protrusio acetabulae deformity is more marked.

The medial wall of the acetabulum also requires careful inspection. There are two cortical lines running side-by-side on the medial aspect of the acetabulum. One is the quadrilateral plate of the ischium, which is the lateral bony wall of the true pelvis. The other is the medial wall of the acetabulum, normally positioned to the lateral side of the quadrilateral plate. These lines should not cross. Protrusio acetabulae deformity is present when the medial wall of the acetabulum is projected medial to the quadrilateral plate by more than 2 mm, indicating protrusion of the acetabular cavity into the pelvis. The quadrilateral plate and the medial wall of the acetabulum join inferiorly, forming a cortical outline known as the 'teardrop' (see Fig. 5.4). This is a constant structure and is a helpful landmark that can be used as a reference point

in the measurement of acetabular angles and femoral head migration. Anterolateral migration of the femoral head is present when the distance from the teardrop to the femoral head is increased by comparison with the normal side.

The femoral head is normally spherical and is completely covered by hyaline cartilage except for the fovea centralis (see below). The hyaline cartilage is thickest over the supero-medial aspect and extends slightly posteriorly. This reflects the primary contact point and load-bearing area of the joint. The general contour of the femoral head and neck should be assessed and the head/neck relationship noted. The epicentre of the femoral head should be coaxial with a line drawn along the centre of the femoral neck. The ligamentum teres runs from the acetabular fossa to the fovea centralis, a localised depression

▼ **Fig. 5.5(a)** This coronal PD-weighted MR image shows a normal hypointense ligamentum teres (arrowhead). **(b)** The ligamentum teres is ruptured and there is an associated effusion, demonstrated on a coronal PD-weighted image with fat saturation.

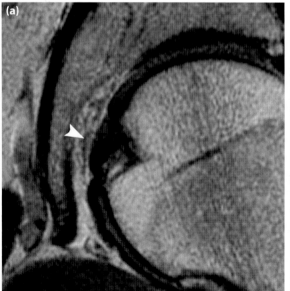
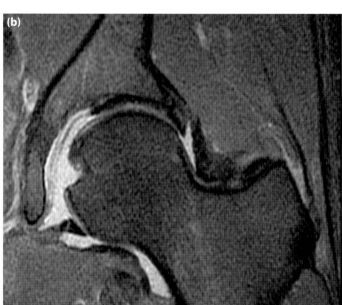

in the femoral head. The function of the ligamentum teres is uncertain, although it is suspected that the ligamentum teres contributes to hip stability as rupture of this ligament causes pain and symptoms of hip instability (see Fig. 5.5).

In the axial plane, the femoral neck is tilted anteriorly from the transcondylar plane of the femur, creating an angle

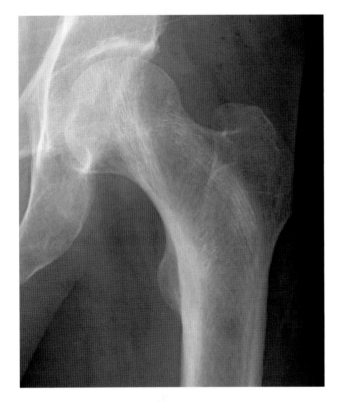

▲ **Fig. 5.6** Because of the physiological forces transmitted through the femoral neck and the trochanteric region, special trabeculae develop in the trochanteric area and femoral neck in orientations best suited to withstand stresses. These trabeculae are best appreciated in an osteopaenic hip.

of 'anteversion'. This angle is about 14° in the adult. The method of measuring this angle is discussed in the section on femoral anteversion on page 372. There is also a twist in the trochanteric region of the femur as the neck joins the shaft. The orientation of the greater trochanter is superolateral and the lesser trochanter points in a posteromedial direction. This asymmetry influences the mechanics of the muscles that insert into the trochanters.

In addition, in the coronal plane, there is an angle of inclination between the femoral neck and the shaft. This is known as the femoral angle and it is normally 125° plus or minus 5° in the adult hip. In the newborn this angle can be as great as 150°. This produces offset loading that creates considerable stress across the femoral neck with the transfer of forces through the hip into the lower limb. It is not surprising that the femoral neck is prone to stress fractures.

During athletic activities, the intertrochanteric and subtrochanteric regions of the femur are subjected to considerable tensile and compressive forces. Trabecular patterns develop in the trochanteric region and the femoral neck in response to stress of these deforming forces (see Fig. 5.6). As a consequence, orientation of these trabeculae indicates the pathway of the stresses affecting the proximal femur.

The hip is enclosed by a strong fibrous capsule, which contributes to hip stability. The capsule attaches to the bony rim of the acetabulum about 6–8 mm from the labrum (Huffman and Safran 2002). Anteriorly, the distal capsule attaches to the intertrochanteric line and greater trochanter, whereas posteriorly the capsule attaches proximal to the intertrochanteric line. Most fibres run in the direction of the femoral neck, although a subset of fibres, the zona orbicularis, encircles the femoral neck reinforcing the labrum. There are three extracapsular ligaments connecting the pelvis and the femur, reinforcing the capsule (see Fig. 5.7):

- The iliofemoral ligament (ligament of Bigelow) is the strongest of the three, extending from the anterior inferior

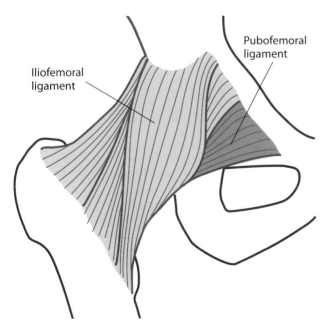

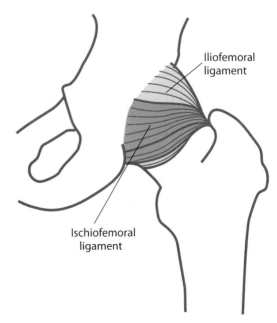

▲ **Fig. 5.7(a)** The iliofemoral and pubofemoral ligaments

▲ **(b)** The ischiofemoral ligament

iliac spine in two bands to the anterior intertrochanteric line. This ligament counters hyperextension of the hip.

- The pubofemoral ligament is attached proximally to the superior pubic ramus and distally to the inferior femoral neck. This ligament resists hyperabduction.

- The ischiofemoral ligament extends from the ischial rim of the acetabulum, across the posteroinferior aspect of the hip to attach to the femoral neck. This ligament stabilises the hip in extension.

Tips on looking at plain films of the pelvis and hips

Radiographic assessment of the pelvis and hip requires a disciplined and systematic approach. A routine should be developed to minimise the possibility of missing pertinent changes. A possible routine for examination of the pelvis and hips might comprise the following:

- assess whether the examination is adequate
- assess overall and relative bone density
- note pelvic tilt, scoliosis or other evidence of leg length discrepancy
- inspect the bony architecture
- assess for localised sclerotic areas

▼ **Fig. 5.8** A pelvic tilt is an important observation to make and is most easily identified by comparing the height of the iliac crests. This is usually indicative of a discrepancy in leg length and is invariably associated with a lumbar scoliosis. Although the lumbar spine is not included in an AP of the pelvis, usually enough of the spine is seen to suggest a scoliosis. An erect film will confirm the tilt and allow an approximate assessment of the degree of leg length discrepancy. Note the bone island in the subtrochanteric region of the right femur.

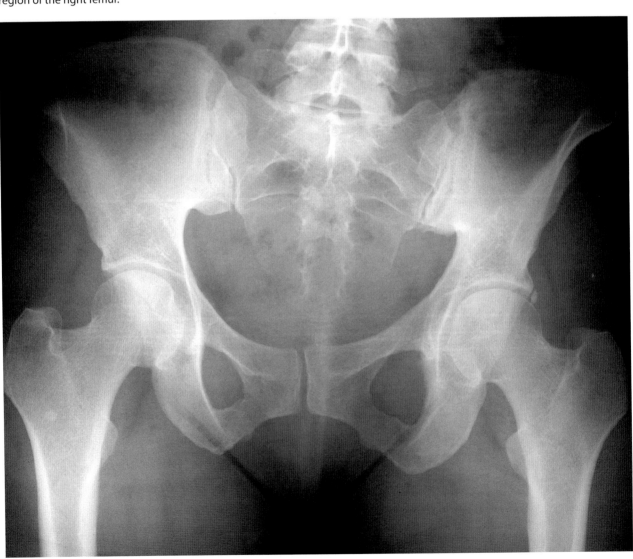

- search for focal lytic areas
- examine the hip joints
- assess the sacroiliac joints and sacrum
- examine the symphysis
- search the soft tissues for evidence of increased density or displacement of fat planes.

The first and probably most important assessment to make is whether the films are adequate. Are the films positioned correctly, and particularly is the pelvis rotated? If rotation is present, comparison of one side with the other is difficult. The other common problem is exposure. Are the iliac crests and anterior superior iliac spines adequately demonstrated? Should extra views have been taken? For example, if there is the suggestion of a fracture of a pubic ramus, an obturator foramen view may be diagnostic.

The general attitude of the pelvis should be noted. A supine film showing a pelvic tilt (see Fig. 5.8), particularly if accompanied by a compensatory lumbar scoliosis, can indicate a discrepancy in leg length and an erect film should then be taken to confirm this finding. Leg length discrepancy may be developmental or acquired and will alter normal biomechanics and exaggerate the stress of athletic performance. If a pelvic tilt is present, there is usually an associated lumbar scoliosis convex to the side of the shorter leg (Walker and Dickson 1984), although pelvic asymmetry can also produce these findings. CT digital radiography is the preferred method of confirming and quantifying the leg length discrepancy. This method is accurate, simple and can be obtained with a low radiation dose (Aitken et al. 1985) (see Fig. 5.9).

The bony architecture of the pelvis and hips is assessed for generalised or focal pathological processes. This can be a difficult task due to overlying gas and faeces. If an area is particularly worrying, an oblique view or a progress film may be required for clarification.

A finding of localised increased bone density is not unusual, as the pelvis and proximal femora are common sites for bone islands. These densities should be carefully examined and a decision made whether these areas warrant further imaging to exclude lesions such as bone stress, a sclerotic metastasis or osteoid osteoma.

Bone islands are areas of compact bone and are a common normal variant with identifying characteristics. They are usually ovoid in shape, have a slightly indistinct margin and are oriented in the direction of the trabeculae (see Figs 5.10

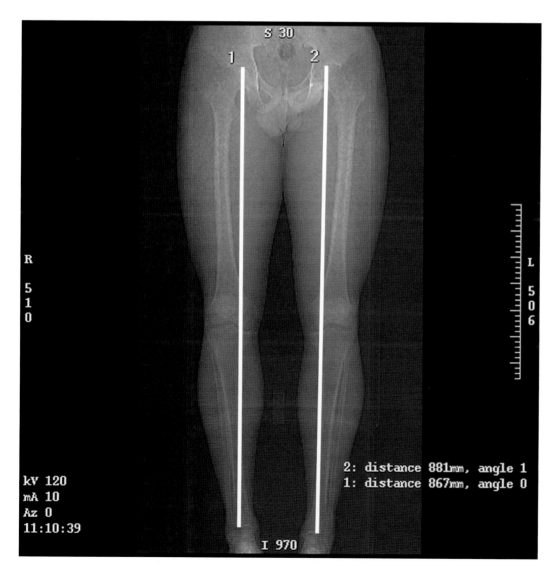

Fig. 5.9 Using a digital CT 'scout film', an accurate measurement of leg length enables any discrepancy to be calculated. The entire leg from the hip to the tibial plafond is measured initially and, if there is a difference, the femora and tibiae are individually measured to determine which bone is responsible for the shortening.

▶ **Fig. 5.10** A large focal density in the ilium (arrowhead) is aligned in the direction of the trabeculae and has an appearance typical of a bone island.

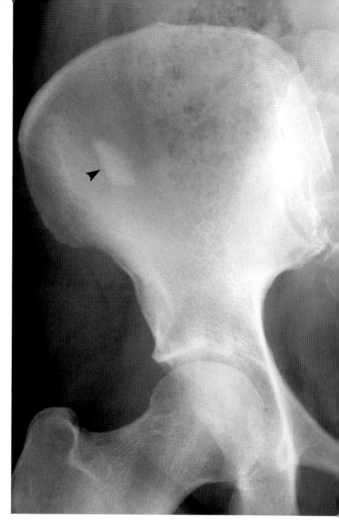

and 5.11). Bone islands are areas of active compact bone that may appear or disappear and increase or decrease in size. When active, bone islands may show increased uptake of isotope on a nuclear bone scan, further confusing their differentiation from bone stress or even a sclerotic metastasis. Bone islands can vary in size from a few millimetres to more than 4 cm.

Bone stress reactions and stress fractures often appear as a vague area of sclerosis, most commonly seen in the femoral neck (see Fig. 5.12), but may also be seen in the pubic rami and sacrum. The sclerosis associated with bone stress is generally less dense than a bone island and often contains a relatively translucent area. Unlike bone islands, the long axis of stress reactions and stress fractures is oriented at 90° to the trabeculae. These areas show a marked increase in uptake of isotope on nuclear bone scans (see Fig. 5.13).

An osteoid osteoma characteristically provokes sclerosis in the surrounding bone (see Fig. 5.14) and has a predilection for the pelvis and upper femora. The area of sclerosis will generally contain a rounded translucent nidus, which has a variable appearance and may be difficult to see on plain films. This benign tumour has to be differentiated from bone stress

▼ **Fig. 5.11** A bone island in the femoral neck shows typical features with orientation in the line of the trabeculae, in contrast to a stress fracture, which is oriented across the trabeculae. The margins of a bone island are characteristically unsharp. A second, smaller bone island should also be noted within the femoral head.

▼ **Fig. 5.12** This is a typical compressive-type stress fracture of the femoral neck. Note the spiculated margin of the sclerotic area and its orientation at right angles to the trabeculae (arrowhead). There is associated periosteal reaction.

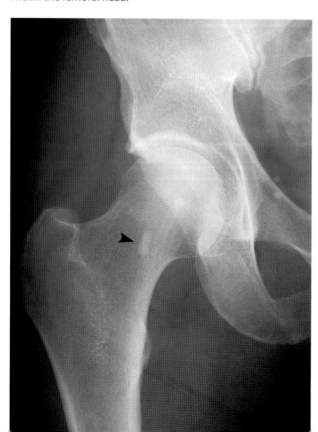

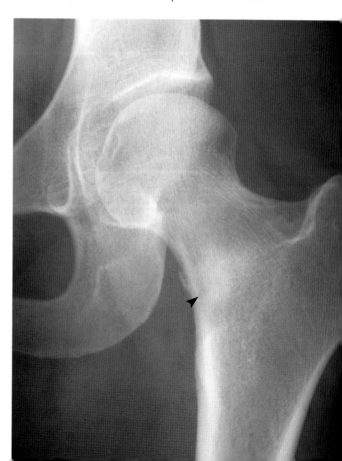

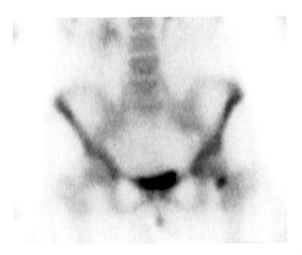

(b)

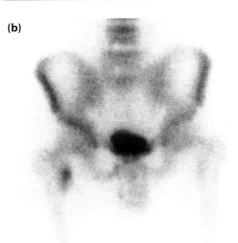

▲ **Fig. 5.13** A nuclear bone scan will show a localised marked increase in isotope uptake and the characteristic orientation of a stress fracture across the femoral neck.

▲ **(b)** A nuclear bone scan shows a corresponding marked uptake of isotope in the lesser trochanter.

▼ **(c)** This characteristic appearance of an osteoid osteoma is demonstrated by CT scanning. There is a translucent nidus containing a small calcific density (arrowhead).

▼ **Fig. 5.14** An osteoid osteoma usually produces reactive sclerosis in the surrounding bone. These benign tumours commonly occur in the upper femur, pelvis and sacrum. This osteoid osteoma has occurred in a favoured site, deep to the lesser trochanter.
(a) The associated bony sclerosis (arrowheads) was only confidently identified after comparison with the asymptomatic side.

(c)

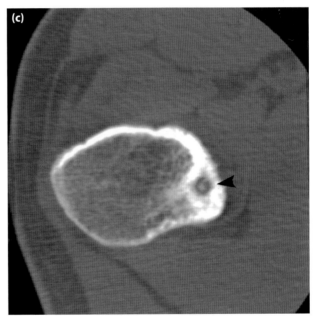

(a)

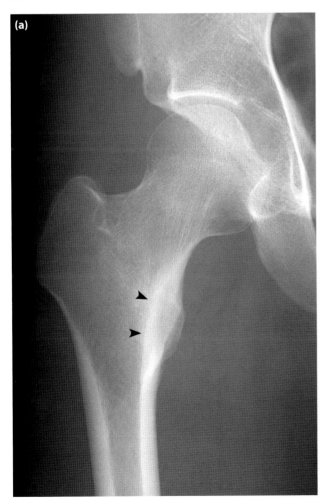

on plain films, remembering that stress fractures may often contain a translucent area within the sclerotic zone. Osteoid osteomata predominantly occur in males (3:1) between the ages of 7 and 25. The typical clinical presentation consists of a dull ache, which is worse at night and is relieved by aspirin. These lesions produce intense focal uptake of isotope on a nuclear bone scan and usually have a characteristic appearance on thin-section CT, with demonstration of a lucent nidus, which may contain calcification (see Fig. 5.15). There can be a great variation in the radiological appearance of an osteoid osteoma (see Fig. 5.16) and this is particularly so if the tumour is intramedullary or intracapsular (see Fig. 5.17), when the sclerosis may not be pronounced. However, the clinical presentation is consistent.

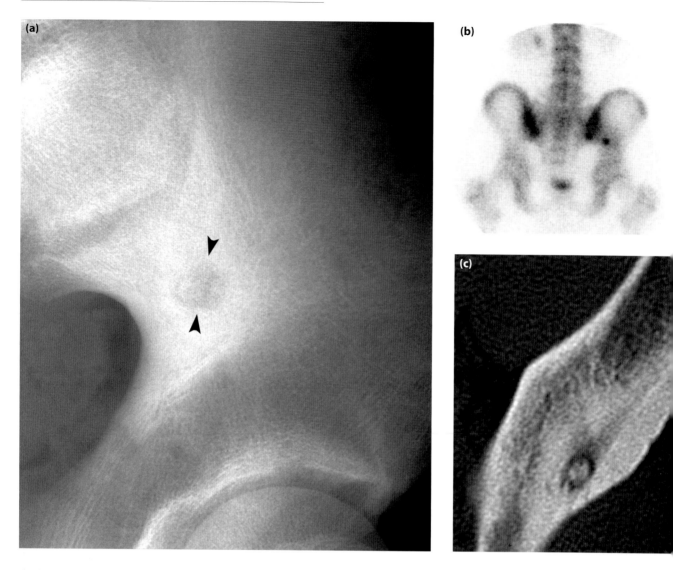

▲ **Fig. 5.15** The radiotranslucent nidus of an osteoid osteoma is characteristically difficult to see on a plain film. When there is an area of surrounding bony sclerosis combined with an appropriate clinical history, a nuclear bone scan and, if positive, a CT scan is advisable.

(a) This area of translucency (arrowheads) is barely discernible within an area of sclerosis in the ilium. This sclerosis could easily be thought to represent osteitis condensans ilii and, if overlying bowel shadows were also present, the task of identification might well be impossible.

(b) A nuclear bone scan shows uptake characteristic of an osteoid osteoma.

(c) A CT scan is diagnostic of an osteoid osteoma, with a translucent nidus containing a sclerotic density.

It is important to remain alert to the possibility of other causes of localised sclerosis, such as a healing fracture, an insufficiency fracture (which occurs fairly commonly in the femoral neck, see Fig. 5.18), Paget's disease, osteoblastic metastasis, avascular necrosis of the femoral head and fibrous dysplasia. These will be seen from time to time. Similarly, lytic changes can occur and overlying bowel gas can cause great difficulty in reaching a confident diagnosis of bone destruction. Common lytic lesions include metastatic carcinoma, multiple myeloma and the osteoporotic stage of Paget's disease. A detailed discussion of these conditions is beyond the scope of this book.

Bony spurs are common at sites of tendon or muscle attachment around the pelvis as a physiologic response to the repetitive stress of contraction. These 'tug' lesions (see Fig. 5.19) are asymptomatic and are clinically unimportant.

In the immature athlete, all apophyses should be routinely assessed for evidence of avulsion or apophysitis. Note should be made of any displacement or change in bony architecture when compared with the opposite side. The growth plate at each apophysis should also be symmetrical (see Fig. 5.20).

No task is more important than performing an accurate assessment of the hip joints. Armed with a knowledge of normal radiographic anatomy, each component of the hip should be examined in turn. A normal acetabular roof is crucial to proper hip functioning. It is important to note its shape and length. The shape of the roof has been discussed

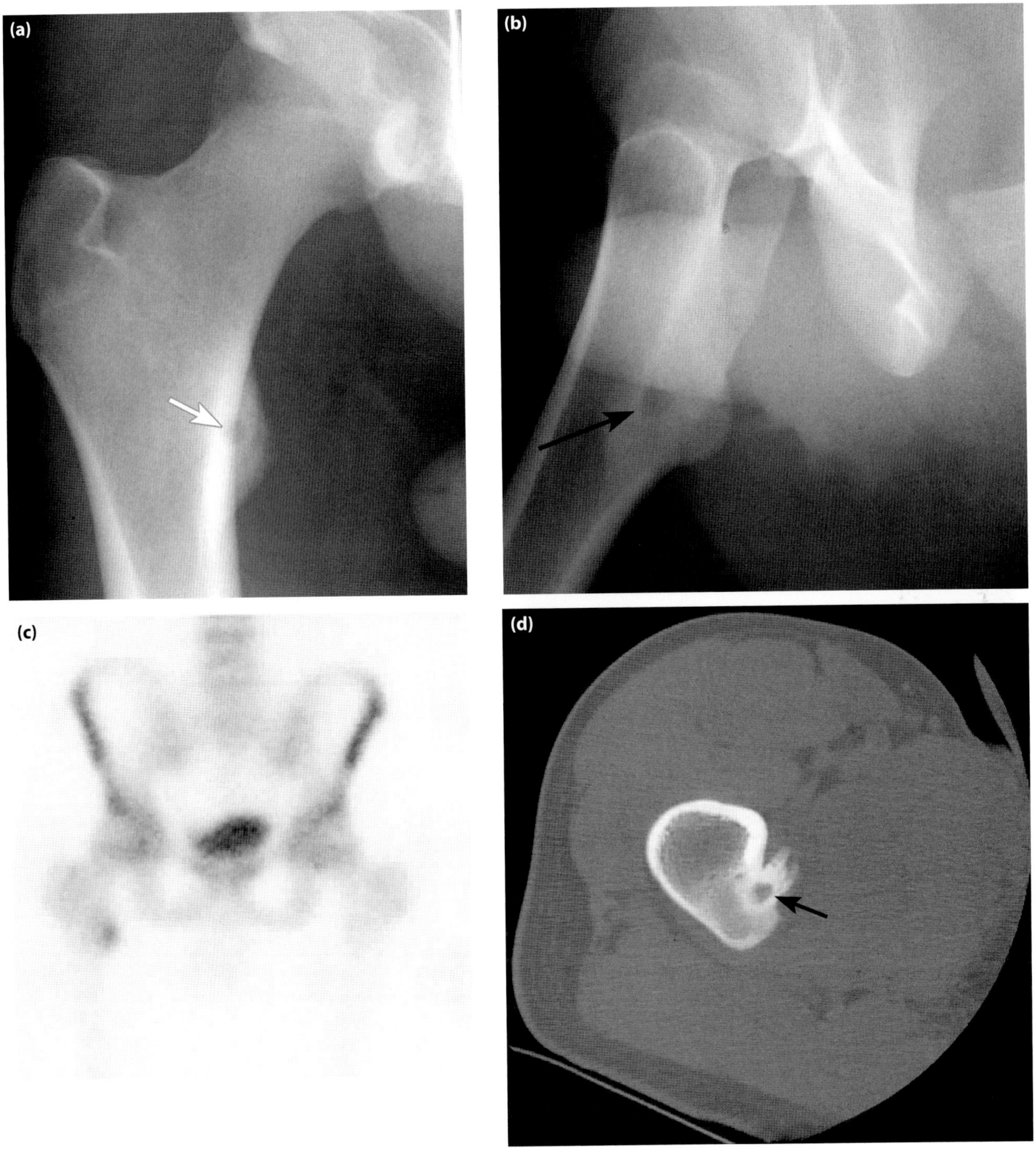

▲ **Fig. 5.16** There is considerable variation in the radiological appearance of an osteoid osteoma. In this example, there is minimal reactive sclerosis

(a) On the AP view, no sclerosis is evident and the translucent nidus is barely visible (arrow).
(b) The nidus is well seen on the lateral view of the hip (arrow).
(c) A nuclear bone scan shows an increased uptake of isotope at the lesser trochanter at the site of the suspected osteoid osteoma.
(d) A CT scan confirms the diagnosis. In this case, the nidus is entirely translucent and is present at the base of a 'tug' lesion at the attachment of the iliopsoas (arrow).

previously and can provide a plain film clue to the presence of hip dysplasia. A small ossicle is often seen at the lateral margin of the acetabular roof and most authorities regard this as an unfused secondary centre of ossification (an os acetabulum) (see Fig. 5.21(a)). However, Klaue et al. (1991) and others believe that some of these ossicles may represent ununited

stress fractures resulting from abnormal lateral loading of the hip associated with dysplasia (see Fig. 5.21(b)). Ossicles at the outer end of the acetabular roof may also result from repetitive impaction of a prominent femoral neck against the acetabular rim in a femoroacetabular impingement syndrome (see Fig. 5.21(c)).

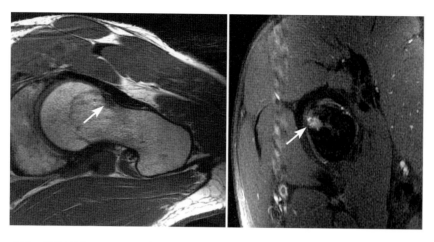

▲ **Fig. 5.17** When an osteoid osteoma is intracapsular, its appearance is altogether different (arrows). No reactive sclerosis occurs and the margins of the lesion are characteristically ragged, as demonstrated on MR images.

The hip joint spaces should be compared for uniformity and symmetry. Even slight narrowing is indicative of articular cartilage loss and the presence of an osteoarthritic process (see Fig. 5.22). To assess femoral head migration, an AP view of the pelvis is required so that the hips can be compared and the distances from the 'teardrops' to both femoral heads measured. In children, a hip joint effusion may cause lateral displacement of the hip (see Fig. 5.23(a)). Anterolateral migration of the femoral head also occurs in dysplastic hips and osteoarthritis (see Fig. 5.23(b) and (c)).

▼ **Fig. 5.19** 'Tug' lesions are spurs of new bone that develop at the bony attachment of tendons and ligaments in response to repetitive traction forces, as seen in Fig. 5.16(d) at the iliopsoas insertion. In this case, a plain film of the pelvis of a sprinter shows that the pelvis has developed 'ears' due to repetitive muscular traction (arrow).

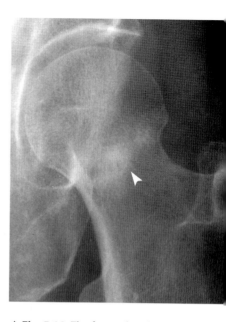

▲ **Fig. 5.18** The femoral neck and the trochanteric region are subjected to considerable stresses, and in a patient with reduced bone mineral and elasticity, insufficiency fractures are relatively common. In this case, a transverse insufficiency fracture (arrowhead) has developed in the subcapital region. The appearance is typical, with a band of poorly defined sclerosis traversing the demineralised femoral neck.

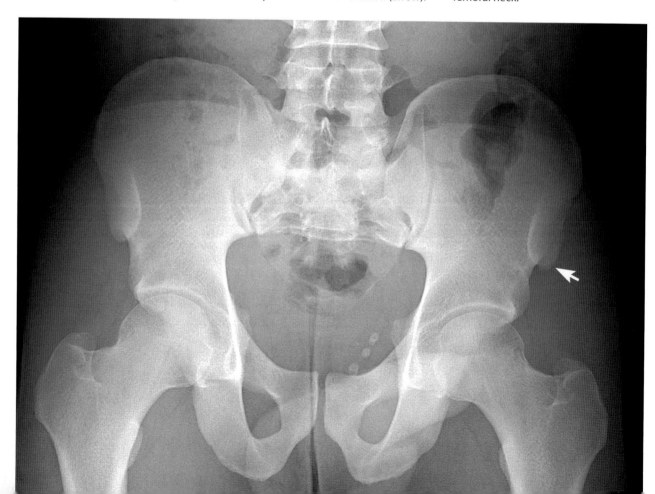

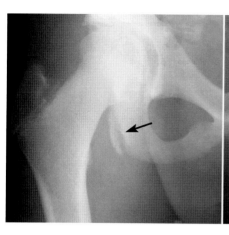
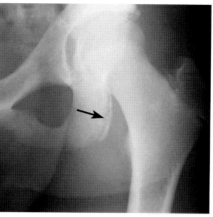

▲ **Fig. 5.20** Apophyses and their growth plates should be symmetrical, although minor individual variations are tolerated as normal. Comparison with the apophysis on the other side is often the only method of confidently determining minor avulsion injuries or apophysitis. In this case, there has been a minor avulsion of the right ischial apophysis (arrows).

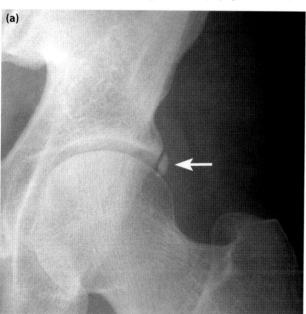

(a)

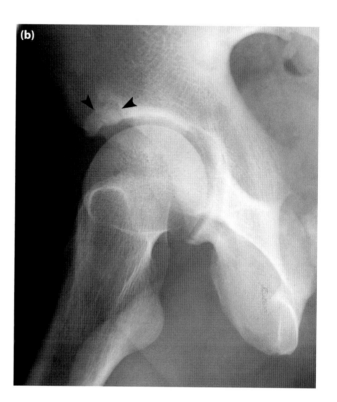

(b)

▲▶ **Fig. 5.21(a)** It is not uncommon to see an ossicle at the outer end of the acetabular roof (arrow). Most of these ossicles are thought to represent unfused secondary centres of ossification.

(b) It is also possible that this atypical os acetabulum (arrowheads) represents a stress fracture.

(c) Dystrophic calcification within an injured acetabular labrum may occur with femoroacetabular impingement and is a further cause of an apparent os acetabulum. In this case, the acetabulum is retroverted. Note the prominence on the lateral margin of the femoral neck (arrow), and joint space narrowing.

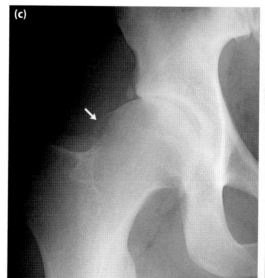

(c)

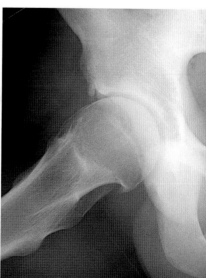

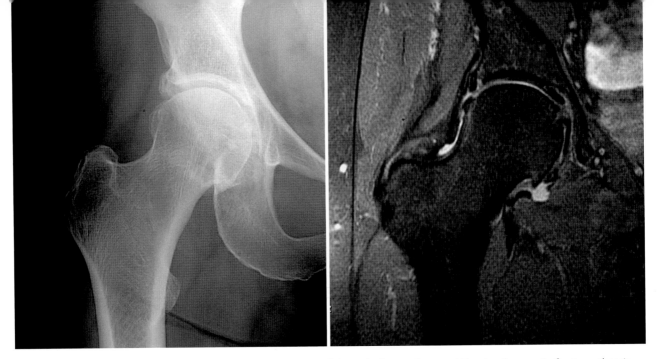

▲ **Fig. 5.22** Narrowing of the hip joint space indicates wearing of the articular cartilage and the development of osteoarthrosis. A plain film shows joint space narrowing most marked superomedially and osteophyte formation is developing at the margins of the femoral articular surface. The coronal fat-suppressed MR image on the right shows generalised loss of the articular cartilage over the femoral head. A small hip joint effusion and synovitis are noted. An ossicle or osteophyte is present at the outer end of the acetabular roof.

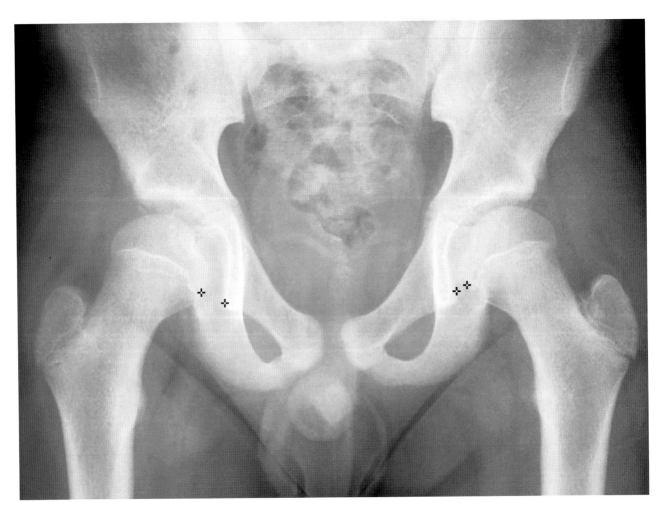

▲ **Fig. 5.23(a)** Anterolateral migration of the femoral head may occur in children when a hip effusion is present. In this case an effusion in the right hip causes lateral displacement of the femoral head, as determined by the relative distance of each femoral head from the 'teardrop' (callipers).

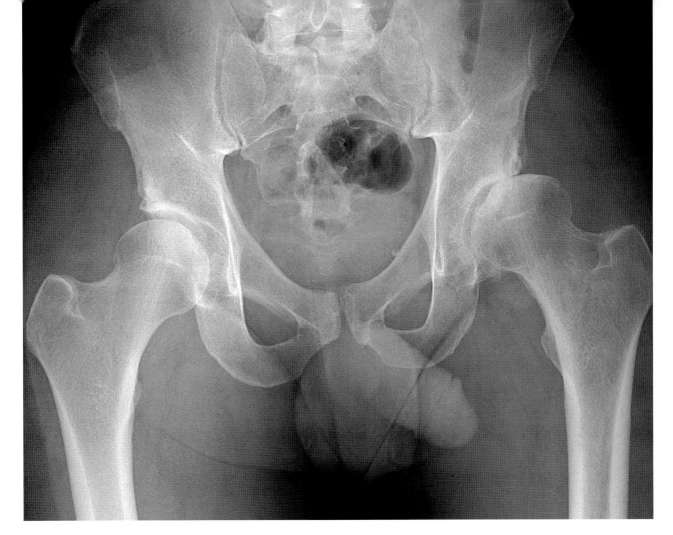

▲▼ Fig 5.23 (b) and (c) Anterolateral displacement of the femoral head also occurs in hip dysplasia and osteoarthrosis. In this case, both hips show dysplastic characteristics, complicated by degenerative changes on the left. Considerable anterolateral displacement of the left femoral head has occurred.

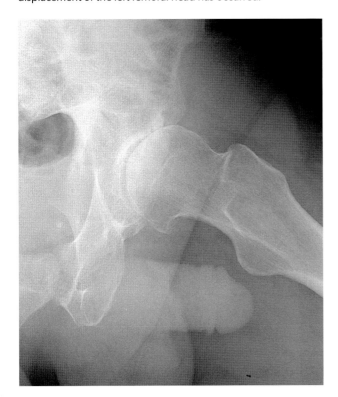

In the adult, a widened joint space following trauma strongly suggests an entrapped fracture fragment and CT imaging should be performed to assess this possibility (see Fig. 5.24).

As previously noted, any abnormality of the shape of the femoral head and its relationship to the femoral neck is an important observation that may predispose to femoro-acetabular impingement and degenerative joint disease. This is discussed later in the chapter.

Cystic-type changes may be seen in the subcapital region of the femoral neck. These may be synovial pits and are of no clinical significance (see Fig. 5.25). However, subcapital cystic changes and sclerosis may also develop from femoro-acetabular impingement and define the site of contact.

Examination of the sacroiliac joints and the sacrum comes next. In the young, the sacroiliac joints can normally show widening and irregularity (see Fig. 5.26). Increased uptake on nuclear bone scanning will also be present. Consequently, sacroiliitis in the developing skeleton is very difficult to diagnose on plain films. In adults, sclerosis is often seen on the ilial side of the sacroiliac joints inferiorly. This change may be bilateral and results from physiological bone stress (so-called 'osteitis condensans ilii'). These changes occur entirely on the ilial side of the joint, and oblique sacroiliac joint views or CT scanning may help to confirm this distribution in difficult cases.

The sacrum is often overlooked and can be difficult to evaluate when overlying bowel shadows are present. In fact, examination of the sacrum requires considerable discipline. This is partly because sacral pathology is unusual

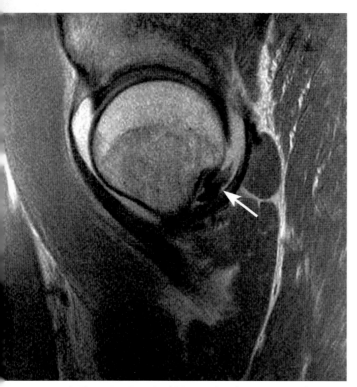

▲ **Fig. 5.24** A sagittal PD-weighted MR image without fat suppression shows an effusion containing a loose body (arrow).

and partly because sacral detail is difficult to appreciate. Stress fractures of the sacrum occur as the result of repetitive strenuous exercise (Volpin et al. 1989) and acute fractures may also occur from direct trauma. A lateral view is essential for detecting and assessing fractures of the sacrum and the coccyx (see Fig. 5.27). Focal alteration in sacral bone density such as may occur with an osteoid osteoma (see Fig. 5.28) would usually require CT scanning for further characterisation.

Changes at the symphysis pubis can be of great significance in an athlete. The cortical margins of the symphysis are normally dense and sharply defined (see Fig. 5.29). A thin layer of hyaline cartilage coats each articular cortex, and the intervening space is occupied by a thick fibrocartilaginous disc. The average radiographic width of the symphysis pubis is 6 mm in males and 5 mm in females, although the width increases with pregnancy. The fibrocartilaginous disc tends to degenerate with age and, particularly in females, a dark line may develop in the midline on plain films. This appearance is known as a 'vacuum' sign. Radiographic changes of athletic osteitis pubis include asymmetric erosion and sclerosis of one or both margins of the symphysis (see Fig. 5.30(a)). There is a corresponding pattern of increased uptake on nuclear bone scanning (see Fig. 5.30(b)). The significance of this radiological appearance is discussed later in the chapter.

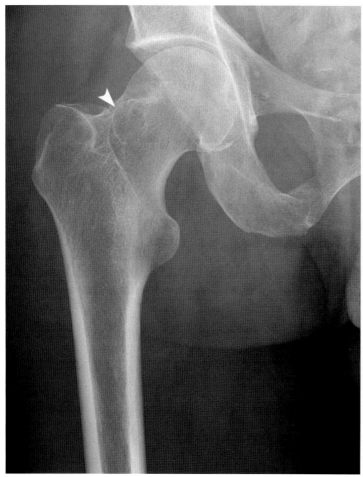

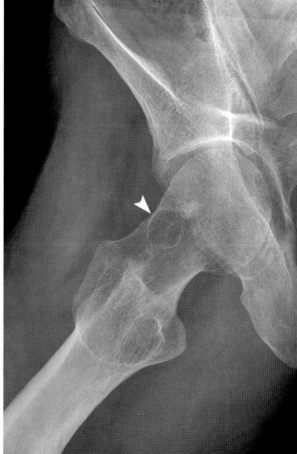

▲ **Fig. 5.25** A giant synovial pit is present (arrowhead). Note the adjacent bone island.

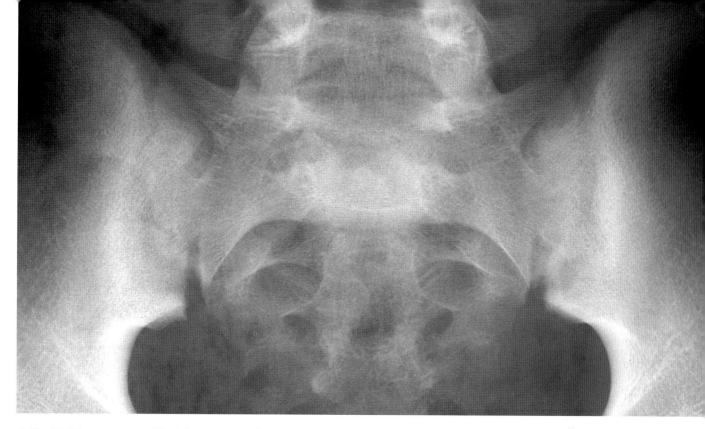

▲ **Fig. 5.26** Immature sacroiliac joints appear widened and eroded, and it is sometimes difficult to accept that this is a normal appearance in children.

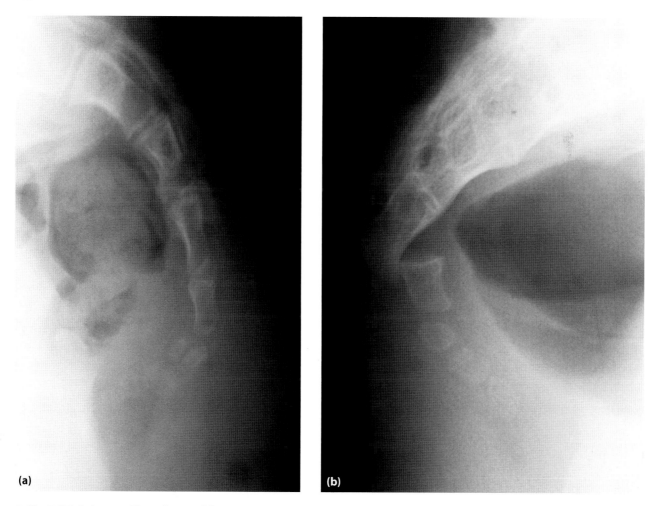

(a)

(b)

▲ **Fig. 5.27(a)** A normal lateral view of the coccyx. This view is sometimes difficult to obtain because an appropriate exposure and coning are crucial. **(b)** An anterior dislocation of the coccyx is well demonstrated on a lateral view of the sacro-coccygeal region.

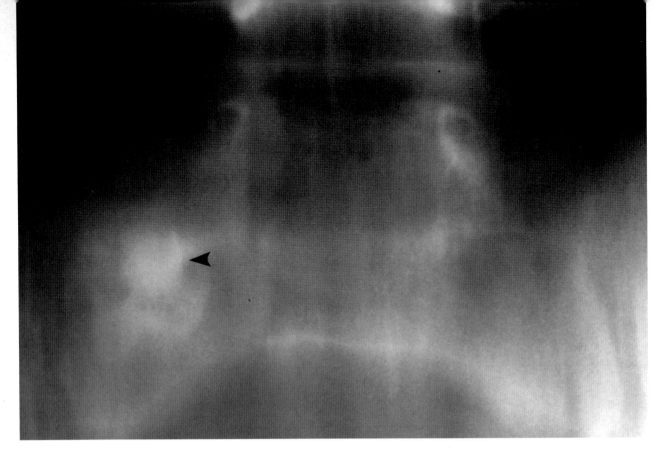

▲ **Fig. 5.28** Finding an osteoid osteoma of the sacrum on a plain film is often difficult. In practice, the search is directed by a characteristic clinical history. This osteoid osteoma (arrowhead) is demonstrated by linear tomography, a superseded technology, but nevertheless a handy imaging method for such a situation if CT is unavailable. This is a good example of the great variation in radiological appearance of an osteoid osteoma. This tumour has limited surrounding sclerosis and, unlike the examples shown previously, has a prominent central sclerotic nidus.

▼ **Fig. 5.29** A normal symphysis pubis has well defined cortical margins. Detail is increased by good coning.

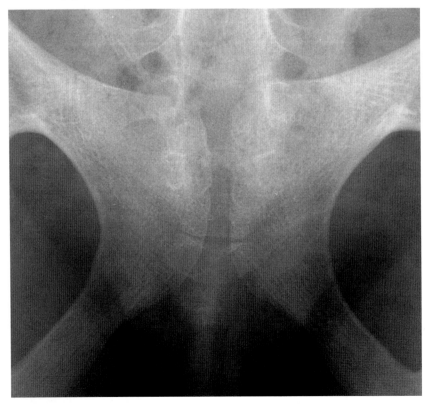

Important clues to pelvis and hip abnormalities can be found by examining the soft tissues around the pelvis and hips. Four fat planes are normally seen (see Fig. 5.31):

- the obturator fat plane
- the psoas fat plane
- the capsular fat plane
- the gluteal fat plane.

Guerra et al. (1978) have shown that the psoas, capsular and gluteal fat planes are quite distant from the hip joint and are consequently often poor indicators of subtle hip pathology. In addition, slight rotation of the pelvis may produce considerable asymmetry of these planes in the normal subject when sides are compared. However, the obturator fat plane is a consistently useful landmark, as unilateral obliteration or displacement usually indicates soft-tissue swelling associated with either a fracture or some other bony process in the ilium (see Fig. 5.32).

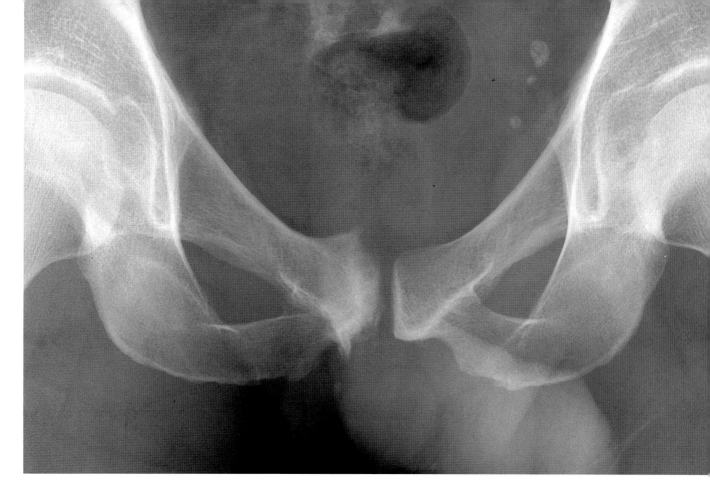

▲ **Fig. 5.30(a)** A soccer player presented with longstanding groin pain. Articular erosion, reactive subarticular sclerosis and new bone formation are demonstrated on the right side of the symphysis pubis. These changes are typical of chronic osteitis pubis. The sclerosis and osteophytes have developed at the adductor and conjoint tendon attachments.
▼ **(b)** A nuclear bone scan of the same case shows an increased uptake of isotope over the right side of the symphysis pubis.

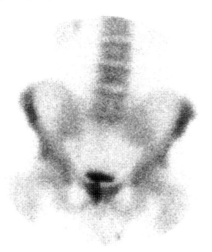

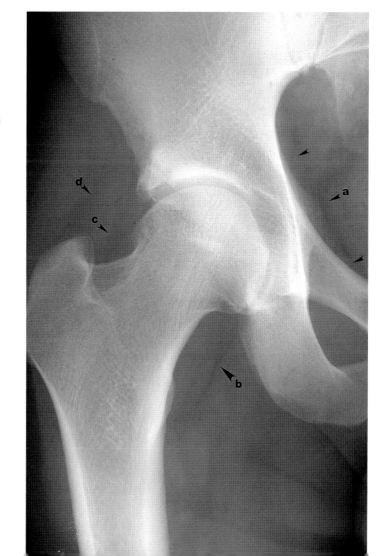

► **Fig. 5.31** Four normal fat planes of the hip should be noted: the obturator fat plane (a), the psoas fat plane (b), the capsular fat plane (c) and the gluteal fat plane (d). Note the large os acetabulum on the lateral aspect of the acetabular roof.

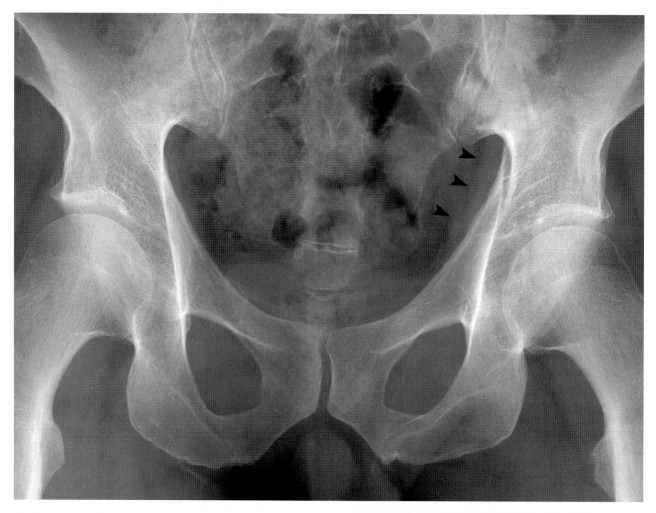

▲ **Fig. 5.32(a)** There is medial displacement of the obturator fat plane (arrowheads), due to a haematoma associated with an ilial fracture.

▼ **(b)** A CT scan shows detail of the ilial fracture and swelling of the adjacent iliacus muscle due to haematoma formation.

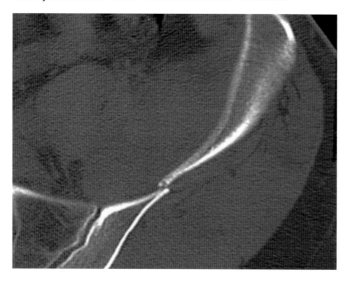

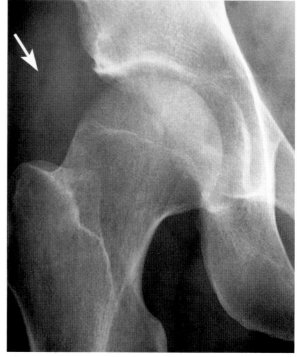

▲ **Fig. 5.33** A case of septic arthritis of the hip demonstrates the diagnostic value of the fat planes. There is displacement of the capsular fat plane (arrow), providing evidence of a large hip effusion.

The psoas, capsular and gluteal fat lines may also indicate underlying hip pathology (see Fig. 5.33), although they are less dependent.

Following muscle injury, an organised intramuscular haematoma may develop dystrophic calcification and heterotopic ossification with associated pain. This condition is called myositis ossificans and occurs most commonly in the thighs, particularly within the vastus intermedius (see Fig. 5.34) and hamstrings (see Fig. 5.35). A more extensive discussion on myositis ossificans can be found in the section on muscle tears (see page 338).

Methods of imaging the pelvis and hips

Routine plain film series

Plain films should always be the first imaging test. There are two projections in the routine hip series:

1. an AP view of the pelvis—this should be a routine part of a hip series even though symptoms may be unilateral
2. a lateral-oblique view of the hip.

An AP view of the pelvis (see Fig. 5.36) is acquired with the patient supine, ensuring that the pelvis is not rotated. The feet are rotated 15° internally to reduce the hip anteversion and optimally profile the femoral neck. This eliminates overlay of the greater trochanter and allows improved examination of the femoral head. The beam is centred 5 cm above the superior border of the symphysis. Gonad shielding is used when appropriate and provided that the area of interest is not obscured.

A lateral or more correctly lateral-oblique view of the hip requires the pelvis to be rolled towards the side of interest. A straight tube is centred on the femoral head (see Fig. 5.37). This view is extremely valuable for examining the femoral head and neck, especially to exclude fractures and to assess the apophyses and femoral capital epiphyses in the immature patient.

Additional plain films

Additional views may be helpful in specific clinical situations. It is important to remember that extra views around the pelvis increase the radiation dose and they

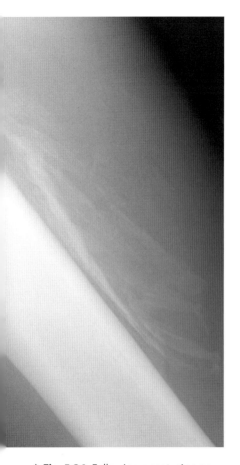

▲ **Fig. 5.34** Following a contusion or compressive rupture injury to the vastus intermedius, myositis ossificans has formed. Note the peripheral distribution of calcification with central lucency and a dense outer margin. This is a key differentiating feature from parosteal osteosarcoma.

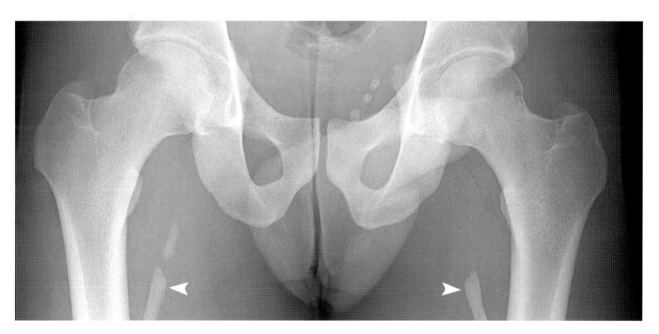

▲ **Fig. 5.35** Dense ossification has formed in both hamstrings following injury (arrowheads).

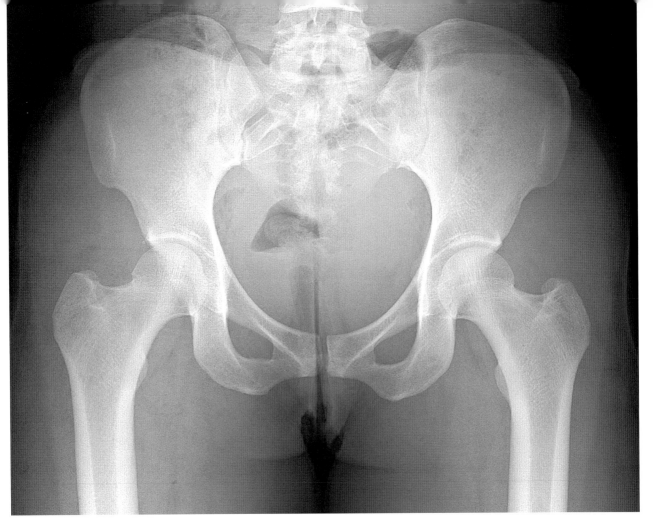

▲ **Fig. 5.36** This is a normal AP pelvis obtained with 15° of internal rotation of the hips to improve assessment of the femoral neck.

▶ **Fig. 5.37** A lateral view is an essential component of the examination of the hip, particularly when the patient is paediatric. In adults, fractures are occasionally seen only in this view.

should be used only in situations where the management may be altered by a positive finding.

Following major trauma and if there is a suspicion of a fracture in the region of the acetabulum, Judet views of the pelvis are useful. These views not only help to demonstrate the fracture, but also are used to assess whether there is involvement of the anterior or posterior columns of the pelvis. Judet views are taken by rolling the patient 40° one way and then the other, acquiring images in both positions. A straight tube is used, centred on the femoral head (see Fig. 5.38).

A prone view of the symphysis pubis will improve detail of the symphysis in patients with groin strain. The pubic rami are also well demonstrated in this view (see Fig. 5.39), which is taken with the patient lying prone to bring the symphysis closer to the film and with

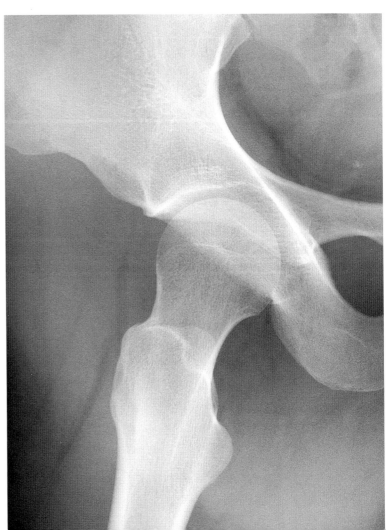

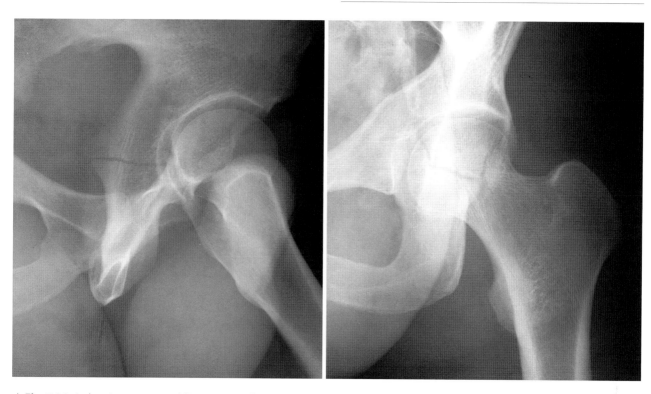

▲ **Fig. 5.38** Judet views are two oblique views taken at 90° to one another showing details of an ilial fracture. The extent of the fracture and involvement of the anterior and posterior columns can be assessed.

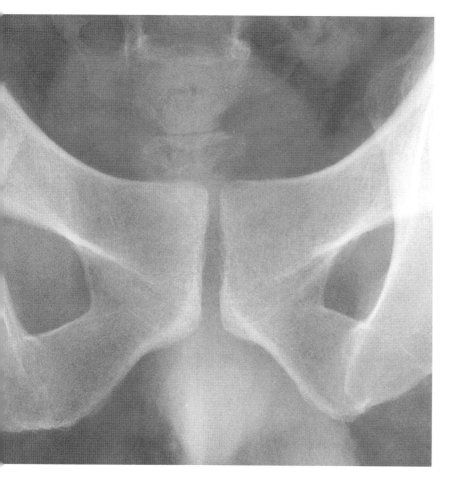

▲ **Fig. 5.39** A specific view of the symphysis is obtained with the patient prone and a cranial tube angulation of 20 to 30°. Coning increases detail. Slight obliquity is present in this case.

20 to 30° of cranial tube angulation. The primary beam is centred on the symphysis and coning further helps to improve detail.

An obturator view improves the examination of the pubic rami and ischial tuberosities. This view can be obtained supine or prone. In the supine position, there is 25 to 30° cranial angulation of the tube and, if the prone position is used, the angulation is caudal. The primary beam is centred just below the inferior margin of the symphysis (see Fig. 5.40). The examination of the margins of the obturator foramen can be further improved by rolling the patient 30° to the symptomatic side into a prone oblique position. A 30° caudal tube angulation is used.

Flamingo views of the symphysis are used in the diagnosis of pelvic instability by demonstrating movement at the symphysis under weightbearing stress. Two PA views of the symphysis are obtained with weightbearing on each leg in turn. Traditionally, the non-weightbearing leg is flexed and the foot of this leg is placed on the knee of the weightbearing side (like a flamingo). Any movement at the symphysis in excess of 2 mm is abnormal (see Fig. 5.41).

An angled and coned PA or AP view of the sacroiliac joints may be helpful

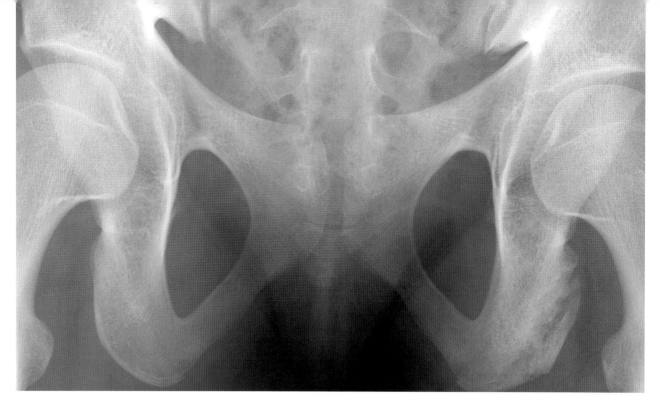

▲ **Fig. 5.40** An obturator view is used to image the pubic rami when there is a clinical suspicion of a fracture of a ramus or ischial apophysitis, as in this case.

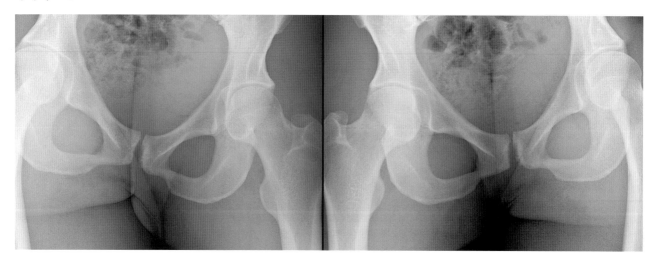

▲ **Fig. 5.41** Flamingo views can be used to confirm pelvic instability in athletes with osteitis pubis or recurrent adductor injuries. In this case, marked changes of osteitis pubis are present bilaterally and more than 2 mm of movement has occurred, suggesting pelvic instability.

when an abnormality of the sacroiliac joints is suspected on a routine view of the pelvis (see Fig. 5.42). A PA view is favoured on the theory that the divergent rays will more closely parallel the orientation of the joints and therefore be better able to show the joint margins. Supporters of the AP technique argue that the joints are closer to the film, increasing detail. A tube angulation of about 30° is used, although this will vary depending upon the lumbar curve. For an AP view the tube is angled in a cranial direction and centred 3 cm above the symphysis. Angulation in the opposite direction is required if the patient is examined prone. Oblique views may also help in assessing the sacroiliac joints. These views may define the complex geometry of the sacroiliac joint

spaces and are particularly useful in differentiating sacroiliitis from physiological sclerosis of the ilium in adults. It must be stressed that there would have to be a high level of suspicion of an abnormality in the sacroiliac joints to warrant the extra exposure to radiation. This is especially so if a CT scan is also being contemplated.

A view of the lesser trochanter (see Fig. 5.43) may be useful if an iliopsoas avulsion injury is suspected. This view is obtained with external rotation of the hip to profile the lesser trochanter.

A view of the anterior superior iliac spine (ASIS) is obtained with the patient rolled steeply onto the affected side and a straight tube is centred on the ASIS (see Fig. 5.44). The most

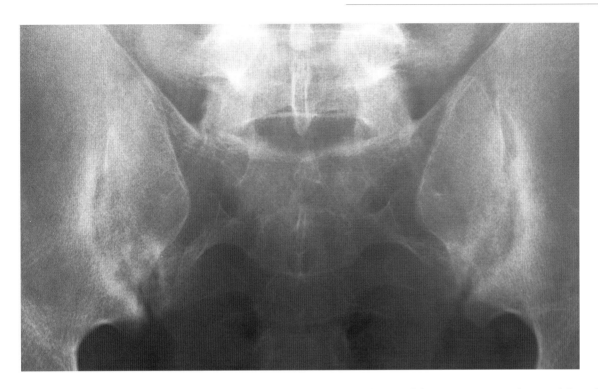

▲ **Fig. 5.42** Specific coned views of the sacroiliac joints improve the definition of the joint margins. In this case, bilateral changes of sacroiliitis are demonstrated. There is erosion of the joint margins and considerable associated sclerosis.

▼ **Fig. 5.43** An external rotation view of the hip is used to better demonstrate the lesser trochanter. A displaced avulsion of the apophysis of the lesser trochanter is demonstrated (arrowhead).

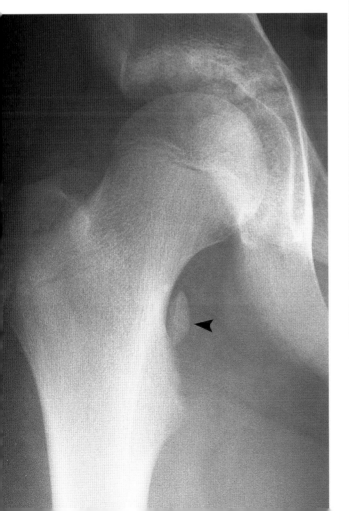

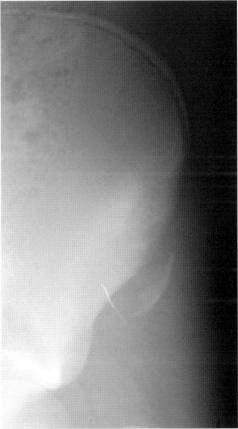

▲ **Fig. 5.44** A specific view of the ASIS is required if an avulsion injury is clinically suspected. The patient is rolled towards the symptomatic side into a steeply obliqued position. A soft-tissue exposure and good coning are important. This image shows avulsion of the ASIS with displacement.

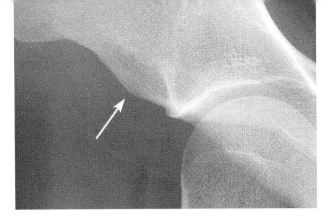

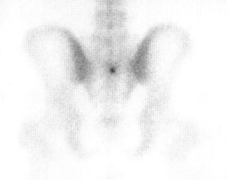

▲ Fig. 5.45 The AIIS (arrow) is clearly shown on a routine lateral hip view, with the primary beam centred on the spine, 3 cm above the hip.

▼ Fig. 5.46 A view of the pubic tubercles shows no abnormality, with no evidence of calcific tendinopathy.

▲ Fig. 5.47 A nuclear bone scan of the pelvis shows an occult fracture of a sacral spinous process. This was an unexpected finding and explained the patient's symptoms.

▶ Fig. 5.48 A nuclear bone scan shows an increased uptake of isotope at the ASIS, indicating an avulsion injury.

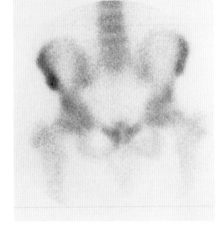

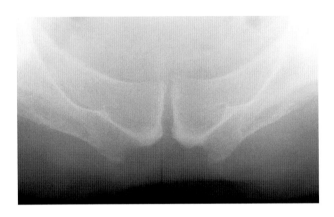

▼ Fig. 5.49 Enthesopathy is present at the hamstring origins on the right side (arrow).

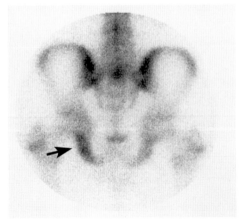

▼ Fig. 5.50 A bone scan demonstrates trochanteric bursopathy and possible gluteal enthesopathy on the left side (arrow).

difficult part of acquiring this view is choosing an appropriate exposure. A soft-tissue exposure is all that is required.

The anterior inferior iliac spine (AIIS) is well demonstrated on a lateral-oblique hip view, with the primary beam centred about 3 cm above the hip joint (see Fig. 5.45).

Imaging of the pubic tubercles may be useful in assessing the adductor origins for evidence of calcific tendinopathy. The patient sits on the side of the x-ray table and leans backwards to 45° inclination, supporting their weight on extended arms. The knees are supported in slight flexion. A straight tube is then centred 4 cm above the symphysis to profile the pubic tubercles (see Fig. 5.46). It must be remembered that the radiation dose for this view is considerable and the gonads are exposed to the primary beam.

Nuclear bone scanning

A nuclear bone scan is a useful screening test for bone or joint pathology when plain films are negative. Bone scans have the advantage of imaging the area from the spine to the knee and may demonstrate unexpected changes that may cause or contribute to the patient's symptoms (see Fig. 5.47). The strengths of bone scanning include the sensitive demonstration of bone pathology, such as acute injury (see Fig. 5.48), bone stress reactions, early slipping of the femoral capital epiphysis, enthesopathy (see Fig. 5.49) and bursopathy (see Fig. 5.50).

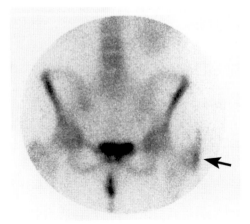

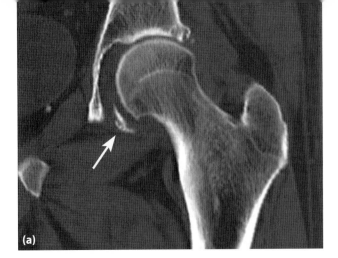

(a)

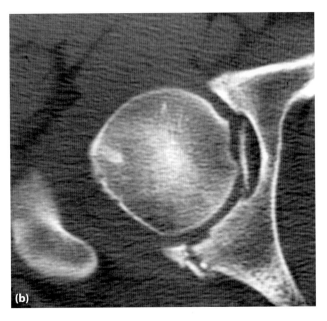

(b)

CT scanning

CT scanning enables the cross-sectional assessment of complex bone and joint anatomy. CT has an important role at the hip joint, where curved surfaces and bony superimposition make assessment of fractures and loose bodies very difficult (see Fig. 5.51). Articular cartilage deficiency can also be accurately evaluated by CT arthrography (see Fig. 5.52). In addition, the complex geometry of the sacroiliac joints is ideally assessed by CT scanning and CT is valuable in the diagnosis of sacroiliitis. CT can also be useful in the diagnosis of osteochondromatosis (see Fig. 5.53).

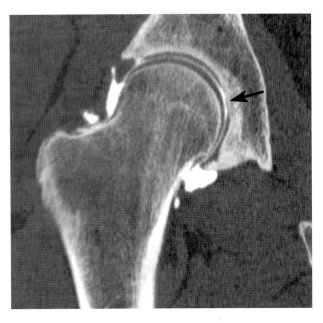

▲ **Fig. 5.51(a)** and **(b)** In two different cases following trauma, CT scanning demonstrates an intra-articular fracture fragment (arrow). In **(b)** there is also a fracture of the posterior lip of the acetabulum.

▲ **Fig. 5.52** Degenerative changes are present with the loss of articular cartilage demonstrated by CT arthrography. Contrast medium occupies the space created by the articular cartilage deficiency (black arrow).

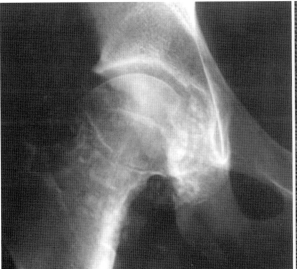

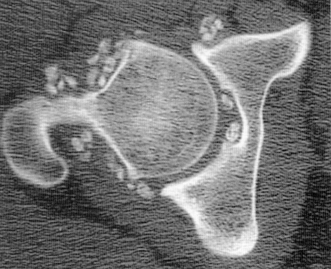

▲ **Fig. 5.53** A CT scan of the hip is valuable for the demonstration of radio-opaque loose bodies or to define osteochondromatosis. A plain film shows numerous calcific densities around the femoral neck and in the acetabular fossa. The 'crushed blue metal' appearance is characteristic of osteochondromatosis. Note the secondary erosions along the femoral neck.

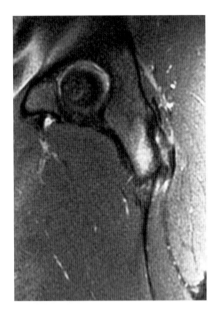

▲ **Fig. 5.54** Enthesopathy at the ischial tuberosity has developed from traction stress of the hamstrings. A sagittal PD-weighted MR image with fat suppression shows high marrow and tendon signal, typical of hamstring enthesopathy, and a complicating partial tear.

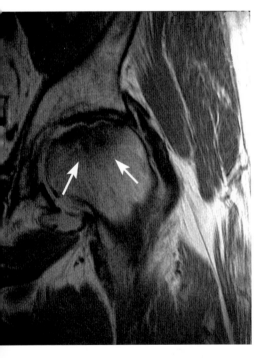

▲ **Fig. 5.55** The changes of femoral head AVN are well demonstrated by MRI. Note the flattening of the femoral head due to bony collapse, and the presence of a mildly serpiginous fluid filled subcortical fracture line. Abnormal marrow signal extends from the weightbearing area (arrows).

MRI

MRI demonstrates abnormal bone marrow changes and at the same time provides a panoramic cross-sectional assessment of complex soft-tissue anatomy. MRI has a useful diagnostic role in many conditions of the pelvis and hip, including enthesopathy (see Fig. 5.54), avascular necrosis (see Fig. 5.55), acetabular labral tears (see Fig. 5.56), hip synovitis (see Fig. 5.57), articular cartilage loss (see Fig. 5.58) and loose bodies (see Fig. 5.59).

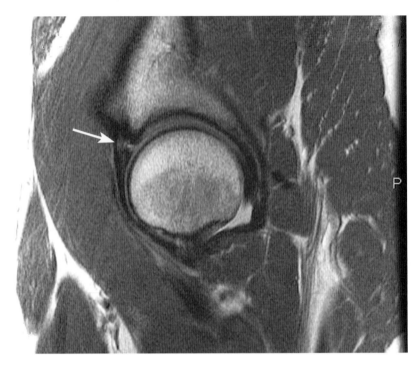

▲ **Fig. 5.56** A non-arthrographic sagittal PD-weighted MR image demonstrates an acetabular labral tear (arrow).

▼ **Fig. 5.57** This STIR coronal MR image shows synovitis in the hip joint. The synovitis is seen as subtle granular hypointensity within a distended hyperintense joint space. Note osteoarthrosis changes involving the hip joint.

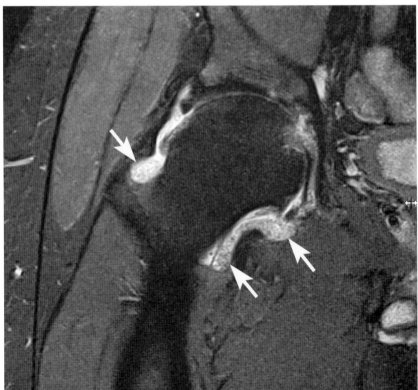

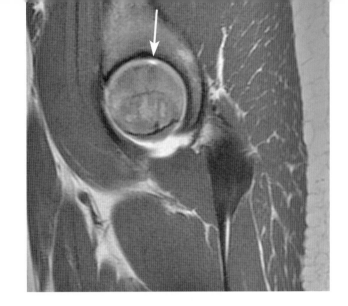

► Fig. 5.58 A small fluid-filled articular cartilaginous deficiency on the femoral head is demonstrated by MRI (arrow). The athlete is 44 years old. This may be a normal variant produced by a development defect in the triradiate cartilage.

▼ Fig. 5.59 An osteochondral fragment separated from the superomedial aspect of the femoral head lies loose within the joint space (arrow). An axial image shows the fracture bed (arrowhead).

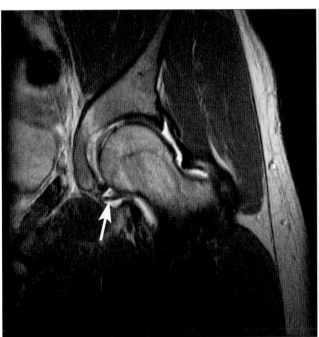

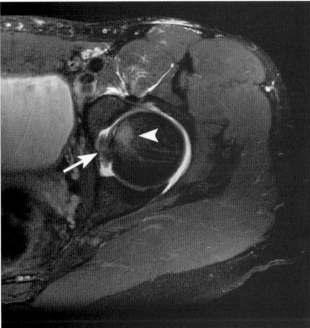

Ultrasound

Ultrasound may be used to assess the major pelvic viscera, detect abnormal fluid collections such as a haematoma following a muscle tear (see Fig. 5.60), demonstrate a hip joint effusion (see Fig. 5.61) and diagnose a paralabral cyst (see Fig. 5.62). In addition, ultrasound is the best method of imaging the scrotum and evaluating injury to the conjoint tendon. Ultrasound also has the unique capability of being able to dynamically assess the inguinal and femoral canals under stress for clinically occult hernias and provides a convenient method of accurately guiding therapeutic injections and aspirations (see Fig. 5.63).

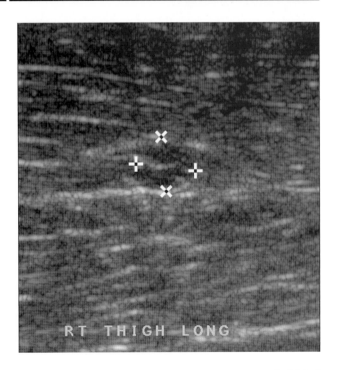

► Fig. 5.60 A small muscle tear is well demonstrated by ultrasound. The tear is defined by callipers.

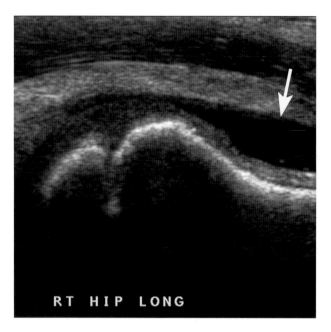

▲ **Fig. 5.61** Ultrasound clearly shows a hip joint effusion in a child, seen as an anechoic space anterior to the femoral neck.

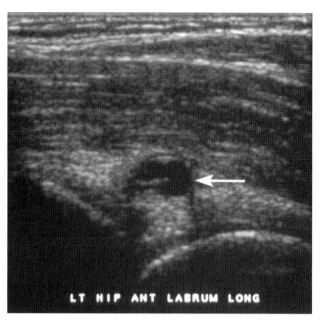

▲ **Fig. 5.62** Long-axis ultrasound image at the anterior aspect of the hip demonstrates a paralabral cyst (arrow).

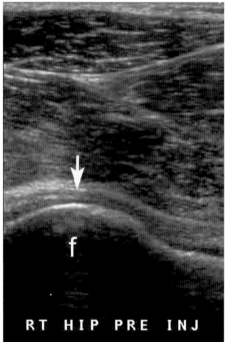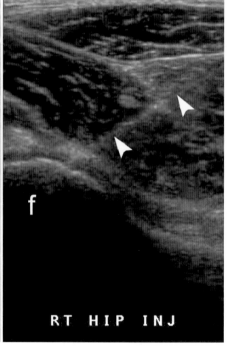

◀ **Fig. 5.63** A hip injection is guided by ultrasound, allowing accurate placement of the needle tip. The needle is identified on the right image (arrowheads). The arrow indicates the echogenic line of the joint capsule. Femoral head = f.

Injuries to the pelvis and hip

Acute bone injury

Major fractures of the pelvis, hip and femur are usually the result of high-energy trauma such as that caused by downhill skiing, waterskiing (see Fig. 5.64) and motor sports. These injuries are well discussed in orthopaedic texts and in general fall outside the field of sports medicine. Our discussion will concentrate on the bony injuries around the pelvis, hip and thigh that are frequently seen in a sports medicine clinic situation.

Avulsion injuries are the most commonly seen acute fractures of the pelvis, occurring in the skeletally immature athlete involving secondary ossification centres, and seen in adults mainly at the hamstring and adductor origins. Apophyseal avulsions are often preceded by a localised ache in the area, which may have been present for some weeks. This suggests that the injury is an acute-on-chronic process, with avulsion occurring at a site of a preceding stress-related apophysitis. Rarely, however, a single strong muscular contraction can avulse a normal apophysis. For example, an avulsion of the apophysis at the ischial tuberosity may result from accidentally doing the 'splits'.

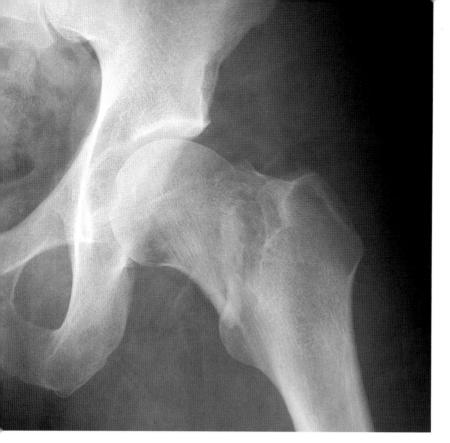

▲ **Fig. 5.64** A waterskier, travelling at high speed, was hit by a wave that violently turned his ski, causing a sudden and forceful external rotation of the hip, and resulting in an oblique fracture of the femoral neck.

Apophyseal avulsions may occur at the following sites:

- *Ischial tuberosity* (see Fig. 5.65) The apophysis of the ischial tuberosity is late in closing. Union usually occurs between 16 and 18 years of age, by which time considerable muscular strength has developed. Maximum hamstring contraction occurs with the hip in flexion and the knee in extension, so, as a consequence, the injury is seen with hurdling, dancing, sprinting and gymnastics. Widely displaced avulsions are prone to non-union and may be associated with exuberant callus formation. Radiographically, this can sometimes be confused with myositis ossificans or a bone tumour (Karlin 1995).

- *ASIS* (see Fig. 5.66) Avulsion of the ASIS is caused by forceful contraction of the sartorius with the hip extended and the knee flexed. This injury classically occurs in sprinters (Khoury et al. 1985). Displacement of the apophysis is usually limited.

▼ **Fig. 5.66** Avulsion of the ASIS (arrowhead) is classically seen in sprinters caused by traction of the sartorius.

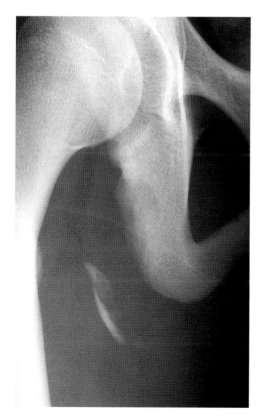

▲ **Fig. 5.65** Avulsion of the apophysis of the ischial tuberosity occurs in adolescent athletes following hamstring traction. The acute avulsion is often superimposed on apophysitis from chronic stress.

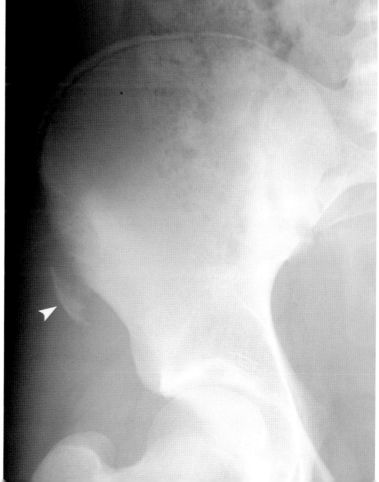

- *AIIS* (see Fig. 5.67) Avulsion of the AIIS occurs as the result of a sudden contraction of the straight head of the rectus femoris. Active hip flexion and knee extension against resistance will reproduce the patient's symptoms. Displacement is invariably minimal and comparison with the other side is sometimes required before making a definite diagnosis. This injury is also seen in sprinters.

- *Iliac crest* (see Fig. 5.68) Avulsion of the iliac crest most commonly presents as a subacute overuse syndrome in runners (Clancy and Foltz 1976). The iliac crest apophysis appears in early adolescence and proceeds to unite from medial to lateral from 14 to 16 years of age. Acute avulsions may result from sudden contraction of the lower abdominal muscles against a fixed planted leg, such as may occur in baseball batting and pitching. Symptoms are produced by abdominal contraction or hip abduction. Separation of the iliac crest may also result from direct trauma.

- *Lesser trochanter* (see Fig. 5.69) A forceful contraction of the iliopsoas muscle with active hip flexion may avulse the apophysis of the lesser trochanter. Clinically, the symptoms are reproduced by resisted hip flexion.

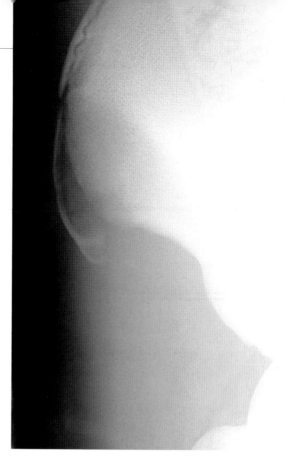

▲ **Fig. 5.68** An iliac crest avulsion is usually a subacute overuse injury in adolescent runners. In this case, forceful traction by the tensor fascia lata and sartorius together has caused avulsion of the anterior segment of the iliac crest apophysis.

▼ **Fig. 5.67** Avulsion of the AIIS (arrowhead) is usually an acute-on-chronic injury. Changes of apophysitis are invariably present. Displacement of the fragment is always limited by an intact reflected head.

▼ **Fig. 5.69** A lesser trochanter apophyseal avulsion has occurred following a forceful iliopsoas contraction.

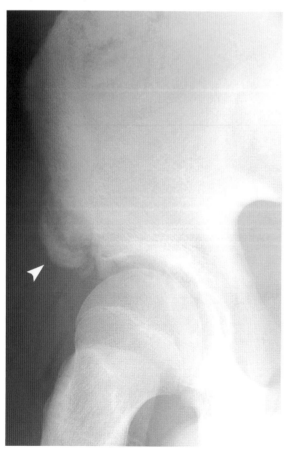

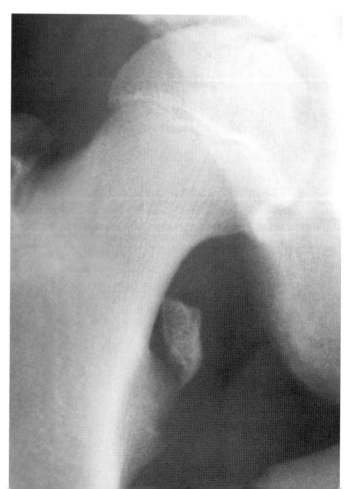

Chronic bone injury

The majority of sports-related injuries around the hip and pelvis result from overuse. In skeletally immature athletes, repetitive forces producing a stress reaction at developing centres of ossification manifest as an apophysitis when involving an apophysis, and as osteochondrosis when involving an epiphysis. At the hip joint, slipping of the femoral capital epiphysis may occur when the growth plate is involved.

In mature athletes, bone stress reactions and stress fractures can cause chronic pain and disability. Stress fractures occur in the femoral neck, pelvis, sacrum and femoral diaphysis. In athletes, the most common conditions causing chronic pain in the pelvis and hips are groin strain and hip joint osteoarthrosis. A more extensive list of causes of chronic groin pain is shown in Table 5.1 on page 328.

Apophysitis

The term 'apophysitis' refers to an acquired condition of pain arising from repetitive traction forces at an apophysis. This process is not uncommon around the pelvis, particularly involving the ischial tuberosity apophysis. Initially, there is apophyseal demineralisation, presumably resulting from locally increased vascularity in response to repetitive stress. At this stage enthesopathy is present (see Figs 5.70 and 5.71). Progression produces irregularity, sclerosis and apophyseal fragmentation, changes that suggest an avascular process (see Fig. 5.72). Healing and remodelling then occur (see Fig. 5.73). Care should be taken in the interpretation of these radiographic signs, as there is considerable variation in the appearance of normal apophyses. For example, discontinuity of the iliac crest apophysis is a normal variation (Lombardo et al. 1983). Comparison with the apophysis on the asymptomatic side is helpful.

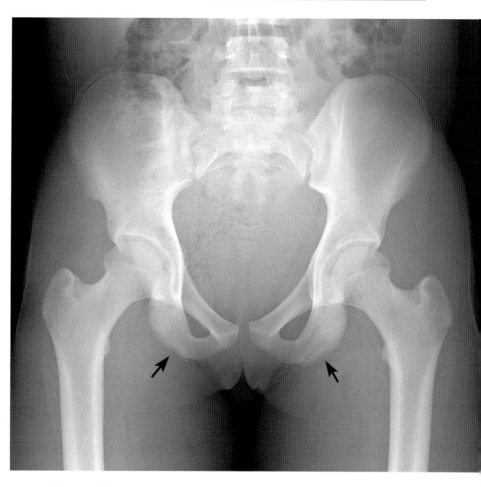

▲ **Fig. 5.70** Early bilateral changes of ischial tuberosity apophysitis are present, with minor bony resorption and loss of definition of the ischial apophyses (arrows).

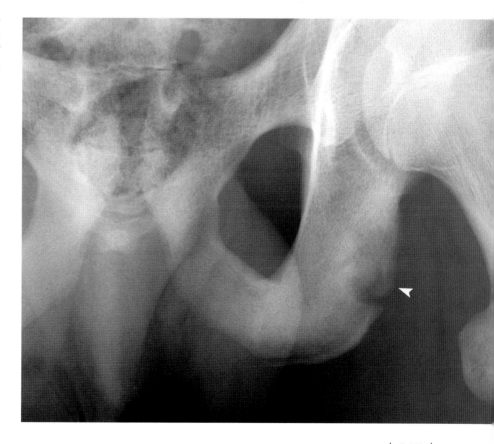

▶ **Fig. 5.71** Demineralisation is developing at the ischial tuberosity apophysis (arrowhead). This is early radiological evidence of apophysitis.

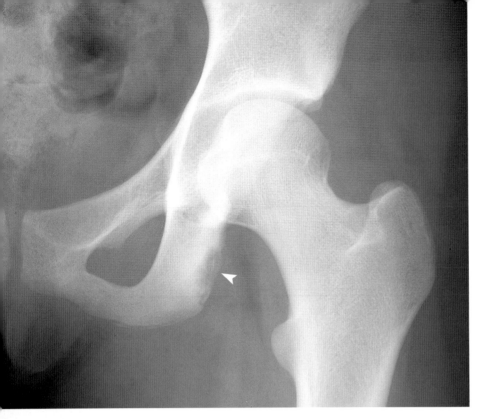

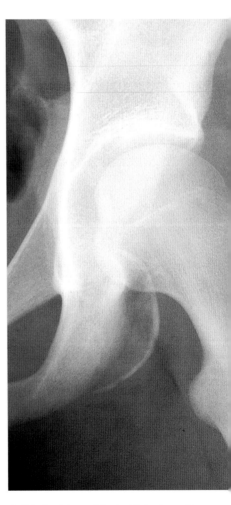

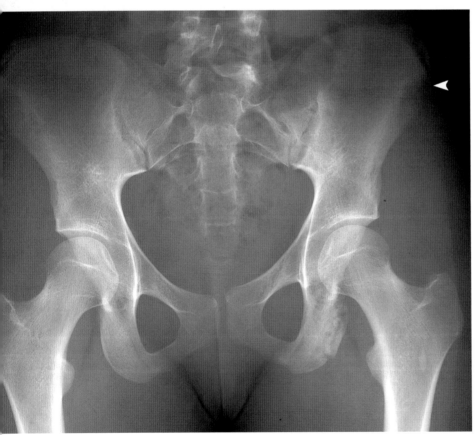

▶**Fig. 5.72** A more advanced stage of apophysitis is present. There is considerable localised demineralisation at the bone/tendon interface (arrowhead) and surrounding sclerosis indicates an attempted healing response. Note the fragmentation of the apophysis.

▲ **Fig. 5.73(a)** Late-stage apophysitis is present at the left ischial tuberosity. Healing is progressing with persisting residual deformity. In addition, there is acute apophysitis involving the ASIS, with bony resorption and deformity of the outer end of the iliac crest apophysis (arrowhead). Slight rotation of the left hemi-pelvis has occurred as a result of an old high-velocity trauma. This has produced asymmetry at the symphysis and widening of the left sacroiliac joint. A bone island is noted in the left subtrochanteric region and both hips show minor dysplastic features. Note the similarity of this case with the case shown in Fig. 5.1 on page 286.

▲ **(b)** Avulsion of the ischial tuberosity apophysis has occurred secondary to pre-existing apophysitis. The athlete had complained of an ache in this area for weeks preceding the avulsion.

Stress fractures of the femoral neck

Athletes with stress fractures of the femoral neck usually present with groin pain of gradual onset, although sometimes pain is referred to the thigh or knee. The pain is worse with weightbearing and is further exacerbated by running. Failure to make an early diagnosis can be devastating, as progression to complete fracture may occur, which carries a risk of serious complications such as avascular necrosis, non-union or malunion in coxa vara.

As a consequence of the offset transmission of force through the femoral angle, normal loading at the hip joint causes compressive stress along the inner concave margin of the femoral neck and tensile stress along the outer margin of the neck. Devas (1965) classified femoral neck stress fractures as compressive and transverse (or distraction).

Compressive fractures are seen in younger athletes and result from activities requiring repetitive stress on the lower limb. Radiographically, these appear as poorly defined areas of sclerosis on the medial side of the neck (see Fig. 5.74). The chance of healing with conservative treatment is reduced if a lucent zone of resorption develops within the sclerotic area (see Fig. 5.75). Progress radiographs are important for the assessment of fracture healing.

Transverse (or distraction) fractures tend to occur in older athletes and develop on the lateral tension side of the femoral neck (see Fig. 5.76). These fractures are seen as subtle lucent lines that occur at 90° to the stress trabeculae in this region. If diagnosis and treatment are delayed, transverse stress fractures are particularly prone to progression and non-union (see Fig. 5.77).

▼ **Fig. 5.74** A compressive-side femoral neck stress fracture is demonstrated by plain film. Periosteal new bone is present (arrow).

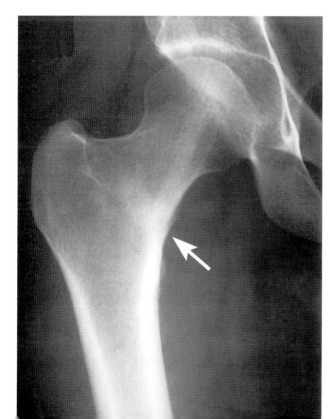

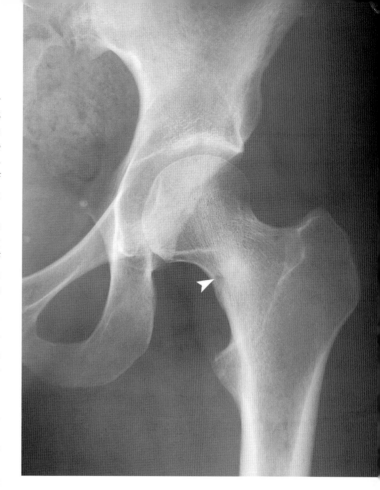

▲ **Fig. 5.75** A plain film of a compressive-side stress fracture shows a small area of bony resorption (arrowhead). This is a poor prognostic sign.

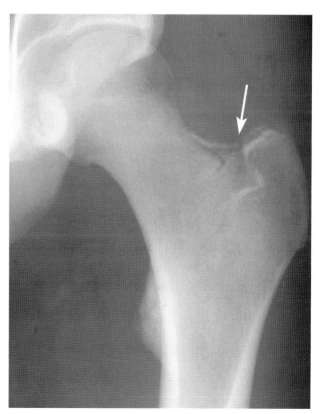

▲ **Fig. 5.76** A plain film demonstrates a distraction-side femoral neck stress fracture (arrow).

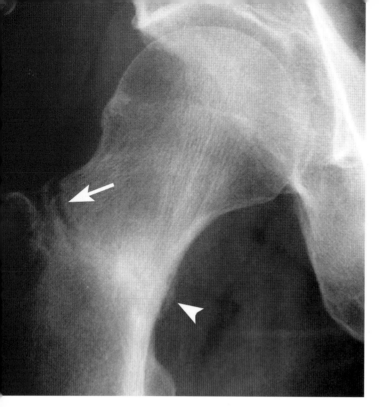

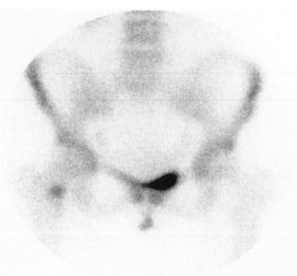

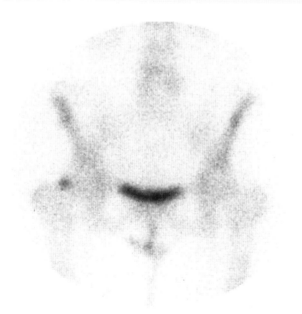

◀**Fig. 5.77** This distraction-side femoral neck stress fracture has a chronic appearance with well-defined margins (arrow). Changes of sclerosis extend across the neck with periosteal new bone present on the compressive side of the neck (arrowhead). These changes are consistent with the imminent progression to a complete fracture and probable displacement.

Imaging begins with a plain film series including an AP pelvis and lateral hip on the symptomatic side. Plain films may be negative for up to three weeks after symptoms commence, so if the plain films are negative and clinical suspicion persists, an early isotope bone scan (see Figs. 5.78 and Fig. 5.79) is mandatory. MRI would appear to be more accurate than bone scanning in the detection of femoral neck stress fractures (Shin et al. 1996). There are reports of both false positive (Shin et al. 1996) and false negative nuclear bone scan results (Keene and Lash 1992; Sterling et al. 1993). An MR image of an established stress fracture will show considerable associated bone marrow oedema (see Figs 5.80 and 5.81).

◀**Fig. 5.78** A nuclear bone scan shows the characteristic appearance of a stress fracture on the compressive side of the right femoral neck.

Stress fractures of the pubic rami

Stress fractures of the pubic rami are relatively uncommon. The cause of this type of stress fracture is unknown, although some authors (Latshaw et al. 1981; Pavlov et al. 1982) believe that repetitive stress at the muscular attachments to the ramus is responsible. This injury is seen most often in female middle- and long-distance runners, in whom osteopaenia may be present. As a result, bone densitometry is an important adjunct to management.

◀**Fig. 5.79** A nuclear bone scan shows a distraction-side stress fracture on the superior aspect of the right femoral neck.

The athlete usually presents with groin pain, which is worse with activity. Noakes et al. (1985) noted that if an athlete is unable to stand on one leg on the affected side without assistance, this is suggestive of a stress fracture of the pubic ramus.

As with all stress fractures, early plain films may be negative. A nuclear bone scan will more reliably demonstrate diagnostic changes and follow-up plain films can then be used to confirm the stress fracture (see Figs 5.82

▶ **Fig. 5.80** A coronal T1-weighted image (top) and a corresponding fat-suppressed T2-weighted image (bottom) demonstrate a femoral neck stress fracture (arrow).

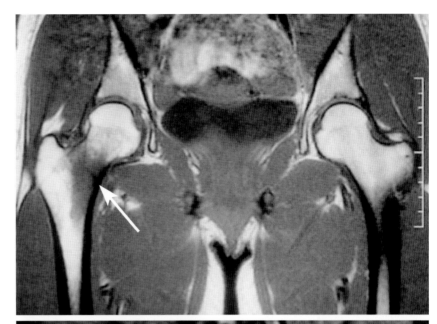

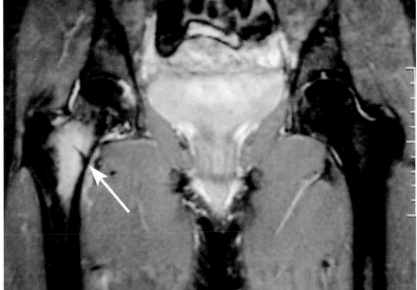

and 5.83). Alternatively, MRI may be helpful in establishing the diagnosis in difficult cases (see Fig. 5.84). An unusual example of a stress fracture in Figs 5.85 and 5.86 shows extension of the fracture line across both the superior and inferior pubic rami. This pattern suggests that muscular imbalance has occurred around this axis. Also, an occasional association between pubic ramus stress fractures and osteitis pubis suggests that forces responsible for a stress fracture may also cause osteitis pubis (see Fig. 5.87). Complete separation of the entire ramus may occur (see Fig. 5.88).

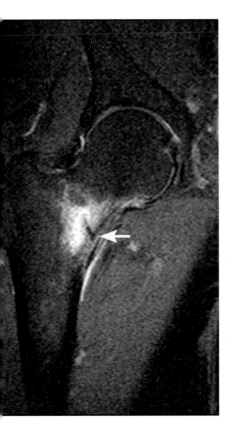

◀ **Fig. 5.81** This coronal fat-suppressed MR image demonstrates considerable high signal representing marrow oedema and localised periosteal reaction associated with a femoral neck stress fracture (arrow).

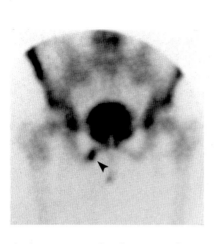

▲ **Fig. 5.82** A nuclear bone scan shows increased uptake of isotope towards the medial end of the inferior pubic ramus at the characteristic site of a stress fracture of the inferior pubic ramus (arrowhead).

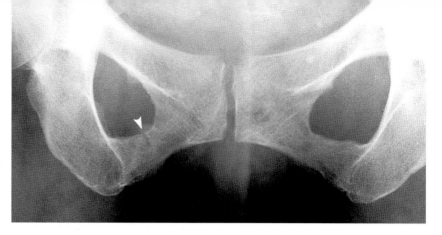

▲ **Fig. 5.83** Following the bone scan shown in Fig. 5.82, a plain film shows a lucent line of an incomplete stress fracture involving the inferior pubic ramus of the pelvis at a site characteristic of this injury (arrowhead). Note the associated periosteal reaction.

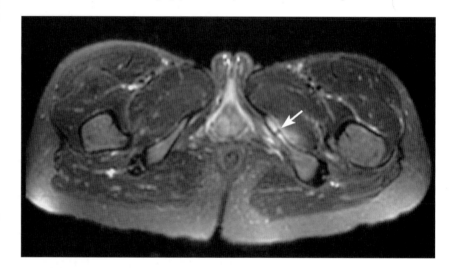

▶ **Fig. 5.84** An MR image demonstrates a stress fracture of the left inferior pubic ramus with associated oedema (arrow).

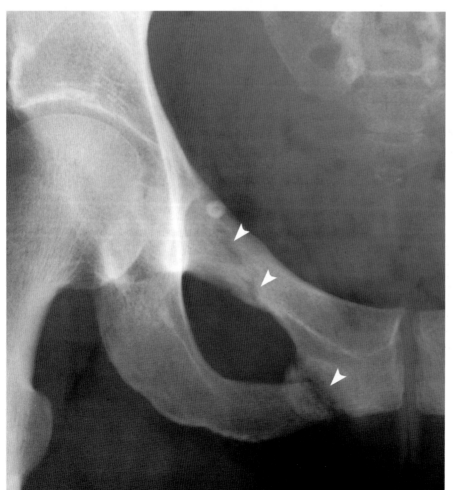

◀ **Fig. 5.85** This interesting case shows stress fractures of both the superior (arrowheads) and inferior pubic rami. These stress fractures are aligned, suggesting that forces on the ischial tuberosity and the superior pubic ramus act to generate a line of continuous stress along the axis of the fractures.

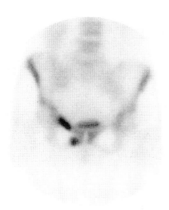

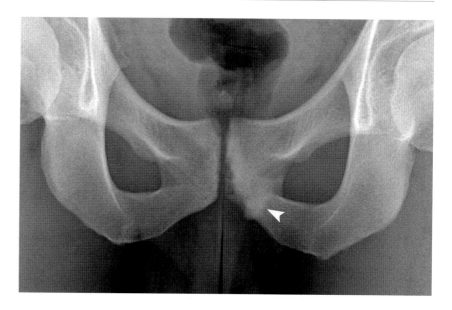

▲ **Fig. 5.86** A nuclear bone scan of the case from Fig. 5.85 shows corresponding increased uptake of isotope in both the superior and inferior pubic rami along the path of both fractures.

▲ **Fig. 5.87** A stress fracture of the inferior pubic ramus (arrowhead) coexists with adjacent osteitis pubis, suggesting that these changes may result from the same stress mechanism.

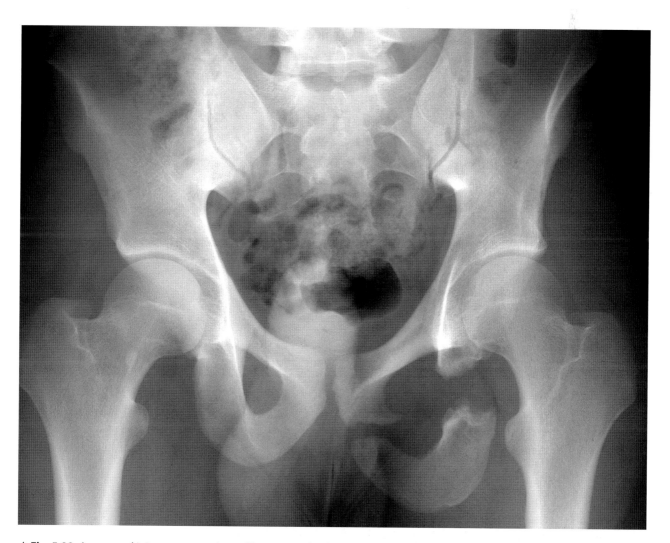

▲ **Fig. 5.88** An unusual injury was experienced by a young footballer, resulting in the separation of the entire inferior pubic ramus. The appearance of the bone ends suggests that the injury is acute-on-chronic and that underlying stress fractures had been present. A forceful hamstring contraction has presumably delivered the final blow.

Stress fractures of the femoral shaft

Stress fractures of the femoral shaft occur in long-distance runners, who usually present with a poorly localised ache. Clinically, the symptoms can be reproduced by stressing the femoral shaft with downward pressure on the knee as the patient sits with their leg hanging over the side of a couch. These stress fractures can occur at any level of the shaft (see Figs 5.89 and 5.90). Progression to complete fracture most often occurs at supracondylar stress fracture sites (see Fig. 5.91).

Plain film changes of periosteal new bone formation occur late (see Fig. 5.92). Nuclear bone scans (see Fig. 5.93(a)) and MRI (see Fig. 5.93(b)) are diagnostic early in the process.

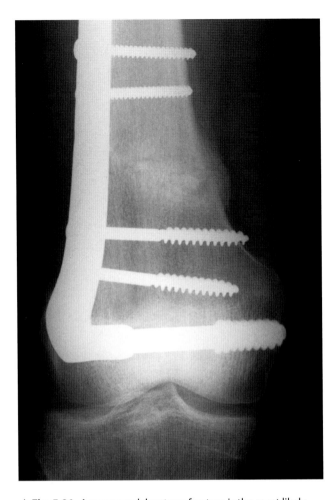

▲ **Fig. 5.91** A supracondylar stress fracture is the most likely femoral stress fracture to progress to a complete fracture. This young footballer chose to ignore pain in the supracondylar region.

▼ **Fig. 5.92** A periosteal reaction on the medial aspect of the mid-shaft of the femoral shaft appeared well after the diagnosis had been established by a bone scan.

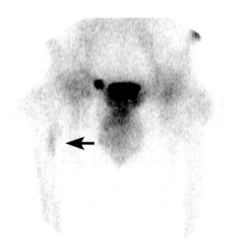

▲ **Fig. 5.89** A nuclear bone scan demonstrates a periosteal reaction due to bone stress on the medial aspect of the subtrochanteric region of the femur (arrow).

▲ **Fig. 5.90** Femoral stress fractures can occur at any level. A nuclear bone scan indicates the presence of a mid-shaft stress fracture.

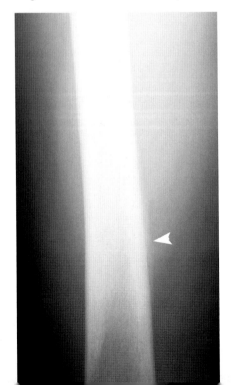

Sacral stress fractures

Sacral stress fractures occur in young runners who train and compete over long distances. The associated sclerotic changes are difficult to see on plain films (see Fig. 5.94) and a nuclear bone scan (see Fig. 5.95) will more reliably detect this injury if there is clinical or radiographic suspicion of a sacral stress fracture. A CT scan or MRI may then further define and characterise the changes (see Figs 5.96, 5.97 and 5.98).

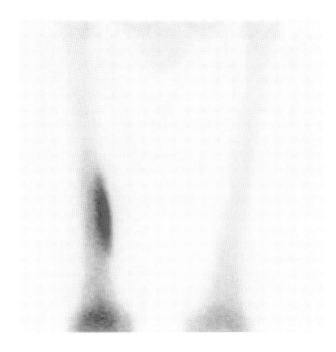

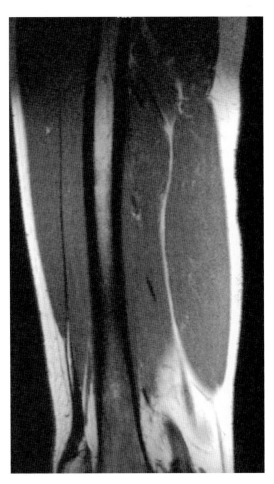

▲ **Fig. 5.93(a)** A nuclear bone scan shows the uptake of isotope that is typical of a stress fracture on the medial aspect of the femur at the junction of its middle and distal thirds.
▶ **(b)** A sagittal T1-weighted MR image shows loss of the normal marrow signal at the junction of the middle and distal thirds of the femoral shaft. There is also thickening of the cortex in this area, a manifestation of the chronic nature of a stress fracture.

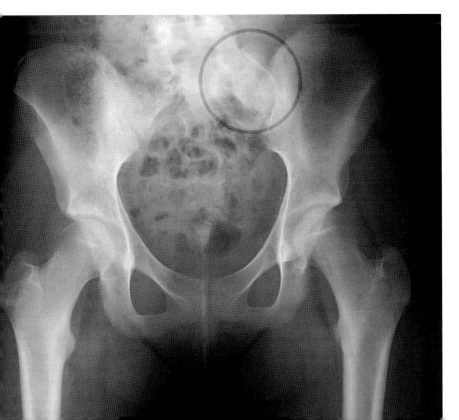

◀**Fig. 5.94** A plain film shows sclerosis associated with a stress fracture involving the left sacral wing in a 14-year-old long-distance runner. The sclerosis (circled) is difficult to appreciate.

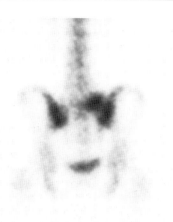

▲ **Fig. 5.95** In the same patient as shown in Fig. 5.94 on page 325, a nuclear bone scan demonstrated corresponding increased uptake of isotope in the left sacral wing.

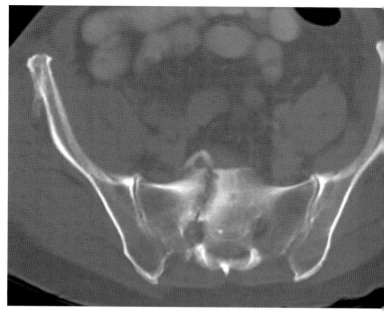

▲ **Fig. 5.97** In another patient a stress fracture of the right sacral wing is well demonstrated by a CT scan.

▼ **Fig. 5.98** A coronal fat-suppressed MR image demonstrates an incomplete stress fracture involving the left wing of the sacrum. Note the associated marrow oedema.

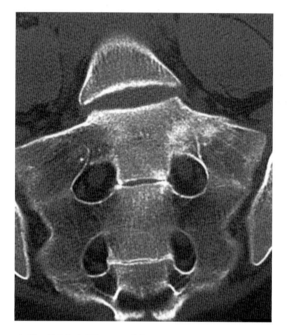

▲ **Fig. 5.96** A CT scan of the patient from Fig. 5.94 shows a stress fracture of the left sacral ala. The fracture is incomplete.

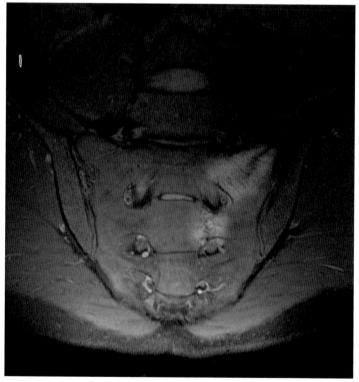

Thigh 'splints'

Thigh 'splints' is a syndrome of regional pain resulting from chronic bone stress, which has a characteristic appearance on both plain films (see Fig. 5.99) and nuclear bone scanning. Invariably there has been excessive and repetitive stress applied to the femur, usually due to faulty athletic technique. There is generally an increase in isotope uptake along the femoral cortex (see Fig. 5.100).

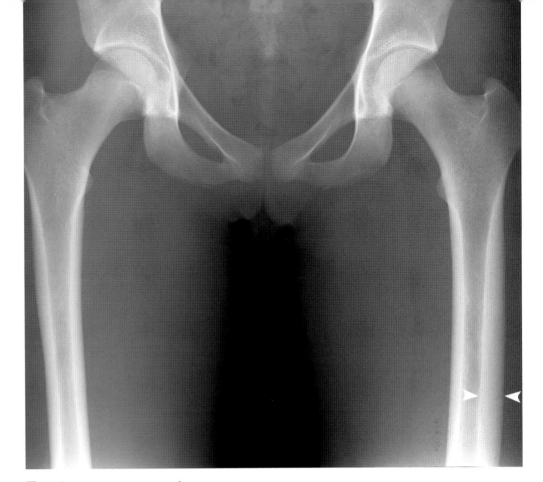

▶ **Fig. 5.99(a)**
A plain film of the pelvis and femora demonstrates a diffuse thickening of the lateral cortex of the left femur when compared with the right. The athlete was a national-level high jumper with a faulty technique, and presented with a constant ache in the left thigh following jumping.

▼ **(b)** The left side is the take-off leg.

▼ **(c)** The appearance on a nuclear bone scan is typical of a 'splint'.

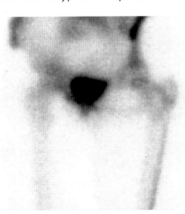

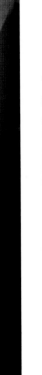

▼ **Fig. 5.100** These bone scans of another athlete complaining of thigh 'splints' show a more localised pattern of isotope uptake. **(a)** Frontal view **(b)** Lateral view

(a)

(b)

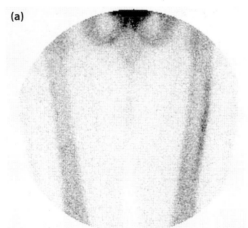

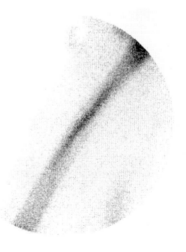

'Groin strain'

'Groin strain' is a general term encompassing the clinical presentation of a number of conditions that may cause chronic groin pain in athletes. The differential diagnosis is extensive (see Table 5.1). Although the various musculoskeletal causes of groin pain may occur in isolation, they may be difficult to differentiate on clinical grounds alone and very frequently coexist. The most frequently encountered are osteitis pubis, conjoint tendon injury, adductor tendon injury, rectus abdominis injury and groin hernias. Less common musculoskeletal sources of groin pain include obturator nerve entrapment and injury to the external oblique.

Table 5.1 Causes of chronic groin pain (abbreviated)

Musculotendinous	Osteitis pubis
	Adductor enthesopathy or tendinopathy
	Sports hernia
	Iliopsoas tendinopathy
	Rectus femoris strain or avulsion
	Rectus abdominis strain or tendinopathy
Bony	Stress fracture of the femoral neck
	Stress fracture of the pubic ramus
Joint	Hip osteoarthritis
	Labral tear
	Femoroacetabular impingement
	T12–L1 pathology
	Sacroiliitis
Nerve entrapment	Ilioinguinal nerve
	Obturator nerve
Genitourinary	Prostatitis
	Epididymitis
	Salpingitis

Groin strain is common and may be career-limiting at any level of sport. Groin strain most commonly occurs in high-impact loading, multidirectional sports such as endurance running, ice hockey and kicking sports like soccer, Australian Rules football, rugby and the martial arts. Groin strain is poorly understood and difficult to diagnose and treat. When multiple injuries simultaneously contribute to symptoms, the failure rate of treatment is high and this is the case with groin strain. The overview presented here is a synthesis of the available published data and the authors' opinions based on clinical experience.

Osteitis pubis

The pubic symphysis is a fibrocartilaginous joint of identical design and construction to the intervertebral discs of the spine. An interpubic disc of fibrocartilage attaches firmly to a thin layer of hyaline cartilage that coats the articular cortex of the joint. The joint capsule is thin and weak both posteriorly and superiorly, but thick and strong inferiorly and anteriorly, where several layers of obliquely oriented fibres decussate and blend with the interlacing sheet-like fibres formed from extensions of the rectus abdominis, conjoint, external oblique and medial adductor tendons.

The pubic symphysis undergoes age- and trauma-related degenerative changes identical to those observed at disc spaces of the spine. As the interpubic disc degenerates, MRI may show features such as joint space narrowing, extrusion and injury of the disc together with subarticular marrow abnormalities including oedema, sclerosis, cyst formation and fatty replacement. Symphyseal joints in both the spine and the pelvis are particularly vulnerable to rotational and shear stresses and it is these exact forces that occur repetitively in kicking sports. The symphysis may be injured either through an isolated high-energy traumatic event (which causes a sudden tear of the interpubic disc, see Fig. 5.101) or by chronic repetitive low-level trauma that

▼ **Fig. 5.101(a)** MR images demonstrate a traumatic rupture of the interpubic disc sustained in a motor vehicle accident 17 months prior to the examination. The tear of the disc is shown as linear high signal (arrows), which involves the full length of the interpubic disc and extends into the left conjoint insertional complex (arrowheads). Marrow oedema is associated with enthesopathy caused by the left conjoint tendon injury.

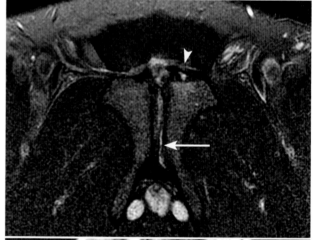

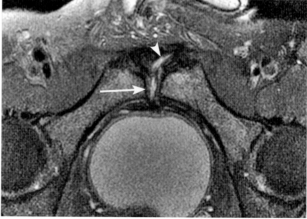

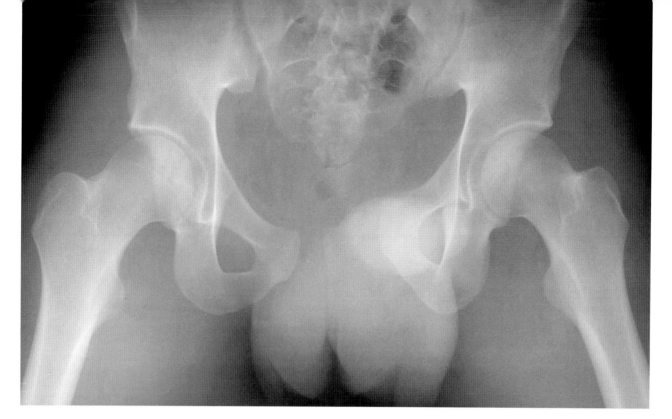

(b) A stockman suffered a complete disruption of the symphysis when his horse was spooked by a feral pig. The pig caused the horse to buck and the stockman experienced a violent groin impact against the saddle. The right sacroiliac joint is also disrupted.

leads to accelerated disc degeneration and an eventual chronic attritional tear. In either scenario, a loss of discal strength or thickness may result in pelvic instability, and this in turn may lead to repetitive mechanical overload of the adjacent supporting soft-tissue structures, producing secondary tendinopathy and tendon tears.

In the characteristic clinical presentation of osteitis pubis, the patient is a male athlete who complains of a gradual onset of central groin pain aggravated by impact-loading activities such as running and kicking. The pain is poorly localised, possibly radiating superiorly into the rectus abdominis, inferiorly into the adductor muscles and often into the scrotum. On physical examination, there may be tenderness over the symphyseal region, with pain produced by both passive adductor stretch and resisted adductor contraction. There is often a restricted range of rotation of one or both hips, the mechanism of which is unclear.

Imaging may include plain films, nuclear bone scans, MRI and ultrasound. The diagnostic features of plain films include cortical erosion along one or both sides of the symphysis in the acute stage, with surrounding sclerosis developing as the process becomes chronic. 'Flamingo' radiographs may be helpful if the routine views are negative, and may confirm the presence of pelvic macroinstability (see Fig. 5.102). This test is often non-contributory, being insensitive to the more common microinstabilities.

▼ **Fig. 5.102** Flamingo views demonstrate macroinstability of the pelvis. The left image was obtained with weightbearing on the left leg, and the right image with the patient standing on their right leg. Changes of osteitis pubis are present, more marked on the right where a subchondral cyst (arrowhead) is also evident. Significant movement of greater than 2 mm has occurred at the symphysis, confirming the clinical suspicion of instability.

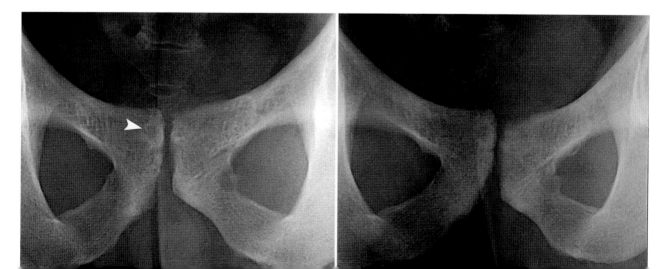

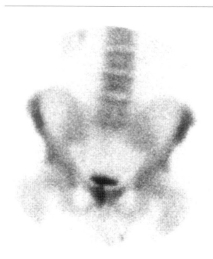

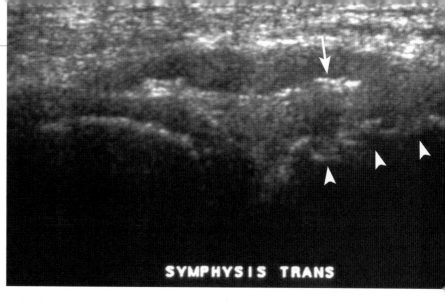

▲ **Fig. 5.103(a)** Osteitis pubis is demonstrated by a nuclear bone scan. Increased isotope uptake is bilateral but asymmetrical, being more marked on the right. Characteristically there is a wide distribution of pubic bone uptake, extending well lateral from the immediate subarticular zone.

▲ **(b)** A transverse ultrasound image shows left conjoint tendon enthesopathy, which may be associated with osteitis pubis. The left conjoint tendon is thickened (arrow) and there is associated marked irregularity of the enthesial bone surface (arrowheads). This bone reaction contributes to the wide lateral distribution of isotope uptake seen on bone scans. The right side is included for comparison and appears normal.

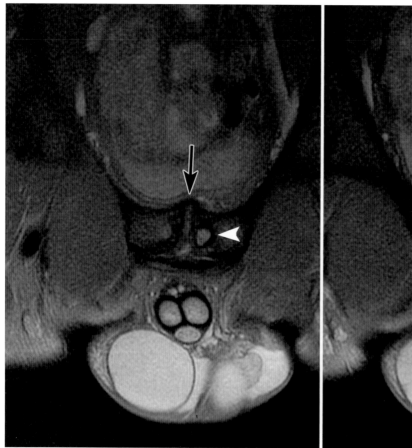
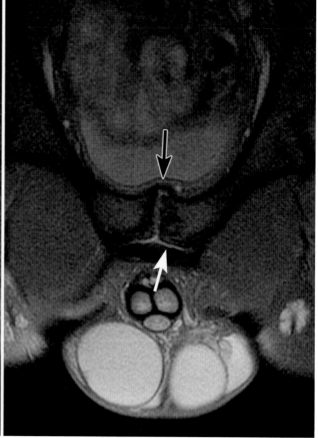

▲ **Fig. 5.104** Short-axis coronal fat-suppressed PD-weighted MR images show predominantly degenerative changes at the symphysis, including articular cortical irregularity, subchondral sclerosis, subchondral cyst formation (white arrowhead) and posterior disc extrusion (black arrows). There is only a minimal degree of patchy subarticular marrow oedema to suggest 'active' osteitis, but note the presence of thin high-intensity fluid lines (white arrow) extending from the anterior margin of the symphysis along the parasymphyseal aspects of both adductor origins, consistent with 'tenoperiosteal' junction tears due to shear stresses associated with pelvic microinstability.

A nuclear bone scan may show increased isotope uptake in the body of pubis that can be either unilateral or bilateral. In sports-related injuries, even though the uptake is bilateral, the appearance is invariably asymmetrical, being more marked on the symptomatic side. The distribution of isotope uptake at the pubic bone is typically wide, reaching well lateral to the joint and consistent with pubic enthesopathy at the adductor and conjoint tendon attachments (see Fig. 5.103). This fits well with a hypothesis of pelvic instability as the primary underlying problem, and accounts for the clinical observation of multiple coexisting pathologies as a common occurrence. Changes consistent with enthesopathy are often seen on a variety of imaging tests, with sclerotic changes present on plain films, irregularity of the enthesial bone surface demonstrated by ultrasound and tendon/bone changes apparent on MRI (see Fig. 5.104).

The primary MRI findings in osteitis pubis are those of degenerative disease at the symphysis occurring in athletes less than 35 years of age, with secondary changes often seen at the adjacent tendon attachments. Changes at the symphysis include subchondral marrow abnormalities, which are identical to the vertebral endplate changes first reported by Modic et al. (1988) as a feature of degenerative disc disease in the spine (see Fig. 5.105(a)). Symptoms of osteitis pubis are generally present when the marrow changes include areas of low T1 and high T2 signal (Modic Type 1 change) (see Fig. 5.105(b)). In the spine, these marrow changes have been shown to correspond to disruption and fissuring of the endplate, vascular granulation tissue sprouting into the bone marrow, and reactive woven bone with thickened trabeculae, prominent osteoclasts and osteoblasts (Modic et al. 1988). Other investigators (Schmid et al. 2004) have also shown that disc extrusions in the spine frequently contain fragments of hyaline cartilage, which can only have arisen from a mechanism of endplate avulsion, and that there is an association between endplate signal abnormality and the amount of chondral material.

When extrapolated to osteitis pubis, these observations would suggest similar underlying mechanisms of avulsion fracturing at the osteochondral junction and degenerative chondral fissuring due to shear stresses across the joint as the source of osteitis. Consequently, signal changes observed in the subchondral marrow may reflect a combination of oedema due to avulsion injury and granulation tissue associated with chondral fissuring. Lovell et al. (2006) have shown that an MRI finding of marrow oedema at the symphysis may be an asymptomatic physiological stress response in young footballers, so it is important to note that an MRI finding of marrow oedema alone may not be clinically significant.

▲ **Fig. 5.105(a)** Long-axis coronal T1 and fat-suppressed T2-weighted MR images of the symphysis pubis demonstrate subarticular marrow changes, including areas of sclerosis (black arrow), fatty change (Modic Type 2 signal abnormality identified by white arrowheads) and osteitis (Modic Type 1 signal abnormality identified by white arrows).

Ultrasound has limited sensitivity for the diagnosis of osteitis pubis, but is nevertheless strongly suggestive whenever distinct irregularity of articular cortex is detected along one or both sides of the symphysis in young athletes (under 35 years of age) (see Fig. 5.105(c)).

▼ **(b)** This case of symptomatic osteitis pubis clearly demonstrates the cardinal MRI feature of active osteitis (Modic Type 1 signal abnormality) involving the subarticular marrow spaces. Note that the abnormality is bilateral but asymmetrical.

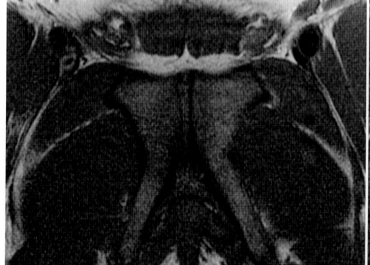
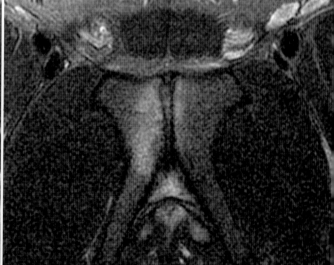

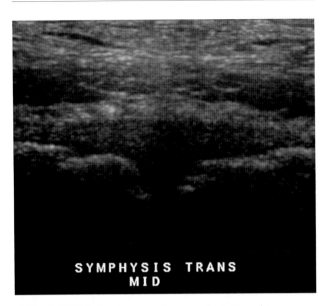

▲ **Fig. 5.105(c)** An ultrasound image of osteitis pubis demonstrates marked irregularity of the articular cortex along both sides of the symphysis.

Tendinopathy and tendon tear

Chronic groin pain may be due to tendon pathology. These cases may present with a history of acute trauma suggesting a musculotendinous tear, or with a more chronic presentation of tendinopathy that often accompanies osteitis pubis as discussed above. The tendons most frequently involved are the conjoint, adductor longus and rectus abdominis. Symptoms of chronic tendinopathy may include pain at rest, initial stiffness that reduces after 'warming up', pain during exercise and stiffness after exercise. Localised tenderness may be present. In most cases, the cause of chronic groin pain following acute tears is presumably an ongoing secondary tendinopathy. In the case of conjoint tendon tears, the development of a secondary 'sports hernia' may alternatively be responsible.

Conjoint tendon injury

The conjoint tendon is a thin, flat structure that attaches at the pubic crest and is formed from the fused inferior fibres of the internal oblique and transversus abdominis. The rectus abdominis also blends with the more superficial fibres of the conjoint tendon and for practical convenience may be regarded as an integral part of the 'conjoint insertional complex'. Overuse associated with repeated contraction of the abdominal muscles, as may occur in gymnastics, kicking sports and sit-ups, may result in conjoint insertion tendinopathy or partial tear. The pain may radiate superiorly into the rectus abdominis or superolaterally along the line of the internal oblique and transversus abdominis. Importantly, conjoint tendon pain may be indistinguishable from that of an inguinal hernia and, to potentially confuse the clinical assessment even further, is often reproduced by coughing and sneezing.

Ultrasound demonstrates the thin and obliquely oriented long-axis fibres of the conjoint tendon quite well, whereas MRI

can only discretely identify the pubic crest insertion of the conjoint tendon on sagittal-plane imaging. The sonographic signs of conjoint insertion tendinopathy may include tendon swelling, heterogeneous hypoechoic echotexture, enthesial bone surface irregularity, intrasubstance calcification and localised tenderness to probing (see Fig. 5.106(a)). MRI may show thickening, mildly increased tendon signal and increased enthesial marrow signal. Tendon tears are not often demonstrated but, when present, they may be appreciated on ultrasound either as linearly marginated interruptions of fibril continuity or, more commonly, as bony avulsions at the pubic crest (see Fig. 5.106(b)). MRI shows most tears as high signal lines at the tenoperiosteal junction, typically extending into the symphysis when background changes of osteitis pubis are present (see Fig. 5.107). Relative atrophy of the lower rectus abdominus muscle belly can be an indirect indicator of a previous conjoint insertion tear. Real-time ultrasound guidance can be used to inject the relevant peritendon spaces in cases of chronic conjoint insertion tendinopathy.

Adductor tendon injury

Adductor origin tendinopathy or partial tear is probably the most frequent cause of chronic groin pain in athletes involved in sports such as soccer, other football codes, fencing, horse riding, ice hockey, skating, skiing and hurdles. Symptoms of tendinopathy usually have a gradual onset. Of the adductor group, the adductor longus is the most commonly affected, but the adductor brevis and the gracilis may also be involved either in isolation or in combination. Pain usually localises to the pubic tubercle region but may radiate inferiorly along the anteromedial thigh. On physical examination, there is localised tenderness over the pubic tubercle, and pain is elicited by both passive adductor stretch and resisted adduction. Radiographs occasionally show associated adductor calcification, but this is much more commonly appreciated on ultrasound, because the overlying pubic bone obscures the x-ray change in most cases. Ultrasound is a reliable means of demonstrating adductor origin tendinopathy. However, MRI is more sensitive and accurate for the detection and characterisation of tendon tears.

Similar patterns of tear are observed on both MRI and ultrasound. These include:

- *Insertional tears*, which involve the tendon/bone junction (see Fig. 5.108(a)) and comprise either transversely oriented defects that typically complicate osteitis pubis and extend into the symphyseal cleft, or longitudinal intrasubstance lines that more typically complicate chronic tendinopathy and may or may not extend into the symphysis.

- *Musculotendinous junction tears*, which occur a little more distally at the level of the musculotendinous junction.

Transverse tenoperiosteal tear components can be relatively inconspicuous on ultrasound and are sometimes difficult to appreciate. On ultrasound, tears are visualised either as linearly marginated and heterogeneously hypoechoic gaps in fibre continuity or, more commonly, as intrasubstance lines of mixed hypo- and hyperechogenicity (see Fig. 5.108(b)).

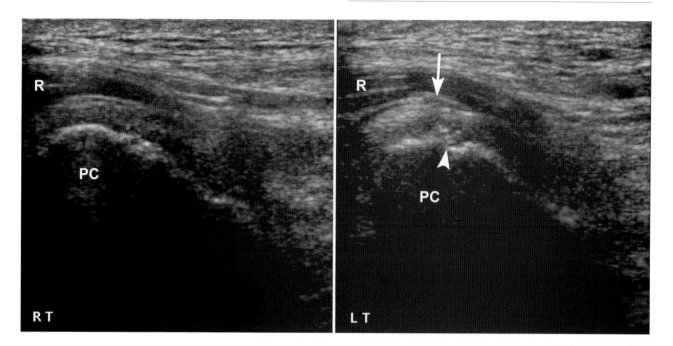

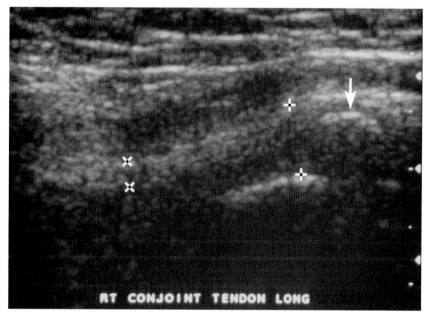

▲ **Fig. 5.106(a)** Ultrasound images obtained over the pubic crests demonstrate left conjoint insertional tendinopathy. Sagittal images of both sides have been obtained for comparison. The left conjoint tendon shows thickening at its insertion (arrow), enthesial bone surface irregularity and intrasubstance microcalcification (arrowhead). Pubic crest = PC. Rectus abdominis = R.
▶ **(b)** An ultrasound image shows an avulsion fracture at the conjoint tendon insertion. A long-axis image of the right conjoint tendon (× callipers) shows an avulsed bone fragment (arrow) and tendon swelling (+ callipers) at the pubic crest insertion.

▼ **Fig. 5.107** Fat-suppressed PD-weighted MR images of the symphysis have been obtained in the sagittal and long-axis coronal planes. A tear is demonstrated at the right adductor origin. Linear high signal is shown at the tendon/bone junction (arrows).

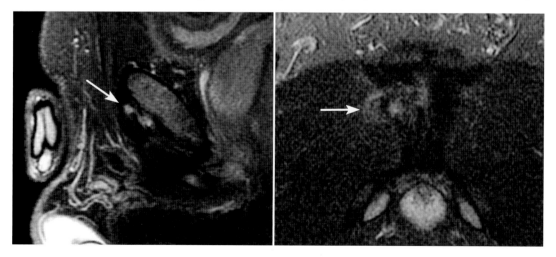

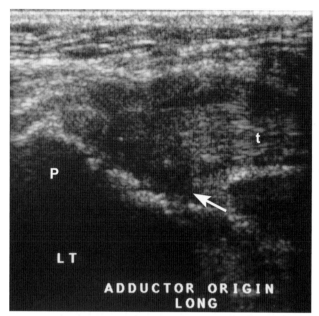

▲ **Fig. 5.108(a)** A transverse tear at the adductor origin is demonstrated by ultrasound. A long-axis image obtained at the pubic bone origin (P) of the adductor longus tendon (t) shows a transverse tear at the tendon/bone junction appreciated as a hypoechoic interruption of normal fibrillar echotexture (arrow). Associated peritendon haemorrhage is present anteriorly.

Groin hernias

Groin hernias can be inguinal or femoral, symptomatic or asymptomatic, bilateral or unilateral. Inguinal hernias occur predominantly in males (ratio 9:1). They are remarkably common, affecting up to 25% of the adult male population (Scott 1984; Skandalakis et al. 1989). Judging from the published findings concerning a team of professional Australian Rules footballers (Orchard et al. 1998), the incidence is probably much higher in adult male athletes. Femoral hernias are much less common (constituting about 4% of groin hernias) and occur predominantly in females (ratio 3:1).

Inguinal hernias are broadly classified as either indirect or direct, depending upon their relation to the inferior epigastric artery and Hesselbach's triangle (a space defined laterally by the inferior epigastric artery, medially by the lateral border of the rectus abdominis muscle and inferiorly by the inguinal ligament). Indirect hernias pass through the deep inguinal ring lateral to the inferior epigastric vessels and are the most common type of hernia in both sexes (see Fig. 5.109). Direct hernias pass through the posterior inguinal wall medial to the epigastric vessels, within the confines of Hesselbach's triangle. Hernias may arise acutely due to a traumatic tear of the inguinal wall or conjoint tendon, or non-acutely due to any combination of chronic exercise-related raised intra-abdominal pressure, developmental predisposition and advancing age.

Femoral hernias are protrusions of intra-abdominal contents that occur through the femoral ring into the anterior thigh, deep to the inguinal canal and usually medial to the femoral vein (see Fig. 5.110). It should be noted that a small protrusion of properitoneal fat through the femoral ring on straining is a

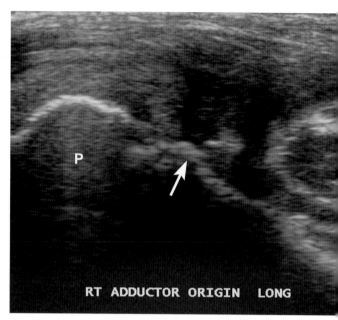

▲ **(b)** A longitudinal intrasubstance tear is demonstrated by ultrasound. A long-axis image obtained at the pubic bone origin (P) of the adductor longus tendon (t) shows the tear as a line of mixed hypo- and hyperechoic appearance (arrow).

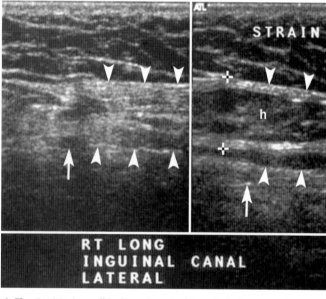

▲ **Fig. 5.109** A small indirect inguinal hernia is demonstrated by ultrasound. Long-axis views of the inguinal canal at the level of the deep ring have been obtained at rest (left image) and while straining (right image). The key anatomical landmark of the inferior epigastric artery is arrowed. The margins of the inguinal canal are indicated by arrowheads. The straining view shows a small finger-like herniation of omental fat (h) through the deep inguinal ring into the outer half of the inguinal canal. Note the associated mild 'ballooning' of the canal.

frequent normal finding on dynamic ultrasound and should not be mistaken for pathology. In this situation, the adjacent femoral vein dilates rather than being compressed. Females may be predisposed to femoral hernia due to a weakness of the pelvic floor musculature after childbirth.

The classical presentation of groin hernia is a lump or localised swelling that may or may not be painful and that often increases in size on coughing or straining, reduces in size or disappears when relaxed or supine, can be manually reduced and has an associated cough impulse. Hernias of this kind are clinically obvious and do not require imaging. However, ultrasound may be useful if the clinical swelling has atypical features and other mass lesions need to be excluded, or if swelling is absent and any cough impulse that may be present is weak and non-diagnostic. This latter scenario typically occurs with the so-called 'sports hernia' (athletic hernia, Gilmore's groin, incipient hernia), an incipient form of direct inguinal hernia that is particularly prevalent in kicking sports such as soccer and Australian Rules football.

Groin pain arising from a sports hernia is usually unilateral, insidious in onset, but associated with an initial tearing sensation in one-third of cases, occurs during exercise and is provoked by coughing, sneezing and sit-ups. The pain tends to be felt more in the lower abdomen than in the leg, is usually centred superior and lateral to the pubic bone, but may radiate to the adductor region, perineum or scrotum. These features overlap with those of conjoint tendinopathy and clinical differentiation of the two conditions is not possible. Despite prolonged rest from sport, the pain returns immediately at full intensity as soon as sporting activities are resumed. On physical examination there may be tenderness over the conjoint tendon insertion, pubic tubercle, superficial inguinal ring and mid-inguinal regions. Any associated cough impulse is often weak and does not generally permit a confident clinical diagnosis.

The imaging findings from either contrast herniography or dynamic ultrasound examination alone cannot be used as an indication for surgery because there is a high background incidence of asymptomatic hernias in the population at large and in the sporting population in particular. Nevertheless, a positive ultrasound finding of a sports hernia (or 'posterior inguinal wall deficiency') is made whenever a convex anterior bulge of the posterior inguinal wall is demonstrated with straining on dynamic real-time examination (see Fig. 5.111).

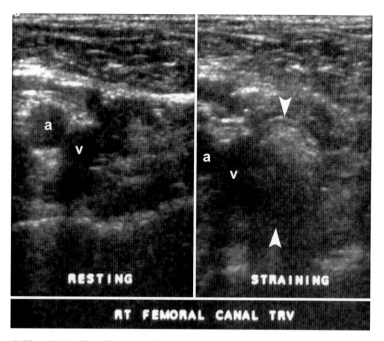

▲ **Fig. 5.110** This ultrasound image shows a small femoral hernia. Transverse images of the femoral canal have been obtained at rest (left image) and while straining (right image). The straining view shows a small herniation of what appears to be bowel (arrowheads) with associated acoustic shadowing and compression of the adjacent femoral vein. Femoral artery = a. Femoral vein = v.

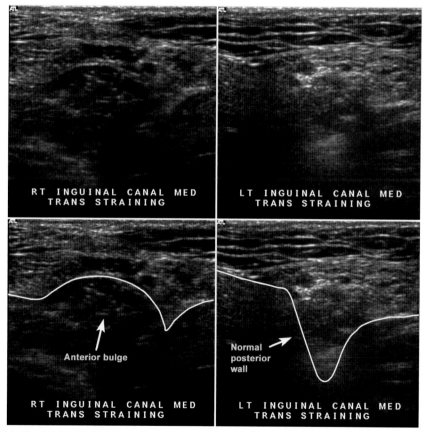

▲ **Fig. 5.111** An incipient direct (sports) hernia is imaged using ultrasound. Comparative short-axis straining images of the inguinal canal have been obtained at the level of the superficial ring. The lower images are identical to those above, but have lines superimposed to more clearly indicate the contours of the posterior inguinal wall (these contours are much easier to appreciate on real-time scanning). The abnormal left side shows a convex anterior bulge of the posterior inguinal wall.

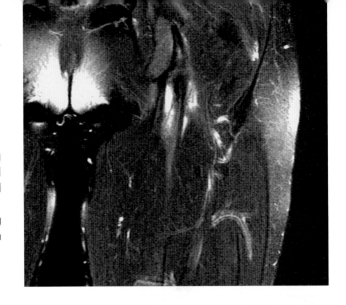

▶ **Fig. 5.112** This coronal fat-suppressed MR image shows minor haemorrhage in and around the proximal semimembranosus tendon.

Interestingly, even though the pain may be unilateral, a strong statistical association with bilateral posterior inguinal wall deficiency has been demonstrated on ultrasound (Orchard et al. 1998).

The determination of the relevance of a positive imaging test requires experienced clinical judgement, correlation with the history and exclusion of other causes of groin pain.

Soft-tissue injuries

Athletic injuries of the pelvis and hip are less common than injuries to other parts of the lower extremity but they may still make a significant contribution to time lost from sport. Diagnosing these injuries by physical examination and by the efficient use of imaging, enables appropriate management to commence sooner, so that athletes lose the least possible amount of time from their sport.

Muscle tears and contusions are the most common sports-related soft-tissue injuries of the pelvis, hip and thigh. Muscle tears most frequently involve the hamstring group of muscles (see Fig. 5.112). Muscle contusions are mostly seen in the vastus intermedius muscle and result from body contact sports such as rugby and gridiron. Contusion may result in a large and partly liquefied haematoma (see Fig. 5.113) (Aspelin et al. 1992), an acute compartment syndrome (see Fig. 5.114) (Gorman and McAndrew 1987; Viegas et al. 1988) or myositis ossificans. Muscle contusions are graded as mild, moderate or severe according to the degree of loss of function. Muscle tears and contusions do not usually require imaging to establish a diagnosis, but imaging may be used to assess the extent of injury and to help establish a prognosis. Imaging may also help to identify large haematoma formation, which may benefit from aspiration.

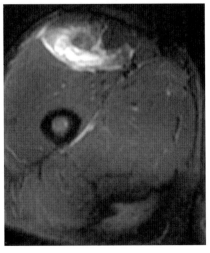

▶ **Fig. 5.113** Contusion of the rectus femoris is demonstrated by axial fat-suppressed MRI. A large intramuscular haematoma is present.

▼ **Fig. 5.114** Coronal and axial fat-suppressed MR images demonstrate a complete rupture of the biceps femoris at the musculotendinous junction with retraction and buckling of the central tendon. This injury with considerable associated haemorrhage may produce an acute compartment syndrome.

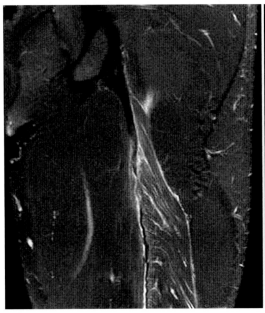

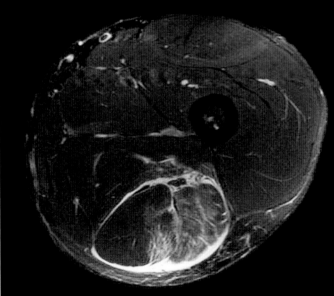

In addition to acute tears and contusions, injuries may be more chronic, producing symptomatic cysts (see Fig. 1.8 on page 8), ossifications, fibrosis and tendinopathies. Examples of these injuries are shown below in the gallery of muscle tears.

Muscle tears

There is a continuum of muscle injury from microscopic tears (strains) to complete rupture. Muscle tears are extremely common and affect athletes at all levels of competition. For example, at the Sydney 2000 Olympics, 80 tears of the musculature of the pelvis and thigh were imaged and an additional large number of athletes with tears would have been treated without recourse to imaging. After having invested years of hard work to reach the Olympics, each tear would have been disastrous to the athlete concerned. Even a Grade I tear can be devastating at this level of competition.

MRI and ultrasound can both be used to establish a diagnosis of muscle tear. MRI produces a more panoramic image and is also more sensitive to the presence of subtle interstitial bleeding. On the other hand, ultrasound can demonstrate the majority of Grade II and III tears.

As discussed in Chapter 1, muscle tears are graded I–III:

- *Grade I* injuries or 'strains' involve micro-tears of muscle fibres. Recovery from a Grade I strain may be possible in seven to ten days. Minor strains tend to become functionally limiting only when the athlete is performing at their peak level. Activity below this level may be possible. Minor strains often develop from overuse. MRI will show muscle oedema and perifascial hyperintensity, but no macroscopic fibre discontinuity or fluid spaces. The appreciation of low-grade muscle injuries by ultrasound can be difficult. MRI is clearly better at detecting oedema associated with low-grade muscle injuries.

- *Grade II* tears involve a partial macroscopic disruption of muscle, with some loss of function at peak performance. Recovery usually takes up to two months. Imaging with MRI demonstrates intramuscular and perifascial muscle spaces with irregular separation of some of the fibres (see Figs 5.115, 5.116 and 5.117).

▶**Fig. 5.115** A Grade II tear of the vastus lateralis demonstrated on a coronal fat-suppressed MR image.

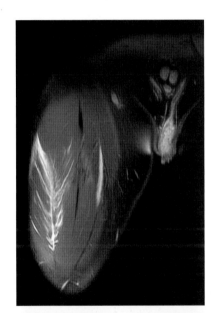

▼**Fig. 5.116** Long-axis ultrasound shows partial loss of muscle fibre continuity and intramuscular haematoma formation in the rectus femoris. The area of disruption is indicated by callipers.

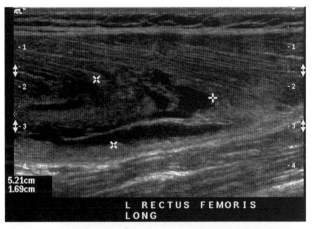

▶**Fig. 5.117** Sagittal and axial MR images demonstrate a complex tear of the semimembranosus tendon (arrow), with only slight separation. The tear shows both transverse and longitudinal components. The lack of any significant retraction favours a Grade II rather than a Grade III injury.

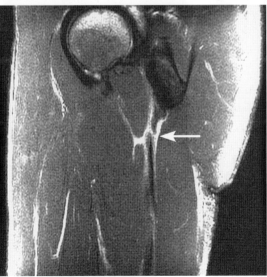
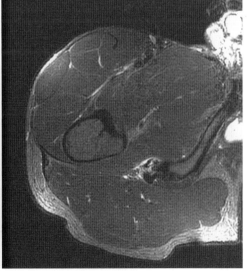

▶ **Fig. 5.118** The ability of MRI to display panoramic changes is demonstrated in this case of injury to the rectus femoris. The extent of the tear and haematoma formation is easily assessed. Sagittal and axial fat-suppressed MR images demonstrate a tear of the rectus femoris, with associated bleeding extending along the length of the fascial compartment.

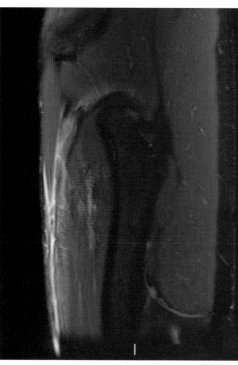
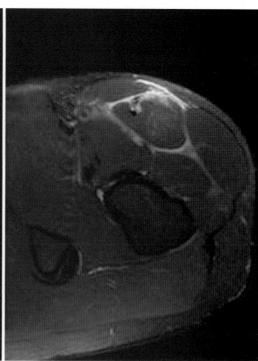

- *Grade III* tears involve complete disruption of the muscle. Recovery may take longer than three months. Imaging with MRI and ultrasound will demonstrate an irregular and complete loss of muscle continuity with retracted tear margins and haematoma filling the resulting gap.

Imaging of muscle tears should begin with plain films, which may disclose unexpected findings such as myositis ossificans from previous injury or evidence of a fracture.

Both MRI and ultrasound can be used to image muscle tears. A recent study compared the ability of both methods to examine hamstring muscle tears in Australian Rules footballers (Connell et al. 2004). This study showed that, although both tests are able to demonstrate the muscle injury in most cases, MRI is better at demonstrating low-grade strains characterised by muscle oedema without macroscopic disruption of muscle architecture. Because of MRI's greater field of view, this method gives a better and more precise understanding of the lesion site and extent. The follow-up evaluation of healing was also found to be easier using MRI.

An additional important finding from this study was that the cross-sectional area and the longitudinal length of the injury are both useful predictors of the time required for the athlete to return to full competition. Furthermore, in contrast to an earlier MRI study (Pomeranz and Heidt 1993), there was no significant correlation between the finding of intramuscular fluid collections or musculotendinous junction tears and the length of convalescence. Connell et al. found that athletes with hamstring tears usually become symptom-free within ten days of injury, and that this often resulted in a return to competition before the healing process had actually completed (probably also explaining the high rate of re-injury). In this study, 35.7% of injuries still had residual imaging abnormality evident on MRI at six weeks.

It must also be stressed that the accuracy of ultrasound is extremely dependent on the operator's skill and experience. Undoubtedly MRI presents a panoramic easy-to-look-at image, the extent of the tear is easily assessed and any associated haematomata is obvious (see Fig. 5.118). At the same time, tears may be elegantly demonstrated by ultrasound (see Fig. 5.119).

Myositis ossificans traumatica

Myositis ossificans is ossification occurring in muscle following a severe muscle contusion or tear where haematoma formation has become organised, resulting in the formation of dystrophic calcification and heterotopic ossification (see Fig. 5.120).

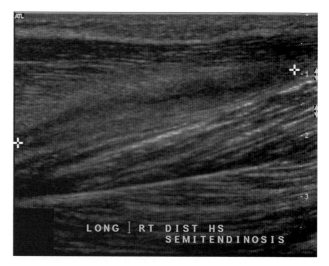

▲ **Fig. 5.119** A long-axis ultrasound image of the semitendinosus muscle shows disruption of the septal architecture and haematoma formation at the site of the tear. The extent of the injury is indicated by callipers.

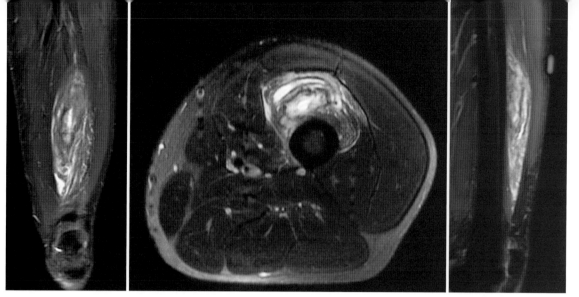

▲ **Fig. 5.120** A 22-year-old male footballer suffered a direct contusional injury to the vastus intermedius. The intramuscular haematoma is becoming organised and myositis ossificans may result. The changes are demonstrated by coronal, axial and sagittal fat-suppressed MR images.

▶ **Fig. 5.121(a)** A nuclear bone scan shows a small area of myositis ossificans developing adjacent to a stress fracture of the subtrochanteric region of the femur. **(b)** A stress fracture involving the medial aspect of the subtrochanteric region of the femur is demonstrated by CT. Calcification is present in the adjacent soft tissues.

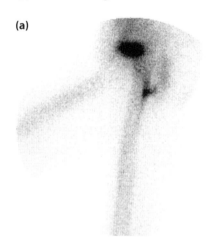

(a)

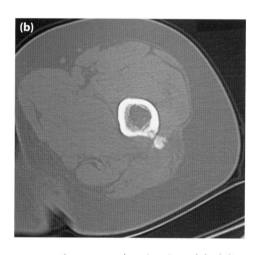

(b)

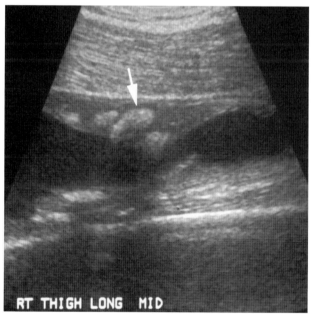

RT THIGH LONG MID

▲ **Fig. 5.122** Early myositis ossificans formation can be recognised by ultrasound. A sagittal ultrasound image at the anterior mid-thigh shows a large haematoma in the vastus intermedius with both solid and large cystic components. Calcification (arrowed) of early myositis ossificans is present.

This condition can sometimes cause chronic pain and disability. The calcification or ossification may become visible on plain radiographs at three to six weeks, although the changes can be seen earlier on nuclear bone scanning, CT scanning (see Fig. 5.121) and ultrasound (see Fig. 5.122). Mature lesions consist of a peripheral zone of dense lamellar bone, a central zone of granulation tissue and fibrosis that is radiolucent and, at some distance from the lesion centre, a zone of osteoid. Myositis ossificans is most commonly seen in the vastus intermedius (see Figs 5.123 and 5.124), the rectus femoris (see Fig. 5.125) and the hamstring muscles (see Figs 5.126 and 5.127).

The athlete commonly presents with a history of an initial injury and a subsequent persisting decrease in the range of motion of the knee. This may be accompanied by a sympathetic knee joint effusion and a palpable mass. Early mobilisation would appear to play an important role in management (Larsen et al. 2002). It has not been conclusively proven that an ultrasound-guided aspiration of the hematoma performed as soon as possible after active bleeding has ceased will reduce the risk of myositis ossificans, although aspiration certainly produces symptomatic relief (see Fig. 5.128). Many cases spontaneously recover with eventual resorption of the ossification to varying degrees. Persistently symptomatic lesions may be excised after they mature, although recurrence rates of up to 67% have been reported (Huss and Puhl 1980).

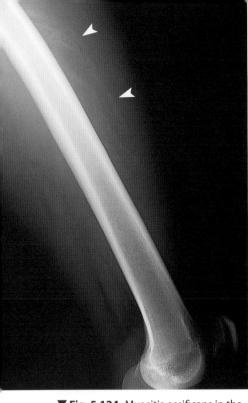

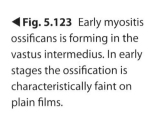

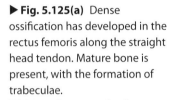

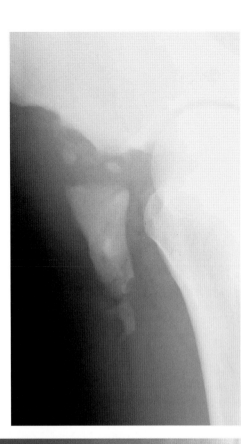

◀ Fig. 5.123 Early myositis ossificans is forming in the vastus intermedius. In early stages the ossification is characteristically faint on plain films.

▶ Fig. 5.125(a) Dense ossification has developed in the rectus femoris along the straight head tendon. Mature bone is present, with the formation of trabeculae.

▼ (b) In this example, the mature bone is continuous with the AIIS origin, preventing movement.

▼ Fig. 5.124 Myositis ossificans in the vastus intermedius is mature and dense. CT is worthwhile if no central lucent zone is evident on plain films.

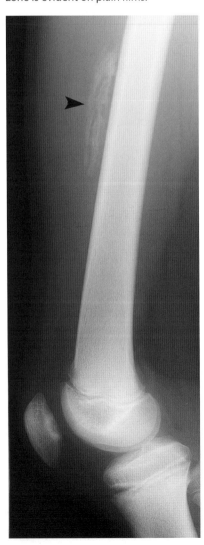

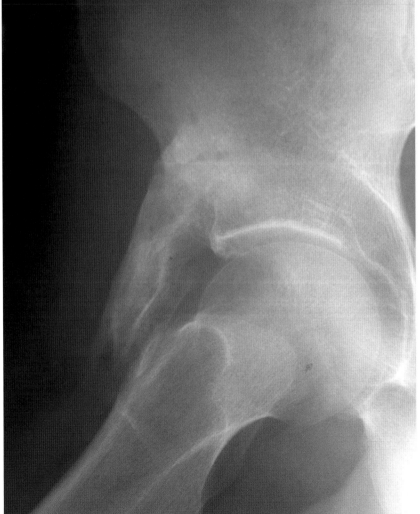

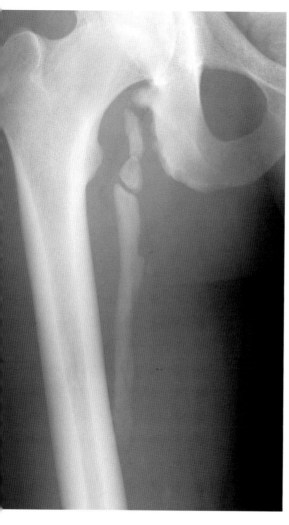

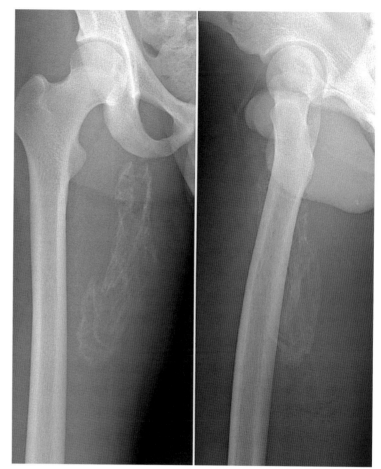

▲ **Fig. 5.127** Extensive myositis ossificans has developed in mid-substance hamstring muscle.

▲ **Fig. 5.126** Following injury, dense ossification has formed in the semimembranosus muscle and tendon.

▶ **Fig. 5.128** An Olympic basketballer fell heavily on her right buttock, resulting in muscle contusion and haematoma formation (left image). Aspiration of the haematoma was performed under ultrasound control for pain relief and hopefully to reduce the possibility of myositis ossificans. The needle is identified (arrowheads). In the long-axis image, the sciatic nerve (SN) is well demonstrated (callipers).

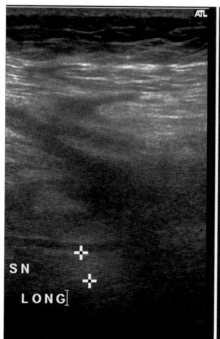

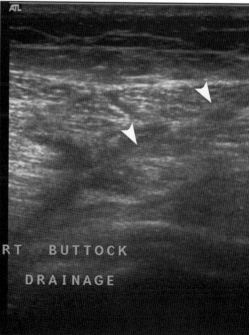

A gallery of muscle tears of the pelvis and thigh

Hamstring injuries

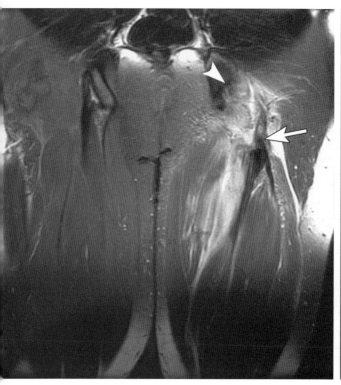

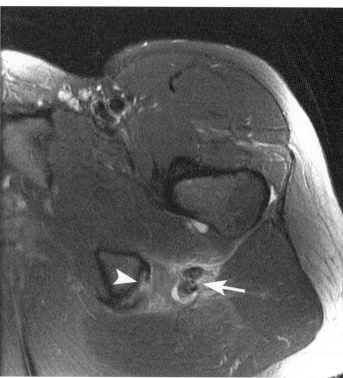

▲ **Fig. 5.129** Coronal and axial fat-suppressed MR images demonstrate a complete avulsion of the hamstring origin (white arrow). There is considerable displacement and associated haematoma formation. A bone fragment has been avulsed, with a bony deficit noted at the ischial tuberosity (white arrowhead). Note the partial tear at the right hamstring origin.

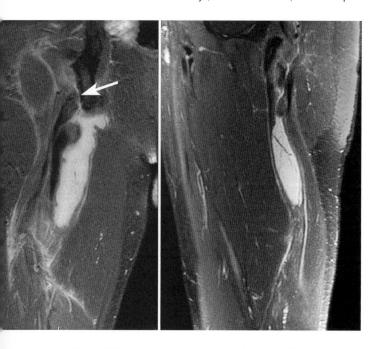

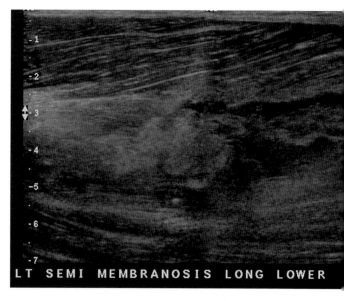

LT SEMI MEMBRANOSIS LONG LOWER

▲ **Fig. 5.130** A hamstring avulsion (white arrow) is demonstrated by MRI, with formation of a large lobulated haematoma. There is only slight displacement at the semimembranosus origin, but moderate retraction of the biceps femoris and the semitendinosus has occurred.

▲ **Fig. 5.131** A 400-metre runner shows considerable disruption of normal muscle architecture in the semimembranosus, shown on a long-axis ultrasound image. There is a haematoma of markedly heterogeneous echotexture. The more echogenic component suggests early calcification due to a previous trauma. Acute tearing is shown adjacent to the previous injury.

▶ **Fig. 5.132** An organising intra-muscular haematoma due to semitendinosus tear is demonstrated on long-axis and transverse ultrasound images.

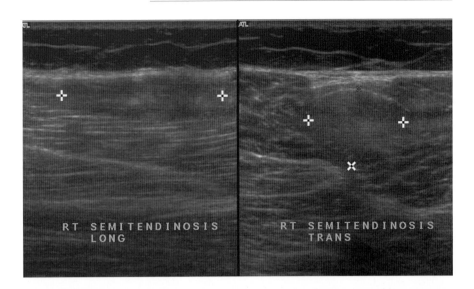

▼ **Fig. 5.133** Coronal and axial fat-suppressed MR images show high signal of a small intrasubstance tear (white arrow) at the origin of the biceps femoris. This injury may appear minor but was sufficient to stop an elite Olympic 100-metre runner halfway through his race.

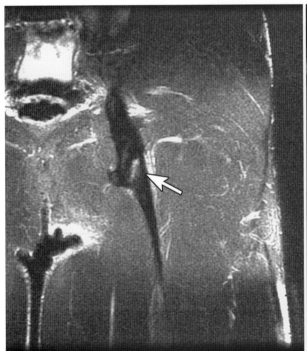

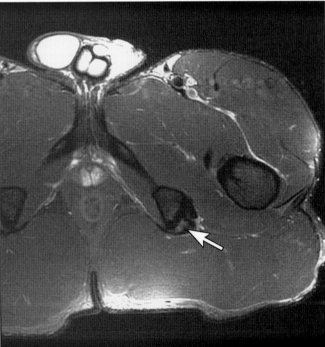

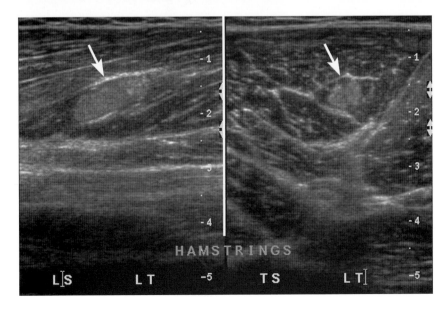

◀ **Fig. 5.134** A small uniformly echogenic intramuscular hamstring haematoma (white arrow) is demonstrated by long-axis and transverse ultrasound imaging.

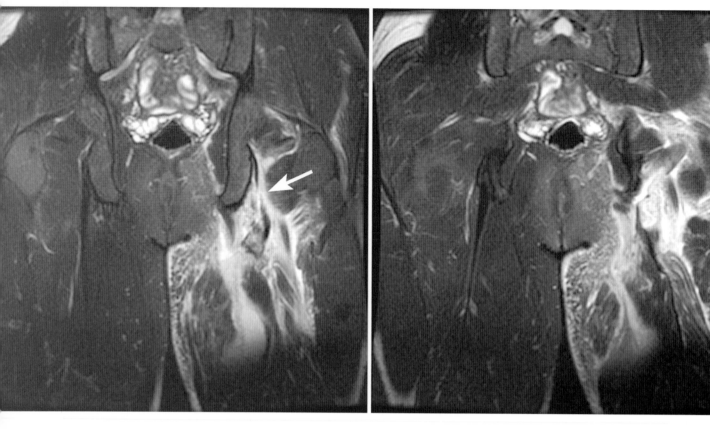

▲ **Fig. 5.135** Coronal fat-suppressed MR images demonstrate a complete rupture of the hamstring tendon origin (white arrow). There is retraction and buckling of the tendon. Considerable bleeding has occurred.

▼ **Fig. 5.136** Coronal and axial fat-suppressed MR images demonstrate a high-grade partial tear of the musculotendinous junction of the semitendinosis.

▼ **Fig. 5.137** A spectacular haematoma has developed in the thigh following a tear of the biceps femoris. Note the close relationship of the haematoma with the sciatic nerve (white arrow).

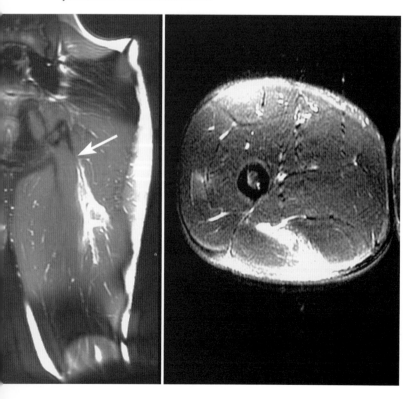

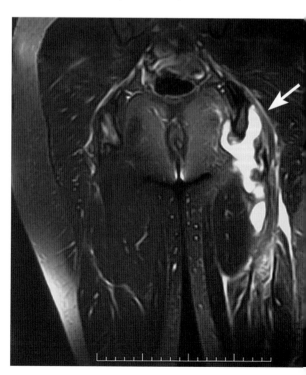

▶ Fig. 5.138 This coronal fat-suppressed MR image shows hyperintense marrow signal in the left ischial tuberosity and a line of bright signal indicating a tear at the adjacent hamstring tendon origin. An accompanying small cortical avulsion cannot be excluded. Haemorrhage outlines the adjacent sciatic nerve.

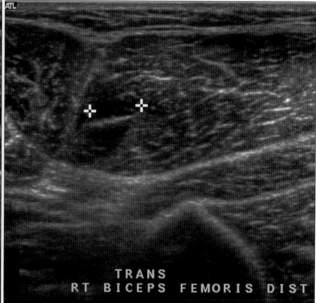

▼ Fig. 5.139 Long-axis and transverse ultrasound images show a small muscle haematoma at the site of a tear in the right biceps femoris (callipers), highlighting this imaging method's capability to demonstrate small fluid collections.

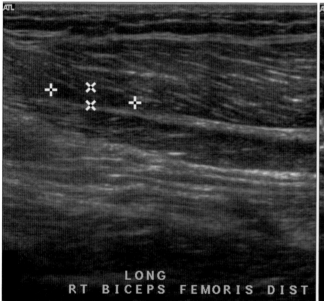

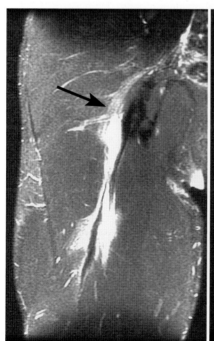

◀ Fig. 5.140 This injury occurred during a 400-metre race at the Sydney 2000 Olympics. Coronal and axial MR images demonstrate a complete tear of the semimembranosus musculotendinous junction. There is only slight separation of the tendon fragments and a haematoma is noted. The sciatic nerve is outlined by surrounding haemorrhage (black arrow).

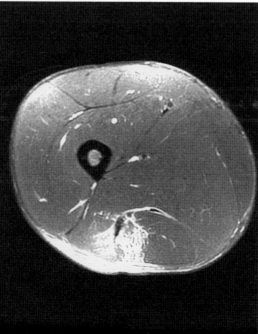

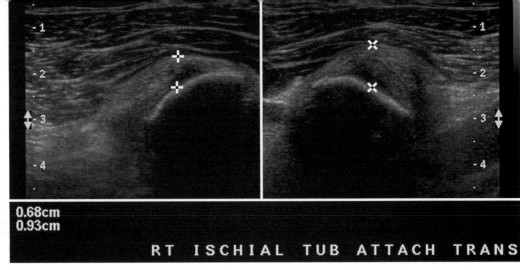

▶ **Fig. 5.141**
Ultrasound demonstrates swelling of the left hamstring origin (× callipers). This appearance is non-specific and indicative of either tendinopathy or a tear. The right side has been imaged for comparison.

0.68cm
0.93cm

RT ISCHIAL TUB ATTACH TRANS

Tears of the quadriceps

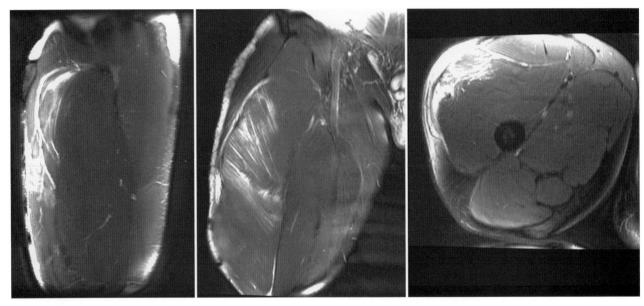

▲ **Fig. 5.142** Sagittal, coronal and axial MR images demonstrate a vastus lateralis muscle tear.

▼ **Fig. 5.143** Coronal and axial fat-suppressed MR images demonstrate a tear of the rectus femoris muscle, with tendon retraction.

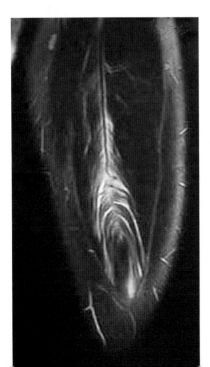

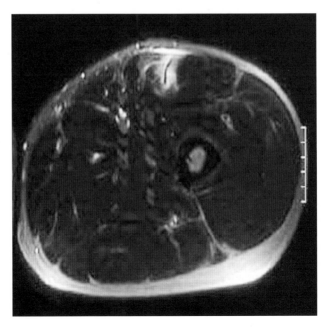

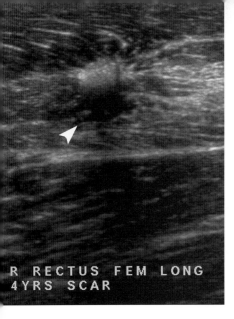

R RECTUS FEM LONG
4YRS SCAR

◀**Fig. 5.144** Ultrasound shows considerable distortion of normal muscle architecture caused by an old rectus femoris scar. A recent tear is also present immediately adjacent to the scar (arrowhead).

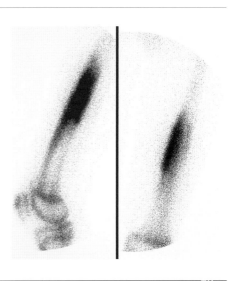

▶**Fig. 5.145** An acute tear at the vastus intermedius insertion in a sprinter is demonstrated as intense periosteal uptake of isotope on a nuclear bone scan.

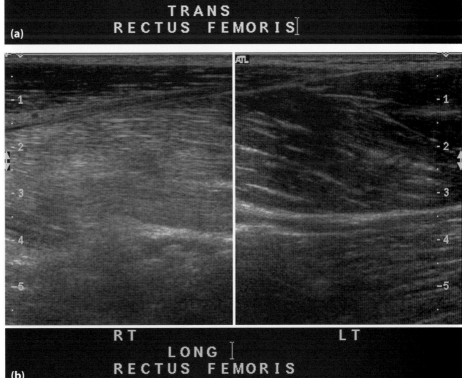

▶**Fig. 5.146** Transverse **(a)** and long-axis **(b)** ultrasound images show the right rectus femoris muscle to be diffusely swollen and echogenic, due to interstitial infiltration by haemorrhage.

(a) RT — LT
TRANS
RECTUS FEMORIS

(b) RT — LT
LONG
RECTUS FEMORIS

▶**Fig. 5.147** Axial fat-suppressed MR images demonstrate a tear of the rectus femoris at the musculotendinous junction. There is moderate associated haemorrhage.

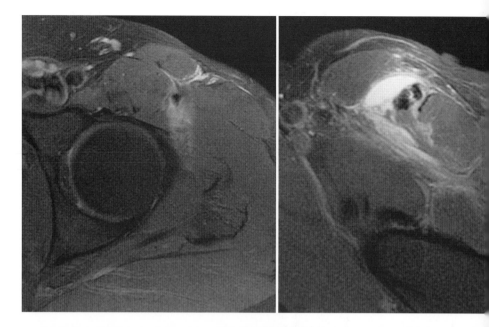

▶**Fig. 5.148** Long-axis and transverse ultrasound images demonstrate a 5 cm haematoma at the site of a tear of the vastus medialis muscle of an Olympic weight-lifter (callipers).

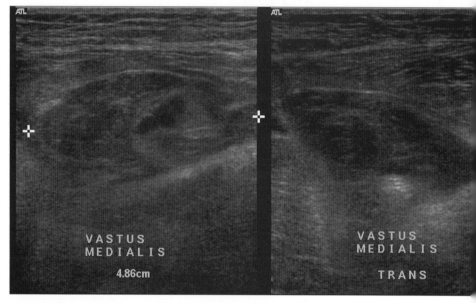

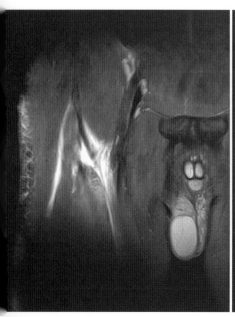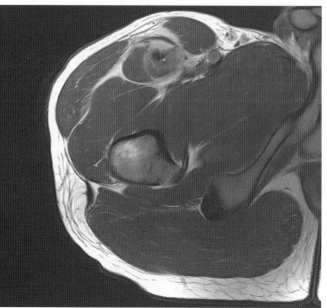

◀**Fig. 5.149** Coronal fat-suppressed and axial PD-weighted MR images demonstrate a tear of the proximal rectus femoris musculotendinous junction with moderate associated bleeding.

▶ **Fig. 5.150** Long-axis ultrasound demonstrates vastus medialis contusion on the right side with the left side for comparison.

▼ **Fig. 5.151** Fat-suppressed MR images obtained in coronal and axial planes demonstrate a tear of the vastus lateralis that occurred in a weight-lifter at the Sydney 2000 Olympics.

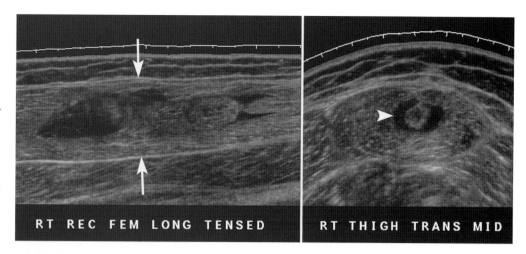

RT REC FEM LONG TENSED

RT THIGH TRANS MID

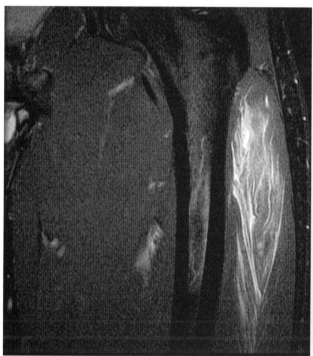

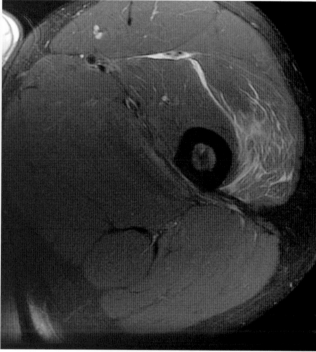

Other interesting pelvic muscle tears

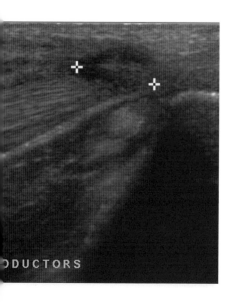

◀ **Fig. 5.152** A subacute adductor origin tear (callipers) is elegantly imaged by long-axis ultrasound. Areas of calcification are noted, indicating a previous injury.

▶ **Fig. 5.153** A coronal MR image demonstrates an organising haematoma in the left adductor brevis (white arrowhead). Note features of osteitis pubis, with bilateral marrow oedema, posterior disc extrusion and osteophyte formation. There is also a small tenoperiosteal junction tear at the parasymphyseal margin of the left adductor longus.

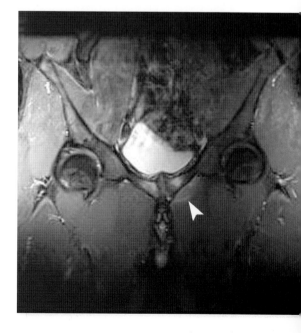

ODUCTORS

▶ **Fig. 5.154** Tendinopathy of the tensor fascia lata is demonstrated by axial fat-suppressed MRI. High signal surrounds the tendon of the tensor fascia lata at its origin (white arrow).

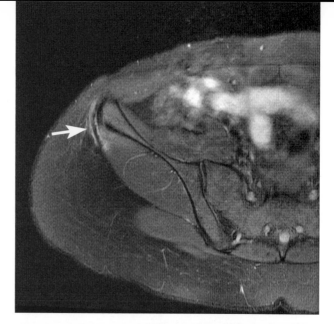

▼ **Fig. 5.155** Hypoechoic swelling of the origin of the left tensor fascia lata shown by ultrasound, with an image of the right origin for comparison. The appearance is consistent with tendinopathy, although an underlying partial tear cannot be excluded.

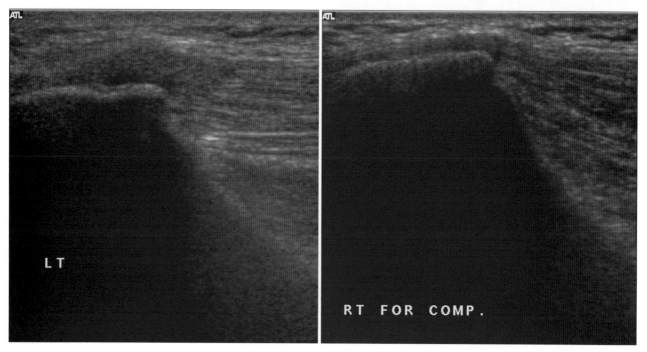

▼ **Fig. 5.156** Coronal and axial fat-suppressed MR images show a tear of the obturator internus, with a diffuse swelling and hyperintensity extending from its origin to mid-substance (white arrow). Perimuscular pooling of blood is noted (black arrowhead).

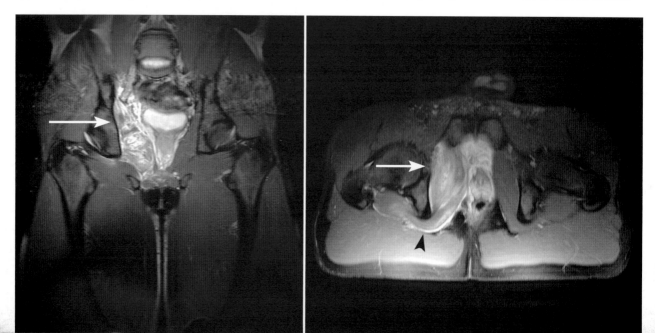

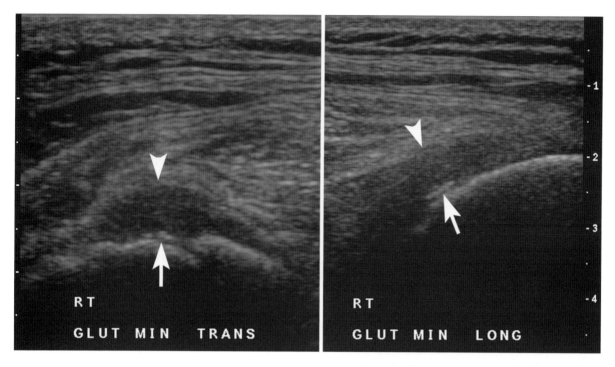

▲ **Fig. 5.157** Transverse and long-axis ultrasound images of the gluteus minimus tendon insertion at the greater trochanter demonstrate tendinopathic changes, which include hypoechoic tendon thickening (arrowheads) and a superimposed echogenic line of complicating partial tear involving the deep fibres (arrows).

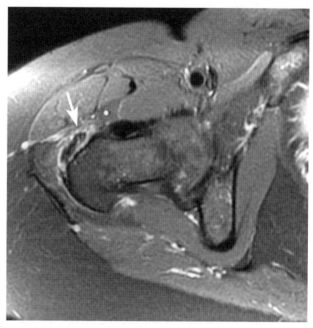

▶ **Fig. 5.158** Gluteus minimus tendinopathy or partial tear is demonstrated by an axial fat-suppressed MR image. High signal surrounds the tendon and a small focus of high signal is noted within the tendon substance.

▼ **Fig. 5.159** A spectacular tear of the left adductor brevis in a 33-year-old soccer player is demonstrated by coronal and axial fat-suppressed MR images. Considerable haemorrhage has occurred.

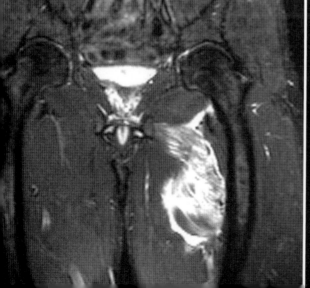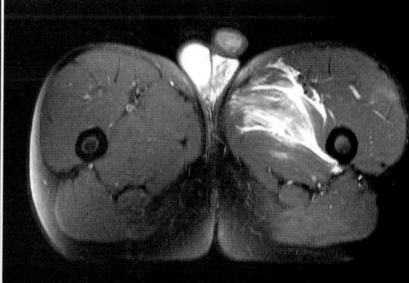

Proximal hamstring injuries

The hamstrings are a group of three muscles: the semi-membranosus, semitendinosus and biceps femoris (see Fig. 5.160). The semimembranosus muscle forms the bulk of the mass of the muscle group. The hamstrings flex the knee and extend the hip joint. As with other frequently injured muscles, the hamstrings span two joints: the hip and the knee. As a consequence, they are subjected to stretching at more than one point. Injury to the proximal hamstring may manifest as an enthesopathy (see Fig. 5.161), tendinopathy (see Fig. 5.162), muscle tear (see Fig. 5.163) or avulsion injury (see Fig. 5.164). The hamstrings are under maximum load during hip flexion and knee extension.

Hamstring injuries can occur gradually from overuse or as the result of a single traumatic incident. Overtraining, especially with repetitive activity, is a common cause of

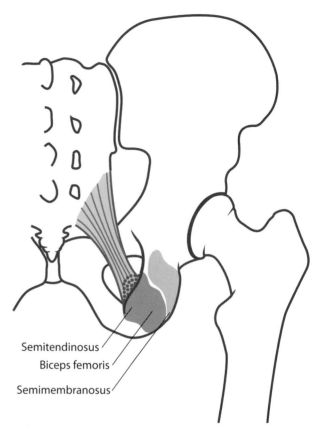

Semitendinosus
Biceps femoris
Semimembranosus

▲ **(b)** This line drawing shows the area of origin of the hamstring group of muscles.

▼ **(c)** This line drawing shows the cross-sectional relationship of the hamstring muscles.

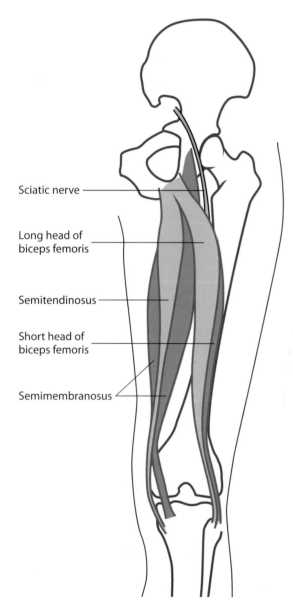

Sciatic nerve

Long head of biceps femoris

Semitendinosus

Short head of biceps femoris

Semimembranosus

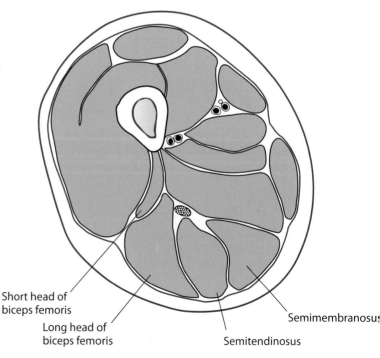

Short head of biceps femoris

Long head of biceps femoris

Semimembranosus

Semitendinosus

▲ **Fig. 5.160(a)** A line drawing shows the hamstring group of muscles.

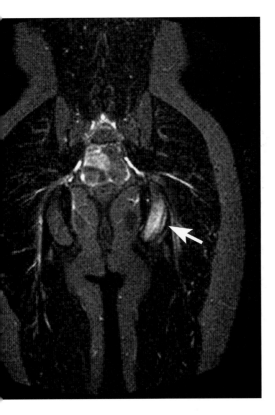

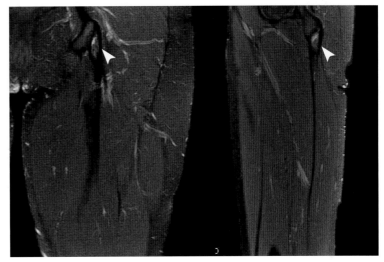

hamstring strain. Initially there is only a slight tightness, which will progress with continuing overload. Overuse injuries to the hamstrings tend to recur. A hamstring tear may also result from an acute overstretching injury, such as may occur with a sudden sprint or a slip with an extended leg. As a consequence, hamstring injuries are associated with track and field sports, soccer, racquet sports and any activity requiring sudden sprinting. A tear may also follow direct trauma to a contracted hamstring.

▲ **Fig. 5.161** A coronal fat-suppressed MR image shows marrow oedema at the left ischial tuberosity with an underlying hypointense line of stress fracture just deep to the hamstring origin (white arrow).

▲ **Fig. 5.162** Coronal and sagittal fat-suppressed MR images show linear high signal at the biceps femoris origin on a background of mild tendon hyperintensity, an appearance consistent with tendinopathy and superimposed tear (white arrowheads). Note the enthesial marrow oedema.

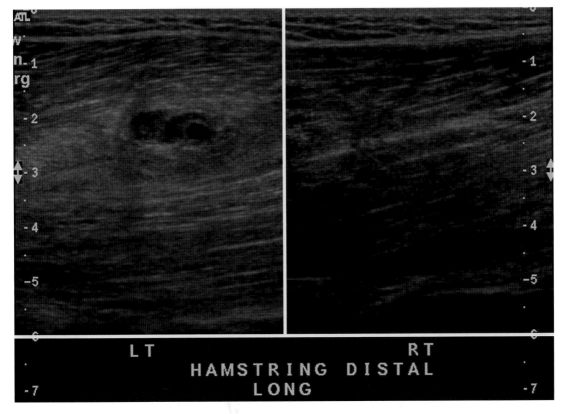

▲ **Fig. 5.163** A long-axis ultrasound image shows a subacute-to-chronic left hamstring tear with possible early cyst formation. A comparison image of the asymptomatic side is also shown.

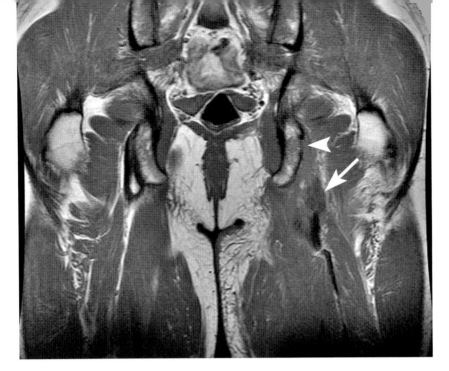

▲ **Fig. 5.164** A coronal TI-weighted MR image shows complete avulsion of the left hamstring origin (white arrow indicates the retracted tendon). A bone fragment has been separated, resulting in a bony deficit at the ischial tuberosity (white arrowhead). Note the focus of intrasubstance ossification indicative of old injury at the right hamstring origin.

Hamstring injuries are common in adult athletes and an avulsed bone fragment will occasionally be seen on plain films (see Figs 5.165 and 5.166). This injury results from a sudden forceful flexion of the hip when the knee is extended and the hamstrings contracted. Power lifting and water-skiing are the most common activities producing a hamstring avulsion injury (Brukner and Khan 2001).

Inefficient muscle function can also contribute to sudden tears in the hamstrings. This may result from an imbalance with quadriceps function. Muscle groups work in pairs. The hamstrings must work in concert with the quadriceps. When the knee is flexed, contraction of the hamstring muscle group will occur as the quadriceps muscles relax. In elite athletes, particularly sprinters, the quadriceps are well developed by a focused gym program and an imbalance with the hamstrings

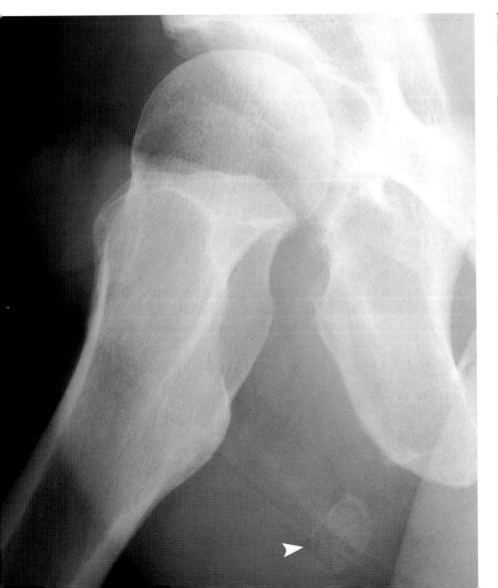

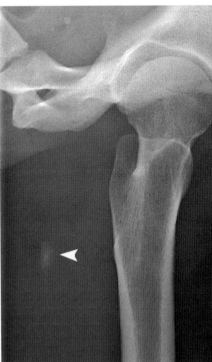

▲ **Fig. 5.165** A bony fragment seen on a plain film (white arrowhead) is the result of an old hamstring avulsion. This Olympic-level athlete presented with re-injury.

◀ **Fig. 5.166** An older athlete performing in a father-and-son race at a school function suffered a hamstring injury with avulsion of a bony fragment.

may be inadvertently produced. The quadriceps muscles are usually much more powerful, so the hamstrings may fatigue faster than the quadriceps, leading to strains.

Quadriceps tears and contusions

Injury to the quadriceps most commonly involves the rectus femoris. Tears of the vastus lateralis, medialis and intermedius are relatively uncommon and these muscles are more prone to contusion from direct trauma. The rectus femoris muscle is thought to be susceptible to injury because it crosses two joints. The straight head of the rectus femoris arises from the anterior inferior iliac spine and unites with the reflected head, which arises from a groove above the acetabulum. A bursa lies deep to the origin of the straight head (see Fig. 5.167). The two heads merge with each other and with the anterior hip joint capsule and the iliofemoral ligament. The quadriceps muscles extend the knee, and the rectus femoris, as it crosses the hip joint, also works synergistically with the other hip flexors to flex the hip. Tears of the rectus femoris usually involve the proximal two-thirds of the muscle (see Fig. 5.168).

Athletes usually remember the specific incident involving a sudden muscle contraction that produced their injury. Initially, all grades of strain will be functionally limiting when attempting to perform activities at maximal speed or when generating force, such as with kicking. The most frequent mechanism of rectus femoris injury occurs during the acceleration phase of sprinting, when maximal contraction of the rectus femoris occurs. Other activities that place a large stress on the rectus femoris include jumping sports

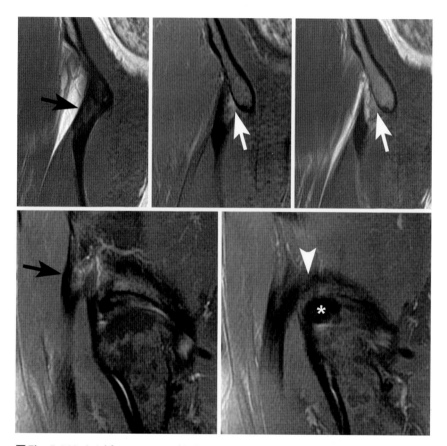

◀**Fig. 5.167** Coronal (top) and sagittal (bottom) MR images show the rectus femoris tendon straight head (black arrow) and reflected head (white arrowhead). Note the hyperintense bursal zone immediately deep to the straight head tendon (white arrows). Acetabular labral chondrocalcinosis is incidentally present (asterisk).

▼**Fig. 5.168** Axial fat-suppressed MR images demonstrate a tear of the rectus femoris tendon or musculotendinous junction in the upper thigh (white arrows).

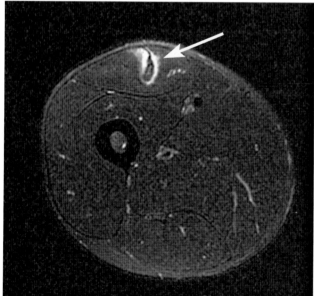
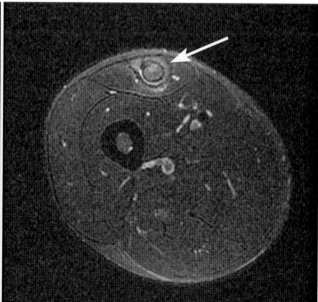

such as the long jump, hurdling and activities involving kicking. A muscle tear is particularly likely to occur when a contracting muscle meets resistance, such as two soccer players simultaneously kicking a ball.

A relevant structure in close relationship to the quadriceps is the femoral nerve, which courses along the anterior femoral triangle and down the anterior thigh. The femoral nerve may become entrapped by scar following rectus femoris injury in a similar way to the sciatic nerve after hamstring injury. The differential diagnosis includes referred pain in the femoral nerve distribution (originating from the L2, 3, 4 nerve roots), psoas pathology and anterior hip joint pathology, including acetabular labral tears, psoas bursopathy or possibly a deep quadriceps haematoma and subsequent myositis ossificans.

Piriformis syndrome

Piriformis syndrome occurs when there is entrapment of the sciatic nerve by the piriformis as the nerve leaves the greater sciatic notch, or by irritation of the piriformis muscle itself, producing sciatica. The relationship between the sciatic nerve and the piriformis muscle is inconstant and seven different anatomic variants have been described (Silver and Leadbetter 1998). The most common variant is when the sciatic nerve passes anterior to the piriformis muscle. The next most common is when the peroneal part of the sciatic nerve passes through the piriformis muscle (Ozaki et al. 1999). Piriformis syndrome has been reported with direct trauma per se, or with resulting myositis ossificans (Beauchesne and Schutzer 1997), excessive exercise (Julsrud 1989), infection (Chen 1992), pseudoaneurysm of the gluteal artery (Papadopoulos et al. 1989) and hypertrophy of the piriformis muscle.

The clinical presentation is often confusing. The athlete may present with an ache in the buttock or cramping and tightness in the hamstrings aggravated by activities requiring hip flexion,

internal rotation of the hip and hip adduction. Motor weakness or sensory loss may also occur. This syndrome is seen in sports such as skiing, gymnastics and dancing. The diagnosis is difficult, requiring a high level of clinical suspicion. Nerve conduction studies and imaging with ultrasound including a diagnostic injection (see Figs 5.169 and 5.170) may occasionally help to confirm the diagnosis. A nuclear bone scan may demonstrate enthesopathy at the piriformis insertion (see Fig. 5.171). Imaging is

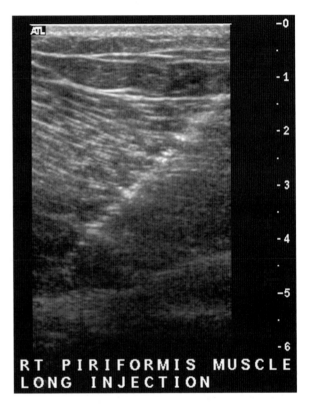

▲ Fig. 5.170 An injection of local anaesthetic into the piriformis under ultrasound control relieved this patient's symptoms. The obliquely oriented echogenic line represents a needle with its tip in the piriformis muscle.

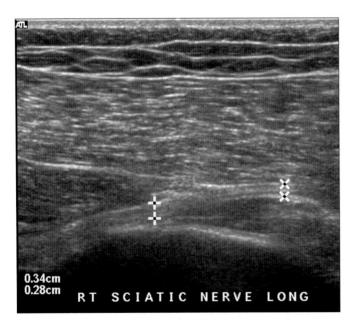

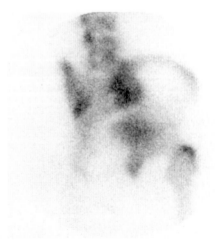

▲ Fig. 5.169 A long-axis ultrasound image demonstrates slight swelling (callipers) of the sciatic nerve in a patient with piriformis syndrome.

▲ Fig. 5.171 A nuclear bone scan demonstrates piriformis enthesopathy, with focal increase in isotope uptake at the greater trochanter.

also used to rule out other causes of sciatica, including disc protrusion, spinal stenosis, lumbar facet syndrome and pelvic tumour.

Interestingly, Melamed (2002) described an association between piriformis syndrome and Morton's foot. If the head of the second metatarsal is prominent, the foot becomes unstable during the push-off phase of the gait cycle. This causes internal rotation of the knee and hip and provoking contraction of the external rotators of the hip, producing piriformis syndrome.

Bursopathy

Three major types of bursopathy are described in the hip region: iliopsoas bursopathy, trochanteric bursopathy and ischial tuberosity bursopathy. Bursal irritation in sport may be produced by direct trauma or soft-tissue friction due to snapping of a tendon over an underlying bursa. Infection and arthritis are other causes that should also be considered.

Iliopsoas bursopathy

Iliopsoas bursopathy is a concept commonly referred to in sports medicine texts. Although an iliopsoas bursal effusion and synovial thickening are not an uncommon finding on imaging tests, these changes are often secondary to hip joint pathology and simply reflect the presence of a communication between the bursa and the hip joint. Iliopsoas bursal effusions are often seen in cases of arthritis or any other hip pathology producing a joint effusion (Underwood et al. 1988) (see Figs 5.172, 5.173 and 5.174).

Frictional bursopathy can also occur in situations of a snapping iliopsoas tendon (see Fig. 5.175) or due to direct bursal

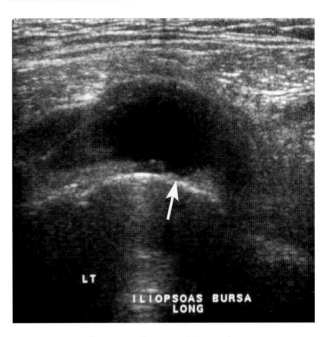

▲ Fig. 5.173 A long-axis ultrasound image demonstrates an echo-free space anterior to the femoral head due to the iliopsoas bursa being distended with fluid. Note the communication with the hip joint via a small opening in the anterior capsule (arrow).

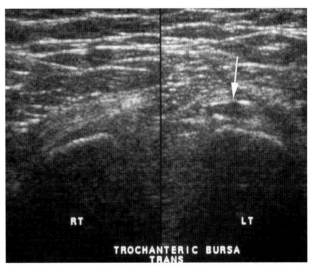

▲ Fig. 5.174 A transverse ultrasound image at the level of the greater trochanter shows a small collection of fluid in the left sub-ITB or sub-maximus trochanteric bursa (arrow). The appearance is consistent with a frictional bursopathy. The asymptomatic side is shown for comparison.

abutment by a hip joint osteophyte, a displaced fracture margin or the proud edge of a joint prosthesis. Such cases contrast with the concept of iliopsoas bursopathy in sport due to overuse, as corresponding bursal changes are not commonly found on imaging in this scenario. When real-time ultrasound confirms the presence of iliopsoas muscle tenderness on transducer pressure, but fails to demonstrate bursopathy change, the underlying pathology is more consistent with iliopsoas muscle soreness, strain or tendinopathy and MRI may be a more definitive test.

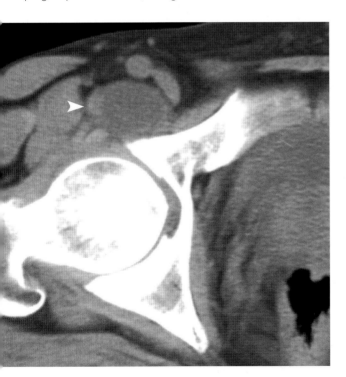

▲ Fig. 5.172 An axial CT image demonstrates distension of the iliopsoas bursa (arrowhead).

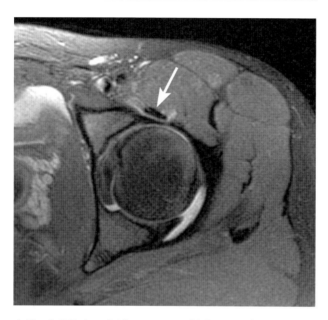

▲ **Fig. 5.175** An axial fat-suppressed MR image demonstrates localised hyperintensity in the line of the iliopsoas bursa deep to the iliopsoas tendon. The appearance is that of iliopsoas bursopathy. Note the small hip joint effusion.

Trochanteric bursopathy

Trochanteric bursopathy (see Fig. 5.176) can arise from frictional overload due to adverse biomechanics such as when dancers adduct beyond the midline, runners have a crossover-style gait or athletes who train in a single direction on a sloped road. Leg-length discrepancy may also cause trochanteric bursopathy. Other associations include a tight iliotibial band or direct trauma. If the clinical diagnosis is uncertain, ultrasound or MRI can differentiate trochanteric bursopathy from a gluteal tear or tendinopathy (see Fig. 5.177). Ultrasound can also be used to accurately guide therapeutic injection of the trochanteric bursae. Calcification may occur in chronic bursopathy (see Figs 5.178 and 5.179).

▼ **Fig. 5.176** A coronal fat-suppressed MR image demonstrates fluid and synovitis within the sub-ITB or sub-maximus trochanteric bursa (arrow). Iliotibial band friction syndrome is present, with fluid on both sides of a thickened and irregular iliotibial band.

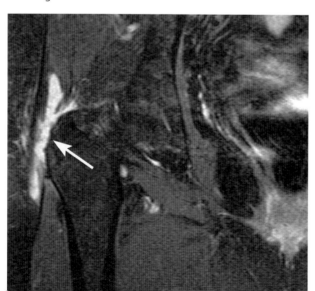

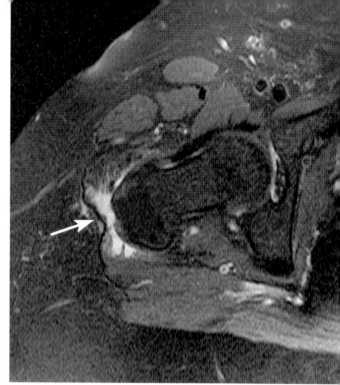

▲ **Fig. 5.177** Trochanteric bursopathy is demonstrated by axial fat-suppressed MRI (arrow). High signal is also noted lateral to the iliotibial band, consistent with iliotibial band friction syndrome.

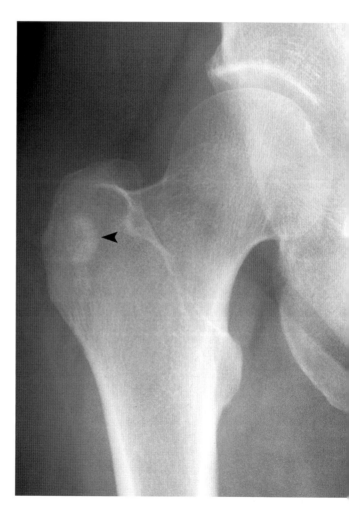

▲ **Fig. 5.178** Calcification is present in the trochanteric bursa, indicating calcific bursopathy (arrowhead).

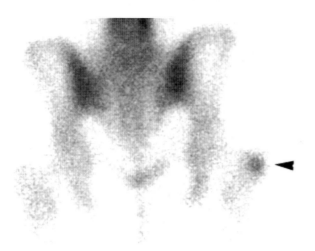

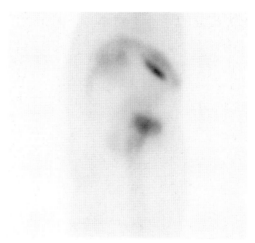

▲ **Fig. 5.179** A nuclear bone scan shows increased uptake of isotope within the calcific bursopathy demonstrated in Fig. 5.178.

▲ **Fig. 5.180** A nuclear bone scan demonstrates an unusual fracture of the ilium below the iliac crest. This injury presented clinically as a hip pointer.

Ischial bursopathy

Ischial bursopathy occurs as a result of a fall or repetitive trauma, such as may occur with horse riding. Other causes of buttock pain include hamstring tendinopathy and gluteal muscle strain (which is seen in cyclists). Buttock pain may also result from piriformis syndrome, referred pain from the lumbar spine or sacroiliac joints, and apophysitis or avulsion of the ischial tuberosity. Imaging has a role to play when the diagnosis is uncertain.

Hip pointer

Localised soft-tissue contusions over the greater trochanter or the iliac crest are called 'hip pointers'. Pointers are caused by direct trauma such as may result from a rugby tackle or from a fall on a hard surface. The athlete presents with localised pain and tenderness, possibly with bruising at the site of the trauma. Other causes of pain in this situation, such as muscle tears, should be excluded. Complications may occur following a hip pointer. Femoral or lateral femoral cutaneous nerve palsy may result from haematoma formation (Melamed 2002) and, after muscle contusion, myositis ossificans can develop.

There are no specific radiographic findings. Plain films or a bone scan may be required to exclude a pelvic fracture (see Fig. 5.180) and ultrasound can assist with aspiration of

a haematoma. Bone bruising could be demonstrated using fat-suppressed MRI but is usually not indicated as the clinical management would be unaltered, whatever the result.

Gluteus medius syndrome

Gluteus medius syndrome is caused by overuse, producing a gluteus medius tendinopathy with pain that simulates and can be mistaken for sciatica. The athlete usually presents with buttock pain or pain in the lateral hip, groin and sacroiliac joints. Numbness on the posterior aspect of the thigh may also be noted and the symptoms are exacerbated by prolonged sitting or hip adduction. These symptoms are non-specific and other conditions such as a lumbar disc protrusion, piriformis syndrome, trochanteric bursopathy, iliotibial band friction syndrome and sacroiliac problems have to be considered in the differential diagnosis. The gluteus medius is the major abductor of the thigh and gluteus medius syndrome is most likely to occur in the martial arts, cycling, aerobics and dancing (Melamed 2002).

Imaging can help to establish the diagnosis. Plain films will be normal, but a nuclear bone scan, ultrasound or MRI may demonstrate the changes of a tendon tear (see Figs 5.181 and 5.182) or tendinopathy (see Figs 5.183 and 5.184).

▶ **Fig. 5.181** Transverse and long-axis ultrasound images obtained over the greater trochanter show a diffusely hypoechoic gluteus medius tendon with associated swelling, most pronounced at the anterior insertion (white arrowheads) where a superimposed echogenic line consistent with complicating partial tear can be seen to involve the deep fibres (arrows). Note the normal echotexture of the gluteus minimus tendon (black arrowhead).

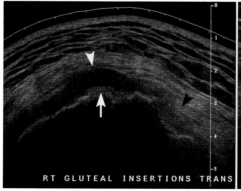
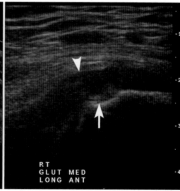

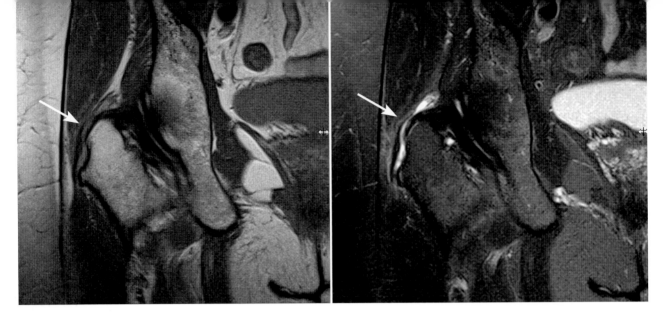

▲ **Fig. 5.182** Coronal MR images demonstrate a chronic partial tear at the gluteus medius tendon insertion with associated sub-medius bursopathy extending proximally (arrows).

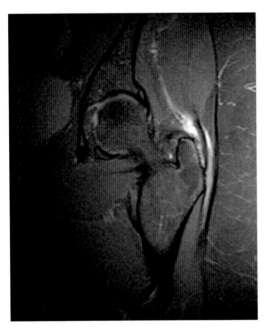

▲ **Fig. 5.183** Gluteus medius insertional tendinopathy and partial tear with accompanying sub-medius and sub-ITB bursopathy are demonstrated on a coronal fat-suppressed MR image.

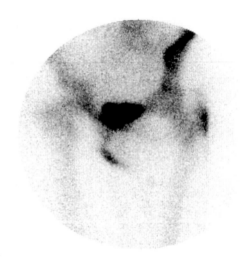

▲ **Fig. 5.184** A nuclear bone scan demonstrates gluteus medius tendinopathy, possibly with accompanying trochanteric bursopathy.

Iliopsoas tendinopathy

The iliopsoas functions as a flexor and external rotator of the hip. The iliopsoas passes anterior to the pelvic brim and hip joint capsule in a groove between the AIIS and the iliopectineal eminence. The musculotendinous junction of the iliopsoas is constantly found at the level of the groove.

Iliopsoas tendinopathy develops as a result of either acute injury or overuse, with the athlete complaining of groin pain that is particularly noticeable when walking up and down stairs. Pain and tenderness are diffuse and poorly localised along the proximal anteromedial thigh area. Overuse iliopsoas tendinopathy may be seen in weight-lifters, snow skiers, uphill runners, soccer players who repetitively shoot for the goal and those with a physical training regimen of sit-ups.

On physical examination, there is pain to resisted hip flexion as well as iliopsoas tightness and irritability to passive stretching. Imaging may show reactive changes in the iliopsoas muscle surrounding the tendon, or there may be a true tendinopathy with associated tendon tenderness and MRI hyperintensity. Imaging with either ultrasound or MRI may demonstrate these changes (see Figs 5.185–5.188). Ultrasound often only reveals tenderness to probing in the line of the iliopsoas muscle-tendon unit and swelling of the tendon by comparison with the opposite side. Recurrent traction of the iliopsoas on the lesser trochanter may produce enthesopathy, which may be demonstrated by either a nuclear bone scan or MRI (see Fig. 5.189).

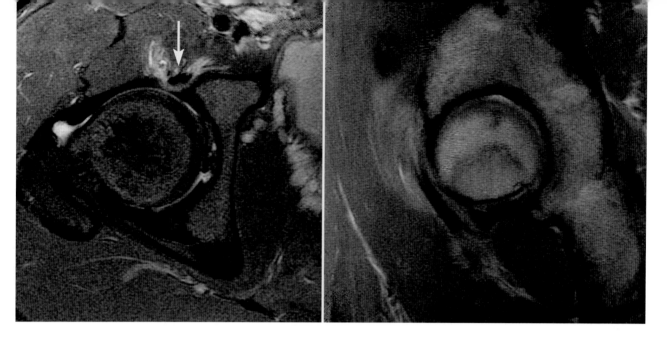

▲ **Fig. 5.185** Axial and sagittal MR images show iliopsoas tendinopathy and bursopathy with the majority of the changes occurring in the tissues surrounding the iliopsoas tendon. The tendon itself (arrow) shows subtle intrasubstance hyperintensity. Note the small hip joint effusion.

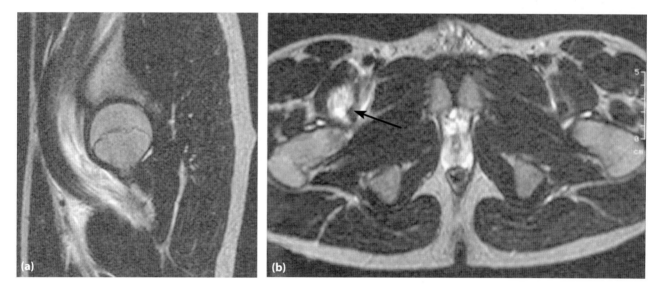

▲ **Fig. 5.186(a)** Iliopsoas tendinopathy and bursopathy are demonstrated on a sagittal fat-suppressed T2-weighted MR image. The changes are marked in the tissues surrounding the tendon. **(b)** An axial MR image in the same case shows that although considerable change is present in the tissues around the tendon, high signal is also seen within the tendon itself (arrow), making a partial tear difficult to exclude.

▶ **Fig. 5.187** Comparison transverse ultrasound images of the right and left iliopsoas tendons at the level of the superior pubic ramus demonstrate subtle thickening of the left iliopsoas bursa (arrow) in an athlete with pain over the anterior aspect of the hip. There was localised tenderness to probing at this location. Note the similarity of this ultrasound appearance to the MRI changes of chronic athletic iliopsoas bursopathy shown in Fig. 5.175. The black asterisk indicates the psoas tendon. Iliopsoas muscle = M.

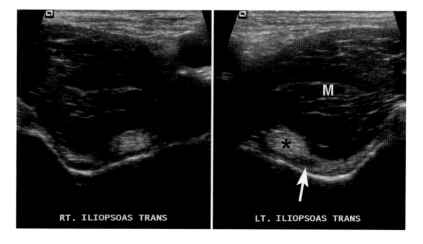

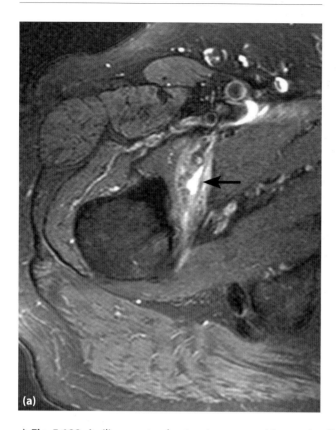

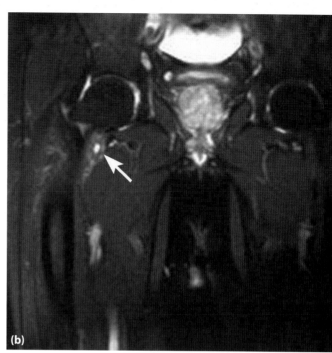

▲ **Fig. 5.188** An iliopsoas tendon tear is present, with non-visualisation of the tendon and replacement by a fluid space on axial (black arrow) **(a)** and coronal (white arrow) **(b)** fat-suppressed MR images.

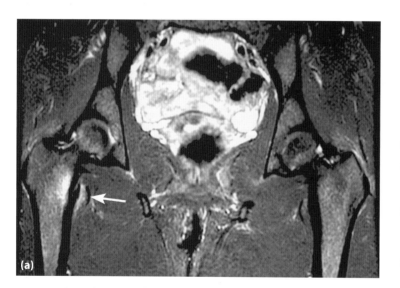

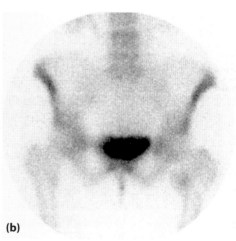

▲ **Fig. 5.189(a)** A coronal fat-suppressed MR image shows high marrow signal at the lesser trochanter and peritendon hyperintensity at the iliopsoas insertion, which would suggest either enthesopathy or an avulsion injury. **(b)** Recurrent traction stress by the iliopsoas has produced enthesopathy at the lesser trochanter, demonstrated by bone scan.

Snapping hip syndrome

Snapping hip syndrome (or coxa saltans) is characterised by an audible snapping sensation that is often accompanied by pain. The two most frequently encountered causes of snapping hip syndrome are an iliopsoas snap (see Fig. 5.190) and snapping of the iliotibial band over the greater trochanter. An iliopsoas snap is common in sports requiring repetitive hip and knee flexion, such as dancing, cycling and running,

with the snap becoming clinically significant when associated with pain. The iliopsoas passes anterior to a bursa, the hip capsule and the pelvic brim, and secondary iliopsoas bursopathy can become the source of pain.

Dynamic ultrasound has been used to confirm the snap of the iliopsoas tendon (Janzen et al. 1996) but may not be helpful if the patient cannot reproduce the snap at the

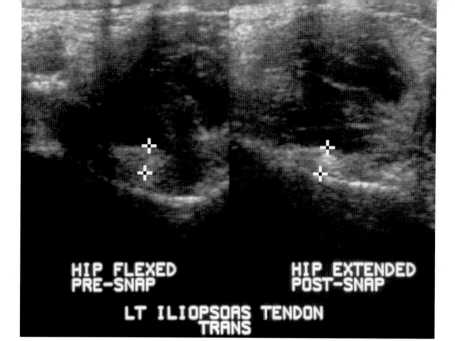

HIP FLEXED
PRE-SNAP

HIP EXTENDED
POST-SNAP

LT ILIOPSOAS TENDON
TRANS

◀ **Fig. 5.190** Transverse ultrasound images show the echogenic iliopsoas tendon (indicated by callipers) suddenly shift as the hip moves from flexion to extension.

Table 5.2 Causes of snapping hip syndrome

Intra-articular causes of snapping hip syndrome	Extra-articular causes of snapping hip syndrome
Acetabular labral tears	**Medial snap**

• Loose bodies
• Synovial chondromatosis
• Exostosis
• Osteochondral injury
• Subluxation of the femoral head
• Villonodular synovitis
• Suction phenomenon in the joint
	• The iliopsoas tendon snaps over
	  – the lesser trochanter
	  – the iliopectineal eminence
	  – the anterior inferior iliac spine
	• The iliofemoral ligament snaps over the femoral head

	Lateral snap
	• The iliotibial band snaps over the greater trochanter • The gluteus maximus snaps over the greater trochanter
	Posterior snap
	• The long head of the biceps femoris snaps over the ischial tuberosity

Source: Adapted from Melamed (2002).

time of the examination or if the snap occurs in a position that does not permit transducer access. Iliopsoas bursography is an invasive method of imaging the same disorder allowing the sudden iliopsoas shift to be identified as the source of the snap as the outline of the iliopsoas muscle can be followed fluoroscopically during hip movements.

Snapping of the iliotibial band occurs when the hip is brought from extension into flexion. There is no restriction to athletic activity and the snap is usually asymptomatic. If pain develops, this is usually due to the development of trochanteric bursopathy.

The causes of snapping hip syndrome are classified as intra-articular and extra-articular, with extra-articular being further divided into medial, lateral and posterior (see Table 5.2).

Acetabular labral tears

The recognition of tears of the acetabular labrum as a cause of hip pain in athletes has occurred only recently. Suzuki et al. (1986) published the first arthroscopic description of a labral tear and since then there have been a number of accounts of labral tears

occurring in athletes (Ikeda et al. 1988; Fitzgerald 1995; Mason 2001). It is now understood that labral tears produce osteochondral lesions on the articular surface of the femoral head, leading to early degenerative joint disease.

There is usually a delay in the diagnosis of a labral tear. There are many reasons for this. The onset of symptoms is insidious. Athletes often have trouble identifying a specific injury leading to their hip discomfort and the symptoms are commonly blamed on muscle strain and groin strain in the first instance. It is important that physicians think of a labral tear as a possible diagnosis and realise that a delayed diagnosis means that important chondral injury is progressing. Not all tears that can be demonstrated are symptomatic, but those with symptoms usually present as groin pain that is catching in quality and that may or may not be associated with a snap or click. Other causes for a snap in this region should also be remembered. Fitzgerald (1995) noted that patients with a tear commonly experience a catch in the hip after sitting for a period. This catch causes only a momentary discomfort on standing up. Difficulty is also experienced with a breaststroke kick and running down stairs.

Injury to the acetabular labrum bears some similarity to meniscal tears in the knee. As in the knee, labral or paralabral cysts may form at the site of a tear. Tears occur in four separate categories: the ageing hip, the dysplastic hip, femoroacetabular impingement and the normal hip.

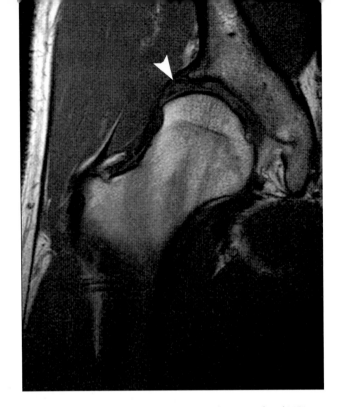

▲ Fig. 5.191 Non-arthrographic coronal PD-weighted MRI demonstrates a labral tear (arrowhead) in a dysplastic hip. Note the anterolateral migration of the femoral head, which increases loading of the labrum.

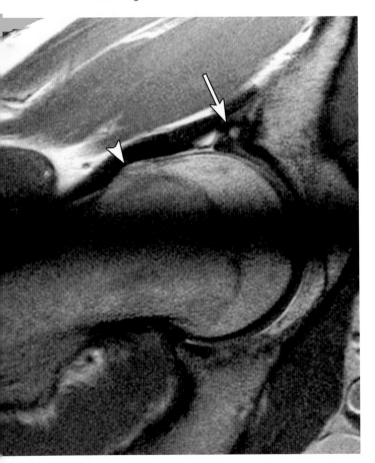

▲ Fig. 5.192 Bony prominence at the femoral head/neck junction (arrowhead) causes femoroacetabular impingement. The impingement occurs against the lateral acetabular rim where labral injury and cyst formation are present (arrow).

- *The ageing hip* The labrum degenerates and weakens with age and by midlife may develop degenerative horizontal cleavage tears. Ageing also brings with it an increasing vulnerability to traumatic tears. MRI studies of the labrum have shown that there is a progressive loss of the triangular cross-sectional shape of the labrum with increasing age (Huffman and Safran 2002). Rounding and irregularities appear in the anterior and superior labrum, findings that are rare before 20 years of age. Labral tears are frequently seen with MRI in osteoarthritic hips.

- *The dysplastic hip* In dysplastic hips the weightbearing forces progressively shift anterolaterally. In response, the labrum becomes hypertrophied as it is exposed to increasing stresses due to the migration of the femoral head. Labral tears and osteoarthrosis are almost inevitable in this patient group (see Fig. 5.191). Radiographic detection of unrecognised minimal hip joint dysplasia is important because it allows an athlete to be counselled about the risks of accelerated osteoarthrosis with sporting activity.

- *Femoroacetabular impingement* Femoroacetabular impingement will cause injury to the labrum, articular cartilage and bone at the anterior or lateral aspect of the acetabular roof in the area of impingement (see Fig. 5.192). See the discussion on page 369.

- *The normal hip* Fitzgerald (1995) reported the diagnostic features and treatment outcomes of 55 patients in the normal hip group. The majority (70%) were less than 40 years of age. The clinical course was usually insidious, with an average of 35 months between symptom onset and presentation. Groin pain was the presenting complaint in 48 cases. Most (93%) had normal plain radiographs. The site of a labral tear was usually anterior (of 49 cases examined arthroscopically, there were 45 anterior tears and 4 posterior tears). Some cases were associated with defects in the articular cartilage of the femoral head where the labral tear had come into contact with the head during hip flexion.

The imaging evaluation of a possible labral tear should begin with a plain film series of the pelvis and hip. Evidence of hip dysplasia is of particular importance. The slope, shape and length of the acetabular roof should be noted and the Wiberg centre-to-edge angle measured to assess acetabular tilt (see the discussion on hip dysplasia on pages 366–9). Also of interest is evidence of prominence at the head/neck junction, which may create a predisposition to anterior femoroacetabular impingement. Note should also be made of degenerative changes and loose bodies.

MRI is the imaging modality of choice, but the preferred examination protocol remains a subject of debate. Non-arthrographic MRI is effective at demonstrating labral tears (see Fig. 5.193), but MR arthrography can further increase the sensitivity and specificity of this imaging method (Czerney et al. 1996) (see Fig. 5.194). At the time of arthrographic injection, bupivacaine should also be instilled into the joint to establish the clinical relevance of any tear. If a tear is symptomatic, pain relief is expected after the injection of local anaesthetic.

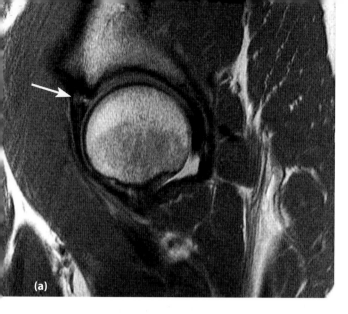

(a)

Ultrasound can also be useful in the detection of labral and paralabral cysts, although MR arthrography remains the imaging 'gold standard' for the detection of tears with or without associated cysts. Ultrasound is also helpful for guiding injections of local anaesthetic and corticosteroid into the joint, a manoeuvre that may be diagnostic and therapeutic (see Fig. 5.195).

◀**Fig. 5.193(a)** A labral tear (arrow) may be well demonstrated without intra-articular gadolinium.
▼ **(b)** MRI satisfactorily demonstrates a labral tear on a sagittal PD-weighted image obtained without intra-articular contrast (arrow).

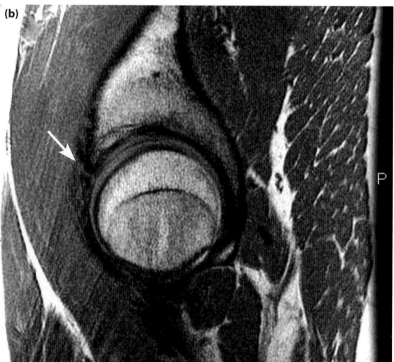

(b)

▼ **(c)** A further example of a labral tear (arrowhead) demonstrated on a non-arthrographic radial PD-weighted MR image.

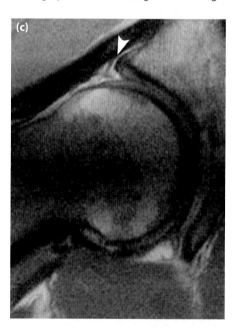

(c)

◀**Fig. 5.194** MR arthrography clearly demonstrates a labral tear (arrowhead).

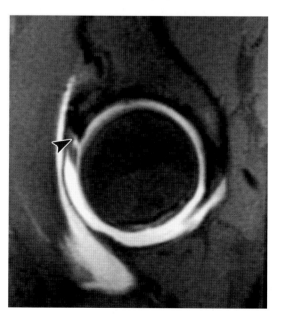

▶ **Fig. 5.195** An ultrasound-guided injection of local anaesthetic into the hip joint may help determine whether the labrum is the source of the symptoms. The obliquely oriented echogenic line traversing the iliopsoas muscle is the needle, with the tip located against the femoral head at the free margin of the acetabular labrum.

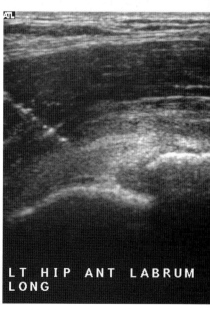

LT HIP ANT LABRUM LONG

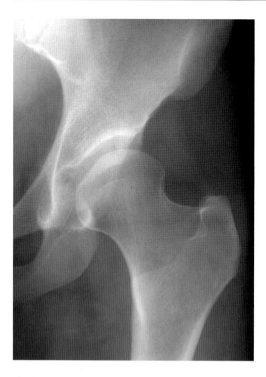

▲ Fig. 5.196 There is a steeply sloped acetabular roof indicating hip dysplasia. Both ends of the 'teardrop' should be at the same horizontal level.

Developmental conditions predisposing to hip injury

Hip joint dysplasia

The incidence of developmental dysplasia of the hip varies in different communities, but across western societies is reported to occur in 1–3% of the newborn population. Minimal degrees of dysplasia may escape clinical detection in early childhood and present later on in early adult life with premature osteoarthrosis. Hip joint osteoarthrosis has been reported to be secondary to dysplasia in as many as 20–47% of cases. In Japan, where hip joint dysplasia is common, a longitudinal prospective study of 86 dysplastic adult hips with no initial radiographic evidence of osteoarthrosis showed a 47% incidence of osteoarthrosis at 7.8 years and a 100% incidence of osteoarthrosis at 9.2 years (Hasegawa et al. 1992).

▼ Fig. 5.197 Bilateral dysplastic changes are present, more marked on the right with degenerative changes progressing on this side. Anterolateral migration of the right femoral head is demonstrated (arrowheads), using the 'teardrop' as a reference point.

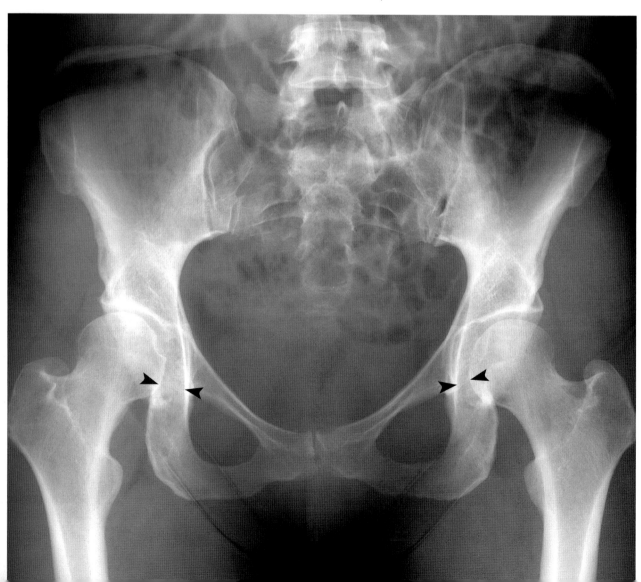

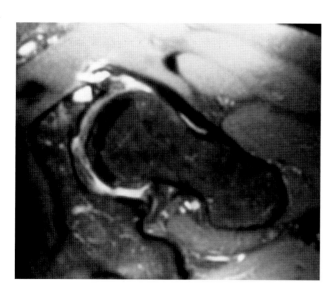

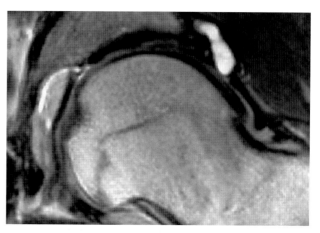

◀▲ **Fig. 5.198** Ganglia are demonstrated by MRI in both bone and adjacent soft tissue at the anterior acetabular rim.

Cooperman et al. (1983) similarly followed 32 dysplastic hips in 20 adult patients for 22 years and found that:

- none of the criteria for dysplasia could be used to predict the severity or age of onset of osteoarthrosis
- males with osteoarthrosis remained symptom-free longer than women
- only two of the 20 patients were free of osteoarthrosis at 20 years of age.

Radiographically, there are two patterns of dysplasia in the adult hip: Type I and Type II.

Type I: Sloping acetabular roof

A line drawn through the medial and lateral ends of the weightbearing area of the acetabular roof is not horizontal. The outer end lies superior to the inner end (see Fig. 5.196). Secondary to this, there is an anterolateral migration of the femoral head, as judged by its distance from the 'teardrop' (see Fig. 5.197). The weightbearing hip distributes acetabular load both laterally and anteriorly. There is a compensatory hypertrophy of the labrum and capsule in an attempt to withstand the abnormal stress. Eventually, being mechanically inferior, the labrum will tear and the hip joint will degenerate. Ganglia may then extend into the bone of the acetabular roof or across the labrum into the periarticular soft tissues (see Fig. 5.198).

Type II: Short acetabular roof (acetabular retroversion)

The femoral head is well positioned but the acetabular roof is short and provides insufficient cover for the femoral head (see Figs 5.199 and 5.200). The degree of cover is determined by the degree of acetabular tilt. A short roof results from a decreased tilt of the acetabulum, so-called acetabular retroversion. The weightbearing load is distributed across

a smaller than normal bone surface area. Over time, large transmitted forces may eventually produce a stress fracture in the acetabular roof. The hypertrophied labrum will inevitably tear and the hip joint will degenerate.

The length of the acetabular roof is assessed on plain films as a part of the routine assessment of the hip. Measurements obtained from an AP view are used to gauge whether the head is adequately covered and if acetabular retroversion is present:

- The femoral head extrusion index (see Fig. 5.201) is the percentage of the femoral head covered by the acetabular roof. If more than 25% of the head protrudes laterally, the head is insufficiently covered.

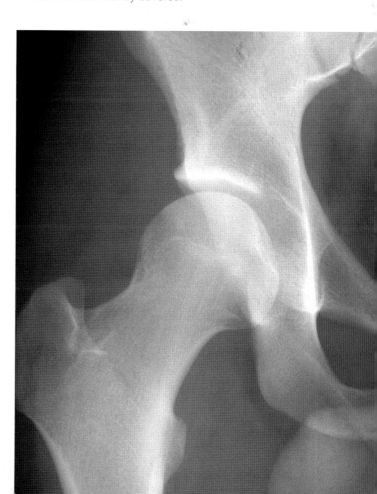

▶ **Fig. 5.199** The acetabular roof is short, with uncovering of the lateral aspect of the femoral head consistent with Type II dysplasia.

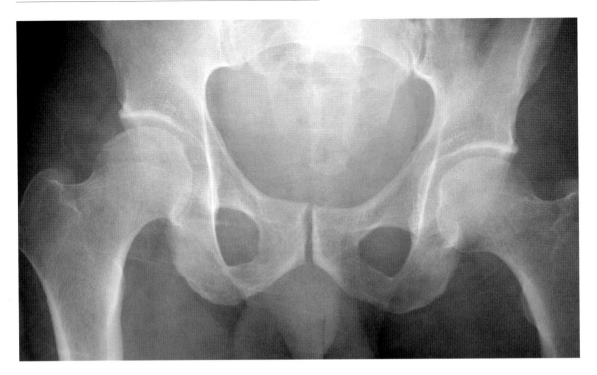

▲ **Fig. 5.200** Both hips show dysplastic changes. There is sloping of the acetabular roof on both sides (Type I dysplasia) and the right acetabular roof is short (Type II dysplasia).

▼ **Fig. 5.201** The femoral head extrusion index calculates how much of the femoral head protrudes lateral to the outer end of the articular surface of the acetabular roof. In excess of 25% is abnormal and indicates acetabular retroversion with a greater risk of injury of the femoral articular surface, particularly during contact sports.

▼ **Fig. 5.202** The Wiberg centre-edge angle assesses the acetabulum for retroversion. It is calculated by measuring the angle between a perpendicular line drawn through the centre of the femoral head and a line drawn through the centre of the femoral head and the outer edge of the acetabular roof. An angle of 25° is normal; less than 20° is definitely abnormal. Acetabular retroversion is present in this case.

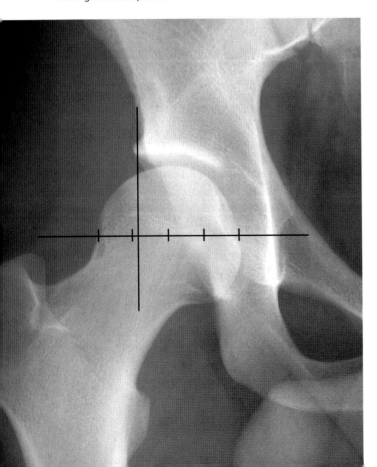

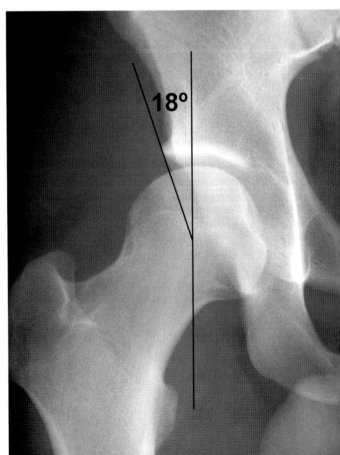

- The Wiberg centre-edge angle (Wiberg 1939) assesses the acetabulum for retroversion. The degree of inferior acetabular tilt is assessed by measuring the angle between a vertical line drawn through the centre of the femoral head and a line drawn through the centre of the femoral head and the lateral edge of the acetabular roof (see Fig. 5.202). An angle of 25° is normal and less than 20° is indicative of acetabular retroversion.

Anterior femoroacetabular impingement: a cause of groin pain

Anterior femoroacetabular impingement is a recently described condition where impingement occurs between the femoral neck and the acetabular rim in a hip with no radiological evidence of hip dysplasia (Ito et al. 2001). This condition causes groin pain and may be seen in young athletes. Injury to the labrum and the anterior acetabular rim results from repetitive abutment on these structures by the femoral neck during forceful hip movements required by particular sports. Ito et al. demonstrated that patients with a reduced femoral anteversion or a reduced femoral head/neck offset at the anterior aspect of the femoral neck were at risk of impingement.

Femoroacetabular impingement also occurs in so-called 'pistol grip' deformity (see Figs 5.203 and 5.204) and is associated with early onset of degenerative hip disease (Murray 1965). The inferior head has a greater radius and there is less space available along the superior aspect of the femoral neck for clearance of the acetabular rim with hip flexion, internal rotation and adduction. Athletes performing these movements include swimmers doing the breaststroke, baseball catchers and batters, and soccer players (Ferguson and Matta 2002). Athletes generally present with an intermittent sharp anterior groin pain, which can be reproduced with flexion, adduction and internal rotation. These movements bring the femoral neck in contact with the labrum and the anterior acetabular rim.

Imaging commences with a plain film series including an AP and lateral view of the symptomatic hip. An AP view of the pelvis is preferred to an AP view of one hip, allowing a comparative assessment to be made (see Fig. 5.205). These films are assessed for evidence of hip retroversion with measurement of the centre-edge angle and careful examination of the acetabular roof. Changes of anterior femoroacetabular impingement syndrome may be seen at the site of impingement on the acetabular roof and femur (see Fig. 5.206). MRI is able to show damage to the articular cartilage, the acetabular labrum and the acetabular rim, and may identify loose bodies (see Fig. 5.207). MR arthrography is reported to be more accurate than MRI alone (Edwards et al. 1995; Anderson et al. 2001). Early changes of osteoarthrosis may also be present on plain films.

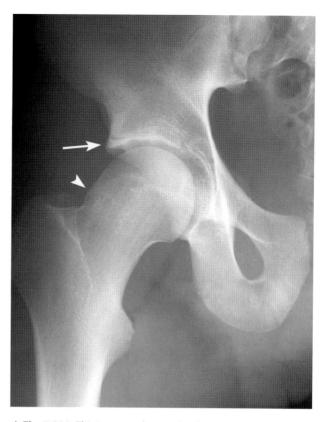

▲ **Fig. 5.203** This is a typical example of 'pistol-grip' deformity of the hip. A bony prominence on the superior aspect of the head/neck junction (arrowhead) impinges on the outer aspect of the acetabular roof with particular hip movements, and sclerotic thickening is developing at the superior acetabular rim (arrow).

▼ **Fig. 5.204** Advanced degenerative changes involving the hip joint of a relatively young athlete. There is an underlying 'pistol-grip' deformity.

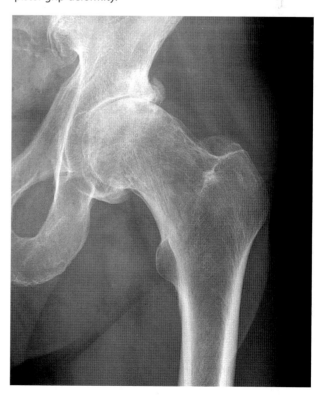

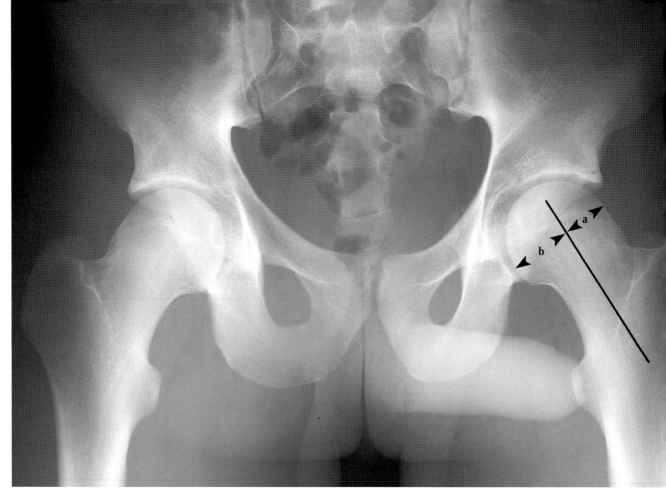

▲ **Fig. 5.205** An AP view of the pelvis with bilateral 'pistol-grip' deformity shows that the femoral heads are not spherical. The upper radius is less than the lower radius and a resulting 'cam' effect on rotation of the femoral head will cause impingement.

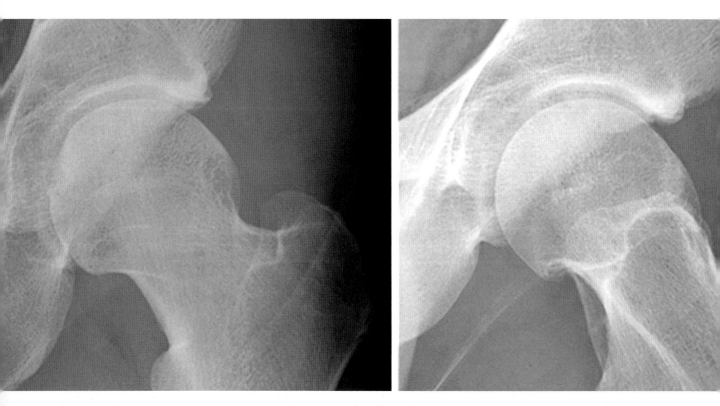

▲ **Fig. 5.206** AP and lateral views of the hip show a bony prominence at the superior head/neck junction and changes at the lateral aspect of the acetabular roof consistent with femoroacetabular impingement. There is bony sclerosis at the anterolateral acetabular rim and joint space narrowing secondary to impingement. Cystic changes at the lateral aspect of the subcapital region indicate the site of bony impingement. Osteophytes are noted at the margins of the femoral articular surface.

If the femoral head/neck angle on the superior apect is obliterated, impingement is likely (see Fig. 5.208). Cystic degeneration at the femoral neck will often indicate the site of impingement. The femoral angle should also be noted and an assessment of femoral anteversion made. A decrease in these measurements may predispose to impingement. Anteversion measurement requires a CT scan and this method is discussed later in the section on anteversion.

▼ **Fig. 5.207** A coronal PD-weighted MR image shows injury to the anterolateral acetabular rim (arrow). There is bony sclerosis, a labral tear and early intra-labral cyst formation. A cystic change on the lateral subcapital aspect of the femoral neck indicates the site of femoral impingement.

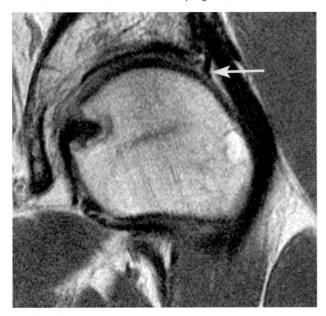

Coxa vara

A decrease in the femoral angle to less than 125° is termed *coxa vara*. Coxa vara can be developmental, due to an ossification defect in the femoral neck, or it can be acquired, secondary to a femoral neck fracture. Coxa vara produces a painless limp or waddling gait, leg-length discrepancy, impaired hip joint abduction and reduced internal rotation. Radiographically, there is a reduced femoral angle, rotation of the growth plate into a more vertical orientation, and a triangular bone fragment on the inferomedial aspect of the proximal femoral neck.

Coxa valga

An increase in the femoral angle beyond the usual 128° is termed *coxa valga*. This is a rare deformity that alters normal hip joint biomechanics and is usually caused by either disruption of the growth plate of the greater trochanter (Taussig et al. 1976) or AVN of the femoral head epiphysis laterally. Occasionally, even with a normal acetabular roof, coxa valgus alignment will cause subluxation of the femoral head. This deformity also predisposes to a femoral neck stress fracture due to altered biomechanics (see Fig. 5.209).

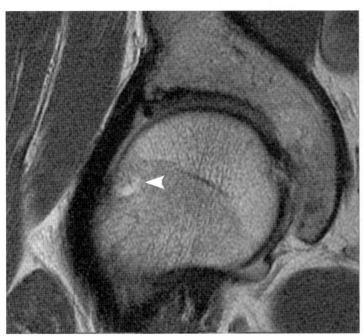
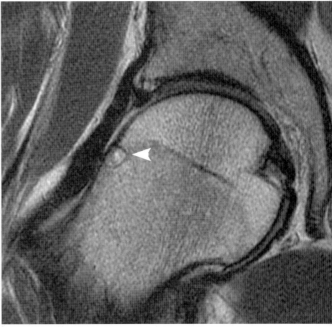

▲ **Fig. 5.208** Cystic changes are demonstrated by MRI at the junction of the femoral head and neck. They occur secondary to impingement. These changes must be differentiated from synovial pits, which commonly occur and are of no clinical significance. The differentiation is made by identifying other evidence of femoroacetabular impingement.

▶ **Fig. 5.209** A developmental coxa valga is present. The biomechanics associated with this anomaly have contributed to the formation of a stress fracture of the femoral neck.

Femoral anteversion

When the normal femur is viewed in a true axial projection, the angle between the neck and the coronal plane is referred to as the femoral anteversion angle (see Fig. 5.210). Excessive femoral anteversion of 30–40° is common at birth but normally reduces to 8–14° at skeletal maturity. If the angle remains excessive, the child will walk with toeing-in and will have an awkward running style. Staheli et al. (1977) found no correlation between increased femoral anteversion and impaired athletic activity. In hip dysplasia, femoral anteversion has been found to be normal (Anda et al. 1991).

The main complication of increased femoral anteversion is limited external rotation at the hip, which is a prime requirement in classical ballet. The dancer is then forced to use compensatory manoeuvres that place increased demands upon the leg, foot and lower spine. Elite ballet dancers have a greater than normal turnout of the hip, but a study by Bauman et al. (1994) showed that in this group femoral anteversion was the same as in a control group. They suggested that the increased turnout might be due to a retroverted acetabular fossa, a shallow acetabular fossa, or laxity of the anterior capsule and Bigelow's ligament (anterior iliofemoral ligament).

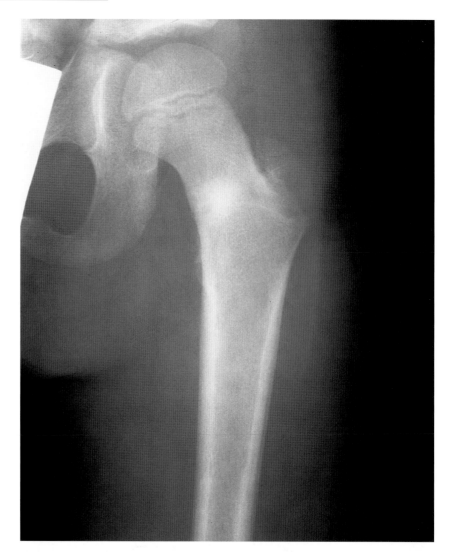

▶ **Fig. 5.210** The femoral anteversion angle is measured by obtaining CT scan images through both the femoral neck and the femoral condyles, without changing the patient's position on the table. A line through the posterior aspect of the femoral condyles is the baseline, and the forward twist of the proximal femur relative to this baseline is the anteversion angle.

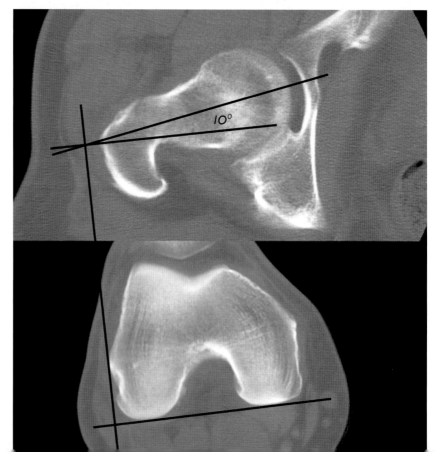

Miscellaneous conditions

Nerve entrapments

Obturator neuropathy has been reported as a cause of chronic groin pain in athletes (Bradshaw et al. 1997). It is suggested that fascial and vascular structures may cause localised entrapment of the obturator nerve. The athlete, usually a footballer, presents with exercise-induced medial thigh pain starting in the region of the adductor origin. Electromyography shows denervation of the adductor muscles, and isotope bone scanning often shows a mild increase in activity at the pubic ramus and at the origins of the adductor longus or adductor brevis on delayed images.

An unusual cause of obturator nerve entrapment in sport was encountered at the Sydney 2000 Olympics. An elite female cyclist presented with medial thigh pain, severe enough to prevent her preparation for competition. The only finding on imaging was an ovarian cyst on the symptomatic side (see Fig. 5.211). It was suspected that the cyst was causing repetitive pressure on the adjacent psoas muscle as the hip flexed and extended with the cycling motion, and that the obturator nerve was being traumatised by this action. The obturator nerve arises in the psoas muscle, derived from the L2, 3 and 4 nerve roots, and passes through the psoas and across the pelvic sidewall to the obturator foramen before entering the thigh. The cyst was aspirated and the athlete's symptoms resolved. Post aspiration, a follow-up MRI showed the intimate relationship between the cyst and the psoas muscle (see Fig. 5.212).

Sciatic nerve entrapment can result from perineural scar formation at the level of the ischial tuberosity or proximal thigh following haemorrhage associated with isolated or recurrent hamstring origin tendon tears. This close relationship between the sciatic nerve and hamstring tears is best assessed with MRI (see Fig. 5.213) and has been demonstrated in Figs 5.137, 5.138 and 5.140 on pages 344 and 345.

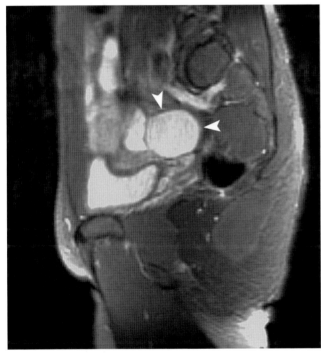

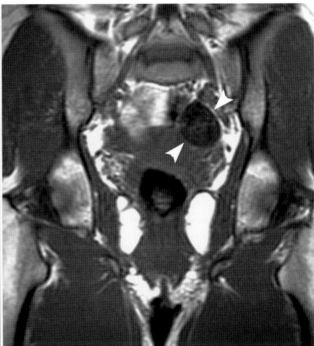

▲ **Fig. 5.211** Sagittal T2 and coronal T1 MR images demonstrate the presence of an ovarian cyst (arrowheads), closely related to the left psoas at the pelvic brim. No other cause for obturator nerve entrapment is evident and it was assumed that the ovarian cyst might have been contributing to the patient's symptoms, by producing pressure on the psoas and entrapping the obturator nerve.

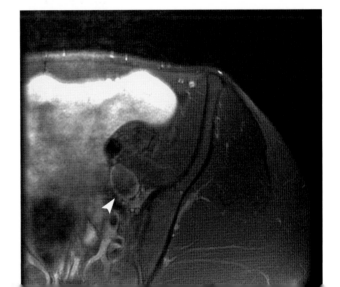

▶ **Fig. 5.212** After aspiration of the ovarian cyst shown in Fig. 5.211, a follow-up fat-suppressed T1-weighted MRI shows the intimate relationship between the cyst (arrowhead) and the psoas, which is noted to be indented by the cyst.

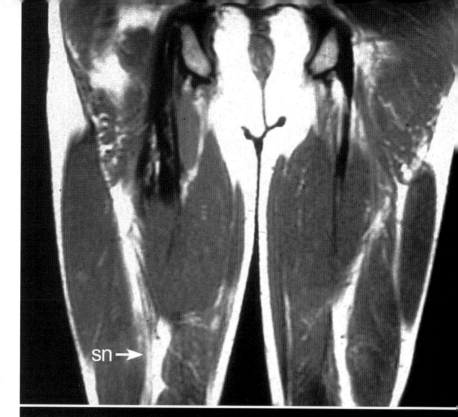

▶ Fig. 5.213 Entrapment of the sciatic nerve has occurred in an area of fibrosis secondary to an old hamstring injury. These changes are demonstrated as an area of hypointense thickening on coronal and axial T1-weighted images.

Meralgia paraesthetica is the most common nerve condition encountered around the pelvis and hip. It is characterised by a burning anterolateral thigh pain and an altered sensation in the same distribution due to lateral femoral cutaneous nerve entrapment beneath the outer end of the inguinal ligament. Weight-lifters and gymnasts are most often affected. The abnormal nerve can be imaged well with ultrasound (see Fig. 5.214) and guided therapeutic perineural injection can also be offered using this modality.

Pudendal nerve entrapment is a condition of chronic perineal pain that may occur in cyclists and horse riders, typically made worse by direct pressure when sitting and relieved by standing. Imaging has a role in guided therapeutic injection, and this is discussed in more detail in Chapter 10.

▼ Fig. 5.214 Transverse and long-axis ultrasound images of the lateral femoral cutaneous nerve demonstrate a short segment of hypoechoic fusiform nerve swelling (arrows) immediately inferior to the inguinal ligament (arrowheads). Normal nerve, both superior and inferior to the swollen segment, is indicated by callipers on the long-axis image.

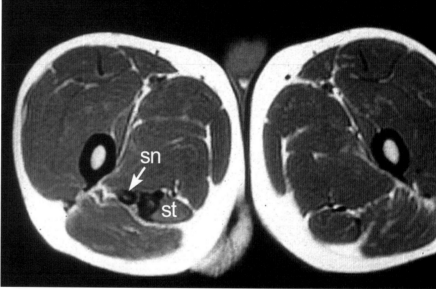

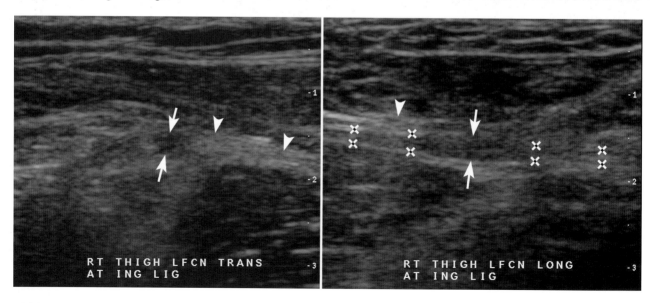

▶ Fig. 5.215 Deformity of the left femoral head is due to a combination of a slipped femoral epiphysis and avascular necrosis, a complication of reduction of a slipped epiphysis. A successful fixation is noted on the right side.

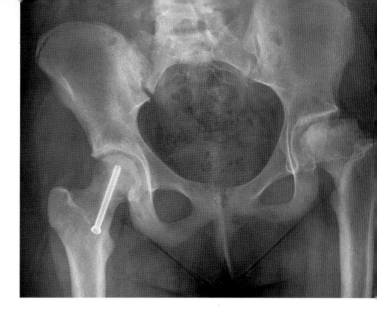

AVN of the femoral head

AVN of the femoral head occurs when the blood supply to the femoral head is interrupted, and is an occasional cause of hip pain.

In adults, AVN may occur spontaneously or as a complication of hip trauma. In the context of sports medicine, AVN may be seen in underwater divers (Amako et al. 1974) and may follow short-term, high-dose corticosteroid therapy (O'Brien and Mack 1992). AVN tends to occur in the 40–70 year age bracket and affects males more frequently than females.

In children, AVN may occur as a primary condition, Perthes disease (see below), and is also seen as a complication of femoral neck fracture or following reduction of a slipped femoral capital epiphysis (see Fig. 5.215). Blood supply to the femoral head in early life is via the ligamentum teres, with the epiphyseal plate acting as a barrier to vessels entering from the femoral neck. Between the ages of four and seven this pattern of supply reverses, and during this time of change the incidence of AVN increases.

Plain films may be normal in the early stages. The earliest plain film change is the so-called 'crescent sign', which is produced by demineralisation of a crescentic area of subchondral bone in the weightbearing area (see Figs 5.216 and 5.217). This area then develops surrounding sclerosis and, with progression of the process, subtle flattening of the femoral head occurs due to the collapse and compression of subchondral bone. Fragmentation occurs (see Figs 5.218 and 5.219), followed by healing with revascularisation. Osteoarthrosis is a late development.

▼ Fig. 5.216 There is a crescent of subchondral demineralisation in the weightbearing area (arrowheads) indicating early AVN. This area has a mildly sclerotic margin. This is the 'crescent' sign.

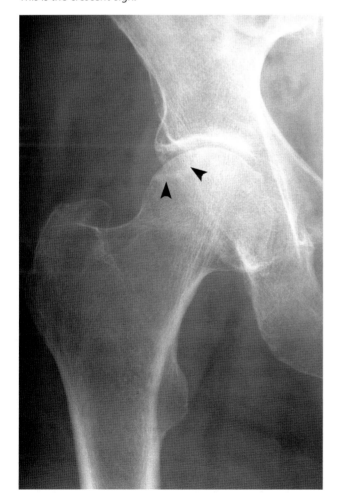

▼ Fig. 5.217 A coronal T1-weighted MR image demonstrates marrow oedema in the subchondral area seen in Fig. 5.215 (arrowhead).

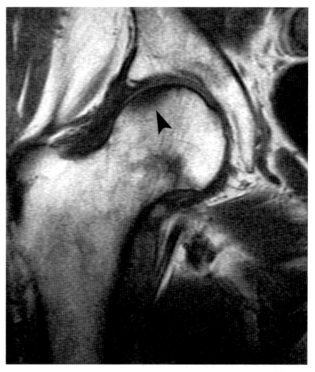

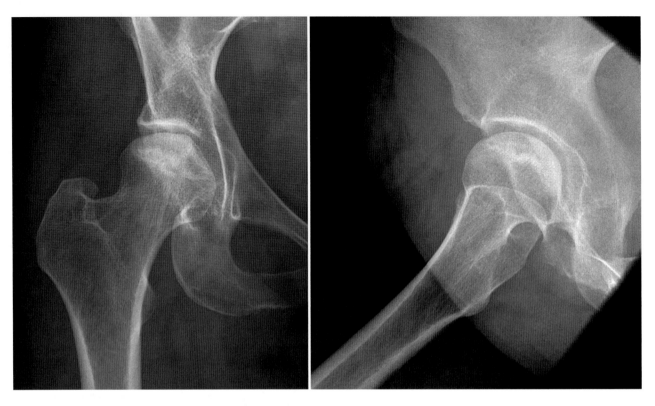

▲ **Fig. 5.518** As healing progresses, the fragmentation unites with flattening of the femoral head persisting together with altered bony architecture in the subchondral bone. Although at this stage there is maintenance of normal joint space, degenerative changes are likely to develop.

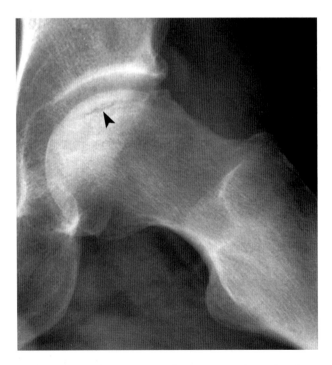

▲ **Fig. 5.219** With progression, fragmentation (arrowhead) and collapse occurs.

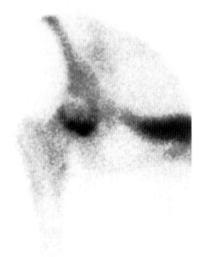

▲ **Fig. 5.220** AVN involves the right hip superiorly in the weightbearing area. This area appears 'cold' on a bone scan, with increased uptake of isotope at the margins of the avascular area.

An isotope bone scan or MRI is required for the early diagnosis of AVN, when plain radiographs are negative. The earliest appearance on bone scanning is an absence of uptake in the avascular area, which looks 'cold' (see Fig. 5.220). In the later stages of revascularisation, the lesion and particularly its margins shows increased uptake of isotope (see Fig. 5.221). MRI is also able to detect early AVN (see Figs 5.222 and 5.223).

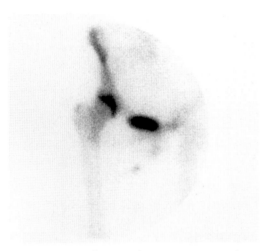

▲ **Fig. 5.221** With revascularisation comes an increase in isotope uptake in the previously 'cold' area.

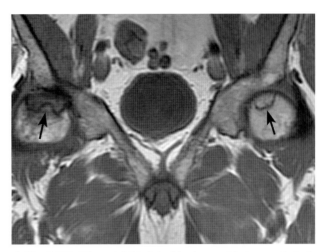

▲ **Fig. 5.222** Bilateral AVN of the hips (arrows) is demonstrated by MRI. These changes followed steroid therapy.

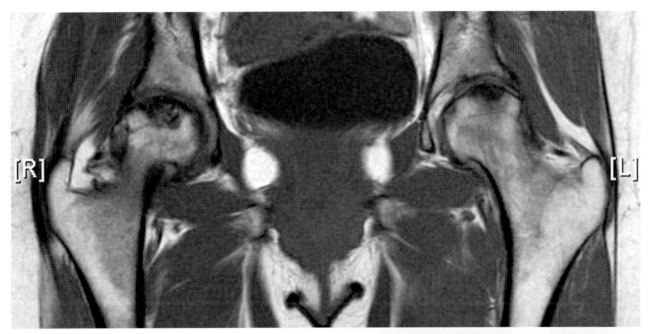

▲ **Fig. 5.223(a)** Coronal TI-weighted MRI shows changes of avascular necrosis of the right hip. The involved area is sharply demarcated from normal bone by a sclerotic margin. The avascular process involves the subchondral bone. Early changes are also noted on the left side.

▶ **(b)** When the avascular area is sharply demarcated from the surrounding bone, the enclosed bone may loosen and become separated, as occurs in osteochondritis dissecans. On the fat-suppressed MR image in the insert, a fluid line is shown beneath the avascular fragment, suggesting that loosening has occurred.

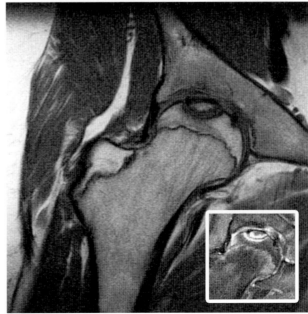

Perthes disease

Perthes disease is an osteochondrosis involving an epiphysis of the femoral head in children between the ages of four and eight, predominantly involving males (with a ratio of 4:1). In 10–12% of cases, Perthes disease involves both hips, but when Perthes is bilateral, the changes do not occur simultaneously. The child will complain of an ache in the hip, thigh or knee, and early diagnosis is important if the optimal management outcome is to be achieved. The process is a spontaneously occurring avascular necrosis, which radiologically passes through the typical avascular stages of sclerosis, fragmentation, compression and healing. The entire epiphysis becomes fragmented. No loose bodies are produced. The process is usually self-limiting.

A clinical suspicion, together with plain films and bone scans, plays a key role in the diagnosis of Perthes disease. Four stages are seen on plain films and the entire process can extend over many months or even years:

1. In the initial stage, the femoral head epiphysis on the symptomatic side appears smaller than the other side and there is apparent widening of the hip joint. The femoral head epiphysis appears denser than the normal hip (see Figs 5.224 and 5.225). At this stage a nuclear bone scan may be helpful in establishing the early diagnosis, and absent or reduced uptake may occur in the femoral head, consistent with avascular changes (see Fig. 5.226).

2. In the second stage (fragmentation), the dense femoral head begins to fragment (see Fig. 5.227). The femoral head progressively shows collapse and irregularity (see Fig. 5.228).

3. In the third stage (reossification), healing begins and the femoral head takes on its final shape (see Figs 5.229 and 5.230).

4. In the fourth stage (healing), there is a continuation of healing, and the deformity of the femoral head and neck remaining at this stage will persist (see Figs 5.231 and 5.232).

Stulberg et al. (1981) and Salter and Thompson (1984) found that four major factors determine the long-term outcome of the disease. These are:

- the child's age at onset: the earlier the onset, the less long-term deformity can be anticipated
- the extent of the femoral head epiphysis that loses its blood supply
- the ability to keep the femoral head in the acetabulum during the disease process. This is called containment. The acetabulum acts as a template or mould for the deformed femoral head and influences its shape as healing progresses
- loss of motion of the hip joint.

Surprisingly, many long-term studies have found that 30–40 years after onset, as many as 90% of children are active and their hips are pain-free in spite of the fact that most do not return to normal shape once they have completely healed.

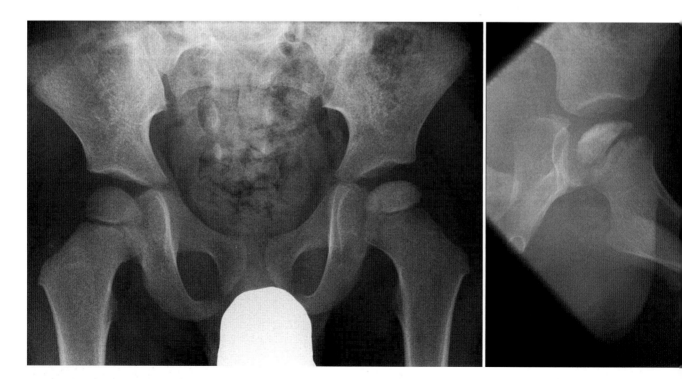

▲ **Fig. 5.224** Early Perthes disease is present on the left side. The left femoral head epiphysis is denser than the right and the left hip also appears 'smaller'.

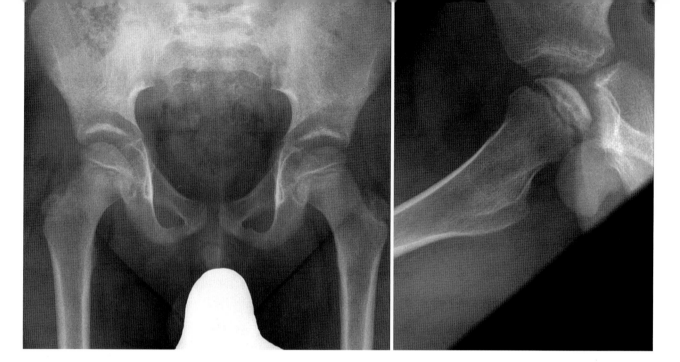

Fig. 5.225 This demonstrates the early sclerotic stage of another case of Perthes disease involving the right hip.

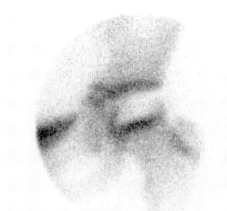

Fig. 5.226 At this early stage, a 'cold area' is demonstrated within the epiphysis, indicating a decreased perfusion.

Fig. 5.227 The fragmentation stage is beginning in this case involving the left hip. This will be followed by progressive compression and irregularity.

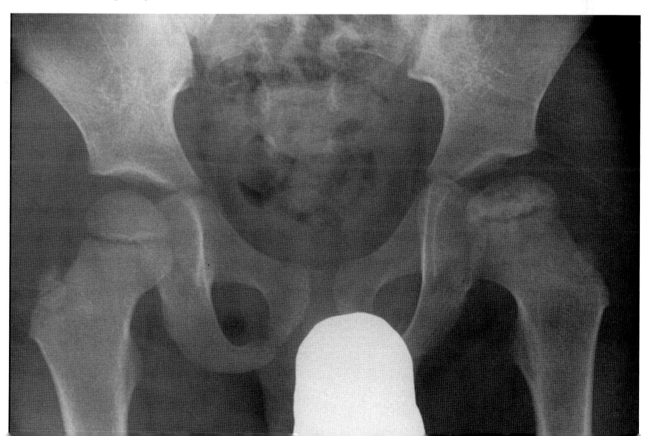

▶ **Fig. 5.228** Fragmentation, compression and irregularity are occurring in another case involving the left hip.

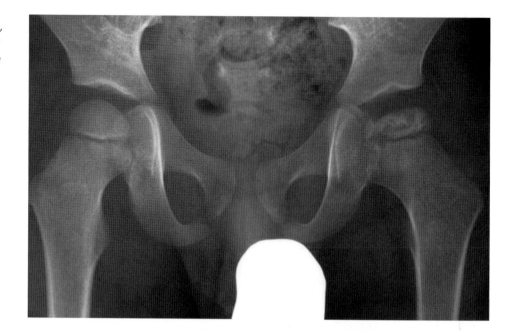

▼ **Fig. 5.229** The reossification stage is occurring on the right.

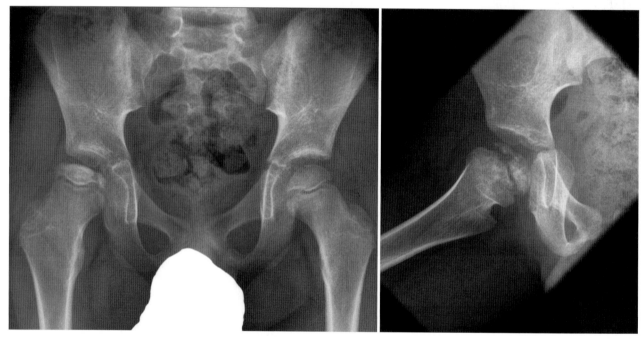

▼ **Fig. 5.230** Healing and reossification are occurring in this case involving the right side.

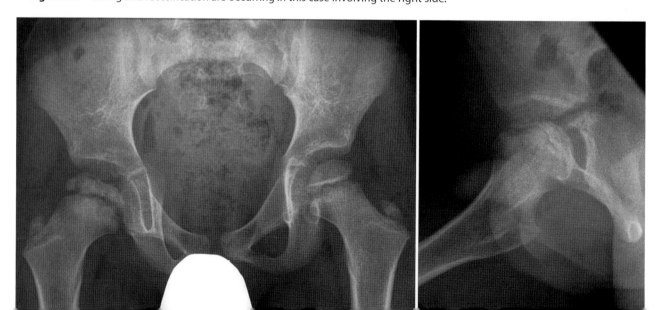

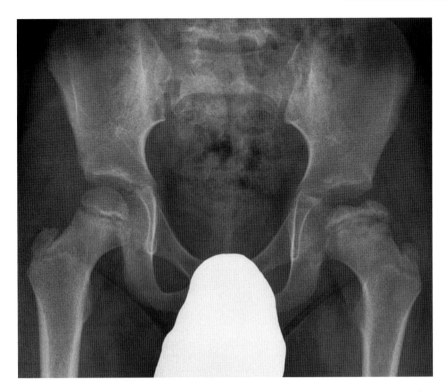

▲ **Fig. 5.231** In this case of Perthes disease, further healing has occurred on the left and the deformity is now permanent.

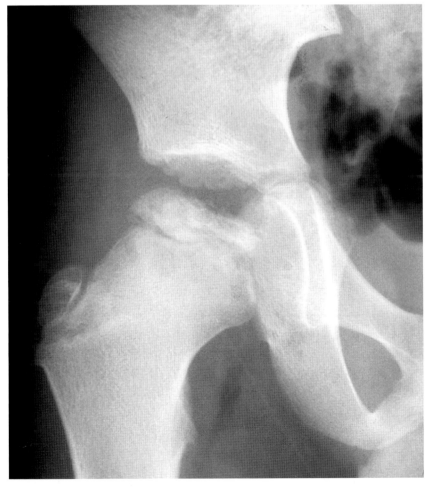

▲ **Fig. 5.232** In this case of Perthes disease, the process on the right side has reached the final stage of healing and permanent deformity.

Slipping of the capital femoral epiphysis

Slipped capital femoral epiphysis (SCFE) occurs during the adolescent growth spurt, most frequently in obese male children (2:1 predominance). Boys typically present between the ages of 14 and 16 and girls between the ages of 11 and 13. About 40% of cases may be bilateral. Classification of SCFE was previously based on duration (Carney, et al. 1991), but is now based on epiphyseal stability (Loder 1995). Up to 90% of cases are stable (Loder 2001) and, if diagnosed early, have a good prognosis. Unstable SCFE has a much poorer prognosis because of the high risk of avascular necrosis. A child with stable SCFE characteristically presents with an intermittent limp and pain of several weeks' duration. The pain is poorly localised to the hip, groin or knee. Unstable SCFE behaves like an acute fracture and the child is unable to walk. This new classification has implications for how imaging is obtained.

The diagnosis of SCFE is usually based on plain film changes. AP and lateral views of both hips are obtained to assess the proximal femoral growth plate and the capital femoral epiphysis. If the hip is stable clinically, an AP and a 'frog-leg' pelvic view are obtained (see Fig. 5.233). If the child presents with an unstable hip, a lateral view of the involved hip is obtained using a cross-table lateral technique. A lateral view of the opposite hip is also obtained. A 'frog-leg' view may be impossible due to pain and carries a theoretical risk of progressing the displacement of the epiphysis. It is important to remember that early in the course of SCFE the AP view is normal, since the initial slipping occurs in a posterior direction. Consequently, a lateral projection must always be obtained. An early slip is seen on the lateral view. There will be a minimal posterior step at the anterior aspect of the growth plate. A nuclear bone scan and/or an MRI scan may be helpful in doubtful cases to establish an early diagnosis (see Figs 5.234 and 5.235).

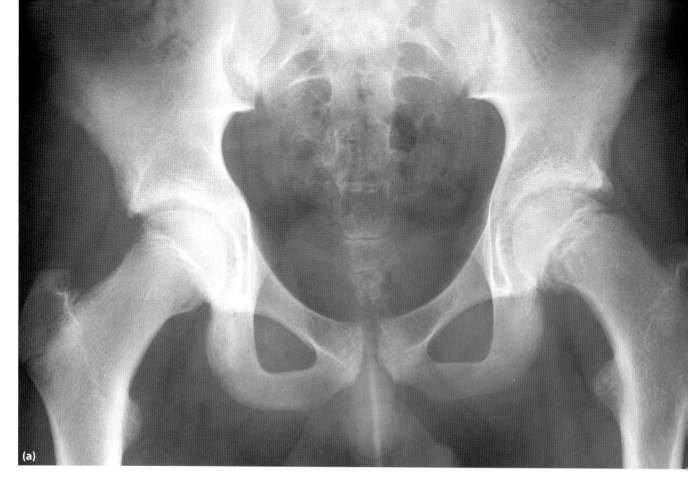

▲▼ **Fig. 5.233** SCFE in the left hip. An AP view **(a)** and a 'frog-leg' image **(b)** were obtained as if the SCFE was clinically stable. The 'frog-leg' view is an efficient way of demonstrating both hips in the lateral position, making comparison simple. A lateral view is an essential part of plain film assessment for possible SCFE. If an early slip is present, there will be a step at the posterior aspect of the growth plate of the femoral head.

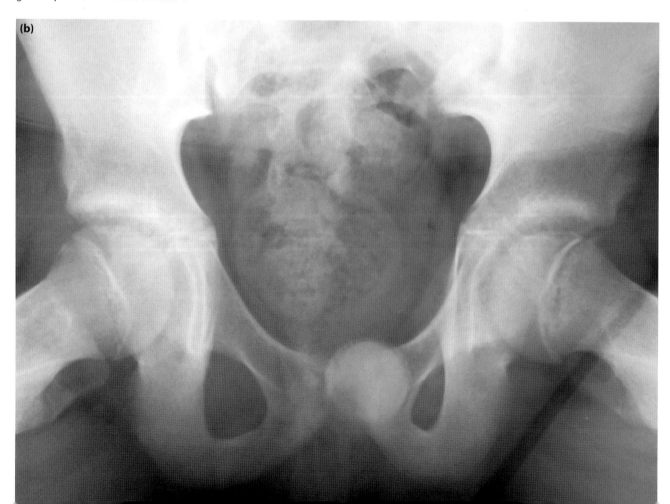

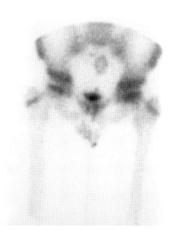

▲ **Fig. 5.234** Early slipping of the left femoral capital epiphysis is present, with a subtle but definite increased uptake of isotope in the left hip growth plate and in the left hip generally.

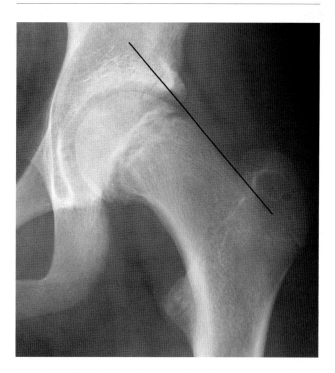

▲ **Fig. 5.236** Klein's line is drawn along the superior border of the femoral neck. Normally a portion of the epiphysis should be projected above this line. This is not the case here and early slipping is present.

▼ **Fig. 5.235** Coronal PD-weighted MR images show early SCFE, with widening of the growth plate of the femoral head and minimal slipping.

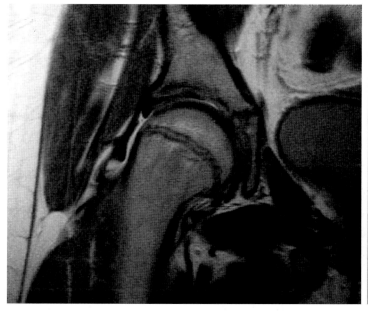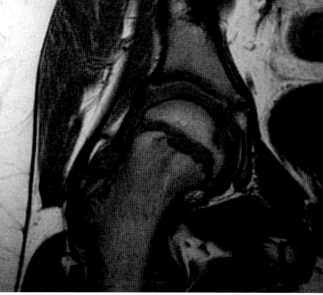

Two radiological signs of early slipping on the AP view have been described:

- Klein's line (Loder 2001) is a line drawn along the superior surface of the femoral neck. The epiphysis should normally project above this line. In early SCFE, the epiphysis is level with Klein's line (see Fig. 5.236).
- The 'blanch sign' of Steel (Steel 1986) is seen in early cases and represents superimposition of the posteriorly displaced epiphysis over the metaphysis (see Fig. 5.237).

As slipping progresses, the capital epiphysis remains within the acetabulum while the femoral neck externally rotates and migrates anterosuperiorly. The degree of slip is graded on the lateral view appearance and is staged as follows:

- *Grade I:* up to one-third of the epiphyseal width (see Fig. 5.238)
- *Grade II:* between one- and two-thirds of the epiphyseal width (see Fig. 5.239)
- *Grade III:* more than two-thirds of the epiphyseal width.

Remodelling then occurs, with callus forming at the inferior and posterior portions of the proximal metaphysis in an attempt to structurally buttress the slippage. Unrecognised or untreated slip in adolescence may present as premature

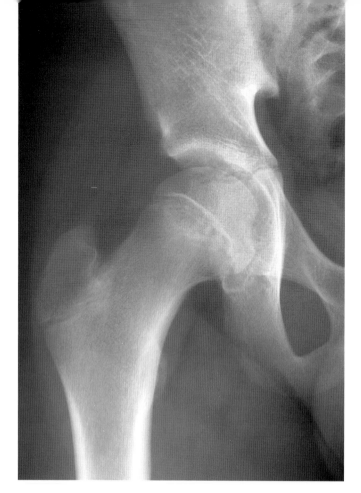

▲ **Fig. 5.237** The 'blanch sign' of Steel occurs in early slipping. The margins of the hip in an AP view may appear normal, but because the epiphysis slips backwards, there is superimposition of the leading margin of the epiphysis over the metaphyseal region, creating the appearance of a widened and irregular growth plate.

▼ **Fig. 5.238** Coronal MR images show a Grade I slip. Note the joint effusion.

hip joint osteoarthrosis in adult life. Minimal degrees of SCFE have been found to underlie so-called primary degenerative disease of the hip joint in up to 40% of cases (Murray 1965).

Following remodelling, this minimal slip produces a radiographic appearance known as 'pistol-grip' deformity (see Fig. 5.240). When seen in the skeletally mature athlete, this deformity can be regarded as a potential, although not an inevitable, precursor to osteoarthrosis. 'Pistol-grip' deformity is found predominantly in males (5.6:1), a statistic used to support the theory that excessive athletic activity in adolescence is a probable cause of 'pistol-grip' deformity and, as a consequence, early osteoarthrosis (Murray and Duncan 1971). The reason for degenerative changes resulting from this deformity is discussed in the above section on anterior femoro-acetabular impingement.

Transient osteoporosis of the hip

Although transient osteoporosis of the hip was originally described in pregnant women (Curtiss and Kincaid 1959; Longstreth et al. 1973), it is now recognised that this condition occurs in middle-aged men and non-pregnant women. Although not aetiologically related to sport, transient osteoporosis of the hip occasionally presents to the sports physician as cryptogenic hip pain. The pain is sufficiently severe during the first month to produce a limp, but a gradual resolution then occurs over the following six to nine months. Once the symptoms have resolved, the other hip or possibly a knee may develop a similar process, although the duration and severity are invariably less severe (Bramlett et al. 1987).

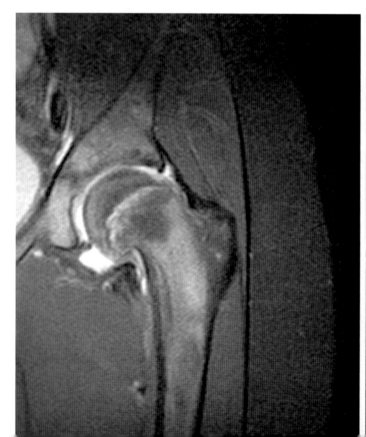

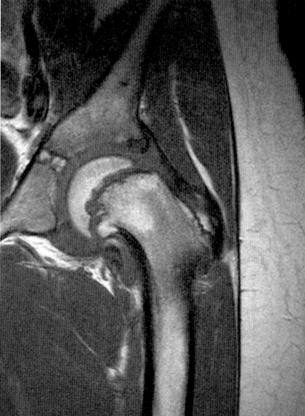

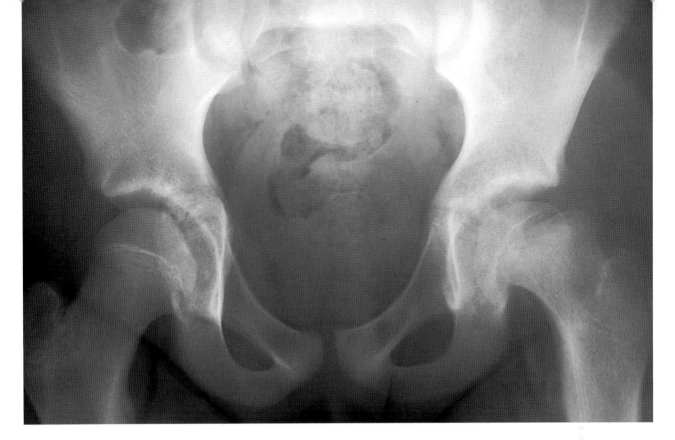

▲ **Fig. 5.239** This is a Grade I-to-II slip.

Imaging with plain films (see Fig. 5.241) and MRI (see Figs 5.242, 5.243 and 5.244) is the key to the diagnosis. A closely related condition is regional migratory osteoporosis, in which the hip is less often involved. Middle-aged men are most commonly affected, presenting with a swollen painful joint, which may last six to nine months and then resolve, only to reappear at another joint or occasionally several joints at a time. Recurrence in an adjacent joint is a distinguishing feature (Banas et al. 1990). Osteoporosis appears radiographically three to four weeks after the symptoms begin. There may be up to two years between joint involvements.

▼ **Fig. 5.240** Healing of a minor slip of the left capital epiphysis is progressing. This will almost certainly remodel as a 'pistol-grip' deformity.

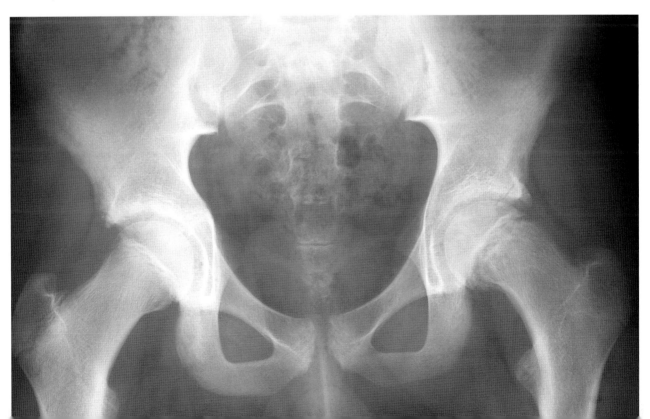

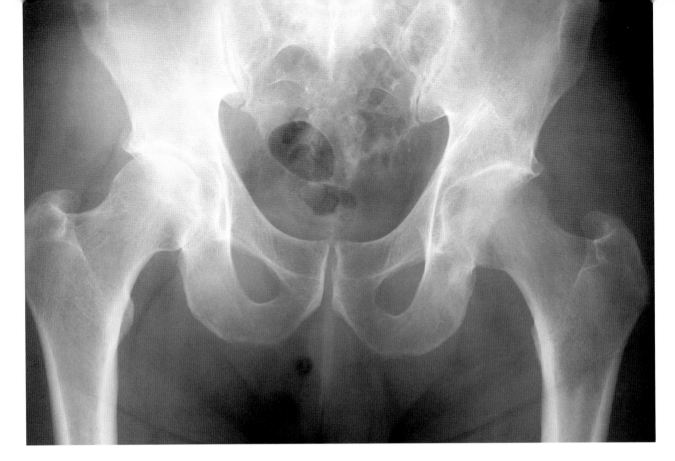

▲ **Fig. 5.241** A plain film shows osteoporosis of the left femoral head and neck when compared with the asymptomatic side.

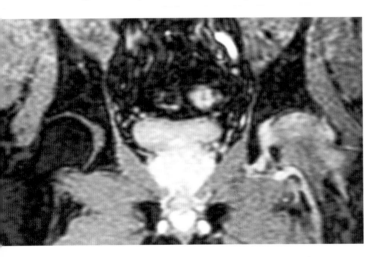

▲ **Fig. 5.242** A coronal fat-suppressed MR image shows increased signal in the left femoral head and neck in exactly the same distribution as the demineralisation demonstrated on the plain film shown in Fig. 5.241. An effusion is present.

Idiopathic chondrolysis

This account is based on a case presentation by Cuce and Dabney (1996). Idiopathic chondrolysis is an uncommon condition, characterised by an acute, rapidly progressive loss of articular cartilage occurring during adolescence and involving the hip. The cause of this condition is unknown. This condition was first described in 1971 and in 1989 42 cases were reported (Daluga and Millar 1989). Idiopathic chondrolysis has an association with SCFE, and this was noted in 8.2% of the 42 cases reported in 1989.

Patients are characteristically adolescent females, aged about 12.5 years, presenting with an insidious onset of pain in the hip producing stiffness and a limp. A contracture develops with fixed flexion, abduction and external rotation.

Plain films show a narrowing of the joint space to less than 3 mm in width (see Fig. 5.245). Demineralisation is associated and osteophyte formation may develop on the lateral aspect of the acetabular roof. A nuclear bone scan will show an increased uptake of isotope on both sides of the joint. As might be expected, CT scanning shows joint space narrowing and osteopaenia.

Sports-related iliac artery flow limitation

Athletes such as cyclists and speed skaters who maintain prolonged hip flexion with a horizontal-back 'aerodynamic' position or repetitive deep hip flexion are susceptible to both kinking and endofibrotic narrowing of the iliac or common femoral arteries (Bender et al. 2004). This may produce claudication, leading to pain in the buttock, thigh or leg occurring at maximal effort. The pain quickly disappears at rest, with the diagnosis requiring clinical suspicion based on the history.

There is relative mobility of the iliac arteries by comparison with the aortic bifurcation and common femoral arteries. As a result, iliac artery lengthening and tortuosity may occur and this predisposes to arterial kinking in hip flexion. Significantly increased peak systolic velocities generated by the kink eventually induce an endofibrotic reaction, which is an entity distinct from arteriosclerosis and fibromuscular dysplasia. Endofibrosis may progress to produce a permanent narrowing in which there is a 10–30% reduction in vessel diameter, with a subsequent

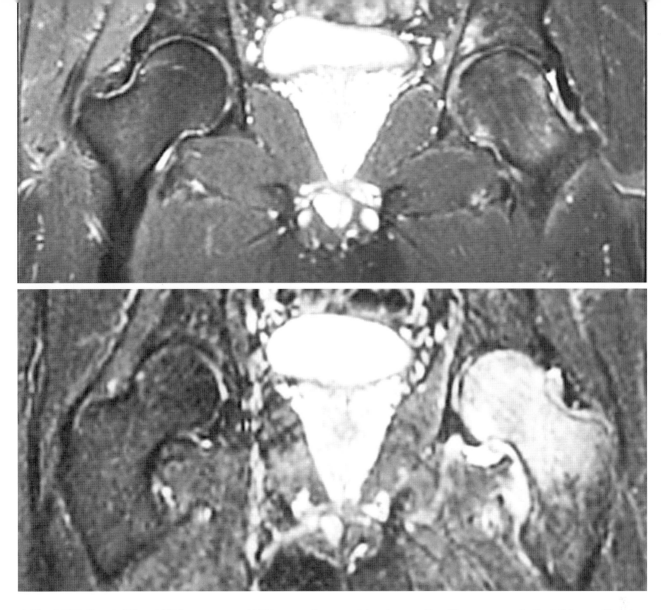

▲ **Fig. 5.243** Coronal T1 and PD fat-suppressed MR images show a patchy abnormality of bone marrow in the left femoral head and neck. The appearance is typical of transient osteoporosis.

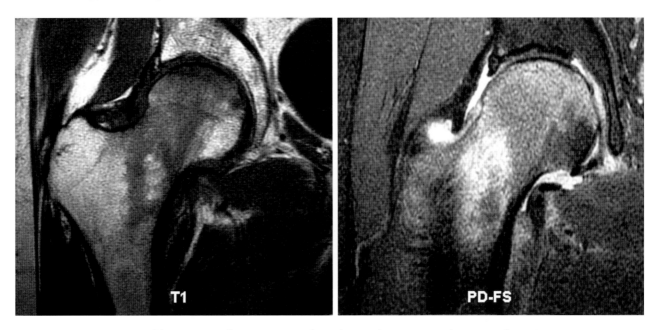

▲ **Fig. 5.244** Coronal T1 and fat-suppressed PD MR images show abnormal marrow signal in a case of transient osteoporosis. Note the hip effusion.

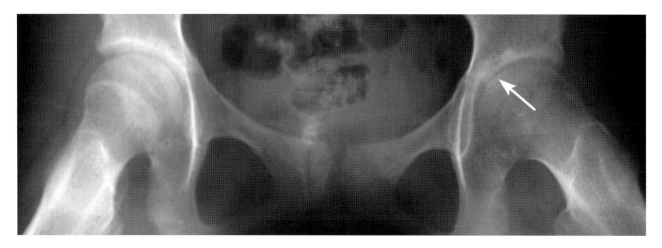

▲ **Fig. 5.245** Demineralisation is present, most marked around the left hip. Considerable narrowing of the left hip space has occurred and the appearance is typical of idiopathic chondrolysis.

risk of arterial dissection and occlusion. The syndrome is bilateral in 20% of cases.

These lesions are subtle and eccentric, most frequently occurring in the proximal external iliac artery just distal to the iliac bifurcation. Imaging plays a vital role in diagnosis and treatment planning, but is technically challenging in terms of demonstrating the functional kinking of the iliac arteries that occurs only with hip flexion. A combination of ultrasound with Doppler and MR angiography with hips extended and flexed may be helpful in identifying the endofibrotic lesion.

References

Aitken AG, Flodmark O, Newman DE, Kilcoyne RF, Shuman WP, Mack LA. 'Leg length determination by digital radiography.' *Am J Roentgenol* 1985, 144: 613–15.

Amako T, Kawashima M, Torisu T, Hayashi K. 'Bone and joint lesions in decompression sickness.' *Semin Arthritis Rheum* 1974, 4: 151–90.

Anda S, Terjesen T, Kvistad KA, Svenningsen S. 'Acetabular angles and femoral anteversion in dysplastic hips in adults: CT investigation.' *J Comput Assist Tomogr* 1991, 15: 115–20.

Anderson K, Strickland SM, Warren R. 'Hip and groin injuries in athletes.' *Am J Sports Med* 2001, 29: 521–2.

Aspelin P, Ekberg O, Thorsson O, Wilhelmsson M, Westlin N. 'Ultrasound examination of soft tissue injury of the lower limb in athletes.' *Am J Sports Med* 1992, 20: 601–3.

Banas MP, Kaplan FS, Fallon MD, Haddad JG. 'Regional migratory osteoporosis. A case report and review of the literature.' *Clin Orthop* 1990, 250: 303–9.

Bauman PA, Singson R, Hamilton WG. 'Femoral neck anteversion in ballerinas.' *Clin Orthop* 1994, 302: 57–63.

Beauchesne RP, Schutzer SF. 'Myositis ossificans of the piriformis muscle: an unusual cause of piriformis syndrome.' *J Bone Joint Surg (Am)* 1997, 79A: 906–10.

Bender MHM, Schep G, de Vries WR et al. 'Sports-related flow limitation in the iliac arteries in endurance athletes: aetiology, diagnosis, treatment, future developments.' *Sport Med* 2004, 34: 427–42.

Bradshaw C, McCrory P, Bell S, Brukner P. 'Obturator nerve entrapment: a cause of groin pain in athletes.' *Am J Sports Med* 1997, 25: 402–8.

Bramlett KW, Killian JT, Nasca RJ, Daniel WW. 'Transient osteoporosis.' *Clin Orthop* 1987, 222: 197–202.

Brukner P, Kahn K. *Clinical Sports Medicine*, 2nd edn, McGraw-Hill, Sydney, 2001.

Carney BT, Weinstein SL, Noble J. 'Long-term follow-up of slipped capital femoral epiphysis.' *J Bone Joint Surg (Am)*, 1991, 73: 667–74.

Chen WS. 'Sciatica due to piriformis syndrome.' *J Bone Joint Surg (Am)* 1992, 74A: 1546–8.

Clancy WG Jr, Foltz AS. 'Iliac apophysitis and stress fractures in adolescent runners.' *Am J Sports Med* 1976, 4: 214–18.

Connell DA, Schneider-Kolsky ME, Hoving JL, Malara F, Buchbinder R, Koulouris G, Burke F, Bass C. 'Longitudinal study comparing sonographic and MRI assessments of acute and healing hamstring injuries.' *Am J Roentgenol* 2004, 183: 975–84.

Cooperman DR, Wallensten R, Stulberg SD. 'Acetabular dysplasia in the adult.' *Clin Orthop* 1983, 175: 79–85.

Cuce F, Dabney KW. 'Idiopathic chondrolysis.' Clinical presentation, Orthopaedic Department, The Alfred I Dupont Institute, Wilmington, Delaware, 1996.

Curtiss PH Jnr, Kincaid WE. 'Transitory demineralization of the hip in pregnancy.' *J Bone Joint Surg (Am)* 1959, 41: 1327–33.

Czerney C, Hofmann S, Neubold A, et al. 'Lesions of the acetabular labrum: accuracy of MR imaging and MR arthrography in detection and staging.' *Radiology* 1996, 200: 225–30.

Daluga DJ, Millar EA. 'Idiopathic chondrolysis of the hip.' *J Pediatr Ortho* 1989, 9: 405.

Devas MB. 'Stress fractures of the femoral neck.' *J Bone Joint Surg (Br)* 1965, 47: 728–38.

Edwards DJ, Lomas D, Villar RN. 'Diagnosis of the painful hip by magnetic resonance imaging and arthroscopy.' *J Bone Joint Surg (Br)* 1995, 77: 374–6.

Ferguson TA, Matta J. 'Anterior femoroacetabular impingement: a clinical presentation.' *Sports Med and Arthro Rev* 2002, 10: 134–40.

Fitzgerald RH Jr. 'Acetabular labrum tears. Diagnosis and treatment.' *Clin Orthop* 1995, 311: 60–8.

Gorman PW, McAndrew MP. 'Acute anterior compartmental syndrome of the thigh following contusion. A case report and review of the literature.' *J Orthop Trauma* 1987, 1: 68–70.

Guerra J Jr, Armbuster TG, Resnick D, Goergen TG, Feingold ML, Niwayama G, Danzig LA. 'The adult hip, Part II: the soft-tissue landmarks.' *Radiology* 1978, 128: 11–20.

Hasegawa Y, Iwata H, Mizuno M, Genda E, Sato S, Miura T. 'The natural course of osteoarthritis of the hip due to subluxation or acetabular dysplasia.' *Arch Orthop Trauma Surg* 1992, 111: 187–91.

Huffman GR, Safran M. 'Tears of the acetabular labrum in athletes: diagnosis and treatment.' *Sports Med and Arthr Rev* 2002, 10: 141–50.

Huss CD, Puhl JJ. 'Myositis ossificans of the upper arm.' *Am J Sports Med* 1980, 8(6): 419–24.

Ikeda T, Awaya G, Suzuki S et al. 'Torn acetabular labrum in young patients: Arthroscopic diagnosis and management.' *J Bone Joint Surg Br* 1988, 70: 13–16.

Ito K, Minka-II MA, Leunig M et al. 'Femoroacetabular impingement and the cam-effect.' *J Bone Joint Surg (Br)* 2001, 83: 171–6.

Janzen DL, Partridge E, Logan PM, Connell DG, Duncan CP. 'The snapping hip: clinical and imaging findings in transient subluxation of the iliopsoas tendon.' *Can Assoc Radiol J* 1996, 47: 202–8.

Julsrud ME. 'Piriformis syndrome.' *J Am Podiatr Med Assoc* 1989, 79: 128–31.

Karlin LI. 'Injuries to the hip and pelvis.' In Nicholas JA, Hershman ER (eds), *The Lower Extremity and Spine in Sports Medicine*, Mosby, St Louis, 1995, pp. 1285–6.

Keene JS, Lash EG. 'Negative bone scan in a femoral neck stress fracture. A case report.' *Am J Sports Med* 1992, 20: 234–6.

Khoury MB, Kirks DR, Martinez S, Apple J. 'Bilateral avulsion fractures of the anterior superior iliac spines in sprinters.' *Skeletal Radiol* 1985, 13: 65–7.

Klaue K, Durnin CW, Ganz R. 'The acetabular rim syndrome. A clinical presentation of dysplasia of the hip.' *J Bone Joint Surg (Br)* 1991, 73: 423–9.

Larsen CM, Almekinders LC, Karas SG, Garrett WE. 'Evaluating and managing muscle contusions and myositis ossificans.' *The Physician and Sportsmedicine* 2002, 30(2): 41–50.

Latshaw RF, Kantner TR, Kalenak A et al. 'A pelvic stress fracture in a female jogger: a case report.' *Am J Sport Med* 1981, 9: 54–6.

Loder RT. 'Unstable slipped capital femoral epiphysis.' *J Pediatr Orthop* 2001, 21: 694–9.

Loder RT. 'Slipped femoral capital epiphysis in children.' *Curr Opin Pediatr* 1995, 7: 95–7.

Lombardo SJ, Retting AC, Kerlan RK. 'Radiographic abnormalities of the iliac apophysis in adolescent athletes.' *J Bone Joint Surg (Am)* 1983, 64A: 444–6.

Longstreth PL, Malink LR, Hill CS Jr. 'Transient osteoporosis of the hip in pregnancy.' *Obstet Gynecol* 1973, 41: 563–9.

Lovell G, Galloway H et al. 'Osteitis pubis and assessment of bone marrow oedema at the pubic symphysis with MRI in an elite junior male soccer squad.' *Clin J Sport Med* 2006, 16: 117–22.

Mason JB 'Acetabular labral tears in the athlete.' *Clin Sport Med* 2001, 20: 779–90.

Melamed H. 'Soft tissue problems of the hip in athletes.' *Sports Med and Arthr Rev* 2002, 10: 168–75.

Modic MT, Steinberg PM, Ross JS, Masaryk TJ, Carter JR. 'Degenerative disk disease: assessment of changes in vertebral body marrow with MR imaging.' *Radiology* 1988, 166: 193–9.

Murray RO. 'The aetiology of primary osteoarthritis of the hip.' *Br J Radiol* 1965, 38: 810–24.

Murray RO, Duncan C. 'Athletic activity in adolescence as an etiological factor in degenerative hip disease.' *J Bone Joint Surg (Br)* 1971, 53: 406–19.

Noakes TD, Smith JA, Lindenberg G, Wills CE. 'Pelvic stress fractures in long distance runners.' *Am J Sports Med* 1985, 13: 120–3.

O'Brien TJ, Mack GR. 'Multifocal osteonecrosis after short-term high-dose corticosteroid therapy. A case report.' *Clin Orthop* 1992, 279: 176–9.

Orchard JW, Read JW, Neophyton J, Garlick D. 'Groin pain associated with ultrasound finding of inguinal canal posterior wall deficiency in Australian rules footballers.' *Br J Sports Med* 1998, 32: 134–9.

Ozaki S, Hamabe T, Muro T. 'Piriformis syndrome resulting from an anomalous relationship between the sciatic nerve and piriformis muscle.' *Orthopaedics* 1999, 22: 771–2.

Papadopoulos SM, McGillicuddy JE, Messina LM. 'Pseudoaneurysm of the inferior gluteal artery presenting as sciatic nerve compression.' *Neurosurg* 1989, 24: 926–8.

Pavlov H, Nelson TL, Warren RF, Torg JS, Burstein AH. 'Stress fractures of the pubic ramus. A report of twelve cases.' *J Bone Joint Surg (Am)* 1982, 64: 1020–5.

Pomeranz SJ, Heidt RS Jr. 'MR imaging in the prognostication of hamstring injury.' *Radiology* 1993, 189: 897–900.

Salter RB, Thompson GH. 'Legg-Calve-Perthes disease: the prognostic significance of the subchondral fracture and a two-group classification of the femoral head involvement.' *J Bone Joint Surg (Am)* 1984, 66: 480–9.

Schmid G, Witteler A, Willburger R et al. 'Lumbar disk herniation: correlation of histologic findings with marrow signal intensity changes in vertebral endplates at MR imaging.' *Radiology* 2004, 231: 352–8.

Scott P. 'External herniae.' In Dudley H, Waxman B (eds), *An Aid to Clinical Surgery*, 3rd edn, Churchill Livingstone, Edinburgh, 1984, p. 231.

Seldes RM, Tan V, Hunt J, Katz M et al. 'Anatomy, histological features and vascularity of the adult acetabular labrum.' *Clin Ortho* 2001, 382: 232–40.

Shin AY, Morin WD, Gorman JD, Jones SB, Lapinsky AS. 'The superiority of magnetic resonance imaging in differentiating the cause of hip pain in endurance athletes.' *Am J Sports Med* 1996, 24: 168–76.

Silver JK, Leadbetter WB. 'Piriformis syndrome: assessment of current practice and literature review.' *Orthopaedics* 1998, 21: 1133–5.

Skandalakis JE, Gray SW, Skandalakis LJ et al. 'Surgical anatomy of the inguinal area.' *World J Surg* 1989, 13: 490–8.

Staheli LT, Lippert F, Denotter P. 'Femoral anteversion and physical performance in adolescent and adult life.' *Clin Orthop* 1977, 129: 213–16.

Steel HH. 'The metaphyseal blanch sign of slipped capital femoral epiphysis.' *J Bone Joint Surg (Am)* 1986, 68: 920–2.

Sterling JC, Webb RF, Meyers MC, Calvo RD. 'False negative bone scan in a female runner.' *Med Sci Sports Exerc* 1993, 25: 179–85.

Stulberg SD, Cooperman DR, Wallensten R. 'The natural history of Legg-Calve-Perthes disease.' *J Bone Joint Surg (Am)* 1981, 63A: 1095–108.

Suzuki S, Awaya G, Okada Y et al. 'Arthroscopic diagnosis of ruptured acetabular labrum.' *Acta Orthop Scand* 1986, 57: 513–15.

Takechi H, Nagashima H, Ito S. 'Intra-articular pressure of the hip joint outside and inside the limbus.' *J Japanese Orthop Assn* 1986, 56: 529–36.

Taussig G, Delor MH, Masse P. 'Growth disturbances of the upper femoral extremity: contribution to knowledge of normal growth in therapeutic trials.' *Rev Chir Orthop Reparatrice Appar Mot* 1976, 62: 191–210.

Underwood PL, McLeod RA, Ginsburg WW. 'The varied clinical manifestations of iliopsoas bursitis.' *J Rheumatol* 1988, 15: 1683–5.

Viegas SF, Rimoldi R, Scarborough M, Ballantyne GM. 'Acute compartment syndrome in the thigh. A case report and a review of the literature.' *Clin Orthop* 1988, 234: 232–4.

Volpin G, Milgrom C, Goldsher D, Stein H. 'Stress fractures of the sacrum following strenuous activity.' *Clin Orthop* 1989, 243: 184–8.

Walker AP, Dickson RA. 'School screening and pelvic tilt scoliosis.' *Lancet* 1984, 2: 152–3.

Wiberg G. 'Studies of dysplastic acetabula and congenital subluxation of the hip joint.' *Acta Chir Scand* 1939, 83: suppl. 58: 7.

Image acknowledgments

The authors wish to thank the following colleagues who kindly offered images for inclusion in this chapter:

- Dr James Linklater (Figures 5.18, 5.21(c), 5.22, 5.33, 5.77, 5.84, 5.147, 5.193(c), 5.206, 5.207 and 5.244)
- Dr Robert Cooper and Dr Stephen Allwright (Figures 5.47, 5.48, 5.49, 5.50, 5.89, 5.90, 5.93(a), 5.100(a), 5.100(b), 5.121(a), 5.145, 5.220, 5.221 and 5.226)
- Dr Bill Breidahl (Figures 5.224, 5.225, 5.227, 5.228, 5.229, 5.230 and 5.231)
- Dr Phil Lucas (Figures 5.95, 5.96, 5.149, 5.188(a) and (b), 5.198(a) and (b), 5.222, 5.238)
- Dr Ruth Highet (Figures 5.85, 5.86 and 5.87)
- Dr Tom Cross (Figure 5.143(a) and (b))
- Dr Paul Bloomfield (Figure 5.156)
- Dr Anthony Smith (Figure 5.213).

These images have significantly added to the quality of the chapter.

The knee and leg

6

Jock Anderson and John Read with Bill Breidahl

The knee

Knee injuries are common in sport, due in part to the exposed position of the knee and also to its constant role in the majority of sporting activities. The knee is subjected to large weightbearing loads and twisting forces that occur during such ordinary and frequent activities as walking, running, jumping and lifting. Furthermore, the functions of the knee are dependent on a complex set of interconnected linkages that transmit and dissipate these loads and forces. This means that trauma causing failure of a single part of a linkage may actually result in more than one structure being injured. Consequently, recognisable and predictable patterns of injuries are seen involving a number of structures. Injury patterns occur in both acute and chronic overuse trauma (see Fig. 6.1).

The patterns of knee injury alter with age and the biomechanics required by particular sports. In the immature athlete, the ligaments are relatively stronger than the developing centres of ossification. Consequently, soft-tissue injuries such as ligamentous and meniscal tears are less likely to occur than disruption of growth plates and avulsion fractures. Symptoms related to problems with the extensor mechanism of the knee are common. Hughston (1968) showed that 65% of subluxations or dislocations of the patella occur before the age of 18 years. In the mature athlete, soft-tissue injuries predominate. Ligamentous injuries are likely to occur as isolated injuries or occasionally in more complex multiligamentous patterns. The incidence of meniscal injuries increases with advancing age.

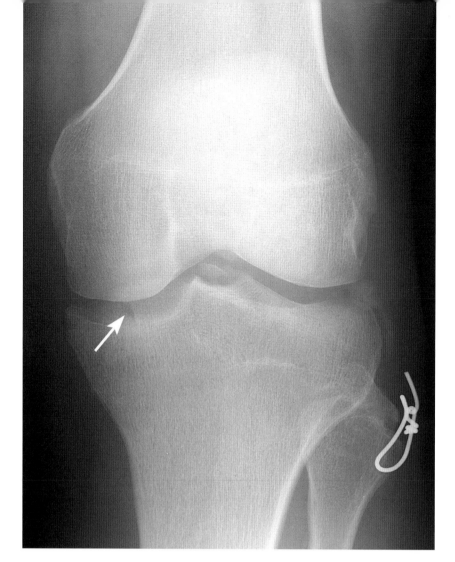

◀ Fig. 6.1(a) Application of a single force to the knee may cause multiple and predictable injuries. A violent varus deformity of the knee has produced traction laterally and compression medially. Lateral traction forces have caused an avulsion fracture of the lateral aspect of the fibular styloid process involving the lateral collateral ligament (LCL) and biceps femoris attachments. Retraction of the separated bone fragment has been reduced and the fragment has been reattached by wiring. Post-traumatic calcific changes extend into the lateral joint space, suggesting that popliteus injury may also have been present. An anterior cruciate ligament (ACL) avulsion has occurred, with separation of a small bone fragment from the intercondylar eminence of the tibia. Compressive force medially has produced a fracture of the medial tibial plateau (arrow). This is a predictable injury pattern that will be discussed later in the chapter.

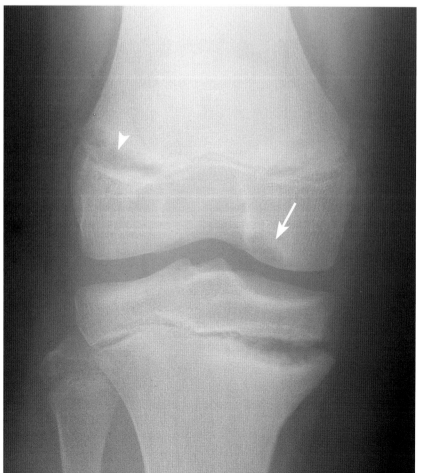

◀ (b) A sports-crazy adolescent is showing the legacy of overuse. Stress reactions involve both the lateral aspect of the distal femoral growth plate (arrowhead) and the medial aspect of the proximal tibial growth plate. There is also an area of osteochondritis dissecans developing in the lateral aspect of the medial femoral condyle (arrow). These injuries are not a specific injury pattern, but generally indicate excessive and chronic stresses being applied to the knee.

Imaging the knee

A number of imaging techniques may play a valuable role in the diagnosis of knee injuries secondary to sporting activities. Over the last decade the investigation of knee injuries has altered. This is due to a number of factors, including the increase in the number of professional athletes requiring an immediate diagnosis, the increased availability of MRI and the more widespread use of arthroscopy as a first-line method of diagnosis and management of knee injuries.

Despite these changes, plain films retain a major role in the diagnosis of knee injuries and in many cases they may be the only imaging method required for a variety of knee problems. However, over the last decade or so the benefit of the routine use of plain films in the diagnosis of knee injury has been questioned (Stiell et al. 1995; Moore et al. 2005). The reasons for requesting many plain film examinations may include fear of litigation and the belief that radiography can be a substitute for adequate history-taking and physical examination. The main reasons for questioning the routine use of plain films are the cost, exposure to radiation and the low yield of significant pathology.

Following acceptance of the 'Ottawa ankle rules' for ankle injuries (Seaberg and Jackson 1994), knee rules have been developed and a prospective validation of 'Ottawa knee rules' published by Stiell, et al. (1996). In this study, the presence of one or more of the findings listed in Table 6.1 would have identified all the patients with fractures in the study group and reduced the number of examinations by 28%. The patient sample was taken from an emergency department and it would be interesting to see the same study carried out on patients passing through a sports medicine centre. In this latter group it might be expected that the standard of history-taking and physical examination might more effectively choose patients whose management would benefit from plain films.

Table 6.1 Ottawa knee rules

- Age 55 years or older
- Tenderness of head of fibula
- Isolated tenderness of the patella
- Inability to flex the knee to 90°
- Inability to walk four weightbearing steps immediately after the injury and in the emergency department

Routine plain film views

If major trauma has occurred, supine anteroposterior (AP) and cross-table lateral views are initially adequate for the exclusion of major trauma. Other imaging methods may then be used, depending on the clinical picture and findings on the initial films. It should also be noted that in the imaging departments of many hospitals, AP and lateral views are routinely the only views taken for all knee injuries, irrespective of their severity. It is important to remember that this practice reduces the value of the examination considerably. If abnormalities are to be excluded, four views should be obtained routinely, as described below. High-quality plain films remain an efficient and cost-effective method of imaging.

The four routine views are the:

1. anteroposterior (AP) view
2. lateral view
3. intercondylar view
4. patellofemoral view.

When both knees are to be examined, each view on each side should be obtained separately to allow correct centring and collimation ('coning').

The AP view

The AP projection provides an overview of the knee and whenever possible should be taken with the patient erect. Weightbearing allows assessment of knee joint alignment and joint space narrowing (see Fig. 6.2). The knee is positioned in a true AP position, which requires the femoral condyles to be equidistant from the film. A straight tube is used, centred on the joint space that corresponds to a level 1 cm below the inferior pole of the patella. An appropriate exposure should demonstrate the surrounding soft tissues while adequately defining trabecular detail. The availability of computed radiography (CR) systems has made this task somewhat easier than in the past. As ever, collimation is essential for acquiring maximum resolution. A posteroanterior (PA) view in flexion is described below and is more sensitive than the routine AP view for the demonstration of compartment narrowing resulting from articular cartilage wear.

The lateral view

The lateral view is particularly valuable in demonstrating the articular surfaces of the femoral condyles, the patella and soft-tissue detail of both the extensor mechanism and the popliteal fossa (see Fig. 6.3). The lateral view should be obtained with the patient lying on their side and the knee flexed no more than 30°. This places the extensor mechanism on mild stretch and allows small joint effusions in the suprapatellar joint recess to be appreciated. If the knee is flexed more than 30°, the joint recess will be compressed and subtle effusions obliterated. Positioning the knee in a true lateral position requires the knee to be examined lying against the tabletop. The pelvis is then rotated into a true lateral position. Palpation of the patellar margins may assist in the accurate positioning of the knee. The primary beam is centred on the joint line with 5° of cranial tube angulation.

The intercondylar view

The intercondylar view profiles the weightbearing articular surfaces of the femoral condyles and allows examination of the intercondylar notch (see Fig. 6.4). An intercondylar view may be obtained with the patient kneeling on the table with the knee flexed to 70°. A straight tube is used, with the beam centred on the inferior pole of the patella. It is also possible to acquire this view in the erect position. The hip is extended and the knee rests on a stool with 70° of knee flexion. This requires the patient to be mobile and supple. An intercondylar view can be taken with the patient supine, the knee flexed

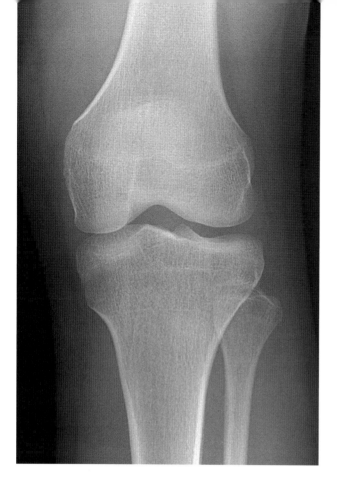

▲ Fig. 6.2 An AP view of the knee has been acquired with weightbearing. This view has been well centred on the joint line allowing the articular surfaces and joint spaces to be examined. The soft tissues on both sides of the knee can be assessed for evidence of localised swelling.

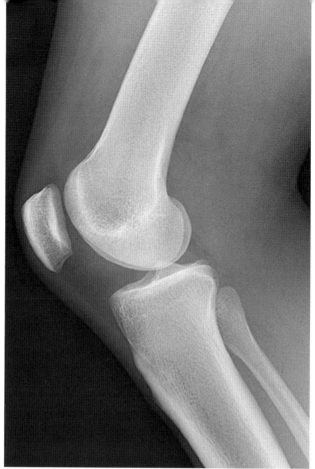

▲ Fig. 6.3 This lateral view is technically pleasing. The condyles are superimposed and the soft-tissue detail of the extensor mechanism is well displayed using an exposure that also demonstrates the bony trabecular pattern.

▶ Fig. 6.4 An intercondylar view adds valuable information to the knee series. Because the primary beam is parallel to the tibial articular surface and the posterior, weightbearing area of the femoral articular surface is profiled, this view is valuable for the demonstration of changes such as osteoarthrosis, osteochondritis dissecans, osteochondral fractures or subchondral avascular changes that occur in the weightbearing region. The walls and roof of the intercondylar notch are also well displayed.

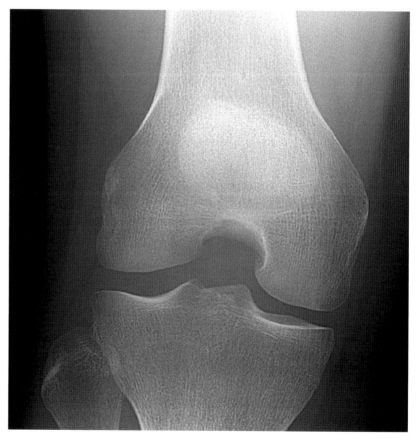

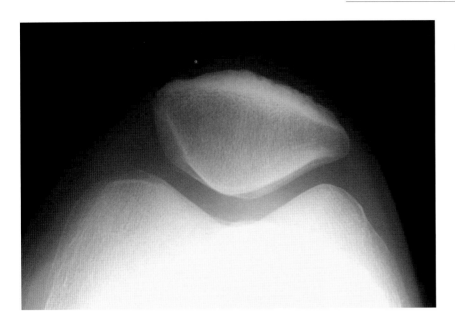

◀**Fig. 6.5** The patellofemoral joint view (or 'skyline' view) is an important knee view. As will be discussed later, the size and shape of the patella and the development of the trochlear groove may provide clues to the cause of patellar subluxations. Often, conditions such as osteochondritis dissecans of the patella and trochlea together with patellofemoral fractures can be well seen only on this view. It is difficult to understand why this view is so often omitted from the knee series.

to 45° and a cranial tube angle of 10°. Whichever method is used, if the positioning is correct, the primary beam will be parallel to the articular surface of the tibial plateau.

The patellofemoral view

The patellofemoral (or 'skyline') view (see Fig. 6.5) is often incorrectly omitted from the routine knee series. A radiographic examination is incomplete without this view, as the patellofemoral joint is a clinically significant articulation of the knee, as shown elsewhere in this chapter.

Many different methods can be used to obtain a patellofemoral view. Hughston (1968), Merchant et al. (1974) and Laurin et al. (1978) have each described ways of obtaining an axial or a 'skyline' radiograph of the patellofemoral joint. Hughston's view is the method preferred by the authors, being simple and reliable. To obtain this view, the patient is prone with the knee resting on the cassette and the tube is angled 45° cranially. The knee is then flexed to allow the foot to rest on the collimator housing. It is essential that the femur and the leg are linear in the sagittal plane so that there is no rotation at the knee. The primary beam is centred on the patellofemoral joint space.

It should also be noted that Minkoff and Fein (1980) pointed out that plain radiography has limited use in the diagnosis of patellofemoral tracking disorders. Plain films can diagnose anomalies of the patella and trochlear groove, but because patellofemoral views cannot be obtained at angles of knee flexion less than 30°, limited information concerning tracking disorders can be obtained as these disorders typically occur during movement between 0 and 30° of flexion. Therefore, axial CT is the preferred method of evaluating patellar malalignment in cases of tracking disorders where conservative treatment has failed and surgery is being considered. This will be discussed later in the chapter.

Additional views

Additional knee views are used when appropriate. The need for these views is usually indicated by the clinical presentation of the patient.

45° oblique views

When a patient has suffered severe trauma, a series may simply include an AP view and a cross-table lateral view. The addition of both 45° oblique views to an acute trauma series has been found to significantly increase the sensitivity of the examination for fracture detection (Gray et al. 1997) (see Fig. 6.6).

Soft-tissue views

Detailed imaging of the extensor mechanism is essential when the clinical presentation suggests a number of conditions (see Fig. 6.7). These conditions include traction apophysitis at the inferior pole of the patella or tibial tuberosity, patellar and quadriceps tendinopathy or rupture, knee joint effusion, fat pad syndrome and deep infrapatellar bursitis. The plain film diagnosis of all these conditions depends on the demonstration of subtle changes, the most important of which is soft-tissue swelling or a change in soft-tissue density. If the soft tissues are not adequately shown on the routine lateral view, a separate soft-tissue lateral view should be acquired.

The proximal tibiofibular joint view

Inspection of the head of the fibula and proximal tibiofibular joint space may be improved by acquiring an oblique view that profiles these structures. Such a view is obtained by using a straight tube centred on the proximal tibiofibular joint with 5 to 10° of internal rotation of the knee. Using this view, subtle subluxations may be detected (see Fig. 6.8(a)). A subluxation is usually confirmed by a comparative CT examination of both sides (see Fig. 6.8(b)).

Assessment of articular cartilage loss (the Rosenberg view)

The plain film assessment of articular cartilage wear has been traditionally dependent on demonstrating narrowing of the medial or lateral compartment joint spaces on a weightbearing AP view. However, an erect film taken with

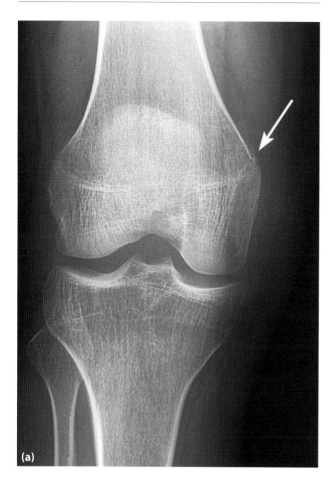

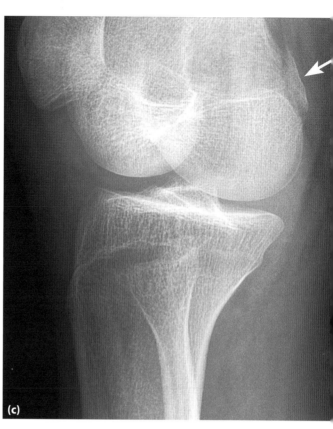

▲▼ **Fig. 6.6(a)** Following severe knee trauma, a supine AP view shows minor irregularity on the medial margin of the distal femoral metaphysis (arrow). This may have been overlooked as residual irregularity associated with growth plate fusion.
(b) However, a cross-table lateral view demonstrates a fluid level (arrow) in a large lipohaemarthrosis, indicating that an intra-articular fracture is present (lipohaemarthroses are discussed below). The site of the fracture is still unknown.
(c) A 45° oblique view was easily obtained by rolling the patient while keeping the leg straight and supported. This view demonstrates a fracture on the posteromedial aspect of the distal femoral metaphysis (arrow).

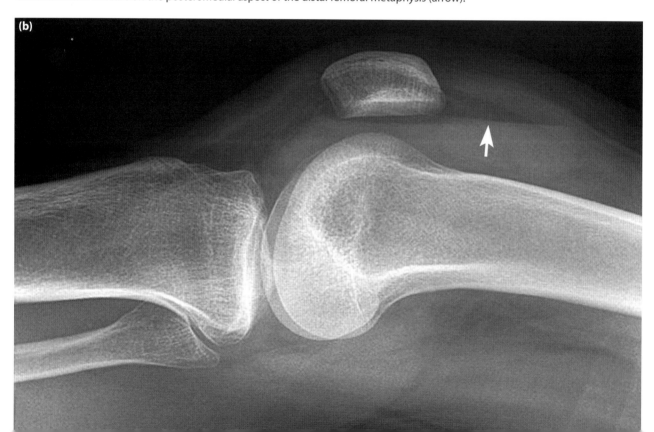

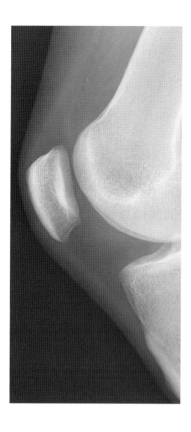

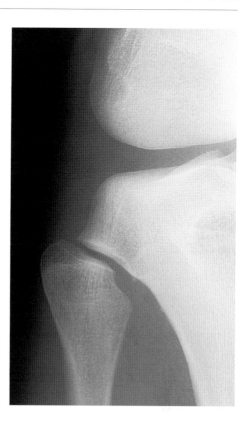

◀ **Fig. 6.7** An appropriate radiographic technique has been able to demonstrate the soft tissues as well as bone detail. The components of the extensor mechanism are well demonstrated. The infrapatellar ('Hoffa's') fat pad should be of homogeneous fat density and similar to the fat density elsewhere in the knee.

▶ **Fig. 6.8(a)** An AP oblique view of the proximal tibiofibular joint assists in the diagnosis of a subluxation. In this case a minor lateral subluxation of the proximal tibiofibular joint is demonstrated in a patient complaining of pain over the joint following a fall. The subluxation is minor and was difficult to see on routine knee views. An AP oblique view requires 5 to 10° of internal rotation of the knee, with the beam centred on the proximal tibiofibular joint.

▼ **(b)** Subluxation of the proximal tibiofibular joint is subtle and CT scans of both the injured and asymptomatic sides are useful for confirming a joint injury. Minor subluxation of the right proximal tibiofibular joint is confirmed by a comparative CT scan.

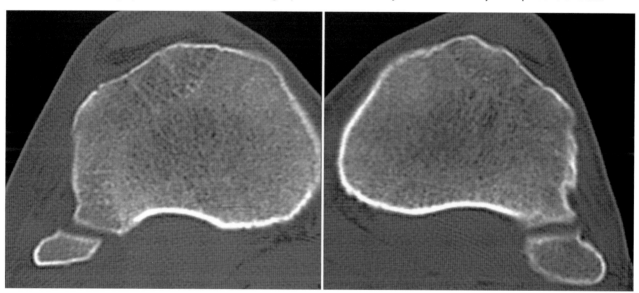

the knee locked straight will assess the cartilage width anteriorly, which is not the major site of cartilage wear. The main wear and tear on the knee occurs more posteriorly and this region is demonstrated by imaging with a Rosenberg view. This view is a weightbearing view in flexion. It gives a far more accurate assessment of early cartilage loss and in addition is useful for profiling other changes such as osteochondritis dissecans (OCD) and subchondral avascular necrosis, which occur in the same area.

A Rosenberg view (Rosenberg et al. 1988) is taken PA, with the patient standing with 45° knee flexion. The beam is centred on the joint space using 10° of caudal tube tilt. If the view has been taken correctly, the primary beam will be parallel to the articular surface of the tibial plateau (see Fig. 6.9).

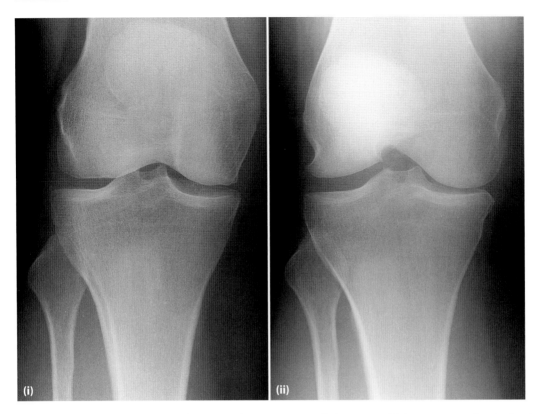

▲ **Fig. 6.9(a)** The Rosenberg view has enjoyed increasing popularity as an addition to a normal series for the assessment of articular cartilage loss in the medial and lateral compartments. As shown in this example, a traditional weightbearing AP view **(i)** may be normal, whereas a Rosenberg view **(ii)** in the same patient demonstrates considerable articular cartilage loss in the medial compartment. This is because the more posterior area of the articular surfaces profiled in a Rosenberg view is the area of the condyles where most wear of the articular cartilage occurs.

▼ **(b)** Occasionally the difference between a routine AP view and a Rosenberg view is extraordinary. In this case a routine view **(i)** shows only minimal lateral compartment narrowing, whereas a Rosenberg view **(ii)** demonstrates a complete loss of articular cartilage.

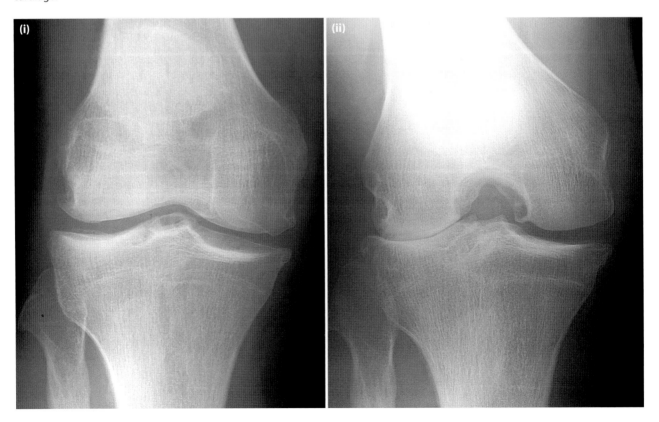

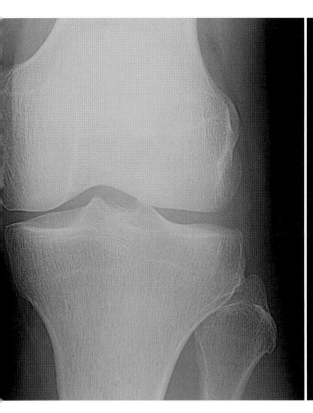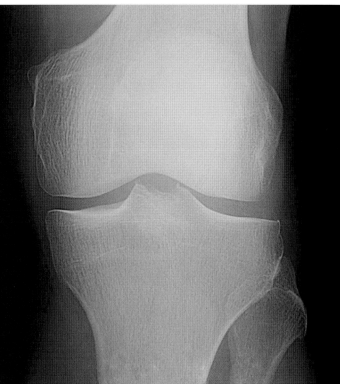

▲ **Fig. 6.10** In most people the tibial plateau slopes downwards from front to back. In a patient with a suspected osteochondral fracture of a tibial condyle, an AP view with 15° of caudal tube angulation is useful for the assessment of fracture depression. The advantage of this view is shown in a normal case. A normal AP view is shown on the left. The image on the right is an AP view with 15° of caudal angulation and the primary beam is now parallel to the articular surface of the tibial plateau.

The tibial plateau view

The examination of the tibial plateau in a patient with a possible plateau fracture should include an AP view with 15° of caudal tube angulation. This is called a Tillman-Moore or tibial plateau view and helps in assessing the degree of depression of a tibial plateau fracture. This view allows for the slope of the tibial plateau when measuring articular depression (McClellan et al. 1999) (see Fig. 6.10). A normal AP view may overestimate depression by as much as 50% compared with the plateau view.

Tips on looking at plain films of the knee

As with all areas, developing a search routine will ensure that all bone, joint and soft-tissue structures are examined in turn and, with this thorough approach, it is hoped that fewer diagnostic errors will occur. In particular, a search should be made for specific fractures that are commonly missed (see Table 6.2).

The authors' routine begins by looking to see whether the patient has an effusion. Absence of an effusion makes an intra-articular abnormality unlikely, and a particularly large effusion following acute trauma would focus attention on the possibility of an anterior cruciate ligament (ACL) rupture, a recent patellofemoral dislocation or an intra-articular fracture.

Table 6.2 Easily missed fractures of the knee

- Tibial plateau fractures
- Segond and reversed Segond fractures
- Stress fractures of the proximal tibia
- Fibular head avulsion fractures
- Vertical patellar fractures
- Avulsion fractures of the patella
- Salter–Harris Type 1 fractures
- Growth plate stress fractures

If there is no effusion present, the suprapatellar recess (or suprapatellar extension of the knee joint) creates an oblique linear soft-tissue density between the prefemoral fat pad and the triangular suprapatellar fat pad, the latter lying immediately posterior to the quadriceps tendon (see Fig. 6.11). The thickness of this soft-tissue density is usually less than 5 mm, although this will vary with the build of the athlete. In the presence of a joint effusion, the suprapatellar recess distends and progressively effaces the prefemoral fat pad (see Figs 6.12 and 6.13). As well as distending the suprapatellar recess, an effusion may also be identified and its size assessed by the degree of distension of the anterior knee joint recess. As the anterior recess distends with larger effusions, there is progressive encroachment on the infrapatellar fat pad (see Figs 6.14 and 6.15).

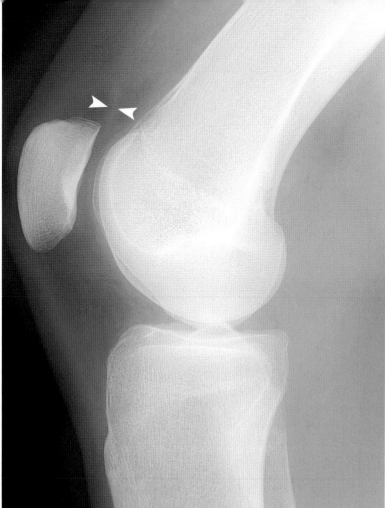

◀ **Fig. 6.11** When there is no effusion present, the two surfaces of the empty suprapatellar recess lie in apposition and produce an oblique linear density separating the prefemoral fat pad from the suprapatellar fat pad (arrowheads).

▲ **Fig. 6.12** When there is an effusion, the synovial layers of the suprapatellar fat pad become progressively separated by fluid density (arrowheads). The thickness of the linear density increases in proportion to the size of the effusion. In this case there is a moderate-sized effusion present.

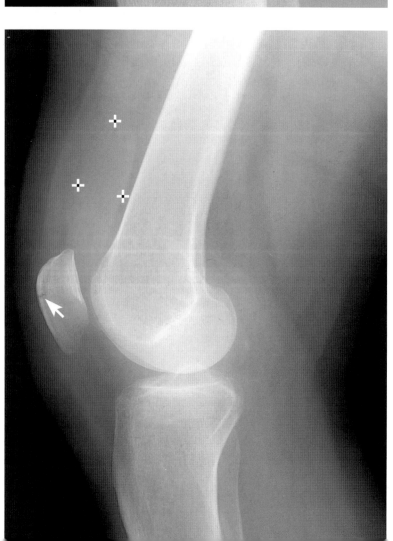

◀ **Fig. 6.13** As the size of the effusion increases, the prefemoral fat pad is progressively effaced and a large soft-tissue swelling becomes apparent (the extent of which is indicated by callipers). In this case, this swelling represents a large haemarthrosis associated with an undisplaced fracture of the patella, the anterior portion of which is demonstrated by an arrow.

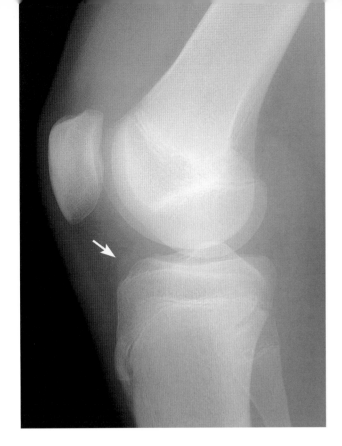

▲ Fig. 6.14 In addition to identifying fluid in the suprapatellar extension of the knee joint, fluid can also be seen in the anterior joint recess on a lateral view. A distended anterior recess becomes silhouetted against the fat density of the infrapatellar fat pad. In this case, there is a moderate collection of fluid present in the anterior recess (arrow).

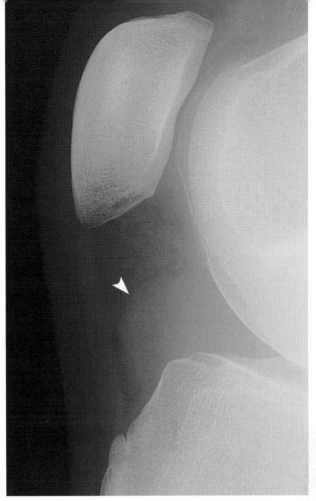

▲ Fig. 6.15 A large effusion is present with considerable distension of the anterior joint recess (arrowhead).

When there has been significant trauma and a fracture is clinically suspected, a cross-table lateral view is obtained to avoid weightbearing and having to move the patient into the lateral position. In this position a fat-fluid level may be seen in the suprapatellar joint recess. This important sign is produced by the escape of marrow fat, which floats on the effusion or haemarthrosis and indicates that a fracture is present (see Fig. 6.16). Occasionally, plain films may show a lipohaemarthrosis with two fluid levels (Lugo-Olivieri et al. 1996) due to the layering of marrow fat, serum and separated red cell sediment (see Figs 6.17 and 6.18).

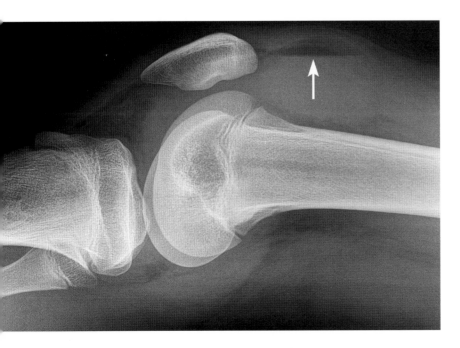

◄ Fig. 6.16 A cross-table lateral view is often necessary when there has been a severe knee injury. A large lipohaemarthrosis is present in this immature athlete. The suprapatellar recess is distended, largely effacing the prefemoral and suprapatellar fat pads. A fat/fluid level within the effusion indicates that there is a fracture present, allowing the escape of fat from the bone marrow. The radiographic appearance is due to fat floating on the haemarthrosis. The fracture is not evident on this view and further imaging will be necessary.

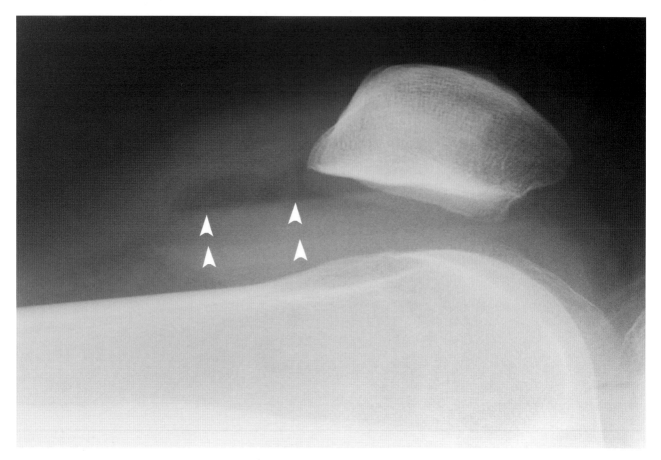

▲ **Fig. 6.17** Following a severe knee injury, a cross-table lateral image has been obtained. A large lipohaemarthrosis has formed with two fluid levels (arrowheads) indicating that a fracture is present, causing bleeding and allowing marrow fat to escape. The upper layer is marrow fat, serum forms the centre layer, and sedimentation of red blood cells creates the third layer.

▼ **Fig. 6.18(a)** An axial fat-suppressed T2-weighted MR image demonstrates a lipohaemarthrosis. Three distinct signal layers are present (the 'parfait' sign). The superficial layer is fat (f), which has been suppressed and is of low signal intensity, there is an intervening high signal intensity layer of serum (s), and a deep layer of intermediate signal intensity is composed of red cell products (r). **(b)** This extraordinary coronal fat-suppressed T2-weighted MR image has captured globules of fat actually escaping from bone marrow at an osteochondral patellar fracture and they are seen floating to the surface. Marrow oedema is associated with the fracture (arrow). Patella = P.

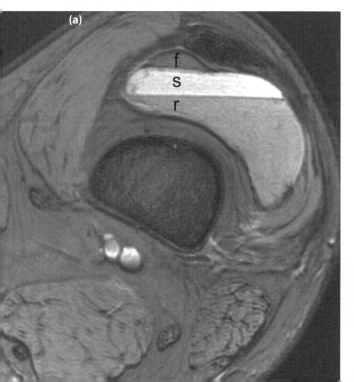

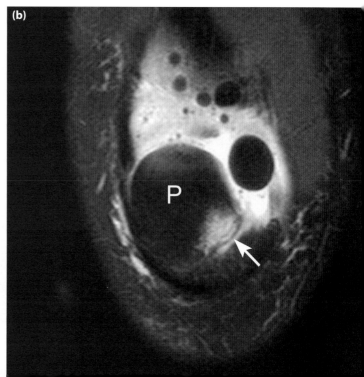

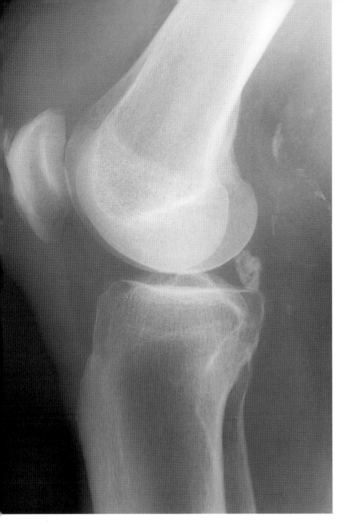

▲ **Fig. 6.19** Considerable information is available in the soft tissues and it is important to assess calcifications. A loose body is present in the knee joint posteriorly and vascular calcification in the soft tissues behind the knee shows an aneurysm at the origin of the popliteal artery. There is a large knee joint effusion, and soft-tissue swelling anterior to the patella and the upper patellar tendon is indicative of pre-patellar bursopathy.

Calcifications may be seen involving soft tissues around the knee and projected over joint spaces. Each of these should be assessed (see Figs 6.19–6.24). Finally, in the examination of soft tissues, localised soft-tissue swelling becomes obvious when there is displacement or obliteration of normal fat lines and anatomical profiles. Other imaging methods are usually used to determine the cause of the swelling. For example, localised soft-tissue swelling may be associated with a medial collateral ligament (MCL) injury (see Fig. 6.25), and bulging at a margin of the joint may be produced by a meniscal cyst (see Fig. 6.26).

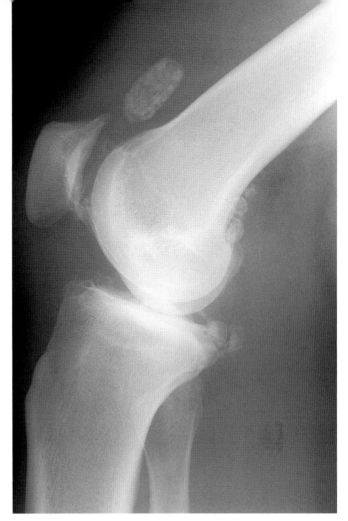

▲ **Fig. 6.20** A large ossicle lies in the suprapatellar recess of the knee joint and an effusion is noted. Other smaller loose bodies are present posteriorly. Moderate degenerative changes are present in the patellofemoral articulation. There is increased density in the infrapatellar fat pad and faint densities are present throughout the fat pad, raising the possibility of Hoffa's disease (this condition is discussed later).

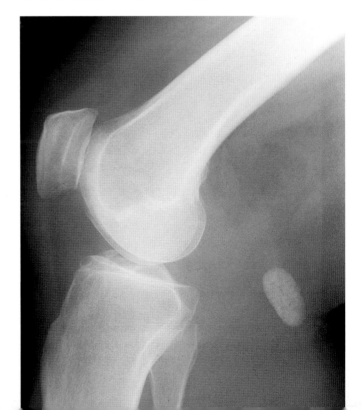

▶ **Fig. 6.21** There is a large ossicle projected over the soft tissues behind the knee. This almost certainly lies within a popliteal cyst.

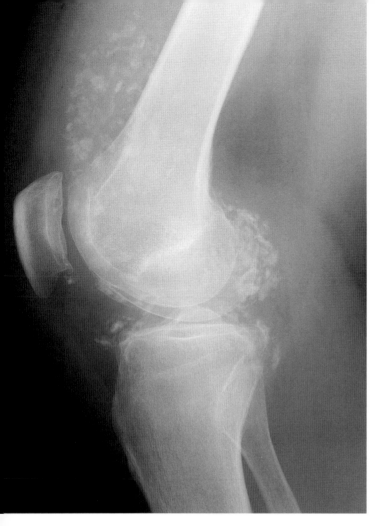

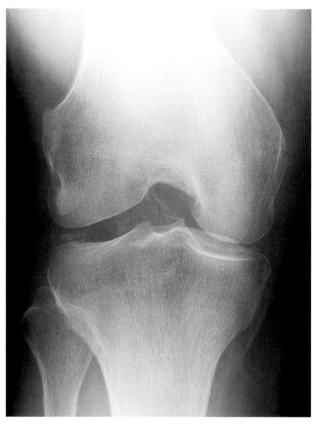

▲ **Fig. 6.22** Multiple ossicles are projected over the knee joint space and its recesses and the appearance is that of synovial osteochondromatosis. The ossicles have an appearance typical of this condition. The majority of ossicles have a jagged, irregular margin like crushed blue metal.

▼ **Fig. 6.23(a)** Changes of chondrocalcinosis involve the articular cartilage of the medial and lateral compartments and calcification is also present in the fibrocartilagenous menisci.

▲ **(b)** There are changes of chondrocalcinosis in the menisci and the ACL.

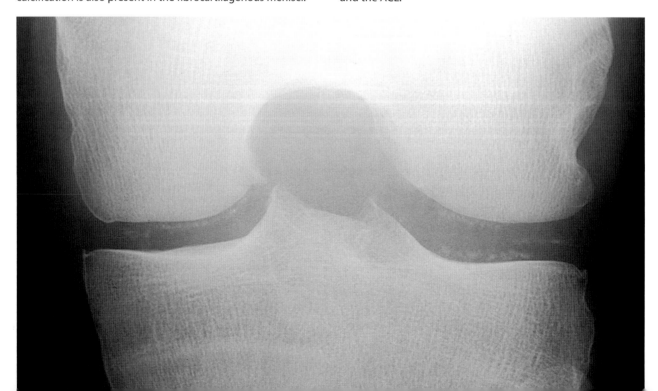

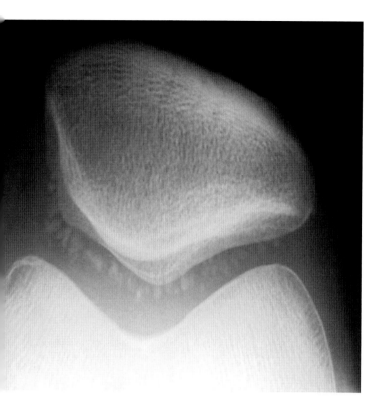

▲ **Fig. 6.24** When chondrocalcinosis involves the articular cartilage of the patella, there is a distinctive pattern of calcification, which has the appearance of a pearl necklace.

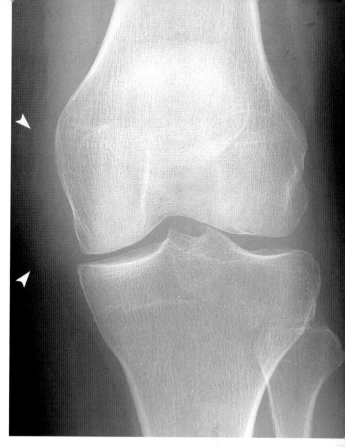

▲ **Fig. 6.25** Soft-tissue swelling is seen in the line of the MCL due to displacement of fat planes. This swelling indicates MCL injury.

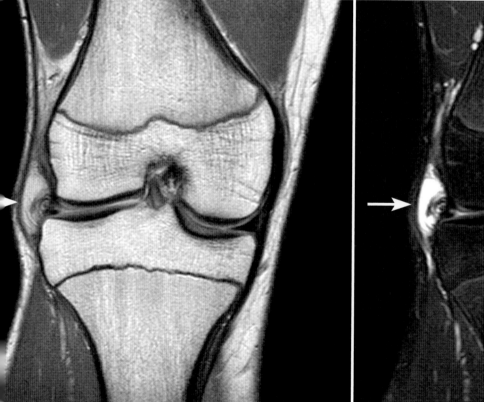

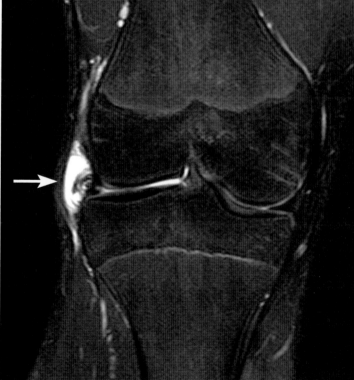

▲ **Fig. 6.26** Coronal T2 and fat-suppressed PD-weighted MR images demonstrate a meniscal and parameniscal cyst producing localised swelling and displacement of the overlying iliotibial band (ITB) at the lateral aspect of the knee (arrow). Note the underlying cleavage tear of the lateral meniscus.

Having completed the examination of the soft tissues, the bones and joints should be scrutinised.

Joint spaces are examined for narrowing, congruity, irregularity of articular margins and alignment abnormalities. Alignment abnormality may indicate a cruciate ligament rupture (see Fig. 6.27). Valgus and varus abnormalities are most often due to degenerative change. Do not forget to check the congruity of the proximal tibiofibular joint! The trabecular pattern and bony cortex throughout the osseous structures of the knee should be carefully examined in a search for pattern disturbances that may provide evidence of injury or other pathology. Fractures may be subtle and fracture diagnosis requires careful examination of all views. Fractures may appear as a linear translucency or sclerosis and, if the cortex is involved, there may be a subtle cortical break or step in cortical alignment (see Fig. 6.28). Particular attention should be paid to the bony structure of the epiphyseal

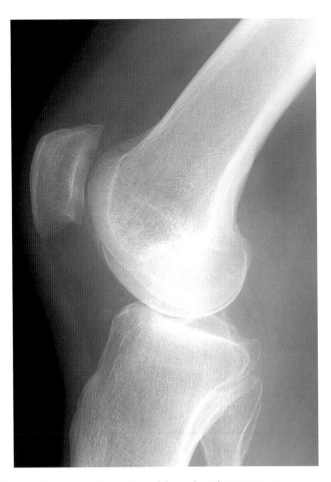

▶ **Fig. 6.27** Femorotibial alignment change may be indicative of a cruciate ligament rupture. With ACL rupture the tibia is able to move forward with respect to the femur, and a posterior cruciate ligament (PCL) deficiency will allow abnormal forward movement of the femur on the tibia, as demonstrated in this case. These alignment abnormalities become more evident in a cross-table lateral film with support beneath the tibia in the case of an ACL rupture and beneath the femur when a PCL rupture is suspected.

▼ **Fig. 6.28** Signs of a fracture are often subtle. When searching for bone injury, any disruption of the trabecular pattern or stepping and buckling of the bony cortex should be noted. This patient experienced a force to the medial side of the knee causing considerable pain and disability.

(a) A cross-table lateral view shows a subtle gap in the cortex on the posterolateral aspect of the distal femoral metaphysis (white arrow) and linear translucency in the subchondral bone of the femoral condyle (black arrow). A fluid level in the suprapatellar recess of the knee joint indicates the presence of a fracture (arrowhead).

(b) The plain film changes are subtle and easily overlooked. In this case, with further imaging by MRI, a sagittal PD image demonstrated a major oblique-coronal fracture traversing the entire lateral femoral condyle (arrow). There is slight displacement with resultant 'step-off' deformities at the fracture margins.

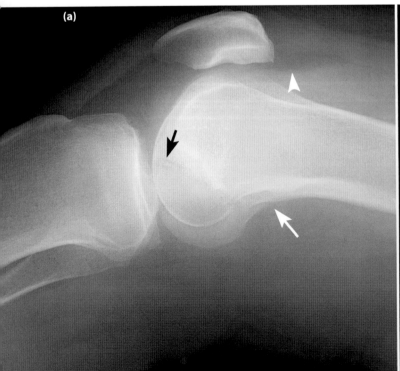

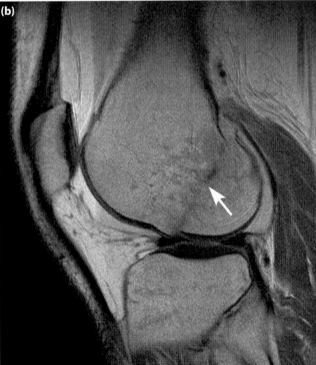

area. Any departure from the normal bony architecture in the epiphyseal region will almost always indicate an important pathological change. In particular, a vague translucency in the epiphysis may be due to a chondroblastoma or osteoid osteoma (see Fig. 6.29), and epiphyseal sclerosis is generally due to a compression fracture or bone stress (see Fig. 6.30).

In examining a series of films, specific radiographic anatomy should be identified. These anatomical landmarks are pertinent to film interpretation. On an AP view, the adductor tubercle, the site of insertion of the adductor magnus, is seen as a localised bony protrusion just above the medial border of the medial femoral condyle. A groove in the lateral profile of the lateral femoral condyle transmits the popliteus tendon (see Fig. 6.31). A normal sesamoid of the popliteus tendon is occasionally present within this notch. This is called the cymella (see Fig. 6.32).

▼ **Fig. 6.29** It is always important to further investigate a small translucent area in the epiphysis such as this. This proved to be an osteoid osteoma. The differential diagnosis of this appearance includes a chondroblastoma.

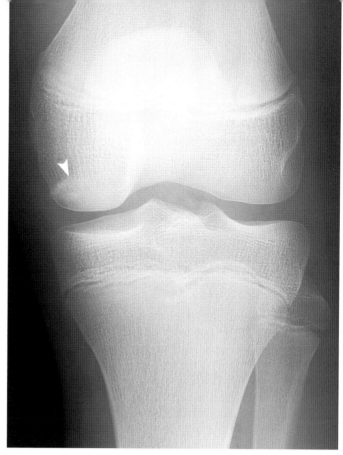

▲ **Fig. 6.30** A small area of sclerosis is present in the femoral epiphysis. The linear sclerosis extends to the medial cortical margin of the medial femoral condyle where minor cortical buckling is apparent. The appearances are those of a compression fracture.

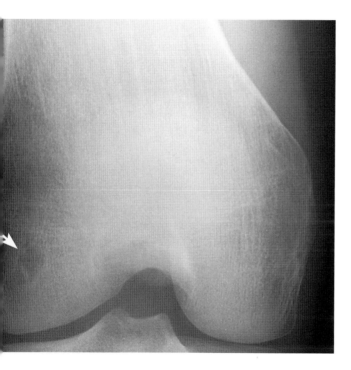

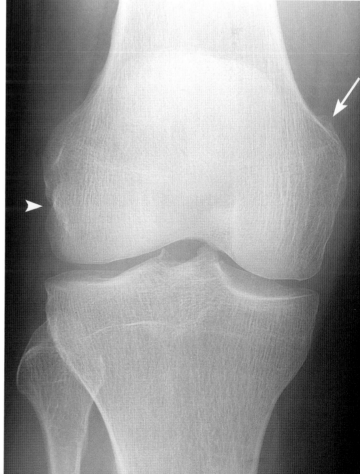

▶ **Fig. 6.31** Anatomical landmarks on an AP image include the adductor tubercle, which is the site of insertion of the adductor magnus (arrow) on the superomedial aspect of the medial condyle. This tubercle is a variable finding. The groove for the popliteus is seen on the lateral profile of the lateral condyle (arrowhead).

▶ **Fig. 6.32** A cymella is a normal ossicle occasionally seen overlying the popliteal groove (arrow). The cymella is a sesamoid in the popliteus tendon. Degenerative changes are noted in the knee joint.

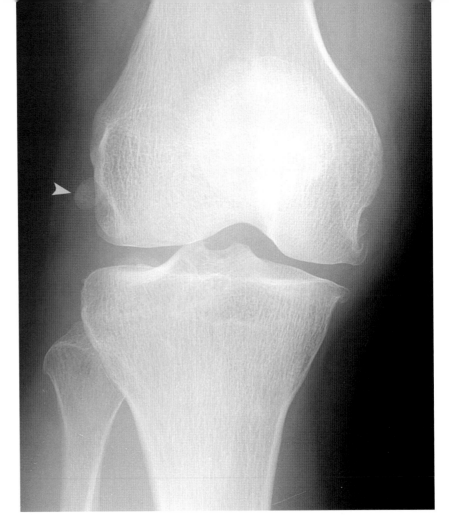

▼ **Fig. 6.33(a)** Profiles of the articular surface of the femoral condyles differ in the lateral view, enabling each condyle to be distinguished. The medial femoral condyle is rounded (white arrowhead) and has a variable slight notch dividing its middle and anterior thirds. The lateral femoral condyle is flattened in its middle third (black arrowhead). There is usually a notch dividing the lateral condyle in halves. This is called the terminal sulcus and should not be confused with an osteochondral fracture associated with an ACL rupture, which may occur in this region. The proximal tibiofibular joint is seen unusually well in the lateral view.

▼ **(b)** The notch in the profile of the medial femoral condyle divides its middle and anterior thirds (arrow). The terminal sulcus of the lateral femoral condyle is indicated by an arrowhead.

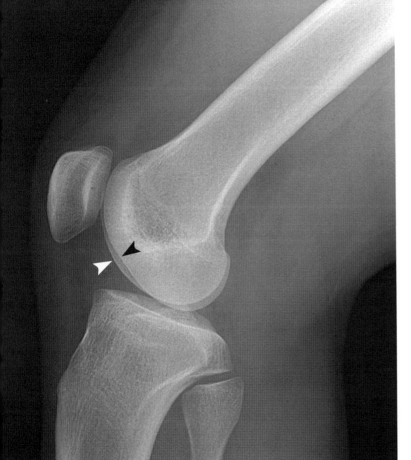

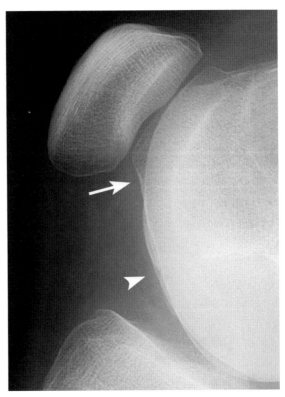

The profile of each femoral condyle should be examined on the lateral view. It is possible to differentiate between the profile of the medial and lateral condyles (see Fig. 6.33). The medial condyle is rounded and may be identified by a groove that separates the anterior and middle thirds of the articular surface. On the other hand, the lateral condyle is flattened in the area of a groove that divides the articular surface into halves. The groove in the lateral condyle is known as the 'terminal sulcus' (see Fig. 6.34). If a defect is found anterior to the normal position of the terminal sulcus in the lateral femoral condyle, it is probable that this is an osteochondral fracture, associated with an ACL rupture (this sign is discussed later).

The bony roof of the intercondylar notch is seen in the lateral view of the knee as a sclerotic line (see Fig. 6.35). This is called Blumensaat's line and is an important landmark for assessment of patella alta, for assessing the placement of the tibial tunnel of an ACL reconstruction and in the investigation of graft impingement. The fabella is a normal sesamoid in the tendon of the lateral head of the gastrocnemius, seen immediately posterior to the lateral femoral condyle (see Fig. 6.36).

The normal patellar tendon is uniform in thickness with sharply defined margins due to contrast with the adjacent subcutaneous and infrapatellar fat. The patellar tendon attaches to the anterior aspect of the inferior pole of the patella and has continuity with the quadriceps tendon through fibres that pass over the anterior surface of the patella. The patella tendon inserts at the tibial tuberosity (syn. tubercle), which is a bony elevation on the anterior aspect of the proximal tibia (see Fig. 6.37). The infrapatellar fat pad (Hoffa's fat pad) lies immediately posterior to the patella tendon and should be uniform in density. Trauma, a mass or inflammation may alter this density.

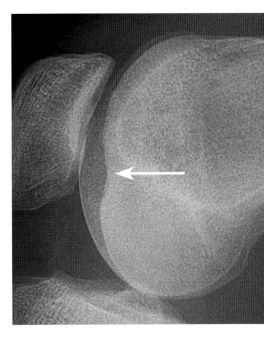

▲ **Fig. 6.34** An unusually prominent terminal sulcus (arrow).

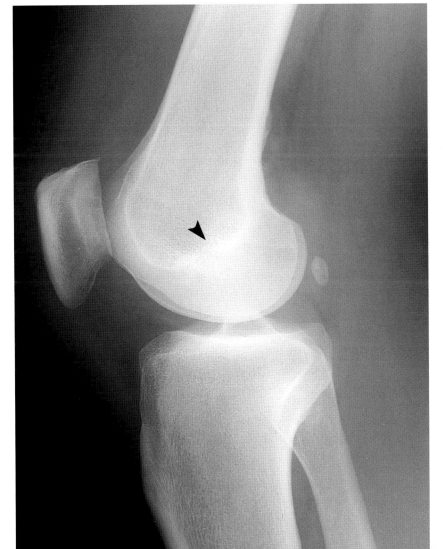

◀ **Fig. 6.35** Blumensaat's line is a sclerotic line (indicated by arrowhead) seen in the lateral view. This represents the roof of the intercondylar notch. If the inferior pole of the patella lies above the level of this line with the knee at 30° of flexion, it is considered to be a patella alta, the significance of which will be discussed later.

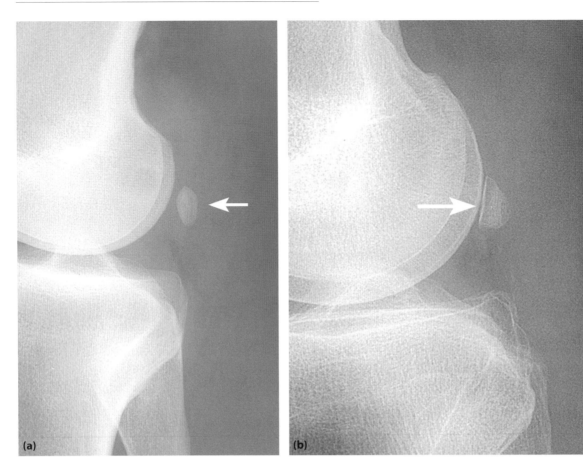

▲ **Fig. 6.36(a)** The ossicle lying posterior to the femoral condyles in the lateral view is a normal sesamoid of the lateral head of the gastrocnemius (arrow). This ossicle is called the fabella. **(b)** One side of the ossicle may be flattened for articulation with the lateral femoral condyle (arrow).

▶ **Fig. 6.37** The normal patellar tendon is of uniform width and there is only minor expansion of a normal tendon at its tibial attachment. The tuberosity is a localised, slightly elevated bony protrusion continuous with the ridge on the anterior surface of the tibia (arrow). At the patella attachment, the tendon is continuous with fibres that pass over the anterior surface of the patella to merge with the quadriceps tendon. The appearances of a normal patella tendon are demonstrated **(a)** by plain film and **(b)** by T1-weighted MR image. Note the uniform density of the infrapatellar fat pad.

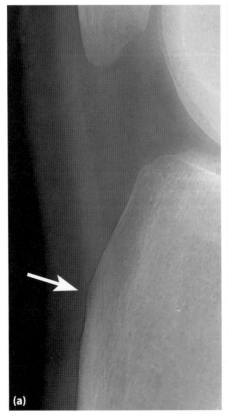

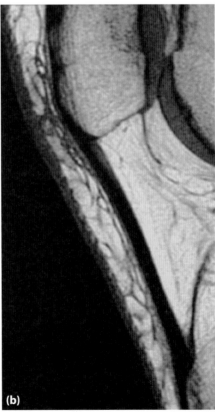

Features of the proximal tibia include the medial and lateral condyles. The articular surface of each condyle is known as a tibial plateau. The intercondylar eminence lies between these articular surfaces and tibial spines are localised prolongations of the articular surfaces that arise from the lateral margins of the eminence. The cruciate ligaments attach to the eminence. The ACL attaches anterior to the tibial spines. The posterior cruciate ligament (PCL) attaches behind the spines and its attachment continues over onto the posterior surface of the proximal tibia for about 1 cm. The medial tibial spine is longer than the lateral tibial spine and lies slightly behind the lateral spine, the spines being separated by an oblique groove (see Fig. 6.38). Gerdy's tubercle is a protrusion on the anterolateral aspect of the lateral tibial condyle and is the site of insertion of the iliotibial band. The posteromedial corner of the upper tibia is grooved for the attaching semimembranosis tendon.

The patella can be evaluated on each of the AP, lateral and patellofemoral views. On the AP view, bipartite or occasionally tripartite deformity may be noted (see Fig. 6.39). A bipartite patella is a developmental anomaly that may be bilateral and occurs when one or more ossification centres at the superolateral corner of the patella remain ununited. Males are affected more than females, 9:1 (Ogden et al. 1982). Although a bipartite patella is usually an incidental finding and asymptomatic, the anomaly can sometimes become painful following trauma due to disruption of the syndesmosis between the fragments. A bone scan or MRI can be used to confirm traumatic disruption.

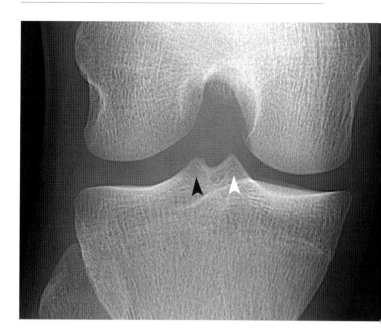

▲ **Fig. 6.38** The articular surfaces of the tibial condyles are separated by the intercondylar eminence. Tibial spines arise from the lateral margins of the eminence. The medial tibial spine (white arrowhead) is longer than the lateral tibial spine (black arrowhead).

In the immature athlete the inferior pole of the patella may be difficult to interpret. Secondary ossification centres are often present and these vary considerably in appearance. The secondary centres may be multiple, rounded or linear (see Fig. 6.40). Often there is a prominent linear secondary centre on the anterior margin of the lower pole. These secondary centres eventually unite to form the tip of the inferior pole (see Fig. 6.41).

Acute fractures

Knee fracture is not a common injury. Only 6% of patients presenting to an emergency department with an acute knee injury have a fracture (Stiell et al. 1995). In the paediatric population, fractures can be expected more often due to the relative strength of ligaments compared to the developing centres of ossification. Assessing the paediatric incidence of knee fractures, Moore et al. (2005) published the results of a prospective study evaluating clinical decision rules for radiography in a paediatric population. This study found that about 10% of patients presenting with an acute knee injury had a fracture. It is interesting to note that of the 15 fractures in their series, 10 had been caused by a trampoline accident.

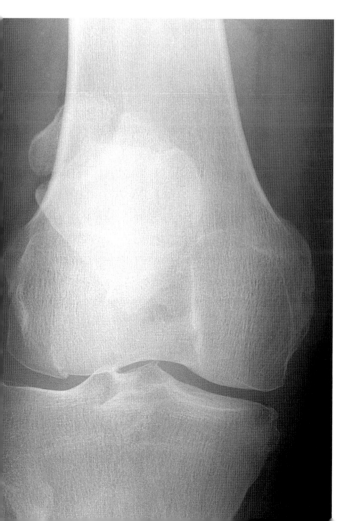

◄**Fig. 6.39** An AP view of the knee shows a separate bone fragment at the superolateral corner of the patella. This is a bipartite patella, which results from a failure of fusion of a secondary ossification centre. Occasionally a tripartite patella is seen. The margins of the syndesmosis are well rounded, defined and smooth, unlike a fracture.

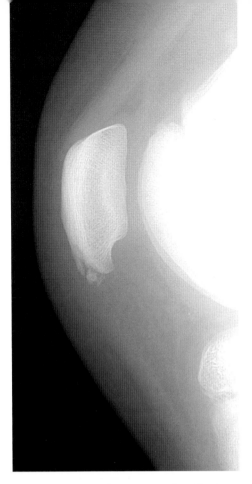

▲ **Fig. 6.40** Secondary centres of ossification at the inferior pole of the patella are often multiple with a mixture of rounded and linear ossicles. Soft-tissue swelling differentiates a traction apophysitis from normal developing secondary centres.

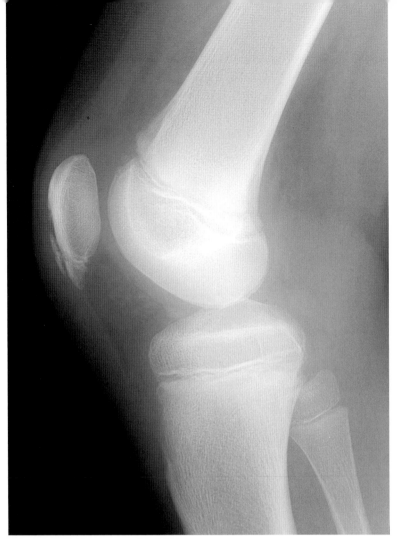

▲ **Fig. 6.41** Fusion of secondary centres at the lower pole of the patella is progressing to form the inferior pole.

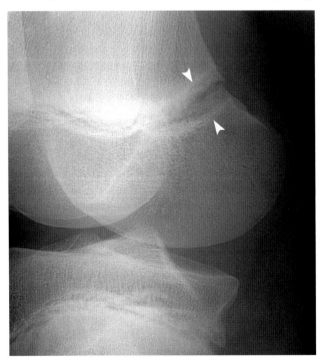

▲ **Fig. 6.42** Disruption of the distal femoral growth plate is demonstrated on an oblique plain film. Widening of the posteromedial aspect of the growth plate has occurred (arrowheads).

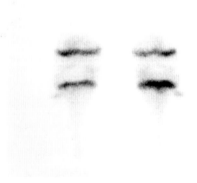

▲ **Fig. 6.43** Nuclear bone scans are helpful in assessing growth plate injury when the plain films are equivocal. There is increased isotope uptake at the proximal tibial growth plate on the left side, indicating a growth plate fracture.

Growth plate fractures

Fractures of the distal femoral and proximal tibial growth plates usually occur between the ages of 10 and 17 and result from hyperextension or valgus stress in sports such as skiing and football. The distal femoral growth plate is the more commonly involved. The Salter–Harris (SH) classification of growth plate injuries has been discussed in Chapter 1.

Growth plate injuries are important to recognise because alignment deformities and premature closure of the epiphysis can occur, resulting in leg-length discrepancy. Plain films may show growth plate widening (see Fig. 6.42). Comparative views of the asymptomatic side are often helpful as the changes are frequently subtle. CT scans may be helpful for identifying fragments and assessing fragment orientation. Bone scans can be of assistance when the diagnosis is uncertain (see Fig. 6.43). MRI allows the most accurate evaluation of injury in the acute and healing phases (see Fig. 6.44).

Distal femoral growth plate fractures

Fractures of the distal femoral growth plate represent 5% of all growth plate fractures and usually result from a hyperextension injury. When displacement occurs in the sagittal plane, neurovascular complications may occur in the popliteal fossa (see Fig. 6.45). Other complications include growth arrest

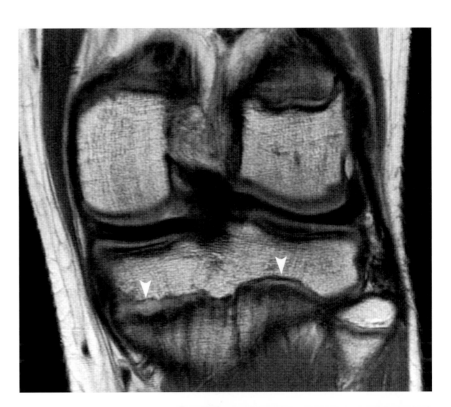

▶ **Fig. 6.44(a)** A coronal PD-weighted MR image demonstrates proximal tibial growth plate widening (arrowheads).

▼ **(b)** A sagittal PD-weighted image of the same case shows growth plate widening and a fat-suppressed T2-weighted image demonstrates high signal in the growth plate (arrows). The appearances are those of a Salter–Harris Type I injury. Bone bruising in the anterior proximal aspect of the tibial epiphysis indicates that a hyperextension injury has occurred.

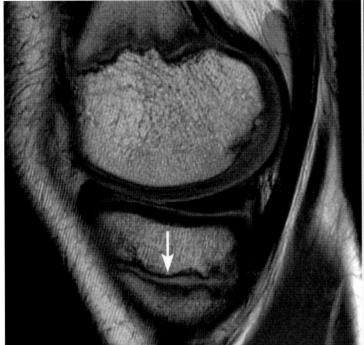

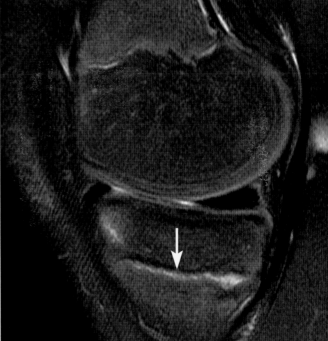

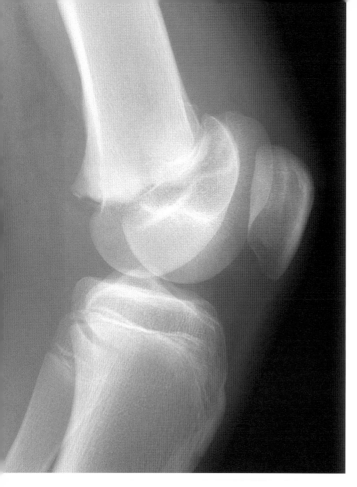

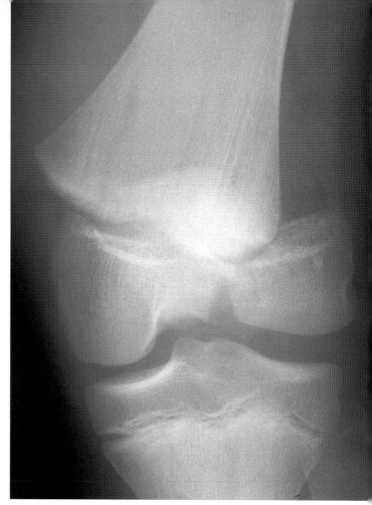

▲ **Fig. 6.45** There has been a fracture of the distal femoral growth plate with anterior displacement and superior rotation of the epiphysis in the sagittal plane. Displacement of the epiphysis in the sagittal plane has an increased incidence of neurovascular complications.

▼ **Fig. 6.47** A Salter–Harris Type II fracture of the proximal tibial growth plate is present with separation of a lateral metaphyseal fragment. There has been medial displacement and lateral angulation of the tibial metaphysis, resulting in a valgus alignment. There is also subluxation of the proximal tibiofibular joint.

▲ **Fig. 6.46** A Salter–Harris Type III fracture of the distal femoral growth plate is present. The fracture extends through the epiphysis into the intercondylar notch, separating the femoral condyles. Lateral displacement and rotation of the epiphysis has occurred, resulting in a valgus alignment.

(growth plate bar formation), which may be partial or complete, angulation and shortening. Growth disturbance has been shown to occur in about 50% of SH Type I and Type II growth plate fractures of the distal femur (Riseborough et al. 1983). Although uncommon, accelerated growth may also occur due to increased vascularity. Angulation in the coronal plane may persist and may not correct spontaneously.

A fracture of the distal femoral growth plate that extends through the epiphysis into the intercondylar notch (see Fig. 6.46) may be associated with an injury to the ACL or MCL (Torg et al. 1981; Bertin and Goble 1983). A widened growth plate following trauma may be the result of soft-tissue interposition, which can be demonstrated by MRI (Whan et al. 2003).

Proximal tibial growth plate fractures

Proximal tibial growth plate fractures are uncommon and have a high rate of complication. Complications include vascular insufficiency and peroneal nerve palsy. Fortunately, these are usually transient. Moore and McKenzie (1996) found that SH Type I fractures occur in a younger age group, with the average being 10 years of age. SH Type II fractures (see Fig. 6.47) are the most common and are usually undisplaced. SH Type III fractures are often associated with a lateral condyle fracture and MCL injury. SH Type IV fractures usually produce an angular deformity.

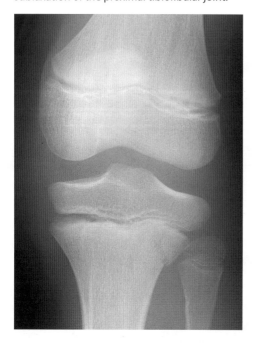

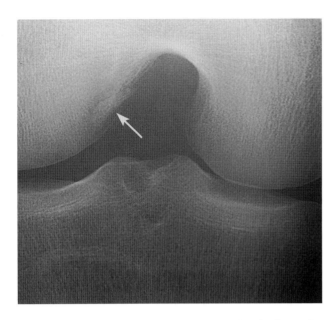

▲ **Fig. 6.48** An avulsion fracture has occurred at the femoral attachment of the ACL at the lateral wall of the intercondylar notch (arrow). A moderate-sized fragment has been separated. This avulsion fracture is an uncommon injury.

Avulsion fractures

ACL avulsion fractures

ACL avulsion fractures are one of the most common injuries in children between the ages of 8 and 14. The avulsion fractures almost always occur at the tibial attachment (Meyers and McKeever 1959; Molander et al. 1981). Rarely, a femoral avulsion will be seen (see Fig. 6.48). ACL avulsions become less frequent with increasing age and in adults the ligament will usually tear before an avulsion occurs. Meyers and McKeever (1959) classified ACL avulsions of the tibial spine into four types:

- *Type I:* An undisplaced partial fracture involves the intercondylar eminence, although often there is slight elevation of the anterior edge of the fragment (see Fig. 6.49).
- *Type II:* The fragment becomes hinged with marked elevation of its anterior edge (see Fig. 6.50).
- *Type III:* The fragment becomes completely separated and lies above the fracture bed (see Fig. 6.51).
- *Type IV:* The fragment is separated from the fracture bed and rotated.

Type III avulsion fractures account for 45% of all avulsions (Sullivan et al. 1989). Rupture of the ACL will be discussed in more detail later in the section on ligament injuries.

▼ **Fig. 6.49** This is a Type I ACL avulsion injury. A fragment has been separated from the intercondylar eminence without displacement (arrowheads).

▼ **Fig. 6.50** A Type II avulsion injury is present, with separation of a bone fragment from the intercondylar eminence. The fragment is hinged, with elevation of its anterior margin (arrow).

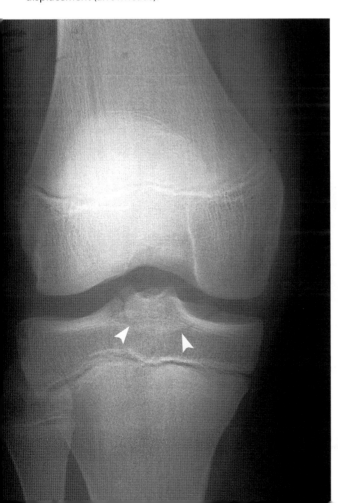

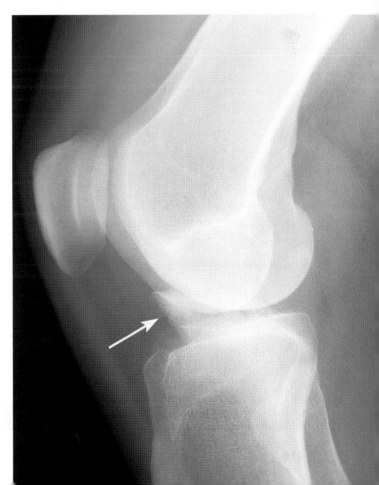

▶ **Fig. 6.51** When the avulsed fragment is completely separated (arrow), the injury is classified as a Type III avulsion injury.

PCL avulsion fractures

PCL avulsions can occur at either the tibial or femoral attachments. Avulsion of the tibial attachment is the fracture most commonly seen and has a characteristic appearance (see Fig. 6.52). It is unusual for injury to occur in isolation and there may be associated injuries including posterolateral corner injury, meniscal injuries, bone bruising and a reversed Segond avulsion (see opposite).

▼ **Fig. 6.52** Proximal PCL avulsions are rarely seen. This case shows a typical tibial PCL avulsion fracture.
(a) The separated fragment is often triangular in profile and is seen to involve the posterosuperior corner of the proximal tibia (arrow).
(b) A linear-shaped fragment is also occasionally seen (arrow). The insert is a sagittal T1-weighted image confirming the plain films finding of a PCL avulsion (arrow). Note the femorotibial alignment abnormality, typical of PCL deficiency.

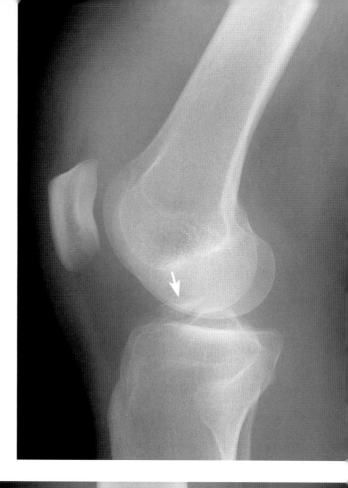

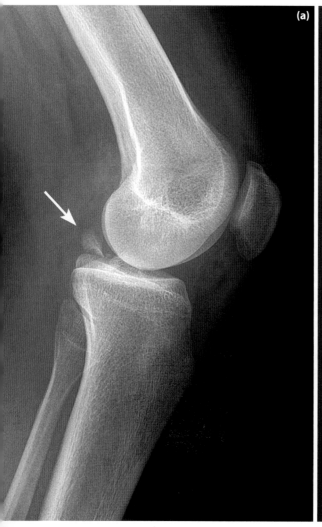
(a)

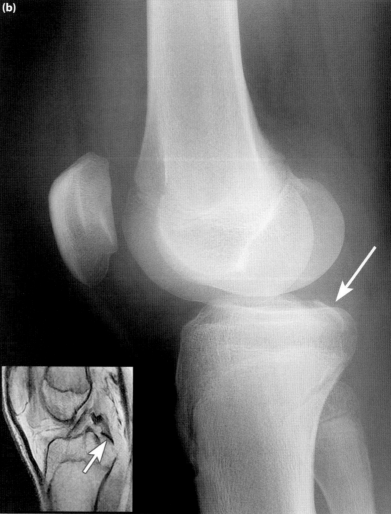
(b)

MCL avulsion fractures

MCL avulsions (see Fig. 6.53) are unusual. Injury to the MCL usually produces an intrasubstance rupture (see the discussion on ligament injuries on page 435).

Avulsion fractures of the proximal fibula

Avulsion fractures of the proximal fibula commonly involve the styloid process of the fibula head and can be due to traction by the arcuate ligament complex, lateral collateral ligament or the biceps femoris tendon (see Fig. 6.54). This avulsion fracture has a high association with multiligamentous injury (Huang et al. 2003). These changes are discussed later in the section on posterolateral corner injuries.

Segond fractures (lateral tibial rim fractures)

A Segond fracture (lateral tibial rim fracture) is the avulsion of a small vertical bone fragment from the lateral aspect of the lateral tibial condyle, just distal to the tibial plateau (see Fig. 6.55). This fracture occurs with internal rotation of the tibia on a flexed knee. It has a high association with ACL rupture (Hess et al. 1994) (see Figs 6.56 and 6.57). It also has an association with meniscal tears and posterolateral corner injuries. The fragment represents a cortical avulsion, usually well seen on an AP view. The actual tissue that attaches to

▼ **Fig. 6.54** It is now recognised that avulsion fractures involving the styloid process of the proximal fibula are important injuries to identify. This avulsion may be an indication that there is a major injury of the posterolateral corner of the knee. In this case, the entire styloid process has been separated (arrowheads). This is unusual.

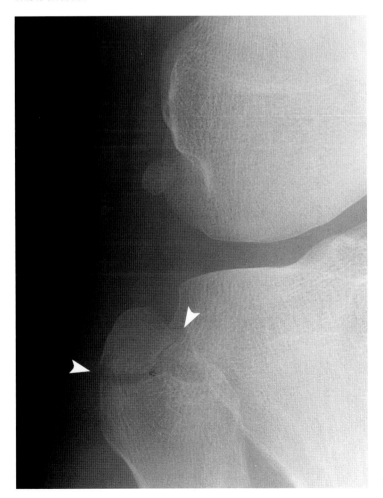

▼ **Fig. 6.53** A valgus force to the knee will commonly produce an MCL injury, and occasionally a small avulsion fracture is separated from its proximal attachment (arrow).

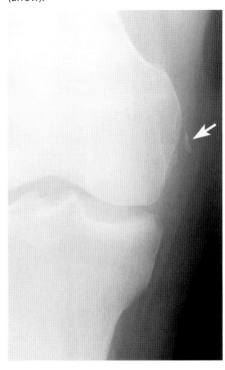

▼ **Fig. 6.55** This bone fragment, separated from the lateral margin of the lateral tibial condyle, is characteristic of a Segond fracture (arrow).

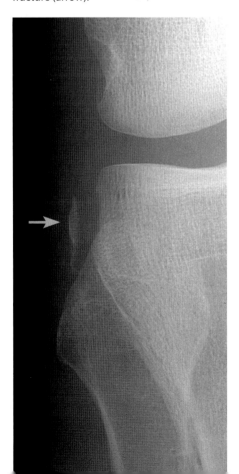

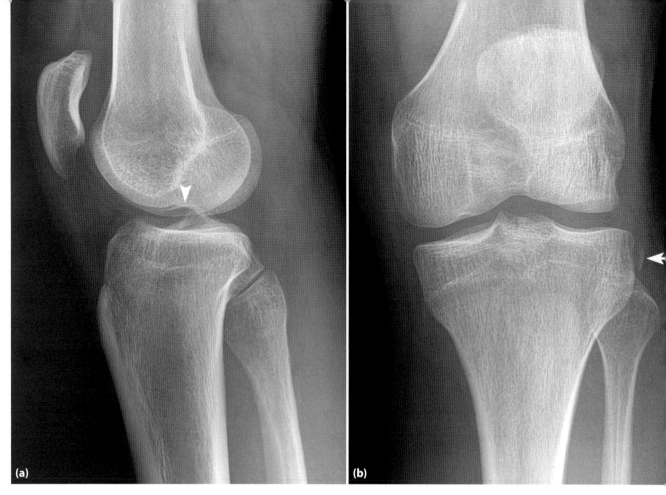

(a)

(b)

▲ **Fig. 6.56** In the lateral view, a depressed osteochondral fracture of the lateral femoral condyle is demonstrated (arrowhead). The pivot-shift displacement and ACL rupture allow impaction of the lateral femoral condyle on the posterior corner of the lateral tibial condyle, producing this fracture. A typical Segond fracture is shown in the AP view (arrow), separated from the lateral margin of the lateral tibial condyle.

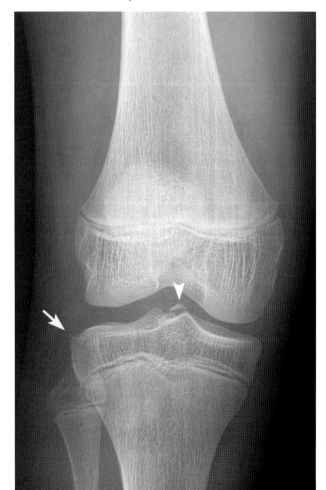

◀ **Fig. 6.57** The association of a Segond fracture and an ACL rupture is again demonstrated. An unusually small Segond fracture is present (arrow) and an avulsion fracture of the intercondylar eminence is demonstrated, indicating an ACL injury (arrowhead).

the avulsed fragment of bone has been a subject of much discussion. A recent cadaver study postulates contributions from posterior fibres of the iliotibial band and the anterior oblique band of the lateral collateral ligament (Campos et al. 2001). MRI may demonstrate marrow oedema in the lateral tibial condyle adjacent to the avulsion and associated injury to the meniscus, ACL and other supporting ligaments.

Avulsion fractures of Gerdy's tubercle

Gerdy's tubercle may be avulsed by the iliotibial band (see Fig. 6.58) and must be differentiated from a Segond fracture. A Segond fracture is separated from the lateral aspect of the proximal tibia and is seen in profile on a true AP view. Gerdy's tubercle, on the other hand, lies on the anterolateral surface and requires slight external rotation to profile the fragment. Isolated tears of the iliotibial band are rare and these tears may be only one component of injuries to multiple ligaments at the posterolateral corner of the knee. The iliotibial band acts as a lateral stabiliser in flexion and extension and remains taut in both positions.

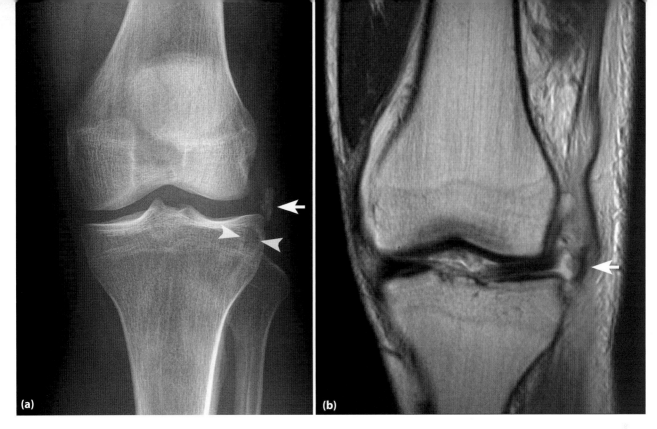

▲ **Fig. 6.58(a)** Avulsion of Gerdy's tubercle has occurred. Retraction of the iliotibial band has caused moderate displacement of the bone fragment (arrow). The fracture bed can be identified on the anterolateral aspect of the proximal tibia (arrowheads). **(b)** A coronal PD-weighted MR image of the same case confirms an avulsion fracture of Gerdy's tubercle (arrow), with retraction and buckling of the iliotibial band.

Reverse Segond fractures

Reverse Segond fractures have been described by Escobedo et al. (2002). In three patients a small cortical fragment was avulsed from the medial margin of the tibial condyle, caused by traction of the deep fibres of the tibial attachment of the medial collateral ligament (see Fig. 6.59). All patients had a PCL tear and peripheral medial meniscal tear.

Posterior capsular ligament avulsions

The posterior capsular ligament may avulse a small fragment from the posterior aspect of the upper tibia due to a hyper-extension injury (see Fig. 6.60).

Medial meniscal avulsion fractures

A small intracapsular bone fragment may be avulsed by the tibial attachment of the posterior horn of the medial meniscus.

Medial retinacular avulsion fractures of the patella

Following lateral dislocation of the patella, an avulsion fracture is commonly seen at the medial border of the patella, caused by traction of the medial patellar retinaculum (see Figs 6.61 and 6.62).

Avulsion fractures of the tibial tuberosity

Fractures of the tibial tuberosity occur mainly in jumping sports following knee flexion against a strong quadriceps contraction with the foot flexed (Ogden et al. 1980), or simply

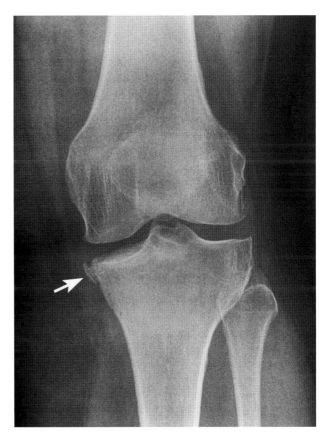

▲ **Fig. 6.59** A reverse Segond fracture is present (arrow). This is an avulsion fracture at the medial border of the medial tibial condyle. An association between this fracture and PCL rupture and meniscal injury has recently been described (see text).

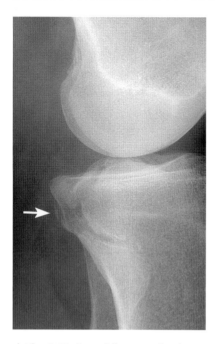

▲ **Fig. 6.60** A small fragment has been avulsed from the posterior surface of the proximal tibia by the posterior capsular ligament (arrow). This avulsion has been caused by a hyperextension injury.

▶ **Fig. 6.61** An avulsion fracture of the medial border of the patella has resulted from traction by the medial retinaculum during dislocation of the patella (arrow). Considerable lateral tilting of the patella is present and orientation of the trabeculae of the patella suggests that excessive lateral pressure syndrome (ELPS) is present (discussed later).

by a violent extension of the knee. The classification of tibial tuberosity avulsion fractures by Ogden et al. (1980) describes three types:

- **Type I:** There is injury to the apophysis of the tubercle, without injury to the proximal tibial epiphysis (see Fig. 6.63).
- **Type II:** A fracture extends across the upper apophysis, parallel to the growth plate. The proximal tibial epiphysis may be incompletely fractured (see Fig. 6.64).
- **Type III:** Traction on the tibial tuberosity causes a vertical fracture at the base of the tuberosity, which extends through the proximal tibial epiphysis into the knee joint. There is anterior hinging of the apophysis (see Fig. 6.65).

Types I and II tibial tuberosity avulsion fractures occur in younger athletes, 12 to 14 years old, whereas Type III fractures occur in 15- to 17-year-old athletes with greater muscular development. There is an increased incidence of pre-existing Osgood–Schlatter's disease (ipsilateral or contralateral) in patients who have an acute tuberosity injury (Ogden et al. 1980).

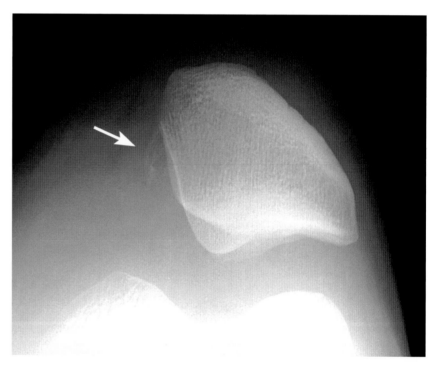

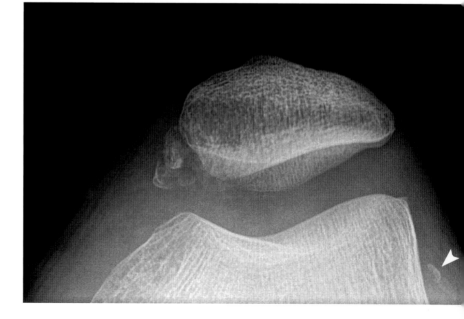

▶ **Fig. 6.62** A comminuted avulsion fracture has occurred at the medial border of the patella secondary to patella dislocation. A small fragment has become a loose body within the joint space and lies lateral to the lateral femoral condyle (arrowhead).

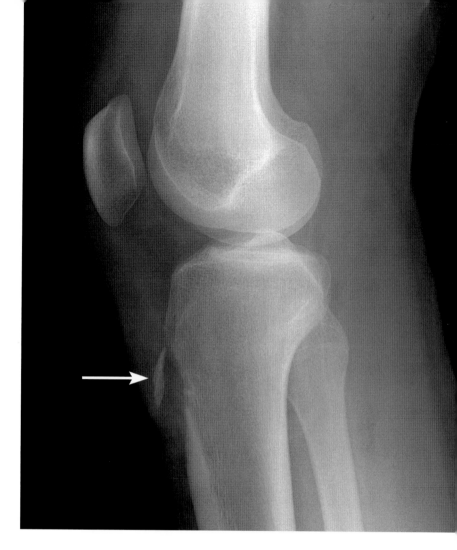

▶ **Fig. 6.63(a)** A Type I injury of the tibial tuberosity involves the tip of the apophysis of the tibial tuberosity with moderate displacement (arrow). There is considerable associated soft-tissue swelling.

▼ **(b)** An old, ununited Type I avulsion fracture is present. Diffuse swelling of the patellar tendon indicates patellar tendinopathy and soft-tissue swelling is also present over the tuberosity.

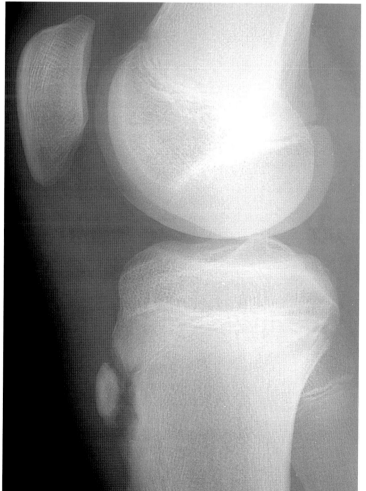

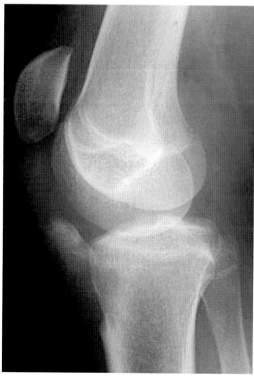

▲ **Fig. 6.64** A Type II avulsion fracture separates the apophysis at the level of the epiphyseal growth plate. There is anterior hinging of the apophysis and patella alta results. The knee joint is not involved.

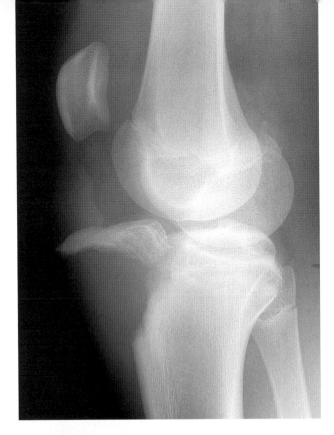

◀ **Fig. 6.65(a)** A Type III tibial tuberosity avulsion fracture extends through the epiphysis into the knee joint with anterior hinging of the apophysis.

▼ **(b)** A Type II tibial tuberosity avulsion fracture has been imaged by MRI. Sagittal PD and fat-suppressed T2-weighted MR images demonstrate a fracture through the base of the apophysis of the tibial tuberosity which involves the anterior epiphysis and extends into the knee joint. Haemorrhage has tracked between the patellar tendon and the infrapatellar fat pad. Patella alta results from anterior hinging of the apophysis. Also note evidence of proximal patellar tendinopathy.

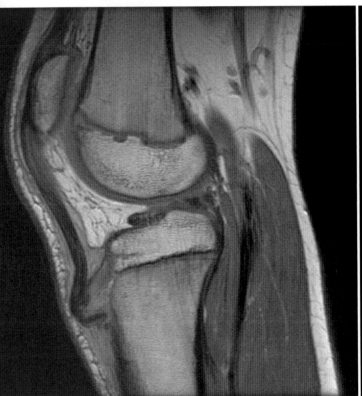
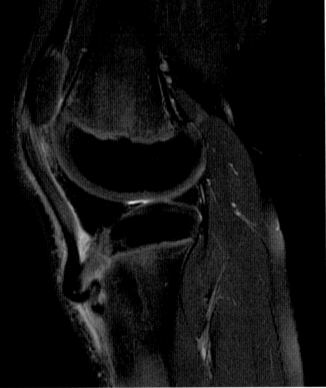

Osteochondral fractures

Osteochondral injuries at the knee most commonly involve:

- the tibial condyles due to compressive and rotational forces
- the lateral femoral condyle associated with an ACL rupture
- the patella during dislocation
- the anterior tibial condyle resulting from an extension injury.

Tibial condyle fractures

Fractures of the tibial plateau result from varus or valgus forces usually in combination with axial loading. There is generally high energy trauma and only 5–10% of tibial plateau fractures occur with a sports-related injury (McClellan et al. 1999). The patient will present with a painful, swollen knee, unable to bear weight.

Valgus stress at the knee may produce a compression fracture of the lateral tibial plateau (see Fig. 6.66). Torsion is more likely to cause a shear fracture of a femoral condyle (see Fig. 6.67). A plain film series is obtained initially and a tibial plateau view (see the section 'Additional views' on page 395) may be helpful for assessing fracture depression. A nuclear bone scan may be helpful when plain films are normal but strong clinical suspicion persists (see Figs 6.68 and 6.69). A CT scan with reformatted images in axial, coronal and sagittal planes, or MRI, is helpful for assessing the degree of depression of the articular surface fragment (see Fig. 6.70).

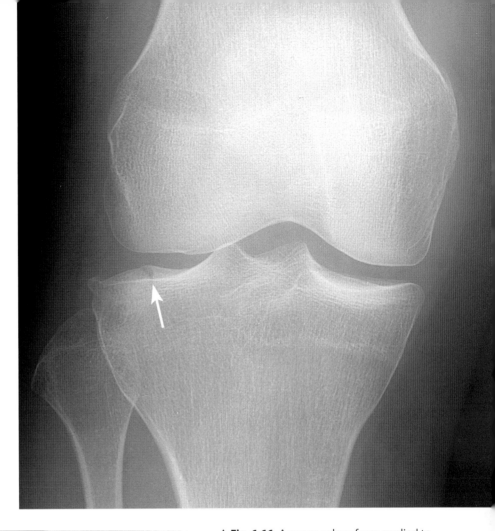

▲ **Fig. 6.66** A severe valgus force applied to the knee has caused compression laterally, resulting in an osteochondral fracture of the lateral tibial condyle (arrow).

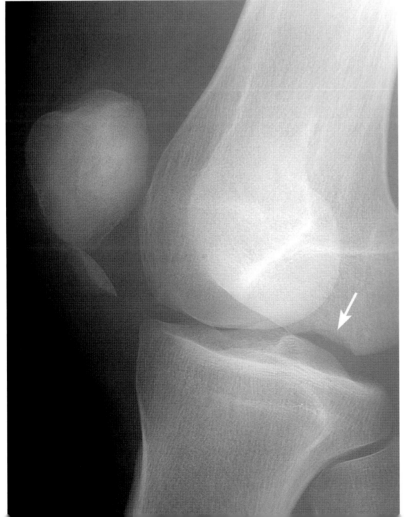

◀ **Fig. 6.67** A shearing force has produced an osteochondral fracture of the articular surface of the lateral femoral condyle (arrow). There has been considerable displacement of the fragment, which now lies in the anterior recess of the knee joint.

▶ **Fig. 6.68** A nuclear bone scan shows an osteochondral fracture of the left lateral tibial condyle. Isotope uptake extends into the subchondral bone.

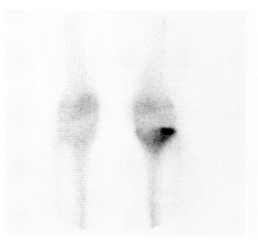
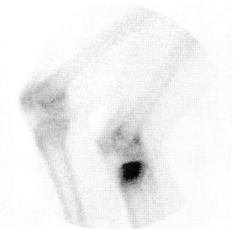

▶ **Fig. 6.69** A nuclear bone scan demonstrates a small osteochondral fracture of the right lateral tibial plateau. The localised horizontal uptake is separate from the growth plate activity.

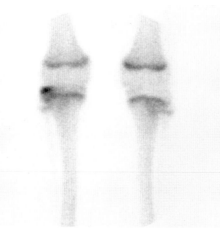
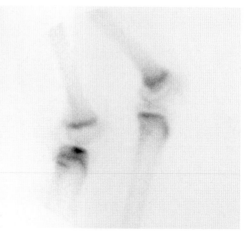

▼ **Fig. 6.70(a)** It is difficult to see any evidence of an osteochondral fracture on plain films. In the lateral view there appears to be minor cortical irregularity of the medial tibial condyle (arrow). This warranted additional imaging.

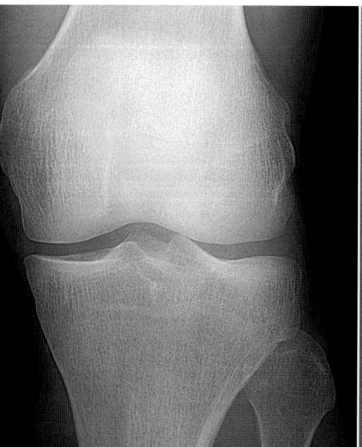
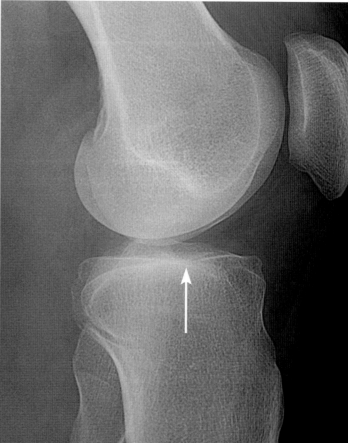

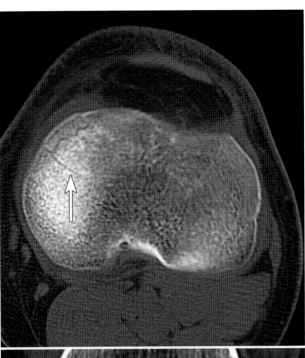

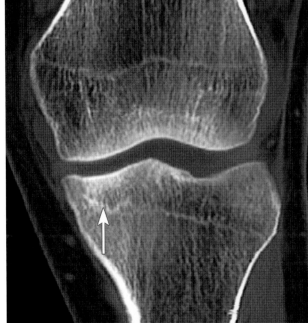

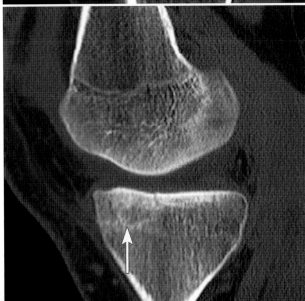

◀**Fig. 6.70(b)** Axial, coronal and sagittal reformatted CT images confirm the presence of a subtle osteochondral fracture of the medial tibial condyle (arrows).

▼ **(c)** The fracture of the anterior aspect of the medial tibial condyle is easily seen by MRI (arrows). The margins of the fracture are well demonstrated on **(i)** a sagittal PD-weighted image, **(ii)** a sagittal fat-suppressed T2-weighted image and **(iii)** an axial fat-suppressed image. Considerable associated bone bruising has occurred (asterisk) and there is a large effusion.

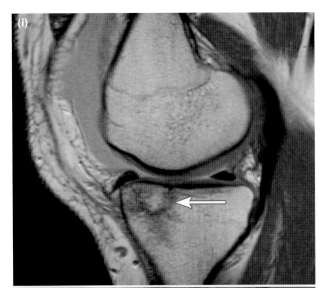

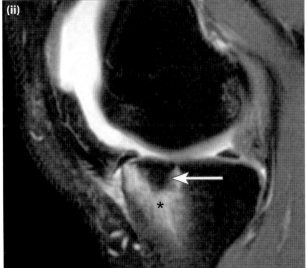

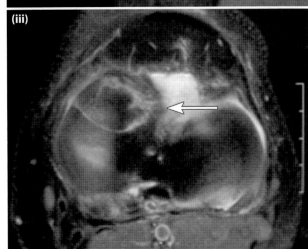

Other soft-tissue injuries may occur with a tibial plateau fracture and, for this reason, MRI plays a valuable role in the pre-operative assessment. Kode et al. (1994) compared the efficacy of MRI and CT in 22 cases of tibial plateau fractures. MRI demonstrated 12 complete ligamentous tears and 15 partial ligamentous tears in 68% of the 22 patients. There were meniscal injuries in 55% of patients and in only three cases was CT superior to MRI in demonstrating the fracture (see Fig. 6.71).

Osteochondral fractures of the femoral condyles

An osteochondral fracture of the articular surface of the femoral condyles may be demonstrated on plain films as a subtle area of subchondral demineralisation (see Fig. 6.72). MRI is necessary to assess overlying chondral damage (see Fig. 6.73). Often a fracture of the subchondral bone is present and the overlying cartilage appears normal (see Fig. 6.74).

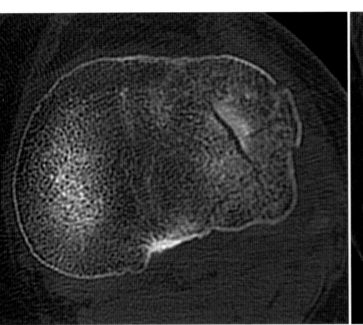
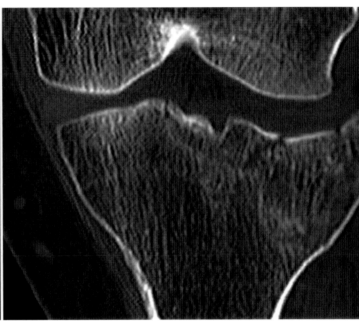

▲ **Fig. 6.71** Tibial condyle fractures are demonstrated in two separate cases.
(a) Axial and reformatted coronal CT images demonstrate a comminuted and depressed fracture of the lateral tibial condyle. The fracture extends below the intercondylar eminence. This imaging method allows an accurate pre-operative assessment of the orientation of the fragments and the degree of depression.
▼ **(b)** Sagittal and coronal T1-weighted MR images demonstrate a fracture of the medial tibial condyle. There is slight separation of the fragments, without depression of the tibial plateau. Note the lipohaemarthrosis.

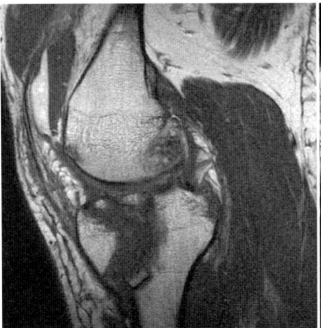
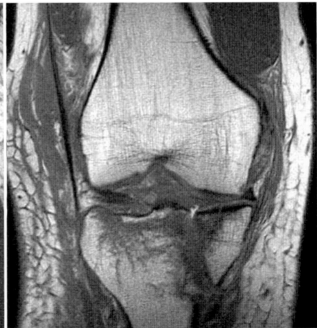

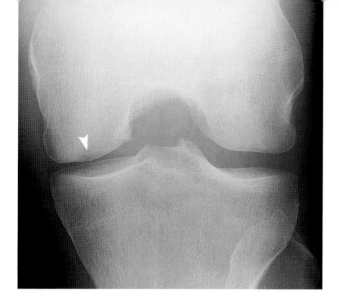

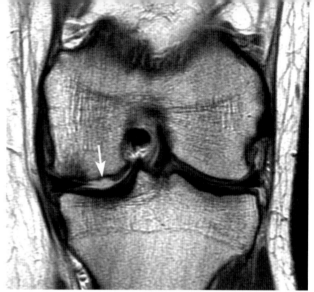

▲ **Fig. 6.72** Plain film changes of an osteochondral fracture may be subtle. In this case an osteochondral fracture of the medial femoral condyle has caused demineralisation of the subchondral bone at the fracture site (arrowhead). An MRI would be necessary to help assess the state of the overlying articular cartilage.

▲ **Fig. 6.73** There has been an osteochondral fracture of the medial femoral condyle. A coronal PD-weighted image shows abnormal signal in the subchondral bone of the medial weightbearing half of medial femoral condyle. There is also subtle flattening of the central articular cortical contour, and overlying chondral deficiency (arrow).

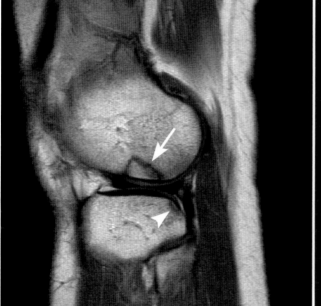

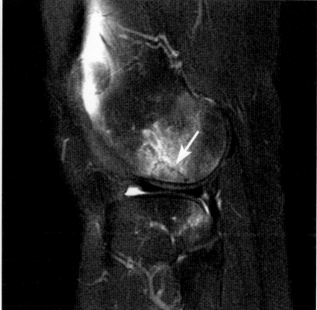

▲ **Fig. 6.74** Sagittal PD and STIR images demonstrate an undisplaced subchondral fracture of the lateral aspect of the lateral femoral condyle (arrows). This was associated with an ACL rupture. A low signal intensity fracture line is demonstrated in the subchondral bone on both sequences. The STIR image demonstrates bone marrow oedema in both the lateral femoral condyle and at the posterior aspect of the lateral tibial condyle. This oedema pattern is typical of the 'translational' mechanism of bone injury that is often associated with ACL rupture. The overlying femoral articular cartilage appears normal and no depression has occurred so the classical 'lateral notch sign' is not present. Also note the hypointense line within the zone of marrow oedema and deep to the articular cortex at the posterior aspect of the lateral tibial condyle (arrowhead). This represents a minimal degree of trabecular impaction fracturing.

A classic osteochondral fracture of the lateral femoral condyle may occur at the time of ACL rupture due to the valgus and rotatory forces causing impaction of the condyle on the apposing posterolateral tibial plateau (Kaplan et al. 1992) and is often accompanied by considerable bone bruising (see Fig. 6.75). This may produce a 'lateral notch sign', which is a depression in the region of the terminal sulcus of the lateral femoral condyle greater than 2 mm in depth. An acute osteochondral fracture may be diagnosed when there is cortical depression of more than 2 mm deep and can be differentiated from the terminal sulcus by its position. An extension of Blumensaat's line will cross the lateral femoral condyle 10 mm anterior to a normal terminal sulcus. If the depression is 20 mm or more posterior to Blumensaat's line, it is pathological (Garth et al. 2000).

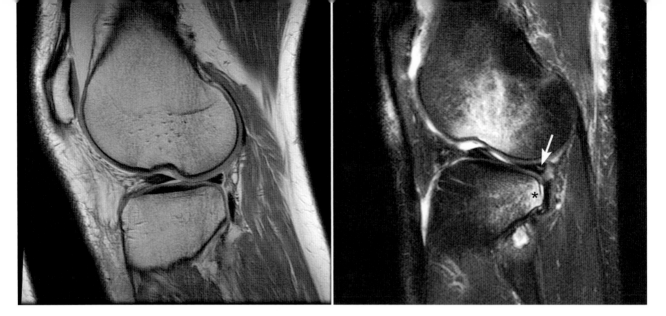

▲ **Fig. 6.75** Following an ACL rupture, sagittal PD and fat-suppressed T2-weighted images in two different patients demonstrate a prominent 'lateral notch sign', which is a depressed osteochondral fracture in the region of the terminal sulcus. Considerable associated marrow oedema is demonstrated on the T2-weighted image. Bone bruising is also demonstrated in the proximal tibial condyle posteriorly (asterisk). There is an accompanying tear of the posterior horn of the lateral meniscus (arrow).

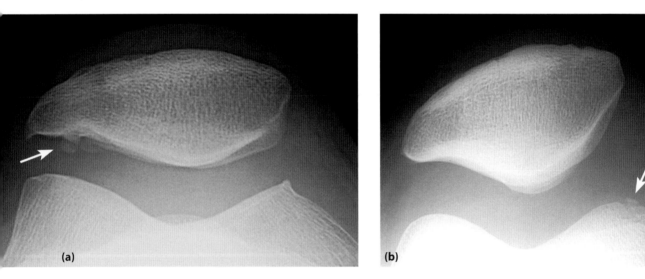

(a)

(b)

▲▼ **Fig. 6.76(a)** Following dislocation of the patella, a patellofemoral view shows an osteochondral fracture of the articular surface of the lateral articular facet of the patella (arrow). **(b)** A patellofemoral osteochondral fracture may also occur due to direct trauma to the patella. A fracture is seen on the anterior aspect of the medial femoral condyle secondary to force transmitted through the patella (arrow). **(c)** Patella dislocation may be complicated by an osteochondral fracture of the median ridge of the patella (arrow). **(d)** The osteochondral fragment separated from the patella in (c) has become displaced and lies above the tibial spines, mimicking an ACL avulsion (arrow).

(d)

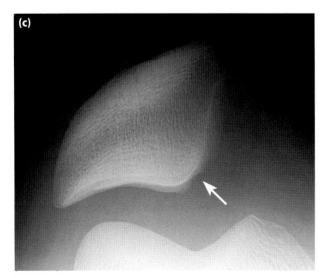

(c)

Osteochondral fractures of the patella

An osteochondral fracture of the lateral articular facet of the patella may occur during lateral dislocation of the patella. This is caused by the patella impacting against the anterior aspect of the lateral femoral condyle. An osteochondral fracture of the femoral condyle may also be produced (O'Donoghue 1984). These fractures may occasionally be seen on the axial view of the patella (see Fig. 6.76). However, often the plain films are negative and MRI is useful for demonstrating bone bruising or an undisplaced fracture (see Fig. 6.77).

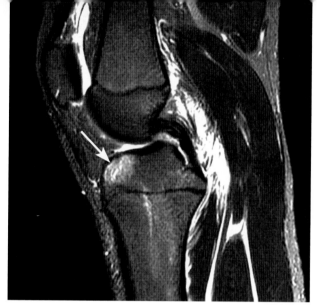

▲ **Fig. 6.78** There has been a violent hyperextension injury of the knee causing the anterior aspect of the tibial condyles to impact against the femoral condyles. A bone bruise has occurred at the point of tibial impaction (arrow). There has also been a rupture of the posterior capsule of the knee joint and injury to the musculotendinous junction of the popliteus, with extensive posterior pericapsular oedema noted.

Osteochondral fractures of the tibial condyle following hyperextension

With violent hyperextension of the knee, the femoral condyles may impact against the anterior aspect of the tibial condyle, producing an area of bone bruising or possibly an osteochondral fracture (see Fig. 6.78). A hyperextension injury may cause multiple injuries including an ACL rupture or a PCL rupture (or both), with its associated osteochondral injuries.

Bone bruising

The term 'bone bruising' represents a spectrum of bone injuries including bleeding, infarction and oedema due to microscopic compression fractures of cancellous bone. Bone bruising may occur as an isolated injury producing clinical symptoms (see Fig. 6.79), or associated with other injuries

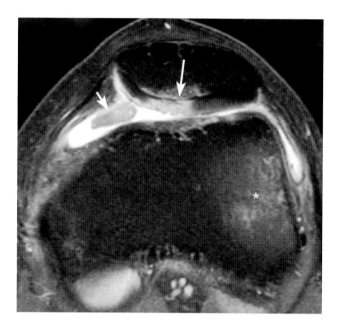

▲ **Fig. 6.77** A recent episode of lateral dislocation of the patella has resulted in impaction of the patella against the lateral femoral condyle, producing an osteochondral fracture at the median eminence of the patella (long arrow). An axial fat-suppressed T2-weighted MR image demonstrates separation and displacement of a large cartilaginous fragment into the medial suprapatellar recess (short arrow). There is subchondral marrow oedema at the patellar fracture site and bone bruising is noted at the lateral aspect of the lateral femoral condyle (asterisk).

◄ **Fig. 6.79** A female surfer was hit by a surfboard on the anteromedial aspect of the proximal tibia. Plain films were normal and persisting symptoms led to an MRI examination. Coronal T1-weighted and STIR images demonstrate extensive bone bruising of the medial tibial condyle.

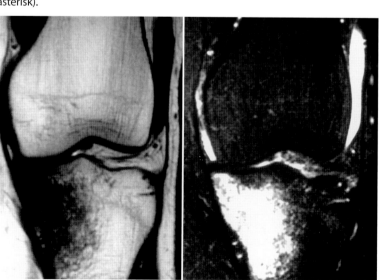

such as an ACL rupture or patellar dislocation, as shown in Figs 6.74–6.78. It is thought that bone bruising may be the main source of pain associated with ACL ruptures.

Plain films and arthroscopy are negative. A nuclear bone scan shows an increased uptake of isotope in the area of the bruise, but cannot grade the contusion or demonstrate other associated injuries. MRI not only reveals the full extent of bone and soft-tissue injury, but can also differentiate diffuse reticular bone contusion (see Fig. 6.80) from focal geographic bone contusion (see Fig. 6.81) and a true osteo-chondral fracture (Lynch et al. 1989). This distinction may have important management and rehabilitation implica-tions for the injured athlete, because inadequate rest of a focal geographic contusion may result in an alteration of the load-bearing properties of subchondral bone, which in turn produces changes in the overlying cartilage (Vellet et al. 1991). There is, however, controversial evidence regarding the prognostic significance of the different types of bone bruising. The reported time for resolution is also quite vari-able, ranging from as early as three weeks up to as much as two years (Mandalia et al. 2005).

Stress fractures of the knee

The most common stress fracture of the knee involves the medial tibial condyle. Initial pain films are usually normal but a nuclear bone scan may demonstrate the presence of bone stress and later plain films will show linear sclerosis, typical of a medial tibial condyle fracture (see Fig. 6.82). Stress fractures

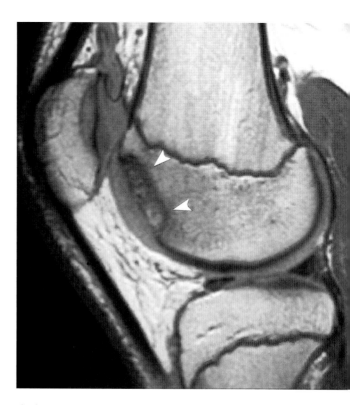

▲ **Fig. 6.81** A sagittal T1-weighted MR image obtained two to three months after direct trauma shows an abnormal area of subchondral bone at the femoral trochlear which has developed a sclerotic margin (arrowheads). Diffuse low signal continues past the margin into the anterior half of the distal femoral epiphysis. This is an example of geographic bone bruising where a sclerotic margin suggests an ischaemic process. Note that the overlying cartilage appears normal and this was confirmed at arthroscopy.

may also affect the patella (see Figs 6.83 and 6.84), second-ary to repetitive stress applied to the extensor mechanism. An unusual stress fracture of the inferior pole of the patella is occasionally seen in the immature athlete, where a stress fracture is associated with an incompletely fused secondary ossification centre (see Fig. 6.85). Also in the immature athlete, stress reactions may involve the growth plates of the distal femur and the proximal tibia. These are not uncommon. There is irregular bone resorption at the margins of the growth plate (see Fig. 6.86). Supracondylar stress fractures of the femur have been discussed in Chapter 5.

Stress fractures of apophyses: traction apophysitis

Osgood–Schlatter disease (OSD) is the better known of the two types of traction apophysitis and occurs at the distal end of the patellar tendon at its attachment to the tibial tuberosity apophysis. Traction apophysitis may also involve the apophysis at the inferior pole of the patella at the patellar tendon attach-ment. This condition is known as Sinding–Larsen–Johannsen (SLJ) disease and occurs most commonly in boys between the ages of 10 and 12.

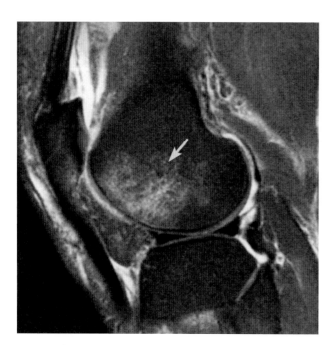

▲ **Fig. 6.80** A sagittal fat-suppressed T2-weighted image demonstrates a bone bruise on the anterior aspect of the lateral femoral condyle from direct trauma (arrow). Also note the high signal and swelling of soft tissues anterior to the patellar tendon and bone bruising at the lower pole of the patella.

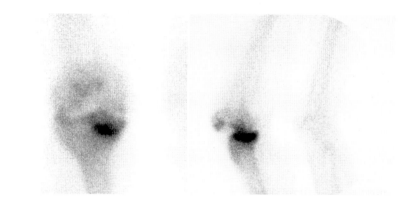

▶ **Fig. 6.82(a)** A nuclear bone scan shows intense isotope uptake in the subchondral bone of the medial tibial condyle. A stress fracture was suspected clinically and the bone scan appearances were consistent with this diagnosis.

▶ **(b)** The diagnosis was confirmed on a progress plain film, which showed linear sclerosis in the medial tibial condyle (arrow). This appearance is typical of a stress fracture of the tibial condyle.

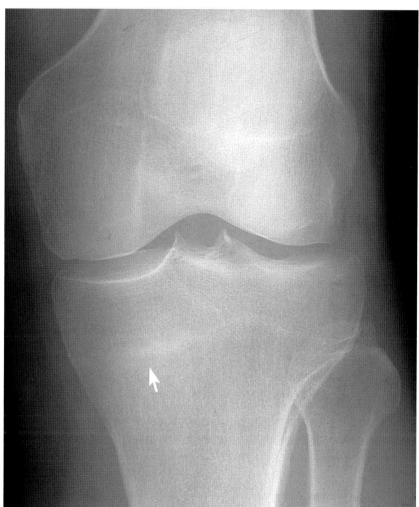

▼ **Fig. 6.83** A 100-metre sprinter at the Sydney 2000 Olympics presented with anterior knee pain. Sagittal PD and fat-suppressed T2-weighted MR images demonstrate a stress fracture involving the inferior pole of the patella (arrows). This athlete had been treated for patellar tendinopathy for a considerable time.

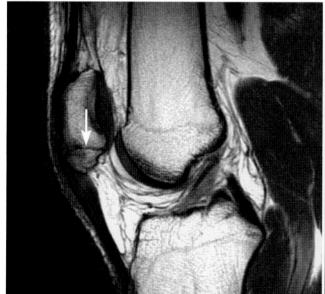
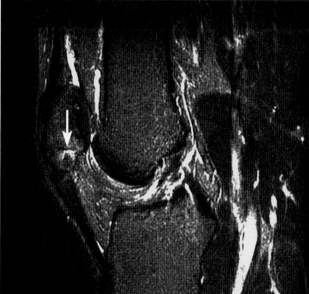

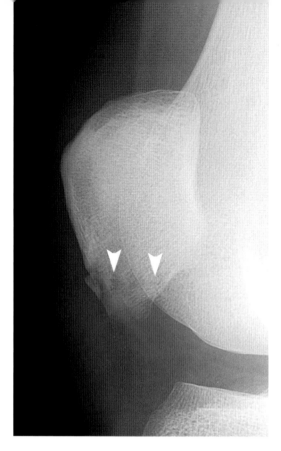

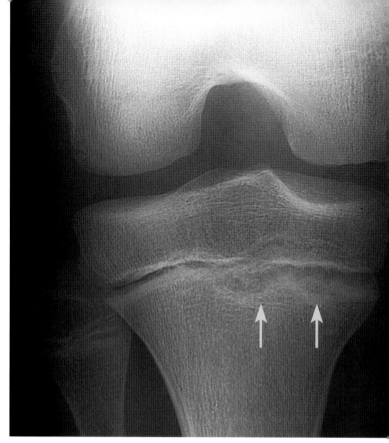

▲ **Fig. 6.84** A stress fracture of the patella is shown by plain film (arrowheads). Although this is a different athlete, the stress fracture involves a similar area of the patella to that seen in Fig. 6.85.

▲ **Fig. 6.86** A stress fracture involves the proximal tibial growth plate. There is irregular widening of the growth plate with marginal sclerosis present on the metaphyseal side of the plate (arrows).

▼ **Fig. 6.85** Two similar cases of stress fractures of the inferior pole of the patella in immature athletes are demonstrated by plain films. In both cases, there is incomplete fusion of the secondary ossification centre for the lower pole of the patella, resulting in a bony defect anteriorly. This has presumably placed additional stress on the fused area, creating bone stress and a stress fracture. Increased uptake of isotope was seen on delayed bone scan images and eventually plain film changes occurred (arrows). In the authors' experience, this fracture is unusual but not rare.

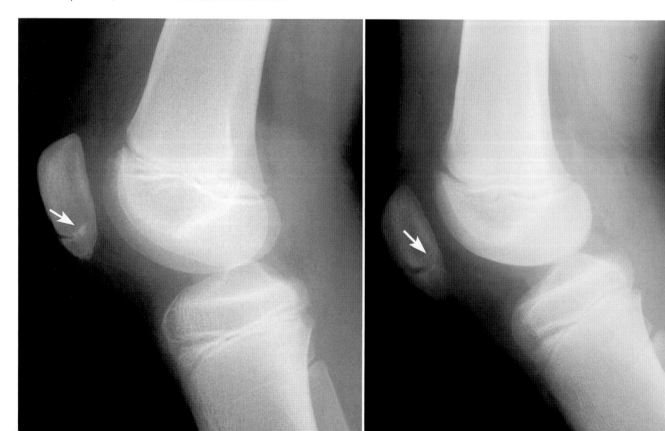

Osgood–Schlatter disease

Osgood–Schlatter disease is a common stress injury of the tibial tuberosity usually occurring in active adolescents between the ages of 11 and 15 (see Fig. 6.87). The incidence of OSD is higher in sports involving jumping, squatting and kicking. This condition presents as pain and swelling over the tibial tuberosity which may extend into the patellar tendon. The symptoms are generally severe enough to interfere with effective training (Kujala et al. 1985). OSD is more common in boys, is often bilateral and almost always follows a growth spurt.

Plain films may show fragmentation of the apophysis of the tibial tuberosity with overlying soft-tissue swelling. Ultrasound demonstrates similar changes (see Fig. 6.88). A comparative view of the opposite side should be included, as the changes are often bilateral, if not symmetrical (see Fig. 6.89). Soft-tissue swelling is the key diagnostic feature, as a normal apophysis may develop from multiple centres and mimic the fragmentation of OSD. Other plain film signs include loss of the sharp angle at the inferior extent of the infrapatellar fat pad, swelling of the distal end of the patellar tendon and soft-tissue changes of infrapatellar bursopathy. Ossification within the patellar tendon is not seen in OSD (Ogden and Southwick 1976). Such ossification results from minor bony avulsion and callus formation. However, anterior bony spurring at the proximal tibia may be seen in adult life secondary to OSD in adolescence, and this can be a cause for deep infrapatellar bursitis or distal patellar tendinopathy (see Fig. 6.90).

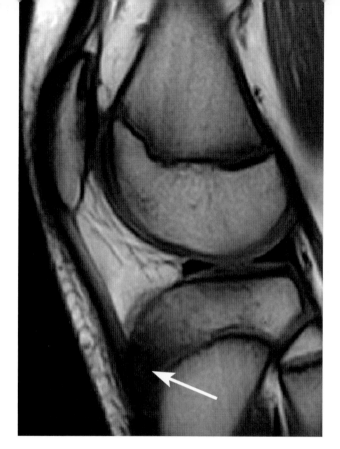

▲ **Fig. 6.87** A sagittal T1-weighted MR image of the patellar tendon shows abnormal marrow signal in the apophysis of the tibial tuberosity in the region of the tendon attachment (arrow). This abnormal marrow signal would almost certainly indicate that abnormal repetitive stress is occurring at the patellar attachment.

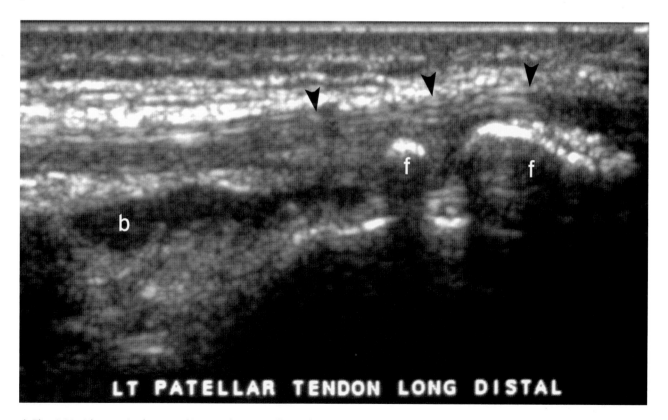

▲ **Fig. 6.88** A long-axis ultrasound image shows swelling of the distal patellar tendon (arrowheads), fragmentation of the tibial tuberosity apophysis (f) and deep infrapatellar bursal effusion/synovitis (b). The appearances are typical of Osgood–Schlatter disease.

▶ **Fig. 6.89(a)** Changes of Osgood–Schlatter disease are present. There is irregularity and demineralisation of the apophysis of the tibial tuberosity on the right side and considerable associated soft-tissue swelling (arrowhead). Swelling of the lower end of the patellar tendon on the right is also noted. A view of both sides is advisable even if only one side is requested. The process is often bilateral and comparison of the shape of both apophyses assists in confirming subtle changes. Soft-tissue swelling can also be compared.

▼ **(b)** Typical changes of Osgood–Schlatter disease are present in an adolescent athlete. There is fragmentation and irregularity of the apophysis of the tibial tuberosity with overlying soft-tissue swelling (arrow). There is also loss of the normal fat density between the patellar tendon and the tibial condyle, suggesting associated deep infrapatellar bursopathy (asterisk). Mild swelling of the distal patellar tendon is also noted.

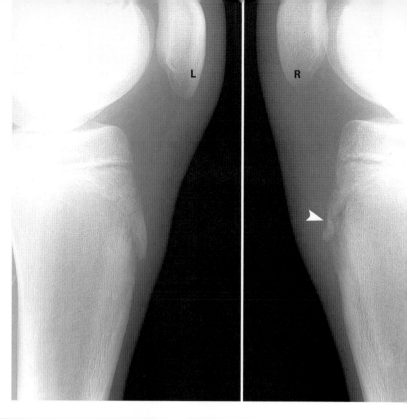

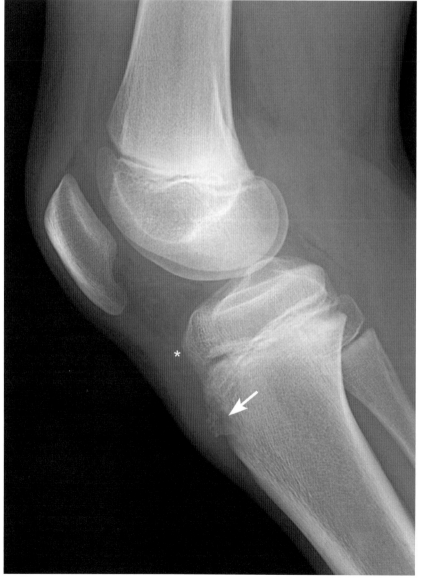

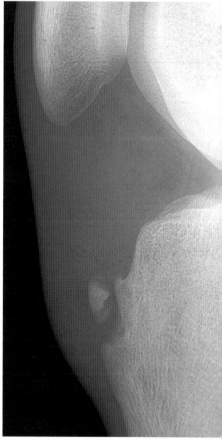

▲ **Fig. 6.90** Spur formation and an ossicle in a mature athlete have resulted from old OSD. There is considerable soft-tissue swelling secondary to these changes, with clouding of the adjacent infrapatellar fat pad, which appears to be due to a combination of infrapatellar bursitis and patellar tendinopathy.

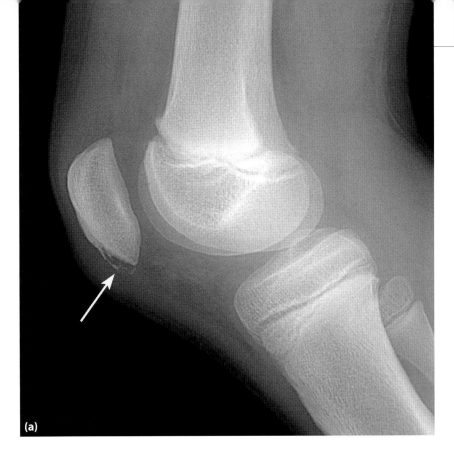

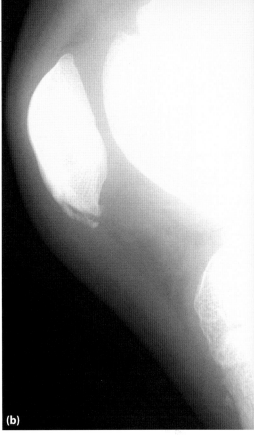

(a)

(b)

▲ **Fig. 6.91(a)** Changes seen on plain films are typical of traction apophysitis at the distal pole of the patella (SLJ disease). There is fragmentation of the secondary ossification centre at the inferior pole of the patella, with overlying soft-tissue swelling (arrow). **(b)** In a more immature athlete, the changes are subtle. The fragmentation is less obvious and the important diagnostic sign is the prominent soft-tissue swelling.

Sinding–Larsen–Johannsen disease

Repetitive micro-trauma at the inferior pole of the developing patella may produce a traction apophysitis stress injury that is the functional equivalent of Osgood–Schlatter disease. Plain films show fragmentation at the inferior pole of the patella and soft-tissue swelling in the adjacent patellar tendon (see Figs 6.91 and 6.92). As with OSD, care must be taken not to confuse secondary ossification centres with fragmentation, and in practice the radiographic diagnosis depends upon the presence of soft-tissue swelling.

Isolated ligament injuries
The medial collateral ligament

The MCL stabilises the knee joint medially, providing the primary restraint against valgus stress (see Fig. 6.93). The ligament has a superficial layer divided into posterior fibres, forming the posterior oblique ligament, and anterior fibres, which are taut with knee flexion. The deep layer is divided into the meniscofemoral and meniscotibial ligaments, which anchor the MCL to the medial meniscus (see Fig. 6.94). There is a bursa between the superficial and deep layers of the MCL (see Fig. 6.95). The MCL attaches proximally to the medial femoral condyle posteromedially and distally on the proximal tibial metaphysis just distal to the pes anserine tendons.

Forceful valgus stress may rupture the MCL (see Fig. 6.96). Injury commonly occurs at its femoral attachment where a small avulsion is occasionally seen.

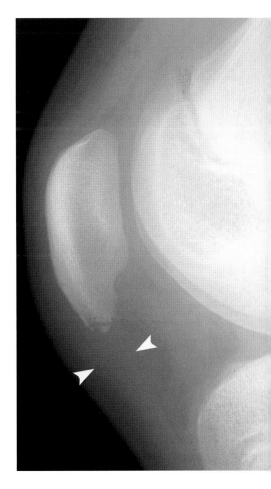

▶ **Fig. 6.92** There is fragmentation of the tip of the inferior pole of the patella with considerable swelling of the proximal patellar tendon (arrowheads). This may well be due to SLJ disease, although the appearance could also be consistent with a small avulsion fracture.

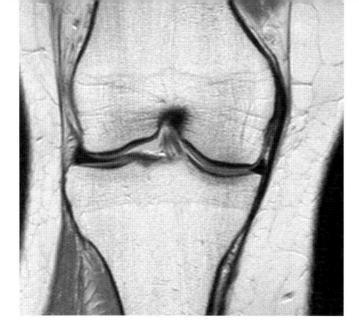

▲ **Fig. 6.93** A coronal PD-weighted MR image shows the normal appearance of an MCL. The ligament is slightly thicker proximally. Note that the most distal point of the MCL attachment to the medial surface of the proximal shaft of the tibia is excluded from the field of view used for most routine MRI examinations of the knee.

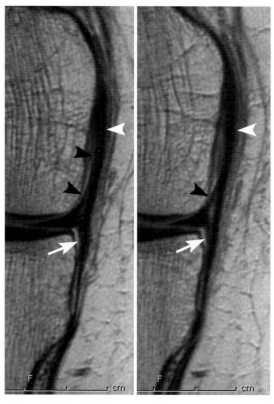

▲ **Fig. 6.94** The MCL has superficial and deep layers and these layers can be appreciated on these coronal PD-weighted MR image (arrowhead). Meniscofemoral and meniscotibial ligaments are also clearly demonstrated (arrows).

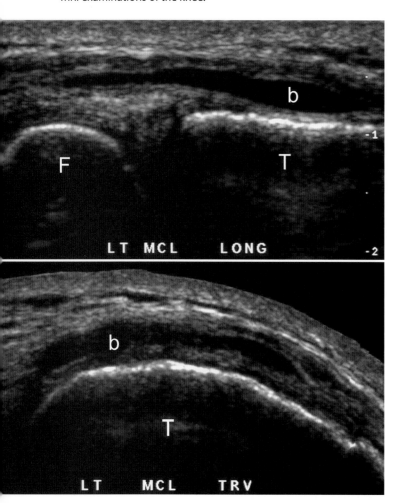

◄ **Fig. 6.95** Long-axis and transverse ultrasound images obtained at the medial margin of the medial compartment show the superficial and deep layers of the MCL separated by fluid within the MCL bursa (b). Femur = F. Tibia = T.

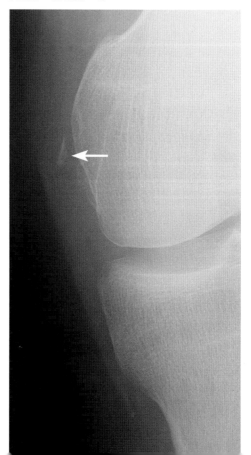

▶ **Fig. 6.96** Femoral MCL avulsion fractures are uncommon. In this case, a small fragment has been avulsed by the proximal MCL attachment (arrow).

A mid-substance tear will usually create a palpable defect in the ligament. Injury may also occur at its distal end, in which case tenderness will be maximal about 6–8 cm from the joint line in the region of the pes anserinus bursa. Plain films can show diagnostic changes, including:

- a femoral avulsion fracture (see Fig. 6.97)
- soft-tissue swelling along the line of the MCL in the acute stage, which is usually most marked at its proximal end
- abnormal opening of the knee joint space medially appreciated on a valgus stress view, confirming the diagnosis of MCL rupture (see Fig. 6.98)
- Pellegrini–Steida ossification occurring in the later stage of healing (see Figs 6.99 and 6.100).

As a consequence of the MCL being extra-capsular, a joint effusion will not occur with MCL rupture alone, although there may be a concurrent intracapsular injury. In 'O'Donoghue's unhappy triad' the ACL, MCL and medial meniscus may all tear in sequence with a valgus stress (Norwood and Cross 1977). Occurring more commonly is the combination of ACL, MCL and lateral meniscal tears (Shelbourne and Nitz 1991; Barber 1992).

▼ Fig. 6.97 Deep fibres of the MCL have avulsed a fragment from the medial margin of the medial femoral condyle (arrow).

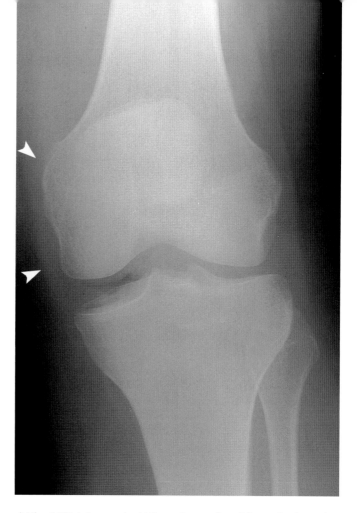

▲ Fig. 6.98 Injury to the MCL can be predicted from a high-quality plain film showing a characteristic soft-tissue swelling along the path of the MCL (arrowheads). In this case, because of the swelling and a clinical suspicion of MCL injury, an AP film was obtained with a valgus force applied to the knee. MCL rupture was confirmed by demonstrating abnormal medial joint space opening.

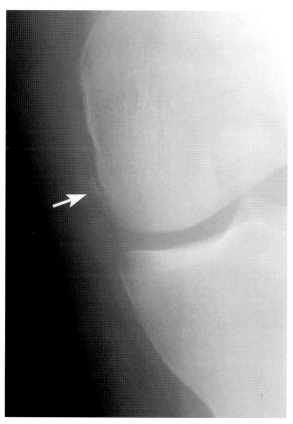

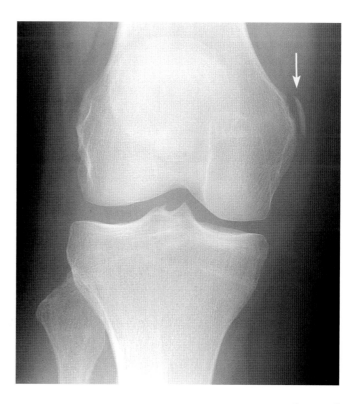

▶ Fig. 6.99 Curvilinear ossification seen at the proximal attachment of the MCL indicates a previous MCL rupture. This is known as Pellegrini–Steida ossification and has a characteristic appearance.

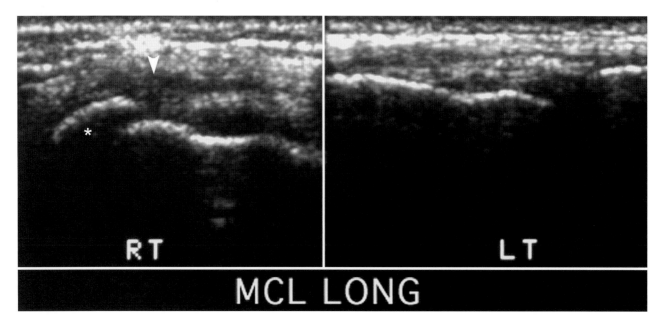

▲ **Fig. 6.100** A long-axis ultrasound image of the femoral attachment of the right MCL shows both hypoechoic ligament swelling (arrowhead) and Pellegrini–Steida ossification (asterisk) in comparison with the normal left side. The appearances are those of an acute-on-chronic injury.

MRI or ultrasound can confirm a tear and determine the grade. MRI is valuable for the assessment of associated bone injury (see Fig. 6.101). Tears are graded I–III both clinically and by MRI. The higher the number, the more severe the injury:

- A *Grade I tear* on MRI appears as periligamentous oedema with intact fibre bundles of normal thickness.
- A *Grade II tear* is present when there is partial disruption of the MCL with periligamentous oedema (see Fig. 6.102).
- A *Grade III tear* is complete disruption of the MCL (see Fig. 6.103).

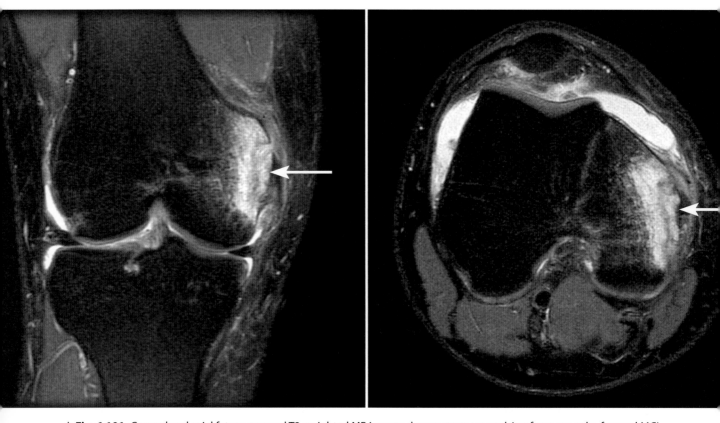

▲ **Fig. 6.101** Coronal and axial fat-suppressed T2-weighted MR images demonstrate an avulsion fracture at the femoral MCL attachment, as the result of a violent traction (arrows). There is separation of a large fragment, and considerable associated bone marrow oedema and a secondary haemarthrosis are noted.

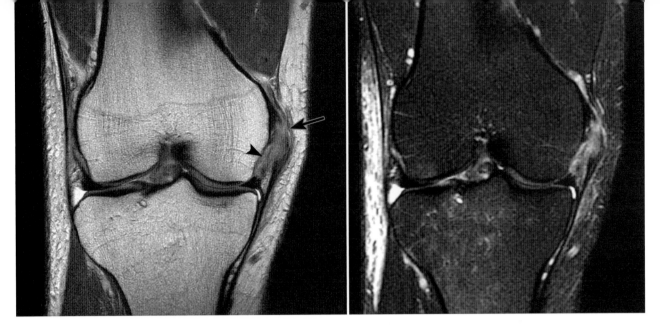

▲ **Fig. 6.102** A high-grade partial tear of the proximal MCL is demonstrated on coronal PD and fat-suppressed T2-weighted MR images. Note that features of fibre discontinuity and increased signal involve both the superficial (arrow) and deep (arrowhead) components of the MCL. There is associated marked ligament swelling but no distal retraction or buckling is present to suggest a Grade III injury. The meniscotibial ligament appears normal.

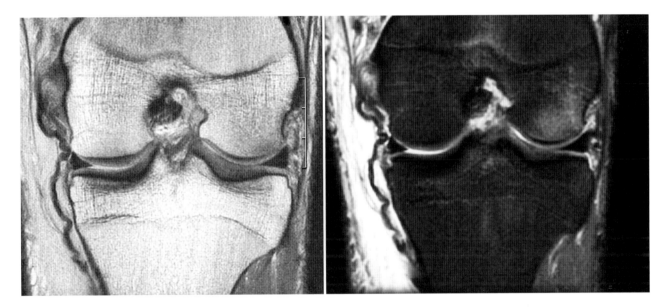

▲ **Fig. 6.103** A violent valgus force to the knee has produced a complete rupture of the MCL due to traction forces on the medial side. A bone bruise at the lateral femoral condyle has resulted from compressive forces on the lateral side. Coronal PD and fat-suppressed T2-weighted images show injury to both the proximal and distal ends of the MCL, with buckling of the ligament indicative of a Grade III tear. There is injury to the deep meniscofemoral and meniscotibial components of the MCL, showing thickening and intermediate signal. Also note the absence of the ACL at the lateral aspect of the intercondylar notch, indicating an accompanying ACL tear.

The anterior cruciate ligament

The ACL is a vital stabiliser of the knee, being the main restraint against anterior translation of the tibia on the femur (see Fig. 6.104). The ACL also acts as a secondary stabiliser against varus–valgus forces and internal and external rotation (Swenson and Harner 1995). Some fibres of the ACL remain taut throughout all movements of the knee (Girgis et al. 1975).

The traditional cause of ACL rupture involves the pivot–shift mechanism of injury with a twisting injury occurring with rapid deceleration and a directional change. The flexed knee undergoes a valgus stress with external rotation of the femur on the tibia. As well as ACL rupture, there may be meniscal injury, collateral ligament injury and lateral patella subluxation. There are other mechanisms of ACL injury, such as hyperextension (Stoller 1997) and a combination of hyperextension and varus stress. Physical examination is extremely accurate at diagnosing an ACL rupture. A skilled clinician can diagnose up to 90% of ACL tears by history and physical examination alone (Lee et al. 1988).

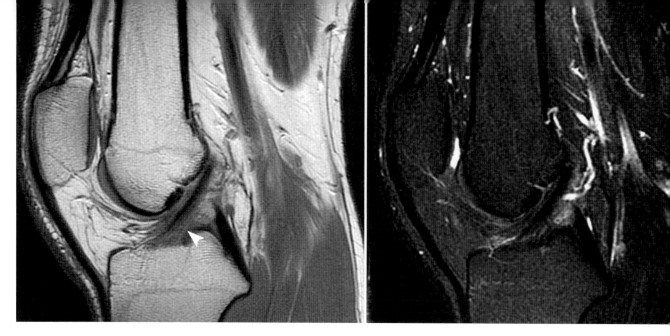

▲ **Fig. 6.104** This is the normal MRI appearance of the ACL demonstrated on sagittal PD and fat-suppressed PD images. The normal ligament appears as a solid or striated low-to-intermediate signal intensity band oriented at 45° to the plane of the tibial condyle. The fascicles are normally straight, although a minimal degree of sag can sometimes be present, especially with the knee in flexion. The ligament fascicles diverge to a footprint of tibial insertion which is larger than the femoral insertion. This divergence of the distal fascicles with interposed loose areolar tissue makes the normal distal segment of the ACL (arrowhead) appear higher in signal than the proximal end.

Following ACL rupture, imaging may show:

- a joint effusion
- abnormal knee alignment, demonstrated by taking a cross-table lateral view with the patient supine, the tibia supported and the femur unsupported. Anterior movement of the tibia with respect to the femur will develop as the patient relaxes. Alignment change may also be shown by stress or weightbearing views (Rijke et al. 1987; Egund et al. 1993) and is occasionally evident on MRI (see Fig. 6.105).
- associated bony injury. There may be a lateral tibial avulsion (Segond) fracture as shown in Figs 6.57–6.59, avulsion of the intercondylar eminence (see Fig. 6.106), a defect in the lateral femoral condyle (see Fig. 6.107) (Stallenberg et al. 1993; Garth et al. 2000) or a fracture or bone bruising of the lateral femoral condyle and posterior aspect of the lateral tibial plateau (see Fig. 6.108).

MRI provides the best investigative method of making this diagnosis and assessing the full extent of associated injury to other structures such as menisci, articular cartilage and bone. Posterolateral ligament injuries are missed with clinical examination and arthroscopy and these associated changes may be well demonstrated by MRI (Miller et al. 1997).

▼ **Fig. 6.105** ACL deficiency may be inferred from an alteration of femorotibial alignment. Without the restraint of a normal intact ACL, the tibia is able to move anteriorly with respect to the femur. A sagittal PD-weighted MR image demonstrates this abnormal alignment in an athlete with chronic ACL deficiency. In this case a normal ACL cannot be seen, although severely atrophic fascicles can still be identified. These show an abnormal horizontal orientation (arrow).

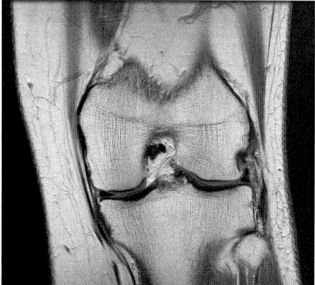
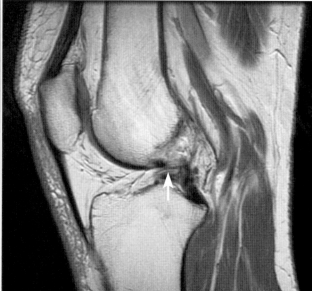

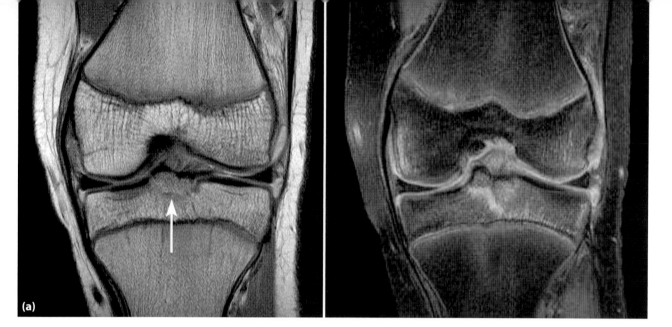

▲ **Fig. 6.106(a)** An undisplaced avulsion fracture of the intercondylar eminence is demonstrated by coronal PD and fat-suppressed T2-weighted MRI (arrow). Note the swelling and hyperintensity at the ACL attachments. Bone bruising is also evident in the femoral and tibial condyles.

▼ **(b)** In another case, using the same MRI sequences in the sagittal plane, a large fragment is shown to be separated from the intercondylar eminence and hinged with elevation of its anterior margin (arrow).

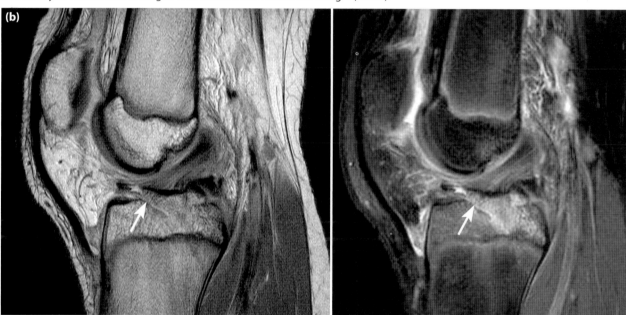

▶ **Fig. 6.107(a)** A 'lateral notch sign' of an ACL rupture is demonstrated on a plain film (arrow). **(b)** A sagittal fat-suppressed T2-weighted MR image demonstrates the pattern of bone bruising that is commonly seen with an ACL rupture. Contusion involves the subchondral bone of the lateral femoral condyle in the region of the terminal sulcus as well as the point of impaction against the posterior aspect of the lateral tibial condyle. In addition, there is often bruising of the inferior pole of the patella, as seen here.

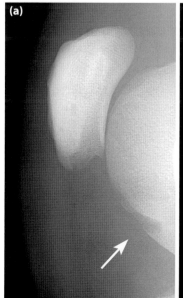

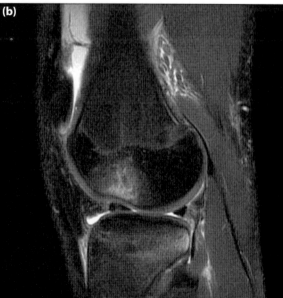

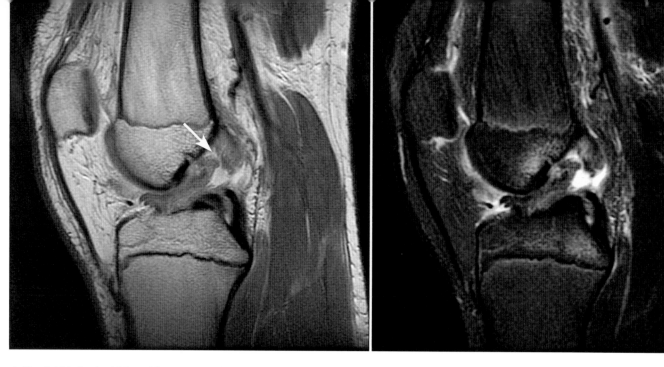

▲ **Fig. 6.108** Sagittal PD and fat-suppressed T2-weighted MR images demonstrate complete rupture of the proximal ACL with retraction of the fibres producing an irregular fluid-filled gap in fibre continuity (arrow). Typical bone marrow oedema is noted.

The primary signs of an ACL tear demonstrated by MRI include tissue disruption and obliteration of the normal fascicles by oedema and haemorrhage (see Fig. 6.109), with increased signal intensity in the substance of the ligament on T2-weighted images (see Fig. 6.110). Interstitial tears will produce increased MR signal with the fascicles appearing grossly intact. In 10–43% of cases ACL tears are partial, being most common in children (Prince 2005). Chronic ACL tears are often associated with osteoarthrosis and meniscal tears. There may be loss of the normal axis and configuration of the ligament (see Fig. 6.111), with abrupt angulation, sagging, wavy appearance or an abnormal ACL axis (see Fig. 6.112). Mellado et al. (2004) noted that an angle of the long axis of the ACL less than 45° relative to a line parallel to the tibial plateau (the ACL angle) is sensitive for an ACL tear.

Secondary signs of ACL injury include pivot shift osteochondral fractures and bone bruising, together with avulsion fractures as previously mentioned.

The posterior cruciate ligament

The primary function of the PCL is to resist posterior displacement of the tibia in relation to the femur (see Fig. 6.113). The ligament has two components: a larger anterior component which is taut in flexion and posterior fibres which tighten in extension. The ligament originates high on the medial femoral condyle in the intercondylar notch and passes posteroinferiorly to attach to the posterior aspect of the tibial condyle. It extends about 1 cm or more below the level of the tibial articular surface on the posterior surface of the condyle.

The mechanism of injury often involves knee hyperextension on a fixed dorsiflexed foot with an anterior force applied to the tibia, as may occur in a rugby tackle. The PCL is also commonly injured when an anteromedial force is applied to the knee and is usually a component of a posterolateral corner injury. The PCL is injured less frequently than the ACL.

An isolated injury to the PCL is an unusual injury. PCL tears are present in only 3% of knee injuries in the general population and 38% of knee injuries in specialised regional trauma centres. Almost 50% of these are associated with another injury (Fanelli et al. 2001).

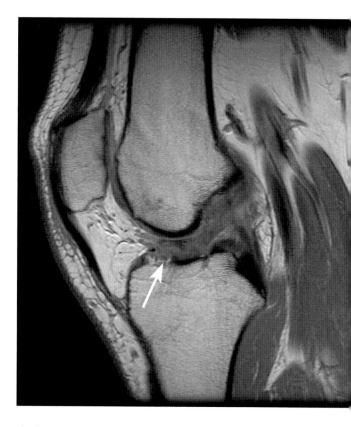

▲ **Fig. 6.109** A sagittal PD-weighted MR image demonstrates a diffuse signal abnormality of oedema and haemorrhage within the ACL. There has been an avulsion fracture at the intercondylar eminence (arrow).

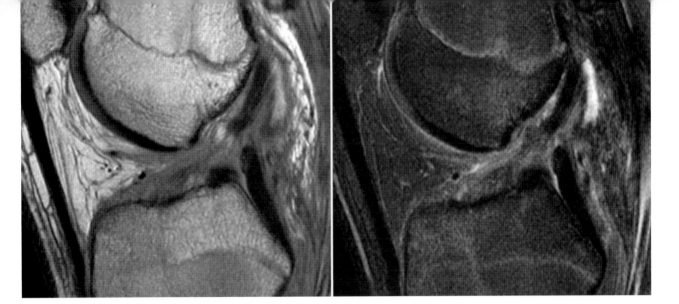

▲ **Fig. 6.110(a)** Sagittal PD and fat-suppressed T2-weighted MR images show a complete mid-segment ACL rupture in a 15-year-old athlete. There is sagging of the middle third of the ligament and increased signal in the distal two-thirds of the ligament, consistent with oedema and haemorrhage.

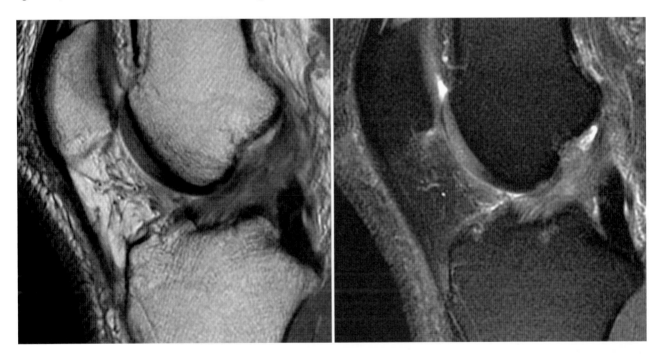

▲ **(b)** In another case of complete ACL rupture, there is a wavy fibre pattern with diffuse ligamentous signal hyperintensity and swelling most pronounced at the mid-segment level.

▶**Fig. 6.111** A sagittal PD-weighted MR image shows an abnormal ACL configuration in a patient with a chronic ACL rupture. The distal stump of the ACL is displaced anteriorly and is folded over with direct abutment against the anterior roof of the intercondylar notch and the proximal tibial surface. Anterior impingement would be anticipated. An absence of both joint effusion and notch haematoma is consistent with the non-acute nature of the ACL tear.

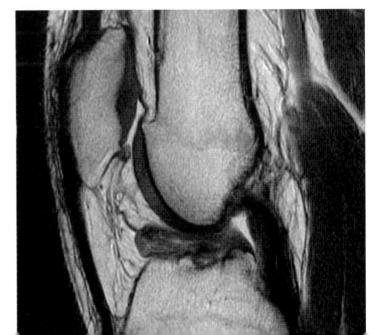

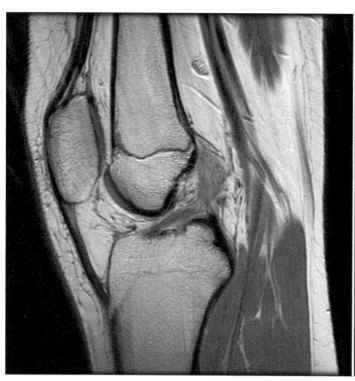
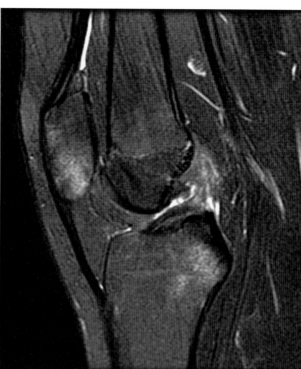

▲ **Fig. 6.112** Sagittal PD and fat-suppressed T2-weighted MR images demonstrate a complete rupture of the proximal ACL. The ligament has detached from the femoral insertion and lies flat along the intercondylar eminence with the long-axis showing an abnormal horizontal orientation. This is an acute lesion with swelling, haemorrhagic signal hyperintensity and loss of fibre visualisation at its femoral attachment. Bone bruising is present at the posterior tibial plateau and the distal pole of the patella.

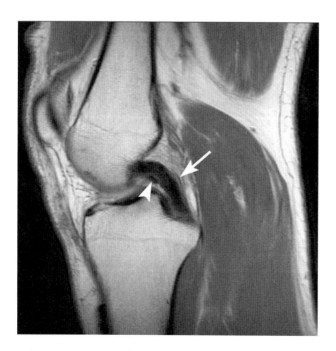

▲ **Fig. 6.113** A sagittal PD-weighted MR image demonstrates the normal appearance of the PCL. The normal PCL appears as a uniformly thick band of homogeneous low signal and continuous smooth configuration. The meniscofemoral ligament of Humphrey lies anterior to the PCL (arrowhead) and the meniscofemoral ligament of Wrisberg lies posterior to the PCL (arrow). These ligaments are considered to be a part of the PCL complex.

Plain films can demonstrate a 'posterior sag' if a lateral film is obtained cross-table. 'Posterior sag' occurs when the tibia loses alignment with the femur and sags posteriorly (see Fig. 6.114). An avulsion fracture may also be seen on plain films. This is seen posteriorly and is usually a characteristic triangular shape. Because the ligament is extra-articular, a haemarthrosis may not be seen as with an ACL injury. There may be associated fractures of the styloid process of the fibula (see Fig. 6.115) and the medial aspect of the proximal tibia (reverse Segond), as demonstrated in Fig. 6.59 on page 419.

MRI is the imaging method of choice for establishing the diagnosis of a PCL rupture. MRI may demonstrate alteration of signal intensity in the ligament, with hyperintensity seen on T2-weighted sequences. There may also be abnormal discontinuity of the ligament (see Fig. 6.116). If hyperextension has occurred, bone bruising on the anterior aspect of the tibia may be demonstrated. As PCL rupture is rarely an isolated event, a search for other injuries should commence as soon as a PCL rupture is recognised. MRI can differentiate between complete and partial PCL tears. PCL injuries are often associated with an MCL tear, meniscal tears and bony injuries (Patten et al. 1994).

The lateral collateral ligament

The LCL is one of a number of structures stabilising the lateral side of the knee. The iliotibial band supplies the majority of lateral support. Other stabilisers resisting joint space opening when the knee is subjected to varus stress include the lateral

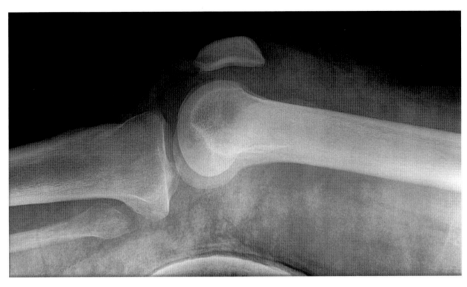

◀ **Fig. 6.114** In a PCL-deficient knee, the restraint against posterior movement of the tibia in relation to the femur is removed and a characteristic alignment abnormality can be produced with the patient supine and relaxed. A cross-table lateral view of the knee shows alignment change indicative of a PCL tear. If a PCL tear is suspected clinically, a support beneath the femur with no tibial support will help to demonstrate a PCL 'sag'.

▶ **Fig. 6.115** A PCL avulsion fracture has occurred with the separated fragment identified at the posterior corner of the proximal tibial condyle (arrow). The configuration of the fragment reflects the extension of the PCL attachment onto the posterior surface of the condyle. Of particular importance is the accompanying avulsion fracture of the styloid process of the fibula (arrowhead). PCL ruptures rarely occur as an isolated injury and in this case it is likely that the PCL rupture is a part of a posterolateral corner injury (see discussion in text overleaf).

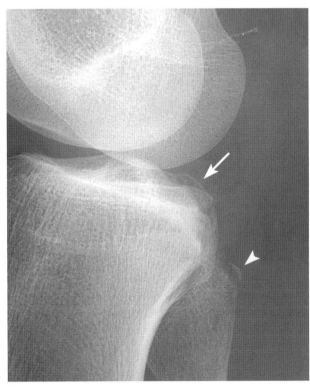

▼ **Fig. 6.116** Sagittal PD and fat-suppressed T2-weighted MR images show a complete rupture of the PCL with fluid separating the tear margins (arrow) and there is high signal within the ligament. Injury of the posterior capsule of the knee is suspected with localised marrow oedema demonstrated at the posterior aspect of the distal femoral metaphysis. The pattern of injuries suggests a hyperextension mechanism. A moderate knee joint effusion is present.

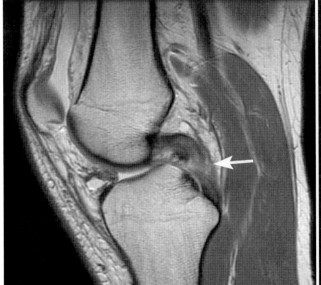

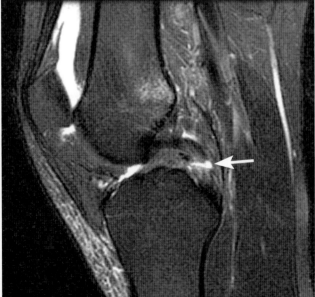

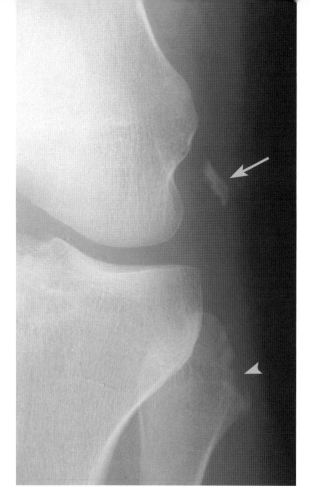

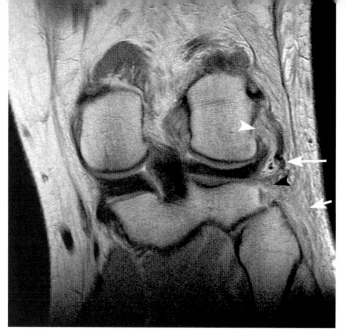

▲ Fig. 6.118 Rupture of the LCL may be only one component of a more extensive posterolateral corner soft-tissue injury. In this case there are multiple injuries including avulsion of the distal biceps femoris and LCL attachments. There is absence of these structures at the fibular head level (short arrow) and a retracted stump of the LCL is also demonstrated (long arrow). There is rupture of the popliteofibular ligament (black arrowhead) and avulsion of the popliteus tendon. The popliteal tendon is absent from the femoral groove (white arrowhead).

▲ Fig. 6.117 There has been an avulsion fracture of the styloid process of the fibula (arrowhead), with considerable retraction of the biceps femoris insertion (arrow). This avulsion is likely to indicate multiligamentous injury at the posterolateral corner of the knee. The LCL is also commonly involved.

capsule, popliteus and biceps femoris. The LCL is injured less frequently than any other knee ligament and is at risk when a varus force is applied to the knee while the leg is abducted and the tibia internally rotated. There is no connection between the lateral meniscus and the LCL, but fascicles extend from the lateral meniscus to create an arcade for the popliteus tendon.

Plain films may show an avulsion fracture of the styloid process of the fibular head (see Fig. 6.117). This avulsion could indicate a posterolateral corner injury and the LCL is usually one of multiple ligamentous injuries involved (see Fig. 6.118). This is discussed in greater detail on page 449. If a fracture of the lateral tibial condyle is present, a tear of the lateral joint capsule and the ACL is more likely than an LCL injury (see Fig. 6.119). Both ultrasound and MRI satisfactorily demonstrate LCL injury (see Fig. 6.120).

▼ Fig. 6.119 Sagittal and coronal PD-weighted MR images demonstrate a transverse fracture of the lateral femoral condyle adjacent to the physeal scar (arrowhead) with an intact LCL (arrows). Note the fluid levels of a lipohaemarthrosis within the anterior recess of the knee joint on the sagittal image.

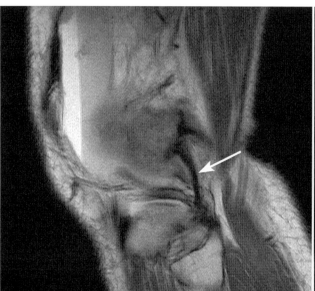

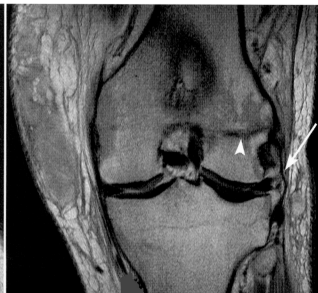

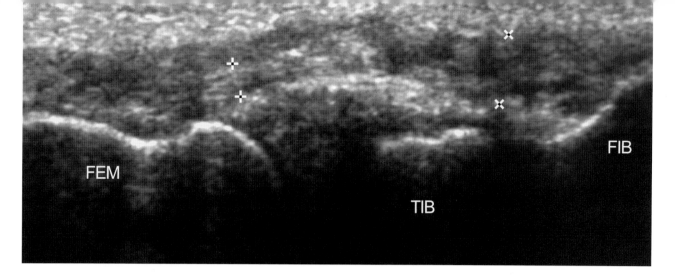

▲ **Fig. 6.120** Rupture of the distal attachment of the LCL has been demonstrated on a long-axis ultrasound image. The intact proximal segment of the LCL shows normal size and fibrillar echotexture (+ callipers), but the distal segment of the LCL shows heterogeneous hypoechoic swelling and fibre disruption (× callipers). Femur = FEM. Tibia = TIB. Fibula = FIB.

Complex ligament injuries

Multiligamentous injuries frequently occur as a result of sport, often in recognisable patterns (see Fig. 6.121). One such pattern is the posterolateral corner injury, which has only recently been recognised.

Knee dislocation and the mutiligament-injured knee

Those involved in sport and sports medicine would like to believe that severe traumas such as knee dislocations are the domain of motor vehicle accidents rather than sport. However, recent articles would suggest otherwise. Twaddle et al. (2003) conducted a prospective study of knee dislocations to identify soft-tissue injury patterns. Of the 60 patients studied, 23 suffered dislocations while involved in sport (38.3%), 34 occurred in motor vehicle accidents and 3 resulted from falls. It is possible that these figures reflect a high involvement in snow sports and a passion for extreme sports in New Zealand, where the research was conducted. However, similar figures were published by Fanelli et al. (2001) in Pennsylvania. In Fanelli's study group of 35 patients, 9 injuries occurred as a result of sport (38.8%).

As these severe multiligamentous knee derangements may occur as sports injuries, it is important that particular patterns of injury should be recognised on imaging. Dislocations may be 'occult' at clinical presentation, the knee having relocated spontaneously, or they may have been reduced at the scene of the trauma. A wide variety of injury patterns were noted by Twaddle et al. (2003) and it is interesting that the soft-tissue injury patterns and vascular and nerve injuries (occurring in 14% of patients) seen in this study were similar for both motor vehicle injuries and sports injuries, suggesting a similar level of force and injury biomechanics.

An extension injury will cause tissue failure in sequence: 30° of hyperextension will cause tearing of the posterior capsule and 50° produces ACL and PCL failure and injury to the popliteal artery (Fanelli et al. 2001). A varus force culminating in a dislocation will rupture the ACL and PCL and produce posterolateral corner (PLC) tears. A dislocation due to a valgus force will rupture the ACL, PCL and MCL (see Fig. 6.122). In regional trauma clinics, 38% of acute knee cases will have a PCL tear. Of these cases, 45.9% will be a combined PCL/ACL injury and 41.2% will be PCL/PLC tears.

In dislocatable knees, Twaddle et al. noted that distal LCL avulsions had a high association with biceps tendon injury (88%) and an association with lateral capsular meniscocapsular avulsions (88%) (see Fig. 6.123). The association of popliteus tendon injury with distal LCL injury was unusual, but there was frequent association with proximal LCL avulsion (75%) (see Fig. 6.124).

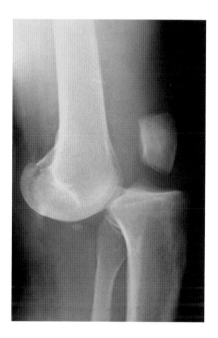

▲ **Fig. 6.121** A lateral plain film shows posterior dislocation of the femur in relation to the tibia. It is important to remember that a large percentage of knee dislocations will result from sporting injuries (Twaddle et al. 2003). Many will have been reduced by the time the patient presents at the clinic. The panoramic ability of MRI is useful for identifying the multiple injuries that have occurred.

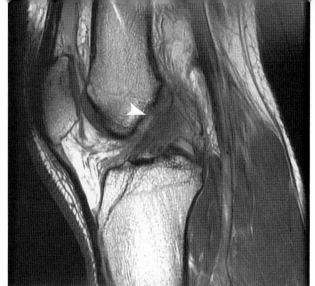

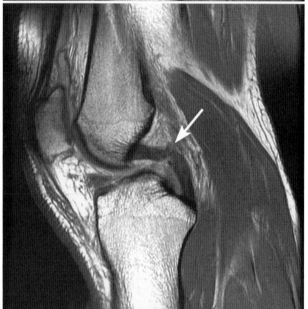

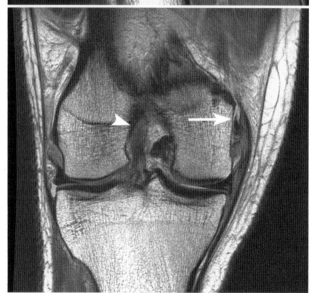

▲ Fig. 6.122 The knee of a wrestler at the Sydney 2000 Olympics was subjected to a powerful valgus force. Sagittal and coronal PD-weighted MR images demonstrate extensive injury, with ruptures of the ACL (top and bottom images), PCL (arrow, middle image) and MCL (arrow, bottom image). Note the knee joint effusion.

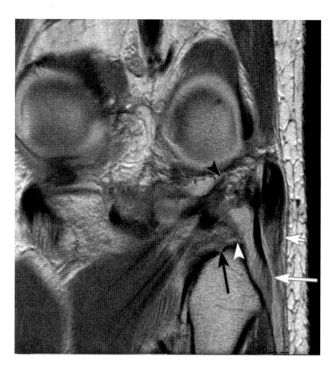

▲ Fig. 6.123 A coronal PD-weighted MR image demonstrates a posterolateral corner soft-tissue injury, including avulsion of the distal LCL (long white arrow) and biceps femoris (short white arrow) attachments and injury to the popliteus tendon (black arrowhead). There is also separation of the arcuate ligament (black arrow) and popliteofibular ligament from the fibula (white arrowhead).

▼ Fig. 6.124 A coronal PD-weighted MR image shows injury to the femoral attachment of the LCL (black arrow), absence of the popliteus tendon due to avulsion (arrowhead) and injury to the tibial attachment of the lateral meniscus (long white arrow). There is also haemorrhage with complete absence of the normal hypointense tendon and ligament structures immediately adjacent to the fibular head. The appearances are in keeping with avulsion of the conjoint insertion of the biceps femoris and distal LCL (short arrow).

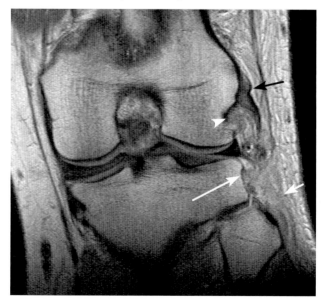

Imaging of ACL and PCL injuries should include plain films to identify associated avulsion fractures. MRI provides an important step in the management of patients with multiple ligamentous injury. In addition, Doppler sonography, MRA and conventional angiography provide methods of assessing associated vascular damage (see Fig. 6.125).

Posterolateral corner injuries: the 'arcuate sign'

The anatomy of the posterolateral corner of the knee is complex. The mechanism responsible for this injury is usually a direct force applied to the anteromedial aspect of an extended knee.

Huang et al. (2003) reported that an avulsion fracture of the head of the fibula may be an important indicator of posterolateral instability of the knee. The term 'arcuate sign' is used to describe an avulsion injury to the insertion of the arcuate complex, which includes the fabellofibular, popliteofibular and arcuate ligaments. Posterolateral instability develops, with posterior subluxation and external rotation of the tibial plateau relative to the femur.

Avulsions of the arcuate ligament complex involve the styloid process of the fibular head and the avulsed fragment is generally oriented horizontally (see Fig. 6.126). Avulsion fractures of the LCL and biceps femoris occur on the lateral aspect of the styloid process of the fibular head. Careful examination of the fibular head on plain films and MR imaging is therefore important to help decide whether the avulsion is likely to involve the arcuate ligament complex (see Fig. 6.127).

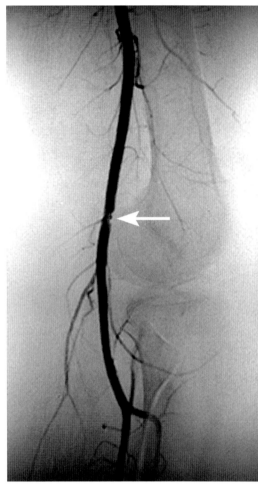

▲ **Fig. 6.125** Following a knee dislocation, conventional angiography demonstrates intimal damage on the anterior wall of the femoral artery at its junction with the popliteal artery.

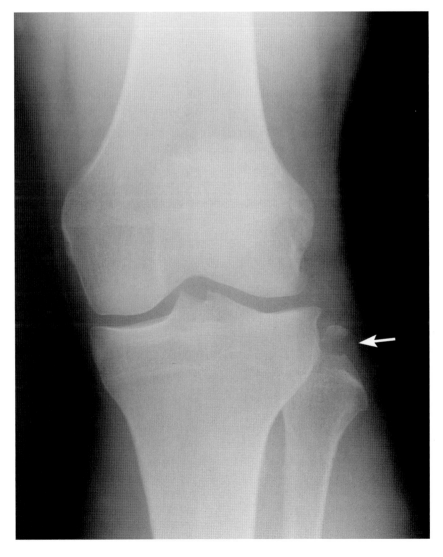

◀ **Fig. 6.126** This avulsion from the tip of the styloid process of the fibula is a classical 'arcuate sign'. The fracture is horizontal and indicates injury to the arcuate ligament complex, which may result in posterolateral instability of the knee.

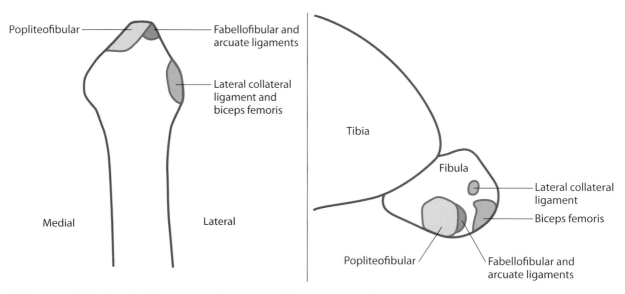

▲ **Fig. 6.127** A line drawing demonstrates the position of the various attachments to the styloid process of the fibula. The popliteofibular ligament inserts on the apex of the fibular head, just medial to the fabellofibular and arcuate ligaments. The LCL and the tendon of the biceps femoris muscle attach to the lateral margin of the head. In the cross-sectional diagram, the LCL attaches just anteromedial to the biceps femoris. The close relationship between the popliteofibular, the fabellofibular and arcuate ligaments is demonstrated.

▶ **Fig. 6.128** Coronal PD and fat-suppressed T2-weighted MR images demonstrate a posterolateral corner injury. There is injury to the arcuate ligament and/or popliteofibular ligament (arrow). Note the bone bruising at the fibular head (asterisk).

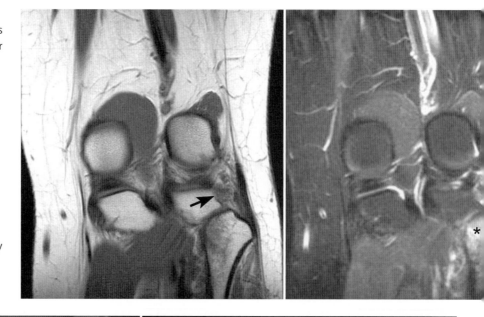

▼ **Fig. 6.129** Coronal PD and fat-suppressed axial T2-weighted MR images demonstrate changes of posterolateral corner instability. Avulsion of the conjoint insertion of the LCL and biceps femoris has occurred (arrow). There is also injury to the popliteus tendon (asterisks). Note the large knee joint effusion (arrowheads).

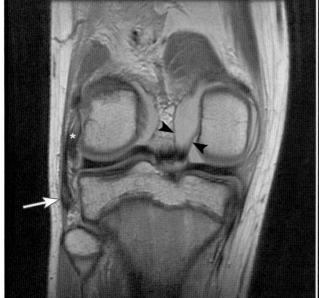
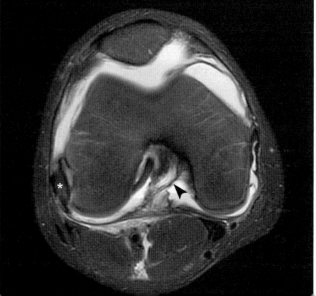

Avulsion of the arcuate ligament complex may be associated with other ligamentous and soft-tissue injuries. The LCL, the tendon of the biceps femoris and the musculotendinous junction of the popliteus may be injured (see Fig. 6.128). The ACL and PCL may also be injured and, in Huang's series, all patients with a fibular head avulsion had injury to the PCL (see Fig. 6.129). All patients also had MCL injury and meniscal tears were common. Bone bruising consistent with hyperextension was also encountered. Any combination of the above injuries may be present.

Plain films are an important starting point, particularly looking for a fracture of the head of the fibula, which may be seen more easily on an AP view with internal rotation. Assessing the extent of possible injury then requires an MRI. In addition to routine sequences, oblique sequences may be useful to examine the arcuate ligament, which is difficult to interpret on a routine examination. Coronal-oblique T2-weighted images have been shown to optimise visualisation of the posterolateral ligamentous structures, and Yu et al. (1996) have demonstrated that the arcuate ligament was visualised 46% of the time, the fabellofibular ligament 48% of the time and fibular origin of the popliteus muscle 48%. With standard sequences the ability to visualise these ligaments successfully was 10%, 34% and 8%, respectively.

The consequences of overlooking an arcuate ligament complex avulsion, or not conducting a careful search for or recognising associated injuries, may be profound.

Tendon and bursal injuries: tendinopathy, rupture and bursopathy

Quadriceps and patellar tendon injuries

Injuries to the quadriceps and patellar tendons are discussed later in the section on the extensor mechanism (see page 462).

Popliteus tendon injuries

Popliteus tendinopathy produces posterolateral knee pain in runners, particularly in sports requiring deceleration such as running or hiking downhill. Popliteus tendinopathy is generally of insidious onset and does not usually follow an acute trauma. Ultrasound (see Fig. 6.130) and MRI (see Fig. 6.131) demonstrate diagnostic changes of popliteus tendinopathy. On examination, posterolateral tenderness is present and the patient's pain is reproduced by external rotation. The popliteus is an internal rotator of the tibia and unlocks the knee from straight alignment. The popliteus also acts to stabilise the knee by contributing to valgus and varus stability and assists the quadriceps and PCL in maintaining normal tibiofemoral orientation.

The anatomy of the popliteus tendon is complex, having three insertions: the popliteal groove, the lateral meniscus and the popliteofibular ligament, a component of the arcuate ligament complex. The popliteofibular ligament is one of

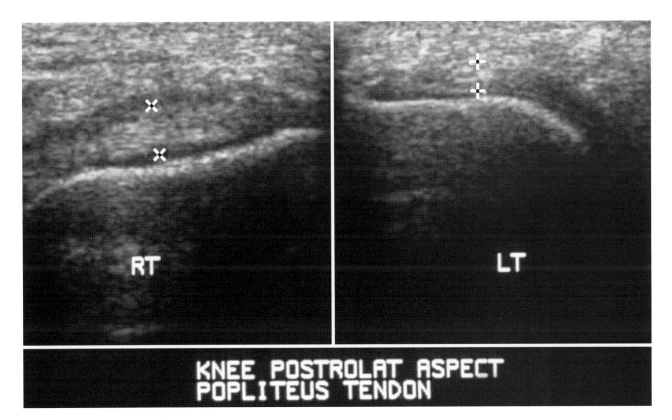

▲ **Fig. 6.130** Comparative long-axis ultrasound images of the popliteus tendons obtained at the femoral groove level demonstrate popliteus tendinopathy on the right side. There is considerable swelling of the tendon of the right popliteus (× callipers) with hypoechoic synovial thickening also surrounding the tendon. Tenderness to probing over the thickened tendon segment is another important feature to elicit during the real-time examination.

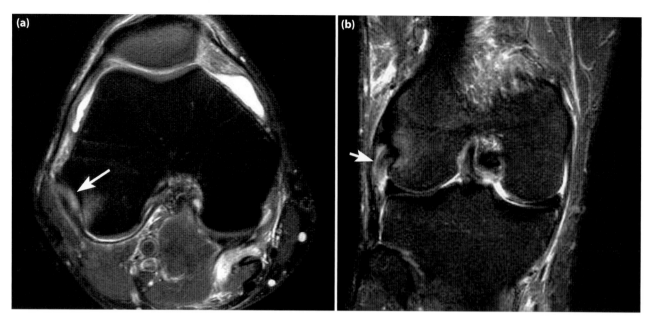

▲ **Fig. 6.131** A middle-aged athlete presented with posterolateral knee pain and tenderness that interfered with his 'stay-fit' program. Fat-suppressed axial **(a)** and coronal **(b)** T2-weighted MR images demonstrate changes of popliteus tendinopathy. The popliteus tendon is swollen and hyperintense (long arrow, axial image). There is a collar of associated peritendon hyperintensity consistent with synovitis (short arrow, coronal image). Reactive bone marrow oedema is shown within the femoral condyle immediately adjacent to the popliteal groove. Note the effusion within the anterior recess of the knee joint and synovitis within the deep recess of semimembranosis-gastrocnemius bursa at the medial aspect of the popliteal fossa.

the important stabilisers in the posterolateral corner (Haimes et al. 2003). The tendon passes through an arcade of struts (popliteomeniscal fascicles) holding the tendon between the capsule and the posterolateral aspect of the lateral meniscus. The tendon is separated from the LCL, femoral condyle and capsule by a bursa and consequently may be associated with bursitis or capsulitis. The differential diagnosis includes iliotibial band syndrome, lateral meniscal tear and biceps femoris tendinopathy.

Popliteus tendon rupture

Rupture of the popliteal tendon may occur as an avulsion injury at its insertion or, more commonly, as a tear at its musculotendinous junction. Injury usually occurs from hyperextension of the knee (see Figs 6.132, 6.133 and 6.134). The avulsion of the popliteus from its insertion is a common component of a high-grade injury to the posterolateral corner (see Fig. 6.135). A tear of the popliteus is seen in association with tears and avulsions of the biceps femoris, arcuate ligament complex and LCL.

Iliotibial band tendinopathy and rupture

The iliotibial band is a combination of tendon and fascia from the deep and superficial fibres of the fascia lata. The superficial layer is the main tendinous component and inserts onto Gerdy's tubercle on the anterolateral aspect of the proximal tibia. Overuse is a common cause of lateral knee pain, usually occurring as the result of activities requiring repetitive knee flexion and extension, such as long-distance running, cycling, rowing and weightlifting. The pain is characteristically

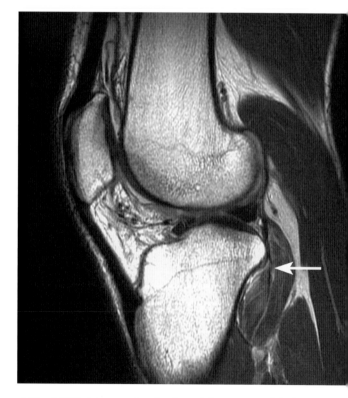

▲ **Fig. 6.132** A hyperextension knee injury occurred during a Taekwondo competition at the Sydney 2000 Olympics. A sagittal PD-weighted MR image shows a subtle localised focus of intermediate signal interrupting the continuity of the central popliteus tendon (arrow) and high signal of oedema and haemorrhage within the adjacent muscle at the popliteus musculotendinous junction. The appearances are those of a low-grade popliteus musculotendinous junction tear.

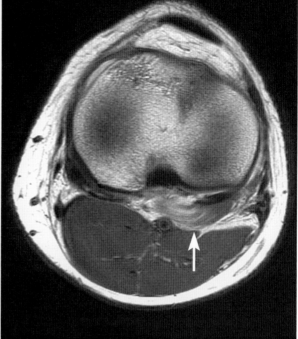

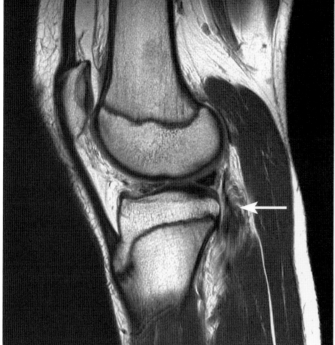

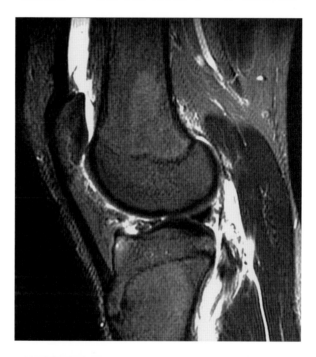

▲ Fig. 6.133 An adolescent athlete playing basketball suffered a hyperextension injury of the knee resulting in a musculotendinous junction tear of the popliteus (arrows). Sagittal and axial PD-weighted MR images show popliteus muscle swelling, fibre irregularity and signal hyperintensity at the level of the musculotendinous junction. Also note evidence of injury to the anterior horn of the lateral meniscus.

▶ Fig. 6.134 A violent hyperextension injury has produced bone bruising of the anterior aspect of the tibial plateau, rupture of the posterior capsule of the knee joint and rupture of the popliteus muscle. Also note injury to the anterior horn of the lateral meniscus and a large knee joint effusion. These changes have been demonstrated on a sagittal fat-suppressed T2-weighted MR image.

▼ Fig. 6.135 Posterolateral corner injuries at the knee commonly involve the popliteus. In this example, sagittal and coronal fat-suppressed T2-weighted MR images show a posterolateral corner disruption that includes injury to the popliteofibular ligament (long arrow), arcuate ligament (short arrow) and musculotendinous junction of the popliteus muscle (arrowheads). Note the haemorrhagic effusion within the popliteus sheath.

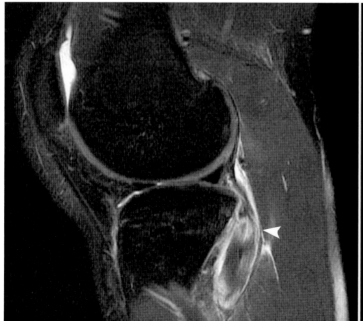

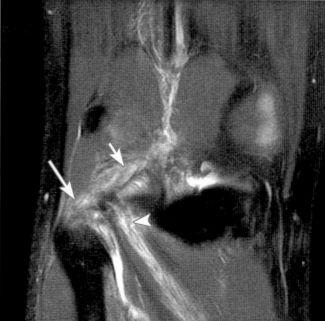

aggravated by running downhill (Taunton et al. 2002). MRI and ultrasound will demonstrate soft-tissue oedema between the ITB and the epicondylar eminence or slightly posterior to it (see Figs 6.136 and 6.137). Occasionally, a fluid collection may be seen with thickening of the ITB (see Figs 6.138 and 6.139). These changes are well demonstrated by both MRI and ultrasound. A varus injury to the knee may cause avulsion of the ITB from Gerdy's tubercle. An example of this injury has previously been shown, imaged by plain films and MRI in Fig. 6.60 on page 420.

Bursopathy

Pre-patellar bursopathy

The pre-patellar bursa is the most commonly injured bursa in the knee. Being anatomically exposed, direct trauma to the bursa is common. The bursa is large and may develop considerable fluid and/or thickening between the skin and the patella (see Fig. 6.140). Imaging is rarely required. Ultrasound will show the changes of bursopathy and can provide imaging control if aspiration is thought necessary (see Fig. 6.141).

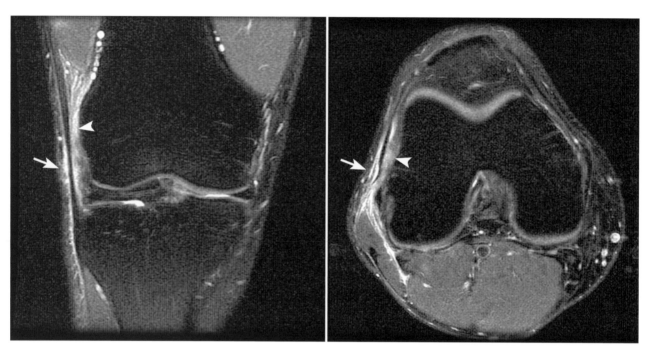

▲ **Fig. 6.136** Coronal and axial fat-suppressed T2-weighted MR images demonstrate changes of frictional ITB peritendinitis. There is oedema in the soft tissues between the ITB and the lateral femoral condyle (arrowheads), and oedema is also noted in the subcutaneous tissues immediately superficial to the ITB (arrows). No thickening or hyperintensity of the ITB tendon itself can be seen.

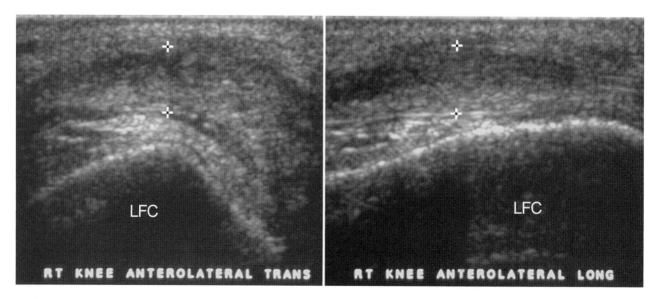

▲ **Fig. 6.137** Transverse and long-axis ultrasound images show changes of ITB friction syndrome producing tendinopathy with marked fusiform thickening of the ITB tendon and associated hypoechoic echotexture (callipers) immediately adjacent to the lateral femoral epicondyle. Lateral femoral condyle = LFC.

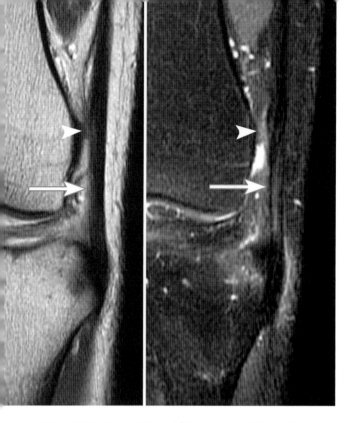

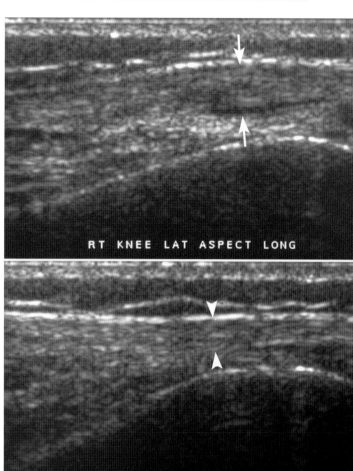

▲ **Fig. 6.138** Coronal PD and fat-suppressed T2-weighted MR images show a thickened ITB (arrows) with intrasubstance increased signal. The appearances are those of ITB tendinopathy. Also note the high signal indicative of frictional bursopathy deep to the ITB at the femoral epicondylar level (arrowheads). In addition, there is peritendon oedema at the ITB insertion and marrow oedema within the tibia just medial to the ITB insertion.

▲ **Fig. 6.139** Long-axis ultrasound images of the ITB tendons obtained at the lateral femoral epicondyle level show features of right ITB friction syndrome. Abnormal fusiform tendon thickening (arrows) can be appreciated by comparison with the normal left side (arrowheads). There is also a thin line of hypoechoic peritendon thickening consistent with associated bursopathy immediately deep to the abnormal segment.

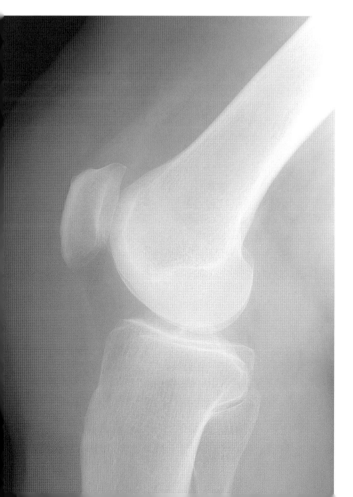

◀ **Fig. 6.140** Pre-patellar bursopathy produces an increase in soft tissues over the anterior aspect of the inferior pole of the patella and over the proximal half of the patellar tendon. When a large effusion occurs due to injury or irritation, a sizable soft-tissue mass can appear on the anterior aspect of the knee.

▶ **Fig. 6.141(a)** A long-axis ultrasound image obtained over the inferior pole of the patella demonstrates a broad area of marked soft-tissue thickening in the pre-patellar space (callipers). The swelling is in the distribution of the pre-patellar bursa extending inferiorly over the proximal patellar tendon. No fluid is present and no foreign body is seen. The patellar tendon (arrowheads) is normal. The patient was a professional ballerina with longstanding symptoms and the appearances are those of chronic pre-patellar bursopathy. Patella = PAT.

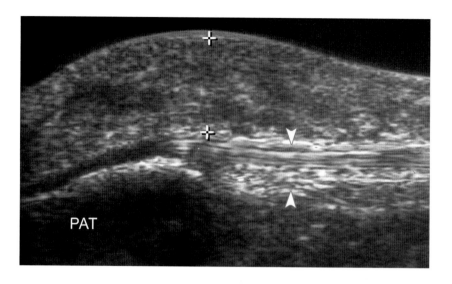

▼ **(b)** Transverse and long-axis ultrasound images of the pre-patellar bursa in a different patient demonstrate an ovoid hypoechoic space with well-rounded margins, consistent with encysted effusion (indicated by callipers).

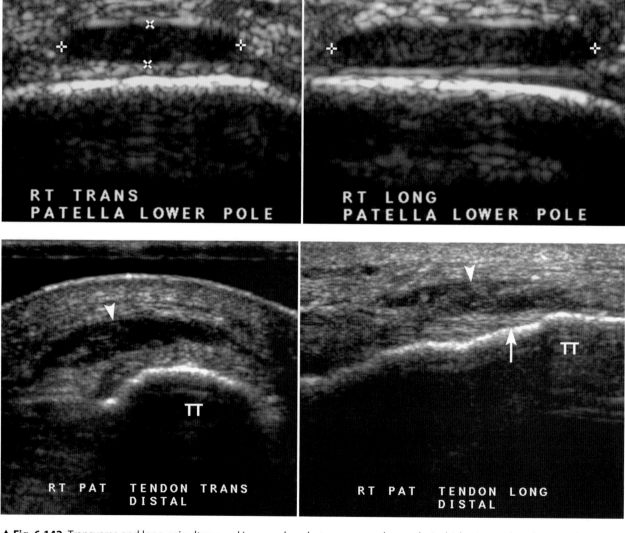

▲ **Fig. 6.142** Transverse and long-axis ultrasound images show heterogeneous hypoechoic thickening within the superficial infrapatellar bursa, overlying the distal insertion of the patellar tendon (arrow). The appearances are those of a chronic pre-tibial bursopathy. Tibial tuberosity = TT.

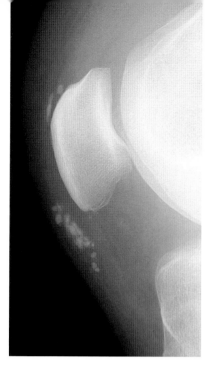

◀ **Fig. 6.143** Multiple small ossicles are present in the superficial infrapatellar bursa resulting from repetitive friction and irritation.

Infrapatellar bursopathy

The superficial infrapatellar bursa is situated between the skin and the proximal patellar tendon (see Figs 6.142 and 6.143). Superficial bursopathy may develop secondary to repetitive trauma and friction from kneeling and is known as 'surfboard rider's knee'. Plain films may show soft-tissue swelling and calcification in the position of the bursa (see Fig. 6.144). The condition is sometimes difficult to differentiate from patellar tendinopathy and Osgood–Schlatter disease. Ultrasound is a useful imaging method for confirming the diagnosis and defining the pathological changes (see Fig. 6.145). Ultrasound is also useful in ruling out an underlying radiolucent foreign body or tendon damage. The deep infrapatellar bursa lies between the patellar tendon and the tibia (see Fig. 6.146).

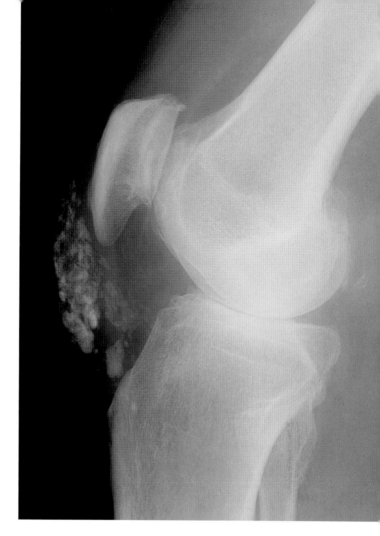

▲ **Fig. 6.144** A large collection of ossicles and calcification are present in and around the superficial infrapatellar bursa. Although the patient had been a keen surfer, his occupation as a carpet layer was most probably the major contributor to this appearance.

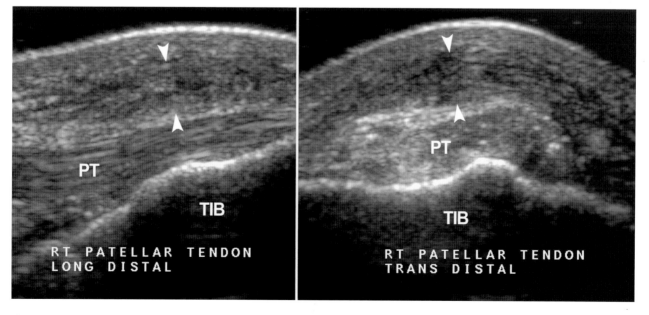

▲ **Fig. 6.145** Long-axis and transverse ultrasound images demonstrate echogenic soft-tissue thickening of chronic pre-tibial bursopathy (arrowheads). No effusion or foreign body can be seen. Tibia = TIB. Patellar tendon = PT.

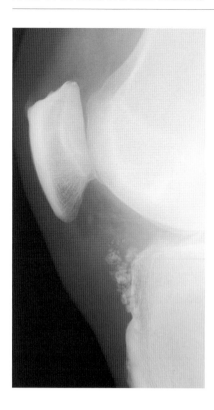

◀ Fig. 6.146 Synovial osteochondromatosis involves the deep infrapatellar bursa. Associated bursopathy is present, with increased density surrounding the ossicles, encroaching on the infrapatellar fat pad. Irregularity of the ossicles is typical of synovial osteochondromatosis.

Anserine bursopathy

The anserine bursa lies between the pes anserinus tendons insertion (a combined insertion of the sartorius, gracilis and semitendinosus tendons) and the MCL insertion. As with other bursae, bursopathy may develop following direct trauma or friction overuse. MRI and ultrasound are able to confirm the clinical suspicion of this condition and characterise the changes (see Figs 6.147 and 6.148).

Iliotibial band bursopathy

Following repetitive flexion and extension of the knee, iliotibial band bursopathy may develop as a result of friction between the iliotibial band and the lateral epicondylar prominence of the distal femur (see Fig. 6.149).

MCL bursopathy

MCL bursopathy is an uncommon cause of medial side knee pain. The bursa is located between the superficial and deep portions of the MCL, along the middle third of the knee (Lee and Yao 1991) (see Fig. 6.150).

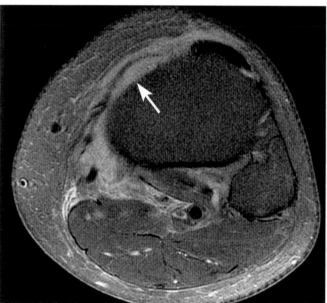
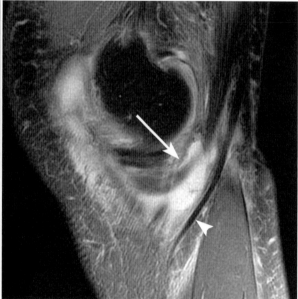

▲ Fig. 6.147(a) Axial and sagittal fat-suppressed T2-weighted MR images demonstrate features of anserine bursopathy. On the axial image, the pes anserinus tendons are elevated away from the tibial surface by hyperintense thickening within the anserine bursa (short arrow). On the sagittal view, a discrete fluid space is also seen within the bursa at a more proximal level (long arrow). This lies deep to the semitendinosus tendon (arrowhead). A knee joint effusion is also present.

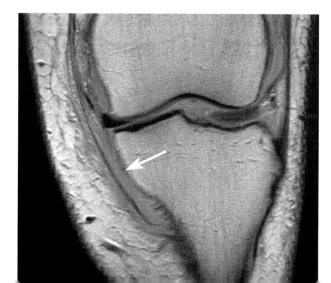

▶ (b) A coronal PD-weighted MR image shows the pes anserinus tendon complex displaced away from the tibia by the fluid signal of anserine bursopathy (arrow).

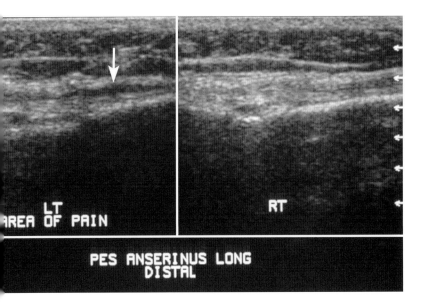

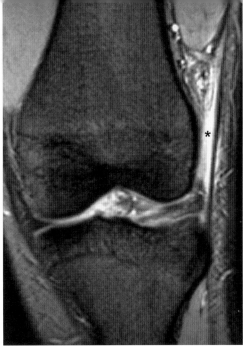

▲ **Fig. 6.148** A long-axis ultrasound image obtained over the site of pain at the medial aspect of the proximal left tibia is compared with the normal right side at the same level. On the symptomatic left side, a line of hypoechoic thickening typical of anserine bursopathy (arrow) separates the more superficial pes anserinus tendon from the subjacent distal end of the MCL.

▲ **Fig. 6.149** A coronal fat-suppressed T2-weighted MR image shows a prominent hyperintense zone of fluid and thickening between the ITB and the lateral femoral condyle (asterisk). The appearances are those of frictional ITB bursopathy.

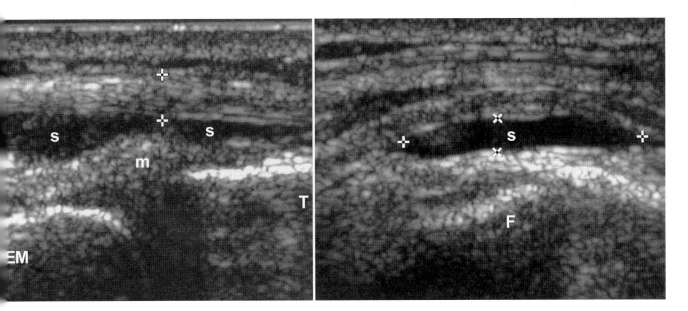

▲ **Fig. 6.150** An example of MCL bursopathy is demonstrated by ultrasound. Long-axis and transverse images have been obtained over the MCL at the level of the tibiofemoral joint. There is thickening of the superficial layer of the MCL (+ callipers). A zone of fluid is shown in the distribution of the MCL bursa, which lies between the superficial and deep layers of the MCL (× callipers). Contained low-level echoes indicate synovitis (s). Femur = FEM/F. Medial meniscus = m. Tibia = T.

Semimembranosus tendinopathy and bursopathy

Semimembranosus tendinopathy and bursopathy can occur as the hamstring tendon passes around the medial tibial metaphysis, and can overlap clinically with pes anserinus tendinopathy and anserine bursitis (see Figs 6.151 and 6.152).

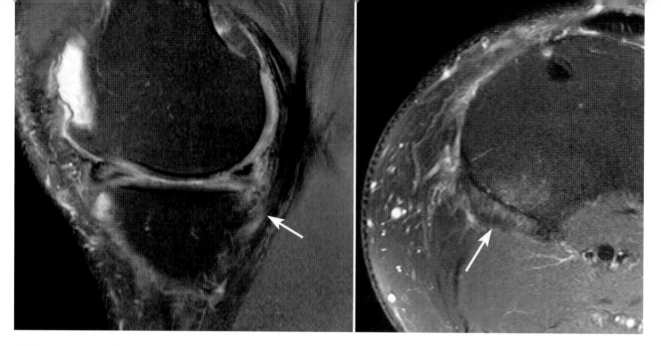

▲ **Fig. 6.151** Sagittal and axial fat-suppressed PD-weighted MR images demonstrate changes of insertional semimembranosus tendinopathy. The abnormal tendon segment shows swelling and hyperintensity (arrows). There is also marrow oedema seen deep to the tibial enthesis on the axial view. Other findings on the sagittal image include a torn medial meniscus, chondral wear over the medial femoral condyle and a knee joint effusion.

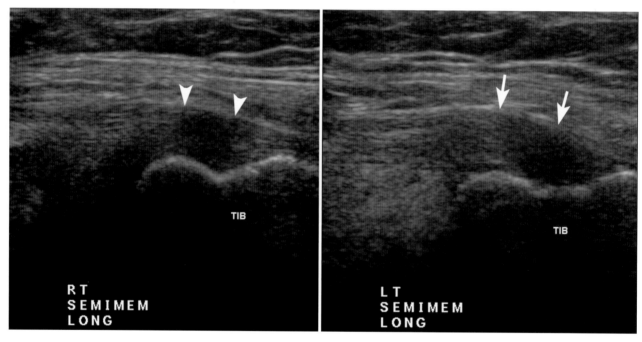

▲ **Fig. 6.152** Comparative long-axis ultrasound images of the semimembranosus tendons at the tibial insertion show features of distal left semimembranosus tendinopathy. The left semimembranosus tendon appears diffusely thickened (arrows) in comparison with the asymptomatic right side (arrowheads) and was also distinctly tender to probing. In this case, tendon echotexture is of limited diagnostic value, as the distal segments of both tendons have a longitudinal curvature producing a similar hypoechoic appearance due to anisotropy. Tibia = TIB.

Baker's cyst (syn. popliteal cyst)

A Baker's cyst is a distended semimembranosus-gastrocnemius bursa (see Fig. 6.153). In children, Baker's cysts arise primarily due to bursal irritation, without associated intra-articular pathology, are usually self-limiting and can be treated conservatively. In adults, they occur as a result of chronic knee joint effusion, usually with a posterior horn medial meniscal tear (Stone et al. 1996). The neck of the bursa arises between the tendons of the semimembranosus and the medial head of the gastrocnemius (see Fig. 6.154). The bursa acts as a sump and often contains radiolucent or radiopaque loose bodies. If synovitis develops, Baker's cysts may be imaged by nuclear bone scan (see Fig. 6.155). Bursal aspiration may be performed under ultrasound control (see Fig. 6.156). An overdistended bursa may suddenly rupture (e.g. at arthroscopy) and produce a clinical syndrome of acute-onset calf pain, which can mimic a deep calf vein thrombosis (see Fig. 6.157).

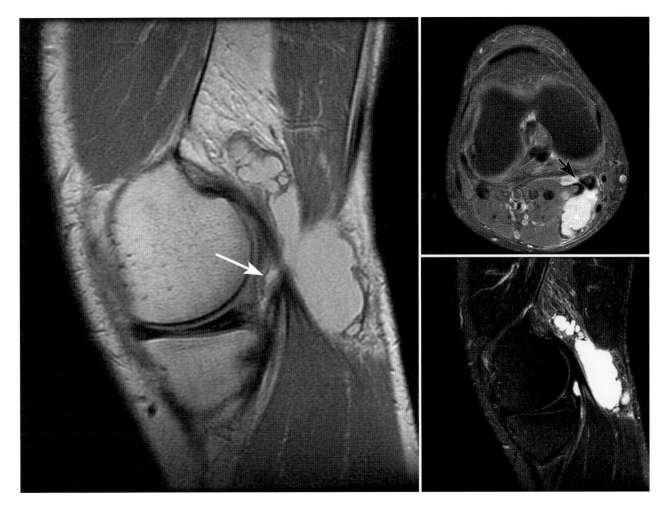

▲ **Fig. 6.153** A large lobulated Baker's cyst is draped along the posterior surface of the medial head gastrocnemius muscle. On the sagittal PD-weighted MR image, a neck of communication with the posterior aspect of the knee joint is demonstrated (white arrow). Note the characteristic appearance of a bursal neck passing between the medial head of the gastrocnemius and the semimembranosus tendon on the axial view (black arrow). A horizontal cleavage tear of the posterior horn of the medial meniscus is also noted.

▼ **Fig. 6.154** An axial T2-weighted MR image shows the neck of a Baker's cyst passing between the semimembranosus (s) and the medial head of the gastrocnemius (m) tendons. The popliteal cyst shows a subtle pattern of intraluminal granularity consistent with contained synovitis.

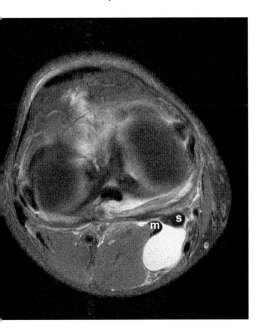

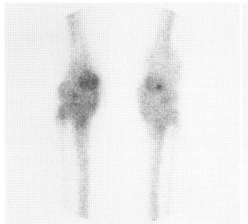

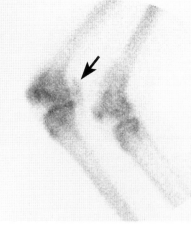

▲ **Fig. 6.155** Delayed images from a nuclear bone scan show low-grade activity within the soft tissues behind the right knee joint (arrow). The appearances are those of a Baker's cyst with contained synovitis.

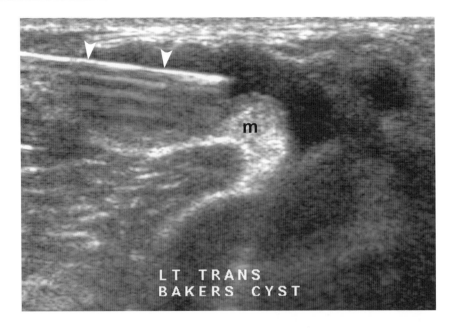

▶ **Fig. 6.156** If a Baker's cyst requires aspiration, this procedure can be performed under ultrasound control. In this example, the strongly echogenic line of an aspirating needle (arrowheads) is demonstrated within the hypoechoic space of a popliteal cyst. Note the presence of a posterior acoustic reverberation artefact deep to the needle. Medial head of gastrocnemius tendon = m.

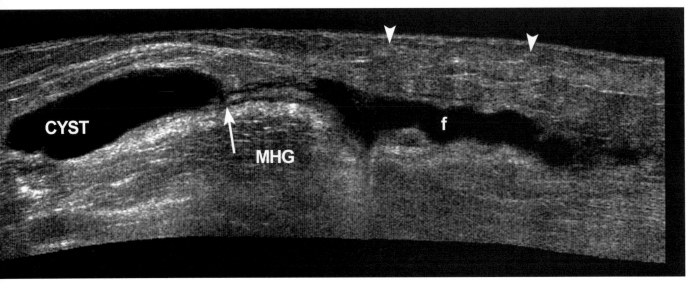

▲ **Fig. 6.157** A long-axis ultrasound image shows a ruptured Baker's cyst with fluid (f) tracking inferiorly from the leak point (arrow) along the superficial surface of the medial head gastrocnemius muscle (MHG). Also note a diffuse increase in echogenicity within the subcutaneous fat at the mid-calf level (arrowheads). This reflects oedema and inflammatory change secondary to fluid dissection from the leaking Baker's cyst, a phenomenon that accounts for the common associated clinical syndrome of 'pseudothrombophlebitis'.

The extensor mechanism

The extensor mechanism begins at the origin of the rectus femoris and extends through the patellofemoral articulation to the insertion of the patellar tendon at the tibial tuberosity. The quadriceps muscle group functions to extend the knee and during walking stabilises the knee on flexion. Injury to the extensor mechanism can occur at any level (see Fig. 6.158).

Quadriceps tendinopathy

Quadriceps tendinopathy occurs far less frequently than patellar tendinopathy and involves the quadriceps tendon at its insertion. Tendinopathy may result from repetitive overuse of the quadriceps muscle group in sports such as weightlifting and sprinting and in jumping and kicking sports.

Quadriceps tendinopathy produces a focal tendon swelling, most marked at the insertion into the patella and extending proximally. Both ultrasound and MRI will demonstrate changes predominantly involving the central one-third of the tendon (see Fig. 6.159). A general loss of the normal lamination of the tendon is usually noted, with structural detail becoming indistinct. MRI can show high signal within tendon substance on T2-weighted MR sequences (see Fig. 6.160), although focal areas of high signal are less common in quadriceps tendinopathy than in patellar tendinopathy. In chronic cases, calcification may develop and this may become evident on plain films.

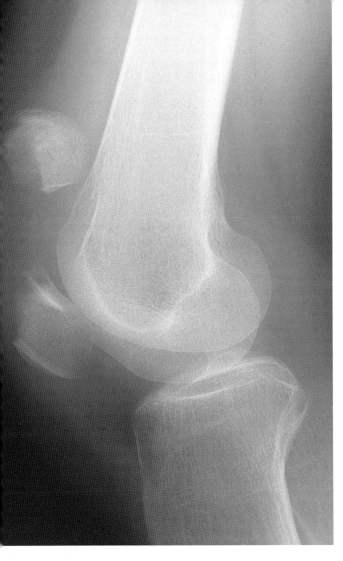

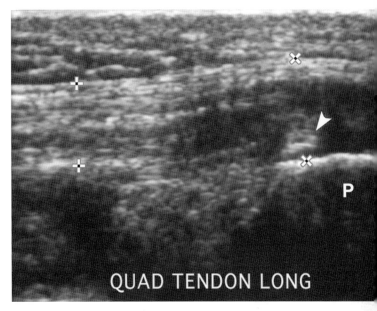

◀**Fig. 6.158** Disruption of the extensor mechanism is caused by a complete transverse fracture of the patella. Displacement of the fragments has occurred due to retraction of the proximal fragment by the quadriceps.

▲**Fig. 6.159** A long-axis ultrasound image shows features of chronic insertional quadriceps tendinopathy. The abnormal tendon segment demonstrates hypoechoic thickening consistent with tendinopathy (× callipers). There is also a small echogenic focus of contained calcification adjacent to the patellar enthesis (arrowhead).

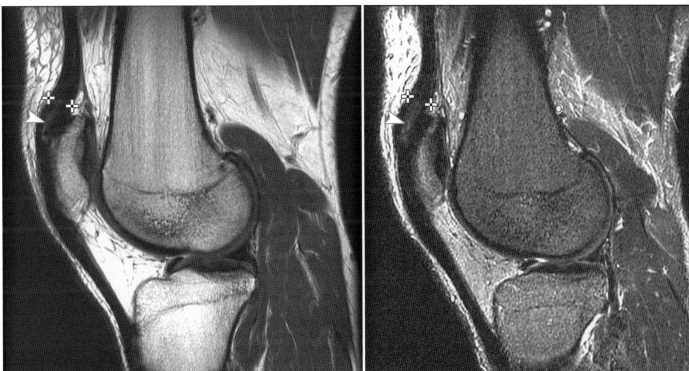

▲**Fig. 6.160** A weightlifter at the Sydney 2000 Olympics presented with pain and tenderness at the upper pole of the patella. Sagittal PD and fat-suppressed T2-weighted MR images demonstrate changes of quadriceps tendinopathy, with thickening of the distal tendon (callipers) and intermediate signal within the tendon (arrowheads).

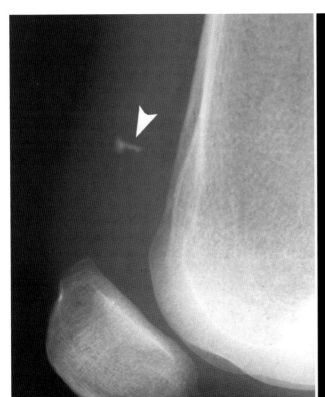

Quadriceps tendon rupture

Rupture of the extensor tendon mechanism can occur at any level, with the quadriceps tendon rupturing more frequently than the patellar tendon.

Quadriceps tendon ruptures tend to occur in part-time athletes from an older age group (40 years plus). Rupture of the quadriceps tendon occurs from overloading the extensor mechanism of the knee on a background of chronic overuse (Siwek and Rao 1981). Tendon rupture is invariably unilateral and characteristically results from falling onto a partly flexed knee, with the foot planted. A violent, eccentric contraction of the quadriceps occurs in an attempt to break the fall. The two major predisposing associations of tendon rupture are previous corticosteroid injection (Kennedy and Willis 1976) and tendinopathy (Kannus and Jozoa 1991).

Complete ruptures, especially when acute, are usually clinically obvious and do not require imaging for diagnosis. Partial tears and, infrequently, chronic complete tears may require imaging to help establish a diagnosis and to assess the extent and exact site of rupture. Partial tears of the quadriceps tendon occur at the patellar insertion and usually involve the superficial rectus femoris fibres. Following a quadriceps tendon rupture, plain films may show a patella baja. Plain films commonly show avulsed bony fragments and invariably there is swelling with disruption of the normal soft-tissue planes (see Figs 6.161 and 6.162).

Confirmation of partial or complete tears of the quadriceps tendon may be obtained with MRI (see Fig. 6.163) or ultrasound (see Figs 6.164 and 6.165) (La et al. 2003). On imaging, there is discontinuity of fibre structure and retraction of the proximal remnant. A haematoma is invariably present.

▲ **Fig. 6.161** A lateral plain film of a quadriceps rupture shows avulsion of bone fragments and associated soft-tissue swelling. The patella has migrated inferiorly (patella baja) with buckling of the patellar tendon. There is anterior rotation of the proximal pole of the patella.

▼ **Fig. 6.162** The avulsed fragments may be subtle (arrow, arrowhead), but the characteristic position of the patella in both cases is an important diagnostic sign.

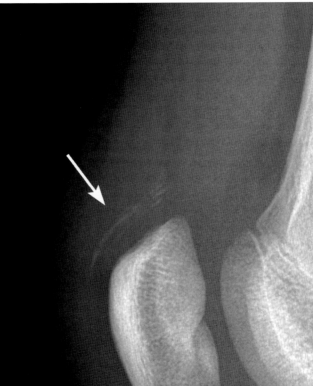

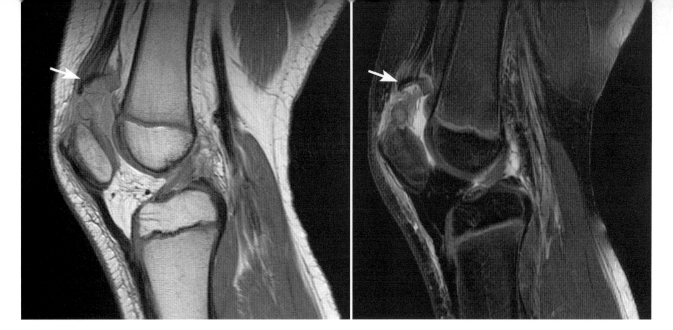

▲ **Fig. 6.163** Sagittal PD and fat-suppressed T2-weighted MR images demonstrate a complete avulsion of the quadriceps tendon insertion with an accompanying cortical fragment detached from the proximal pole of the patella (arrows). The tendon has retracted proximally and haemorrhage fills the gap between the patella and the torn end of the tendon. The patella has moved distally and there is characteristic anterior rotation of the proximal pole of the patella and buckling of the patellar tendon.

▶ **Fig. 6.164** A long-axis ultrasound image demonstrates an acute partial-thickness rupture of the quadriceps tendon. There is mild retraction of the torn superficial tendon layer with a fluid-filled cleft (asterisk) separating the margins of the tear, and fluid extending proximally as a laminar intrasubstance defect (e). Arrowheads indicate the margins of the quadriceps tendon. Note the intact deep tendon layer. Patella = PAT.

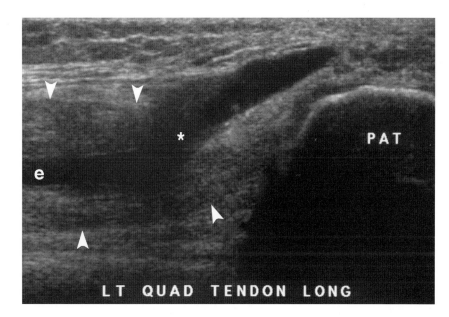

▶ **Fig. 6.165** A composite long-axis ultrasound image demonstrates a subacute complete tear at the patellar attachment of the quadriceps tendon. Arrowheads indicate the superficial and deep surfaces of the quadriceps tendon. The retracted tendon edge (arrow) shows a focus of contained calcification (c) and the tendon gap is filled with heterogeneous echotexture of organising haemorrhage (h). Patella = P.

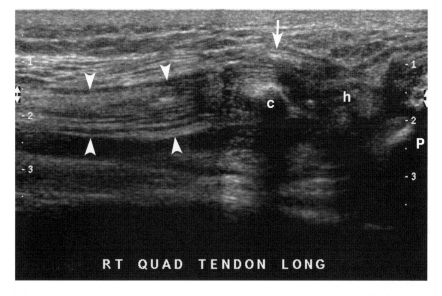

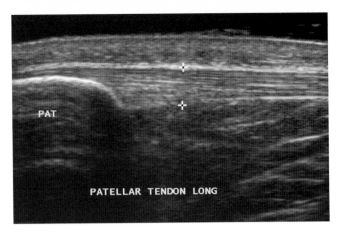

▲ **Fig. 6.167** A long-axis ultrasound image demonstrates the appearance of a normal patellar tendon (callipers) with a uniform compact fibrillar echopattern. Patella = PAT.

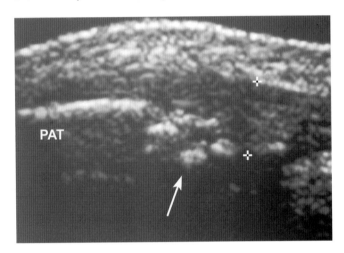

▲ **Fig. 6.168** Long-axis ultrasound shows swelling of the proximal patellar tendon (callipers). Multiple calcifications are also noted (arrow) and the appearances are those of chronic calcific patellar tendinopathy. Patella = PAT.

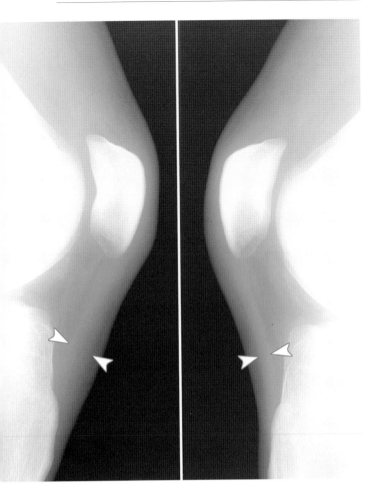

▲ **Fig. 6.166** The patellar tendon is well seen on lateral plain films with the anterior and posterior surfaces contrasted against subcutaneous fat and the infrapatellar fat pad (arrowheads). Comparative views in this case show a diffuse swelling of the patellar tendon in the left image when compared with the normal right image. The appearances are characteristic of patellar tendinopathy.

Patellar tendinopathy

Patellar tendinopathy ('jumper's knee') results from repetitive loading of the extensor mechanism, particularly in sports requiring jumping and kicking, such as basketball, volleyball and football. Plain films may show swelling of the tendon (see Fig. 6.166). Ultrasound is a valuable imaging method for demonstrating the patellar tendon (see Fig. 6.167) and is best able to distinguish swelling, calcifications (see Fig. 6.168) and confluent mucoid degenerative change (see Fig. 6.169).

Ultrasound can also detect cystic changes and micro-tears from surrounding degeneration and correlates well with surgical findings (Kalebo et al. 1991) (see Fig. 6.170). In addition, ultrasound has the potential to assess neovascularisation associated with patellar tendinopathy rapidly and non-invasively (see Fig. 6.171). The area of the tendon with structural tendon changes and neovascularisation is most often the symptomatic area on which the clinical diagnosis of patellar tendinopathy is based (Gisslen and Alfredson 2005).

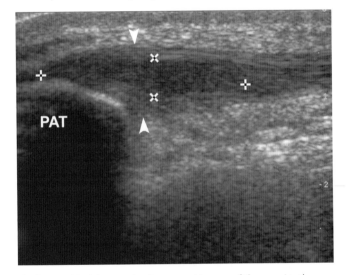

▲ **Fig. 6.169** A long-axis ultrasound image of the proximal patellar tendon demonstrates chronic patellar tendinopathy. The proximal tendon is swollen (arrowheads) and there is an area of central intrasubstance hypoechoic change, which shows a subtle preservation of fibrillar echopattern, consistent with mucoid degeneration. This area is demarcated by callipers. Patella = PAT.

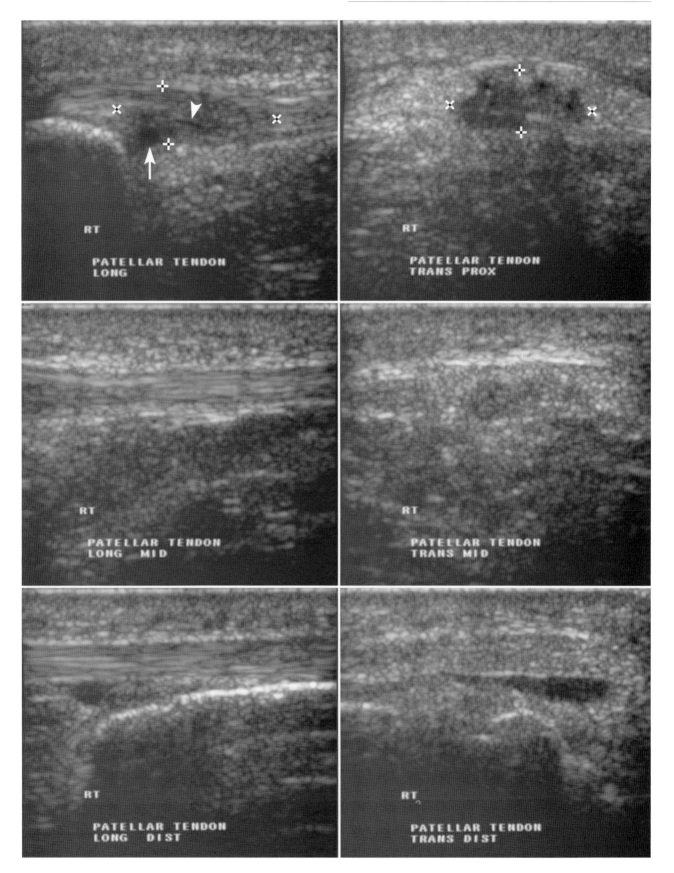

▲ **Fig. 6.170** The entire patellar tendon has been imaged with both longitudinal and transverse ultrasound images. Just below the inferior pole of the patella, the tendon is thickened by a central zone of hypoechoic mucoid degeneration (indicated by callipers). Within the area of degeneration there is a rounded focus of anechoic cystic change (arrow) and a linear defect consistent with an intrasubstance tear (arrowhead). Note the increased echogenicity within the adjacent portion of the deep infrapatellar fat pad. A normal ultrasound appearance is demonstrated in the distal tendon.

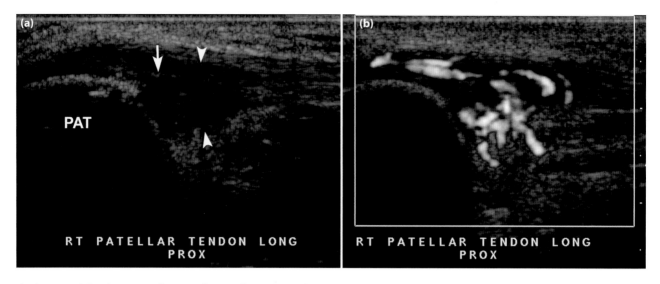

▲ **Fig. 6.171(a)** A long-axis ultrasound image from a case of 'jumper's knee' demonstrates an area of mucoid degeneration at the proximal end of the patellar tendon (arrowheads). There is also a superimposed line of mixed hypo-hyperechoic appearance due to a complicating central intrasubstance tear extending from a focus of localised enthesial bone reaction at the inferior pole of the patella (arrow). Patella = PAT. **(b)** A corresponding Power Doppler image shows considerable tendon neovascularity associated with the zone of mucoid degeneration. The patient's symptoms were centred on this area.

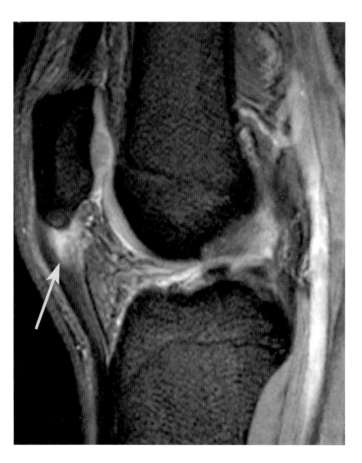

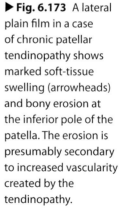

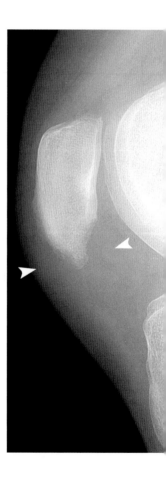

◄**Fig. 6.172** A sagittal GRE MR image demonstrates florid changes of proximal patellar tendinopathy. There is marked tendon swelling and signal hyperintensity (arrow). A small area of high signal is also present in the adjacent inferior pole of the patella.

▶ **Fig. 6.173** A lateral plain film in a case of chronic patellar tendinopathy shows marked soft-tissue swelling (arrowheads) and bony erosion at the inferior pole of the patella. The erosion is presumably secondary to increased vascularity created by the tendinopathy.

MRI may show focal thickening of the proximal tendon with increased signal on both T1- and T2-weighted MR sequences (see Fig. 6.172). Oedema may also be seen in the paratenon, the infrapatellar fat pad, the inferior pole of the patella and subcutaneous fatty tissues. If the process is acute, high signal may be seen without tendon thickening.

In chronic cases, bony erosion can occur at the inferior pole of the patella secondary to the increased vascularity (see Fig. 6.173). Patellar tendinopathy is less commonly triggered by a direct blow, surgery (e.g. arthroscopic portal surgery (see Figs 6.174 and 6.175) or ACL graft harvest site) or, rarely, by a crystal deposition disease such as gout.

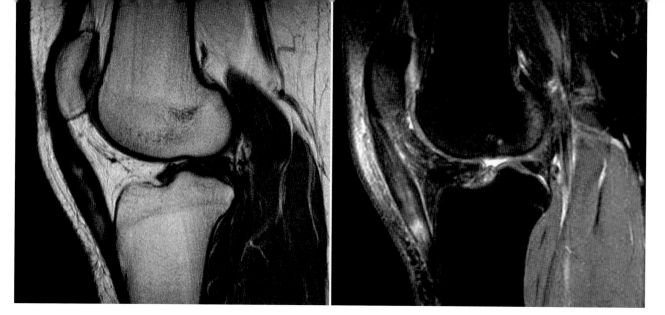

▲ **Fig. 6.174** Marked patellar tendinopathy has occurred secondary to trauma caused by a knee arthroscopic portal. The patellar tendon shows diffuse fusiform swelling and hyperintensity most marked in the mid and distal patellar tendon on both PD and fat-suppressed T2-weighted MR sequences. There is also high signal in the inferior pole of the patella and the infrapatellar fat pad.

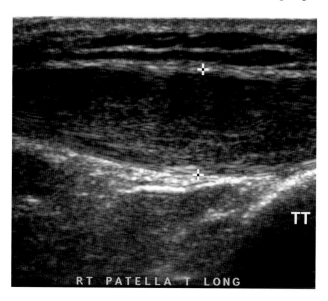

RT PATELLA T LONG

◀ **Fig. 6.175** A long-axis ultrasound image of the case demonstrated in Fig. 6.174 shows marked fusiform swelling and a hypoechoic echotecture typical of a tendinopathy involving the mid patellar tendon (callipers). Tibial tuberosity = TT.

Patellar tendon rupture

A study by Kelly et al. (1984) noted that 60% of patients who sustained a patellar tendon rupture had previously received two to three steroid injections around the patellar tendon. Patellar tendon ruptures will present as patella alta on a lateral plain film (see Fig. 6.176) due to quadriceps retraction. An avulsed fragment is often identified (see Fig. 6.177). Ultrasound (see Fig. 6.178) and MRI (see Fig. 6.179) will provide further information and determine whether the rupture is partial or complete.

▼ **Fig. 6.176** A cross-table lateral view of the knee shows patella alta resulting from retraction of the patella following a tear of the patellar tendon (arrowhead).

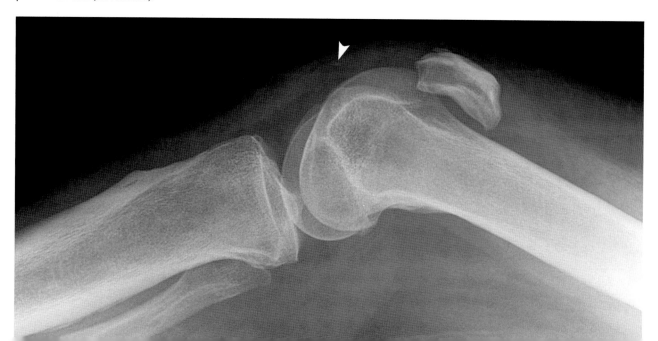

▶ **Fig. 6.177** There has been an avulsion fracture at the inferior pole of the patella with separation of a small fragment (arrowhead). There is moderate anterior displacement of the fragment and the patella–patellar tendon alignment is abnormal. No retraction of the patella has occurred, suggesting that the avulsion is incomplete.

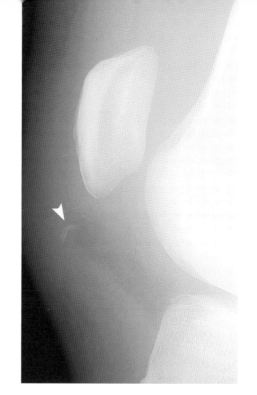

▼ **Fig. 6.178** This athlete presented with acute pain and swelling at the inferior pole of the patella. Long-axis ultrasound images of the symptomatic left knee are shown with the asymptomatic right side for comparison. There is marked swelling of the proximal segment of the left patellar tendon (callipers) and a bone fragment is noted to be avulsed from the inferior pole of the patella (arrow). In addition, on the clinically asymptomatic right side, note the localised enthesial bone surface irregularity with shallow pitting. There is also subtle hypoechoic texture in the adjacent patellar tendon indicative of chronic tendinopathy at the inferior pole of the patella. Patella = P.

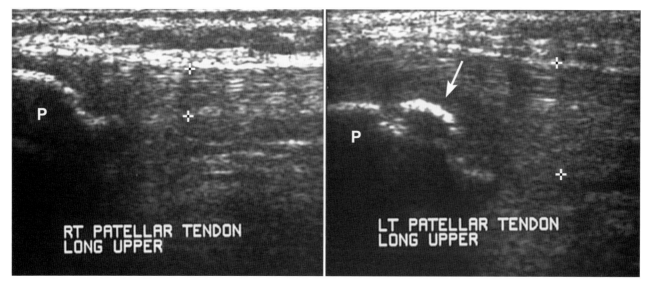

▼ **Fig. 6.179** Sagittal PD and fat-suppressed T2-weighted MR images demonstrate a complete transverse rupture of the proximal patellar tendon. There is retraction and buckling of the distal patellar tendon stump and patella alta results from quadriceps retraction.

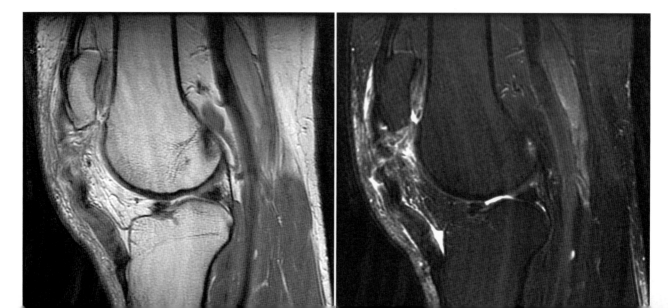

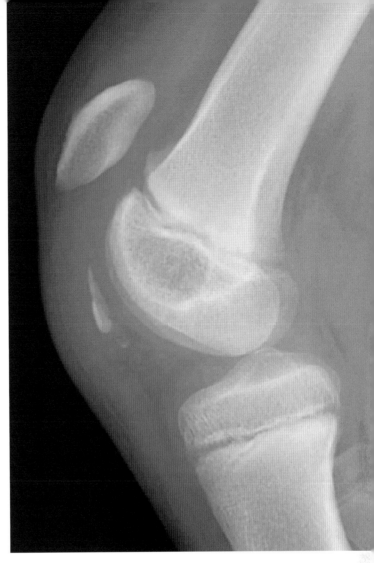

▶ **Fig. 6.180** A sleeve avulsion fracture of the inferior pole of the patella has separated the dorsal lower pole secondary ossification centre together with unossified lower pole centres and articular cartilage. Retraction of the patella has resulted in patella alta.

Patellar sleeve fractures

In the immature athlete, forceful contraction of the quadriceps against a partially flexed knee may cause an avulsion fracture of the inferior pole of the patella. Bony fragments may be separated together with articular cartilage, secondary ossification centres, periosteum and retinaculum (Houghton and Ackeroyd 1979). Bony fragments may be seen on plain films, with MRI necessary to assess whether soft tissues have also been avulsed (see Fig. 6.180). The superior fragment, which may be devoid of much of its articular cartilage, is retracted superiorly (see Figs 6.181–6.184).

The patella and patellofemoral joint

Patellofemoral articulation is the pivotal component of the extensor mechanism of the knee. With flexion, the patella begins to engage the femoral sulcus at about 20° of knee joint flexion. The area of the patella that is in contact with the femur increases as the knee flexes up to 90°. In the first 20° of flexion, soft tissues alone will stabilise the patella, whereas after engagement, bone contact and a compressive force add stability. Kaplan (1962) described static and dynamic stabilisation. Static stability is created by the bony anatomy of the patella and the femoral sulcus, while dynamic stability is provided by the muscles, tendons and ligaments. Laterally the iliotibial band is an important stabiliser of the patellofemoral articulation through fibres that connect the iliotibial tract to the patella, the iliopatellar band. The patellar retinaculum is a further stabiliser of the patellofemoral joint, with medial and lateral components. The lateral retinaculum, the thicker of the two, merges with the patellofemoral ligament and iliopatellar band. On the medial side there are focal thickenings of the capsule referred to as the medial patellofemoral, patellomeniscal and patellotibial ligaments.

The quadriceps pulls the patella in the anatomic axis of the femur and creates a 'Q' angle with the forces acting from the patella to the tibial tuberosity (see Fig. 6.185 on page 473). The Q angle changes from supine to standing in normal subjects (Woodland and Francis 1992). In males the Q angle is 12.7° supine and 15.8° standing, and in females it is 13.6° supine and 17.0° standing. There is an increased incidence of patellar subluxation in knees with a supine Q angle of more than 15°. The quadriceps tendon acts as an anchor to the quadriceps mechanism.

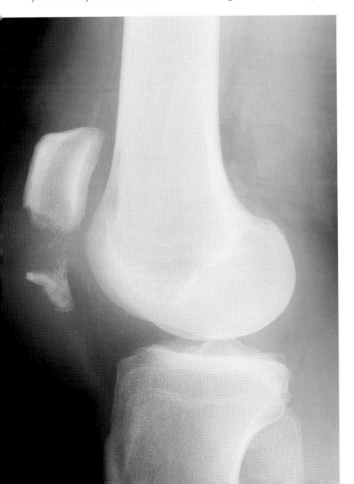

◀ **Fig. 6.181** A further example of a sleeve fracture is demonstrated, with avulsion of a fragment from the lower pole of the patella. This fragment incorporates the secondary ossification centres of the lower pole and a significant segment of articular cartilage. There is separation of the fragments, resulting in buckling of the patellar tendon and superior retraction of the proximal fragment.

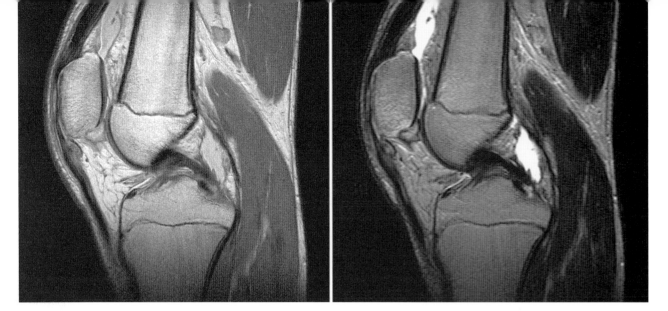

▲ **Fig. 6.182** Sagittal PD and T2-weighted MR images show avulsion of a bony and cartilaginous sleeve from the inferior pole of the patella. A fragment of articular cartilage is also noted to be involved. No retraction of the patella has occurred, presumably due to fibres passing from the patellar tendon over the anterior surface of the patella remaining in continuity with the quadriceps tendon. A moderate effusion is noted.

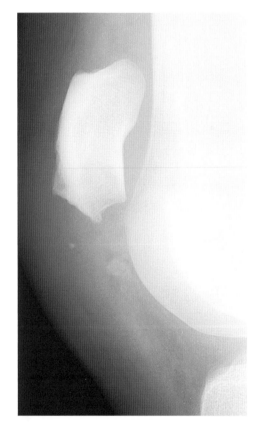

▶ **Fig. 6.183** A number of bone fragments have been avulsed from the inferior pole of the patella, with moderate displacement and considerable resultant soft-tissue swelling. The secondary ossification centre of the dorsal aspect of the inferior pole of the patella has been separated and the appearances are those of a sleeve fracture.

▼ **Fig. 6.184** Sagittal T1-weighted FSE and T2*-weighted GRE MR images show partial avulsion of a secondary ossification centre at the inferior pole of the patella.

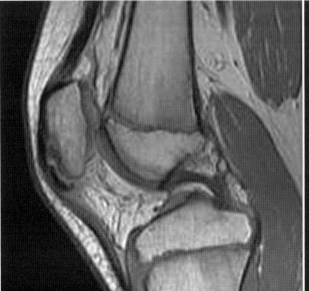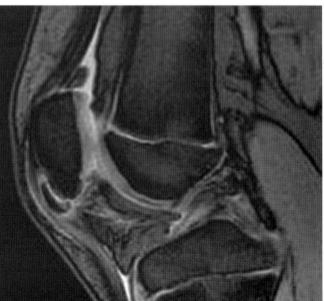

It is important to recognise that many patients with patellar malalignment present with clinically non-specific anterior knee pain and prompt investigation may prevent degenerative changes. Patellofemoral CT (see Fig. 6.186) can be used to accurately select those patients with anterior knee pain who will benefit from realignment surgery and help to select the type of procedure most suited (Shea and Fulkerson 1992; Guzzanti et al. 1994).

If MRI is used to image these patients, oedema may be seen in the infrapatellar fat pad, particularly on axial and sagittal T2-weighted images, immediately deep to the proximal patellar tendon laterally (see Fig. 6.187) (Chung et al. 2001). Fat pad impingement is discussed in greater detail later in the chapter (see page 507).

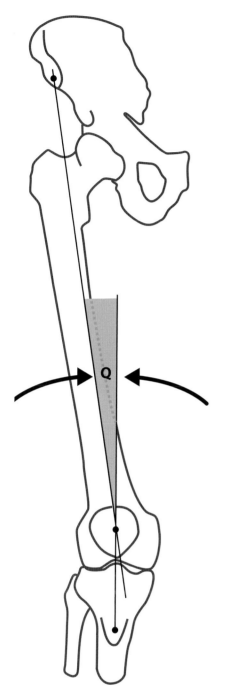

▲ **Fig. 6.185** This line drawing indicates how the Q angle is assessed. The Q angle is the angle between a line joining the anterior superior iliac spine and the patella and a line joining the patella and tibial tubercle.

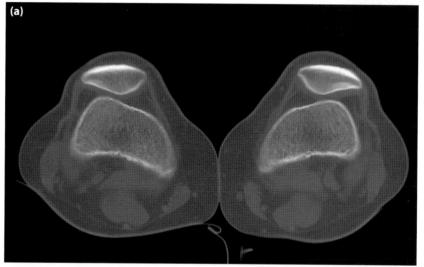

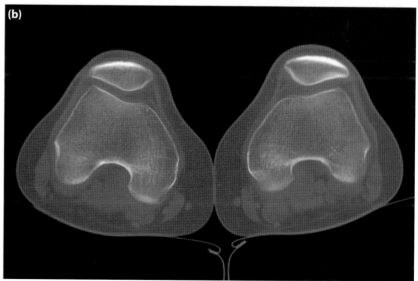

▲ **Fig. 6.186** Patellofemoral CT is particularly useful for assessing patellar subluxation and lateral tilting at knee flexion angles that are too small to be demonstrated by axial plain films. The images shown here have been acquired before the patella engages the femoral sulcus (at less than 30° of knee flexion).
(a) The patellae are horizontal, with lateral subluxation present bilaterally with the quadriceps muscles at rest.
(b) When the quadriceps muscles are contracted, the lateral subluxation is reduced and the patellae remain horizontal. Prominent anteversion is noted.

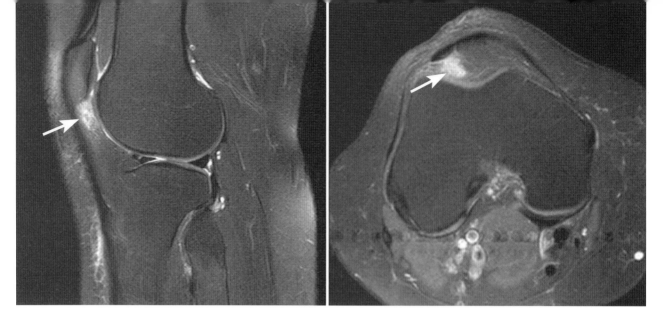

▲ **Fig. 6.187** Sagittal and axial fat-suppressed T2-weighted MR images show localised high signal within the deep infrapatellar fat deep to the inferolateral margin of the patella (arrows). This appearance is typical of fat pad impingement.

Patellar subluxation and dislocation

Patellar instability may be due to bony or soft-tissue causes. Bony causes include anomalies such as a dysplastic patella (see Fig. 6.188), patella alta (see Fig. 6.189), a hypoplastic femoral sulcus (see Fig. 6.190) or an exaggerated Q angle. Soft-tissue causes include a torn medial retinaculum and tight lateral structures. A hypoplastic patella may be a manifestation of 'nail-patella' syndrome (Fong 1946). This syndrome consists of hypoplastic patellae, nail dysplasia, iliac horns, elbow dysplasia and nephropathy (see Fig. 6.191). These anomalies of patella tracking decrease the stability of the patellofemoral articulation and predispose to lateral patellar instability. Patellar subluxation or dislocation can also be the result of acute direct trauma and torsion or valgus stresses applied to the knee.

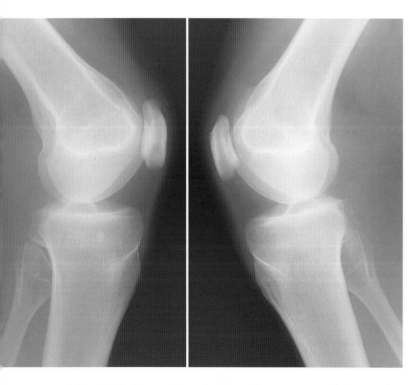

▲ **Fig. 6.188** Bilateral hypoplastic patellae are present. This anomaly predisposes to patellar instability.

▶ **Fig. 6.189** A patella alta is present.

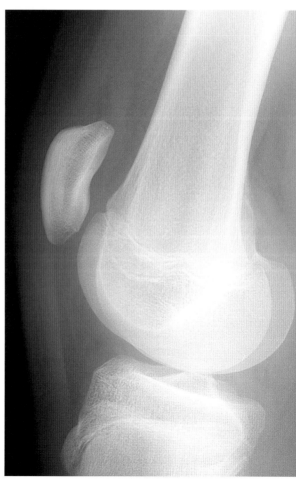

▶ **Fig. 6.190** Hypoplasia of the medial facet of the femoral sulcus will contribute to patellar instability. There is also hypoplasia of the patella and lateral tilting and subluxation of the patella.

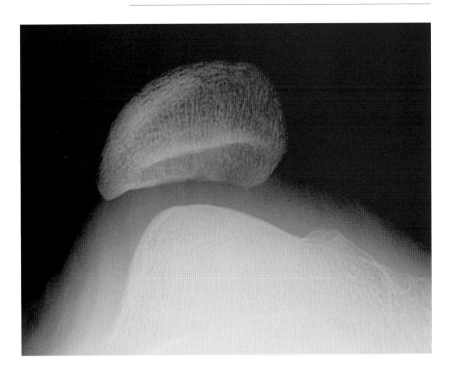

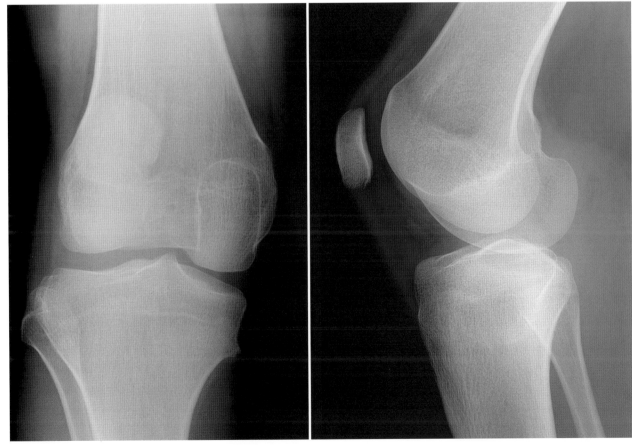

▲ **Fig. 6.191(a)** There is hypoplasia of the patella and the medial femoral condyle.

▶ **(b)** In addition iliac 'horns' are seen on a plain film of the pelvis, indicating that the hypoplastic patella is a manifestation of Fong's Syndrome.

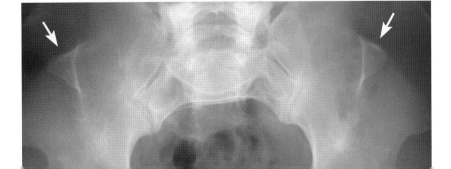

▶ **Fig. 6.192** With 30° of knee flexion, considerable lateral patellar tilting and subluxation is present. As the degree of knee flexion increases from 30 to 60°, the patella progressively engages the femoral sulcus and patellar tilting and subluxation reduce. A traction spur is evident at the patellar attachment of lateral retinaculum. Also note that the orientation of the major stress trabeculae in the patella in this case suggests excessive lateral pressure syndrome.

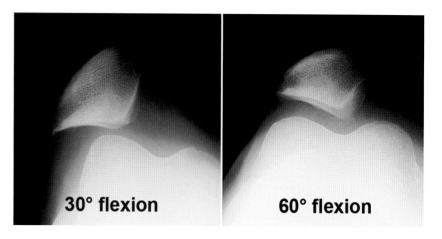

Subluxation of the patella is a transient displacement of the patella, which may occur in early knee flexion and may be accompanied by a lateral patellar tilt. The subluxation commonly occurs in a lateral direction, although medial displacement may also occur (see Fig. 6.192). Subluxation and/or lateral tilting of the patella can be demonstrated by axial CT of the patellofemoral joints obtained at varying degrees of knee flexion at rest with and without quadriceps contraction (see Fig. 6.193). Medial subluxation is uncommon but may be seen as a complication of patellar realignment surgery. Guzzanti et al. (1994) suggested that axial CT with quadriceps contraction should be used to identify those cases of lateral patellar subluxation where lateral release surgery may be complicated by a medial patellar subluxation. On a pre-operative CT examination, this group of patients will show a reduced degree of lateral subluxation with quadriceps contraction when compared with resting images.

Imaging of patellar dislocation is usually requested after relocation of the patella to confirm a successful reduction or residual injury, or to confirm the clinical impression that a transient dislocation has in fact occurred. As previously discussed on pages 419 and 420, following a patellofemoral dislocation, a 'skyline' view of the patella may demonstrate fractures of the medial border of the patella, an osteochondral fracture of the medial articular facet of the patella or an osteochondral fracture of the anterior aspect of the lateral femoral condyle.

▼ **Fig. 6.193** CT can be used to assess patellofemoral alignment at varying degrees of knee flexion and quadriceps contraction.

(a) The patellae show lateral tilt and subluxation at 10° of knee flexion.

(b) At 20° of knee flexion and with the quadriceps muscles relaxed, the right patella returns to normal alignment while the left patella still shows slight lateral tilt and subluxation.

(c) With the knees still flexed to 20° and the quadriceps muscles now contracted, both patellae show normal alignment.

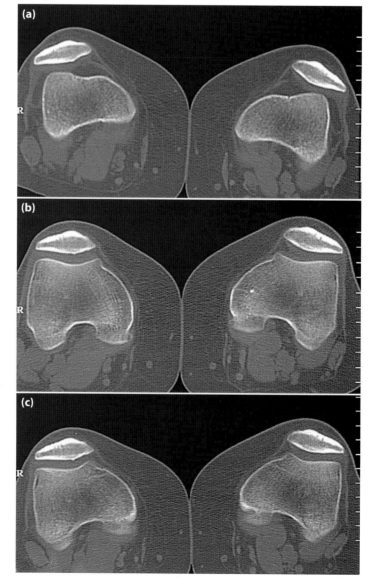

MRI may show changes that are diagnostic of a recent patellofemoral dislocation, including:

- residual subluxation or dislocation (see Fig. 6.194)
- partial or complete rupture of the medial retinaculum (see Fig. 6.195)
- a bone bruise or avulsion fracture of the medial border of the patella and the lateral margin of the lateral femoral condyle (see Fig. 6.196)
- an osteochondral fracture of the medial articular facet of the patella (see Fig. 6.197)
- strain or tear of the vastus medialis
- a large joint effusion.

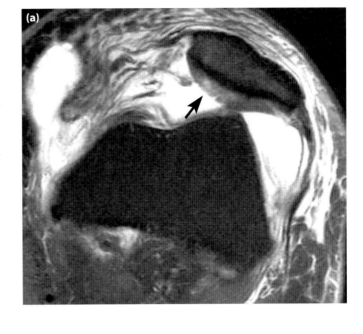

▶ **Fig. 6.194(a)** An axial fat-suppressed T2-weighted MR image shows persisting lateral patellar subluxation with the patella perched on the lateral articular rim of the femoral trochlear groove. The medial patellar retinaculum is torn and there is injury to the articular cartilage of the medial facet of the patella evidenced by hyperintensity and swelling of the chondral segment (arrow). This segment also shows chondral fissuring.

▶ **(b)** Imaging is occasionally performed if reduction is difficult, rather than as an aid to the diagnosis. It is possible that a fracture fragment could prevent relocation. In this case, no cause for a difficult reduction can be seen.

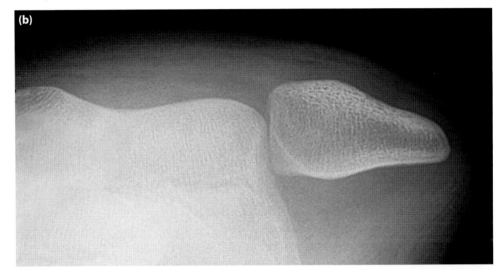

▶ **Fig. 6.195** An axial fat-suppressed PD-weighted MR image demonstrates complete rupture of the medial patellar retinaculum (arrow), resulting from a previous dislocation.

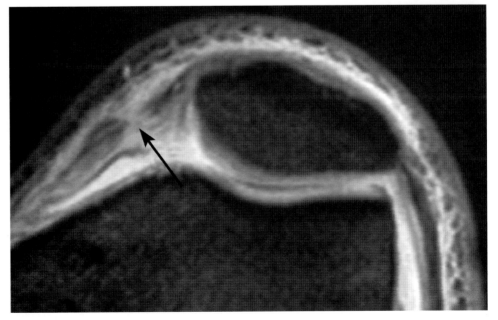

Meniscal pathology

Meniscal anatomy

The menisci are 'C'-shaped discs of fibrocartilage located within the medial and lateral compartments of the knee. Both menisci effectively increase the tibial articular surface area and contribute to stability by supplying a congruent surface for the femoral condyles. The menisci move with flexion and extension of the knee, moving posteriorly with flexion and anteriorly with extension. The semimembranosus and popliteus are thought to contribute to and stabilise this movement.

The medial meniscus is semicircular, attached to the tibia through both its anterior and posterior horns, and the more posterior fibres of the anterior horn are attached to the transverse ligament. The lateral aspect is attached to the deep medial ligament, which is a condensation of the joint capsule and semimembranosus tendon sheath. The lateral meniscus is almost circular, is also attached to the tibia anteriorly and posteriorly, and is loosely attached to the joint capsule peripherally by meniscocapsular ligaments. The lateral meniscus is not attached to the LCL. With advancing age, myxoid degeneration of fibrocartilage is commonly demonstrated by ultrasound or MRI, seen as an inhomogeneity in the meniscus (see Fig. 6.198). The meniscus may appear swollen, with the degenerative changes producing bulging.

Discoid meniscus

A discoid meniscus is an anomalous thickened disc-like meniscus, which occurs most frequently in the lateral compartment of the knee (see Fig. 6.199), but may occasionally be seen involving the medial meniscus (see Fig. 6.200). This anomaly is seen in approximately 3% of people, and when present may be bilateral. As a result of its abnormal morphology, a discoid meniscus is prone to tears. These usually present with the features of a meniscal tear, but a discoid meniscus may also be the source of an audible 'snap', which may indicate a Wrisberg's variant of a discoid meniscus, in which the posterior horn is not attached to the joint capsule and, as a result, is excessively mobile. A tear in a discoid meniscus should be remembered as a cause of pain in the adolescent knee. The radiographic diagnosis is suspected when there is widening of the lateral compartment and flattening of the lateral femoral condyle on an AP view of the knee (see Fig. 6.201).

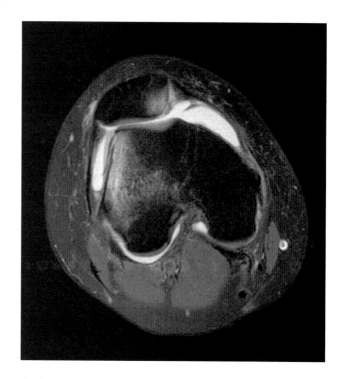

▲ **Fig. 6.196** An axial fat-suppressed T2-weighted MR image shows the typical pattern of bone contusion seen following patellofemoral dislocation. The dislocating patella impacts against the lateral surface of the lateral femoral condyle, as seen in Fig. 6.194(b). This impaction may produce bone bruising of both the medial border of the patella and the anterior aspect of the lateral femoral condyle. No discrete fracture line can be seen. Also note the hypoplastic femoral groove and medial patellar facet. There is also mild injury to the patellar attachment of the medial retinaculum and a large knee joint effusion has developed.

MRI will establish the diagnosis of a discoid meniscus (Silverman et al. 1989). It is present when the transverse width of a meniscus is greater than 14 mm (Araki et al. 1994). MRI is less accurate at diagnosing tears in discoid menisci than in normally shaped menisci (Ryu et al. 1998) (see Figs 6.202 and 6.203).

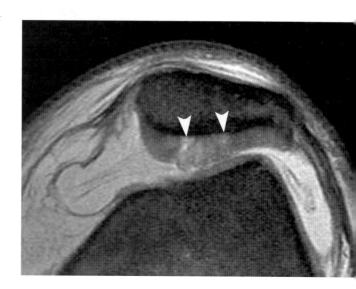

▶ **Fig. 6.197** Following lateral patellar dislocation, an axial fat-suppressed PD-weighted MR image shows injury to the articular cartilage of the patella. There is chondral swelling and variable hyperintensity with a bright linear focus of fluid signal at the median patellar ridge indicating deep chondral fissures (arrowheads). The subchondral bone appears normal. Note the hypoplastic medial patellar facet, knee joint effusion and mild persisting lateral patellar subluxation.

▶ **Fig. 6.198** On this sagittal T1-weighted MR image, an area of intermediate signal in the posterior horn of the medial meniscus indicates myxoid degeneration (arrow). The abnormal intra-meniscal signal does not extend to the articular surface. This is a key imaging feature that helps to differentiate meniscal degeneration from a tear. Meniscal degeneration is a common MRI finding.

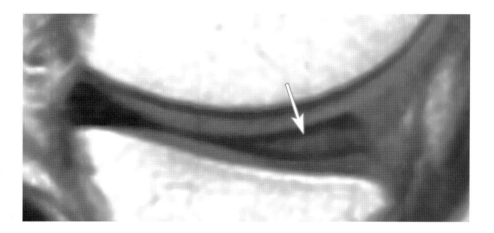

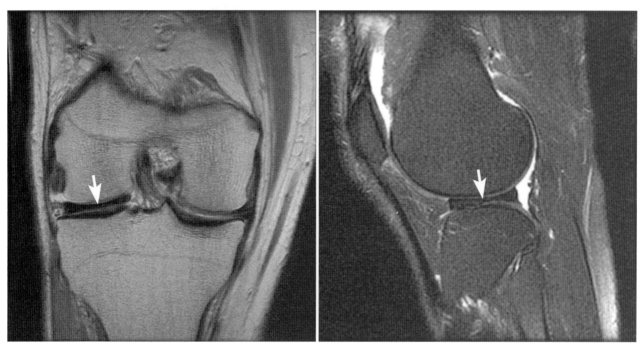

▲ **Fig. 6.199** **(a)** Coronal PD and sagittal fat-suppressed T2-weighted MR images demonstrate a discoid lateral meniscus (arrows). This case also shows the features of a Wrisberg variant (see text). The sagittal image shows a fluid space posterior to the meniscus with no identifiable bridging meniscocapsular attachments.

▶ **(b)** A lateral discoid meniscus is demonstrated by CT arthrography. A reformatted coronal image shows the meniscal silhouette traversing the full width of the central joint space (arrowheads).

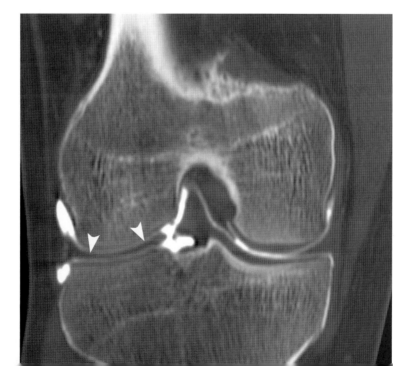

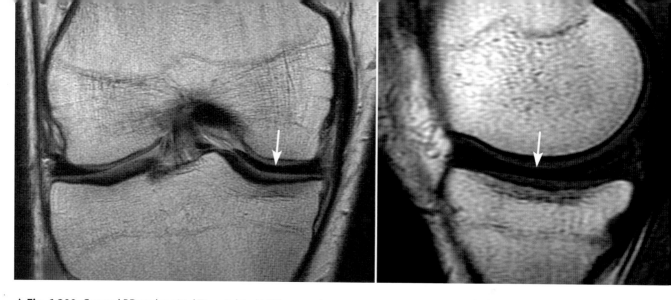

▲ **Fig. 6.200** Coronal PD and sagittal T1-weighted MR images demonstrate an uncommon medial compartment discoid meniscus (arrows). On the sagittal image, note the myxoid degeneration in the posterior horn, which does not extend to a meniscal surface.

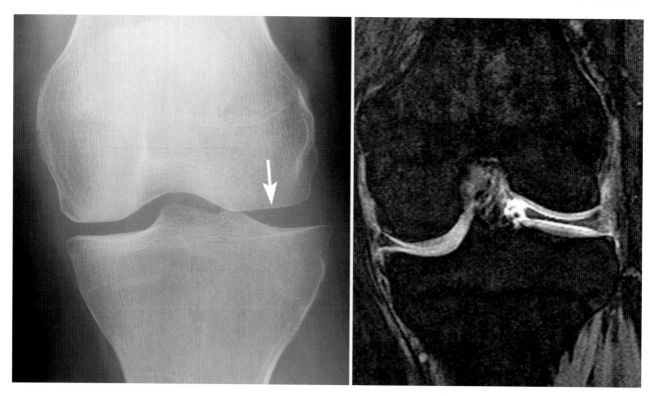

▲ **Fig. 6.201** The presence of a discoid meniscus can be suspected on plain films when the lateral femoral condyle shows a flattened articular surface (arrow) together with slight widening of the lateral compartment joint space. In this case, the discoid lateral meniscus is confirmed by a coronal fat-suppressed T2-weighted MR image. There is increased signal within the meniscus, consistent with mucoid degeneration. No tear can be seen.

▶ **Fig. 6.202** This sagittal PD-weighted MR image demonstrates another example of a Wrisberg variant lateral meniscus, with discoid morphology and developmental posterior horn meniscocapsular separation. There is an oblique tear involving the anterior horn (arrow).

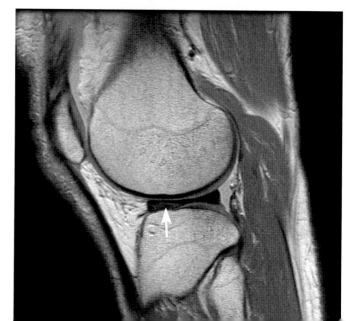

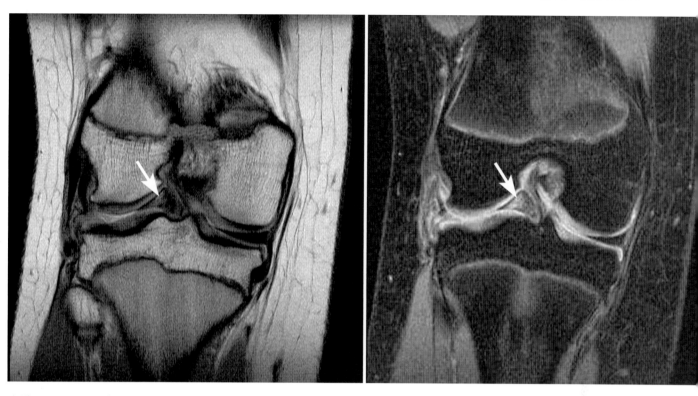

▲ **Fig. 6.203 (a)** In this case, discoid lateral and medial menisci are present. The medial meniscus has a transverse meniscal dimension exceeding the normal upper limit of 14 mm suggested by Araki et al. (1994) (see text). Coronal PD and fat-suppressed T2-weighted MR images show a bucket-handle tear of the discoid lateral meniscus in which the entire meniscus has become displaced into the intercondylar notch (arrow).

▼ **(b)** In another case, sagittal and coronal fat-suppressed T2-weighted images demonstrate extensive mucoid degeneration in a discoid lateral meniscus with a complicating horizontal cleavage tear (arrow). Note both intrameniscal and parameniscal cyst formation (arrowhead).

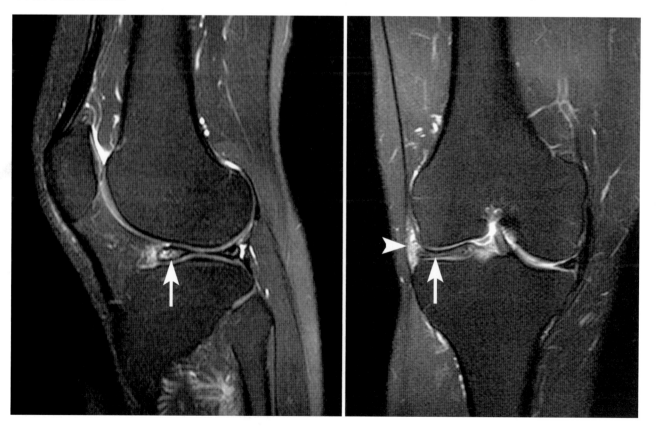

Meniscal ossicles

A rounded focus of post-traumatic or possibly developmental ossification is occasionally found within a meniscus (see Fig. 6.204). Meniscal ossicles may occur in any position, but are most common at the posterior horn of the medial meniscus. They are clearly differentiated from loose bodies or osteochondral fragments by MRI (Schnarkowski et al. 1995) (see Fig. 6.205).

Meniscal tears

Meniscal tears are classified by type and position.

- A degenerative meniscus has a frayed edge.
- When a meniscal tear develops at the medial edge and extends along the line of the radius of the circular meniscus, this is known as a radial tear.
- If a radial tear becomes chronic and the tear margins become worn and rounded, the tear may become

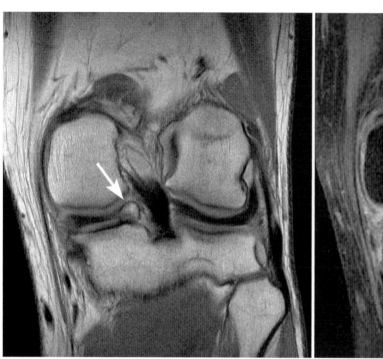
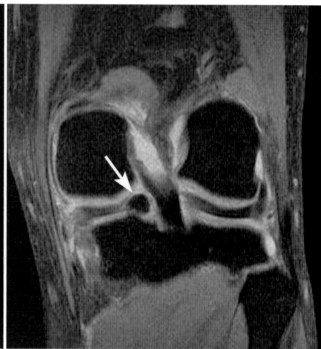

▲ **Fig. 6.204** Coronal PD and fat-suppressed T2-weighted MR images demonstrate a meniscal ossicle in the lateral aspect of the medial meniscus (arrow).

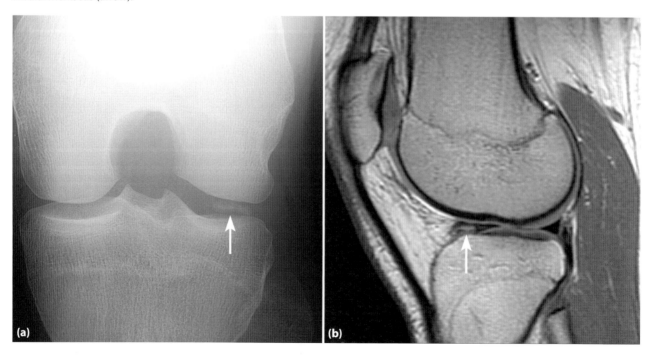

▲ **Fig. 6.205(a)** Linear ossification is projected over the lateral compartment of the knee on an intercondylar plain film (arrow).
(b) This is a meniscal ossicle in the anterior horn of the lateral meniscus, confirmed by a sagittal T1-weighted MR image (arrow).

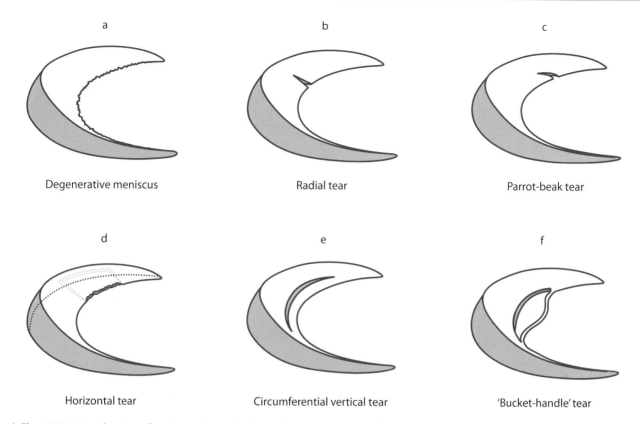

a	b	c
Degenerative meniscus	Radial tear	Parrot-beak tear

d	e	f
Horizontal tear	Circumferential vertical tear	'Bucket-handle' tear

▲ **Fig. 6.206** Line drawing of patterns of meniscal tears demonstrate the various orientations and nomenclature.

more oblique and develop a hard, rounded edge, like a parrot's beak.

- A circumferential tear follows the curvature of the meniscus and may extend from one surface to the other. If this occurs, displacement of the free-edge fragment may occur and this creates a so-called 'bucket-handle' tear.
- A split through the meniscus in the horizontal plane is known as a cleavage tear. Until a cleavage tear extends to an articular surface, the meniscus will appear normal to arthroscopy, although the cleavage tear is evident on MRI.

Degenerative tears become more frequent with advancing age and are usually horizontal in type, whereas traumatic tears are common in younger patients and are usually vertical in type, although sometimes there are longitudinal, radial or oblique extensions along the meniscus (see Fig. 6.206). It is the clinical setting rather than the imaging appearance that determines the significance of a tear, as asymptomatic tears are common (Zanetti et al. 2003). However, tears that are vertical, radial, complex, displaced or associated with adjacent bone marrow oedema are more likely to be symptomatic.

The role of imaging in the management of a clinically symptomatic meniscal tear is to help exclude other pathology, such as an osteochondral fracture which can mimic or accompany an injured meniscus. Imaging also assists the surgeon to decide between primary meniscal repair and partial meniscectomy as a treatment option, by accurately describing the type, position and extent of the tear. The goal is to preserve meniscal tissue whenever possible. Tears involving the outer two-thirds of a meniscus, such as peripheral vertical or radial tears and meniscocapsular separations, may be candidates for surgical repair.

Meniscocapsular separation may occur at the posterior horn of the lateral meniscus, where fascicles (or struts) normally attach the lateral meniscus to the lateral capsule coursing around the popliteal tendon sheath (see Fig. 6.207). Usually,

▼ **Fig. 6.207** A sagittal fat-suppressed T2-weighted MR image shows the popliteus tendon (arrow) passing between two struts (arrowheads). The struts secure the lateral meniscus to the lateral capsule.

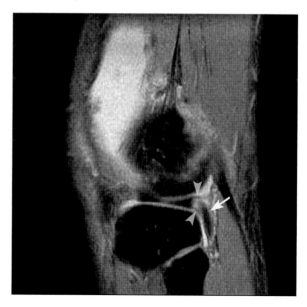

ruptured struts will heal during a minimum six-week trial of conservative management. However, when this approach fails, a small percentage requires reattachment. Patients will usually complain of mechanical locking episodes (Simonian et al. 1997).

Although CT arthrography can demonstrate meniscal tears (see Fig. 6.208), MRI is a better imaging test because it is less invasive, more accurate and can demonstrate displaced meniscal fragments, intrasubstance meniscal changes, parameniscal cysts and other associated injuries.

MRI's sensitivity and specificity for the detection of meniscal tear are decreased in the presence of meniscal chondrocalcinosis. Chondrocalcinosis may appear as intra-meniscal high signal intensity on T1-weighted, proton density and STIR sequences, and correlation of MRI with plain films is required to avoid this potential error (Kaushik et al. 2001).

A gallery of meniscal tears

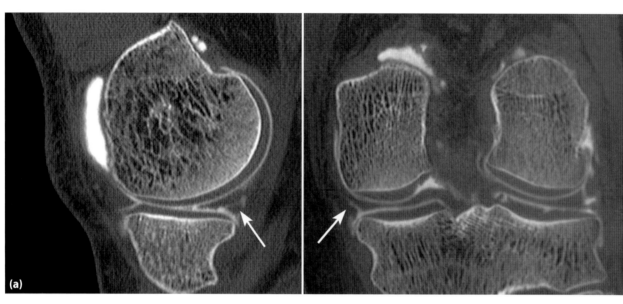

(a)

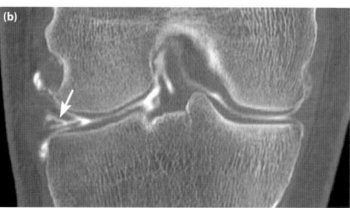

(b)

▲▶▼ **Fig. 6.208** CT arthrography is an effective imaging method for demonstrating meniscal tears. **(a)** Reformatted sagittal and coronal images show a tear in the posterior horn of the medial meniscus extending to the inferior meniscal surface (arrows). **(b)** A cleavage tear of the lateral meniscus (arrow) is demonstrated on a coronal CT arthrographic image. **(c)** CT arthrography, with sagittal and coronal reformations, demonstrates a radial tear of the body of the lateral meniscus (arrowheads). An additional horizontal component of the tear extends towards the capsular surface.

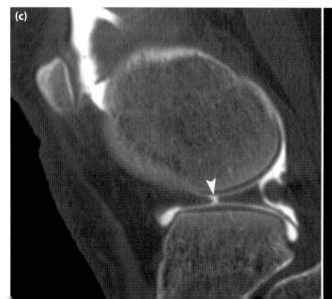

(c)

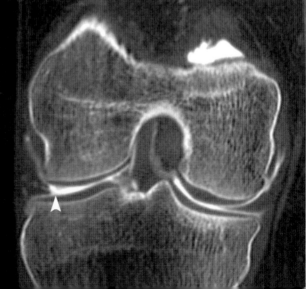

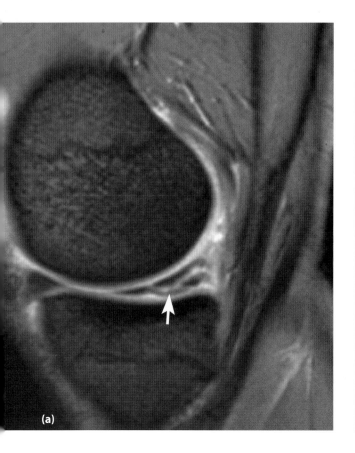
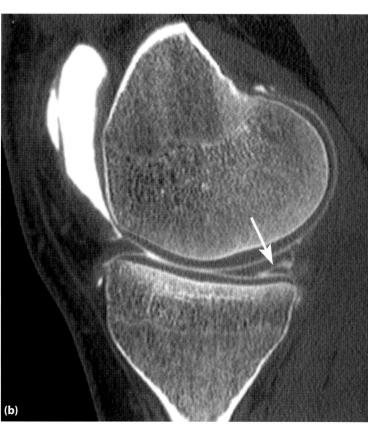

▲ **Fig. 6.209(a)** A sagittal T2*-weighted GRE MR image demonstrates an oblique tear of the posterior horn of the medial meniscus which involves both the superior and inferior meniscal surfaces (arrow). **(b)** Another example of an oblique tear of the posterior horn of the medial meniscus is demonstrated using a sagittal reformation from a CT arthrogram (arrow).

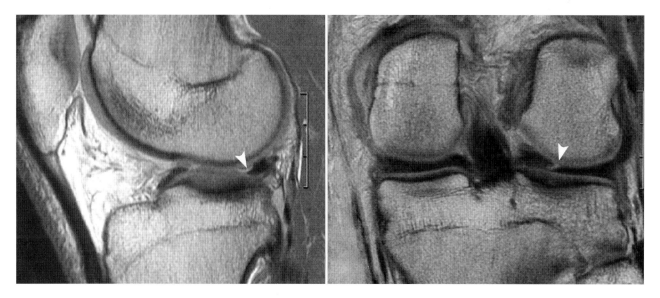

▲ **Fig. 6.210** Sagittal and coronal PD-weighted MR images show a small oblique radial (or parrot-beak) tear of the posterior horn of the lateral meniscus (arrowheads).

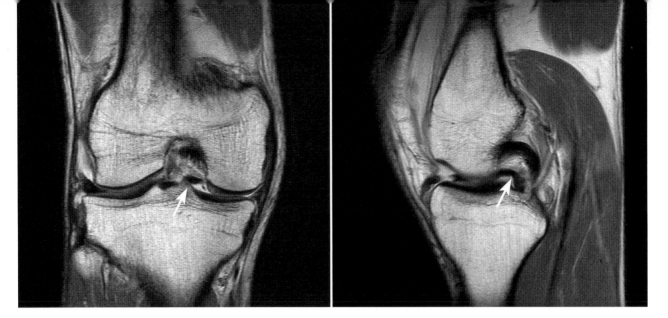

▲ **Fig. 6.211** Coronal and sagittal PD-weighted MR images demonstrate the typical appearances of a displaced 'bucket-handle' tear of the medial meniscus. In the coronal image, the bucket-handle fragment is shown to be displaced into the intercondylar notch (arrow), and on the sagittal image there is a diagnostic 'double PCL' sign present. The apparent second (inferior) PCL is the 'bucket-handle' fragment (arrow).

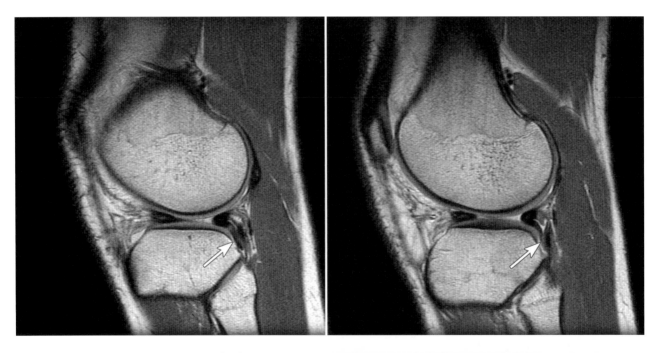

▲ **Fig. 6.212** Contiguous sagittal PD-weighted MR images show a tear of the posterior horn of the lateral meniscus. A meniscal fragment has become displaced into the sheath of the popliteus (arrows).

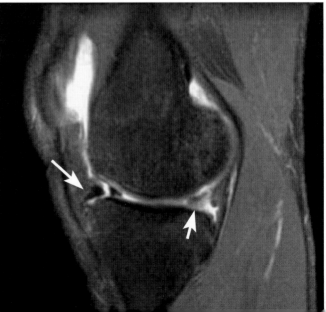

▶ **Fig. 6.213** A sagittal fat-suppressed T2-weighted MR image shows a flipped meniscal fragment (long arrow), which has become separated from the posterior horn of the medial meniscus and lies in a displaced position adjacent to the native anterior horn. Note the abnormal remnant 'ghost' of the native posterior horn (short arrow).

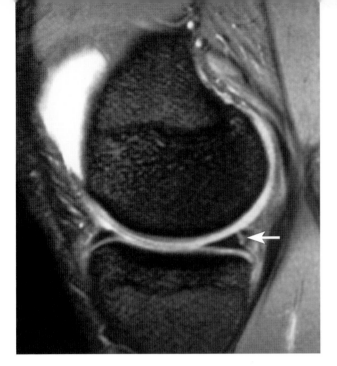

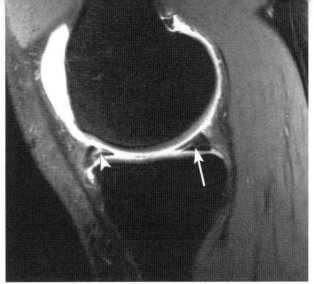

▲ Fig. 6.215 There are complex tears of the medial meniscus. The anterior horn shows both horizontal and vertical tear components (arrowhead), while the posterior horn shows a horizontal cleavage tear (arrow). The tears contain fluid and are well resolved on this fat-suppressed and heavily T2-weighted sagittal image.

▲ Fig. 6.214 A peripheral vertical tear of the posterior horn of the medial meniscus (arrow) is demonstrated on a sagittal T2*-weighted GRE MR image.

▶ Fig. 6.216 Saggital PD-weighted MR images have been obtained nine months apart through the same segment of the posterior horn of the medial meniscus. The initial image on the left shows an undisplaced vertical tear at the base of the mid-posterior horn (arrow). The progress image on the right shows a healed tear with scar tissue now bridging the previous defect (arrowhead). This illustrates the potential of the vascularised meniscal periphery for repair. It also shows the subtlety of signal change which, in the absence of previous imaging for comparison, may be the only clue to an old healed or more recent healing meniscal tear.

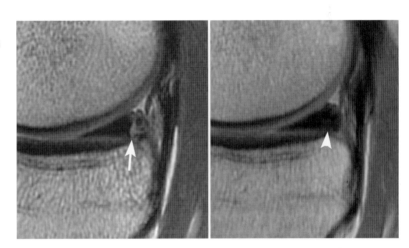

▼ Fig. 6.217 A seven-year-old boy suffered a valgus injury to the medial side of the knee. Coronal PD-weighted images show irregular thickening and intermediate signal indicative of injury to the meniscofemoral ligament (arrows). The meniscotibial ligament and superficial fibres of the MCL appear intact.

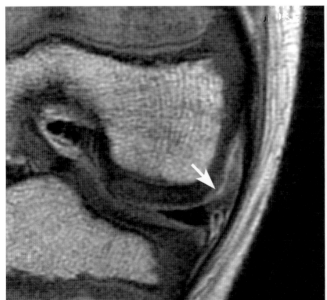

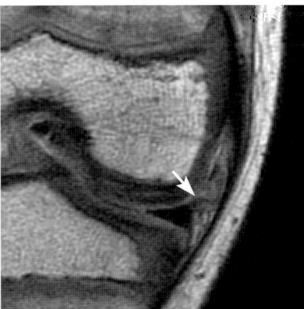

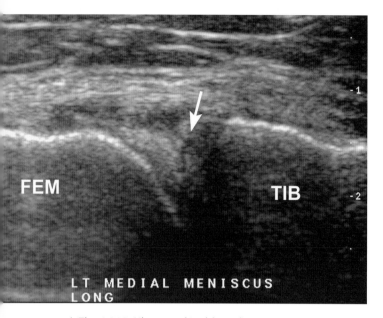

▲ **Fig. 6.218** Ultrasound is able to demonstrate some peripheral meniscal tears. A coronal image demonstrates a horizontal cleavage tear of the medial meniscus. The tear is shown as a linear hypoechoic cleft within an otherwise echogenic meniscal background (arrow). FEM = femur. TIB = tibia.

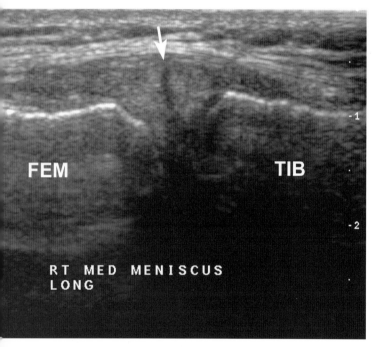

▲ **Fig. 6.219** A further example of a cleavage tear demonstrated by ultrasound (arrow). Also note the associated mild degenerative meniscal bulge in this case. FEM = femur. TIB = tibia.

Meniscal and parameniscal cysts

Meniscal and parameniscal cysts contain mucinous material and usually arise from degenerative meniscal tears of the horizontal cleavage type. They can be imaged by either ultrasound (see Fig. 6.220) or MRI (see Fig. 6.221). They occur with similar frequency medially and laterally. The most important

imaging feature is the connection of the cyst to a meniscal tear. This distinguishes it from other fluid collections such as a pes anserine bursa on the medial side. They are frequently septated and although usually anechoic on ultrasound and of fluid signal intensity on MRI, they may have echogenic areas on sonography and complex signal characteristics on MRI due to the presence of haemorrhage or proteinaceous fluid (see Fig. 6.222). Occasionally, a longstanding parameniscal cyst will erode the adjacent femoral or tibial bone surface (see Fig. 6.223).

Meniscal and parameniscal cysts should be differentiated from synovial cysts and Baker's cysts. Synovial or ganglion cysts may arise from a defect in the knee joint capsule and possess a 'neck' of communication with the joint space which can be well demonstrated by MR arthrography. Synovial cysts are not associated with meniscal tears (Burk et al. 1988).

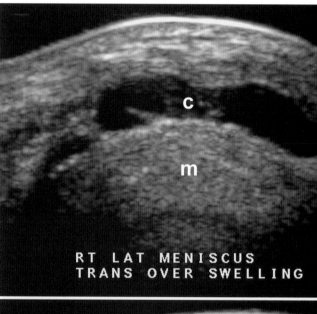

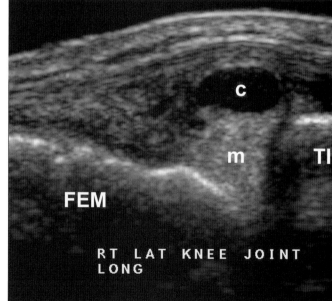

▲ **Fig. 6.220** Transverse and long-axis ultrasound images demonstrate a parameniscal cyst (c) at the lateral joint line. Lateral meniscus = m. Femur = FEM. Tibia = TIB.

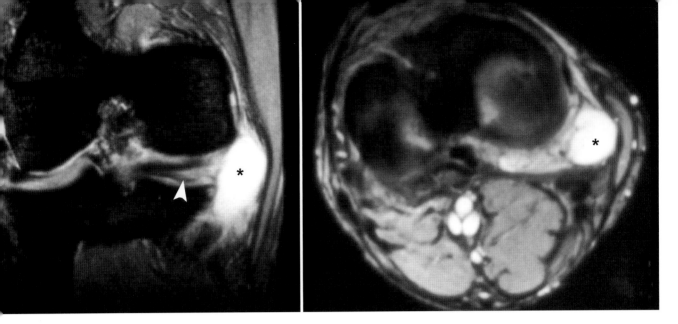

▲ **Fig. 6.221(a)** Coronal and axial T2*-weighted GRE images show a cleavage tear of the medial meniscus with an associated intrameniscal cystic change (arrowhead) and communication with an unusually large parameniscal cyst at the posteromedial joint line (asterisk). High signal extending inferiorly from the cyst suggests either leakage or recent aspiration.

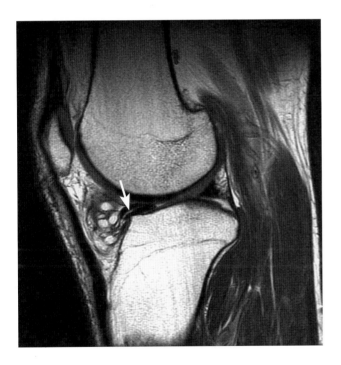

▲ **(b)** A sagittal PD-weighted MR image demonstrates a multiloculated parameniscal cyst associated with a cleavage tear of the anterior horn of the lateral meniscus (arrow).

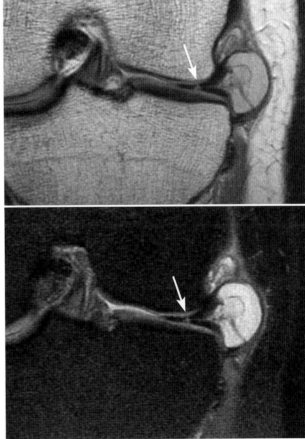

▶ **Fig. 6.222** Coronal PD and fat-suppressed T2-weighted MR images demonstrate a parameniscal cyst associated with a complex tear of the lateral meniscus. The meniscal tear shows both vertical and horizontal components (arrows). The cyst shows internal septation.

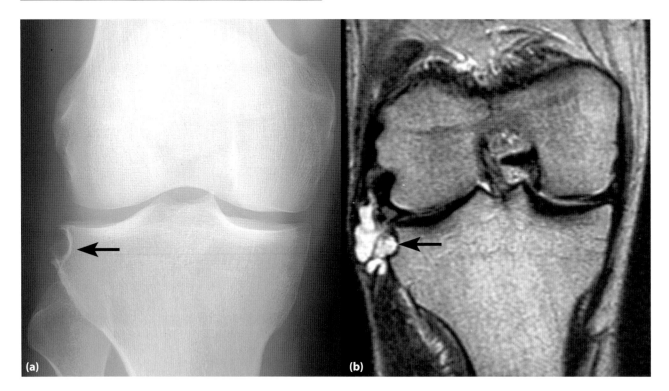

▲ **Fig. 6.223(a)** A plain film shows a cortical defect in the lateral margin of the lateral tibial condyle (arrow). This erosion has resulted from pressure from a parameniscal cyst and is a favoured site of such erosions. The margin of the defect is well corticated, indicating the chronic nature of the process. **(b)** The presence of a lobulated parameniscal cyst is confirmed on a coronal T2-weighted MR image (arrow). The cyst is associated with a cleavage tear of the lateral meniscus.

Disorders of the articular cartilage

Osteoarthrosis (OA) and chondromalacia patellae are important disorders of the articular cartilage of the knee. Chondral and osteochondral fractures may also occur in the knee and result from trauma that is often sports related.

Osteoarthrosis of the knee

The earliest and most characteristic radiographic feature of osteoarthrosis is loss of joint space due to wearing and thinning of the articular cartilage. Later features may include bony sclerosis, subchondral cyst formation associated with

▼ **Fig. 6.224** Sagittal PD and fat-suppressed T2-weighted MR images demonstrate changes of an osteochondral injury on the anterior aspect of the lateral femoral condyle due to trauma six months previously. A large full-thickness chondral defect is present (long arrows) with associated subchondral cyst formation and marrow oedema. Fluid extends beneath an unstable chondral flap at the superior margin of the full-thickness cartilage defect (arrowhead). There is also subchondral cystic change associated with a chondral fissure on the lateral tibial condyle (short arrow).

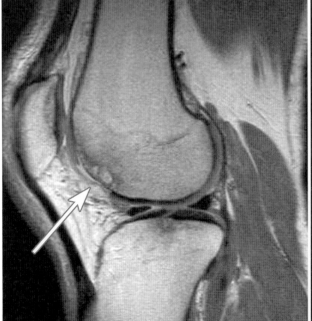
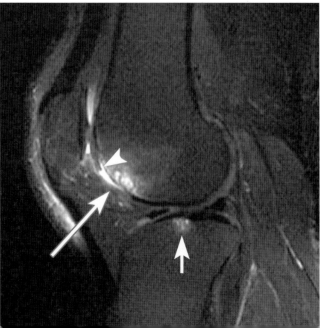

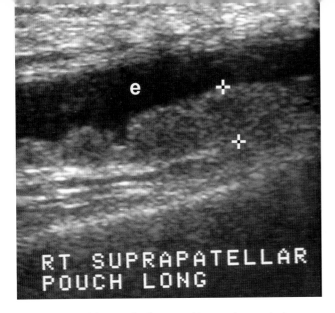

RT SUPRAPATELLAR POUCH LONG

▲ **Fig. 6.225** A long-axis ultrasound image demonstrates effusion (e) and synovitis (callipers) in the suprapatellar recess of the knee joint.

weightbearing areas of the joint and osteophyte formation at the joint margins (see Fig. 6.224). Synovial proliferation may also occur in OA and is sufficiently pronounced in some cases to be imaged by ultrasound or MRI (see Figs 6.225 and 6.226).

The plain film assessment of cartilage is limited to the indirect evidence of cartilage thinning, resulting in joint space narrowing. As discussed previously, a standard weightbearing AP view does not give a true indication of cartilage wear in the knee. A PA weightbearing view of each knee, as described by Rosenberg et al. (1988), should be a routine part of any knee series assessing degenerative changes. The method of acquiring this view is discussed on pages 397–8.

Arthrography and CT arthrography (see Fig. 6.227) are able to define the surface features of the articular cartilage, but are not commonly used in clinical practice. Arthroscopy, which allows direct probing of the cartilage in addition to direct visualisation, is often used for diagnostic purposes. MRI has

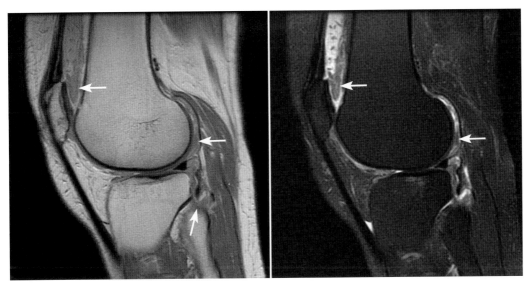

▲ **Fig. 6.226** Sagittal PD and fat-suppressed T2-weighted MR images demonstrate a generalised synovitis extending throughout the knee joint and also involving the proximal tibiofibular joint (arrows).

▼ **Fig. 6.227** Reformatted coronal and sagittal CT-arthrographic images demonstrate marked wear of the articular cartilage along the central weightbearing area of the medial femoral condyle (arrows).

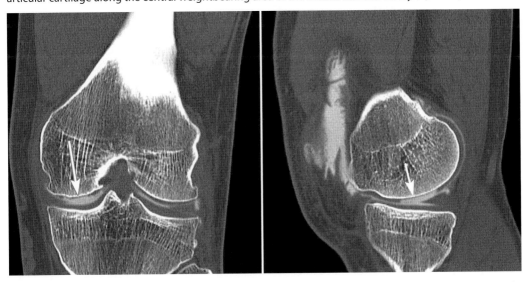

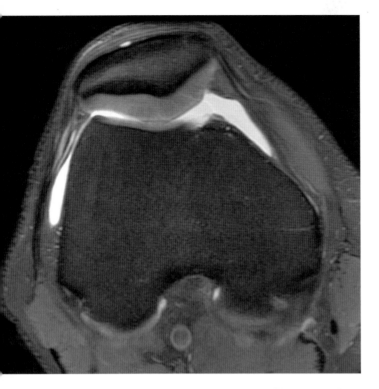

▲ Fig. 6.228 The normal layered anatomy of hyaline cartilage is well demonstrated on this axial fat-suppressed PD-weighted MR image of the patella. The lamina splendans is a thin superficial layer of low signal intensity that constitutes the normal gliding surface of the joint (see the section on chondral fractures on page 494). Deep to this is the transitional layer, a thin subsurface zone of high signal that is designed to resist compressive forces. Beneath this, the deep radial layer is a thick zone of intermediate signal that distributes loading and resists compression. Finally, a calcified cartilage layer separates the deep radial layer from bone. This cannot be differentiated on MR imaging.

also been used to examine the profile of cartilage. However, recent developments in MRI technology offer a method of imaging the internal structure of the cartilage as well as the surface contours.

On MRI, normal cartilage has a trilaminar appearance on PD and T2-weighted sequences, with a higher signal transitional layer separating a thin low signal intensity superficial layer (the lamina splendans) and a thicker low signal intensity zone adjacent to the subchondral bone (see Fig. 6.228). The appearances of the articular cartilage are influenced by its orientation to the main magnetic field (the magic angle effect). Numerous pulse sequences have been advocated for the assessment of the articular cartilage, including fat-saturated 3D SPGR imaging and FSE PD and T2-weighted imaging sequences with and without fat suppression. Sensitivities of greater than 90% have been described for both techniques (Bredella et al. 1999). Degenerative disease is seen as cartilage thinning of variable degree. Alteration in cartilage signal intensity includes basal layer foci of high signal on PD and T2-weighted sequences, together with both subchondral sclerosis and oedema. Traumatic chondral lesions appear as solitary defects with acute angles (see Fig. 6.229).

New techniques in MR imaging have shown sensitivity to specific structural and biochemical components of the articular cartilage. Variations in T2 relaxation times may be related to local alterations in collagen, with T2 values increasing with the severity of OA (Dunn et al. 2004). A delayed imaging technique following injection of IV gadolinium measures the glycosaminoglycan content within cartilage, with abnormal regions of cartilage having relatively high glycosaminoglycan content (Williams et al. 2004).

Multislice CT following the injection of intra-articular contrast has also shown promise for the assessment of cartilage (Vande Berg et al. 2002). The high spatial resolution allows accurate detection of subtle changes to the superficial layer

▼ Fig. 6.229 Sagittal PD and fat-suppressed T2-weighted MR images show a deficiency of articular cartilage along the weightbearing area of the medial femoral condyle, and joint fluid directly abuts the articular cortex of the condyle (arrows). Subchondral bone marrow oedema is present. There is also thinning of the articular cartilage over the anterior third of the medial tibial condyle (arrowheads).

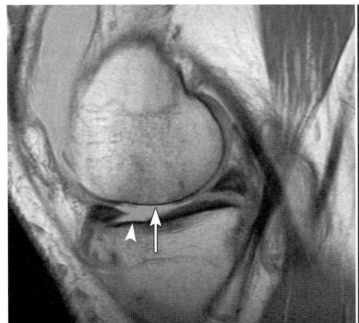
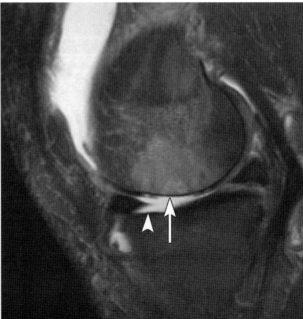

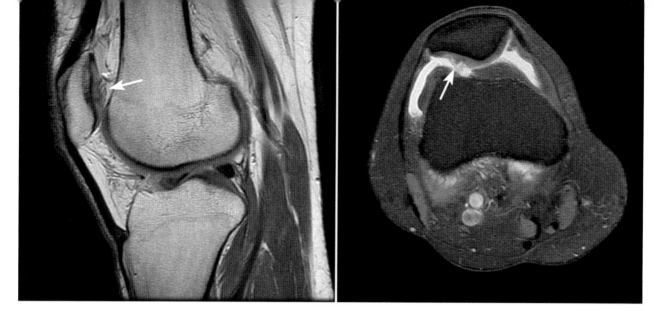

▲ **Fig. 6.230** Sagittal PD and axial fat-suppressed T2-weighted MR images demonstrate Grade II–III changes of chondromalacia patellae. There is deep chondral fibrillation and a focus of chondral ulceration on the lateral patellar facet (arrows). The trochlear cartilage is normal. The MRI grading system for chondromalacia patellae is discussed in Chapter 1 (see page 5).

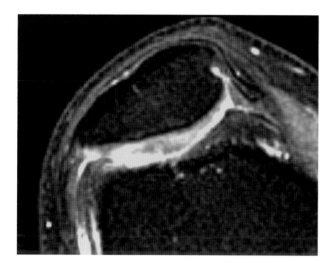

▲ **Fig. 6.231(a)** Changes of chondromalacia patellae are displayed on an axial fat-suppressed T2-weighted MR image. There is a variable degree of chondral wear and softening with deep ulceration on both the medial and lateral patellar facets.

of articular cartilage. However, the changes in the basal layer cannot be visualised. These changes may precede superficial cartilage ulceration.

Chondromalacia patellae

Chondromalacia patellae, or 'softening' of the articular cartilage, is poorly understood. This condition may be a source of anterior knee pain but is not always symptomatic. The articular cartilage of the patella may develop fibrillation, fasciculation, blistering and ulceration. These chondral changes may ultimately lead to secondary OA. However, Radin (1979) suggests that chondromalacia patellae does not inevitably result in OA. Chondromalacia patellae may be localised or global, and there are a large number of possible aetiological factors. Changes confined to the lateral patellar facet are often due to excessive lateral pressure syndrome or reflex sympathetic dystrophy. The causes of medial facet chondromalacia patellae are more obscure, but a history of trauma can be elicited in about 50% of cases. MRI may show subchondral bone changes or joint space narrowing at the site of chondromalacia patellae due to compressibility or erosion of the soft articular cartilage (see Figs 6.230 and. 6.231).

▶ **(b)** An axial fat-suppressed T2-weighted MR image demonstrates advanced chondral wear along the articular surfaces of the patella.

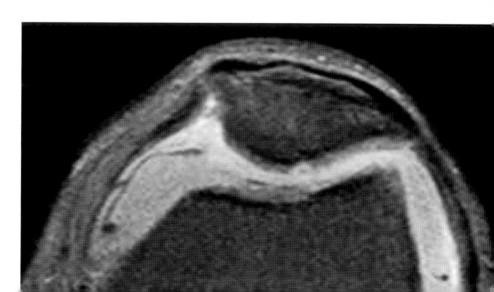

Chondral fractures

Chondral and osteochondral injuries are commonly the result of direct trauma or rotational forces. These fractures almost always involve the weightbearing areas of the articular cartilage, and the medial compartment is involved four times as often as the lateral compartment.

Hyaline (articular) cartilage provides a cushion of protection to the subchondral bone and a lubricated surface to permit easy movement of opposing articular surfaces. Nutrition is provided by synovial fluid and a narrow surrounding rim of perichondrium.

Articular cartilage consists of four zones:

1. *The superficial layer* represents 10% of the articular cartilage. This layer is composed of two sub-zones: the lamina splendans, which is the more superficial and is a clear film composed of small fibrils, and the cellular layer of flattened chondrocytes. This superficial layer resists shearing forces and provides a gliding surface for the joint. This surface is where the first changes of osteochondrosis become evident.
2. *The transitional layer* is important for the resistance of compressive forces.
3. *The deep radial layer* is the largest part of the articular cartilage, distributes loads and is resistant to compression.
4. *The calcified cartilage layer* contains the tidemark zone, which separates hyaline cartilage from the subchondral bone.

In adults, the tidemark zone is a weak link between the overlying cartilage and the subchondral bone. Shearing injuries most often produce a chondral rather than a subchondral injury (see Figs 6.232, 6.233 and 6.234).

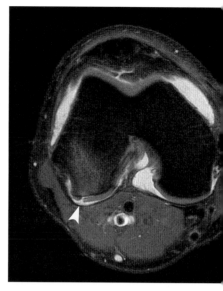

▲ **Fig. 6.233** An axial fat-suppressed PD-weighted image demonstrates a deep chondral flap at the posterior aspect of the lateral femoral condyle (arrowhead). Fluid is seen undermining the articular cartilage and there is associated subchondral bone marrow oedema. Also note the moderate-sized effusion, ruptured PCL and thickened MCL.

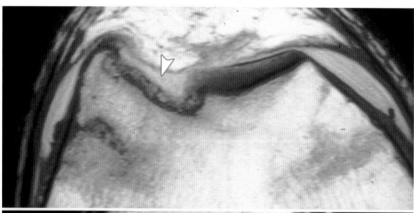

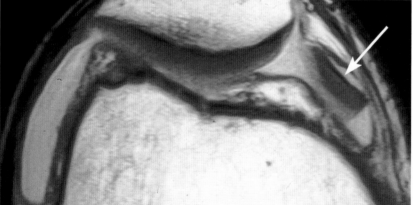

▲ **Fig. 6.232** Axial PD-weighted images demonstrate a chondral fracture of the lateral facet of the trochlear groove (arrowhead). The displaced chondral fragment has become a loose body in the medial recess and displays the layered structure of cartilage (arrow).

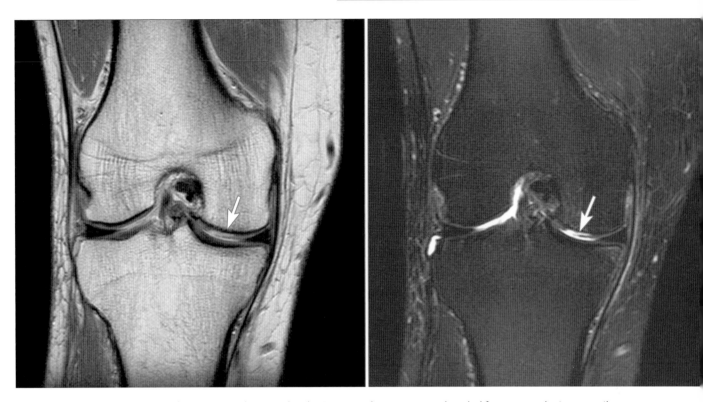

▲ **Fig. 6.234** **(a)** Coronal PD and fat-suppressed T2-weighted MR images demonstrate a chondral fracture producing a cartilage flap on the medial femoral condyle (arrow). The subchondral bone appears intact. Note the accompanying low-grade injury of the MCL.

▼ **(b)** Sagittal and coronal reformatted CT images show a fracture of the articular cartilage on the medial femoral condyle (arrowheads). The fracture extends along the tidemark zone, without injury to the subchondral bone, creating a chondral flap.

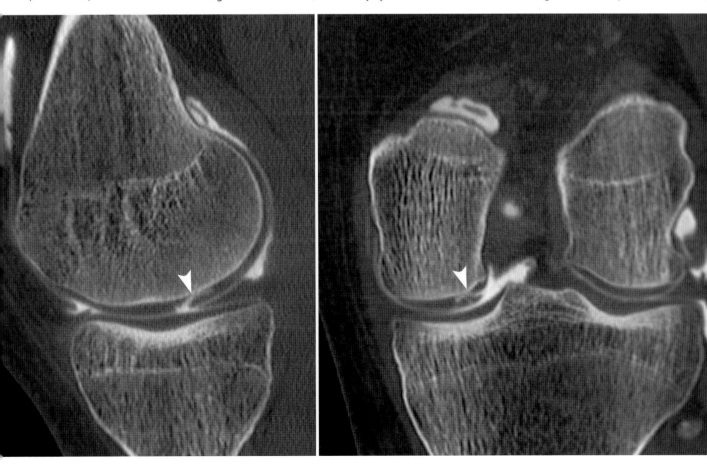

Patella alta and patella baja

Patella alta describes a patella that is abnormally high in position, while patella baja is a low-lying patella. In 1936 Blumensaat stated that the inferior pole of the patella should touch the continuation of Blumensaat's line (the roof of the intercondylar notch) with the knee flexed at 30° (Resnick and Niwayama 1988). Patella alta is present if the inferior pole lies above this level (see Fig. 6.235). Another method of diagnosis described by Insall and Salvati (1971) defines patella alta as a ratio of patellar tendon length to patellar bone length of more than 1.2:1. This method has been criticised for not taking into account cases with an elongated inferior pole of the patella. Patella alta can be associated with lateral patellar subluxation, chondromalacia patellae, Sinding–Larsen–Johannsen disease and quadriceps atrophy (Lancourt and Cristini 1975; Fulkerson 1990).

When the patella is relatively low lying and the patellar tendon to bone ratio is less than 0.8:1, this is termed patella baja (or patella infera). The most common cause of this is prior surgery or arthrofibrosis. It may also be the sequela of Osgood–Schlatter disease. In addition, patella baja may occur following a quadriceps tendon rupture, as previously seen in Figs 6.164 and 6.165.

A recent assessment of patella alta and patella baja measured on sagittal MR images was proposed by Shabshin et al. (2004) and differs from the traditional ratios. These ratios of patellar bone length to patellar tendon length found that in patella alta the tendon length to bone length ratio is greater than 1.50:1, while for patella baja it is less than 0.74:1.

Excessive lateral pressure syndrome

Abnormal tracking of the patella within the trochlear groove can produce focal areas of increased stress on the patellofemoral joint. One such tracking abnormality is known as excessive lateral pressure syndrome (ELPS), a condition where increased loading across the lateral patellofemoral joint occurs during flexion and extension. ELPS is also known as lateral hyper-compression syndrome and patellofemoral pain syndrome (Thomee et al. 1999).

The symptoms are characterised by joint pain that is accentuated by flexion. This condition may be clinically silent for many years before the development of anterior knee pain due to superimposed acute trauma or secondary OA. Causes for ELPS include a developmentally thickened or 'tight' lateral retinaculum, developmental dysplasia resulting in a convex lateral patellar facet or protuberant lateral trochlear facet, a lax or torn medial patellar retinaculum and vastus medialis muscle atrophy. Another important mechanism is increased anteversion of the hip, which may cause the patient to internally rotate the hip and bring the patella into a medial alignment. This increases the lateral pull on the patella, resulting in lateral patellar tilt (Reikeras 1992; Eckhoff et al. 1994).

Plain films usually show thickening of the articular cortex and perpendicular orientation of related stress trabeculae along the lateral patellar facet. Lateral patellar tilt may be seen but it is generally better demonstrated at shallow angles of knee flexion by axial CT. There may also be traction spurring at the patellar attachment of the lateral retinaculum, soft-tissue thickening in the line of the lateral retinaculum, underlying bony dysplasia, patellofemoral OA and slight lateral patellar subluxation due to cartilage loss (see Fig. 6.236). In addition, abnormalities of the trochlear sulcus and patella dysplasia may be seen. MRI techniques for dynamic scanning of patellofemoral tracking have recently been reviewed by Spritzer (2000) and Shellock and Powers (2001).

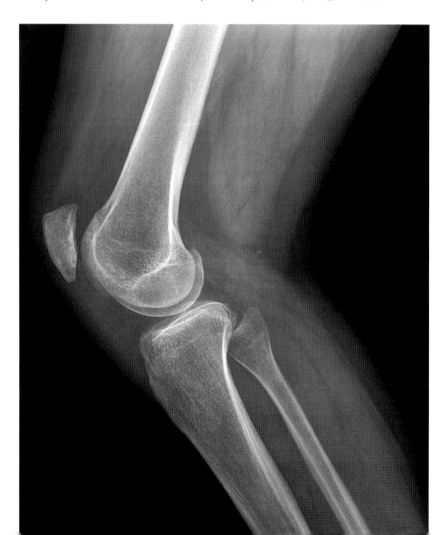

◀ **Fig. 6.235** Patella alta is present. Subchondral cyst formation is shown beneath the articular surface of the femoral sulcus, almost certainly indicating chondromalacia patella, a condition that has an association with patella alta.

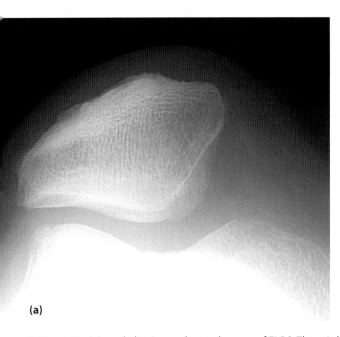

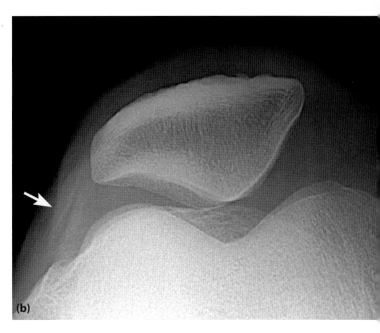

(a)

(b)

▲ **Fig. 6.236(a)** A 'skyline' view shows changes of ELPS. There is lateral tilting of the patella and sclerotic changes in the subchondral bone of the lateral facet of the patella. Another important observation to make is the orientation of the patellar trabeculae, which are at 90° to the lateral facet. These have altered in response to excessive lateral pressure. **(b)** Thickening of the lateral retinaculum is demonstrated on a 'skyline' patellofemoral view (arrow).

The key to effective treatment of ELPS is the early surgical release of the lateral retinaculum, before significant damage to the articular cartilage has taken place. Shea and Fulkerson (1992) have shown a 92% satisfactory outcome for lateral release surgery in cases where CT identifies lateral patellar tilt and only minimal articular cartilage damage.

Other conditions

Osteochondritis dissecans

The precise aetiology of this process remains unknown, but it is likely that the process is due to a combination of trauma and microvascular compromise. Subchondral bone is the site first affected, identified by an area of demineralisation on plain films (see Fig. 6.237) or high signal on MRI. Secondary changes then occur in the overlying articular cartilage (see Fig. 6.238). The abnormal area may revascularise and heal, or alternatively it may become increasingly well demarcated from the surrounding normal bone, behaving as a necrotic fragment. The fragment can destablise, and loosening, separation and displacement of the fragment may occur (see Fig. 6.239). An understanding of the basic pathology helps in the interpretation of MRI appearances at the various stages of this process.

OCD affects males more than twice as commonly as females. The maximum incidence in both sexes occurs between the ages of 10 and 20 years (Linden 1976). The juvenile form occurring with open epiphyses differs from the adult form on the basis of treatment and prognosis.

▼ **Fig. 6.237** Well-defined zone of subchondral demineralisation is demonstrated on a lateral plain film (arrow) and the appearance is almost certainly due to OCD.

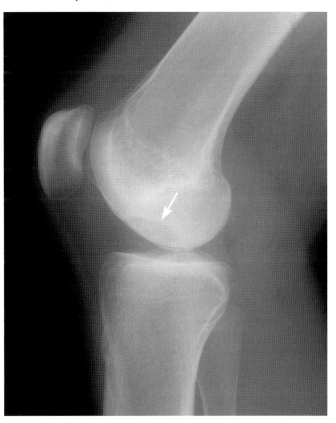

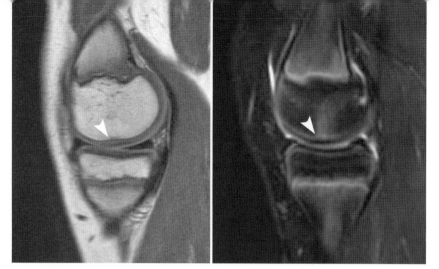

▶ **Fig. 6.238** Sagittal PD and fat-suppressed T2-weighted images show the early changes of OCD. There is altered signal in the subchondral bone and swelling of the overlying articular cartilage (arrowhead). Also note the increased chondral signal on the PD-weighted image.

▶ **Fig. 6.239** A plain film shows OCD involving the lateral aspect of the medial femoral condyle. There is a well-demarcated area of demineralisation in the subchondral bone. Two separated bone fragments are present. One has remained in the defect, while the other has become a loose body and lies in the neck of the suprapatellar recess.

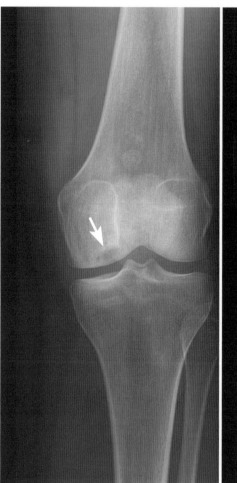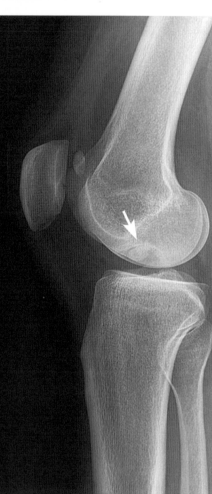

▼ **Fig. 6.240** Sagittal and coronal PD-weighted MR images show an area of OCD involving the lateral weightbearing aspect of the medial femoral condyle (arrow). The overlying articular cartilage shows an irregular surface contour and heterogeneous signal. No definite fluid line can be seen beneath the lesion to indicate separation. A T2-weighted image would provide a more confident assessment of loosening versus healing.

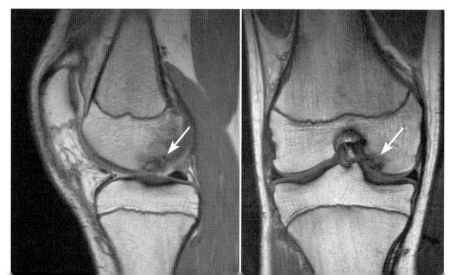

Imaging of areas of OCD may involve the use of plain films, nuclear bone scans, CT scanning and MRI. MRI is playing an increasing role due to its ability to accurately assess loosening of the fragments and healing, and to image the overlying articular cartilage (see Fig. 6.240).

Imaging plays an important role in the initial diagnosis and is also valuable in the management of OCD. As mentioned above and seen in Fig. 6.242, subchondral bone is involved in the acute stage, and a well-demarcated area of demineralisation is seen on plain films. This area will become increasingly demarcated by a sclerotic border as the process progresses. Four sites that are commonly involved (DiStefano 1995):

- 75–80% of cases occur in the lateral aspect of the medial femoral condyle, 20% of which extend medially (see Fig. 6.241)
- 15–20% of cases develop in the lateral femoral condyle, usually at the central weightbearing surface (see Fig. 6.242)
- 5% of cases occur on the articular surface of the patella (Schwartz et al. 1988); OCD defects occur in the distal half of the articular surface (see Fig. 6.243)
- 2% of cases are seen in the femoral sulcus (Obedian and Grelsamer 1997; Boutin et al. 2003) (see Fig. 6.244).

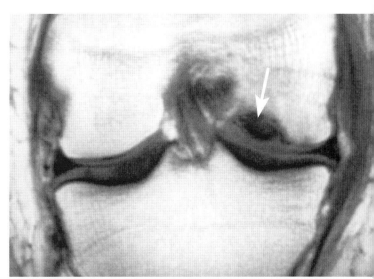

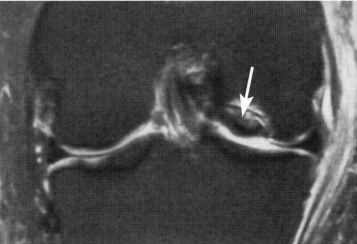

▶ **Fig. 6.241** Changes of OCD are demonstrated at the lateral weightbearing aspect of the medial femoral condyle on coronal T1- and fat-suppressed T2-weighted MR images (arrows). The presence of undermining fluid signal indicates loosening of the OCD fragment. Also note the predominantly hypointense appearance of the fragment on both imaging sequences, suggesting avascular changes within the fragment. A mid-segment MCL tear is also noted.

▼ **Fig. 6.242** Bilateral and symmetrical changes of OCD involve the lateral femoral condyles. The process on the right remains active, with a sclerotic border clearly demarcating the changes from the surrounding condyle (arrow). There is fragmentation, mixed sclerosis and demineralisation, and slight displacement of the separated ossicle. The process on the left has healed and the separated fragment has either been removed or become a loose body.

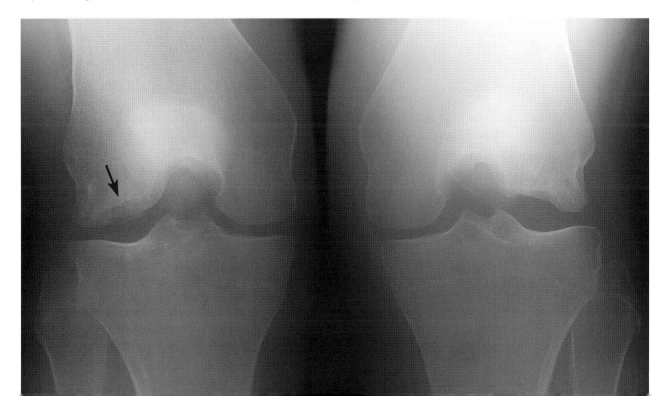

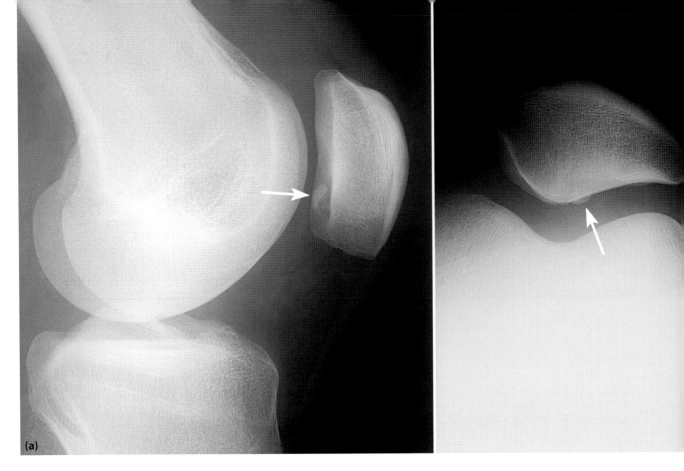

▲▼ Fig. 6.243 OCD involving the patella is well demonstrated by plain films.

(a)–(c) In all three cases, the OCD process involves the distal half of the lateral articular facet, towards the median ridge. In **(a)** and **(b)**, the separated ossicles remain within the OCD defect with only slight displacement. In **(c)** (opposite), the fragment has become displaced and is a loose body in the suprapatellar recess.

(d) (opposite) With the fragment displaced, the defect persists and this appearance would have to be differentiated from a developmental bone defect, which may occur on the articular surface of the patella. Ossification defects occur in the superolateral surface of the patellar articular surface, although occasionally these may be seen more centrally (Van Holsbeek et al. 1987).

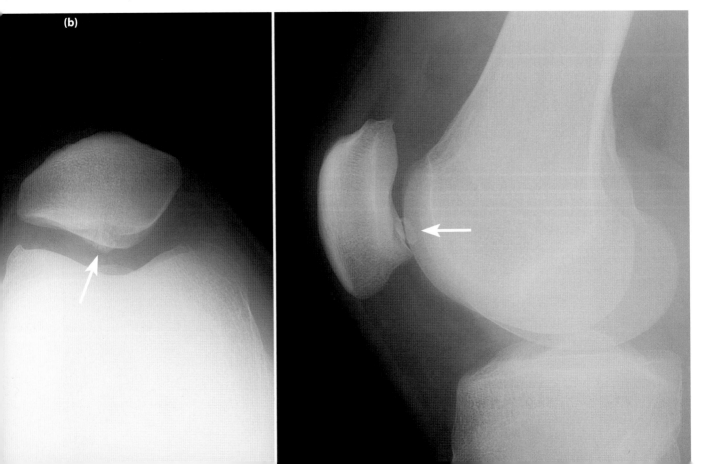

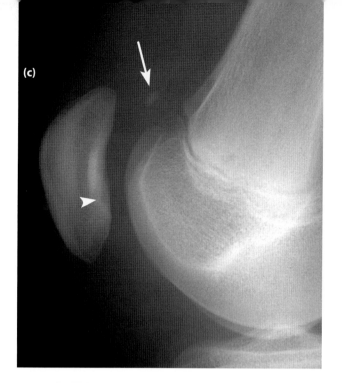

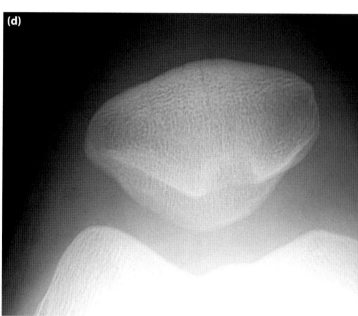

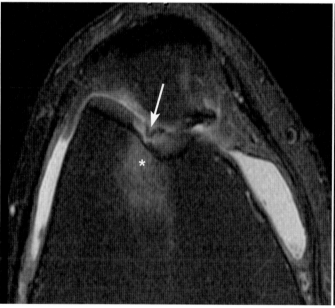

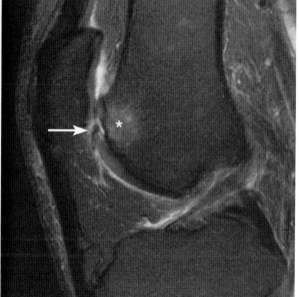

▲ **Fig. 6.244 (a)** Axial and sagittal fat-suppressed T2-weighted MR images show OCD involving the lateral trochlear facet, with a characteristic hypointense margin. There are displaced osteochondral fragments (arrows) and subchondral marrow oedema (asterisks). Note the associated joint space effusion.

▶ **(b)** An area of OCD has developed in the lateral facet of the femoral sulcus, demonstrated on a 'skyline' view of the patellofemoral articulation (arrows). A small fragment has become displaced.

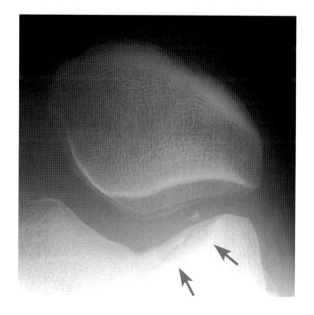

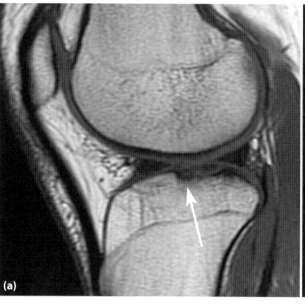

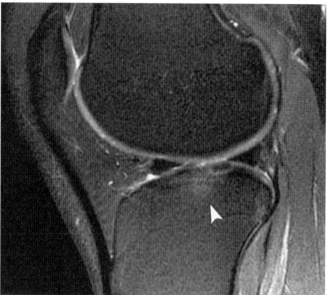

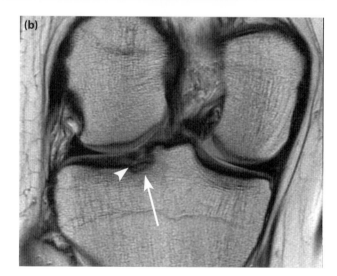

▲▶ Fig. 6.245 An OCD lesion involves the mid-medial margin of the lateral tibial condyle near its junction with the intercondylar eminence. This is an unusual site.
(a) Sagittal PD and fat-suppressed PD-weighted MR images clearly show a discrete hypointense line of demarcation at the margin of the lesion (arrow). There is adjacent bone marrow oedema (arrowhead).
(b) A coronal PD-weighted MR image of the same case shows the OCD lesion (arrow) and demonstrates an associated fluid line of chondral fissuring and early loosening (arrowhead).

Rarely, an area of OCD will develop on the tibial condyle (see Fig. 6.245).

A nuclear bone scan may be useful when there is doubt about the plain film changes, or when the area is difficult to demonstrate, such as when the OCD involves the patella or femoral sulcus. There is usually intense uptake of isotope (see Fig. 6.246). Mesgarzadeh et al. (1987) noted that the greater the intensity of isotope uptake, the greater the chance of loosening of a fragment.

MRI demonstrates OCD well (see Fig. 6.247). The abnormal area is progressively demarcated on heavily T2-weighted images. The area has a margin of linear low signal, which in turn is surrounded by high signal, reflecting oedema (see Fig. 6.248). Other MRI criteria that have been associated with instability of OCD lesions include a discrete surrounding area of homogeneously high signal intensity on T2-weighted images measuring at least 5 mm in diameter, a focal defect in the articular cartilage measuring at least 5 mm, and a high signal intensity line traversing the cartilage and subchondral bone plate on T2-weighted images (De Smet et al. 1997) (see Figs 6.249 and 6.250).

▶ Fig. 6.246 A nuclear bone scan shows increased uptake of isotope in the subchondral bone of the right medial femoral condyle. The appearances are consistent with OCD.

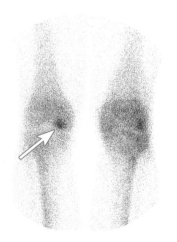

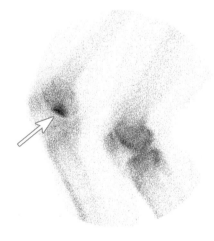

► **Fig. 6.247** A sagittal PD MR image demonstrates characteristic changes of OCD involving the medial femoral condyle. There is an unusually elongated osteochondral fragment that has become separated and slightly displaced (arrow). The fragment is hypointense, consistent with avascular change. Fluid is present deep to the fragment and the adjacent bone shows a discrete hypointense line of demarcation with accompanying marrow oedema and cystic change.

▼ **Fig. 6.248** Sagittal PD and fat-suppressed T2-weighted MR images demonstrate features of OCD in the trochlear groove with a separated osteochondral fragment. The fragment is surrounded by a rim of bright fluid signal and the femoral defect is in turn demarcated by a discrete hypointense line. There is marrow oedema in the surrounding femoral epiphysis. A chondral fragment has been displaced and lies in the suprapatellar recess (arrows). The fragment demonstrates the typical layered appearance of articular cartilage. An effusion is noted.

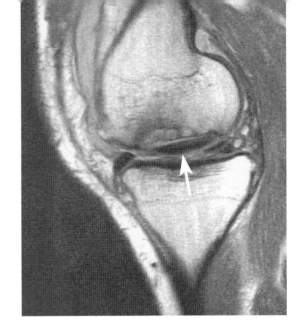

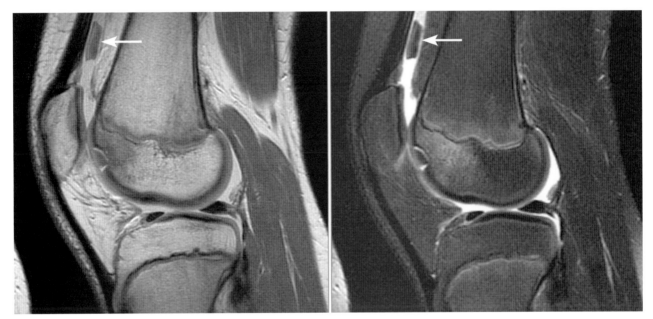

▼ **Fig. 6.249** Coronal PD and fat-suppressed T2-weighted MR images demonstrate classical changes of OCD involving the lateral aspect of the medial femoral condyle. The process extends laterally to involve the medial wall of the intercondylar notch. An oval osteochondral fragment has separated and become slightly displaced. This lesion shows the MRI features of instability, being entirely surrounded by bright fluid signal intensity on the T2-weighted image. Also note subchondral marrow oedema within the medial femoral condyle on the medial side of the OCD lesion.

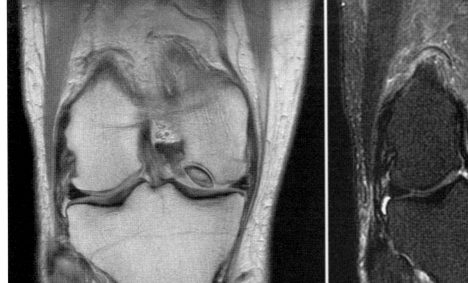

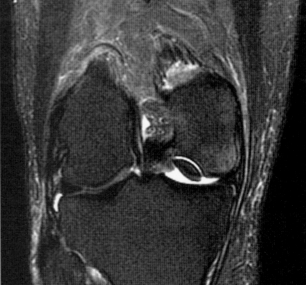

▶ **Fig. 6.250** An axial fat-suppressed T2-weighted MR image shows an area of OCD at the posterior margin of the lateral femoral condyle. The separated osteochondral fragment has loosened and become inverted (arrow). Note the surface layer of articular cartilage along the deep border of the fragment.

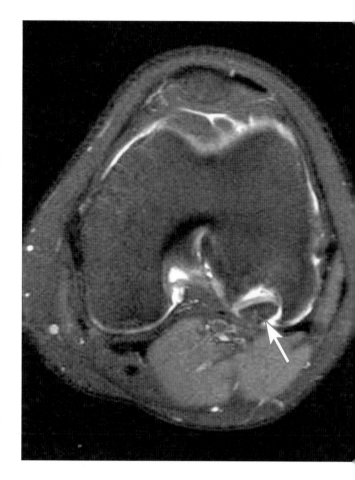

A study has suggested that the accuracy of MRI in predicting OCD instability is increased from 45% to 85% when the high signal line at the base of the lesion on T2-weighted sequences is accompanied by a breach in the articular cartilage on a T1-weighted image (Connor et al. 2002). Another group had similar findings following a small cohort longitudinally. Despite extensive subchondral changes on MRI, all cases with intact articular cartilage showed improvement with conservative treatment (Hughes et al. 2003). A CT or an MRI arthrogram can help to confirm or exclude fragment separation (see Fig. 6.251).

Subluxation and dislocation of the proximal tibiofibular joint

Stabilisers of the proximal tibiofibular joint include the joint capsule, tibiofibular ligaments, arcuate ligament complex, popliteus, LCL and biceps femoris tendon. In 10% of the population the proximal tibiofibular joint communicates with the knee joint. The proximal tibiofibular joint is responsible for about 17% of axial loading of the leg and resists torsion and lateral bending of the fibula. Injury to the proximal tibiofibular joint is commonly confused with a lateral meniscal tear.

The proximal tibiofibular joint is inherently stable, being in an anatomically protected position, supported by ligaments and stabilised by the LCL in extension. Subluxation and dislocation of the proximal tibiofibular joint usually occur in an anterolateral direction and are uncommon. Approximately 10% of subluxations are posteromedial. Dislocation mostly results from a fall when the leg is hyperflexed, with the foot inverted and extended (Falkenberg and Nygaard 1983).

A tibiofibular joint dislocation is usually diagnosed on plain films (see Fig. 6.252), although a comparative CT will be helpful in doubtful cases (see Fig. 6.253). On the other hand, subluxations may be extremely subtle and easily overlooked unless inspection of the proximal tibiofibular joint is a part of a search routine. Nuclear bone scans may be helpful in confirming injury to the proximal tibiofibular joint (see Fig. 6.254).

▼ **Fig. 6.251** Sagittal and coronal reformatted images from a CT arthrogram demonstrate a contrast-filled OCD defect at the lateral aspect of the medial femoral condyle (arrowhead). A large separated chondral fragment has become displaced in the intercondylar notch anterior to the ACL (arrows).

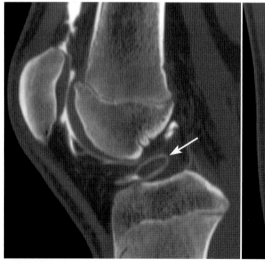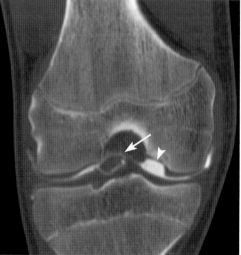

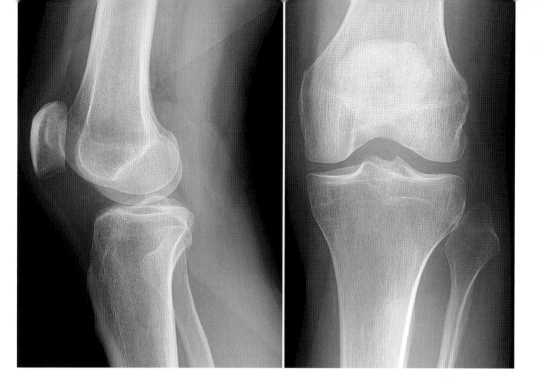

▲ **Fig. 6.252** Dislocation of the tibiofibular joint is seen on plain films. There is anterolateral displacement of the fibular head.

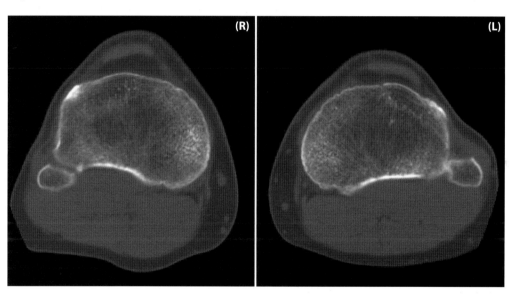

(R) (L)

◀ **Fig. 6.253** A dislocation of the left proximal tibiofibular joint is demonstrated by a CT scan, comparing the symptomatic side with the normal right side. The fibular head has displaced anterolaterally. No associated fracture can be seen.

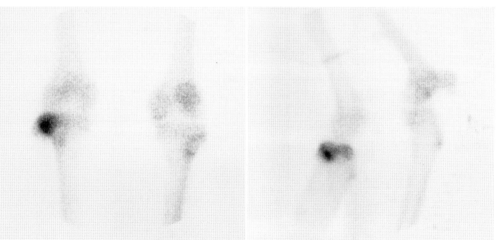

▲ **Fig. 6.254** Traumatic synovitis is demonstrated in the proximal tibiofibular joint. Abnormal uptake of isotope in the joint is seen on a delayed nuclear bone scan image.

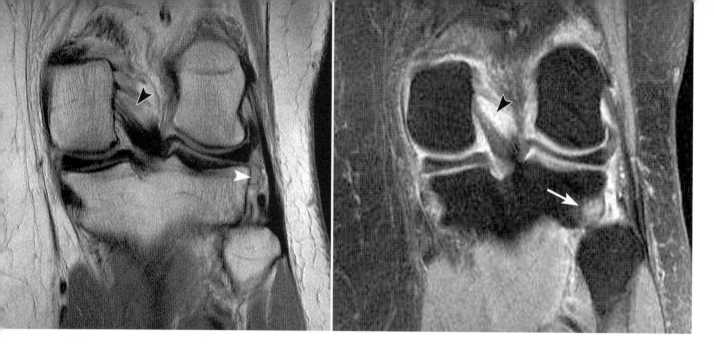

▲ **Fig. 6.255** Coronal PD and fat-suppressed T2-weighted MR images show subluxation of the proximal tibiofibular joint. There is bruising of the tibia adjacent to the joint (arrow) and disruption of the neighbouring posterolateral corner soft-tissue structures including the arcuate ligament complex (white arrowhead). A partial tear of the PCL is demonstrated (black arrowheads). The LCL is intact.

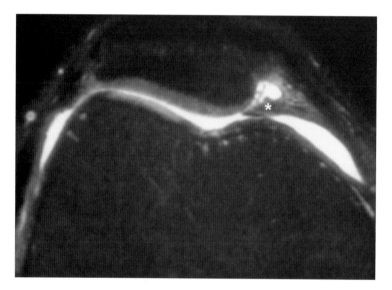

▲ **Fig. 6.256** An axial fat-suppressed T2-weighted MR image shows a thickened medial plica (asterisk) contacting the medial patellofemoral articular surfaces. Synovitis is noted adjacent to the medial patellar articular surface.

A subluxation may be an indicator of a posterolateral corner injury and associated posterolateral instability (see Fig. 6.255). Twisting on a fixed foot with external rotation can also cause subluxation of this joint (Thomason and Linson 1986). As previously seen in Figs 6.8 and 6.9 on pages 397–8, minor subluxations may require an additional oblique view and a comparative CT examination to help in making a confident diagnosis.

Peroneal nerve entrapment at the proximal tibiofibular joint

Entrapment of the peroneal nerve may occur as the result of compression of the nerve by a synovial cyst arising from the proximal tibiofibular joint. The peroneal nerve is most commonly compressed as it courses around the lateral aspect of the fibular head, adjacent to the origin of the peroneus longus.

Plica syndrome

Plicae are synovial folds or cords in the knee and are persisting embryological remnants of normal joint development. Various types may occur but the suprapatellar, medial patellar and infrapatellar plicae are the most common. The medial patellar plica, which may be found in up to 60% of the population, can abrade the medial femoral condyle (see Fig. 6.256) or the

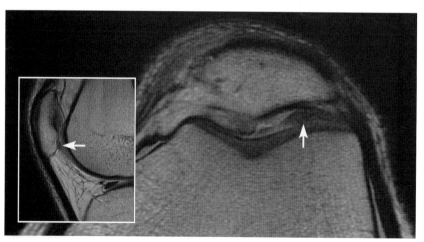

◀ **Fig. 6.257** Lateral plicae are unusual. This infrapatellar plica seen on axial and sagittal PD-weighted MR images (arrows) shows considerable thickening and is interposed between the lateral patellar and lateral trochlear facets.

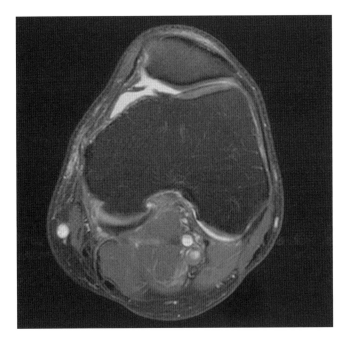

▲ **Fig. 6.258** A medial patellar plica has eroded the articular surface of the medial facet of the patella. The plica shows a focal perforation.

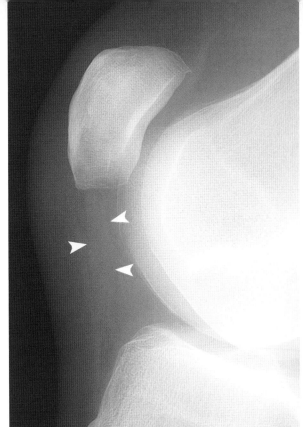

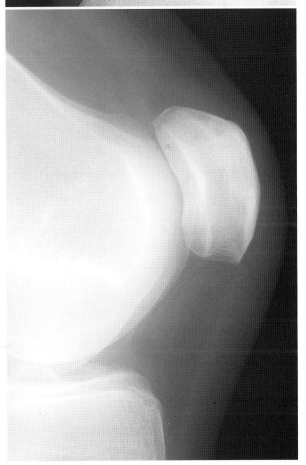

medial patellar facet during knee flexion (see Fig. 6.257). A normal plica is smooth in contour and no more than 1–2 mm thick (Ghelman and Hodge 1992). An abnormal plica may thicken, become fibrotic and perforate or cause pain with or without clicking, catching or locking. MR arthrography can show the thickened plica as a band of low signal intensity, and may also reveal erosion of the articular cartilage along the medial patellar facet or the anterior aspect of the medial femoral condyle (see Fig. 6.258). Plicae should not be confused with post-surgical adhesions.

Infrapatellar fat pad impingement and fat pad changes of Hoffa's disease

Infrapatellar fat pad impingement describes a condition of anterior knee pain characterised by pain and tenderness behind and to either side of the patellar tendon. Acute cases are invariably post-traumatic and occur after forced extension of the knee, producing fat pad contusion. These cases may present with anterior knee pain, swelling and disability suggestive of patellar tendon injury. Chronic cases commonly present with recurrent effusions, joint weakening and discomfort below the patella resulting from repetitive impingement of the infrapatellar fat pad. There is an increased incidence of the condition in patients with patella baja (a patella that is low in position, usually due to previous soft-tissue injury or surgery) or genu recurvatum.

Plain films may demonstrate patella baja or posterior tilt of the inferior pole of the patella. Plain films demonstrate an abnormality of the infrapatellar fat pad with loss of the normally homogeneous fat density (see Fig. 6.259). Ultrasound may show a focal fat pad hyperaemia just below the patella in a small percentage of cases. MRI demonstrates the infrapatellar fat pad extremely well and in the presence of fat pad impingement (see Figs 6.187 and 6.260). There is a diffuse replacement of normal fat signal intensity within Hoffa's fat pad by material of

▲ **Fig. 6.259** On the symptomatic right side (upper image), there is increased density in the infrapatellar fat pad (arrowheads). The appearance is due to Hoffa's disease. In this case, the process commenced with trauma. The asymptomatic side (lower image) has the normal plain film appearance of an infrapatellar fat pad.

▶ **Fig. 6.260** Sagittal and axial fat-suppressed T2-weighted MR images demonstrate a localised area of high signal within the deep infrapatellar fat pad adjacent to the inferolateral margin of the patella (arrow). This appearance is typical of infrapatellar fat pad impingement.

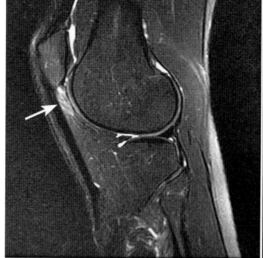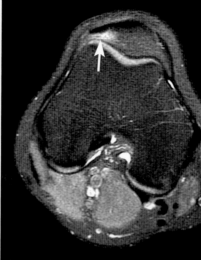

▶ **Fig. 6.261** Sagittal PD and fat-suppressed T2-weighted MR images show substantial replacement of Hoffa's fat pad with a circumscribed area of variable signal intensity compatible with haemorrhage and fibrosis (Hoffa's disease).

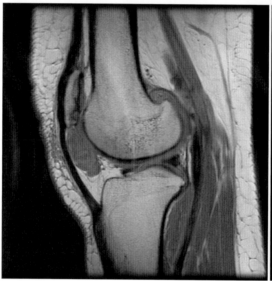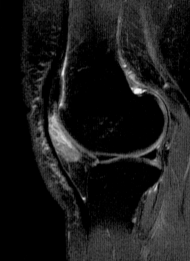

▼ **Fig. 6.262** A sagittal T2-weighted MR image shows bands of low signal intensity fibrosis replacing the normally homogeneous infrapatellar fat pad.

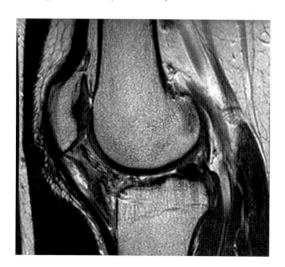

variable signal intensity representing haemorrhage interspersed with fibrosis (Hoffa's disease) (see Figs 6.261 and 6.262). Morini et al. (1998) found MRI changes to be specific for Hoffa's disease, particularly in its acute stage, and were able to differentiate other hypertrophic conditions such as chondromatosis, pigmented villonodular synovitis and systemic diseases like rheumatoid arthritis from chronic Hoffa's disease.

Subchondral stress fractures

A subchondral stress fracture is a subchondral lesion classically seen in the medial femoral condyle, and was initially described as a distinct form of osteonecrosis (spontaneous osteonecrosis, SONC) (Ahlback et al. 1968). The avascular segment in this entity tends to involve a small subchondral crescentic area, as opposed to the larger wedge-shaped areas in classical osteonecrosis. These changes are evident on plain films (see Fig. 6.263), although considerably more information is available on MRI (see Figs 6.264, 6.265 and 6.266). A recent review of histopathological findings indicates that the primary event is a subchondral insufficiency fracture, and the localised osteonecrosis is a result of the fracture (Yamamoto and Bullough 2000). This is often precipitated by abnormal loading secondary to a radial tear of the posterior horn of the medial meniscus near its central root attachment.

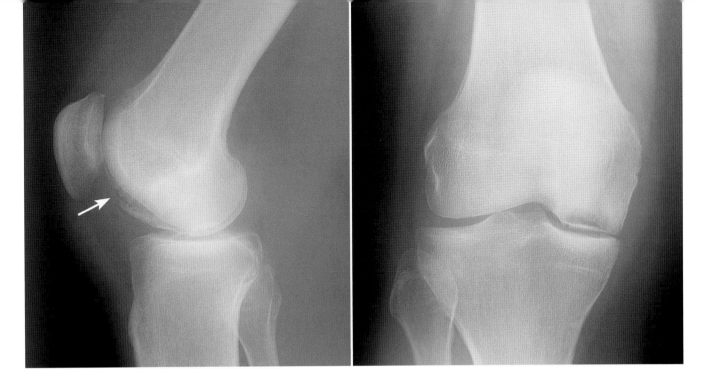

▲ **Fig. 6.263** Lateral and AP plain films show abnormality in the subchondral bone of the medial femoral condyle. There is demineralisation, and a fracture line is seen deep to the cortex. This is best seen in the lateral view (arrow). Compression of the cortex has occurred over this area. This process was previously thought to originate from avascular changes, but is now believed to follow a subchondral insufficiency fracture.

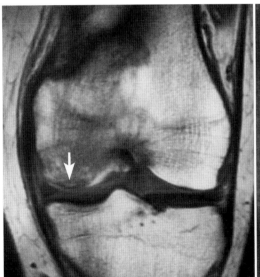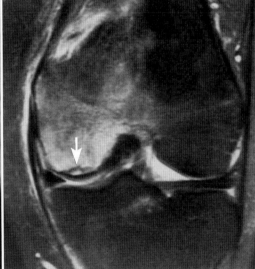

◀**Fig. 6.264** Coronal T1- and fat-suppressed T2-weighted MR images show a hypointense subchondral stress fracture line (arrows) in the medial femoral condyle, with considerable associated bone marrow oedema extending through the condyle.

▶**Fig. 6.265** More advanced findings are demonstrated by coronal PD and fat-suppressed T2-weighted MR images, in a patient with persistent pain following a partial medial meniscectomy. There is a fluid-filled subchondral crescent at the central weightbearing area of the medial femoral condyle with a sclerotic line of demarcation (arrows). Extensive adjacent marrow oedema and a hypointense subchondral bone fragment are also noted. These changes represent a completed fracture with loosening of an avascular osteochondral fragment.

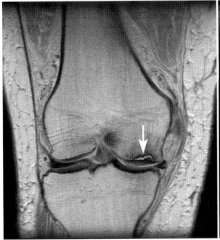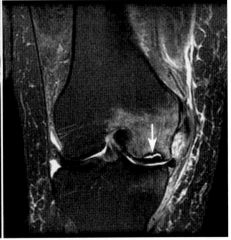

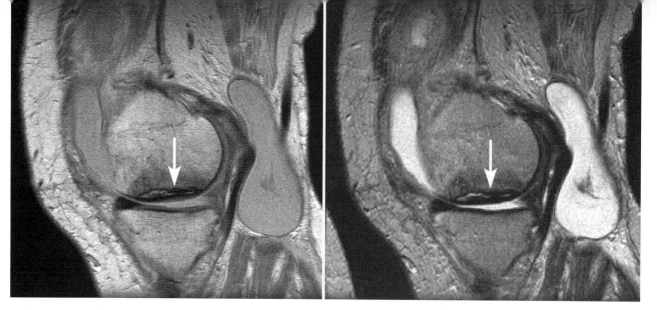

▲ **Fig. 6.266** In a further case of a subchondral stress fracture, sagittal PD and fat-suppressed T2-weighted MR images demonstrate a thin fluid line adjacent to a sclerotic line of fracture demarcation (arrows). The osteochondral fragment appears to be avascular. Note the subtle flattening of the overlying articular cortical contour indicative of associated bony collapse. An effusion is present and a popliteal cyst is also noted.

Ganglia of the knee

Intra-articular ganglia are most commonly seen associated with the ACL and PCL in the intercondylar notch. ACL ganglia and mucoid degeneration commonly coexist but are not associated with ligament instability (Bergin et al. 2004). Ganglia are occasionally seen associated with the ACL or PCL (see Figs 6.267 and 6.268) or between the ACL and PCL (see Fig. 6.269). Although prior trauma has been a suggested aetiology, the relationship is uncertain. On MRI, ACL tears need to be distinguished from the entity of mucoid degeneration, which may coexist with ACL ganglia (Bergin et al. 2004). Mucoid degeneration generally occurs in people over 40 years of age. Criteria for mucoid degeneration include poor visualisation of the ligament bundles on T1-weighted and PD MR images. The ACL appears thickened and ill-defined but some intact fibre bundles are usually seen on T2-weighted images (see Figs. 6.270, 6.271 and 6.272) (McIntyre et al. 2001). There is often associated oedema and cystic change within the lateral wall of the intercondylar notch. Ganglia may also occur in Hoffa's fat pad (see Fig. 6.273).

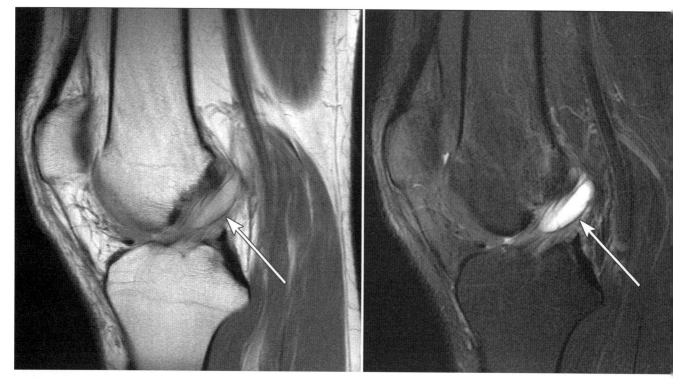

▲ **Fig. 6.267** Sagittal PD and fat-suppressed T2-weighted MR images demonstrate an elongated intrasubstance ACL ganglion (arrows) separating ACL fibres of normal appearance.

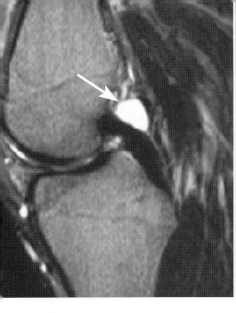
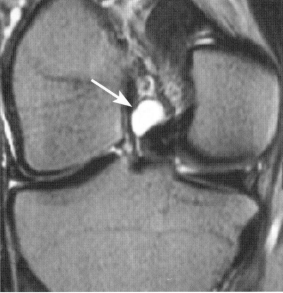

◀ **Fig. 6.268** Sagittal and coronal T2-weighted images show a ganglion (arrows) lying between the posterolateral aspect of the PCL and the proximal ACL.

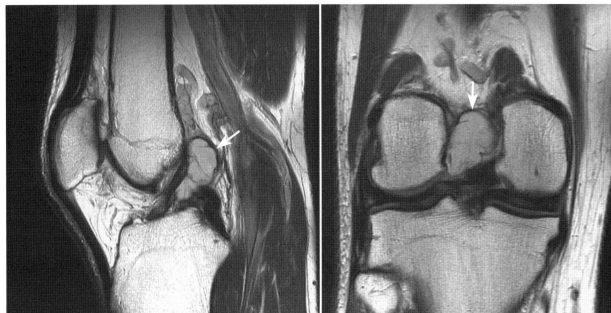

▲ **Fig. 6.269** Sagittal and coronal PD-weighted MR images show a large multiloculated ganglion lying between the ACL and the PCL (arrow).

▼ **Fig. 6.270** Sagittal PD and fat-suppressed T2-weighted MR images show changes typical of mucoid degeneration involving the ACL. There is generalised ligament swelling with increased interstitial signal separating the normal fascicles, creating a 'celery stalk' appearance. This is a degenerative process occurring with advancing age (40+ years). A small- to moderate-sized joint effusion is noted.

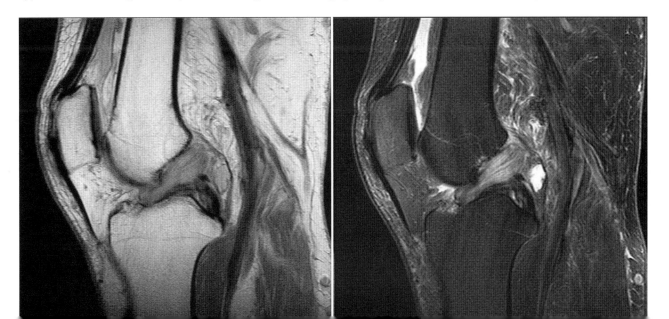

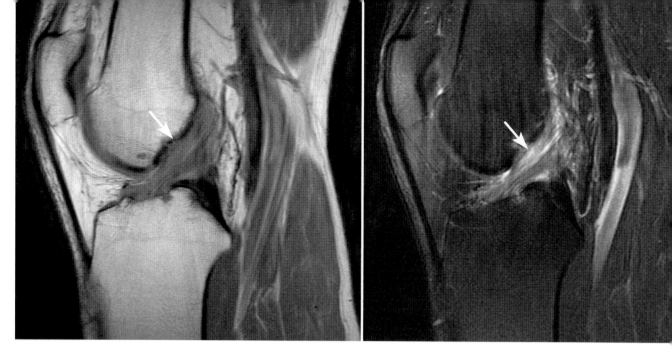

▲ **Fig. 6.271** This case of mucoid degeneration of the ACL could easily be mistaken for a recent incomplete tear. Sagittal PD and fat-suppressed T2-weighted MR images show intrasubstance signal hyperintensity (arrows). The fascicles are intact and the patient's presentation and history would further help to differentiate between mucoid degeneration and a tear.

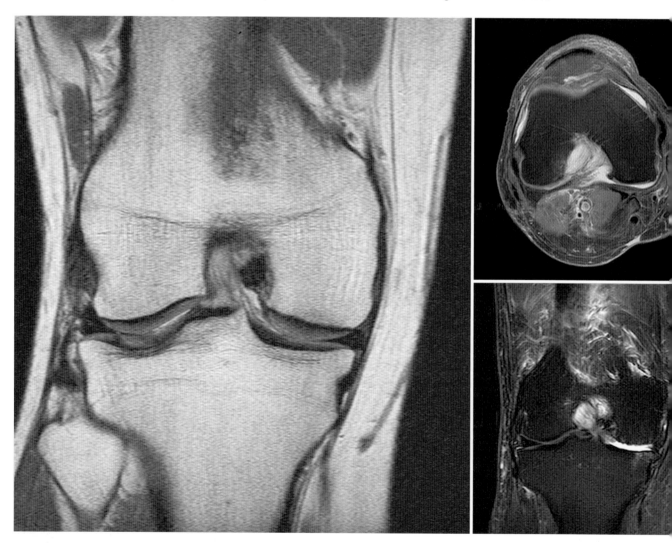

▲ **Fig. 6.272** A coronal PD MR image and axial and coronal fat-suppressed T2-weighted MR images demonstrate MRI changes of mucoid degeneration of the ACL. The swollen ACL shows increased signal with separated but intact fibres on all images. There is minor marrow oedema of the adjacent lateral wall of the intercondylar notch, which is not an uncommon finding.

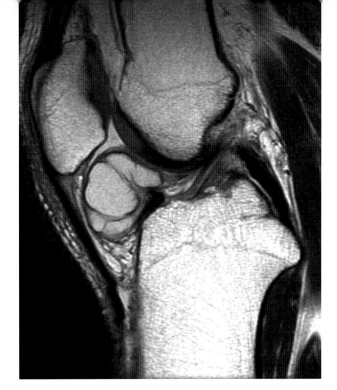

▶ **Fig. 6.273** A sagittal PD-weighted MR image demonstrates an extremely large multiloculated ganglion encroaching on the infrapatellar fat pad of an Olympic athlete competing at the Sydney 2000 Olympics. No communication with a meniscal tear can be identified, although the cyst was based against the anterior horn of the medial meniscus, which shows changes of mucoid degeneration.

The leg

Leg pain is a common problem in sport, particularly for athletes involved in running and jumping activities. Imaging plays an important role in helping to identify the origin of the pain. Common causes of leg pain in athletes include stress fractures, compartment syndromes and 'shin splints'. Other less common conditions that need to be considered are a muscle tear, tendinopathy, muscle hernia, peripheral nerve entrapment and other neurovascular causes secondary to spinal canal stenosis and popliteal artery entrapment.

Imaging of the leg

Routine plain views include an AP view and a lateral view (see Fig. 6.274):

- The AP view is obtained with the patient supine, the foot vertical and the ankle at 90°. The knee must also be in an AP position and, if possible, the knee and ankle should be included on the same film. A second film is usually required for an adult. A straight tube is centred on the midpoint of the leg.

- The lateral view is obtained with the lateral border of the leg lying on the cassette. The knee and ankle must be in a lateral position. Inclusion of the knee and ankle on the one film is desirable. If the patient has problems lying on their side, a cross-table lateral is a satisfactory alternative.

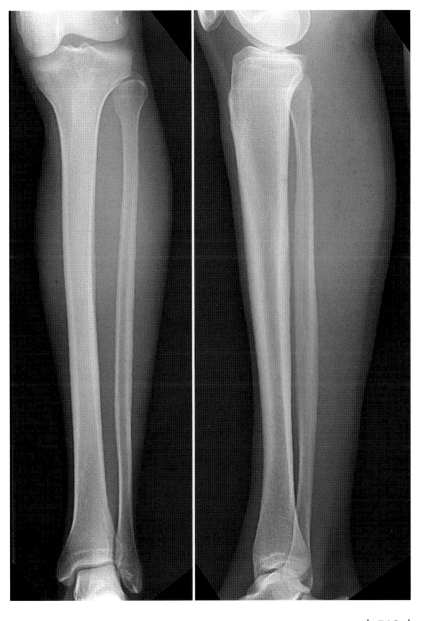

▶ **Fig. 6.274** A plain film examination of the leg consists of AP and lateral views that should include both the proximal and distal articular surfaces of the tibia and the entire fibula.

Acute fractures of the leg

Acute fractures of the tibia and fibula are common, usually occurring in the distal leg or at the ankle (which will be discussed in Chapter 7).

Acute fractures of the tibia

The tibia is the most commonly fractured long bone in the body. Many of these fractures involve the tibial condyles and tuberosity and have been discussed earlier in this chapter. Other fractures occurring around the ankle joint are reviewed in Chapter 7.

Tibial shaft fractures are usually due to high-speed activities such as motor sports, skiing and equestrian activities. Shaft fractures are also seen in sports such as soccer, where a direct blow to the leg is common. In infants, spiral fractures occur in the distal shaft.

A classification of these fractures is used as a guide for treatment and to predict union. This discussion lies outside the scope of this book and can be found in orthopaedic texts. It is important to remember that occasionally acute fractures of the tibial shaft may result from the progression of a stress fracture (see Fig. 6.283 on page 518).

Imaging with plain films plays a role in establishing the configuration of the fracture and a nuclear bone scan may be useful occasionally for confirming the presence of a subtle undisplaced fracture. MRI is useful for assessing associated soft-tissue injury and demonstrating complications such as a compartment syndrome.

Acute fractures of the fibula

Acute fractures of the fibula mostly occur at the ankle joint and these will be discussed in Chapter 7. Other acute fibular fractures do not offer a particular challenge in diagnosis or management, but are extremely valuable as indicators of important injuries elsewhere. It has already been shown that an avulsion fracture at the fibular head may indicate major disruption of the posterolateral corner of the knee.

In a similar way, a spiral fracture of the fibular shaft may indicate important injury at the ankle joint. The usual fracture mechanism involves the foot being planted on the ground with the leg internally rotating around the foot, resulting in external rotation of the foot. Many injuries occur at the ankle joint in sequence, culminating in disruption of the distal tibiofibular joint (syndesmosis injury). The rotational force then continues up the leg, tearing the interosseous ligament and producing a spiral fracture of the fibular shaft. This fibular fracture is known as a Maisonneuve fracture and usually involves the proximal shaft of the fibula (see Fig. 6.275). Maisonneuve-type fractures may also be seen in the more distal fibular shaft if there is external rotation with the foot in pronation, in which case the fracture is often 6–8 cm above the distal tibiofibular joint (see Fig. 6.276). The ankle pain and disability often overshadow the pain associated with the fibular fracture and, as a consequence, the fibular fracture may be missed or diagnosed late. The many injuries occurring at the ankle joint are reviewed in Chapter 7.

Stress fractures of the leg

Bone stress in the leg is a common cause of leg pain in sport, generally resulting from overuse and often involving faulty technique. Bone stress itself may be a cause of pain, but in the tibia a stress fracture is usually found at presentation, whereas in the fibula a periosteal reaction is the common finding at presentation. Stress fractures are common in the medial condyle and these have been demonstrated in the preceding section on the knee. There are three different areas of the tibial shaft where stress fractures commonly occur (see below) and in the more distal tibia bone stress is a component of 'shin splints', a less well-defined cause of exercise-induced pain in the leg.

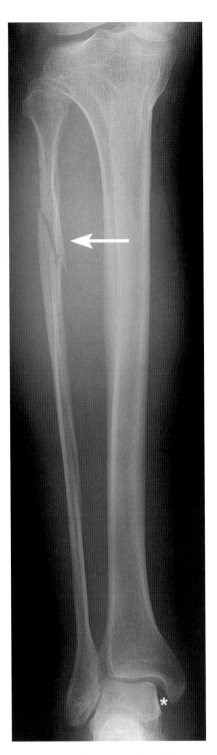

▲ **Fig. 6.275** This is the classical appearance of a Maisonneuve fracture, which is a spiral fracture of the proximal shaft of the fibula (arrow). Note the widened medial clear space at the ankle joint (asterisk) and widening of the distal tibiofibular joint produced by a syndesmosis injury.

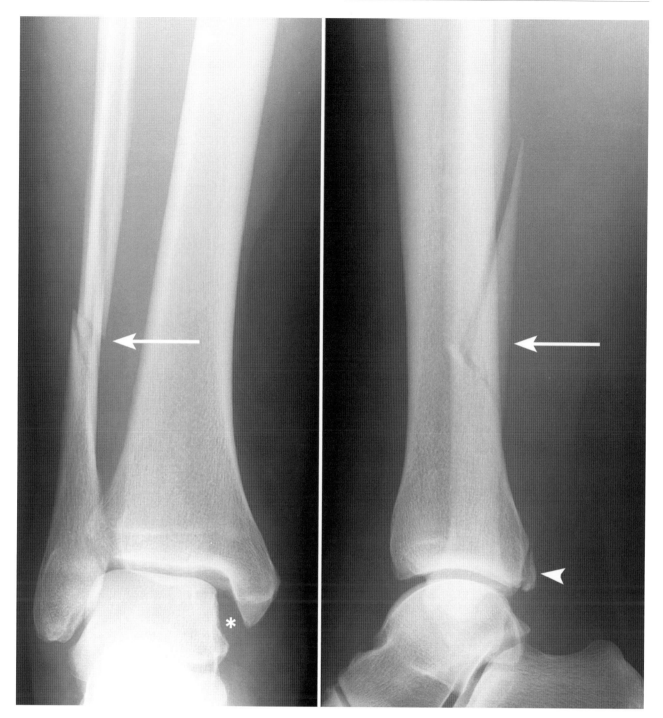

▲ **Fig. 6.276** The spiral fracture is not always at the proximal end of the shaft. This Maisonneuve-type fracture (arrows) has been caused by the foot being externally rotated. Widening of the medial clear space of the ankle (asterisk) and the fracture of the posterior lip of the distal tibia (arrowhead) have resulted from a syndesmosis injury.

Tibial shaft stress fractures

The incidence of tibial stress fractures in athletes varies from 19% to 63% (Brukner et al. 1996). Stress fractures occur in both elite and recreational athletes and are seen at all ages (see Fig. 6.277).

Stress fractures may develop in any area of the tibial shaft, but characteristically involve:

1. the proximal tibial shaft
2. the anterior tibial cortex
3. the junction of the middle and distal thirds of the tibia, usually involving the posteromedial aspect of the tibia ('shin splints')
4. stress fractures involving the distal tibia (discussed in Chapter 7).

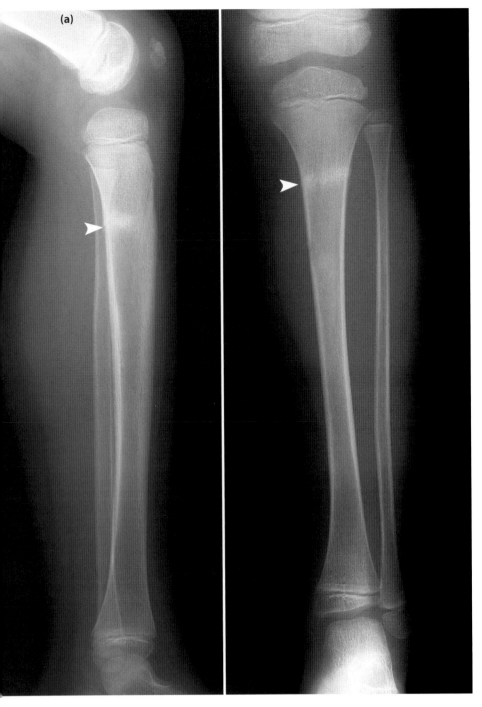

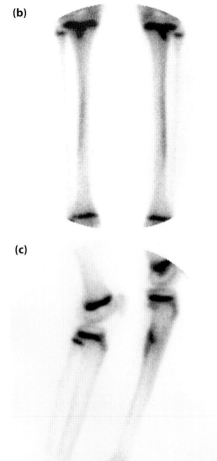

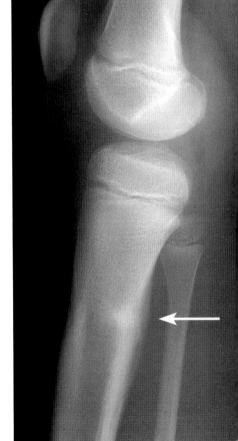

▲▶ **Fig. 6.277(a)** Tibial stress fractures occur at any age. Plain film changes typical of a proximal tibial stress fracture are demonstrated in an immature athlete. Periosteal elevation is noted posterolaterally.

(b) Bilateral anterolateral tibial stress reactions are demonstrated in an elite 15-year-old high jumper. The degree of uptake exceeds that accepted as normal and indicates pathological bone stress.

(c) This adolescent athlete was a national representative in the World Youth Games in walking. Following the development of leg pain with exercise, a bone scan demonstrated increased isotope uptake involving the proximal posterior tibial cortex, extending into the medulla. The appearances are those of a stress fracture.

(d) Following the positive bone scan shown in **(c)**, plain film changes of a stress fracture became apparent within two weeks (arrow).

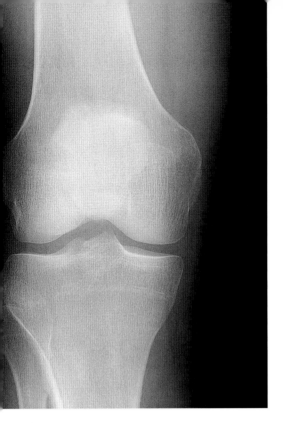

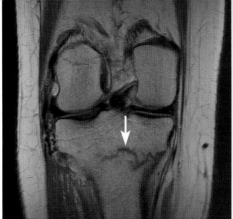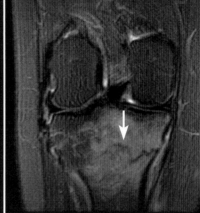

▲ **(b)** Coronal PD and fat-suppressed T2-weighted MR images obtained on the same day as the plain film demonstrate the presence of a fracture extending almost all the way across the proximal tibial metaphysis (arrows), with considerable associated marrow oedema. This is an acute presentation of a stress fracture, which is almost a complete fracture on presentation.

Proximal tibial shaft stress fractures

Stress fractures of the proximal tibial shaft present in much the same way as all stress fractures in weightbearing bones. Pain is of gradual onset and is aggravated by running and jumping, particularly on hard surfaces. As the tibia bears considerable body weight, these injuries carry a significant risk of progression to complete fractures. Conversion to a complete fracture may occur as an acute event (see Fig. 6.278). Although the appearances on plain films and nuclear bone scans suggests that the activity is localised to the posterior cortex (see Fig. 6.279), a CT scan will often show fracturing extending across the entire shaft (see Fig. 6.280).

▲ **Fig. 6.278(a)** No sign of the proximal tibial stress fracture can be seen on the AP view of the knee. No discernible bony sclerosis is evident.

▶ **Fig. 6.279(a)** A plain film demonstrates periosteal new bone on the posterior cortex of the proximal tibial shaft. Sclerosis extends into the medullary cavity.

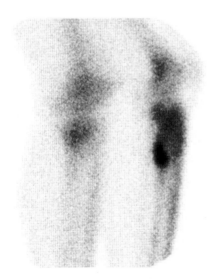

▲ **(b)** A delayed nuclear bone scan image shows an extensive abnormal uptake of isotope, typical of a stress fracture of the proximal tibia.

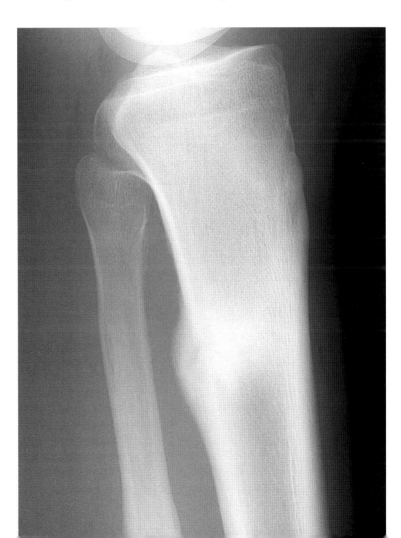

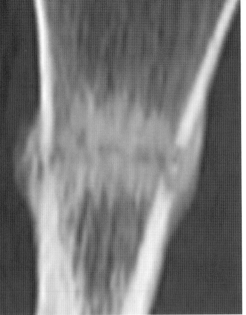

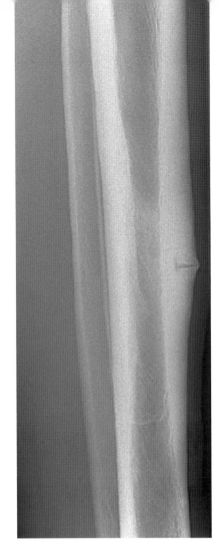

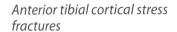

Anterior tibial cortical stress fractures

Anterior cortical stress fractures (see Fig. 6.281) occur in jumping sports and are called the 'dreaded black line of ballet' because of their frequency of occurrence in ballet dancers and the difficulty and considerable time required for the process to heal (see Fig. 6.282). Rarely, they are also seen in runners, volleyball players and cricketers (fast bowlers). These fractures frequently progress to complete fractures of the mid-shaft of the tibia (Brahms et al. 1980; Green et al. 1985) (see Fig. 6.283). Delayed healing probably relates to the fact that these fractures are on the tension side of the physiologically bowed tibial shaft, which means that any axial loading causes distraction at the fracture site (Lanyon and Smith 1970).

▲ **Fig. 6.280** A reformatted coronal CT image of the stress fracture shown in Fig. 6.179 shows that the fracture already extends across the shaft and the potential for conversion to a complete fracture is quite understandable.

▶ **Fig. 6.281** This advanced anterior cortical stress fracture was diagnosed in an athlete on their arrival at Sydney for the Olympics. The athlete was involved in a jumping activity and had not previously disclosed the injury. This caused the medical team great concern, being fearful that conversion to a complete fracture was a real possibility. Fortunately, the athlete progressed through the event without mishap.

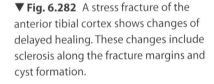

▼ **Fig. 6.282** A stress fracture of the anterior tibial cortex shows changes of delayed healing. These changes include sclerosis along the fracture margins and cyst formation.

▼ **Fig. 6.283** Anterior cortical stress fractures are difficult to heal and deserve respect due to their inclination to progress to a complete fracture. This case involved a classical dancer who, having rested a stress fracture for more than 12 months, suffered a complete tibial fracture on return to limited activity. Note in the pre-fracture film on the left, cystic changes are associated with the fracture. This is a sign signifying a poor prognosis.

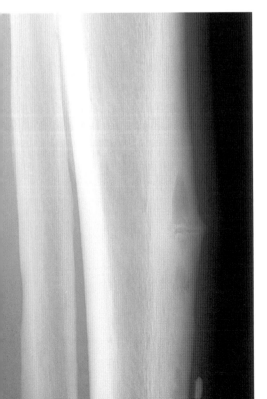

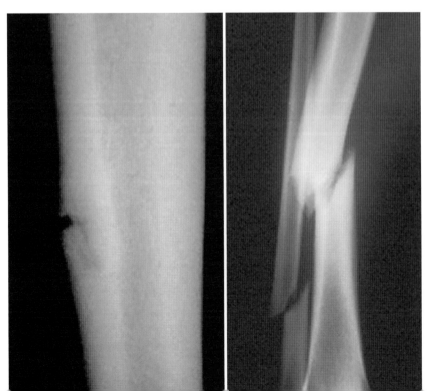

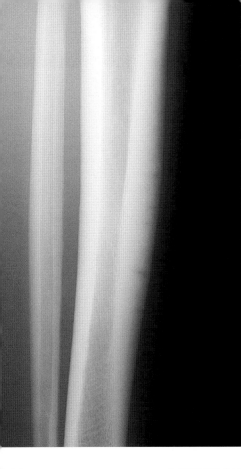

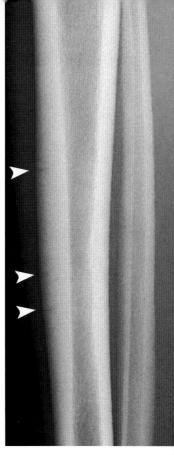

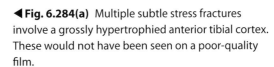

◄ Fig. 6.284(a) Multiple subtle stress fractures involve a grossly hypertrophied anterior tibial cortex. These would not have been seen on a poor-quality film.

► (b) The requirement for high-resolution films for the diagnosis of anterior tibial cortex fractures must be stressed. Whenever hypertrophy of the anterior cortex is present, a careful examination of the cortical margin is imperative. The cortical hypertrophy is evidence of recurrent stress over a long period.

▼ Fig. 6.285 A delayed nuclear bone scan image shows bilateral multiple anterior tibial cortex stress fractures.

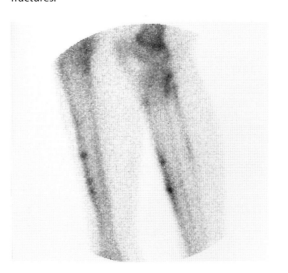

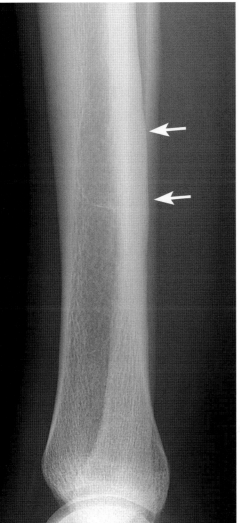

The fractures are often multiple, and high-quality, high-definition films are usually required to see these fractures in the early stage (see Fig. 6.284). A nuclear bone scan may assist in doubtful cases (see Fig. 6.285).

Shin splints

'Shin splints' is an umbrella term that has been loosely used to describe a number of different conditions (Batt 1995). Although the term refers broadly to exertional pain in the leg, it is best reserved for the more specific entity of posteromedial stress syndrome. This commonly occurs at the posteromedial tibial border and is probably caused by traction of the soleus muscle and its investing fascia (Michael and Holder 1985). Plain films are often negative but a characteristic linear pattern of increased isotope uptake is seen on delayed bone scan images. The angiogram and blood pool phases of the bone scan are negative.

Prior to the availability of MRI, Detmer (1986) classified the plain film and bone scan appearances of 'medial tibial stress syndrome' as follows:

- *Type I:* Plain film changes occur within the tibial cortex posteromedially and show cortical thickening (see Fig. 6.286). A nuclear bone scan shows an uptake typical of a bone stress reaction or stress fracture (see Fig. 6.287).

◄ Fig. 6.286 This is a Detmer Type I stress reaction. Thickening of the cortex has occurred on the posteromedial aspect of the distal tibial shaft. This corresponded with the area of the athlete's symptoms.

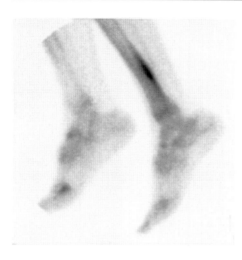

◀ **Fig. 6.287** In a Type I stress reaction, delayed nuclear bone scan images show an uptake of isotope typical of a stress fracture in the area of the thickened cortex.

▶ **Fig. 6.288** A Type II stress reaction occurs at the junction of muscle and the periosteum and on a nuclear bone scan has a normal angiogram and blood pool phase, but has characteristic linear isotope uptake posteromedially on delayed bone scan images.

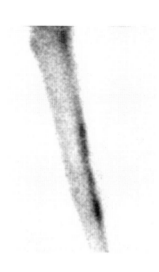

- *Type II:* Changes occur at the junction of the periosteum and muscle. Plain films are normal. Linear uptake is seen on isotope bone scanning along the posteromedial aspect of the lower third of the tibia (see Fig. 6.288).

- *Type III:* Changes occur within the muscle and/or its fascial constraints (this is possibly chronic posterior compartment syndrome). Plain films are normal. No consistent findings are present on isotope bone scanning.

This disorder was then referred to as a 'shin splint' occurring along the posteromedial aspect of the distal third of the leg.

A continuum of MR imaging findings and a classification of stress injuries demonstrated by MRI has been described by Fredericson et al. (1995):

- *Grade I injuries* are present when there is a mild periosteal oedema on T2-weighted images (see Fig. 6.289).

- *Grade II injuries* have more severe periosteal oedema with associated bone marrow oedema on T2-weighted sequences (see Fig. 6.290).

- *Grade III injuries* demonstrate periosteal and bone marrow oedema on both T1 and T2 sequences.

- *Grade IV injuries* have a low signal fracture line on all sequences with severe associated oedema (see Fig. 6.291(a)). The fractures associated with posteromedial stress syndrome have a vertical orientation and can be shown by axial imaging to extend over consecutive levels (see Fig. 6.291(b)).

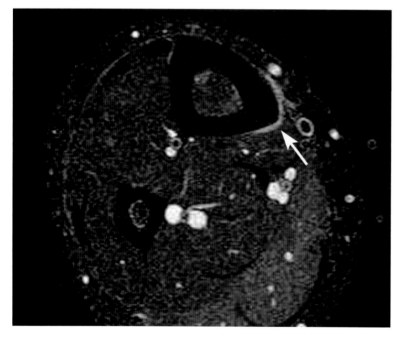

▲ **Fig. 6.289** An axial fat-suppressed T2-weighted MR image demonstrates a Grade I–II posteromedial tibial stress injury. There is periosteal reaction along the posteromedial aspect of the distal tibia (arrow) and minor subtle high signal involving the adjacent endosteal marrow. Also note the mild diffuse increase in gastrocnemius muscle signal. This 18-year-old athlete is a member of a state Track and Field Development Squad as a middle-distance runner. The examination was performed immediately after training.

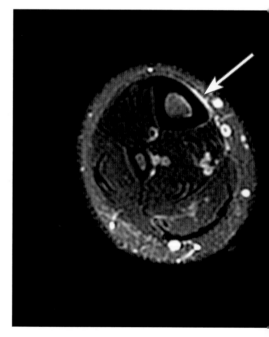

▲ **Fig. 6.290** An axial fat-suppressed T2-weighted MR image shows a Grade II injury, with definite bone marrow oedema and posteromedial periosteal oedema (arrow).

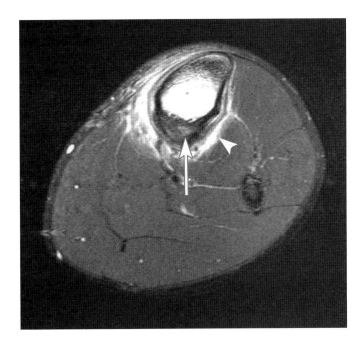

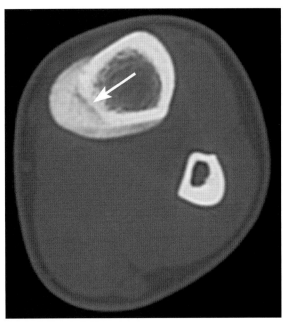

▲ **Fig. 6.291(a)** At the other end of the spectrum of severity is a Grade IV posteromedial tibial stress injury. An axial fat-suppressed T2-weighted MR image demonstrates high signal in the marrow and cortex (arrow), with considerable oedema surrounding the posteromedial and to a lesser extent the posterolateral aspects of the tibia. This change is in the mid-tibial diaphysis. Associated oedema within the deep posterior compartment of the leg (arrowhead) could potentially produce a compartment syndrome, which may contribute to the patient's symptoms.

▲ **(b)** The fractures associated with posteromedial stress syndrome are characteristically vertical in orientation (see discussion below). Axial imaging will demonstrate the cortical fracture extending over many levels. This CT image demonstrates a chronic Grade IV fracture extending through the posterior tibial cortex (arrow). There has been extensive periosteal reaction, which has now become mature bone.

While it has been assumed that a normal bone scan effectively rules out a stress injury, there have been a number of reports of early cortical stress fractures detected by CT or MRI that had normal bone scans. This has been explained by osteopaenia and the absence of a significant osteoblastic response in early stress reactions (Gaeta et al. 2005). Consequently, some authors consider MR imaging to be the single best technique for the assessment of suspected tibial stress injuries.

Proximal fibula stress fractures

Stress fractures of the proximal and mid-shaft of the fibula are uncommon (see Figs 6.292, 6.293 and 6.294). Having little weightbearing function, upper and mid-shaft stress fractures are secondary to powerful muscle forces applied by the soleus, peroneus longus, tibialis posterior and flexor hallicus longus (Symeonides 1980).

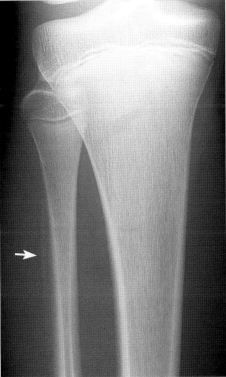

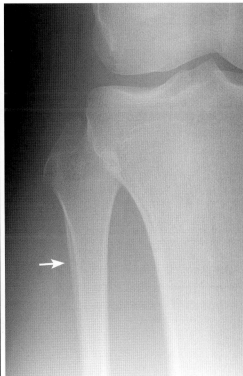

▲ **Fig. 6.292(a)** There is periosteal reaction on the lateral border of the proximal fibula. This stress reaction is due to repetitive overuse at the origin of the peroneus longus.

▲ **(b)** In this case, the reaction is at a higher level, reflecting the extension of the origin of the peroneus longus onto the neck of the fibula.

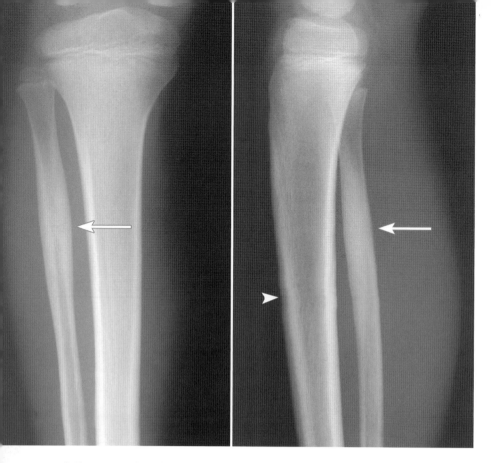

▲ **Fig. 6.293** This adolescent dancer shows evidence of a stress fracture of the proximal fibula, with considerable periosteal and endosteal new bone formed. There are also stress fractures involving the anterior cortex of the tibia.

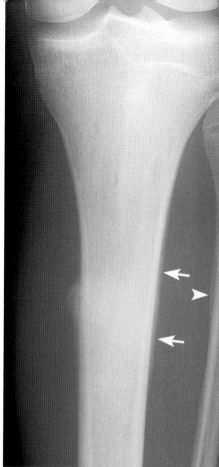

▲ **Fig. 6.294** Stress fractures involve the tibia and fibula at the same level.

Vertical stress fractures of the leg

Vertical stress fractures may involve the distal tibia or fibula. The fractures are confined to the bone cortex, which appears thickened and shows periosteal new bone formation (see Figs 6.295 and 6.296). The reason for the vertical orientation is unclear, but it would seem likely that the force of muscular traction at 90° to the axis of the fracture may produce such a fracture. With cross-sectional imaging, a cleft in the cortex is usually best appreciated on consecutive axial images (see Fig. 6.297). Eccentric oedema within the soft tissues, periosteum and bone marrow on MRI reflect the vertical nature of the stress fracture, as has been shown in Fig. 6.288. A relationship between the site of the stress fracture and a nutrient foramen has also been described (Craig et al. 2003). In other cases, the linear translucency appears to extend along the original cortical margin and the overlying periosteal new bone (see Fig. 6.298).

Plastic bowing of the fibula

Plastic bowing is a further manifestation of trauma, producing a bending fracture due to plastic deformation of bone and is also characteristically seen in children (see Fig. 6.299). Plastic bowing is usually seen in the forearm bones, clavicle and fibula. A nuclear bone scan will demonstrate a uniform increase in isotope uptake throughout the bone, without a discrete fracture (see Fig. 6.300).

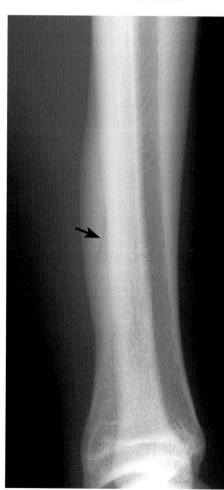

▶ **Fig. 6.295** A vertical tibial stress fracture is present in markedly thickened cortex on the posterior margin of the tibia at the junction of its middle and distal thirds (arrow). There is also considerable endosteal new bone formation.

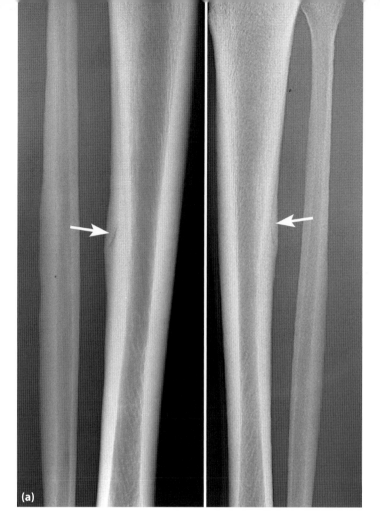

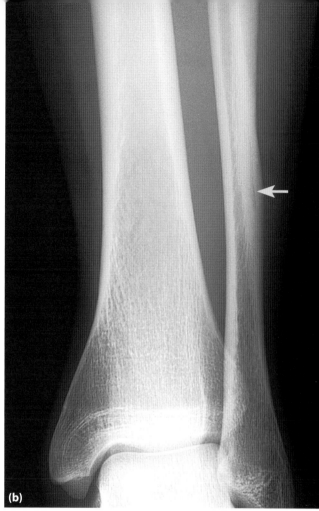

▲ ▼ **Fig. 6.296(a)** Bilateral, roughly symmetrical vertical stress fractures (arrows) are seen at the junction of the proximal and middle thirds of the tibial shaft in a 1500-metre runner at the Sydney 2000 Olympics. Associated periosteal thickening is present. **(b)** A vertical stress fracture involves the lateral aspect of the distal shaft of the fibula. Endosteal and periosteal new bone formation is noted. **(c)** A nuclear bone scan demonstrates bilateral longitudinal stress fractures.

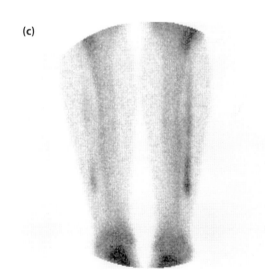

▶ **Fig. 6.297** Reformatted sagittal CT images show a vertical tibial stress fracture at the junction of its proximal and middle thirds. There is associated periosteal and endosteal new bone formation.

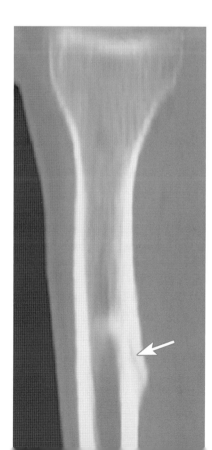

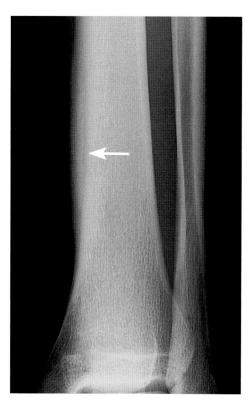

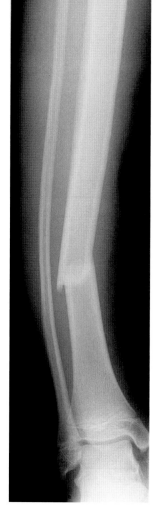

▲ **Fig. 6.299** A force to the medial side of the leg has caused a fracture of the tibial shaft at the junction of its middle and distal thirds and plastic bowing of the fibula. As usually occurs, the bowing resisted straightening. The bowed deformity prevented reduction of the tibial fracture and the fibula had to be fractured to obtain a satisfactory tibial fracture reduction.

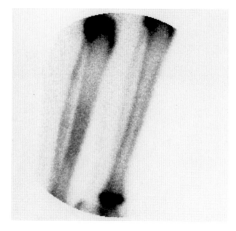

▲ **Fig. 6.298** In some cases of vertical stress fractures, the fracture largely extends along the line between the original tibial or fibular shaft and the overlying periosteal new bone.

▲ **Fig. 6.300** In another case of plastic bowing of the fibula, there is uniform uptake of isotope throughout the fibula with no localised fracturing apparent.

Compartment syndrome

The leg is divided into four main functional fascial compartments: the superficial posterior, deep posterior, anterior and lateral compartments (see Fig. 6.301):

1. The superficial posterior compartment contains the gastrocnemius and soleus muscles.
2. The deep posterior compartment contains the tibialis posterior, flexor hallicus longus and flexor digitorum longus muscles.
3. The anterior compartment contains the tibialis anterior, extensor hallicus longus and extensor digitorum longus muscles. The interosseous ligament separates the anterior and deep posterior compartments.
4. The lateral compartment contains the peroneus longus and brevis muscles. The anterior and lateral intermuscular septa are the boundaries of the lateral compartment.

Other compartments may also exist, such as the tibialis posterior compartment described by Davey et al. (1984).

Compartment syndrome (CS) occurs when perfusion pressure falls below tissue pressure in an enclosed anatomical space. So increased tissue pressure in a myofascial compartment compromises blood flow to the tissues and nerves in that compartment, which may result in tissue injury. CS may be acute or chronic (also known as exertional CS). In sport, acute CS may result from injury causing bleeding or swelling (see Figs 6.302 and 6.303). Chronic CS was first described in

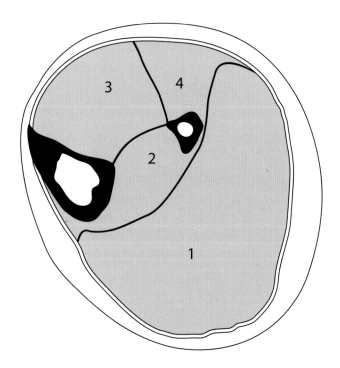

▲ **Fig. 6.301** This line drawing shows the major compartments of the leg:
1. The superficial posterior compartment
2. The deep posterior compartment
3. The anterior compartment
4. The lateral compartment

1956 and was thought to be a form of enthesopathy. With the popularity of endurance sports and the pursuit of personal fitness, chronic CS has become the focus of research and there is now an understanding of this phenomenon. Simply by exercising, muscle volume can increase by up to 20%, and increased compartment pressure and pain can result.

Exertional CS is most commonly seen in long-distance runners and other endurance sportspeople. Clinically, the symptoms are like claudication. The pain is commonly bilateral and starts within about 15 minutes of commencing running. The pain may be too severe to keep running and will subside within one hour of stopping. Unlike acute CS, the pathophysiology of exertional CS is probably not related to ischaemia (Amendola et al. 1990).

Imaging may help to diagnose predisposing anatomical anomalies such as an accessory flexor digitorum longus or an accessory soleus muscle (Buschman et al. 1991). Plain films may identify an acute or stress fracture. Ultrasound can be used for demonstrating compartment swelling, fascial thickening and other space-occupying encroachments that may contribute to CS (see Fig. 6.304). Ultrasound may also be used for imaging guidance during needle placement, and to accurately identify the deep posterior compartment during compartment pressure measurement studies (Wiley et al. 1990). The role of MRI in the assessment of chronic exertional CS remains to be defined. A number of studies have demonstrated increased signal intensity on T2-weighted sequences in anterior compartment muscles when compared to those of the superficial posterior compartment post-exercise. Following fasciotomy, there is no difference in signal intensity on T2-weighted images between the compartments (Verleisdonk et al. 2001). However, as discussed in Chapter 1, increased muscle signal on T2-weighted sequences can be a physiological finding following exercise.

Fascial defects may develop with compartment syndrome, leading to the herniation of muscle and potentially causing nerve entrapment. Styf (1989) described this mechanism as a cause of superficial peroneal nerve entrapment (see Fig. 6.305). Trauma and weakness in the overlying fascia have been implicated in the development of muscle hernias, which most commonly involve the tibialis anterior. Clinically, they present with a focal swelling apparent on standing or when the affected muscle is contracted. Ultrasound is particularly useful in the diagnosis, with a focal defect evident within the normally continuous echogenic line of the enveloping crural fascia. The herniated muscle often has a 'mushroom-like' appearance where it overlaps the fascial defect and has a convex superficial contour (Beggs 2003).

Muscle tears in the leg

The gastrocnemius originates from medial and lateral heads on the posterior aspect of the femoral condyles, which join with the soleus to form the Achilles tendon, inserting on the posterior aspect of the calcaneal tuberosity. The soleus arises from the upper tibia and fibula and runs deep to the gastrocnemius, contributing to the Achilles tendon.

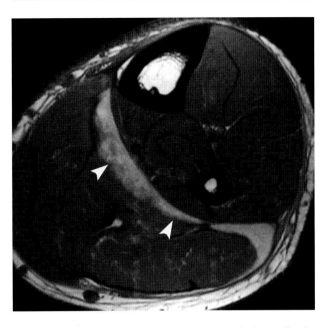

▲ **Fig. 6.302** An elite soccer player complained of superficial posterior compartment symptoms that were shown to be due to haemorrhage (arrowheads) on this axial PD-weighted MR image.

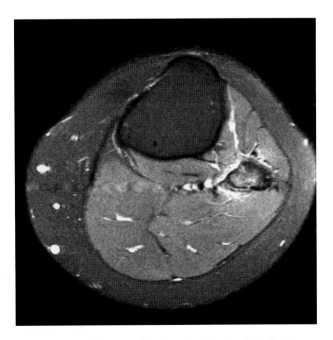

▲ **Fig. 6.303** A fracture of the head and neck of the fibula was evident on plain films. An axial fat-suppressed PD-weighted MR image shows high signal of haemorrhage associated with the fracture in the deep posterior compartment and extending along the fascial plane between the anterior and deep posterior compartments. Acute deep compartment syndrome could be anticipated.

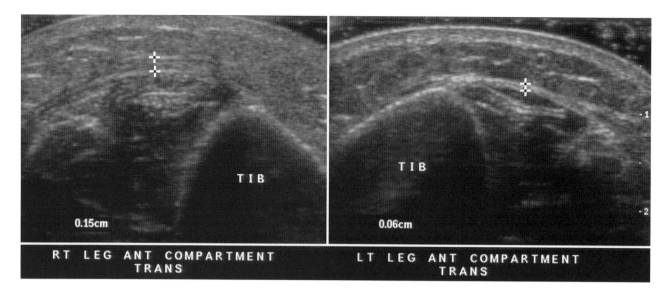

▲ Fig. 6.304(a) Ultrasound demonstrates acute anterior compartment syndrome of the right leg. The patient developed anterior leg pain and swelling of the right leg during a long hiking trip. Comparison transverse ultrasound images at rest have been obtained over the anterior compartments of both legs. The epicentre of the imaging abnormality is the investing fascia of the right anterior compartment, which shows thickening and an exaggerated anterior bulge by comparison with the normal left side (callipers). Also note the associated acute inflammatory features of diffusely increased echogenicity within the overlying sub-cutaneous fat, dermal oedema and increased echogenicity within the contiguous portion of the tibialis anterior muscle. Tibia = TIB.

▶ (b) Chronic anterior compartment syndrome of the left leg is demonstrated by ultrasound. The patient presented with a long history of left-sided anterior leg pain provoked by exercise. Comparison transverse ultrasound images at rest have been obtained over the anterior compartments of both legs. There is distinct thickening of the investing fascia of the left anterior compartment (arrowheads) when compared with the normal right side (arrows). Note the equivalence of resting anterior compartment muscle volumes and normal muscle echotexture.

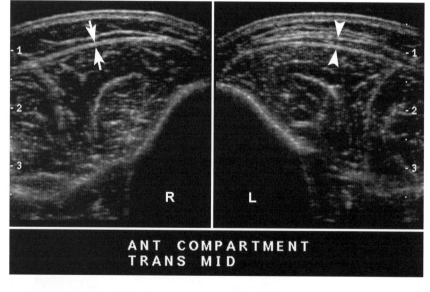

▶ Fig. 6.305 A long-axis ultrasound image obtained over a site of clinical swelling demonstrates herniation of muscle (arrow) through a defect in the investing fascia of the anterior compartment at the point of the superficial peroneal nerve passage. In this case there was little change with muscle contraction. The hernia was responsible for symptoms of superficial peroneal nerve entrapment.

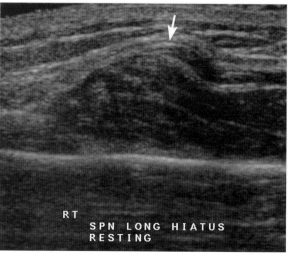

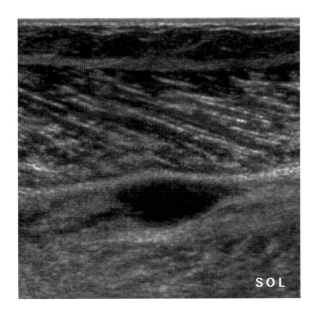

▲ Fig. 6.306 A long-axis ultrasound image of an athlete at the Sydney 2000 Olympics shows a tear of the soleus adjacent to the soleal tendon.

Tears of the medial head are more common than those on the lateral side and usually occur at the musculotendinous junction of the medial head following sudden dorsiflexion of the foot, which stretches the calf muscle. This is usually associated with sudden acceleration and is a common injury in men over 40 years of age. The injury is known as 'tennis leg' and is common in racquet sports, skiing and running.

The most frequent pattern of injury is a partial tear of the medial head of the gastrocnemius muscle at its distal attachment to the gastrocnemius tendon. Less commonly, the injury is a gastrocnemius–soleus aponeurosis tear, in which a fluid collection splits the aponeurosis between the two muscles and no discrete intrasubstance muscle defect is visualised (see Fig. 6.306). A 'pop' is felt or heard and the athlete invariably looks to see what has hit the back of their leg. Swelling and disability follow.

The diagnosis of muscle tears is usually established clinically, but ultrasound (see Fig. 6.307) and MRI can be used to confirm a clinical suspicion (Kane et al. 2004). Rarely, a rupture of the plantaris tendon is responsible for calf muscle pain, and produces a tubular fluid collection extending along the muscle junction and bunching of the plantaris muscle belly.

Popliteal artery entrapment syndrome

Popliteal artery entrapment syndrome (PAES) is an important cause of severe intermittent claudication in young adults (20–40 years old). PAES is due to an anomalous relationship between the popliteal artery and the surrounding musculotendinous structures.

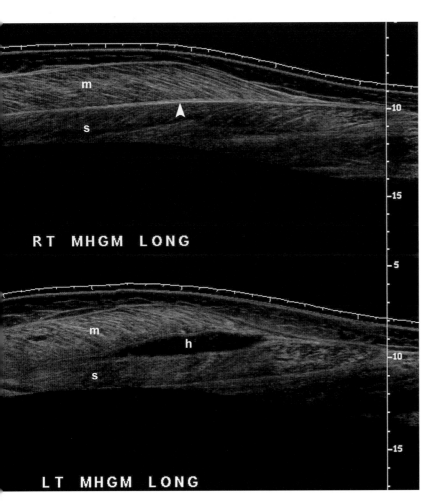

◄ Fig. 6.307 A long-axis panoramic ultrasound image demonstrates a tear of the aponeurosis between the left gastrocnemius and soleus (lower image). In this type of injury, no intrasubstance muscle tear is present. The normal right side (upper image) was imaged for comparison. An arrowhead indicates the normal intact medial head of the gastrocnemius–soleus aponeurosis on the asymptomatic right side. Medial head of gastrocnemius muscle = m. Soleus muscle = s. Haematoma = h.

The condition was first described by Stuart (1879) and has since been classified into five types by Whelan (1984):

- *Type I* is present when a normally developing medial head of the gastrocnemius displaces the popliteal artery medially. This is the most common type, accounting for 50% of cases.
- *Type II* occurs with an arrested migration of the medial head of the gastrocnemius, resulting in a variable anomalous origin from the lateral surface of the medial femoral condyle. The displacement of the popliteal artery is less marked than with Type I.
- *Type III* occurs when the popliteal artery develops within the muscle mass.
- *Type IV* occurs when the artery develops deep to the popliteus.

- *Type V* involves the popliteal vein as well as the artery.

Types II–V may also involve the tibial nerves, producing a paraesthesia in addition to the claudication. In some athletes, simple hypertrophy of the medial head of the gastrocnemius may cause impingement on the popliteal artery and a functional claudication may result. Other causes of claudication in the young athlete include early onset atherosclerosis, adventitial cystic disease and arterial embolism (Pillai 2002).

Imaging with ultrasound and Colour Doppler with and without muscle contraction is an efficient method of making a diagnosis of PAES (see Fig. 6.308). MRI may also demonstrate anomalous relationships between the popliteal artery and the surrounding structures. Angiography may demonstrate the narrowing, but will not demonstrate the cause, possibly leading to unsuccessful intervention.

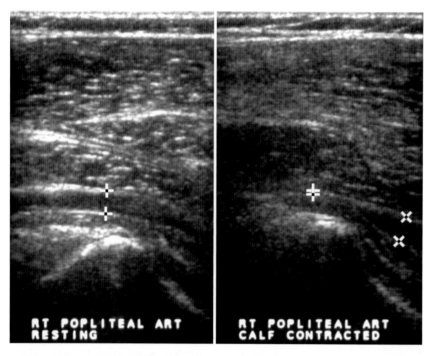

◄Fig. 6.308(a) Popliteal artery entrapment is demonstrated by ultrasound. Long-axis ultrasound images have been obtained over the popliteal artery at the level of the tibial plateau (callipers), with the calf at rest and with maximal contraction. Contraction is produced by standing in a tip-toe position. With the calf muscle contracted, the popliteal artery shows a short segment of severe narrowing (+ callipers)

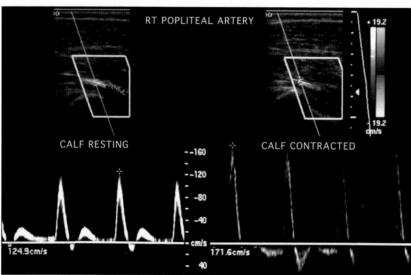

◄(b) Doppler interrogation of the narrowed popliteal artery segment shows a corresponding increase in the measured peak systolic velocity when compared with the resting vessel.

References

Ahlback S, Bauer GC, Bohne WH. 'Spontaneous osteonecrosis of the knee.' *Arthritis Rheum* 1968, 11(6): 705–33.

Amendola A, Rorabeck CH, Vellett D, Vezina W, Rutt B, Nott L. 'The use of magnetic resonance imaging in exertional compartment syndromes.' *Am J Sports Med* 1990, 18: 29–34.

Araki Y, Yamamoto H, Nakamura H, Tsukaguchi I. 'MR diagnosis of discoid lateral menisci of the knee.' *Eur J Radiol* 1994, 18(2): 92–5.

Barber FA. 'What is the unhappy triad?' *Arthroscopy* 1992, 8: 19–22.

Batt ME. 'Shin splints: a review of terminology.' *Clin J Sport Med* 1995, 5: 53–7.

Beggs I. 'Sonography of muscle hernias.' *Am J Roentgenol* 2003, 180(2): 395–9.

Bergin D, Morrison WB, Carrino JA, Nallamshetty SN, Bartolozzi AR. 'Anterior cruciate ligament ganglia and mucoid degeneration: coexistence and clinical correlation.' *Am J Roentgenol* 2004: 182(5): 1283–7.

Bertin KC, Goble ME. 'Ligament injuries associated with physeal fractures about the knee.' *Clin Orthop* 1983, 177: 188–95.

Boutin RD, Januario JA, Newberg AH, Gundry CR, Newman JS. 'MR imaging features of osteochondritis dissecans of the femoral sulcus.' *Am J Roentgenol* 2003, 180(3): 641–5.

Brahms MA, Fumich RM, Ippolito VD. 'A typical stress fracture of the tibia in a professional athlete.' *Am J Sports Med* 1980, 8: 131–2.

Bredella MA, Tirman PF, Peterfy CG, Zarlingo M, Feller JF, Bost FW, Belzer JP, Wischer TK, Genant HK. 'Accuracy of T2-weighted fast spin-echo MR imaging with fat saturation in detecting cartilage defects in the knee: comparison with arthroscopy in 130 patients.' *Am J Roentgenol* 1999, 172(4): 1073–80.

Brukner P, Bradshaw C, Khan KM, White S, Crossley K. 'Stress fractures: a review of 180 cases.' *Clin J Sport Med* 1996, 6: 85–9.

Burk DL Jr, Dalinka MK, Kanal E, Schiebler ML, Cohen EK, Prorok RJ, Gefter WB, Kressel HY. 'Meniscal and ganglion cysts of the knee: MR evaluation.' *Am J Roentgenol* 1988, 150: 331–6.

Buschman WR, Cheung Y, Jahss MH. 'Magnetic resonance imaging of anomalous leg muscles: accessory soleus, peroneus quartus and the flexor digitorum longus accessorius.' *Foot Ankle* 1991, 12: 109–16.

Campos JC, Chung CB, Lektraul N, Pedowitz R, Trudell D, Yu J, Resnick D. 'Pathogenesis of the Segond fracture: anatomic and MR imaging evidence of an iliotibial tract or anterior oblique band avulsion.' *Radiology* 2001, 219(2): 381–6.

Chung CB, Skaf A, Roger B, Campos J, Stump X, Resnick D. 'Patellar tendon-lateral femoral condyle friction syndrome: MR imaging in 42 patients.' *Skeletal Radiol* 2001, 30(12): 694–7.

Connor MA, Palaniappan M, Khan N et al. 'Osteochondritis dissecans of the knee in children: a comparison of MRI and arthroscopic findings.' *J Bone Joint Surg (Br)* 2002, 84B: 258–62.

Craig JG, Widman D, van Holsbeek M. 'Longitudinal stress fracture: patterns of edema and the importance of the nutrient foramen.' *Skeletal Radiol* 2003, 32(1): 22–7.

Davey JR, Rorabeck CH, Fowler PJ. 'The tibialis posterior muscle compartment. An unrecognized cause of exertional compartment syndrome.' *Am J Sports Med* 1984, 12: 391–7.

De Smet AA, Ilahi OA, Graf BK. 'Untreated osteochondritis dissecans of the femoral condyles: prediction of patient outcome using radiographic and MR findings.' *Skeletal Radiol* 1997, 26(8): 463–7.

Detmer DE. 'Chronic shin splints. Classification and management of medial tibial stress syndrome.' *Sports Med* 1986, 3: 436–46.

DiStefano VJ. 'Skeletal injuries of the knee.' In: Nicholas JA, Hershman EB (eds), *The Lower Extremity and Spine in Sports Medicine*, Mosby, St Louis 1995, p. 776.

Dunn TC, Lu Y, Jin H, Ries MD, Majumdar S. 'T2 relaxation time of cartilage at MR imaging: comparison with severity of knee osteoarthritis.' *Radiology* 2004, 232(2): 592–8.

Eckhoff DG, Montgomery WK, Kilcoyne RF, Stamm ER. 'Femoral morphometry and anterior knee pain.' *Clin Orthop* 1994, 302: 64–8.

Egund N, Friden T, Hjarbaek J, Lindstrand A, Stockerup R. 'Radiographic assessment of sagittal knee instability in weight bearing. A study of anterior cruciate-deficient knees.' *Skeletal Radiol* 1993, 22: 177–81.

Escobedo EM, Mills WJ, Hunter JC. 'The "reverse Segond" fracture: association with a tear of the posterior cruciate ligament and medial meniscus.' *Am J Roentgenol* 2002, 178(4): 979–83.

Falkenberg P, Nygaard H. 'Isolated anterior dislocation of the proximal tibiofibular joint.' *J Bone Joint Surg (Br)* 1983, 65: 310–11.

Fanelli GC, Edson CJ, Maish DR. 'Combined anterior/posterior cruciate ligament/medial/lateral side injuries of the knee.' *Sports Med. Arth. Rev.* 2001, 9(3): 208–18.

Fong EE. '"Iliac horns" (symmetrical bilateral central posterior iliac processes): a case report.' *Radiology* 1946, 47: 517–18.

Fredericson M, Bergman AG, Hoffman KL, Dillingham MS. 'Tibial stress reaction in runners. Correlation of clinical symptoms and scintigraphy with a new magnetic resonance grading system.' *Am J Sports Med* 1995, 23(4): 472–81.

Fulkerson JP, Shea KP. 'Disorders of patellofemoral alignment.' *J Bone Joint Surg (Am)* 1990, 72: 1424–9.

Gaeta M, Minutoli F, Scribano E, Ascenti G, Vinci S, Bruschetta D, Magaudda L, Blandino A. 'CT and MR imaging findings in athletes with early tibial stress injuries: comparison with bone scintigraphy findings and emphasis on cortical abnormalities.' *Radiology* 2005, 235(2): 553–61.

Garth WP Jr, Greco J, House MA. 'The lateral notch sign associated with acute anterior cruciate ligament disruption.' *Am J Sports Med* 2000, 28(1): 68–73.

Ghelman B, Hodge JC. 'Imaging of the patellofemoral joint.' *Orthop Clin North Am* 1992, 23: 523–43.

Girgis F, Marshall J, Monajem A. 'The cruciate ligaments of the knee joint: anatomical, functional, and experimental analysis.' *Clin Orthop* 1975, 106: 216–31.

Gisslen K, Alfredson H. 'Neovascularisation and pain in jumper's knee: a prospective clinical and sonographic study in elite junior volleyball players.' *Br J Sports Med* 2005, 39(7): 423–38.

Gray SD, Kaplan PA, Dussault RG, Omary RA, Campbell SE, Chrisman HB, Futterer SF, McGraw JK, Keats TE, Hillman BJ. 'Acute knee trauma: how many plain film views are necessary for the initial examination?' *Skeletal Radiol* 1997, 26(5): 298–302.

Green NE, Rogers RA, Lipscomb AB. 'Non-union of stress fractures of the tibia.' *Am J Sports Med* 1985, 13: 171–6.

Guzzanti V, Gigante A, Di Lazzaro A, Fabbricianni C. 'Patellofemoral malalignment in adolescents. Computerized tomographic assessment with or without quadriceps contraction.' *Am J Sports Med* 1994, 22: 55–60.

Haimes AH, Medvecky MJ et al. 'MR imaging of the anatomy and injuries to the lateral and posterolateral aspects of the knee.' *Am J of Roentgen* 2003, 180: 647–53.

Hess T, Rupp S, Hopf T, Gleitz M, Liebler J. 'Lateral tibial avulsion fractures and disruptions to the anterior cruciate ligament. A clinical study of their incidence and correlation.' *Clin Orthop* 1994, 303: 193–7.

Houghton G, Ackeroyd C. 'Sleeve fractures of the patella in children.' *J Bone Joint Surg (Am)* 1979, 165–8.

Huang GS, Yu JS, Munshi M, Chan WP, Lee CH, Chen CY, Resnick D. 'Avulsion fracture of the head of the fibula (the "arcuate" sign): MR imaging findings predictive of injuries to the posterolateral ligaments and posterior cruciate ligament.' *Am J Roentgenol* 2003, 180(2): 381–7.

Hughes JA, Cook JV, Churchill MA, Warren ME. 'Juvenile osteochondritis dissecans: a 5-year review of the natural history using clinical and MRI evaluation.' *Pediatr Radiol* 2003, 33(6): 410–7.

Hughston JC. 'Subluxation of the patella.' *J Bone Joint Surg (Am)* 1968, 50: 1003–26.

Insall J, Salvati E. 'Patella position in the normal knee joint.' *Radiology* 1971, 101: 101–4.

Kalebo P, Sward L, Karlsson J, Peterson L. 'Ultrasonography in the detection of partial patellar ligament ruptures (jumper's knee).' *Skeletal Radiol* 1991, 20: 285–9.

Kane D, Balint PV, Gibney R et al. 'Differential diagnosis of calf pain with musculoskeletal ultrasound.' *Ann of Rheum Diseases* 2004, 63: 11–14.

Kannus PA, Jozoa L. 'Histopathological changes preceding spontaneous rupture of a tendon. A controlled study of 891 patients.' *J Bone Joint Surg (Am)* 1991, 73(10): 1507–25.

Kaplan EB. 'Some aspects of functional anatomy of the human knee joint.' *Clin Orthop* 1962, 23: 18–29.

Kaplan PA, Walker CW, Kilcoyne RF et al. 'Occult fracture patterns of the knee associated with anterior cruciate ligament tears: assessment with MR imaging.' *Radiology* 1992, 183(3): 83–8.

Kaushik S, Erickson JK, Palmer WE, Winalski CS, Kilpatrick SJ, Weissman BN. 'Effect of chondrocalcinosis on the MR imaging of knee menisci.' *Am J Roentgenol* 2001, 177(4): 905–9.

Kelly DW et al. 'Patellar and quadriceps tendon rupture: jumper's knee.' *Am J Sports Med* 1984, 12(5): 375–80.

Kennedy JC, Willis RB. 'The effects of local steroid injections on tendons: a biomechanical and microscopic correlative study.' *Am J Sports Medicine* 1976, 4(1): 11–21.

Kode L, Mota A. 'Evaluation of tibial plateau fractures: efficacy of MR imaging compared with CT.' *Am J Roentgenol* 1994, 163: 141–7.

Kujala UM, Kvist M, Heinonen O. 'Osgood–Schlatter's disease in adolescent athletes. Retrospective study of incidence and duration.' *Am J Sports Med* 1985, 4: 236–41.

La S, Fessell DP, Femino JE, Jacobsen JA, Jamadar D, Hayes C. 'Sonography of partial-thickness quadriceps tendon tears with surgical correlation.' *J Ultrasound Med* 2003, 22(12): 1323–9.

Lancourt JE, Cristini JA. 'Patella alta and patella infera. Their etiological role in patellar dislocation, chondromalacia and apophysitis of the tibial tubercle.' *J Bone Joint Surg (Am)* 1975, 57: 1112–15.

Lanyon LE, Smith RN. 'Bone strain in the tibia during normal quadrupedal locomotion.' *Acta Orthop Scand* 1970, 41: 238–48.

Laurin CA, Levesque HP, Dussault R, Labelle H, Peides JP. 'The abnormal lateral patellofemoral angle: a diagnostic roentgenographic sign of recurrent patellar subluxation.' *J Bone Joint Surg (Am)* 1978, 60: 55–60.

Lee JK, Phelps CT et al. 'Anterior ligament tears: MR imaging compared with arthroscopy and clinical tests.' *Radiology* 1988, 166: 861–4.

Lee LK, Yao L. 'Tibial collateral ligament bursa: MR imaging.' *Radiology* 1991, 178: 855–7.

Linden B. 'The incidence of osteochondritis dissecans in the condyles of the femur.' *Acta Orthop Scand* 1976, 47: 664–7.

Lugo-Olivieri CH, Scott WW Jr, Zerhouni EA. 'Fluid levels in injured knees: do they always represent lipohemarthrosis?' *Radiology* 1996, 198: 499–502.

Lynch TC, Crues JV 3rd, Morgan FW, Sheehan WE, Harter LP, Ryu R. 'Bone abnormalities of the knee: prevalence and significance at MR imaging.' *Radiology* 1989, 171: 761–6.

McClellan R, Trigg MD et al. 'Evaluation and treatment of tibial plateau fractures.' *Current Opin in Orthop* 1999, 10(1): 10–21.

McIntyre J, Moelleken S, Tirman P. 'Mucoid degeneration of the anterior cruciate ligament mistaken for ligamentous tears.' *Skeletal Radiol* 2001, 30: 312–15.

Mandalia V, Fogg AJ, Chari R, Murray J, Beale A, Henson JH. 'Bone bruising of the knee.' *Clin Radiol* 2005, 60(6): 627–36.

Mellado JM et al. 'Magnetic resonance imaging of anterior cruciate ligament: re-evaluation of quantitative parameters and imaging findings including a simplified method of measuring the anterior cruciate ligament angle.' *Knee Surg Traumatol Arthrosc* 2004, 12(3): 217–24.

Merchant AC, Mercer RL, Jacobsen RH, Cool CR. 'Roentgenographic analysis of patellofemoral congruence.' *J Bone Joint Surg (Am)* 1974, 56: 1391–6.

Mesgarzadeh M, Saprega AA, Bonakdarpour A, Revesz G, Moyer RA, Maurer AH, Alburger PD. 'Osteochondritis dissecans: analysis of mechanical stability with radiography, scintigraphy, and MR imaging.' *Radiology* 1987, 165: 775–80.

Meyers MH, McKeever FM. 'Fracture of the intercondylar eminence of the tibia.' *J Bone Joint Surg (Am)* 1959, 41A: 209–22.

Michael RH, Holder LE. 'The Soleus syndrome. A cause of medial tibial stress (shin splints).' *Am J Sports Med* 1985, 13: 87–94.

Miller TT, Gladder P et al. 'Posterolateral stabilizers of the knee: anatomy and injuries assessed with MR imaging.' *Am J Roentgenol* 1997, 169(6): 1641–7.

Minkoff J, Fein L. 'The role of radiography in the evaluation and treatment of common anarthrotic disorders of the patellofemoral joint.' *Clin Sports Med* 1980, 8: 203–60.

Molander ML, Wallin G, Wikstad I. 'Fracture of the intercondylar eminence of the tibia: a review of 35 patients.' *J Bone Joint Surg (Br)* 1981, 63–B: 89–91.

Moore BR, Hampers LC, Clark KD. 'Performance rule for radiographs of paediatric knee injuries.' *J Emerg Med* 2005, 28(3): 257–61.

Moore MS, McKenzie WG. 'Fracture of the proximal tibial epiphysis. Clinical case presentation: Alfred I', Dupont Institute, 4 April 1996.

Morini G, Chiodi E et al. 'Hoffa's disease of the adipose pad: magnetic resonance versus surgical findings' *Radiol Med (Totino)* 1998, 95: 278–85.

Norwood LA Jr, Cross MJ. 'The intercondylar shelf and the anterior cruciate ligament.' *Am J Sports Med* 1977, 5: 171–6.

Obedian RS, Grelsamer RP. 'Osteochondritis dissecans of the distal femur and patella.' *Clin Sports Med* 1997, 16(1): 157–74.

O'Donoghue DH. *Treatment of Injuries to Athletes*, 4th edn, W.B. Saunders, Philadelphia, 1984, p. 524.

Ogden JA, McCarthy SM, Jokl P. 'The painful bipartite patella.' *J Pediatr Orthop* 1982, 2: 263–9.

Ogden JA, Southwick WO. 'Osgood-Schlatter's disease and tibial tuberosity development.' *Clin Orthop* 1976, 116: 180–9.

Ogden JA, Tross RB, Murphy MJ. 'Fractures of the tibial tuberosity in adolescents.' *J Bone Joint Surg (Am)* 1980, 62: 205–15.

Patten RM, Richardson ML, Zink-Brody G, Rolfe BA. 'Complete vs partial-thickness tears of the posterior cruciate ligament: MR findings.' *J Comput Assist Tomogr* 1994, 18: 793–9.

Pillai A. 'Popliteal artery entrapment: diagnosis by MRI.' *Ind J Radiol Imag* 2002, 12: 91–3.

Prince JS, Lalor T, Bean JA. 'MRI of anterior cruciate ligament injuries and associated findings in the paediatric knee: changes with skeletal maturity.' *Am J Roentgenol* 2005, 185: 756–62.

Radin EL. 'A rational approach to the treatment of patellofemoral pain.' *Clin Orthop* 1979, 144: 107–9.

Reikeras O. 'Patellofemoral characteristics in patients with increased femoral anteversion.' *Skeletal Radiol* 1992, 21: 311–13.

Resnick D, Niwayama G. *Diagnosis of Bone and Joint Disorders*, 2nd edn, W.B. Saunders, Philadelphia, 1988, p. 727.

Rijke AM, Tegtmeyer CJ, Weiland DJ, McCue FC 3rd. 'Stress examination of the cruciate ligaments: a radiologic Lachman test.' *Radiology* 1987, 165: 867–9.

Riseborough EJ et al. 'Growth disturbances following distal femoral physeal fracture separations.' *J Bone Joint Surg (Am)* 1983, 65(7): 885–93.

Rosenberg TD, Paulos LE, Parker RD, Coward DB, Scott SM. 'The forty-five degree posteroanterior flexion weightbearing radiograph of the knee.' *J Bone Joint Surg (Am)* 1988, 70: 1479–83.

Ryu KN, Kim IS, Kim EJ, Ahn JW, Bae DK, Sartoris DJ, Resnick D. 'MR imaging of tears of discoid lateral menisci.' *Am J Roentgenol* 1998, 171(4): 963–7.

Schnarkowski P, Tirman PF, Fuchigami KD, Crues JV, Butler MG, Genant HK. 'Meniscal ossicle: radiographic and MR imaging findings.' *Radiology* 1995, 196: 47–50.

Schwartz C, Blazina ME, Domenick JS et al. 'The results of operative treatment osteochondritis dissecans of the patella.' *Am J Sports Med* 1988, 16: 522–9.

Seaberg DC, Jackson R. 'Clinical decision rule for knee radiographs.' *Am J Emerg Med* 1994, 12: 541–3.

Shabshin N, Schweitzer ME et al. 'MRI criteria for patella alta and baja.' *Skeletal Radiol* 2004, 33(8): 445–50.

Shea KP, Fulkerson JP. 'Preoperative computed tomography scanning and arthroscopy in predicting outcome after lateral retinacular release.' *Arthroscopy* 1992, 8: 327–34.

Shelbourne KD, Nitz PA. 'The O'Donoghue triad revisited. Combined knee injuries involving anterior cruciate and medial collateral ligament tears.' *Am J Sports Med* 1991, 19: 474–7.

Shellock FG, Powers CM. 'Kinematic MRI of the patellofemoral joint. Kinematic MRI of the joints: functional anatomy.' *Kinesiology and Clinical Appli.* 2001, 165–202.

Silverman JM, Mink JH, Deutsch AL. 'Discoid menisci of the knee: MR imaging appearance.' *Radiology* 1989, 173: 351–4.

Simonian PT, Sussmann PS, Wickiewicz TL, Potter HG, van Trommel M, Weiland-Holland S, Warren RF. 'Popliteomeniscal fasciculi and the unstable lateral meniscus: clinical correlation and magnetic resonance diagnosis.' *Arthroscopy* 1997, 13(5): 590–6.

Siwek CW, Rao JP. 'Ruptures of the extensor mechanism of the knee joint.' *J Bone Joint Surg (Am)* 1981, 63: 932–7.

Spritzer CE. '"Slip sliding away": Patellofemoral dislocation and tracking.' *Magn Reson Imaging Clin N Am* 2000, 8(2): 401–11.

Stallenberg B, Gevenois PA, Sintzoff SA, Matos C, Andrianne Y, Struyven J. 'Fracture of the posterior aspect of the lateral tibial plateau: radiographic sign of anterior cruciate ligament tear.' *Radiology* 1993, 187: 821–5.

Stiell IG, Greenberg GH, Wells GA et al. 'Prospective validation of a decision rule for the use of radiography in acute knee injuries.' *JAMA* 1996, 275: 611–15.

Stiell IG, Wells GA et al. 'Use of radiography in acute knee injuries: need for clinical decision making.' *Academic Emerg Med* 1995, 2: 966–73.

Stoller DW. *Magnetic Resonance Imaging in Orthopaedics and Sports Medicine*, 2nd edn, Lippincott-Raven, 1997.

Stone KR, Stoller D, Carli AD, Day R, Richnak J. 'The frequency of Baker's cysts associated with meniscal tears.' *Am J Sports Med* 1996, 24: 670–1.

Stuart TPA. 'A note on a variation in the course of the popliteal artery.' *J Anat Physiol* 1879, 13–162.

Styf J. 'Entrapment of the superficial peroneal nerve. Diagnosis and results of decompression.' *J Bone Joint Surg (Br)* 1989, 71: 131–5.

Sullivan D, Dines D, Hershon S. 'Natural history of a type III fracture of the intercondylar eminence of the tibia in an adult.' *Am J Sports Med* 1989, 17: 132–3.

Swenson TM, Harner CD. 'Knee ligament and meniscal injuries. Current concepts.' *Ortho Clin North Am* 1995, 26(3): 529–46.

Symeonides PP. 'High stress fractures of the fibula.' *J Bone Joint Surg (Br)* 1980, 62–B: 192–3.

Taunton JE, Ryan MB, Clements DB et al. 'A retrospective case: control analysis of running injuries.' *Br J Sports Med.* 2002, 36: 95–101.

Thomason PA, Linson MA. 'Isolated dislocation of the proximal tibiofibular joint.' *J Trauma* 1986, 26: 192–5.

Thomee R, Augustsson J, Karlson J. 'Patellofemoral pain syndrome: a review of current issues.' *Sports Med* 1999, 28(4): 245–62.

Torg JS, Pavlov H, Morris VB. 'Salter-Harris type III fracture of the medial femoral condyle occurring in the adolescent athlete.' *J Bone Joint Surg (Am)* 1981, 63: 586–91.

Twaddle BC, Bidwell TA, Chapman JR. 'Knee dislocations: where are the lesions? A prospective evaluation of surgical findings in 63 cases.' *J Orthop Trauma* 2003, 17(3): 198–202.

Van Holsbeek M, Vandamme B, Marchal G et al. 'Dorsal defects of the patella: concept of its origin and relationship with bipartite and multipartite patella.' *Skeletal Radiol* 1987, 16(4): 304–11.

Vande Berg BC, Lecouvert FE, Poilvache P, Jamart J, Materne R, Lengle B, Maldague B, Malghelm J. 'Assessment of knee cartilage in cadavers with dual-detector spiral CT arthrography and MR imaging.' *Radiology* 2002, 222(2): 430–6.

Vellet AD, Marks PH, Fowler PJ, Munro TG. 'Occult post-traumatic osteochondral lesions of the knee: prevalence, classification, and short-term sequelae evaluated with MR imaging.' *Radiology* 1991, 178: 271–6.

Verleisdonk EJ, van Gils A, van der Werken C. 'The diagnostic value of MRI scans for the diagnosis of chronic exertional compartment syndrome of the lower leg.' *Skeletal Radiol* 2001, 30(6): 321–5.

Whan A, Breidahl W, Janes G. 'MRI of trapped periosteum in a proximal tibial physeal injury of a pediatric patient.' *Am J Roentgenol* 2003, 181(5): 1397–9.

Whelan TJ. 'Popliteal artery entrapment.' In Haimovici H (ed.), *Vascular Surgery: Principles and Techniques*, 2nd edn, Appleton-Century-Crofts, New York, 1984, pp. 557–67.

Wiley JP, Short WB, Wiseman DA, Miller SD. 'Ultrasound catheter placement for deep posterior compartment pressure measurements in chronic compartment syndrome.' *Am J Sports Med* 1990, 18: 74–9.

Williams A, Gillis A, McKenzie C, Po B, Sharma L, Micheli L, McKeon B, Burstein D. 'Glycosaminoglycan distribution in cartilage as determined by delayed gadolinium-enhanced MRI of cartilage (dGEMRIC): potential clinical applications.' *Am J Roentgenol* 2004, 182(1): 167–72.

Woodland LH, Francis RS. 'Parameters and comparisons of the quadriceps angle of college-aged men and women in the supine and standing positions.' *Am J Sports Med* 1992, 20: 208–11.

Yamamoto T, Bullough PG. 'Spontaneous osteonecrosis of the knee: the result of subchondral insufficiency fracture.' *J Bone Joint Surg (Am)* 2000, 82A: 858–66.

Yu JS, Salonen DC, Holder J et al. 'Posterolateral aspect of the knee: improved MR imaging with a coronal oblique technique.' *Radiology* 1996, 198: 199–204.

Zanetti M, Pfirrmann CW, Schmid MR, Romero J, Seifert B, Hodler J. 'Patients with suspected meniscal tears: prevalence of abnormalities seen on MRI of 100 symptomatic and 100 contralateral asymptomatic knees.' *Am J Roentgenol* 2003, 181(3): 635–41.

Image acknowledgments

The authors wish to thank the following colleagues who kindly offered images for inclusion in this chapter:

- Dr James Linklater (Figs 6.29, 6.37(b), 6.44(a), 6.44(b), 6.87, 6.111, 6.121, 6.125 and 6.230)
- Dr Bill Breidahl (Figs 6.56, 6.57, 6.58, 6.74, 6.93, 6.102, 6.105, 6.108, 6.112, 6.116, 6.153, 6.154, 6.186(a) and (b), 6.199(a), 6.209(b), 6.212, 6.221(b), 6.226, 6.228, 6.239, 6.251, 6.252, 6.253, 6.258, 6.270, 6.271, 6.272, 6.278(b) and 6.279(b))
- Dr Phil Lucas (Figs 6.18(a), 6.18(b), 6.59, 6.65(b), 6.71(b), 6.101, 6.106(a), 6.106(b), 6.124, 6.136, 6.163, 6.174, 6.194(a), 6.196, 6.197, 6.202, 6.203(a), 6.204, 6.224, 6.208(b), 6.221(a), 6.232, 6.238, 6.247, 6.250, 6.255, 6.256, 6.257, 6.261, 6.268 and 6.285)
- Dr Robert Cooper and Dr Stephen Allwright (Figs 6.43, 6.68, 6.69, 6.82(a), 6.246, 6.254, 6.277(b), 6.277(c), 6.288, 6.296(c) and 6.300)
- Gosford Hospital (Figs 6.6(b), 6.6(c), 6.28, 6.63(a) and 6.266).

These images have significantly added to the quality of the chapter.

The ankle and foot

Jock Anderson and John Read with James Linklater

7

The ankle

The ankle is commonly injured at all levels of sport and becomes particularly vulnerable during agility activities. The ankle is a hinge joint creating a stable linkage between the body and the foot. The talus is held in a rigid mortise created by the malleoli and the tibial plafond, with added stability provided by strong supporting ligaments. The design of the joint restricts ankle movement to flexion, extension and slight anterior glide of the talus, providing stability even when subjected to large dynamic loads. The component of internal rotation required for walking is provided by rotation of the entire lower limb. The ankle ligaments provide an essential constraint against inversion, eversion, anteroposterior translation and torsion.

The lateral ligament complex is the most common site of sporting injury (Garrick 1982) and accounts for 16–21% of all athletic injuries (Mangwani 2001). Lateral ligament complex injuries or 'sprains' occur at all ages and every level of fitness. Although these injuries are usually minor, occasionally the ligament damage is severe or there are associated fractures, significantly delaying a return to sporting activity. Whether the injured athlete is recreational or professional, a rapid return to sport is a priority, and this depends on the early implementation of appropriate management. Referral for diagnostic imaging is an important part of this management, as the complexity of ankle anatomy and the potential for multiple concurrent sites of injury can make an accurate clinical diagnosis difficult (Anzilotti et al. 1996).

Imaging the ankle

The imaging assessment of the ankle begins with plain films of a high technical standard. As discussed below, each view of this series is required to demonstrate specific anatomical structures. As a consequence, if these films are technically poor, these structures cannot be assessed and diagnostic changes will be missed. Clinicians who bypass plain films for more sophisticated imaging tests will inevitably make embarrassing errors. Plain films may provide unexpected information about the ankle. There may be a coalition or other developmental anomalies, evidence of old injury, degenerative changes, bone stress or possibly a tumour (see Fig. 7.1).

Other imaging methods commonly used around the ankle include nuclear bone scans, ultrasound, CT and MRI. The use of these methods is discussed below.

Plain films

Although the ankle is the most injured and imaged joint in the body, plain films of the ankle are often technically unsatisfactory. The radiographer needs to understand the basic anatomical structure of the ankle joint and to remember that the talus is oriented 10 to 15° to the long axis of the foot. This influences the positioning required to achieve adequate views and, in particular, affects the lateral and 'mortise' views.

Standard plain film views of the ankle

The standard ankle series includes anteroposterior (AP), 'mortise' and lateral views, with additional views used when clinically indicated, or if there is doubt about an abnormality on the initial series. Generally, the routine series is non-weightbearing, with weightbearing views obtained as additional functional views. However, in a specialised sports medicine environment, views are often obtained with weightbearing in the first instance because of the valuable additional information supplied. The advantage of weightbearing views is discussed later, in the section 'Additional plain film views of the ankle'. The initial series is acquired as outlined below.

AP view

The routine AP view is obtained with the patient supine, the toes pointing directly upwards and the ankle dorsiflexed. Using a straight tube, the primary beam is centred on the ankle joint space, midway between the malleoli. The anterior tubercle of the tibia overlies the medial margin of the distal fibula and, because of the obliquity of the talus in this view, the lateral clear space of the ankle joint and the lateral corner of the talar dome are obscured by the lateral malleolus (see Fig. 7.2).

'Mortise' view

The 'mortise' view is an extremely important view and is an essential part of any ankle series. The ankle is internally rotated 15 to 20° to bring the talus into its true AP alignment. If the position is correct, the malleoli will be equidistant from the cassette and the lateral border of the foot will be roughly perpendicular to the tabletop. A straight tube is used, centring on the joint space midway between the malleoli. A clear space surrounds the talus, allowing the medial and lateral clear spaces and the talotibial joint space to be compared and the entire profile of the talar dome to be assessed. This is essential for the identification of talar dome fractures and in the diagnosis of a tibiofibular syndesmosis injury (see Fig. 7.3). It is important that the ankle is positioned in dorsiflexion to avoid the tip of the lateral malleolus being obscured by

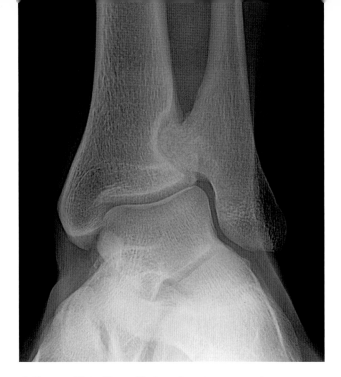

▲ **Fig. 7.1** Plain films will often show important changes and remain the cornerstone of imaging diagnosis. The information is sometimes unexpected, as in this case, where an osteochondroma arises from the lateral margin of the distal fibula and erodes the adjacent tibia, disrupting the function of the distal tibiofibular syndesmosis.

calcaneal superimposition (see Fig. 7.4). Unfortunately, this is a common and important radiographic fault, as the tip of the lateral malleolus is a frequent site of an avulsion fracture.

▼ **Fig. 7.2** The AP view is obtained with the long axis of the foot at right angles to the cassette. In this position, the intrinsic external angulation of the talus will cause the lateral corner of the talar dome and the anterior tubercle of the tibia to be superimposed over the medial border of the fibula and to obliterate the lateral gutter of the ankle. Nevertheless, this view is valuable in the assessment of soft-tissue swelling, bony architecture, malleoli fractures and both the distal tibiofibular and ankle joint spaces.

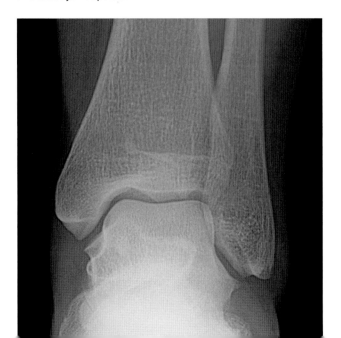

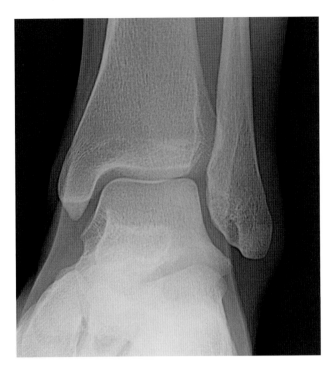

▲ Fig. 7.3 The 'mortise' view is a true AP projection of the talus and is an extremely important component of an ankle series. The margins of the talus are clearly displayed in their entirety and the spaces surrounding the talus are easily assessed. This view is particularly important for identification of talar dome fractures and the subtle changes of a syndesmosis injury.

Lateral view

Substandard lateral views are common. A correctly positioned lateral view is required for the assessment of important features of both bone and soft-tissue anatomy. For the ankle to be correctly positioned, the medial and lateral malleoli should be superimposed and the joint space clearly demonstrated to enable examination of its articular surfaces. This is achieved by centring the primary beam with a straight tube on the joint space. Preferably, the lateral view is obtained with the medial border of the foot against the cassette and a small pad placed beneath the anterior aspect of the knee to rotate the ankle into a true lateral position. An appropriate exposure will allow examination of the soft tissues around the ankle joint as well as important bony structures. The presence of an ankle joint effusion, subtle pathological changes in the pre-Achilles (Kager) fat pad and any abnormality in the profile of the Achilles tendon should be detectable on a correctly exposed lateral view (see Figs 7.5 and 7.6).

▶ Fig. 7.5 This is a technically correct non-weightbearing lateral view of the ankle, demonstrating superimposition of the malleoli and the articular surfaces of the tibiotalar articulation. Soft tissues to be examined include the Achilles tendon, the plantar fascia and the various fat planes anterior to the ankle. A small spur is noted at the anterior margin of the distal tibial articular surface and there is prominence of the anterior joint soft tissues, consistent with a small effusion or synovitis (arrow). This appearance is discussed later in the chapter.

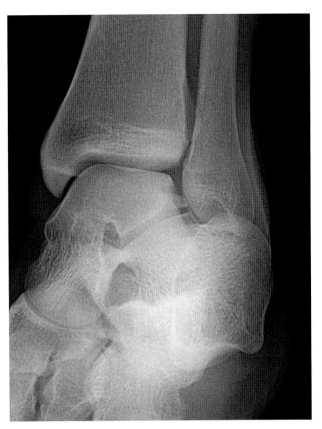

▲ Fig. 7.4 In acquiring a 'mortise' view of the ankle, it is important that the ankle is dorsiflexed, to prevent superimposition of the tip of the lateral malleolus over the calcaneum, as shown in this case. Unfortunately, this is a common radiographic fault and prevents proper assessment of the tip of the lateral malleolus.

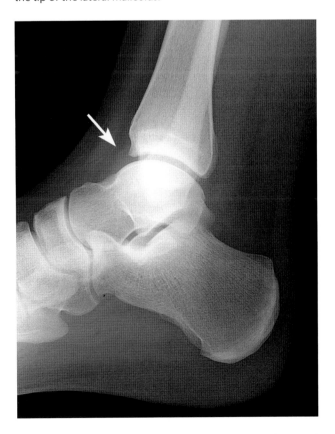

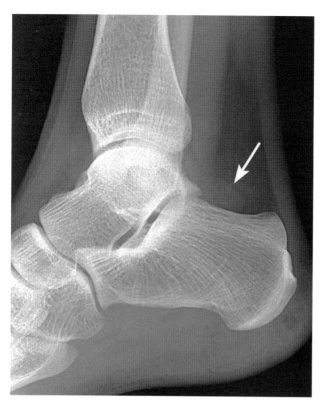

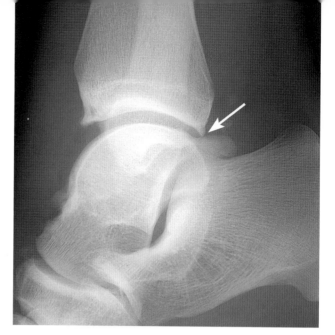

▲ Fig. 7.7 With plantar flexion of the ankle, bony abutment occurs between a small spur on the posterior tip of the distal tibia and the prominent posterior process of the talus (arrow). Small ossicles lying behind the ankle are almost certainly loose bodies, possibly lying in a distended posterior joint recess, or within a ganglion or in the FHL tendon sheath. There is also a spur on the anterior aspect of the distal tibia and it is likely that this athlete experiences anterior as well as posterior impingement symptoms.

▲ Fig. 7.6 An oval opacity encroaches on the pre-Achilles fat pad (arrow). The appearance is likely to be due to a ganglion, although an effusion distending the posterior recess of the subtalar joint may also produce this appearance.

The lateral view should be non-weightbearing when there is a clinical suspicion of a foreign body or localised soft-tissue swelling on the plantar aspect of the foot.

Additional plain film views of the ankle

Often an extra view at the time of the initial imaging visit will confirm a diagnosis and avoid the need for a return visit or the use of more expensive imaging methods. Extra views that are often provided to complement the routine views include impingement, oblique tarsal, Harris-Beath, weightbearing and 'lazy' lateral views, views of the proximal fibula, stress views of the tibiofibular syndesmosis, other stress views and reversed oblique views.

Impingement view

To assess bony contribution to posterior impingement, a lateral film is obtained with the ankle in extreme plantar flexion. Posterior impingement commonly results from direct bony abutment between the posterior rim of the tibia and an os trigonum or a prominent posterior process of the talus (see Fig. 7.7). An anterior impingement view is obtained with weightbearing and maximum dorsiflexion. This is also known as a 'lunge' view. Anterior impingement is commonly seen in kicking sports and is usually caused by the development of a bone spur at the anterior margin of the distal tibia. This spur impinges on an area of new bone formation on the dorsal aspect of the neck of the talus (see Fig. 7.8).

Although these views help determine the degree to which bony factors contribute to the clinical syndrome of ankle

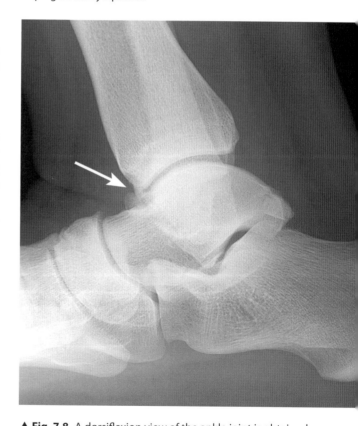

▲ Fig. 7.8 A dorsiflexion view of the ankle joint is obtained to detect anterior bony impingement. This is easily performed with weightbearing using the 'lunge' position. In this case, bony abutment is demonstrated between an anterior tibial spur and new bone formation on the dorsal surface of the neck of the talus (arrow). A large os trigonum is noted.

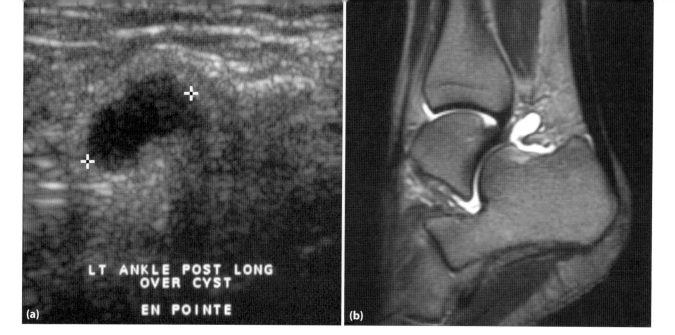

LT ANKLE POST LONG
OVER CYST

EN POINTE

(a)

(b)

▲ **Fig. 7.9** Soft-tissue causes for impingement may be suspected on plain films, but characterisation of these changes generally requires ultrasound or MRI.

(a) Ultrasound demonstrates a ganglion cyst as a cause of posterior impingement in a ballerina (callipers). The cyst was aspirated and injected under ultrasound control.

(b) Another ballerina with posterior impingement syndrome has a loculated collection of fluid on the posterior aspect of the ankle, demonstrated by a T2-weighted MR image. It is difficult to be certain whether this is a ganglion or a distended posterior recess of the subtalar joint. Degenerative changes involve the subtalar joint, with an effusion, minor joint space narrowing and sclerosis beneath the talar articular surface.

▶ **Fig. 7.10** Joint instability may predispose to impingement. There is a chronic lateral ligament complex insufficiency, resulting in marked varus angulation of the talus. The talus impinges on the tibial plafond and will eventually erode its articular surface. The lateral corner of the talar dome impinges on the lateral malleolus. There is also evidence that there has been impingement between a spur arising from the tip of the lateral malleolus and the lateral process of the talus. Flattening of the impinging surfaces has developed. An ossicle at the tip of the medial malleolus has resulted from a previous injury.

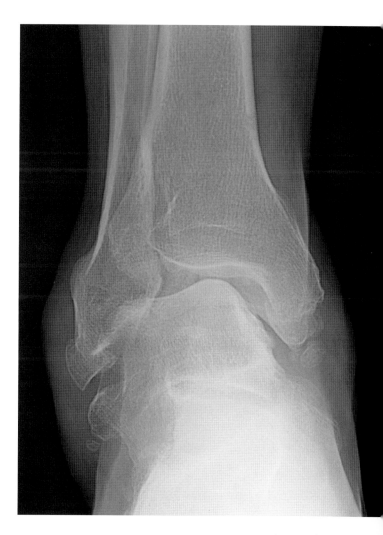

impingement, it must be remembered that both anterior and posterior impingement may be due to soft-tissue changes, which may often be identified on a correctly exposed plain film. Usually, accurate characterisation of these soft-tissue abnormalities will require further imaging by ultrasound or MRI (see Fig. 7.9). Lateral and medial bony impingement at the ankle may also be demonstrated using weightbearing AP and oblique views (see Fig. 7.10).

Oblique tarsal view

An oblique tarsal view is an important additional view to include in all ankle series requested for injury assessment following an inversion injury of the ankle (see Fig. 7.11). A fracture of the anterior process of the calcaneum is known as the 'missed fracture' because it is notorious for being over-looked (see Table 7.1 on page 547). An oblique tarsal view is included as an additional view in the ankle series purely to demonstrate this fracture. All post-traumatic ankle series at the Sydney 2000 Olympics contained this view routinely

▼ **Fig. 7.11** An oblique view of the foot demonstrates two key structures often injured as the result of an ankle inversion injury: the base of the fifth metatarsal and the anterior process of the calcaneum. Fractures of these structures are commonly missed if an ankle series alone is requested following an inversion injury. Consequently, if initial films are normal but there is a high level of clinical concern, this extra view is invaluable. There is a strong argument to support the routine inclusion of this view in an ankle series for trauma in the sports medicine environment.

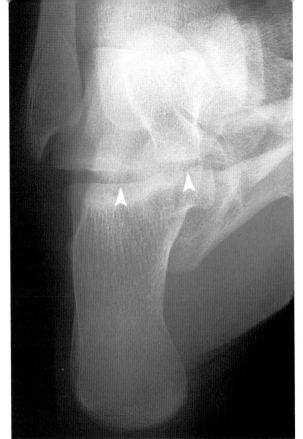

▲ **Fig. 7.12** A Harris-Beath view is simple to obtain and is a useful extra view to demonstrate the posterior and middle subtalar joints (indicated by arrowheads).

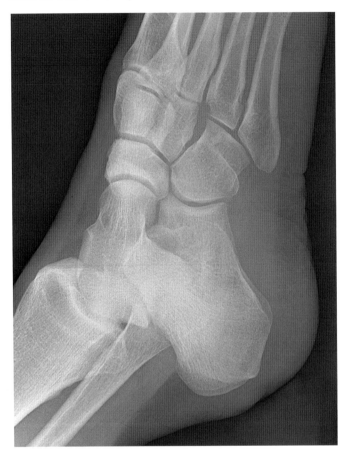

and many anterior process injuries were demonstrated that may have otherwise been missed. In addition, this oblique view will demonstrate fractures of the base of the fifth metatarsal, which are also caused by inversion injury.

Harris-Beath view

The Harris-Beath view demonstrates the articular surfaces of both the posterior and middle subtalar joints. This view is obtained with the patient sitting on the x-ray table, leg extended and the heel resting on the cassette. The ankle is extended and held in this position by the patient applying traction to the forefoot with a bandage or strap. A 45° cranial tube angle is used, with the primary beam entering the sole of the foot at the level of the base of the fifth metatarsal. Minor internal rotation of the foot will improve the view by bringing the sustentaculum tali into profile (Anderson 2000) (see Fig. 7.12).

▶ **Fig. 7.13** A fracture of the sustentaculum tali is well demonstrated by a Harris-Beath view (arrow).

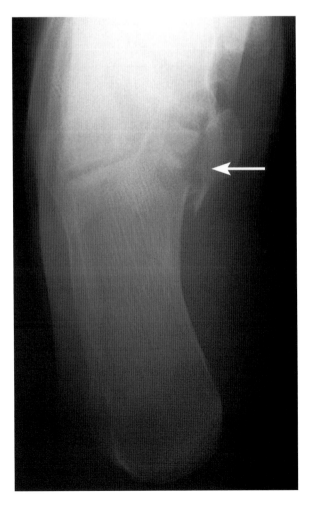

A Harris-Beath view is useful for the diagnosis of talo-calcaneal coalition and to demonstrate fractures of the sustentaculum tali (see Fig. 7.13). These conditions will be discussed later in the chapter.

Weightbearing views

Weightbearing views can help in the assessment of articular cartilage loss (see Fig. 7.14), subluxation of the ankle joint (see Fig. 7.15) and diastasis of the distal tibiofibular syndesmosis (see Fig. 7.16). Weightbearing accentuates changes in alignment, such as in valgus and varus hindfoot deformities (see Fig. 7.17).

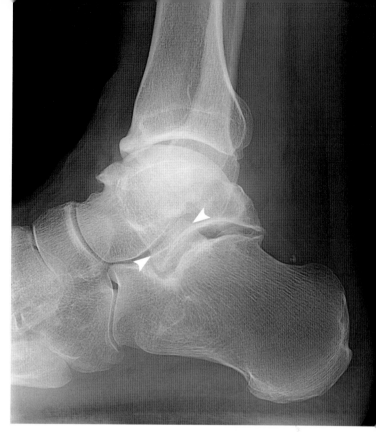

▼ **Fig. 7.14** A weightbearing view of the ankle is useful for the assessment of degenerative disease of the ankle, with joint space narrowing indicating loss of articular cartilage. In this case, in addition to joint space narrowing, there is minor lateral subluxation of the talus and narrowing of the lateral gutter. The inferior tibiofibular joint space shows widening and the appearance suggests degenerative changes occurring following an untreated diastasis injury.

▲ **Fig. 7.15** A lateral weightbearing view of the ankle joint shows changes occurring with functional loading. In this case, degenerative changes become obvious, with anterior joint space narrowing as well as anterior subluxation of the talus. These changes were not appreciated on a non-weightbearing series of films. A large spur has developed at the anterior margin of the distal tibial articular surface and anterior impingement would occur with dorsiflexion of the ankle. There is also a medial middle subtalar joint coalition present, with a characteristic 'hump' on the posterior profile of the body of the talus. Note the bony bar passing across the middle subtalar joint (arrowheads). This condition is discussed later in the chapter.

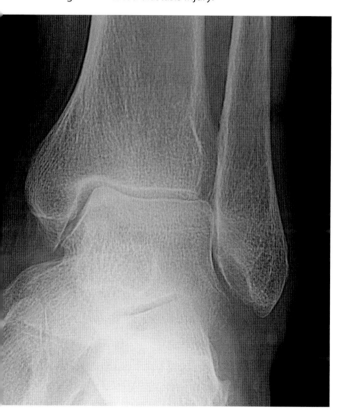

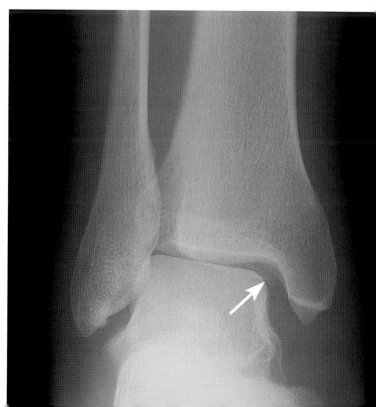

▶ **Fig. 7.16** A weightbearing AP view of the ankle joint shows changes diagnostic of an inferior tibiofibular syndesmosis injury. Weightbearing may accentuate widening of the tibiofibular joint space as well as widening of the medial clear space of the ankle joint. A small bone fragment projected over the medial aspect of the ankle joint (arrow) is an avulsion fracture separated from the posterior lip of the distal tibia by deltoid ligament traction.

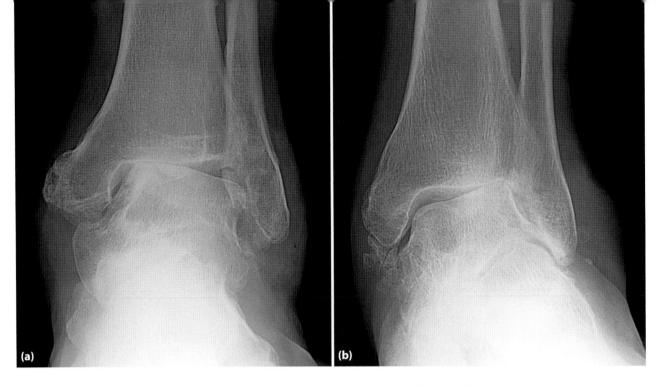

▲ **Fig. 7.17** Using weightbearing reproduces functional deformities due to chronic ligament injuries.

(a) Chronic lateral ligament insufficiency produces varus angulation of the talus. There is excavation of the medial tibial plafond by the medial corner of the talar dome, and the lateral talar dome impinges on the fibula. Post-traumatic spur formation or ossicles are present at both malleoli and the lateral process of the talus.

(b) Valgus tilting of the talus results from an old deltoid ligament injury. Multiple large ossicles are noted below the medial malleolus, and the lateral corner of the talar dome is eroding the lateral tibial plafond. There is a large subchondral cyst in the medial body of the talus.

'Lazy' lateral view

A 'lazy' lateral view is a specific view used for assessment of the lateral tubercle of the talus and identification of an os trigonum. A lateral view with 10 to 15° external rotation of the foot will project the lateral malleolus behind the medial malleolus, profiling the lateral tubercle of the posterior process of the talus or os trigonum (see Fig. 7.18). This view is called a 'lazy' lateral because the rotated lateral view is the view produced by a lazy radiographer who allows the ankle to lie naturally on its lateral side without placing a pad under the anterior aspect of the knee to rotate the ankle into a true lateral position. An os trigonum or a prominent posterior tubercle of the posterior process may cause posterior impingement of the ankle. This condition is discussed later in the chapter.

▼ **Fig. 7.18(a)** A true lateral view demonstrates what appears to be a moderately prominent posterior process of the talus (arrow). **(b)** With 15° of external rotation of the foot, the posterolateral structures are profiled and an os trigonum becomes apparent (arrow). An os trigonum is a common cause of posterior impingement. This rotated view is known as a 'lazy' lateral view (see text).

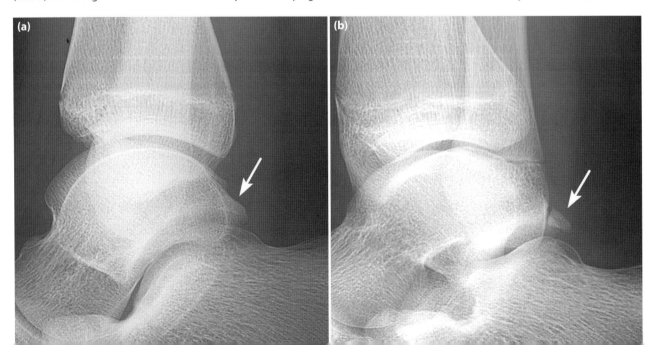

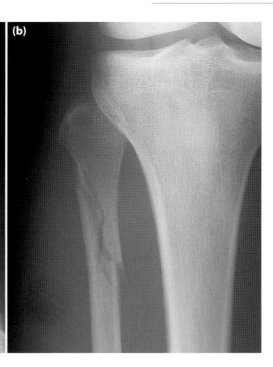

◀ **Fig. 7.19(a)** An AP view demonstrates changes diagnostic of a diastasis injury of the syndesmosis. There is widening of both the medial clear space of the ankle and the tibiofibular syndesmosis (arrowheads).
(b) Tenderness of the proximal fibula was initially overshadowed by ankle pain. When eventually discovered, a view of the proximal fibular demonstrated a Maisonneuve fracture.

View of the proximal fibula

If diastasis of the distal tibiofibular syndesmosis has been demonstrated on the initial routine films, the possibility of a Maisonneuve fracture should be considered. The fibula should be clinically examined and, if tender, a film showing the proximal shaft of the fibula is advisable (see Fig. 7.19). The mechanism of a Maisonneuve fracture is discussed later in the chapter.

Stress view of the distal tibiofibular syndesmosis

When a diastasis injury of the distal tibiofibular syndesmosis is suspected clinically and the plain film changes are equivocal, a stress view can be diagnostic. An AP view is obtained with maximum external rotation stress applied to the foot against a firmly held tibia. If there is injury to the tibiofibular syndesmosis, the width of the medial clear space and tibiofibular syndesmosis will increase (see Fig. 7.20).

▼ **Fig. 7.20** If there is a clinical suspicion of a diastasis injury, but the initial plain films are inconclusive, a stress view is often helpful. To stress the inferior tibiofibular joint, the mid-shaft of the tibia is held firmly, with the ankle in an AP position. The foot is then rotated laterally and stressed against the firmly held tibia, and an AP film is acquired. Clinically, if there is a diastasis injury no firm end-point is detected. A film obtained with stress maintained will show widening of the medial clear space and the distal tibiofibular joint. In this case, **(a)** is the unstressed ankle view with the suspicion of a widened clear space. In **(b)** there are definite diagnostic changes following stress.

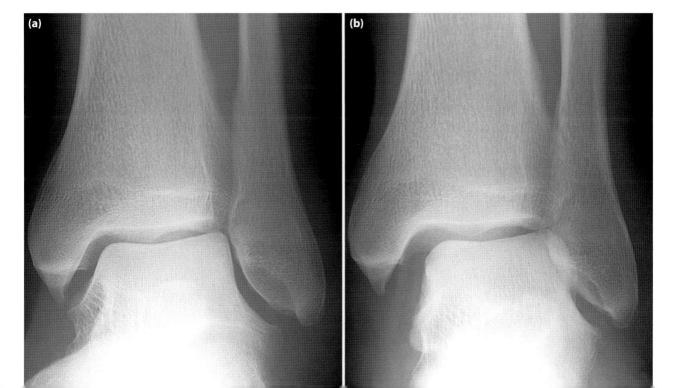

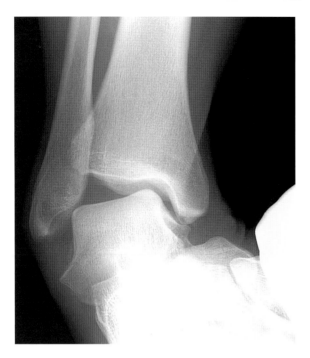

▲ Fig. 7.21 Inversion stress demonstrates abnormal laxity, with the degree of medial talar tilting diagnostic of lateral ligament complex insufficiency.

The tibiofibular syndesmosis can also be stressed with weight-bearing and this may be further increased by dorsiflexion of the ankle. The anterior width of the talus is greater than its posterior width, so as ankle dorsiflexion increases, a wedge is driven between the malleoli.

Other stress views

When the clinical problem is one of chronic ankle joint instability, additional imaging with stress radiographs may be helpful. Instability can be diagnosed when inversion stress produces a talar tilt that is 7° greater than can be produced on the uninjured side (see Fig. 7.21). However, the use of stress radiography remains controversial, as reliability may be compromised by the large range of normal variation (Rubin and Witten 1960). Disagreement exists as to the amount of laxity considered significant, and many physicians regard instability as a clinical assessment. Liu and Baker (1994) have suggested that a combination of talar tilt and anterior draw be used to grade instability.

Reversed oblique view

The reversed oblique view is particularly helpful for assessing fractures of the medial malleolus. This is an AP view with the ankle turned laterally through 45°. This angulation tends to highlight the plane of a medial malleolus fracture (see Fig. 7.22).

▼ Fig. 7.22 A reversed oblique view of the ankle may be useful for assessing an injury of the medial malleolus. The plane of a fracture of the medial malleolus is often well demonstrated in this position.
(a) This is a normal reversed oblique view.
(b) In a different case this view shows the usual plane of an oblique fracture of the medial malleolus.

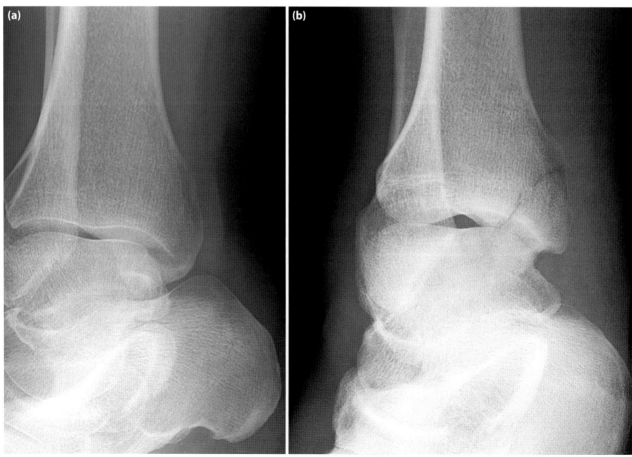

Tips on looking at plain films of the ankle

A routine of looking at plain films should be developed and repeated for every ankle series examined, so that all important structures are assessed, soft-tissue indicators of injury noted and injury patterns recognised. The authors' search pattern begins with identification of soft-tissue swelling and checking for an effusion, the presence of which may indicate a possible intra-articular fracture or intra-articular ligamentous injury (see Fig. 7.23). A post-traumatic effusion measuring 13 mm or more in diameter at the anterior recess of the ankle joint in an otherwise normal examination has a positive predictive value of 82% for an intra-articular fracture (Clark et al. 1995).

Soft-tissue swelling is an important marker of injury, which will immediately draw the experienced eye to assess the swelling and the adjacent structures (see Fig. 7.24). Swelling over the lateral side of the ankle joint and lateral malleolus is common following a 'sprain' injury to the lateral ligament complex (see Fig. 7.25). When soft-tissue swelling is present, note changes in skin contour, the thickness of the subcutaneous tissues, and obliteration or displacement of fat planes (see Figs 7.26 and 7.27). Important soft-tissue changes are occasionally present in the pre-Achilles fat pad and may indicate a variety of abnormalities.

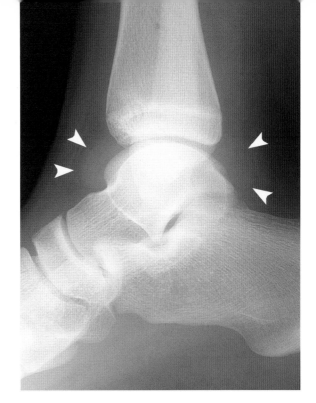

▲ **Fig. 7.23** Arrowheads indicate the margins of a large ankle joint effusion. The presence of a traumatic large effusion such as this calls for a particularly careful inspection of bony structures, as an intra-articular fracture is likely. Large effusions may also be seen with injury to the intra-articular anterior talofibular ligament.

▼ **Fig. 7.24** This young surfer was hit by a surfboard on the lower leg. **(a)** In the lateral view of the ankle, the eye is drawn to soft-tissue swelling on the anterior surface of the leg, just above the ankle. The area of concern is obvious and a careful examination of the adjacent bone is important.

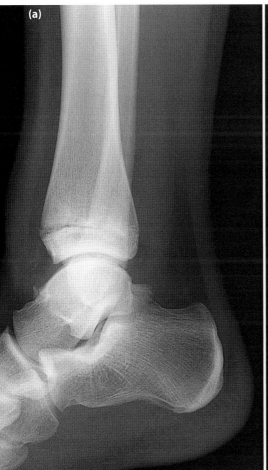

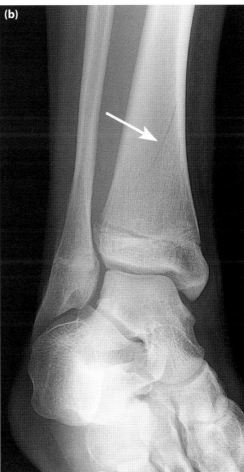

◀**(b)** In the 'mortise' view, a fracture of the distal tibial shaft can be seen (arrow), and there is disruption of the anterolateral aspect of the distal tibial growth plate, suggesting that an undisplaced Salter–Harris Type II injury has occurred.

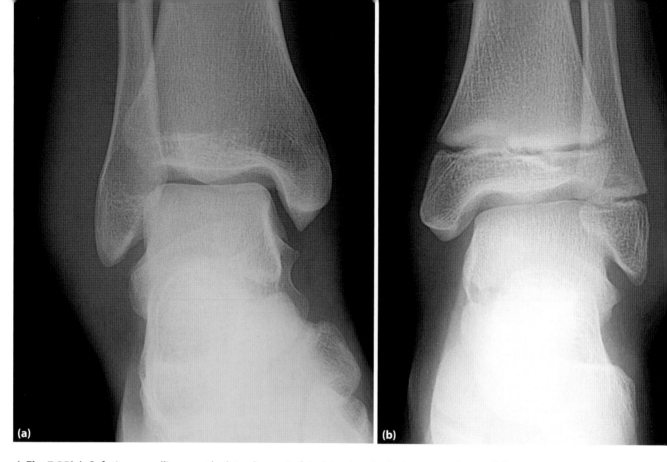

▲ Fig. 7.25(a) Soft-tissue swelling over the lateral aspect of the lateral malleolus is commonly seen following an inversion injury to the lateral ligament complex. A careful inspection of both the lateral malleolus and the lateral process of the talus is important. **(b)** If the patient is skeletally immature and the soft-tissue swelling is centred slightly higher, disruption of the distal fibular growth plate should be considered.

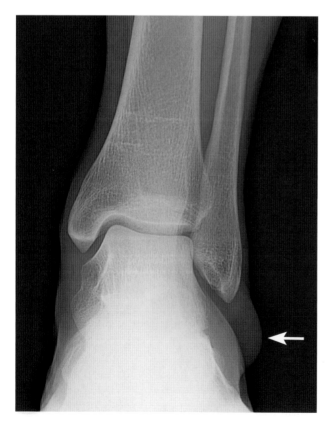

▲ Fig. 7.26 In this case, soft-tissue swelling is centred at a lower level, and this appearance was due to a tendon sheath ganglion (arrow).

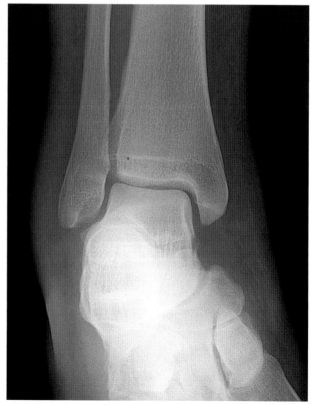

▲ Fig. 7.27 When soft-tissue swelling is diffuse with thickening of the subcutaneous tissues, the process is likely to be due to cellulitis or lymphoedema.

Following trauma, the presence of generalised ankle swelling without an ankle effusion is a red flag situation, which should immediately raise the possibility of an injury to the tibiofibular syndesmosis. The lack of effusion with this injury is due to tearing of the joint capsule allowing fluid to run out into the surrounding tissues (see Fig. 7.28). It is also important to remember that cortical deformity without adjacent soft-tissue swelling is more likely to represent old rather than recent injury. Other abnormal soft-tissue densities include foreign bodies and calcifications. It is important to identify vascular calcification, which in athletes under 50 years of age may be the first indication of diabetes (see Fig. 7.29).

Having examined the soft tissues, the bones and joints are then carefully examined. Hind-foot morphology and alignment should be routinely assessed on a lateral view of the ankle and this is best achieved with weight-bearing films. Recognition of cavus hind-foot morphology (see Fig. 7.30) is relevant because it may predispose to chronic lateral ankle instability and ankle osteoarthropathy (Sugimoto et al. 1997; Fortin et al. 2002). A valgus hind-foot may be a sign of tibialis posterior dysfunction.

When examining the bones and joints of the ankle for signs of acute or chronic trauma, a general search pattern should be developed that not only assesses each bone and joint in turn but particularly looks for signs of the five most commonly missed fractures (see Table 7.1). These fractures occur commonly and are notorious for being overlooked both clinically and radiologically. Poor film quality is one of the leading causes contributing to these fractures being missed (Anderson et al. 1989). Consequently, the standard of the film series obtained should be assessed, and views repeated if necessary. For example, a talar dome fracture cannot be excluded without an adequate 'mortise' view that shows the complete contour of the talar dome. A talar dome fracture is often subtle and may be a small bony flake adjacent to the medial or lateral corner of the talar dome (see Fig. 7.31). The base of the fifth metatarsal should also be examined

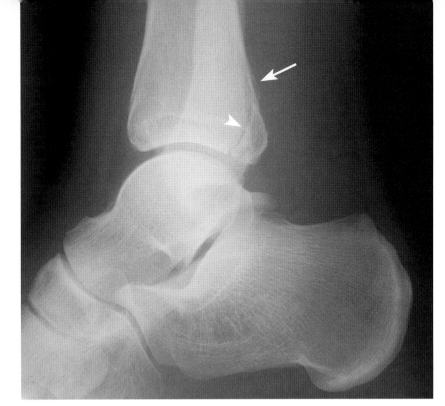

▲ **Fig. 7.28** With a diastasis injury to the tibiofibular syndesmosis, there is diffuse soft-tissue swelling, without any discrete ankle joint effusion. This is due to capsular tearing allowing fluid to escape into the surrounding tissues, as seen in this case. The presence of a fracture of the posterior lip of the distal tibia (arrowhead) and periosteal reaction (arrow) confirms the presence of a recent diastasis injury.

▼ **Fig. 7.29** Extensive arterial calcification is seen in the ankle film of a 41-year-old athlete (arrows). At this age, diabetes must be considered likely.

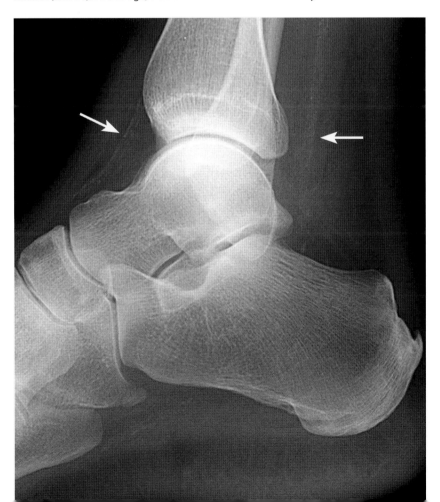

▶ **Fig. 7.30** A weightbearing lateral view shows a cavus foot. This deformity predisposes to chronic ankle instability, metacarpal stress fractures, sesamoiditis and stress fractures of the navicular. A weightbearing lateral view is necessary to assess the degree of this deformity.

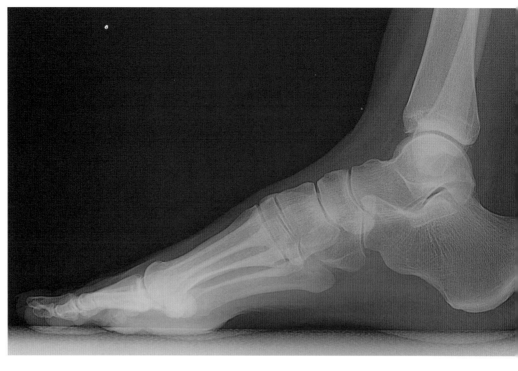

routinely. Although this fracture may be easily identified on an oblique view of the foot, if the examination is limited to an ankle series, a fracture of the base of the fifth metatarsal is often difficult to see (see Fig. 7.32).

Searching for commonly missed fractures is important and should be performed *every* time on *every* ankle examined. Before removing the films from the viewing box, ask: 'Have I really examined the talar dome, anterior process of the calcaneum, posterior process of the talus, lateral processes of the talus and base of the fifth metatarsal carefully for a fracture?' If there is any remaining suspicion, think of using appropriate additional plain film views to confirm the diagnosis, preferably while the patient is still in the imaging department.

▼ **Fig. 7.31** The majority of talar dome fractures are subtle and easily overlooked. In this case a medial talar dome fracture is present, with the detached fragment remaining within the fracture bed (arrow).

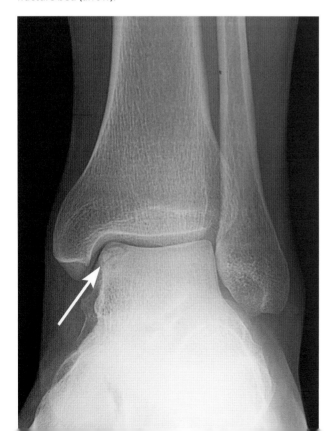

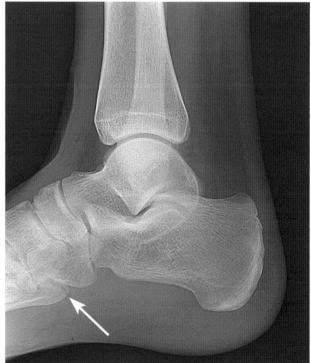

▲ **Fig. 7.32** Every time an ankle is examined, a disciplined search must be made for the commonly missed fractures. In this case, a fracture of the base of the fifth metatarsal was visible only on the lateral view of the ankle series (arrow).

Table 7.1 Easily missed fractures around the ankle joint

1. Fractures of the talar dome and tibial plafond
2. Fractures of the anterior process of the calcaneum
3. Fractures of the lateral tubercle of the talar posterior process
4. Fractures of the lateral process of the talus
5. Fractures of the base of the fifth metatarsal (on an ankle series)

The role of isotope scanning of the ankle

The major role of nuclear medicine imaging around the ankle is to identify bone injuries and other processes that are difficult or impossible to see on plain films. In this regard, nuclear imaging offers an alternative to MRI. Occult fractures are common at the ankle due to complex anatomy and curved surfaces (see Fig. 7.33). Nuclear bone scans are also valuable for demonstrating marrow changes that may be associated with a bone bruise, an overuse injury, an impingement syndrome or traction by a ligament or tendon.

In the highly trained athlete, areas of increased isotope uptake are incredibly common and may therefore be considered almost 'normal' (see Fig. 7.34). This is particularly so in the adolescent athlete (Cooper et al. 2003). Consequently, the clinical history and presentation must be carefully considered before interpreting the significance of an area of increased isotope uptake. Bone injury produces an increase in uptake on the delayed images. Injuries that are more severe and acute will also show an increase in uptake during the flow and blood pool phases. Low-grade injury will show a lesser degree of uptake on delayed images. Synovitis may be demonstrated as mild increased uptake throughout the joint on delayed images (see Fig. 7.35).

CT of the ankle joint

CT is used to assess bony detail and MDCT technology is able to provide high-resolution images in any plane, helping in the assessment of complex fractures (see Fig. 7.36). For complex trauma, surface-rendered 3D images can provide an improved understanding of fragment displacement.

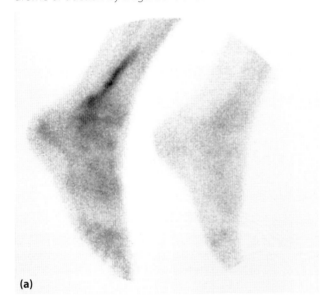

(a)

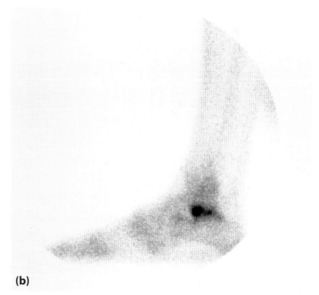

(b)

▲ **Fig. 7.33(a)** A radiographically occult vertical fracture of the distal fibula is clearly demonstrated by a nuclear bone scan.
(b) A fracture of the body of the talus adjacent to the posterior subtalar joint is demonstrated by a nuclear bone scan. This fracture could not be seen on plain films. Note the sharp inferior margin of the area of isotope uptake due to the subtalar joint.

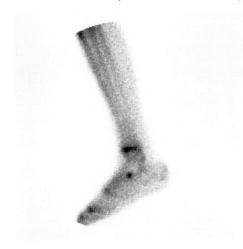

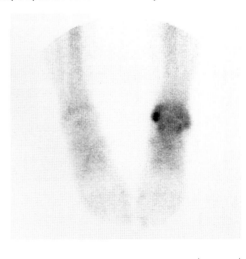

◀ **Fig. 7.34** Multiple areas of increased uptake of isotope are seen in the foot of this young athlete.

▶ **Fig. 7.35** A moderate diffuse increase in uptake of isotope indicates traumatic synovitis of the ankle, with an additional well-defined area of marked uptake indicating ligamentous injury and fracture at the tip of the left medial malleolus.

▶ **Fig. 7.36** MDCT technology allows the acquisition of high-resolution images in any plane. However, the complexity of an injury may be difficult to appreciate on planar images alone. In this case a fracture is demonstrated passing obliquely through the distal tibia to involve the growth plate and distal tibial epiphysis.

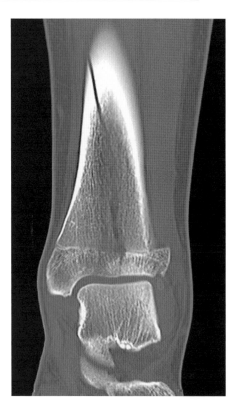

This can be important if surgery is contemplated (see Figs 7.37 and 7.38). CT is also used to define loose bodies, avulsed fragments and to assess the tibiofibular syndesmosis for disruption.

Imaging the ankle with ultrasound

Ultrasound is an alternative to MRI, or may complement MRI as an imaging method for some soft-tissue conditions around the ankle. In particular conditions, most notably those that affect tendons, ultrasound may be preferred (see Fig. 7.39). Ultrasound is most effective when well localised symptoms permit a focused examination that attempts to answer a specific clinical question. Particular strengths of ultrasound include the ability to compare the imaging appearances of a point of tenderness with the asymptomatic side, the ability to demonstrate abnormal soft-tissue dynamics such as tendon subluxation and the ability to guide various percutaneous interventions with great accuracy. Common therapeutic interventions include injections of joints and tendon sheaths (see Fig. 7.40), aspiration of ganglia, and guided injections for posterior ankle impingement.

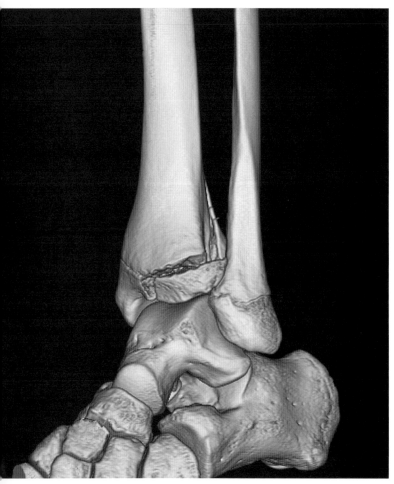

▲ **Fig. 7.37** In the same case as Fig. 7.36, a 3D image of fracture geometry is far easier to interpret. This 3D surface-rendered image clearly shows the injury to be a triplane fracture.

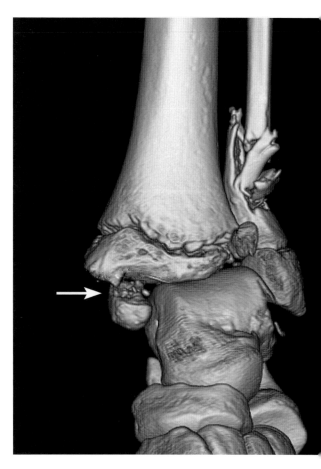

▲ **Fig. 7.38** A 3D image with surface rendering graphically demonstrates fractures of the distal fibula and medial malleolus (arrow) with subluxation of the ankle joint and diastasis at the distal tibiofibular joint. There is also an avulsion fracture of the distal tibial epiphysis laterally.

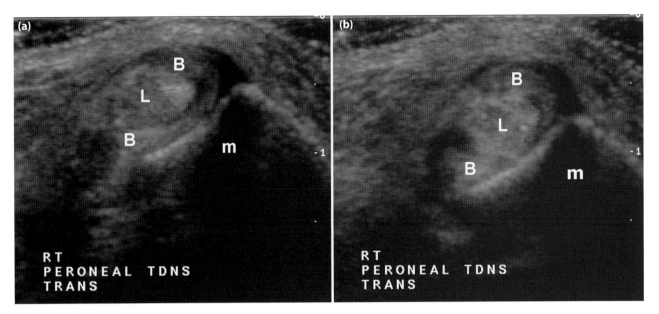

▲ **Fig. 7.39** A longitudinal tear of the peroneus brevis is demonstrated by dynamic ultrasound. Two frames are shown from a cine clip of the peroneal tendons viewed in transverse section at the level of the retromalleolar groove during active circumduction of the foot. Note the 'C'-shaped configuration of the peroneus tendon (B), which separates the peroneus longus tendon (L) from the lateral malleolus (m). Frame **(a)** represents the tendon position with the foot in plantar flexion and inversion. Although this shows a very subtle hypoechoic line traversing the peroneus brevis at its midpoint, the appearance is not convincing for a tear. However, frame **(b)** clearly demonstrates complete separation of the anterior and posterior halves of the peroneus brevis tendon by the peroneus longus as it moves towards the lateral malleolus during dorsiflexion and eversion of the foot.

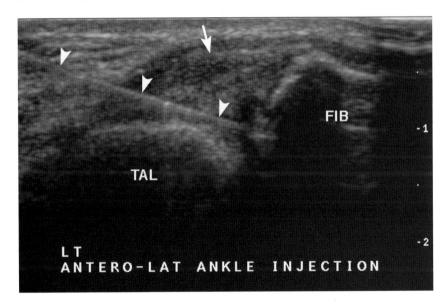

◀**Fig. 7.40** An ankle injection has been performed under ultrasound control for anterolateral impingement syndrome. Post-traumatic thickening and scarring of the ATFL is noted (arrow). The in-situ needle is indicated by arrowheads. Fibula = FIB. Talus = TAL.

Ankle joint MRI

MRI provides a comprehensive overview of ankle anatomy and its use is now well established. One recent study demonstrated a significant improvement in clinical diagnostic confidence in almost two-thirds of cases assessed by MRI and a consequent change to proposed surgical management in about one-third of cases (Bearcroft et al. 2006). MRI is particularly useful in the detection and characterisation of a number of conditions including ligamentous injuries (see Fig. 7.41), bone bruising (see Fig. 7.42), bone stress, chondral and osteochondral lesions (see Fig. 7.43) and impingement syndromes (see Fig. 7.44). MRI is often a useful clinical problem-solving tool in situations of unexplained ankle pain due to its comprehensive and panoramic demonstration of bone and soft-tissue anatomy. MRI can also be helpful in the work-up of nerve entrapments such as tarsal tunnel syndrome.

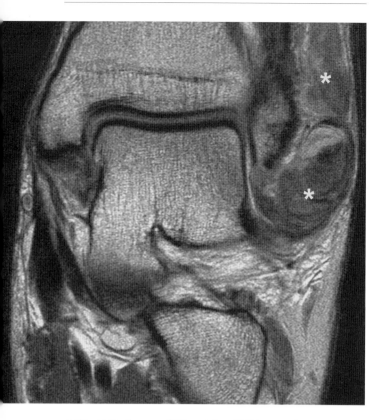

▲ **Fig. 7.41** A coronal PD-weighted MR image shows an acute ATFL tear, with ligament swelling, disruption at the anterolateral gutter and an associated subcutaneous haematoma (asterisks).

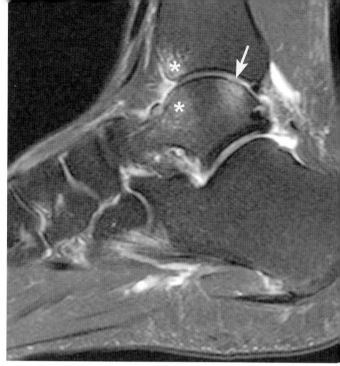

▲ **Fig. 7.42** MRI is an extremely useful imaging method for the identification of bone marrow oedema at the ankle. Following trauma to the anterior ankle, a sagittal fat-suppressed image demonstrates bone bruising at the anterior lip of the distal tibia and the anterior body of the talus (asterisks) associated with an osteochondral fracture of the posterior talar dome (arrow).

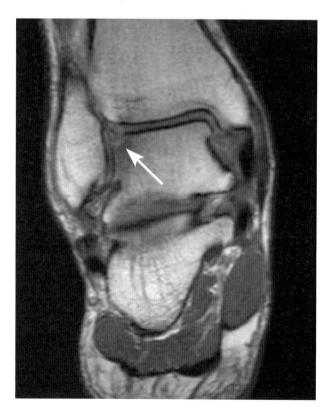

▲ **Fig. 7.43** A small osteochondral fracture of the lateral talar dome is demonstrated on a coronal T1-weighted MR image (arrow). Note the abnormal marrow signal associated with the osteochondral fracture.

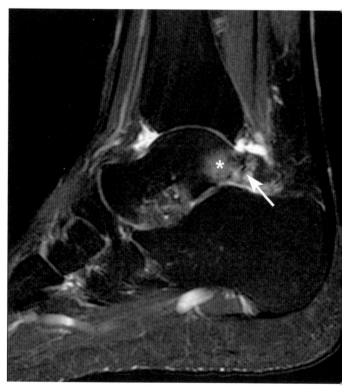

▲ **Fig. 7.44** A sagittal STIR MR image of the ankle in a patient with posterior impingement syndrome demonstrates a prominent os trigonum and abnormal high marrow signal in the posterior body of the talus (asterisk) and in the os trigonum adjacent to the synchondrosis (arrow). No disruption of the synchondrosis is apparent. A moderate-sized ankle joint effusion is present.

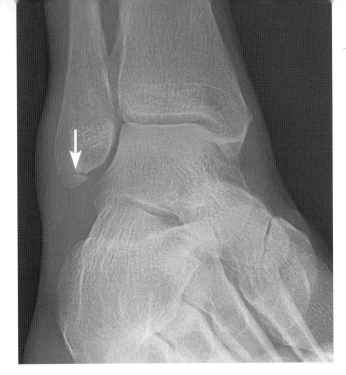

▲ **Fig. 7.45** If a distal fibular fracture involves the lateral malleolus below the level of the mortise, the fracture is classified as a Weber A fracture. These fractures are typically horizontal avulsion fractures (arrow).

Ankle joint injuries

Sports-related conditions involving the ankle joint include a variety of bone, joint and soft-tissue abnormalities resulting from either acute or overuse trauma. Old injuries can also produce symptoms in the sporting population, due to the development of spurs and osteophytes that may cause impingements, or due to degenerative processes such as tendinopathies and arthropathies. Imaging plays an important role in the diagnosis and management of these injuries. High-quality plain films remain the cornerstone of accurate imaging. Nuclear bone scans, ultrasound, MRI and MDCT can all play specific roles in identifying and characterising particular abnormalities.

Distal fibular fractures

These common fractures are almost invariably diagnosed on plain films. The Danis-Weber classification is the simplest and most widely used method of guiding management, and is a good predictor of the outcome of fractures that involve only the distal fibula (Kennedy et al. 1998):

- *Weber A fractures* are horizontal in orientation and involve the lateral malleolus below the level of the mortise (see Fig. 7.45). These are avulsion fractures arising from lateral collateral ligament traction and are generally stable, unless accompanied by a displaced medial malleolus fracture. Isolated Weber A fractures are never associated with distal tibiofibular syndesmosis injuries.
- *Weber B fractures* are spiral or oblique fractures that start at the level of the mortise and extend superiorly. They result from an external rotational force and are associated with distal tibiofibular syndesmosis injuries in about 50% of cases (see Fig. 7.46). These fractures may be unstable.

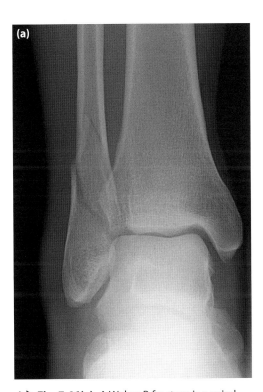

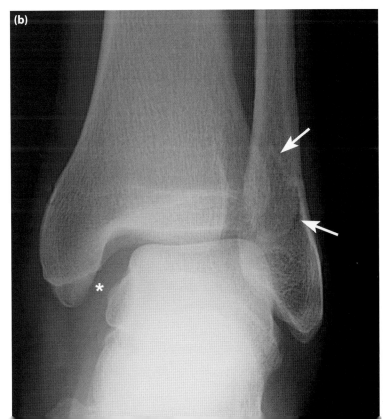

▲▶ **Fig. 7.46(a)** A Weber B fracture is a spiral fracture at the level of the distal tibiofibular syndesmosis. This fracture is associated with a diastasis injury in about 50% of cases.
(b) There is a subtle undisplaced Weber B fracture (arrows). Widening of the medial clear space of the ankle (asterisk) indicates an associated diastasis injury.

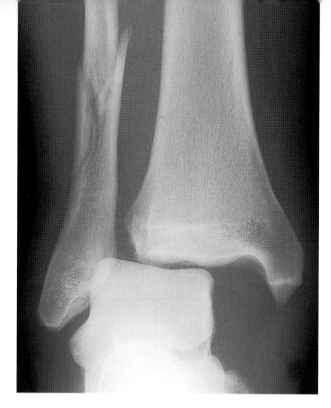

▲ Fig. 7.47 A spiral fracture of the distal shaft of the fibula, 4–10 cm above the level of the mortise, is classified as a Weber C fracture and is invariably associated with a syndesmosis diastasis injury. This case shows marked widening of both the distal tibiofibular joint space and the medial clear space. This is the low equivalent of a Maisonneuve fracture.

- *Weber C fractures* involve the fibular shaft 4–10 cm above the mortise. These fractures are always associated with distal tibiofibular syndesmosis disruption and tearing of the interosseous membrane (see Fig. 7.47).

Posterior malleolar fractures

The posterior lip of the distal tibia is known as the posterior malleolus. A fracture of the posterior malleolus is always associated with an injury of the distal tibiofibular syndesmosis. These fractures are often undisplaced and, unless the lateral view of the ankle is well positioned, may be easily missed (see Fig. 7.48).

Medial malleolar fractures

There are three types of medial malleolar fractures. The most common is an oblique fracture due to an ankle eversion mechanism with deltoid ligament traction producing an avulsion injury. If the fracture of the medial malleolus is transverse, there is often an associated syndesmosis injury (see Fig. 7.49). The transverse fracture plane is indicative of the axial rotary force of a syndesmosis injury. The third type is a stress fracture that is characteristically vertical (see Fig. 7.50). Most medial malleolar fractures are seen on routine plain films. If there is any doubt about a fracture on the routine views, a reversed oblique view of the ankle will often define the fracture plane.

▼ Fig. 7.48 Unless a lateral view is correctly positioned, a fracture of the posterior lip of the distal tibia is easily missed. This is an important fracture to identify, as it is indicative of injury to the distal tibiofibular syndesmosis and represents an avulsion caused by posterior tibiofibular ligament traction. The left image **(a)** is a 'lazy' lateral and the posterior malleolus appears normal. **(b)** In the same case, when the view was repeated with correct positioning, a fracture of the posterior malleolus is demonstrated (arrow).

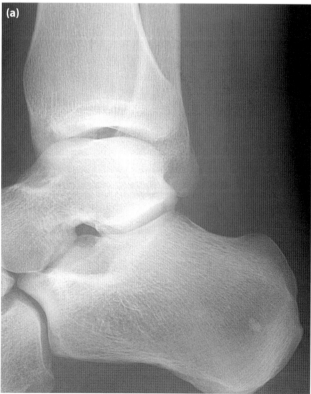

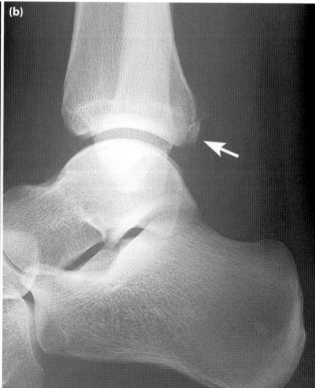

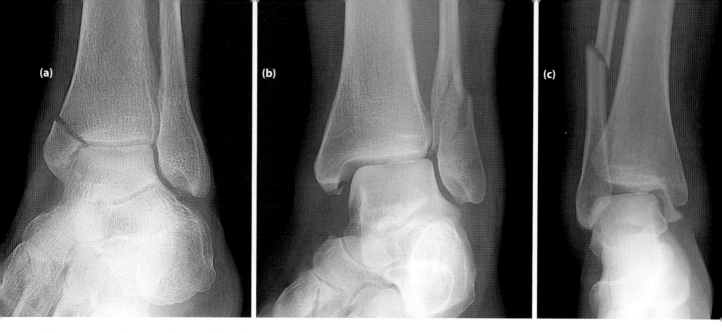

▲ Fig. 7.49(a) A fracture of the medial malleolus is usually the result of ankle eversion, and characteristically extends obliquely from the medial corner of the tibial plafond.

(b) If the fracture passes transversely across the medial malleolus, a syndesmosis injury is likely. In this case there is a transverse fracture of the tip of the medial malleolus and also a Weber B fracture of the fibula. Widening of the medial clear space confirms a diastasis injury.

(c) Rotational eversion forces to the foot produce a transverse fracture of the medial malleolus and a Weber C fracture of the fibula. There is a tibiofibular diastasis injury, widening of the lateral ankle joint space, and the interosseous membrane is almost certainly torn up to the level of the fibular fracture. There is also a fracture of the posterior lip of the distal tibia, and the fracture line can be faintly seen on this view.

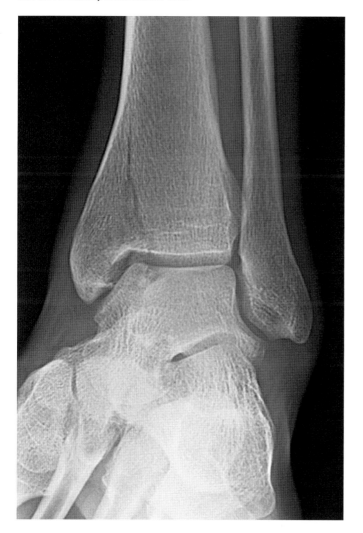

◀ Fig. 7.50 The third type of fracture of the medial malleolus is a stress fracture, which characteristically has a vertical orientation. Note that in this case the line of force has extended across the ankle joint, resulting in a fracture of the talar dome, and there is also a fracture extending across the base of the medial malleolus. Stress fractures of the medial malleolus are discussed later in the chapter.

Fractures of the lateral tubercle of the posterior process of the talus

The posterior process of the talus consists of lateral and medial tubercles, separated by an oblique groove for the flexor hallucis longus (FHL) tendon. A fracture of the lateral tubercle occurs during severe plantar flexion, which causes the lateral tubercle of the posterior process to impact against the posterior lip of the tibia (see Fig. 7.51). Apparent separation of the lateral tubercle may be due to developmental non-union of the tubercle's apophysis (os trigonum) and care must be taken not to confuse this normal variant with a fracture. An os trigonum has a well-defined cortical margin rather than a fracture margin. It should also be remembered that traumatic separation of an os trigonum with disruption of the synchondrosis may cause persistent posterior ankle pain (see Fig. 7.52).

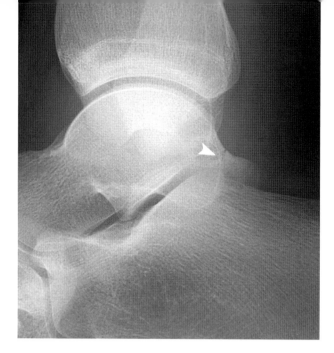

▲ Fig. 7.51 A fracture of the lateral tubercle of the posterior process of the talus is invariably subtle and is usually difficult to differentiate from an os trigonum. A fracture has a sharply defined margin without a cortical edge, as demonstrated in this case (arrowhead).

Fractures of the medial tubercle of the posterior process of the talus

A fracture of the medial tubercle of the posterior process of the talus may occur with combined ankle dorsiflexion and pronation. This is an avulsion fracture at the insertion of the posterior talotibial fibres of the deltoid ligament (Kim et al. 2003). These fractures are difficult to detect on plain films. Diagnosis usually requires a nuclear bone scan and CT or MRI (see Fig. 7.53). Stress fractures may also occur at this site and will be discussed later in the chapter.

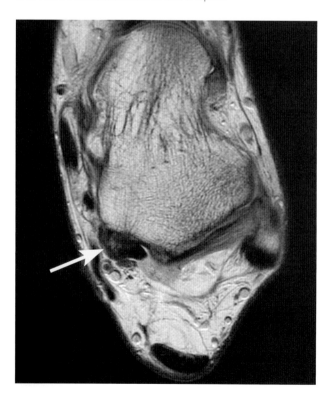

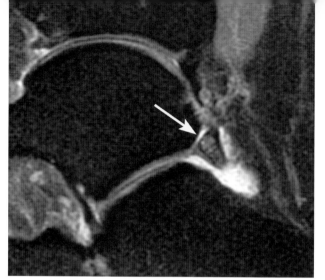

▲ Fig. 7.52(a) A sagittal STIR MR image demonstrates traumatic disruption of the synchondrosis between the os trigonum and the body of the talus (arrow). High marrow signal is noted in the os and there is an associated effusion present.

▼ (b) A destabilised os trigonum is demonstrated on a lateral plain film. Note the cortex on the margin of the ossicle that would have adjoined the synchondrosis. The lack of associated effusion indicates an old injury.

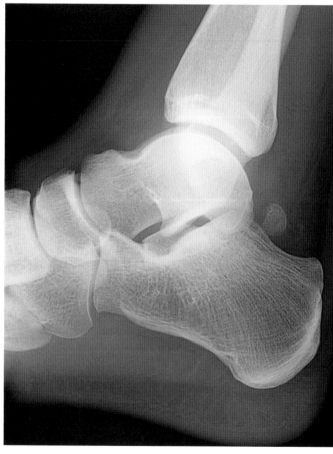

◀ Fig. 7.53 An axial PD-weighted MR image demonstrates a chronic avulsion of the medial tuberosity of the posterior process of the talus and hypertrophic scarring of the associated fibres of the deltoid ligament attachment (arrow). This causes a posteromedial impingement syndrome.

Talar neck fractures

A talar neck fracture (see Fig. 7.54) is incredibly difficult to detect on plain films and it is not uncommon for an undisplaced fracture of the talar neck to be missed. A delayed diagnosis may increase the risk of complicating avascular necrosis (AVN). The talar body is particularly susceptible to AVN because of its retrograde blood supply. AVN is usually manifest as an area of increased density on plain x-ray, often with a zone of demarcation seen on CT or MRI. There may be subsequent subchondral bony collapse and secondary osteoarthropathy in up to 50% of talar neck fractures, the risk increasing in displaced fractures and those associated with a subtalar dislocation. Imaging of AVN of the talus is discussed later (see pages 618 and 619).

Fractures of the lateral process of the talus

Fractures of the lateral process of the talus are thought to result from an external rotation or axial force applied to a dorsiflexed and everted foot (Funk et al. 2003). McCrory and Bladin (1996) have described this fracture in snowboarders. Fractures of the lateral process of the talus can be seen on a lateral view, a 'mortise' view or a 45° internal oblique view, depending on the fracture plane (see Figs 7.55 and 7.56). It has been suggested that a lateral view of the ankle obtained in dorsiflexion and inversion may be helpful for demonstrating a lateral process fracture (Bladin and McCrory 1995). Fractures of the lateral process of the talus may remain occult, requiring nuclear bone scanning, CT or MRI for diagnosis (see Figs 7.57, 7.58 and 7.59). Fracture assessment, including the extent of subtalar joint involvement and the presence of loose intra-articular bodies, is best provided by CT scanning.

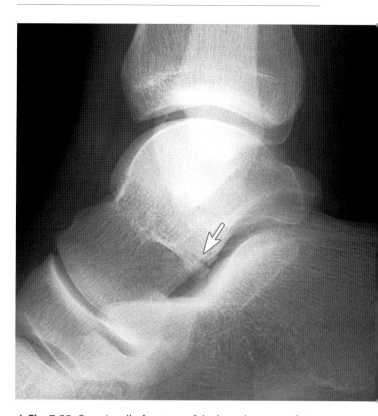

▲ **Fig. 7.55** Occasionally, fractures of the lateral process of the talus can be detected on a lateral view of the ankle. In this case, an acute fracture of the lateral process is seen following a waterskiing accident (arrow) (see also Fig. 7.358 on page 683).

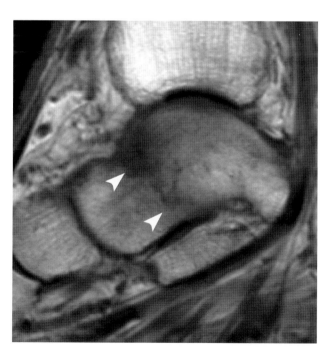

▲ **Fig. 7.54** MRI demonstrates an incomplete fracture of the talar neck on a sagittal T1-weighted image (arrowheads). No changes of AVN are evident.

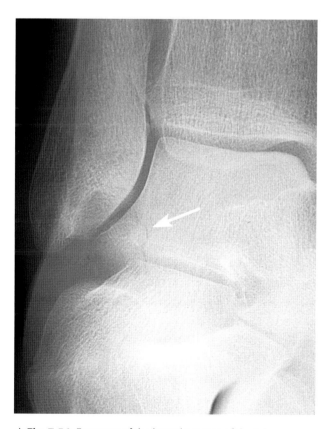

▲ **Fig. 7.56** Fractures of the lateral process of the talus are best seen in a 'mortise' view or an internal oblique view. This case shows an acute undisplaced fracture (arrow).

▶ **Fig. 7.57** A nuclear bone scan demonstrates a fracture of the lateral process of the talus on the right (arrow). Also note the fracture of the right third metatarsal base.

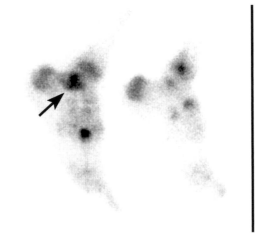
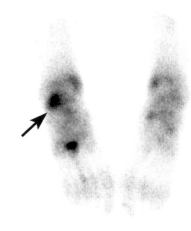

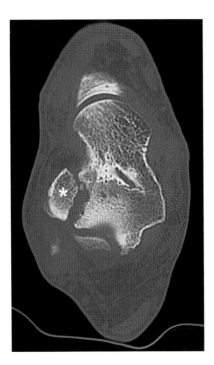

▲ **Fig. 7.58** An axial CT image demonstrates complete separation of the lateral process of the talus (asterisk).

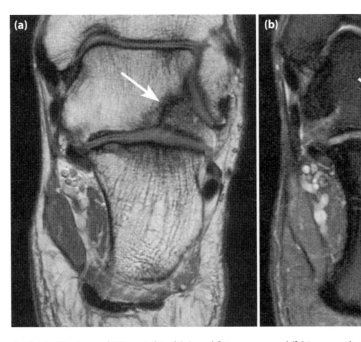

▲ **Fig. 7.59** Coronal PD-weighted **(a)** and fat-suppressed **(b)** images demonstrate a stress fracture extending across the base of the lateral process of the talus from the talar articular surface of the posterior subtalar joint (arrows).

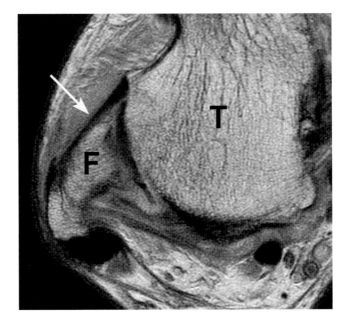

▶ **Fig. 7.60** A normal ATFL is demonstrated on an axial PD-weighted MR image (arrow). The normal ATFL is homogeneously hypointense and is often visualised along its full length on a single axial image, acquired with the ankle in a neutral position. Talus = T. Fibula = F.

Ankle ligament injuries

Stability is required for normal function of the ankle, with alignment maintained by the ligaments. There are three ligament complexes, each composed of three components. The three ligament complexes are the lateral ligament complex, the deltoid ligament complex and the distal tibiofibular syndesmosis. Approximately 85% of ankle joint injuries involve the lateral ligament complex (Cardone et al. 1993).

Injury to the lateral ligament complex

The lateral ligament complex consists of three parts: the anterior talofibular ligament (ATFL), the calcaneofibular ligament (CFL) and the posterior talofibular ligament (PTFL). This complex is frequently injured in activities requiring a combination of running with rapid change in direction and jumping. These activities occur in sports such as basketball, volleyball, netball and the various codes of football.

The ATFL

The ATFL provides the primary restraint to ankle inversion in plantar flexion, and also resists anterolateral translation of the talus within the mortise, becoming taut with ankle plantar flexion. It is an intra-articular band comprising two fascicles which extend from the anteroinferior margin of the lateral malleolus to the talar body at its junction with the talar neck. The ATFL forms the superficial margin of an articular recess at the ankle joint known as the anterolateral gutter (see Fig. 7.60). Functionally, the ATFL is the weakest component of the lateral ligament complex, with the most frequent mechanism of injury being plantar flexion and inversion (supination-adduction). A concomitant tear of the CFL may then occur with increasing force.

The CFL

The CFL runs vertically from the tip of the lateral malleolus to the posterior tubercle of the calcaneum, deep to the peroneal tendons (see Fig. 7.61). The CFL is extra-capsular and crosses both the ankle and the subtalar joints. The CFL is taut is dorsiflexion and inversion, and with continuing inversion and plantar flexion is the next ligament to rupture after the ATFL. Occasional isolated CFL tears are recognised (Usami et al. 1997). Acute injury to the CFL is most commonly interstitial, manifesting as a diffuse ligament swelling with increased signal on MRI or reduced echogenicity on ultrasound. However, localised avulsion injuries can also occur at the fibular or calcaneal insertions (see Fig. 7.62). A complete tear of the CFL may produce a communication between the ankle joint and the peroneal tendon sheath, allowing fluid from the ankle joint to decompress into the sheath (Freiberger et al. 1979).

The PTFL

The PTFL acts as a constraint against posterior displacement of the talus within the mortise as well as external rotation of the talus, and is the strongest ligament of the lateral ligament complex. The PTFL also acts against inversion when the ankle is in the neutral or dorsiflexed position. It originates on the digital fossa of the fibula and inserts into the lateral tubercle of the posterior process of the talus (see Fig. 7.63). Tears of the PTFL are rare and occur only in combination with ATFL and CFL tears in the context of a transient subluxation or dislocation of the talus (see Fig. 7.64). When an os trigonum is present, force transmitted by the PTFL may disrupt and destabilise the synchondrosis, resulting in posterior impingement symptoms (see Fig. 7.65).

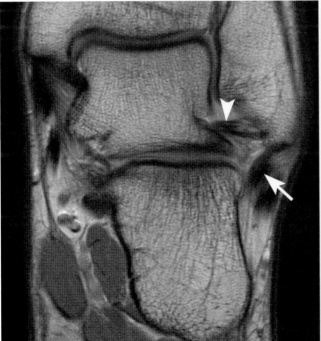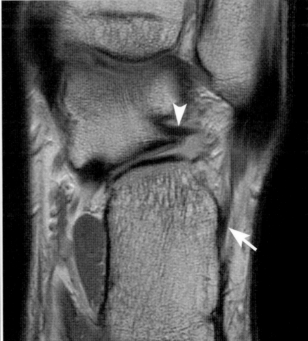

▲ **Fig. 7.61** Coronal PD-weighted MR images demonstrate a normal CFL (arrows) and a normal PTFL (arrowheads).

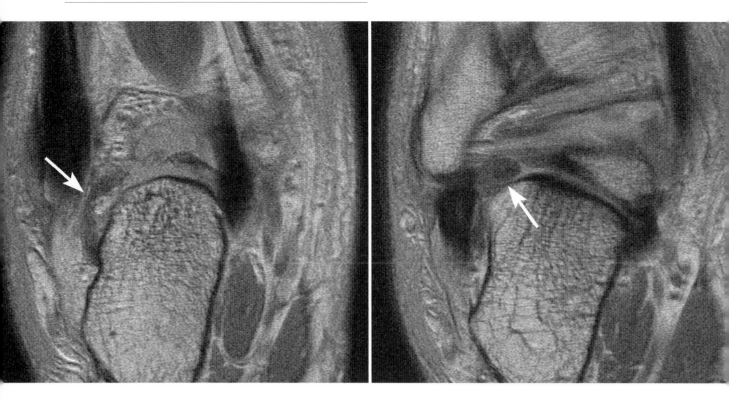

▲ **Fig. 7.62** Coronal PD-weighted MR images demonstrate avulsion of the CFL from the fibula. There is diffuse marked ligamentous thickening (arrows). The free end of the ligament projects into the posterolateral recess of the subtalar joint.

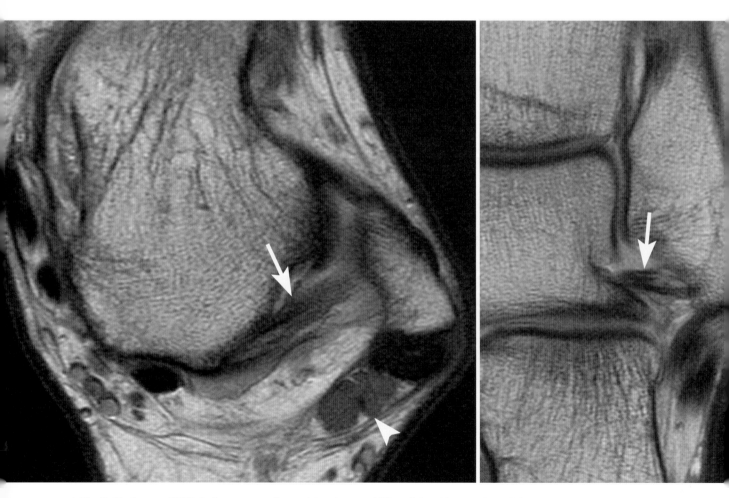

▲ **Fig. 7.63** A normal PTFL is demonstrated on axial and coronal PD-weighted images (arrows).

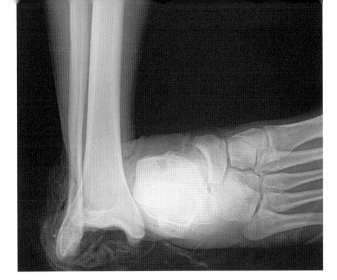

▲ Fig. 7.64 Rarely, a tear of the PTFL may follow rupture of the ATFL and CFL. At this point, dislocation of the ankle may occur. No bone injury can be seen, and the dislocation is due to sequential ligamentous injury.

A 'meniscoid' lesion

Following an inversion sprain, a 'meniscoid' lesion, which is a mass of hyalinised post-traumatic synovitis, may develop within the anterolateral gutter of the ankle joint (Wolin et al. 1950). This may become fibrotic and simulate the appearance of a knee meniscus at arthroscopy. It is a common cause of chronic or recurring pain due to anterolateral ankle impingement. Meniscoid lesions may develop following injury to either the ATFL or AITFL (see Fig. 7.66).

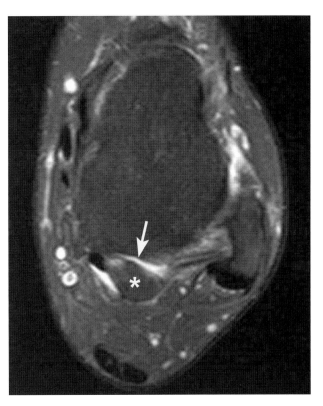

▲ Fig. 7.65 An axial fat-suppressed T2-weighted MR image demonstrates a subacute destabilisation of the os trigonum (asterisk), seen as a fluid line traversing the full width of the synchondrosis (arrow). Note the mildly increased marrow signal in the os trigonum.

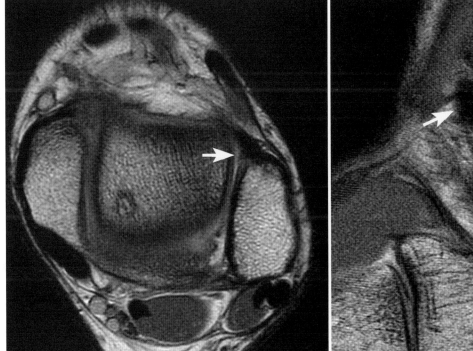
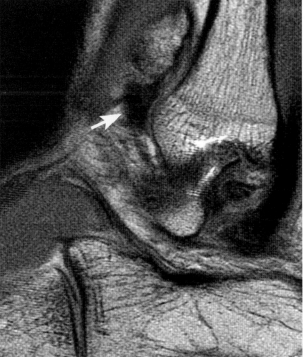

▲ Fig. 7.66 A mature meniscoid lesion is demonstrated by axial and sagittal PD-weighted MR images. There is a well-defined hypointense thickening of the inferior fascicle of the anterior inferior tibiofibular ligament (arrow). The axial image shows a triangular projection of this thickening into the anterolateral ankle gutter. Note the posteromedial osteochondral lesion in the talar dome.

Imaging of lateral ligament complex injuries and the Ottawa ankle rules

Most acute ankle sprains settle without significant complication, and the role of imaging in the acute stage is to exclude injuries that might require early intervention. To assist the clinician, the Ottawa ankle rules were developed to help decide whether a plain film should be requested (Stiell et al. 1994). These guidelines state that an examiner is unlikely to miss a clinically significant fracture if there is no bony tenderness and the patient is able to bear weight for at least four steps. Failing this, or if symptoms and signs persist more than four weeks after injury, a plain x-ray examination should be performed.

Plain films

Acutely, plain films may show features of ankle joint effusion, soft-tissue swelling around the lateral malleolus, and avulsion fractures at the fibular attachments of the ATFL or CFL (see Fig. 7.67). Avulsion fractures commonly proceed to non-union. Perimalleolar ossicles with rounded and corticated margins are often found on plain radiographs as an incidental indicator of previous avulsion injuries.

Stress radiography

Stress views have been advocated for assessment of ligament disruption (Rijke and Vierhout 1990). It has also been suggested that athletes with negative stress radiographs after an acute ankle sprain may return to sport earlier than those with positive stress tests (Mazur and Bartolozzi 1999). Stress radiography is not widely requested because its use remains controversial, not only due to its questionable diagnostic value, but also because the surgical treatment of acute sprains is rarely indicated (Raatikainen et al. 1992). Most physicians would instead argue that decisions about joint laxity, initial management and return to sport should be guided by clinical assessment. The criteria of a positive stress examination have been discussed in the section 'Additional plain film views of the ankle'.

Ultrasound and MRI

Although more sophisticated imaging tests are generally not indicated in the assessment of acute ankle injuries, the elite or professional athlete can occasionally benefit from an early MRI if there is persisting inability to bear weight, increasing the probability of an underlying fracture. There may also be clinical difficulty differentiating a lateral collateral ligament injury from injury to the tibiofibular syndesmosis. MRI is indicated for the athlete who has a joint effusion or pain and loss of function persisting more than six weeks after an ankle sprain.

Ultrasound examination is a valid alternative to MRI for the differentiation of a lateral collateral ligament injury from a syndesmosis injury (see Fig. 7.68). Ultrasound provides an accurate demonstration of the ATFL and allows dynamic assessment during combined plantar flexion and inversion stress or with an anterior drawer test (Campbell et al. 1994;

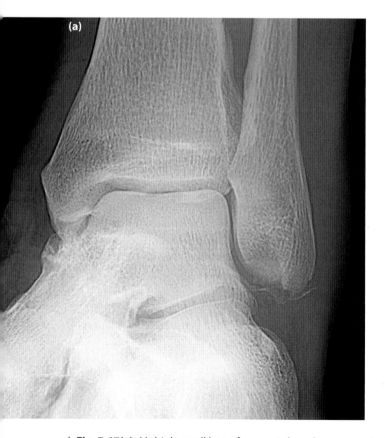

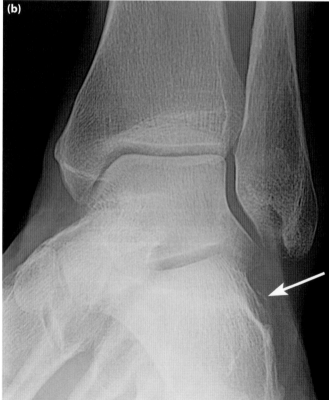

▲ **Fig. 7.67(a)** Multiple small bone fragments have been separated from the tip of the lateral malleolus by ATFL traction.
(b) The CFL has avulsed a small bone fragment from the posterior tubercle of the calcaneum (arrow).

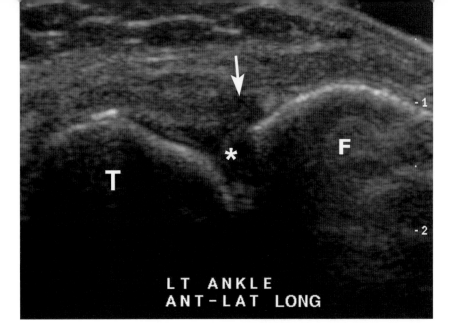

▶ **Fig. 7.68** A long-axis ultrasound image demonstrates a late subacute healing tear in the ATFL. Hypoechoic texture at the fibular end of the ATFL denotes the point of injury with evolving scarring (arrow). Note the localised synovitis in the adjacent anterolateral gutter of the ankle joint (asterisk). Talus = T. Fibula = F.

Milz et al. 1999). When oriented perpendicular to the ultrasound beam, the normal ATFL is mildly echogenic and demonstrates compact uniform fibrillar architecture (see Fig. 7.69). Using ultrasound, an acute complete ATFL tear is seen as an anechoic cleft in ligament continuity, with redundancy of the torn fibres (see Fig. 7.70). The point of tear may become more obvious on plantar flexion and inversion. An acute diffuse interstitial tear will manifest as hypoechoic thickening of the ligament with accompanying hyperaemia on Doppler interrogation. Associated small avulsion fractures are much more conspicuous on ultrasound than MRI.

▶ **Fig. 7.69** A long-axis ultrasound image of a normal ATFL has been obtained using a liberal amount of ultrasound gel to stand the transducer off the skin surface and allow insonation perpendicular to the path of the ligamentous fibres. This allows optimal demonstration of the uniform compact fibrillar echotexture that characterises a normal ligament (arrow). Talus = TAL. Fibula = FIB.

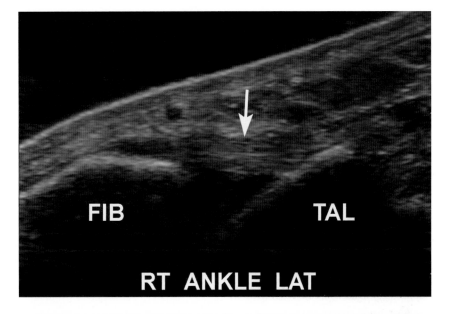

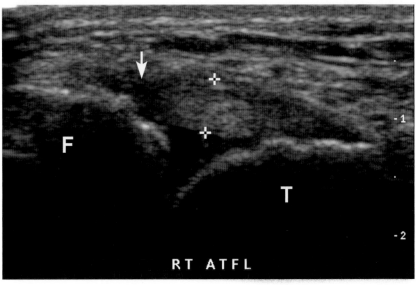

▶ **Fig. 7.70** A long-axis ultrasound image shows a full-thickness tear at the fibular attachment of the ATFL as an anechoic gap in fibre continuity (arrow). Note the thickened mid-segment fibres of the ATFL (callipers). Talus = T. Fibula = F.

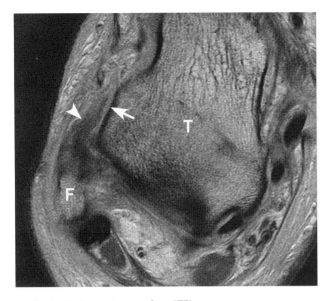

Characteristic MRI changes of a low-grade acute ATFL injury include loss of definition of the ligament structure, mild signal hyperintensity and periligamentous oedema (see Fig. 7.71). High-grade acute injuries may produce focal ligamentous attenuation or complete fibre discontinuity (see Fig. 7.72). MRI studies suggest that ATFL tears assessed clinically as Grade II are often in fact complete. Although cadaveric studies have found almost all ATFL tears to be mid-substance or distal, clinical experience would suggest that tears towards the fibular attachment are not uncommon (Siegler et al. 1988). Associated proximal or distal cortical flake avulsion fractures often remain attached to the ATFL (Berg 1991) and may proceed to atrophic non-union (see Fig. 7.73).

Most ATFL tears have a good prognosis. At 6–12 weeks post-injury, complete tears commonly show ill-defined bridging scar tissue of intermediate signal on MRI with no clinical evidence of residual laxity. Nevertheless, laxity of the ankle

▲ **Fig. 7.71** An acute complete ATFL tear is demonstrated on an axial PD-weighted MR image. The ligament shows diffuse thickening and hyperintensity (arrowhead) with abrupt discontinuity at the distal end (arrow). Talus = T. Fibula = F.

▶ **Fig. 7.72** An ATFL avulsion fracture is demonstrated by MRI. Axial PD and sagittal fat-suppressed PD-weighted images show a separated fragment or 'flake' of fibular cortex that corresponds with the footprint of the ATFL attachment. Arrowheads point to the fracture line. The ATFL itself appears intact (arrow). There is surrounding haemorrhage. Note the presence of only mild bone marrow oedema, a finding that is often seen with avulsion-type fractures and can sometimes render them inconspicuous.

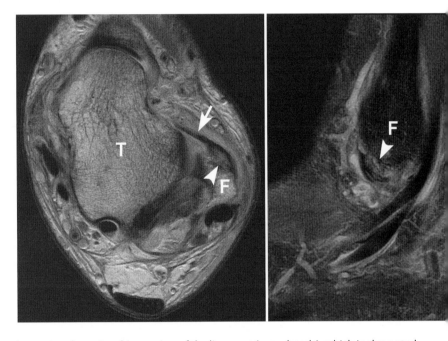

▼ **Fig. 7.73** An old ATFL injury is demonstrated as mature hypertrophic scarring of the ligament (arrowheads), which is also noted to contain an avulsed bone fragment (a) showing a well-defined smooth cortical margin. A fluid line separates the ossicle from the adjacent fibula (arrows). This appearance is indicative of chronic non-union.

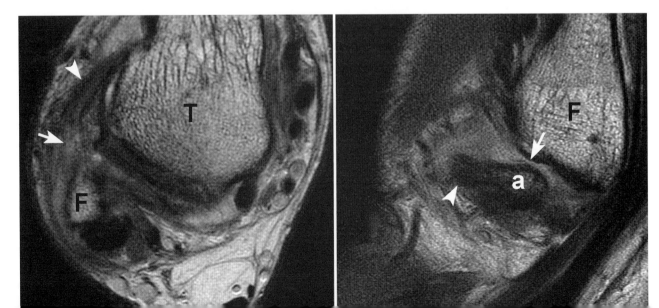

▶ **Fig. 7.74** As previously seen in the discussion on impingement, varus tilting of the talus may result from chronic lateral ligament instability, leading to ankle impingement and osteoarthropathy.

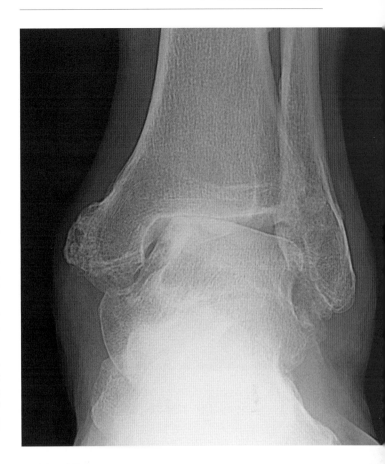

joint may occur in 10–20% of athletes after ankle sprains (De Simoni et al. 1996) and, infrequently, a varus pattern of degenerative osteoarthropathy of the ankle can develop related to underlying chronic lateral ligament instability (Valderrabano et al. 2006) (see Fig. 7.74). The majority of injured ligaments remodel with mature scarring and appear as well-defined structures of homogeneously low signal (see Fig. 7.75 and Fig. 1.22(b) on page 18). When laxity develops, MRI may demonstrate a range of appearances from attenuation to immature hypertrophic scarring (see Fig. 7.76). Hypertrophic scarring at the anterolateral ankle gutter can cause persistent impingement pain.

The oblique-coronal orientation of the CFL makes full-length demonstration on a single MR image difficult. The normal ligament is homogeneously hypointense on all MRI pulse sequences (Muhle et al. 1999). Ultrasound of the CFL is limited by difficulties in visualising the fibular attachment (Lagalla et al. 1994), but interstitial and avulsion injuries at the calcaneal insertion can be readily identified. Dorsiflexion of the ankle places the ligament under tension and is helpful during ultrasound assessment.

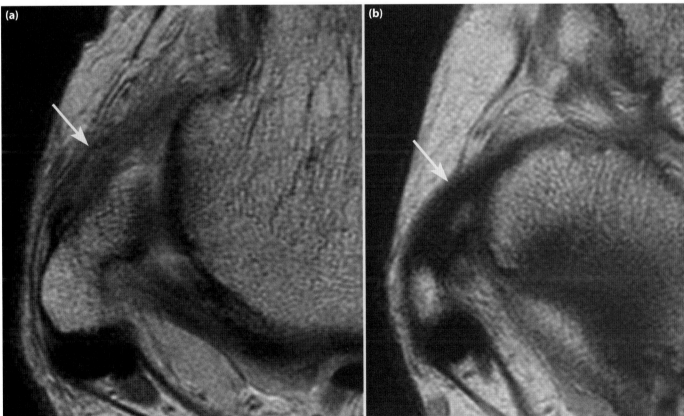

▲ **Fig. 7.75** Axial PD-weighted images demonstrate satisfactory healing of an injured ATFL.
(a) This is the appearance six weeks after the injury, showing thickening of the ligament and signal hyperintensity (arrow).
(b) Twenty months after the injury, the ligament has remodelled and formed a uniform mature scar of homogeneously low signal (arrow).

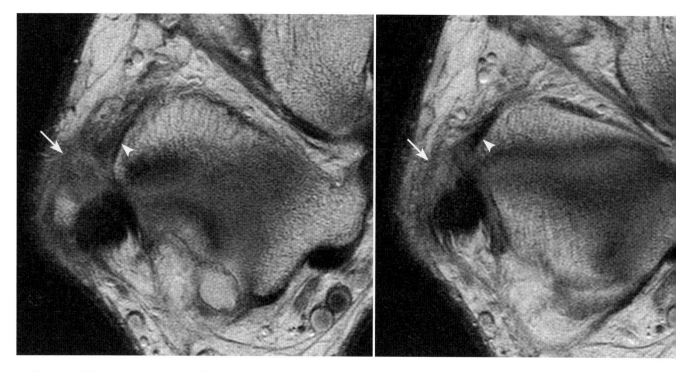

▲ **Fig. 7.76** MRI demonstrates an ineffective ATFL healing response. This patient had a previous history of ankle sprain and, in the clinical context, an axial PD-weighted MR image shows features of an old ATFL rupture at the fibular attachment with immature hypertrophic scarring at the site of tear (arrows). Also note the distal stump of the ATFL (arrowheads).

Injury to the deltoid ligament complex

The deltoid ligament complex of the ankle is much stronger than the lateral ligament complex. Injury requires large eversion and abduction forces, and bony avulsion of the medial malleolus will occur more often than a tear of the deltoid ligament (see Fig. 7.77). The deltoid ligament consists of three main components:

1. the tibionavicular ligament runs from the apex of the medial malleolus to the navicular tuberosity
2. the tibiocalcaneal ligament attaches to the medial aspect of the medial malleolus and passes inferiorly to attach to the sustentaculum tali
3. the tibiotalar band passes from the posterior aspect of the medial malleolus to the medial talus.

The deltoid ligament complex is a large, fan-shaped structure with both deep and superficial components. The deep fibres extend from the medial malleolus to the posterior aspect of the talar body. The superficial fibres course from the medial malleolus to the sustentaculum, dorsomedial talar neck, spring ligament and medial process of the navicular. Medial ankle injury is an initial stage of a syndesmosis injury, either as a rupture of the deltoid ligament or as a transverse fracture of the medial malleolus.

▶ **Fig. 7.77** The deltoid ligament is robust, and fractures of the medial malleolus will occur more readily than tearing of the ligament. Subtle changes suggestive of a fracture of the posterior malleolus are seen projected over the distal tibial metaphysis.

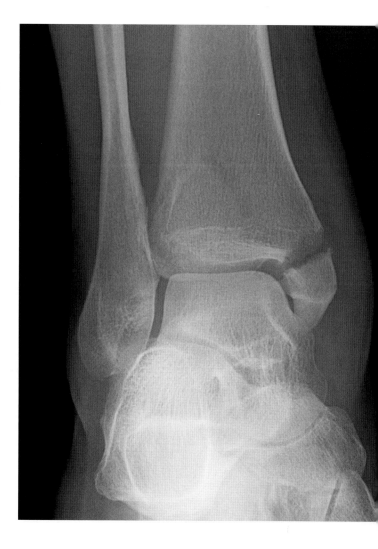

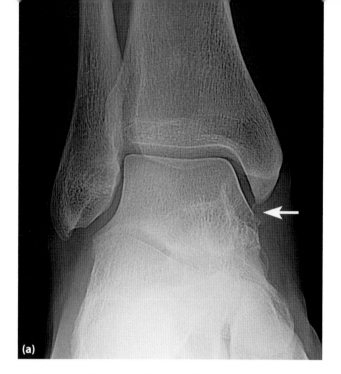
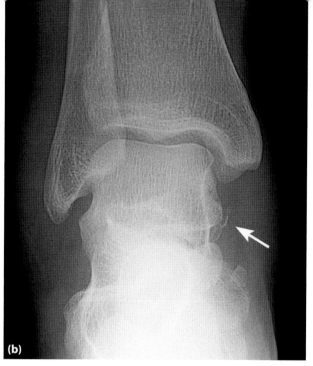

▲ **Fig. 7.78(a)** The deltoid ligament has avulsed small fragments from its talar attachment (arrow).
(b) In a different case, deep fibres of the deltoid have avulsed small fragments from the talus (arrow).

Imaging of deltoid ligament complex injuries

Deltoid ligament tears are uncommon, reflecting the inherent strength of this structure. Acute tears of the deltoid ligament may be partial or complete.

Plain films

Plain radiographs are usually of limited value for assessing injury of the deltoid ligament, but widening of the medial clear space indicates deep fibre disruption and is best assessed on weightbearing AP and 'mortise' views. Avulsion fractures may occasionally be present at the attachment of the deep fibres to the talus (see Fig. 7.78).

Ultrasound and MRI

Deep fibre deltoid ligament tears are identified by MRI as linear defects in continuity and may be quite subtle (see Figs 7.79 and 7.80). In most cases scar tissue will bridge the tear and impart reasonable stability, provided anatomical alignment is maintained at the ankle mortise (Harper 1988). Occasionally, ineffective scar response can result in valgus instability with or without hind-foot valgus deformity (Hintermann et al. 2004) (see Fig. 7.81). Interposition of the ruptured deltoid ligament may prevent the reduction of extra-articular ankle fractures (Feldman 1997). Corticated ossicles that project over the medial ankle gutter on plain films are indicative of old deltoid ligament injury. Although some ossicles may

▼ **Fig. 7.79** A deltoid ligament tear is demonstrated by axial and coronal PD-weighted MR images. There is fibre discontinuity indicating an acute tear at the talar attachment of the deep fibres (arrows).

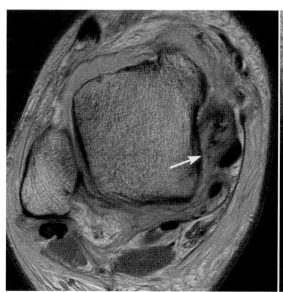
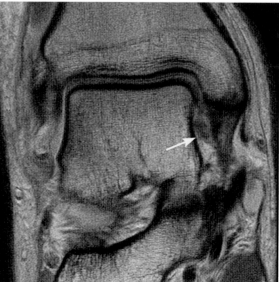

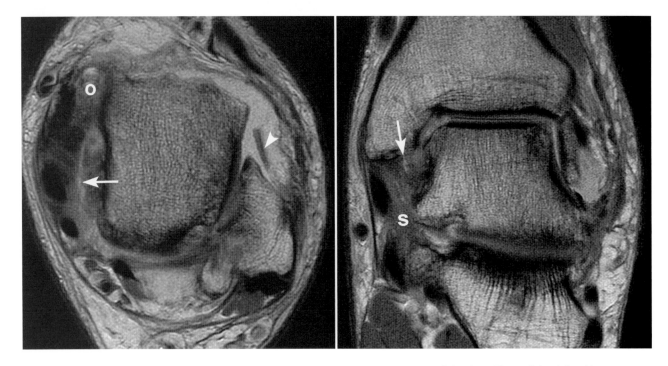

▲ **Fig. 7.80** Axial and coronal PD-weighted images show a subacute incomplete tear of the deep fibres of the deltoid ligament (arrows) and an interstitial tear of the superficial tibiocalcaneal fibres (s). Note the adjacent chondral defect at the medial corner of the talar dome, with the chondral fragment displaced into the anterolateral gutter (arrowhead). There is also an ossicle in the medial ankle gutter anteriorly (o).

be the result of an avulsion, most are due to post-traumatic dystrophic ossification.

Acute or subacute injuries of the superficial fibres of the deltoid ligament are shown by MRI as ligament thickening, hyperintensity and associated periligamentous oedema (see Fig. 7.82). Macroscopic fibre discontinuity may or may not be evident. This should be distinguished from an injury to the anterior insertion of the flexor retinaculum at the medial malleolus (which may accompany a deltoid ligament injury). Injuries to the superficial fibres of the deltoid ligament, particularly the anterior tibiotalar fascicle, may result in chronic anteromedial ankle impingement (Mosier-La Clair 2000).

▼ **Fig. 7.81** A late subacute-stage complete tear of the deep fibres of the deltoid ligament is demonstrated by axial and coronal PD-weighted MR images. There is a persisting thin fluid intensity cleft at the site of the tear (arrows). Also note concomitant injury to the tibial end of the flexor retinaculum with maturing hypertrophic scar response (f), tearing of the CFL with subsequent immature hypertrophic scar response (c), and an osteochondral fracture at the lateral corner of the talar dome (arrowhead). The corresponding chondral fragment is displaced into the posterior recess of the ankle joint (asterisk).

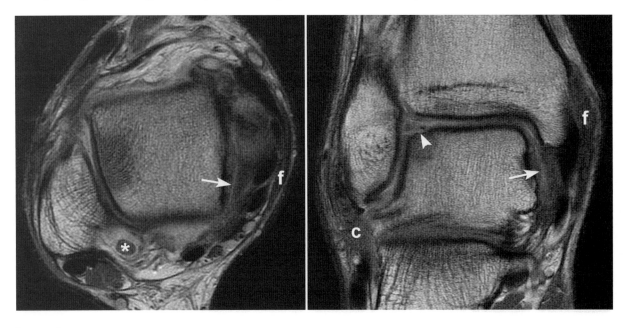

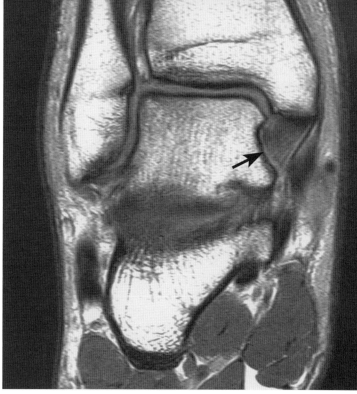

▶ Fig. 7.82 A coronal T1-weighted image shows a high signal line, consistent with a high-grade tear at the talar attachment of the deep tibiotalar fibres of the deltoid ligament (arrow).

Deltoid ligament tears should be distinguished from ligament contusions, which do not result in ligament fibre discontinuity but instead produce diffuse deltoid swelling with hyperintensity and loss of normal fatty striation on MRI, or hypoechoic echotexture with accompanying hyperaemia on ultrasound (see Fig. 7.83). There may be associated protrusion of the thickened ligament into the adjacent ankle gutter with accompanying synovitis. This mechanism of ligament impact may be associated with posteromedial ankle impingement, medial talar dome osteochondral fractures (Paterson and Brown 2001) and degenerative arthropathy at the medial ankle gutter in cases of chronic lateral ligament instability.

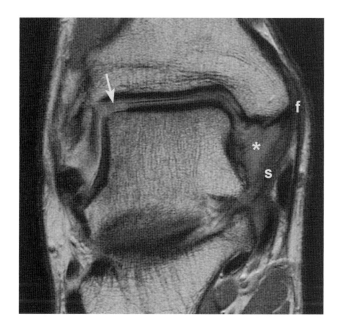

◀ Fig. 7.83(a) A deltoid ligament contusion is demonstrated by a coronal PD-weighted MR image, showing changes of late subacute stage medial rotational impaction injury to the deep tibiofibular fibres (asterisk). Note the loss of normal fat signal between the ligament fascicles. The superficial tibiocalcaneal fibres are also mildly scarred (s) and there is scarring of the overlying segment of the flexor retinaculum at the tibial attachment (f). A chondral defect is present at the lateral corner of the talar dome (arrow).

▼ (b) In the same case as **(a)**, diffuse hypoechoic swelling and hyperaemia of the deltoid ligament are demonstrated by transverse and long-axis Power Doppler ultrasound images (arrows).

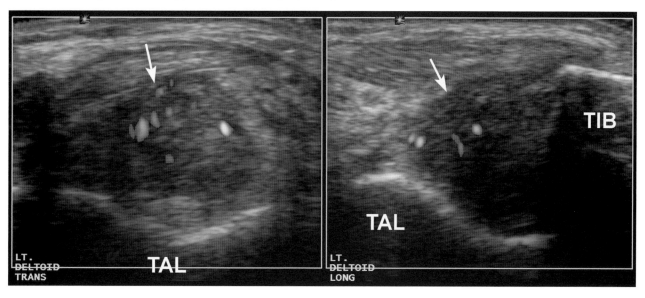

Injury to the distal tibiofibular syndesmosis (diastasis injury)

Injuries to the supporting ligaments of the distal tibiofibular syndesmosis are sometimes referred to as 'high' ankle sprains. They constitute about 1% of all ankle sprains (Hopkinson et al. 1990). The true incidence is higher in the sporting population and studies suggest that the injury is under-recognised. For example, Gerber et al. (1998) reported an incidence rate in excess of 30% in those athletes involved in high-impact sports.

It is important to diagnose and treat a syndesmosis injury early, as recovery time is longer than with other ankle sprains. Pain and loss of push-off power are the major factors preventing a return to athletic activity (Nussbaum et al. 2001). If a syndesmosis injury goes unrecognised or untreated, chronic distal tibiofibular joint instability may develop and a rapid-onset osteoarthropathy may result. The imaging findings can be subtle and it is important that the many clues to the presence of a syndesmosis injury be recognised and an appropriate imaging protocol followed.

Anatomy of tibiofibular syndesmosis injuries

The inferior tibiofibular ligament complex is an important stabiliser of the ankle joint and consists of three components:

1. *The anterior inferior tibiofibular ligament (AITFL):* this is a flat band passing obliquely, laterally and distally from the distal tibia to the adjacent fibula.
2. *The posterior inferior tibiofibular ligament (PITFL):* this component runs obliquely from the posterior lip of the distal tibia to the posterior aspect of the adjacent fibula and has deep and superficial components.
3. *The inferior interosseous ligaments:* these consist of a number of short strong bands passing between the adjacent surfaces of the tibia and the fibula.

Studies have shown that the inferior tibiofibular ligaments and the posterior tibiotalar component of the deltoid ligament are stronger than the ligaments of the lateral ligament complex, and the PITFL has been shown to be stronger than the AITFL. The posterior tibiotalar component of the deltoid ligament may also rupture in syndesmosis injuries (Beumer et al. 2003).

Biomechanics of tibiofibular syndesmosis injuries

The mechanism of syndesmosis injury is usually external rotation of a dorsiflexed foot. Commonly this occurs in collision sports such as football when a player is tackled or collides with another player and the ankle is forcibly dorsiflexed while the foot is planted and externally rotated (Nussbaum et al. 2001).

Non-contact syndesmosis injuries usually involve catching the toe on the ground while running, with a resultant external rotation force to the ankle. A variation of this mechanism is seen in skiers when a ski tip catches at high speed, resulting in a sudden external rotation force (Fritschy 1994). An internal rotation force to the tibia with a fixed planted foot is another less common mechanism of injury.

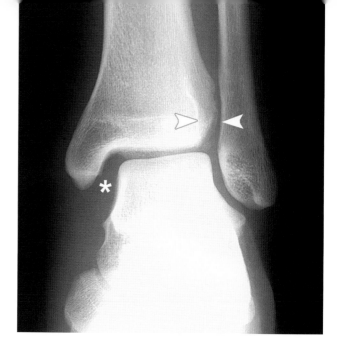

▲ **Fig. 7.84** Widening of the medial clear space of the ankle joint (asterisk) is a diagnostic sign of diastasis of the inferior tibiofibular joint. This widening is due to rupture of both the deep fibres of the deltoid ligament and the distal tibiofibular syndesmosis. In this case there is also widening of the inferior tibiofibular joint space (arrowheads).

Pure abduction injuries to the ankle are rare and are usually accompanied by deltoid ligament disruption or a medial malleolus fracture.

There are a number of different classifications of syndesmosis injuries, the details of which are beyond the scope of this book. In general, ligaments and fractures occur in sequence and the progression of disruption, as described by Pankovich (1976), is discussed in the section on Maisonneuve fracture later in this chapter.

Imaging of tibiofibular syndesmosis injuries

Plain films

The starting point of any imaging investigation is a high-quality plain film series. Plain films detect only 64% of syndesmosis injuries, reflecting the fact that not all syndesmosis injuries are unstable and not all unstable injuries demonstrate malalignment on unstressed plain films (Takao et al. 2001). It is important to remember that low-grade injuries also occur, producing pain and swelling without fracture or instability. These injuries have no plain film signs apart from non-specific soft-tissue swelling. Nevertheless, the plain film series should be examined carefully, as diagnostic clues may be subtle.

Changes of alignment due to ligamentous injury

Widening of the medial clear space occurs due to disruption of the deep fibres of the deltoid ligament (see Fig. 7.84). Although radiographic positioning may not be crucial to the measurement of the width of the distal tibiofibular joint, the width of the medial clear space varies dramatically with rotation and correct positioning is very important. Consequently, this sign is dependent on a technically satisfactory 'mortise' view, allowing comparison of the lateral and medial clear spaces.

The most reliable finding is widening of the distal tibio-fibular syndesmosis, which is a width greater than 5.5 mm (see Fig. 7.85). This measurement is made from the medial border of the fibula to the vertical sclerotic line representing the base of the fibular notch of the tibia (see Fig. 7.86). Pneumaticos et al. (2002) demonstrated that the position of the ankle was not crucial to measuring the width of the tibiofibular syndesmosis. The study found that the width of the syndesmosis did not vary significantly with rotation from 5° external rotation to 25° internal rotation.

Associated fractures

Certain fractures commonly occur in association with syndesmosis injuries and include:

- a transverse fracture of the medial malleolus (see Fig. 7.87)
- Weber B and C distal fibular fractures—50% of Weber B fractures are associated with diastasis of the distal tibiofibular joint, whereas a diastasis is always present when a Weber C fracture has occurred (see Fig. 7.88)
- a Maisonneuve fracture, which is discussed below
- avulsion fractures, which may occur at the tibial insertions of the AITFL or PITFL (the latter constituting a 'posterior malleolus' fracture (see Fig. 7.89))
- syndesmotic injuries are also associated with an increased incidence of ankle joint chondral injuries when compared with lateral collateral ligament injuries (Loren and Ferkel 2002).

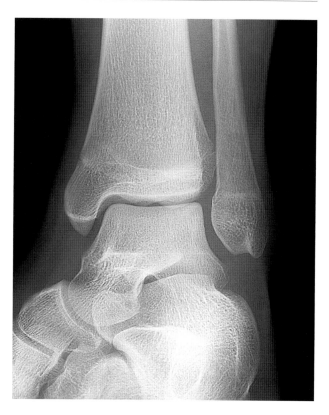

▲ **Fig. 7.86** The base of the fibular notch of the tibia is well demonstrated in this case of a diastasis injury.

▼ **Fig. 7.87** A transverse fracture of the medial malleolus (arrow) is produced by a screwing rotational force in the axial plane rather than an eversion injury and usually indicates a diastasis injury of the distal tibiofibular syndesmosis. A subtle Weber B fracture is also present and widening of the medial clear space is noted.

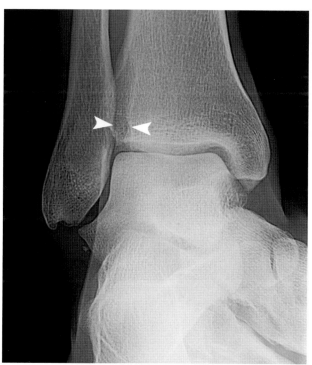

▲ **Fig. 7.85** The width of the inferior tibiofibular joint space is measured from the medial border of the fibula to the base of the fibular notch of the tibia, shown as a vertical sclerotic line (arrowheads).

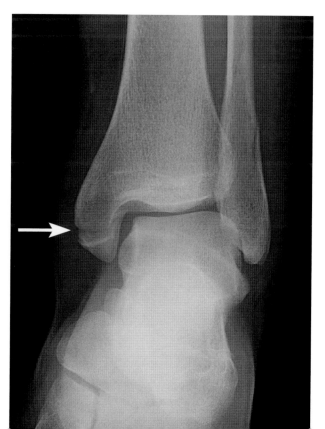

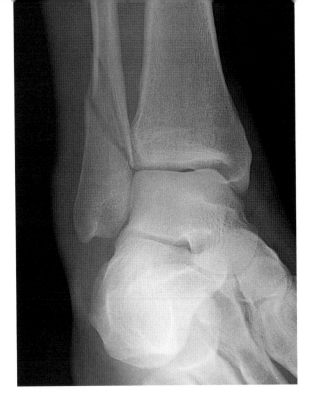

▲ **Fig. 7.88** A Weber B fracture of the distal fibula is associated with a diastasis injury in 50% of cases.

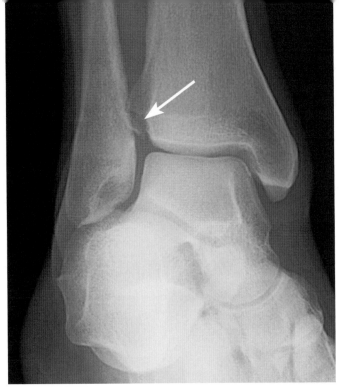

▲ **Fig. 7.89** An avulsion fracture has been produced by PITFL traction (arrow).

Soft-tissue changes

The following soft-tissue changes may be seen.

- A swollen ankle without any ankle joint effusion may indicate a syndesmosis injury. The effusion leaks into the surrounding tissues through a capsular tear (see Fig. 7.90).
- A progress examination may show periosteal reaction at the syndesmosis or calcification in the interosseous ligament two to three weeks after the injury (see

Fig. 7.91). In the subacute setting, periosteal reaction may appear on the posterior margin of the tibia, above the posterior malleolus (see Fig. 7.92). Later, heterotopic ossification may also develop in the interosseous membrane between the distal tibia and the fibula (see Fig. 7.93). Heterotopic ossification at a site of old syndesmosis injury is a relatively common radiographic finding in athletes, and is occasionally a source of persistent pain requiring excision (Veltri et al. 1995; Kennedy et al. 2000).

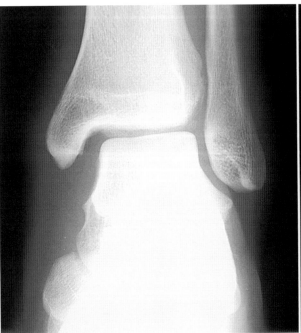
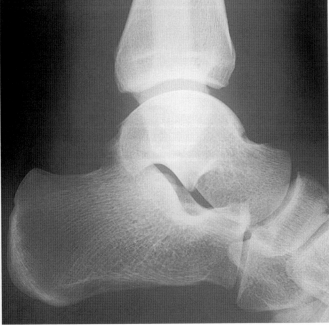

▲ **Fig. 7.90** Following a diastasis injury, diffuse soft-tissue swelling may be present rather than a discrete ankle joint effusion. Note the widening of both the medial clear space and the inferior tibiofibular joint space.

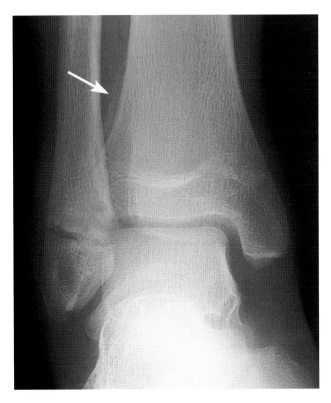

▲ **Fig. 7.91** Calcification of the torn interosseous membrane is appearing two weeks after a diastasis injury (arrow).

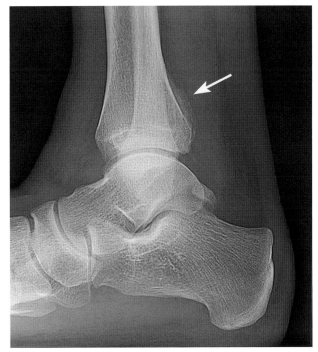

▲ **Fig. 7.92** Periosteal new bone on the dorsal margin of the distal tibia may appear following a diastasis injury due to periosteal stripping or bone injury at the PITFL attachment (arrow). An ankle joint effusion is noted.

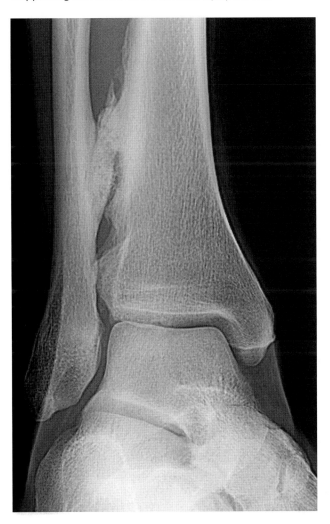

◀ **Fig. 7.93** Following a recent syndesmosis injury, ossification has developed in the inferior interosseous ligament and interosseous membrane. Cross union is developing.

Stress views

Stress radiographs can help in the detection of syndesmosis instability. If clinical suspicion is high but the routine views are normal or equivocal, stress views with comparison views of the normal side may provide evidence of diastasis.

Stress views may be obtained in two ways (see 'Additional plain film views of the ankle'). Stress may be applied:

1. with forced abduction and external rotation of the foot, while holding the tibia in an AP position (see Fig. 7.94)
2. with weightbearing and ankle dorsiflexion (which stresses the syndesmosis because the talar dome widens anteriorly).

Nuclear bone scans

A nuclear bone scan can detect a diastasis injury, if increased uptake of isotope is demonstrated at the tibiofibular syndesmosis (see Fig. 7.95), and can demonstrate a tear of the interosseous membrane (see Fig. 7.96). A CT scan or MRI is then useful for defining bone detail and assessment of associated fractures.

CT

Axial CT of both ankles can demonstrate subtle abnormalities of syndesmosis alignment that are not evident on plain films (Ebraheim et al. 1997) (see Fig. 7.97). Axial CT images can also detect ligamentous swelling (see Fig. 7.98).

▶ **Fig. 7.94** A stress view of the inferior tibiofibular joint has confirmed the presence of a diastasis injury. The method of applying stress has been described in the text. Stress has opened the medial clear space, demonstrating both deltoid ligament injury and distal tibiofibular syndesmosis injury.

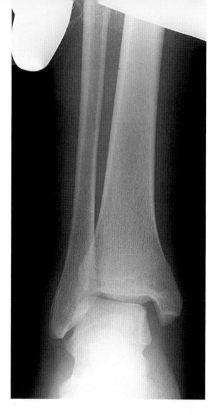

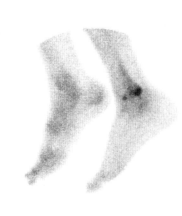

▲ **Fig. 7.95** There is increased uptake of isotope at the inferior tibiofibular joint, particularly associated with the PITFL, suggesting that an avulsion fracture may be present.

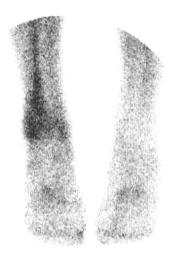

▲ **Fig. 7.96** Tearing of the interosseous membrane is well demonstrated as linear uptake of isotope in the blood pool phase of a nuclear bone scan.

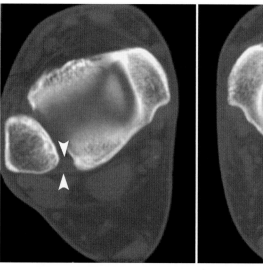

▲ **Fig. 7.97** An axial CT examination of the left ankle has been obtained, with an image of the right ankle included for comparison. The left ankle remains painful and swollen three weeks after a twisting trauma. On the left, there is soft-tissue swelling obscuring detail of the AITFL and marked swelling of the PITFL, appreciated by comparison with the right side (arrowheads). Calcification has developed over the attachment of the PITFL, but is separated from the periosteal surface.

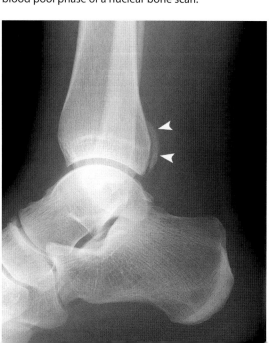

◀ **Fig. 7.98** Curvilinear calcification is occasionally seen over the posterior surface of the posterior malleolus two to three weeks following a diastasis injury (see Fig. 7.97). The position of the calcification suggests that it may be secondary to a PITFL injury (arrowheads).

Ultrasound and MRI

MRI is the method of choice for imaging the changes associated with a syndesmosis injury. Axial images must extend 4–5 cm above the plafond in order to evaluate the entire inferior interosseous ligament and the inferior margin of the interosseous tibiofibular membrane (see Fig. 7.99). The normal AITFL is visualised as a hypointense multifascicular structure on axial and coronal PD-weighted images (see Fig. 7.100). Acute complete tears are shown as a ligament defect of fluid intensity, redundancy of the ligament fibres and infiltration of the adjacent fat plane (see Fig. 7.101). There may also be widening of the syndesmosis anteriorly and anterior fibular subluxation. Subacute tears generally show immature scar response of intermediate-to-low signal bridging the fibre gap and producing a thickened ligament (see Fig. 7.102). Over time, maturing scar will remodel the ligament to produce a more hypointense structure with less thickening (see Fig. 7.103). The thickened ligament may protrude into the anterolateral ankle gutter as a meniscoid lesion. Bony spurs may develop at the tibial or fibular attachments.

Old injuries manifest as a chronically scarred ligament (see Figs 7.103 and 7.104). Tears of the PITFL usually occur at the tibial insertion, with associated bone marrow oedema and periosteal stripping at the adjacent posterior tibial malleolus (see Fig. 7.105). Adjacent chondral lesions at the posterolateral tibial plafond are also common (Loren and Ferkel 2002). Synovitis and scar tissue may form around the injured PITFL and protrude into the posterior syndesmotic recess causing impingement symptoms (Harper 2001).

Ultrasound can also demonstrate the AITFL (Milz et al. 1998). Acute tears of the AITFL are usually manifest as an anechoic cleft (see Fig. 7.106). Avulsion bone flakes may be seen at the tibial or fibular attachments. The syndesmosis may be widened anteriorly compared to the contralateral side or there may be dynamic widening with applied external rotation stress (van Holsbeek and Powell 1995). At the subacute stage, immature scar produces a thickened, hypoechoic appearance (Fessell and van Holsbeek 2001) (see Fig. 7.107), and there may be an associated increase in vascularity on Power Doppler scanning, extending inferiorly into the anterolateral gutter. Sonographic visualisation of the inferior interosseous ligament is not possible and visualisation of the PITFL is limited. Nevertheless, careful side-to-side comparison can usually establish whether the PITFL has been injured.

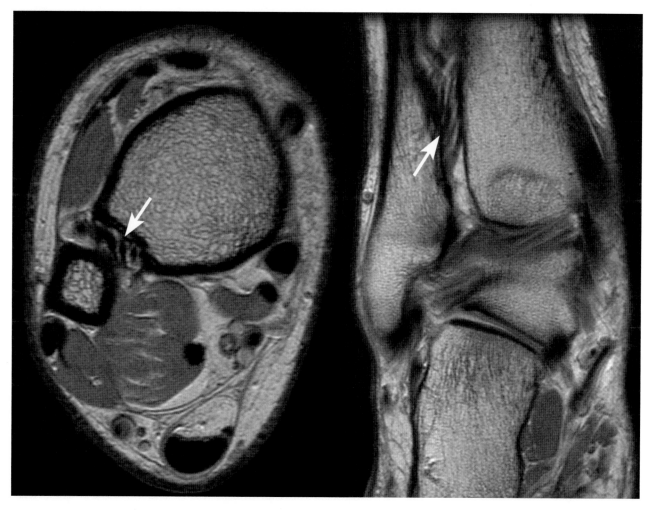

▲ **Fig. 7.99** Axial and coronal PD-weighted MR images demonstrate a normal interosseous ligament (arrows). To examine the interosseous ligament in its entirety, the field of view must extend 4–5 cm above the ankle joint.

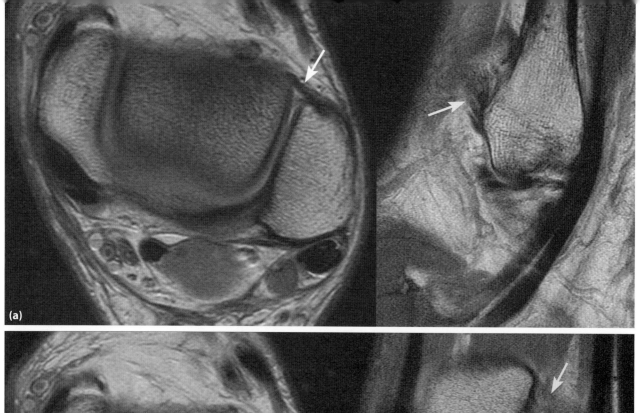

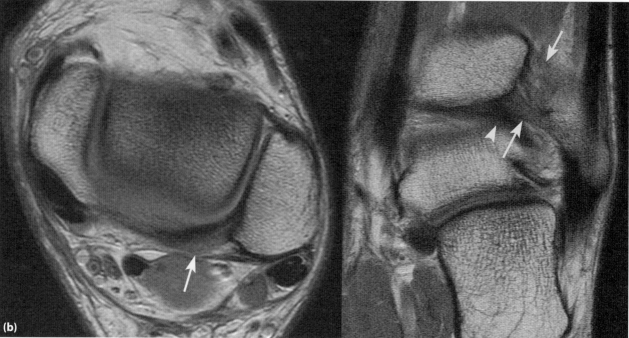

▲ **Fig. 7.100(a)** The MRI appearance of a normal AITFL is shown on axial and sagittal PD-weighted images (arrows).
(b) Axial and coronal PD-weighted images demonstrate a normal PITFL (arrows) and transverse tibiofibular ligament (arrowhead).

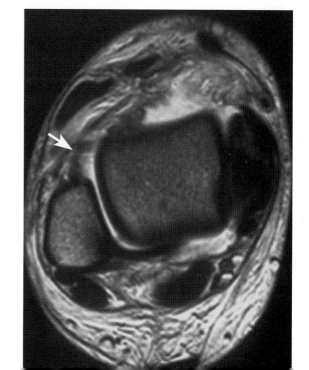

▶ **Fig. 7.101** A T2*-weighted MR image obtained following an acute ankle injury shows a redundant swollen and hyperintense AITFL, consistent with a complete rupture (arrow). Note the ankle joint effusion.

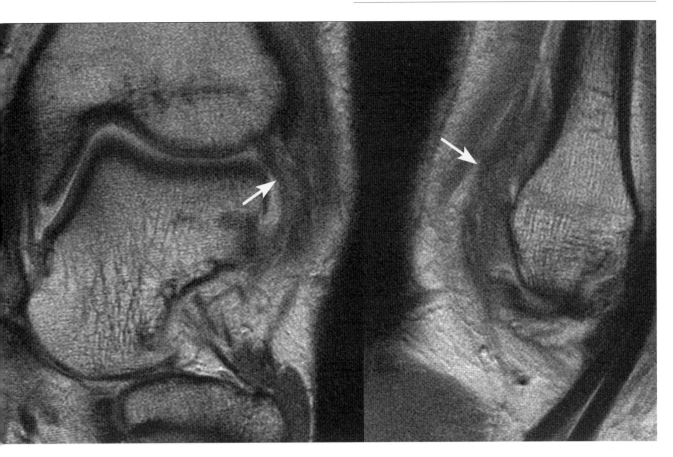

▲ **Fig. 7.102** A subacute AITFL tear is demonstrated on coronal and sagittal PD-weighted MR images. There is diffuse immature AITFL hypertrophic scarring, which bridges and obscures the site of fibre disruption (arrows).

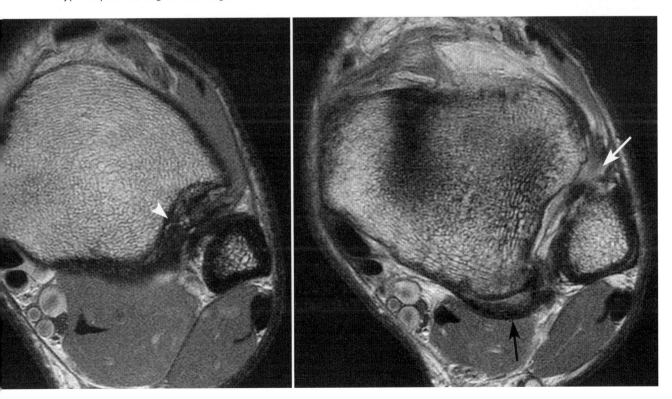

▲ **Fig. 7.103** A chronic syndesmosis injury is demonstrated on axial PD-weighted MR images, showing ineffective AITFL scar response (white arrow), a densely scarred inferior interosseous ligament (arrowhead) and scarred PITFL with a residual component of periosteal detachment (black arrow). Note the predominantly low signal intensity of the torn ligaments and stripped periosteal attachment of the PITFL.

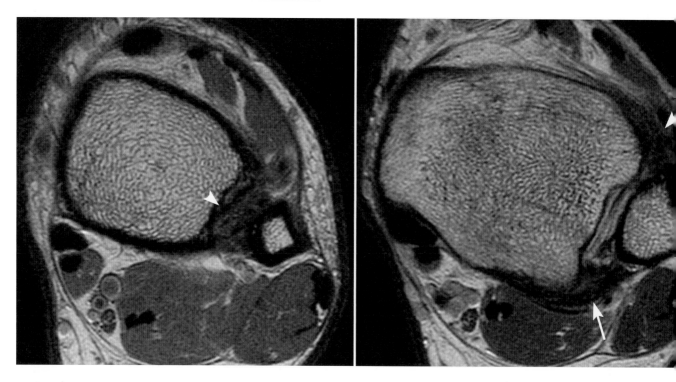

▲ **Fig. 7.104** A late subacute to chronic syndesmotic ligament injury is demonstrated on axial PD-weighted MR images, which show hypertrophic scar response along the injured AITFL and PITFL (arrows), and a thick densely scarred interosseous ligament (arrowhead).

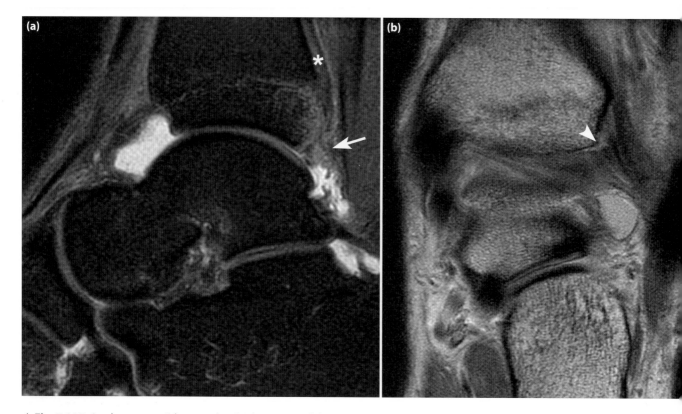

▲ **Fig. 7.105** A subacute partial tear at the tibial insertion of the PITFL is demonstrated by sagittal fat-suppressed PD and coronal PD-weighted MR images.

(a) The sagittal fat-suppressed image demonstrates a hyperintense PITFL with periosteal reaction extending along the posterior surface of the tibia (asterisk), and adjacent tibial bone marrow oedema. There is hyperintense thickening of the adjacent injured transverse tibiofibular ligament (arrow). Also note the ankle joint effusion.

(b) On the coronal image, there is a cleft of fluid signal indicating detachment at the tibial insertion of the deep fibres of the PITFL (arrowhead).

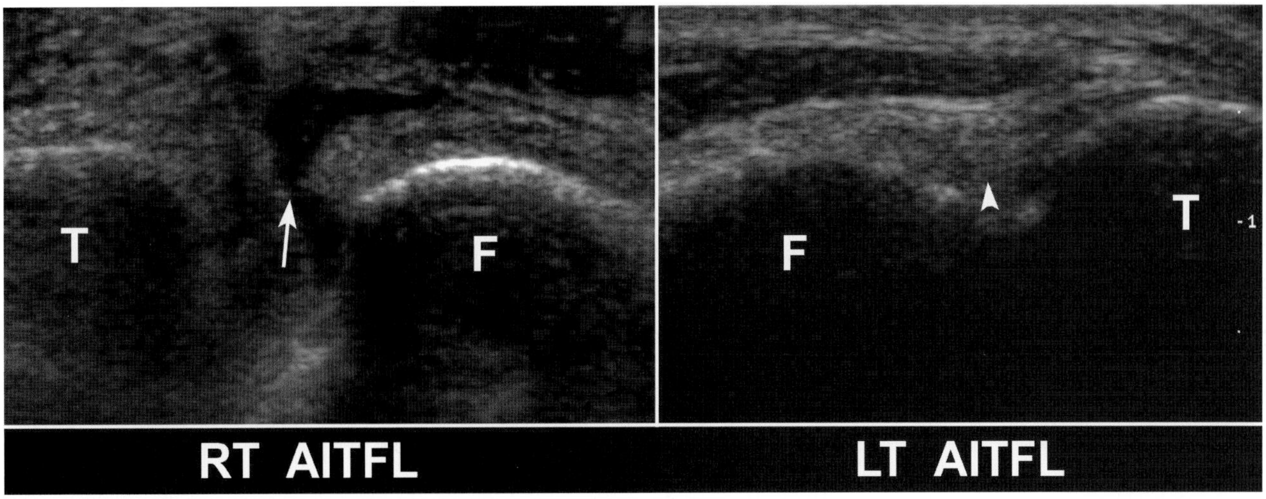

RT AITFL

LT AITFL

▲ Fig. 7.106 An acute tear of the right AITFL is demonstrated by ultrasound. Comparison long-axis images show a transverse hypoechoic defect in fibre continuity on the right (arrow). This represents haemorrhage in the gap between the slightly distracted margins of a complete mid-segment ligament rupture, and contrasts with the normal appearance of an intact ligament on the left side (arrowhead). Tibia = T. Fibula = F.

▶ Fig. 7.107 A long-axis ultrasound image demonstrates the AITFL nine weeks after a 'high' ankle sprain. The ligament is diffusely thickened and hypoechoic (callipers), with changes most marked at the fibular attachment. There is no discrete tear plane. Tibia = T. Fibula = F.

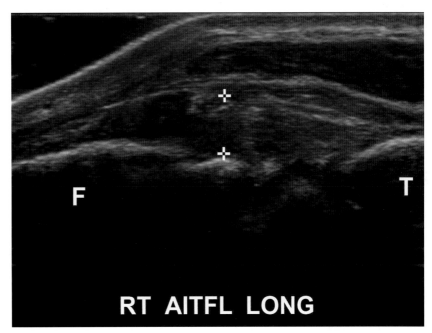

RT AITFL LONG

Maisonneuve fractures

Pankovich (1976) described the Maisonneuve fracture as a spiral fracture of the proximal fibular shaft, usually occurring in association with diastasis of the tibiofibular syndesmosis (see Fig. 7.19). A Maisonneuve fracture is a manifestation of the spiral force that begins with the failure of medial structures at the ankle joint and travels up the lateral side of the leg, tearing the interosseous ligament. It is now realised that a Maisonneuve-type fracture may occur anywhere in the fibula from just proximal to the level of the distal tibiofibular joint to the superior tibiofibular joint (see Figs 7.108 and 7.109). Kumar et al. (2004) described rotational forces associated with a syndesmosis injury causing a dislocation of the proximal tibiofibular joint as a variation of the Maisonneuve fracture. This is clinically important as this can result in instability of the knee joint.

Pankovich described the sequence of events. First there is rupture of the AITFL, followed by strain and rupture of the interosseous ligament and fracture of the posterior tibial tubercle or rupture of the PITFL. Rupture of the anteromedial aspect of the capsule of the ankle joint, fracture of the proximal fibular shaft and rupture of the deltoid ligament or fracture of the medial malleolus then follow. Rupture of the distal tibiofibular ligaments is rarely an isolated injury. The interosseous membrane may tear all the way up to the level of the Maisonneuve fracture. The Maisonneuve-type fracture is not specific to a tibiofibular syndesmosis injury and has also been reported occurring in association with a 'triplane fracture' (Dhukaram et al. 2003). A Maisonneuve fracture is generally diagnosed on plain films. A nuclear bone scan may be helpful if the plain films are inconclusive (see Fig. 7.110).

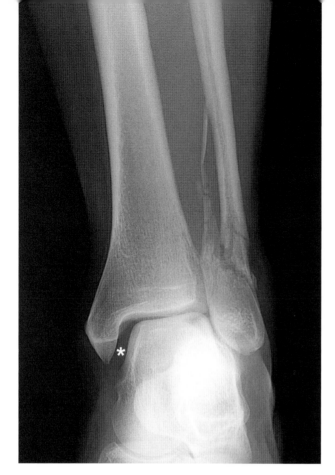

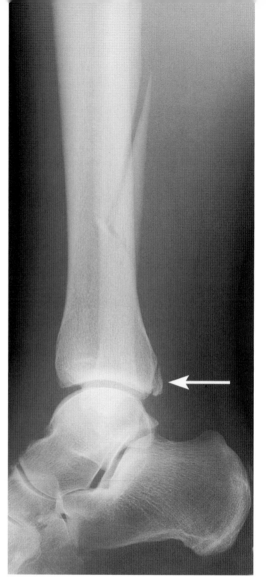

▲ **Fig. 7.108** A Maisonneuve-type spiral fracture may occur anywhere along the fibular shaft, with fractures in the distal fibula merging with the Weber C fracture at the ankle. This is an exceptionally low Maisonneuve-type fracture, showing manifestations of a spiral force produced by external rotation of the foot. The interosseous ligament and interosseous membrane have avulsed an elongated cortical fragment from the medial margin of the distal fibula. There has been a diastasis injury to the inferior tibiofibular joint with widening of the medial clear space indicating deltoid ligament disruption (asterisk).

▲ **Fig. 7.109** In this case, a spiral fracture involves the fibula at the junction of its middle and distal thirds. There are changes of a diastasis injury at the ankle, with an avulsion of the posterior lip of the distal tibia (arrow).

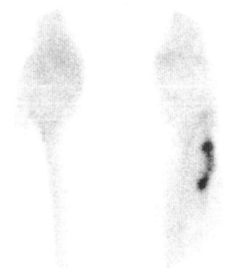

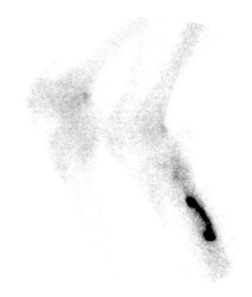

▲ **Fig. 7.110** A nuclear bone scan demonstrates a Maisonneuve fracture.

Ankle impingement

Ankle impingement is a common painful condition that results from abutment of bony structures or 'pinching' of soft tissue in an ankle joint recess. Impingement can be acute or chronic, anterior, posterior, medial or lateral in combination or alone. The affected joint recess usually demonstrates localised tenderness, and the pain is typically relieved by an injection of a local anaesthetic. Bony causes for impingement include osteophytes, exostoses (see Fig. 7.111), ossicles such as an os trigonum, ankle instability (see Fig. 7.112) and intra-articular loose bodies (see Fig. 7.113). Ganglion cysts and synovial proliferations are common soft-tissue causes of impingement. Trauma is the leading cause of ankle impingement, and can occur as either an acute episode or chronic repetitive low-level stress.

Anterolateral ankle impingement

Anterolateral ankle impingement usually results from ankle inversion trauma, sustained in sports such as basketball, soccer and volleyball. A tear of either the ATFL or the inferior fascicle of the AITFL may produce a haemarthrosis, which predisposes to post-traumatic synovitis and the possible development of a 'meniscoid' lesion in the anterolateral gutter. Post-traumatic impingement pain may also be caused by capsuloligamentous scarring. Ongoing impingement can produce chondral lesions as a consequence of repetitive abrasion at the anterolateral

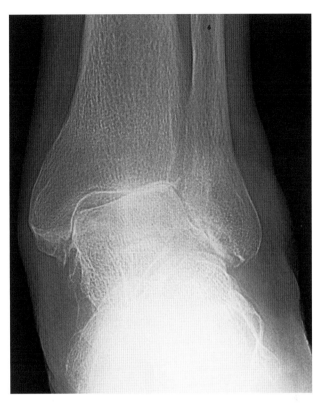

▲ **Fig. 7.112** Ankle instability due to chronic deltoid ligament insufficiency has produced osteoarthropathy, with both medial and lateral bony impingement.

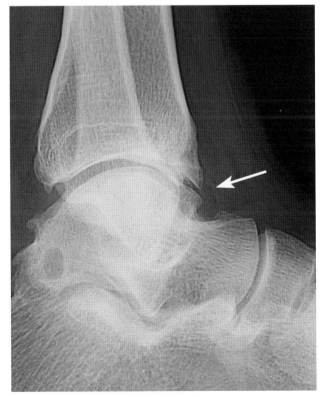

▲ **Fig. 7.111** Spur formation at the anterior aspect of the ankle produces anterior impingement with dorsiflexion of the ankle (arrow). A talar cyst is noted related to the talar articular surface of the posterior subtalar joint.

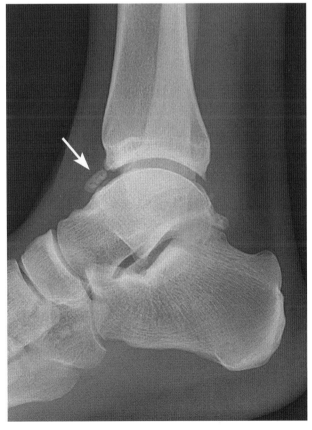

▲ **Fig. 7.113** Anterior impingement is due to a loose body in the anterior joint recess (arrow).

▶ **Fig. 7.114** With the ankle maximally dorsiflexed, bone-on-bone abutment occurs between the anterior lip of the distal tibia and the talar neck (arrowheads).

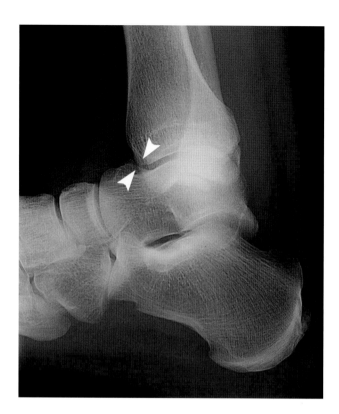

corner of the talar dome (Bassett et al. 1990). Symptoms can also be caused by plafond osteophytes and ossicles in the anterolateral gutter.

Imaging of anterolateral ankle impingement

Imaging assessment should begin with a routine plain film series with an additional lateral view obtained in ankle dorsiflexion (the 'lunge' view) (see Fig. 7.114). Plain films may show contributing factors such as ossicles or loose bodies in the anterolateral gutter or spurs at the anterolateral margin of the tibial plafond. It is also important to note any inferior prolongation of a bone spur, as this can abrade the chondral surface of the talar dome and predispose to the development of a sagittally oriented gouge defect known as a 'tram track' lesion.

The reported diagnostic accuracy of MRI for anterolateral ankle impingement is variable. On high-resolution PD-weighted MRI, post-traumatic anterolateral gutter synovitis is demonstrated as either linear or lobulated foci of intermediate signal intensity on both axial and coronal images. As a meniscoid lesion matures, this synovial thickening becomes more confluent and shows a lower signal intensity (see Fig. 7.115). The absence of an accompanying ankle joint effusion on MRI can make anterolateral impingement lesions difficult or impossible to detect (Rubin et al. 1997). Only about 60% of synovial impingement lesions demonstrate contrast enhancement (Bagnolesi et al. 1998).

Although MR arthrography and CT arthrography are both more accurate than conventional MRI, these tests are not commonly performed (Hauger et al. 1999). Interestingly, arthrography has been shown to correctly detect scarring or synovitis in more than 50% of patients without clinical features of anterolateral impingement (Robinson et al. 2001). This highlights the fact that anterolateral impingement remains a clinical diagnosis and that imaging is able to demonstrate only predisposing abnormalities and is unable to predict whether these changes are symptomatic.

Ultrasound is not helpful in diagnosis but can be used to guide therapeutic injections.

Anteromedial ankle impingement

Injuries to the superficial fibres of the deltoid ligament, particularly the anterior tibiotalar fascicle, may produce anteromedial ankle impingement due to localised synovitis or hypertrophic scarring (Egol and Parisien 1997). Patients typically complain of chronic anteromedial ankle pain, localised tenderness and sometimes snapping or 'popping' with ankle dorsiflexion. Post-traumatic ossicles (see Fig. 7.116), bone spurring (see Figs 7.117 and 7.118) and chondral damage to the anteromedial corner of the talar dome are also common findings (Mosier-La Clair et al. 2000).

▼ **Fig. 7.115** Axial PD-weighted MR images show changes of a mature meniscoid lesion. There is well-defined hypointense thickening of the inferior fascicle of the AITFL (arrow), with 'meniscoid' projection of this thickening into the anterolateral ankle gutter.

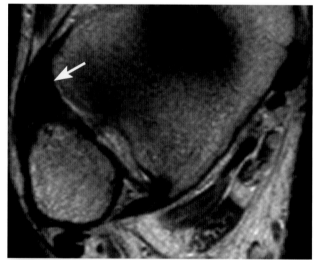

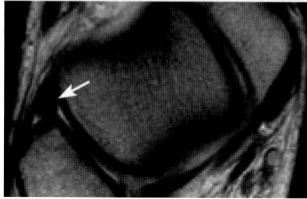

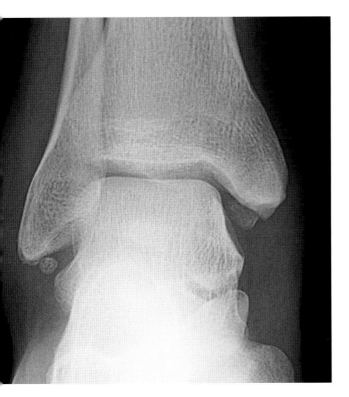

▲ **Fig. 7.116** Old post-traumatic ossicles are present adjacent to both malleoli. The ossicle originating from the medial malleolus is likely to contribute to anteromedial impingement.

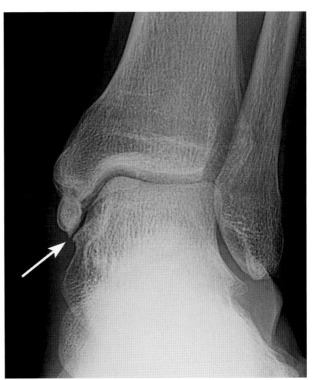

▲ **Fig. 7.117** There is a large spur originating from the tip of the medial malleolus. This spur impinges against the medial margin of the talus (arrow).

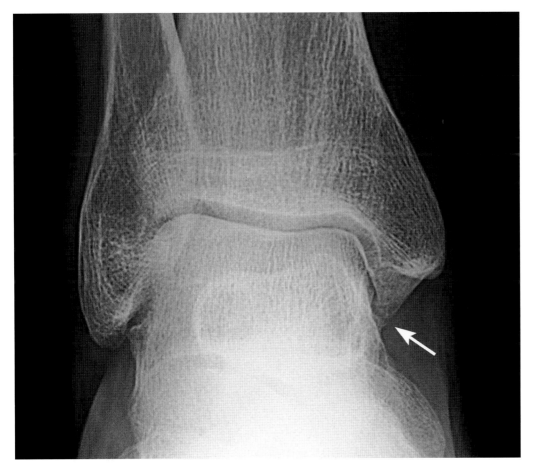

▲ **Fig. 7.118** A prominent spur extending from the medial malleolus abuts another spur on the medial margin of the talus (arrow).

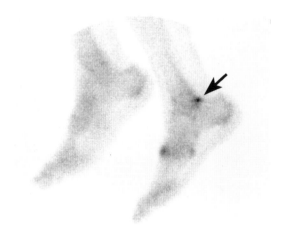

▲ **Fig. 7.119** Posterior impingement has produced focal uptake of isotope in the posterior process of the talus (arrow). There is also increased uptake in the first TMT joint due to degenerative changes.

Imaging of anteromedial ankle impingement

On true lateral radiographs of the ankle, it is difficult to tell whether anterior bone spurs are medial or lateral, and a supplementary oblique view may clarify. Soft-tissue causes of impingement in the anteromedial gutter are often difficult to appreciate with MRI (Mosier-La Clair et al. 2000). However, ultrasound can readily detect capsulosynovial and ligamentous thickening by simple side-to-side comparison. Ultrasound can also accurately guide corticosteroid injections.

Posterior (or posterolateral) ankle impingement

Posterior impingement generally produces ankle pain associated with forced plantar flexion and push-off manoeuvres and usually has a lateral predominance. These activities are seen in female dancers, soccer players, cricket fast bowlers, javelin throwers, divers, figure skaters, downhill runners and gymnasts (DeAsla et al. 2002). In ballet dancers this may occur in the demi-pointe or en pointe positions and can be disabling. The clinical suspicion of posterior impingement can be confirmed by a nuclear bone scan (see Fig. 7.119).

Variations in bony anatomy may predispose an athlete to posterior impingement. These variants include an os trigonum of any size (Hamilton et al. 1996) and a prominent posterior process of the talus as gauged by projection beyond the sagittal arc of curvature of the talar dome on a lateral plain film, MRI or CT (see Fig. 7.120). Many other causes have been reported, including ganglion cysts, chronic synovitis and a scarring associated with ligament tears at the posterior margin of the ankle joint (Rosenberg et al. 1995) (see Fig. 7.121). Ganglionic change within the FHL tendon sheath may also present with posterior impingement, and additional causes to be considered include a fracture of the posterior process of the talus (see Fig. 7.122), spurs, loose bodies within the posterior recess of the ankle or subtalar joint, and acquired capsular laxity (see Fig. 7.123). Peroneal tendon pathology, retrocalcaneal bursopathy and Achilles tendon pathology should also be considered as possible causes of posterior impingement. FHL tenosynovitis is a separate clinical entity that frequently coexists with posterior ankle impingement and is reported in more than 60% of dancers with impingement (Hamilton et al. 1996). This will be discussed in detail later in the chapter.

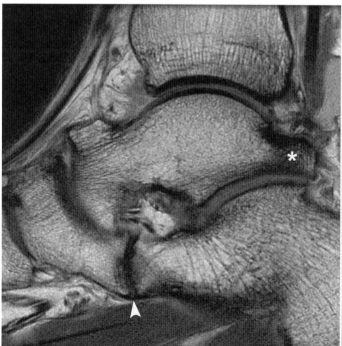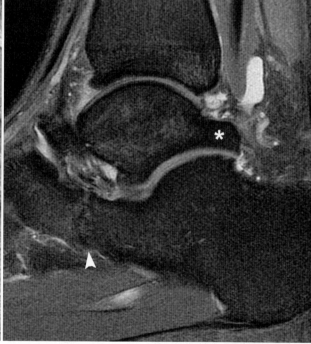

▲ **Fig. 7.120** Posterior ankle impingement symptoms in a first-grade cricketer are due to tibial impingement against a prominent posterior process of the talus (asterisks). There is mild marrow oedema at the articular corner of the posterior malleolus. Also note the presence of a calcaneonavicular coalition (arrowheads).

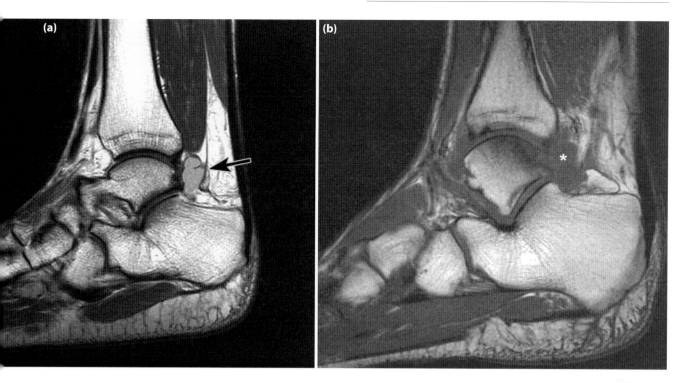

▲ **Fig. 7.121(a)** MRI demonstrates the cause of posterior impingement in a dancer. A sagittal PD-weighted MR image demonstrates a moderate-sized ganglion posterior to the ankle and subtalar joints (arrow).
(b) In another patient with a posterior impingement syndrome, a T1-weighted MR image demonstrates extensive synovitis causing impingement (asterisk). Synovitis is also present in the anterior joint recess. Degenerative changes involve the ankle joint.

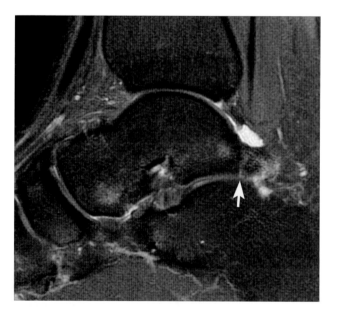

▲ **Fig. 7.122** A sagittal STIR MR image demonstrates a fracture of the posterior process of the talus (arrow). There is an adjacent small ankle effusion. Areas of high signal in other tarsal bones are a common finding in athletes involved in heavy training.

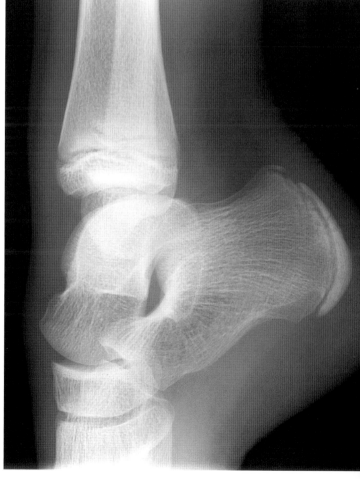

▶ **Fig. 7.123** Joint laxity is demonstrated in a dancer. This allows posterior bony impingement to occur with plantar flexion.

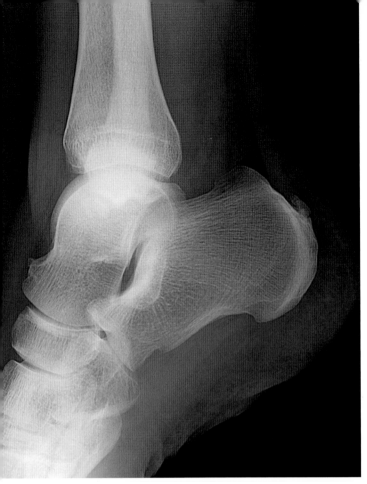

▲ **Fig. 7.124** Posterior ankle impingement is demonstrated on a lateral view in extreme plantar flexion showing bony abutment.

Imaging of posterolateral ankle impingement

When impingement symptoms become chronic, imaging tests are used to determine the cause and to guide management. Plain films, nuclear bone scanning, CT scanning, ultrasound and MRI can all play a role in diagnosis. The imaging assessment should begin with routine plain films and a 'lazy' lateral view to detect an os trigonum, as discussed above in the section 'Additional plain film views of the ankle'. A lateral view with the ankle in extreme plantar flexion may demonstrate posterior bony abutment (see Fig. 7.124).

Bone scans are non-specific in the assessment of posterior ankle pain, as they may demonstrate increased osteoblastic activity in active individuals with an os trigonum who do not have posterior impingement symptoms (Sopov et al. 2000).

CT scanning is occasionally used for fracture assessment, or the identification of an os trigonum or loose body if the MRI findings are equivocal (see Fig. 7.125).

In most cases high-resolution MRI is the imaging test of choice for the demonstration of all relevant anatomical features and pathological changes. MRI evaluation should not only include a search for the cause, but should also aim to identify associated effects of impingement such as marrow oedema (see Figs 7.126 and 7.127), effusion or synovitis. Enhancement with intravenous contrast is generally not required. Any os trigonum should be evaluated for fluid signal suggesting disruption of the synchondrosis, or bone marrow oedema at the margins of the synchondrosis, which may be caused by active impingement in the absence of

▲ **Fig. 7.125** CT is a useful imaging method for the examination of the posterior process of the talus, enabling comparison of the sides. In the case of posterior impingement on the left, an old fracture of the posterior process of the left talus is demonstrated (arrow). Surrounding soft-tissue thickening is presumably due to synovitis.

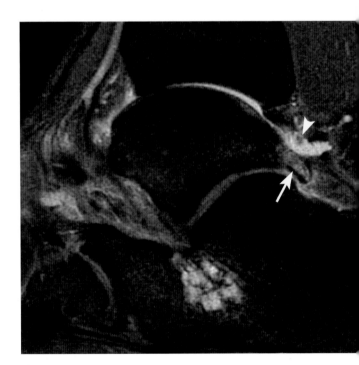

▲ **Fig. 7.126** MRI demonstrates changes of posterior ankle impingement. A fat-suppressed sagittal PD-weighted MR image shows a mildly prominent posterior process of the talus with marrow oedema (arrow). There is synovitis in the posterior recess of the ankle joint (arrowhead). An intra-osseous ganglion is incidentally present at the angle of the calcaneum.

▶ **Fig. 7.127** A sagittal STIR MR image shows increased marrow signal in the posterior body of the talus of an athlete at the Sydney 2000 Olympics. This change had resulted from repetitive bony impingement (arrow).

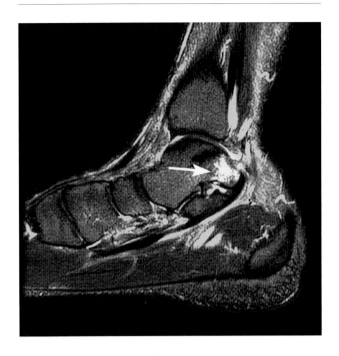

an acute injury. A small os trigonum can be subtle on MRI, being visible only on a single axial or sagittal image. Identifying fatty marrow signal and corticated margins on a T1- or PD-weighted sequence may confirm the presence of an os trigonum, although a small sclerotic os will occasionally lack a central marrow component. It is important to confirm loose bodies in all three imaging planes in order to avoid confusion with other structures such as the deep fibres of the PITFL or a fibrous synovial band.

Ultrasound can also be helpful in posterior impingement cases and is often requested with a view to guided therapeutic injection. The examination should include the FHL tendon and tendon sheath, the PTFL, the PITFL and the posterior joint recesses. Careful side-to-side comparison is required to appreciate hypoechoic thickening in the PTFL, which may indicate myxoid change. Real-time ultrasound can usefully differentiate a true ganglion cyst from a distended but otherwise normal posterior joint recess, a distinction which is not always easy on MRI (see Fig. 7.128).

Subject to the type of underlying lesion, imaging-guided injections can be performed under ultrasound or fluoroscopic control. Potential targets include ganglia, the synchondrosis of an os trigonum, the posterior recess of an ankle or subtalar joint, and the extra-articular surface of the talus. If performed immediately prior to sport, an extra-articular approach is advisable to minimise any proprioceptive loss.

Posteromedial ankle impingement

Following a medial rotational impaction injury of the ankle, hypertrophic capsuloligamentous scar and synovitis overlying the posteromedial corner of the talar dome and medial tubercle of the talus may protrude into the posteromedial ankle gutter, causing posteromedial impingement symptoms. This has been called a 'Poster-o-Medial Impingement', or 'PoMI', lesion (Liu and Mirzayan 1993; Paterson and Brown 2001).

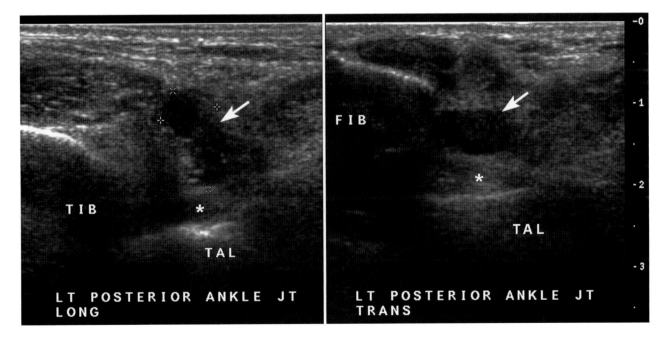

▲ **Fig. 7.128** Long-axis and transverse ultrasound images show a typical posterolateral ankle ganglion in a patient with posterior ankle impingement. The ganglion (arrows) directly overlies the PTFL (asterisks). Note the rounded contours in the two planes of view, a feature that helps to differentiate a ganglion from a fluid-distended posterior joint recess. Other features of differentiation include resistance to compression with transducer pressure, and failure to disperse with plantar and dorsiflexion manoeuvres of the ankle.

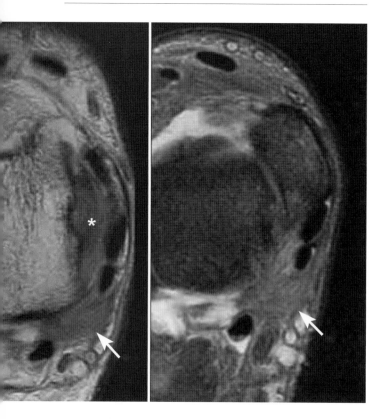

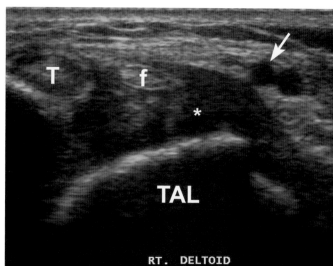

◀ **Fig. 7.129** Axial PD and fat-suppressed PD MR images demonstrate features that would predispose to posteromedial impingement following a medial rotation impaction injury. There are diffusely thickened deep fibres of the deltoid ligament (asterisk) and pronounced focal capsular thickening of intermediate signal overlying the medial tubercle of the posterior process of the talus (arrows).

▲ **Fig. 7.130** Ultrasound demonstrates posteromedial ankle impingement. A transverse greyscale image has been obtained over the margin of the deltoid ligament at the level of the posteromedial process of the talus. There is focal hypoechoic thickening of the deep posterior fibres of the deltoid ligament (asterisk) and posteromedial ankle capsule resulting in posterior protrusion between the FDL tendon (f) and the posterior tibial artery (arrow). Talus = TAL. Posterior tibial tendon = T.

Imaging of posteromedial ankle impingement

It is important to recognise that the discovery of a PoMI lesion on imaging does not necessarily predict posteromedial impingement symptoms.

The posterior deep fibres of the deltoid ligament can be visualised by both MRI and ultrasound (see Fig. 7.129). On ultrasound, a PoMI lesion appears as focally pronounced hypoechoic ligamentous thickening or 'bulge' with associated hyperaemia (see Fig. 7.130). Post-traumatic ossicles are also well demonstrated by ultrasound, and a guided injection of the posteromedial ankle gutter may be therapeutic. Occasionally an avulsion fracture at the medial tubercle of the talus may mimic a soft-tissue impingement lesion.

Osteochondral and chondral ankle fractures

Osteochondral lesions of the talar dome

Osteochondral injuries of the ankle may be secondary to acute or repetitive trauma, with a history of trauma being identified in the vast majority of cases (Anderson et al. 1989). These are a common cause of persistent pain, swelling and instability following an ankle sprain. The underlying pathology may range from a bone bruise representing microtrabecular impaction, to a partial or complete undisplaced or displaced osteochondral fracture, to a fracture confined to the articular cartilage. An osteochondral injury of the talar dome should be suspected clinically whenever ankle pain or an ankle joint effusion persists for more than six weeks after a sprain.

Osteochondral fractures of the talar dome most commonly involve the anterior third of the lateral margin of the dome and the middle or posterior third of the medial margin of the dome (see Fig. 7.131). Lateral fractures occur following inversion of a dorsiflexed ankle due to the lateral border of

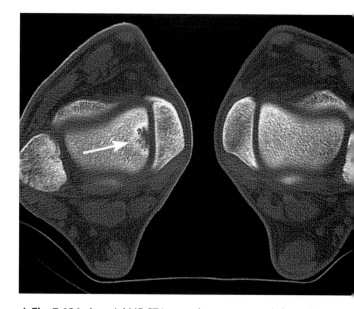

▲ **Fig. 7.131** An axial MDCT image demonstrates a left medial osteochondral fracture involving the middle third of the talar dome. A surrounding ring of sclerosis indicates that healing is progressing at the margins of the lesion (arrow). No loose body is evident.

the dome impacting against the fibula. These fractures are generally shallow with separation of a thin fragment (Burns et al. 1992). There is often an associated injury to the lateral ligament complex.

Posteromedial talar dome fractures result from inversion, plantar flexion and external rotation of the ankle with the talar dome impacting against the tibial articular surface. Medial lesions are deeper and more cup-shaped (see Fig. 7.132).

Berndt and Harty (1959) developed a classification system for osteochondral lesions, identifying four stages. Although other classifications have been suggested, the Berndt and Harty system of staging remains the basis of current systems. Other systems have incorporated outcomes of a Stage I injury that may be complex and depend on the availability of MRI (Anderson et al. 1989; Loomer et al. 1993).

- *Stage I* Initially described as a compression fracture of subchondral bone with normal overlying articular cartilage, this injury is now regarded as a bone bruise, and the outcome of this injury depends on the vascularity of the area involved. The majority of bone bruises heal, with a satisfactory clinical outcome. However, some bone bruises do not resolve and may instead develop avascular changes due to disruption of the tenuous retrograde blood supply of the talar dome. Initially, plain films and a CT scan of a Stage I injury are normal (see Fig. 7.133), requiring either a nuclear bone scan or MRI to demonstrate the subchondral changes (see Fig. 7.134). The MRI pattern of the bone bruise may heal or progress to become 'geographic' and a line of demarcation is seen separating avascular from viable bone (see Fig. 7.135). Occasionally, a subchondral cyst may develop in an area of osteonecrosis (see Figs 7.136 and 7.137). Ischaemic changes may also progress to a true osteochondritis dissecans (see Fig. 7.138) (discussed on page 593).

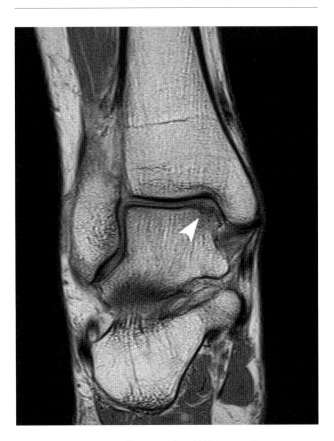

▲ **Fig. 7.132** A coronal PD-weighted MR image shows a medial talar dome fracture demonstrating a typical cup-shaped configuration (arrowhead). The appearance of a sclerotic margin denotes a chronic rather than a recent injury.

- *Stage II* This stage describes a partially detached osteochondral fragment, which usually remains hinged on the articular cartilage (see Figs 7.139 and 7.140).

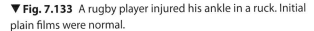

▼ **Fig. 7.133** A rugby player injured his ankle in a ruck. Initial plain films were normal.

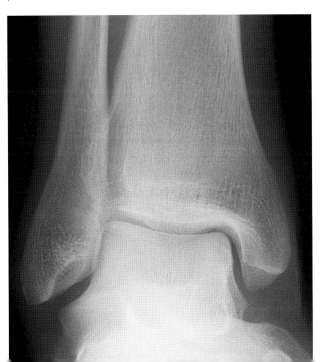

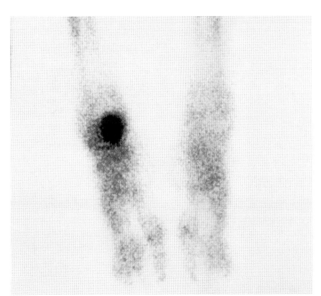

▲ **Fig. 7.134** Following persisting symptoms in the same case as in Fig. 7.133, further investigation with a nuclear bone scan showed increased uptake of isotope in the medial talar dome, suggesting a medial talar dome injury.

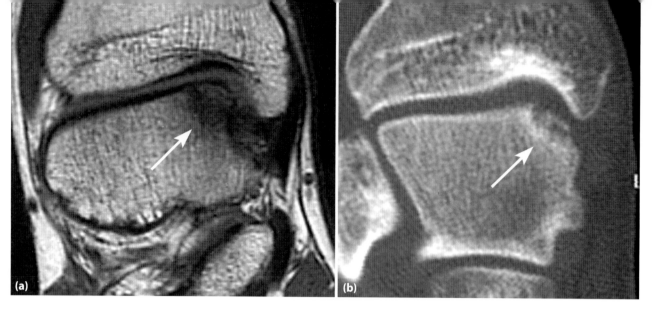

▲ **Fig. 7.135** In the same case as in Fig. 7.133, an MRI was also performed.
(a) A coronal T1-weighted MR image demonstrates a thick sclerotic line indicating the margin of an avascular area at the medial corner of the talar dome (arrow). **(b)** A follow-up CT scan shows progression of an avascular process, with compression and fragmentation of the abnormal bone (arrow).

▶ **Fig. 7.136** Subchondral cystic changes may develop in areas of osteonecrosis (arrows).
(a) Subchondral cysts are demonstrated on an AP view of the ankle (arrow). Minor irregularity of the cortical margin is also noted.
(b) A coronal T1-weighted MR image shows subchondral cystic change (arrow).

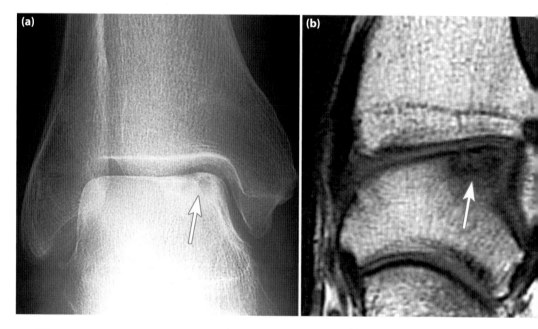

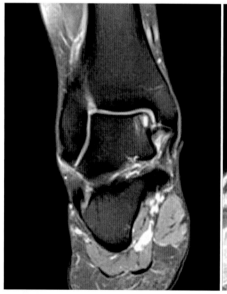
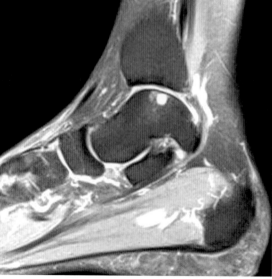

◀ **Fig. 7.137** Coronal and sagittal STIR MR images show subchondral cyst formation in the medial talar dome. High signal is noted in the surrounding marrow.

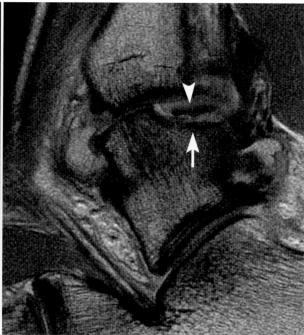

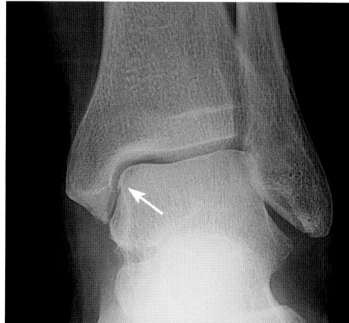

▲ Fig. 7.138 Coronal and sagittal PD-weighted MR images show a chronic talar dome fracture. In this case a chronic devascularised osteochondral fragment (arrowheads) at the lateral corner of the talar dome has displaced from its fracture bed (arrows). The fracture bed has well-defined sclerotic margins. This is a Stage IV osteochondral lesion (see below) and is indistinguishable from osteochondritis dissecans.

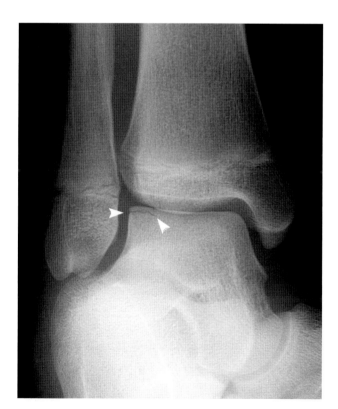

- *Stage II(a)* Although cystic changes may develop in an area of osteonecrosis, the vast majority of cysts are associated with an overlying chondral fracture and develop secondary to a 'ball-valve' effect of synovial fluid being pumped into the subchrondral bone through the fracture line (Anderson et al. 1989).

- *Stage III* A Stage III injury is present when there is a completely detached osteochondral fragment, which remains undisplaced within the fracture bed (see Fig. 7.141).

- *Stage IV* A Stage IV injury is present when there is a completely detached and displaced osteochondral fragment (see Fig. 7.142).

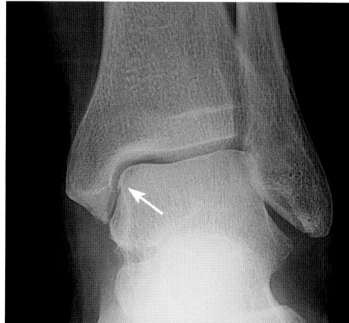

▲ Fig. 7.139 A Stage II osteochondral fracture is incomplete. The medial extent of this lateral osteochondral fracture remains attached (arrowheads).

▶ Fig. 7.140 This fracture of the medial corner of the talar dome appears to be incomplete and would be classified as Stage II (arrow).

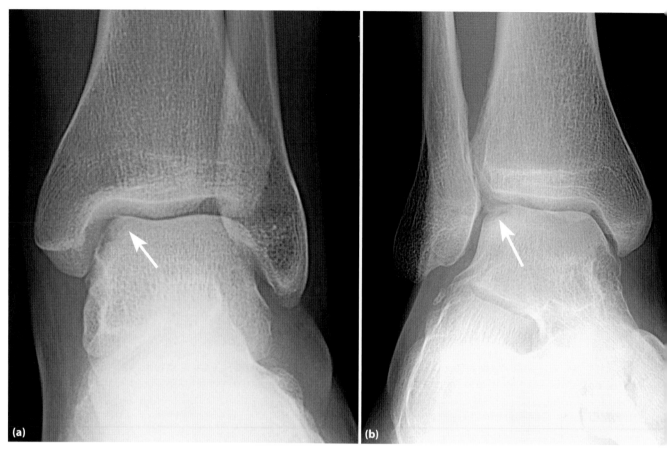

▲ **Fig. 7.141** Two different cases demonstrate examples of a Stage III talar dome fracture, one medial **(a)** and one lateral **(b)**. The fracture fragments are detached, but remain undisplaced within the fracture bed (arrows).

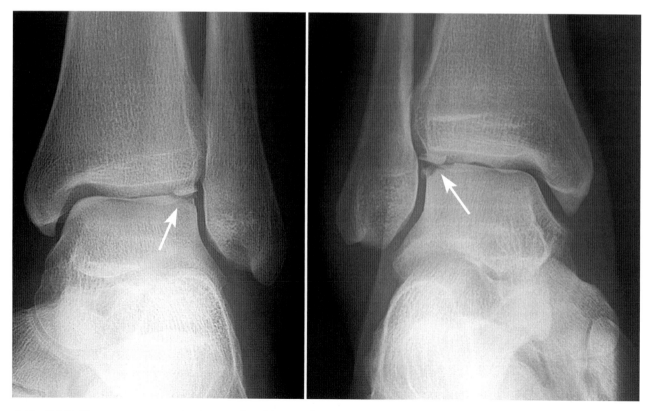

▲ **Fig. 7.142** These two cases are classic examples of Stage IV lesions, where the fragments have flipped upside down within their respective fracture beds (arrows). Any fracture with displacement of the fragment from the fracture bed is classified as a Stage IV.

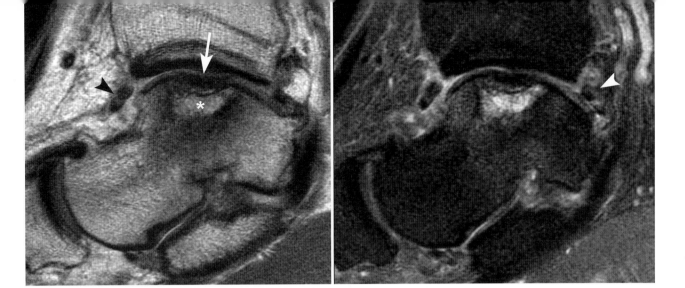

▲ Fig. 7.143 A chronic Type IV osteochondral talar dome lesion with spontaneous fibrocartilage repair is demonstrated by sagittal PD and fat-suppressed PD-weighted MR images showing displaced osteochondral fragments in the anterior recess (black arrowhead) and posterior recess (white arrowhead). There has been spontaneous filling of the osteochondral crater by reparative fibrocartilage (arrow). Note the adjacent subchondral cystic change (asterisk) with surrounding sclerosis and marrow oedema.

Loosening at the interface between normal bone and an osteochondral fragment may be assessed by MRI. Destabilisation typically occurs along a well-defined sclerotic fracture bed, which is best depicted on a T1-weighted image. Hyperintensity of the interface on PD or T2-weighted images usually indicates a line of undermining fluid in continuity with the joint space (see Fig. 7.143). However, this finding alone is not entirely specific, as reparative granulation tissue can give a similar appearance. An osteochondral fragment is likely to be viable if the marrow space on MRI demonstrates fat signal, oedema or contrast enhancement. Fragmentation of an osteochondral lesion, which may be obvious on CT, can often be difficult to appreciate on MRI, and non-fat-suppressed T2*-weighted gradient echo sequencing may be helpful in this regard. The presence of adjacent bone marrow oedema generally indicates an 'active' (symptomatic) osteochondral lesion.

Although multislice CT is able to confirm a frank talar dome fracture or show chronic bone changes such as sclerosis or a subchondral cyst, MRI is the preferred imaging modality as this provides a more comprehensive assessment including details of the chondral surface, the viability of the bone fragment and the presence of marrow oedema. CT arthrography is an accurate alternative for assessment of the chondral surface, but is invasive and therefore not often performed.

Chondral injuries of the talar dome

Acute post-traumatic chondral lesions typically occur at the medial or lateral talar dome margins and are seen as small fissures, flaps or chondral fractures (see Fig. 7.144). Sometimes there is an associated delamination component

▼ Fig. 7.144 There is a displaced chondral fracture at the posteromedial talar dome. Coronal PD and sagittal fat-suppressed PD-weighted MR images show a chondral defect involving the medial gutter and weightbearing surfaces, with displaced chondral fragments in the medial gutter (arrow) and posterior recess (arrowhead). Note the intact subchondral plate and presence of only mild subchondral bone marrow oedema (asterisk).

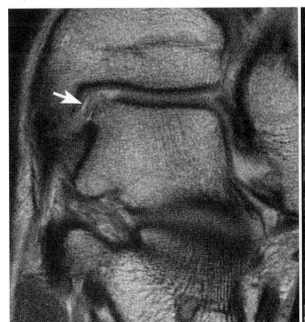
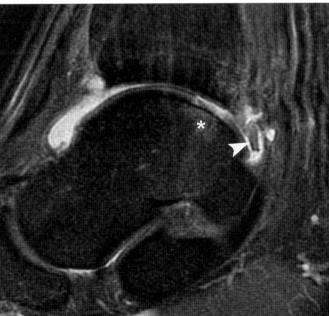

▶ **Fig. 7.145(a)** A basal chondral delamination injury of the talar dome is demonstrated by a coronal PD-weighted MR image. There is subtle linear hyperintensity involving the basal layer of the medial talar dome articular cartilage (arrow), consistent with a chondral delamination injury. Also note the small crack in the chondral surface at the medial gutter.
(b) A sagittal fat-suppressed PD-weighted MR image shows accompanying extensive subchondral bone marrow oedema (asterisk).

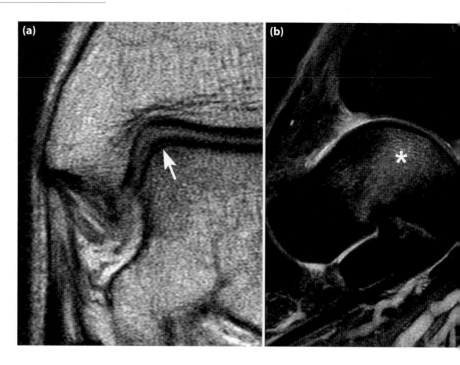

(see Fig. 7.145). Interestingly, chondral fibrillation is uncommon at the ankle. On MRI, subchondral bone marrow oedema is commonly demonstrated, although this finding alone does not necessarily predict an overlying chondral lesion. A synovial fringe at the posteromedial or posterolateral aspect of the ankle may simulate a chondral lesion and is a potential pitfall in diagnosis.

'Kissing' osteochondral and chondral injuries

Kissing injuries are matching traumatic lesions seen on apposing articular surfaces. 'Kissing' bone contusions are common on MRI after an ankle sprain and do not necessarily indicate a poor prognosis (Alanen et al. 1998; Sijbrandij et al. 2000) (see Fig. 7.146).

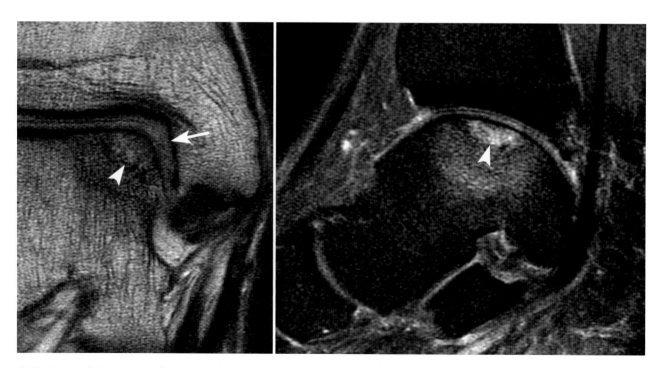

▲ **Fig. 7.146** A chronic talar dome osteochondral lesion is demonstrated by coronal PD and sagittal fat-suppressed PD-weighted MR images showing subchondral cystic change at the medial corner of the talar dome (arrowheads). Also note the crack in the overlying chondral surface (arrow), the presence of subtle basal chondral delamination, and the broad zone of perifocal marrow oedema.

Tibial plafond injuries

Chondral injuries involving the tibial plafond are most common at the anterior and posterior rim (see Fig. 7.147). Anterior rim chondral lesions often produce a subtle chondral flap. An MRI finding of marrow oedema in association with an anterior plafond impingement spur is common and does not necessarily predict an overlying chondral defect. Posterior rim chondral lesions are often associated with syndesmosis injury and are usually situated towards the tibial insertion of the PITFL where posterior malleolar fractures also occur. Isolated osteochondral fractures involving the tibial plafond are substantially less common than those involving the talar dome. As with the talar dome, subchondral cystic change may be associated with symptomatic chondral fractures.

Osteochondritis dissecans of the talar dome and tibial plafond

In the past, the term 'osteochondritis dissecans' has been used as a synonym for an osteochondral fracture. A true osteochondritis dissecans may rarely occur in the talar dome and tibial plafond. As in the knee, this process is thought to be due to post-traumatic avascular change (see Figs 7.148, 7.149 and 7.150).

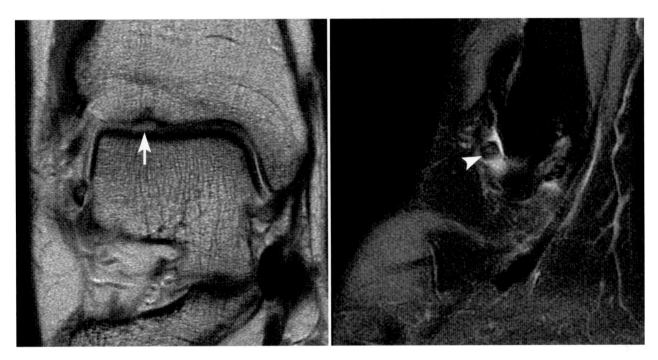

▲ **Fig. 7.147** An osteochondral lesion at the anterior rim of the tibial plafond is demonstrated on a coronal PD-weighted MR image. A sagittal fat-suppressed PD-weighted image shows the corresponding osteochondral fragment displaced into the anterolateral ankle gutter (arrowhead).

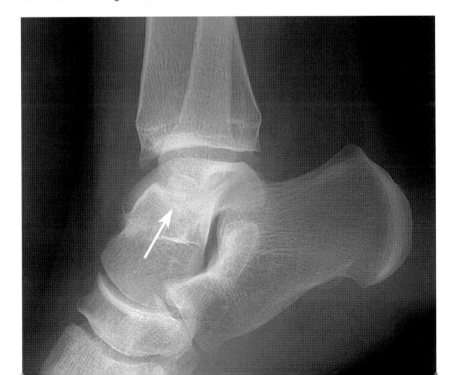

◀**Fig. 7.148** A lateral plain film demonstrates a large bony defect in the talar dome and body (arrow). The deformity is the end result of osteonecrosis leading to an area of osteochondritis dissecans.

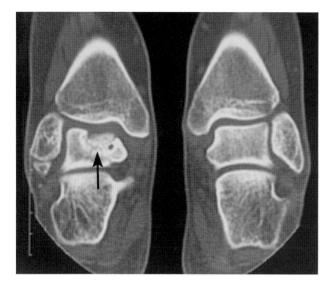

▲ Fig. 7.149 Bilateral coronal CT images of the same case as in Fig. 7.148 define the large bony defect in the talar dome, with the contained ossicle (arrow). The appearance is that of an old osteochondritis dissecans.

Ossification defects in the talar dome and tibial plafond

Developmental ossification defects can occur in the talar dome and tibial plafond and these may be difficult to differentiate from an osteochondral fracture or area of osteochondritis dissecans (see Figs 7.151 and 7.152). These defects are often 'kissing' lesions (see Figs 7.153 and 7.154).

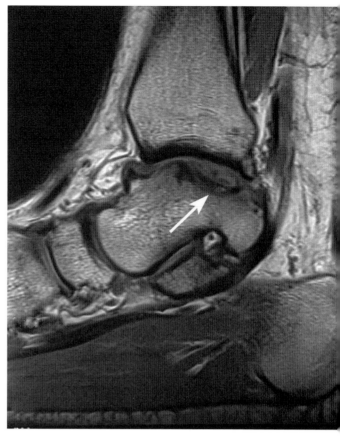

▲ Fig. 7.150 In another case, a T1-weighted MR image demonstrates a large defect in the talar dome, with a prominent, well-defined sclerotic margin (arrow), suggesting that the deformity is the end result of osteonecrosis.

▶ Fig. 7.151 Developmental ossification defects occasionally occur in the tibial plafond and talar dome. These are perfectly round, with a cortical margin (arrows). The appearance suggests a developmental defect rather than osteochondritis dissecans, although the differentiation is not simple. This defect contains an ossicle, adding to the difficulty in differentiation.

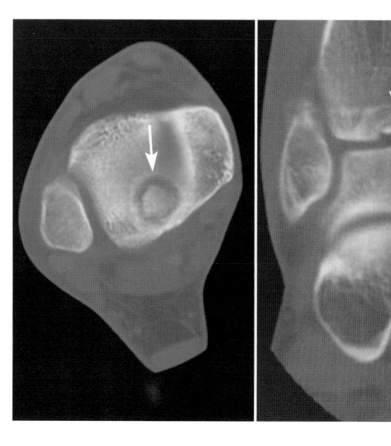

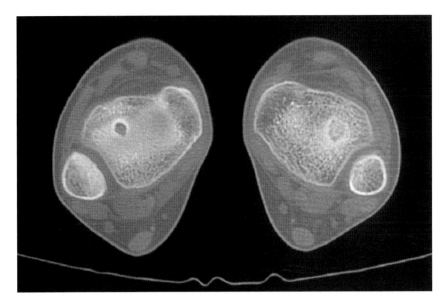

▲ **Fig. 7.152** Bilateral tibial plafond ossification defects are present. Both defects have cortical margins and contain calcified material or ossicles.

The role of MRI in the assessment of articular cartilage repair

Talar dome chondral injuries may spontaneously heal or be surgically assisted using either chondral grafts or arthroscopic stimulative techniques such as debridement, curettage and drilling. Spontaneous repair and stimulative techniques both attempt to fill a chondral or osteochondral defect with reparative fibrocartilage. However, this cartilage lacks the resilience and durability of normal hyaline cartilage (see Fig. 7.155). Additionally, the bony component of an osteochondral defect will often fail to spontaneously fill with new bone. Autologous osteochondral grafting (e.g. mosaicplasty) and autologous chondrocyte implantation (ACI)

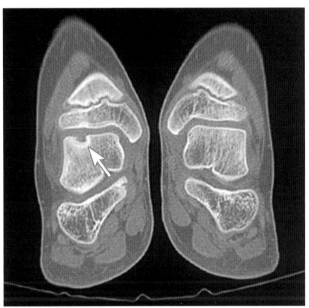

▲ **Fig. 7.153** Often these ossification defects can be 'kissing' lesions. In this case, there is an ossification defect in the talar dome (arrow) and focal cortical thickening at the apposing tibial plafond.

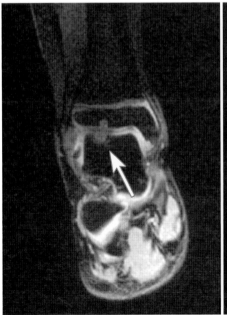
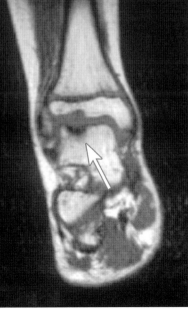

◄ **Fig. 7.154** Coronal STIR and T1-weighted MR images demonstrate 'kissing' defects in the tibial plafond and talar dome (arrows).

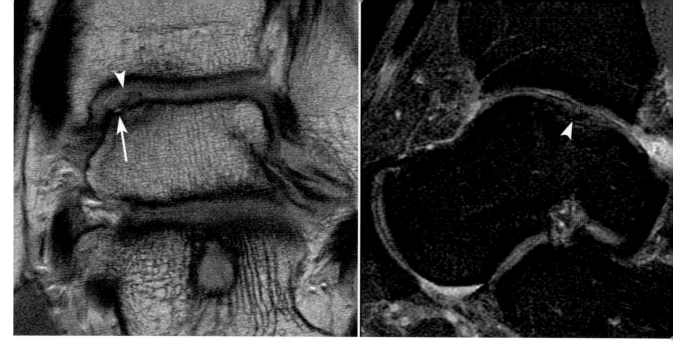

▲ **Fig. 7.155** Reparative fibrocartilage fills a previously debrided chronic medial talar dome osteochondral lesion. Note the focal destabilisation (arrow) and heterogeneous signal (arrowheads) of the reparative fibrocartilage.

are alternative surgical techniques that attempt to deliver a more physiological, stable and durable reconstruction of the joint surface. MRI provides the best assessment of progress following these surgical procedures (see Fig. 7.156), although the MR signal characteristics of a graft do not allow reparative fibrocartilage to be differentiated from hyaline-like articular cartilage. Experimental techniques such as dGEMRIC and T2 mapping show some promise in this regard.

Ankle arthrofibrosis

'Arthrofibrosis' describes a thickening of the joint capsule due to excessive scar response after trauma or surgery (Lindenfeld et al. 2000). This may result in joint stiffness, pain and impingement symptoms. The response of tissue to injury may lead to a subsequent fibroblastic and myofibroblastic proliferation with exuberant collagen synthesis. The end result both clinically and pathologically

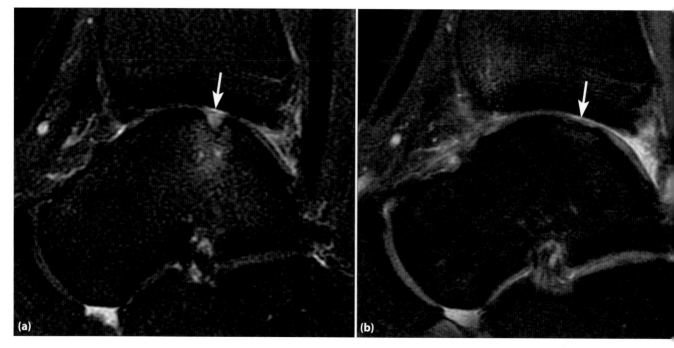

▲ **Fig. 7.156** A chronic osteochondral lesion has been treated with a matrix autologous chondrocyte implantation (MACI) graft.
(a) An initial sagittal fat-suppressed PD-weighted MR image demonstrates friable reparative fibrocartilage in a shallow osteochondral crater following previous arthroscopic debridement (arrow).
(b) A subsequent sagittal fat-suppressed PD-weighted MR image obtained one year post-chondrocyte graft demonstrates 100% fill of the lesion, good peripheral integration, a smooth graft surface and resolution of the pre-operative cystic change and bone marrow oedema (arrow).

is excessive fibrosis. Immobilisation following trauma or surgery is a recognised risk factor (Enneking and Horowitz 1972). The likelihood of arthrofibrosis is also related to the severity of the initiating injury, with several reports demonstrating an increased incidence occurring if multiple ligaments have been injured or multiple procedures performed (Noyes and Barber-Westin 1997). The diagnosis is usually clinical, although MRI can be helpful in atypical or unsuspected cases, or when there is concomitant pathology that may confuse the clinical picture. The MR imaging findings in cases of established ankle arthrofibrosis are those of a thickened joint capsule (usually over 3 mm) of low signal intensity (see Figs 7.157 and 7.158 and Fig. 1.26 on page 20).

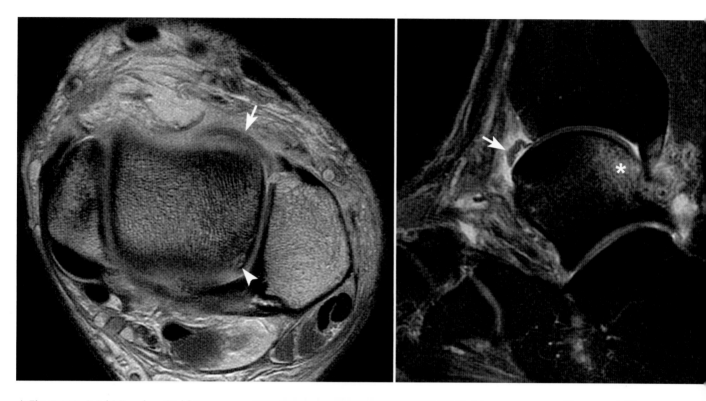

▲ **Fig. 7.157** Axial PD and sagittal fat-suppressed PD-weighted MR images showing a thick band of intermediate signal intensity in the anterolateral recess of the ankle joint (arrows). The differential diagnosis here would include a fibrinous or fibrous synovial band and, less likely, an immature or evolving arthrofibrosis. Note also a posterolateral talar dome fracture (arrowhead) with associated marrow oedema (asterisk).

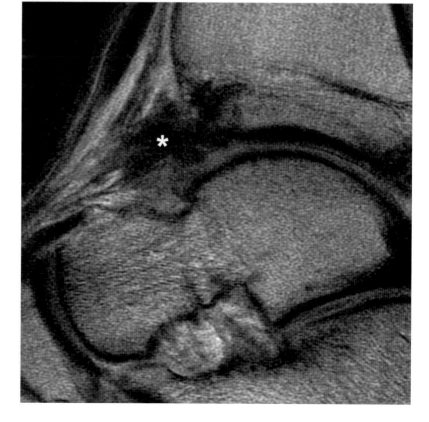

▶ **Fig. 7.158** Mature ankle arthrofibrosis is demonstrated by a sagittal PD-weighted MR image showing focal thickening of the anterior ankle capsule (asterisk), consistent with arthrofibrotic change.

Stress fractures of the ankle

The reaction of bone to stress ranges from a painless physiological osteoblastic response associated with increased loading, to a painful stress reaction, and eventually to bone failure and fracturing if stress continues.

Imaging stress reactions and fractures

The stress reaction that precedes a fracture can be confidently detected only by nuclear bone scanning and MRI. On a nuclear bone scan, there is increased uptake of isotope in the area of bone stress on delayed images, and on MRI bone stress is demonstrated as intra-medullary bone marrow oedema and often non-mineralised periostitis without any frank fracture (see Fig. 7.159). MRI may occasionally produce a false negative result for a stress fracture which is purely intracortical.

Plain radiographs are initially normal and the early changes may be extremely subtle with localised demineralisation and a faint periosteal reaction seen prior to a visible fracture line developing. The fracture may not become visible until two to three weeks after the onset of symptoms.

Distal fibular stress fractures

The most common stress fracture of the ankle involves the distal fibula, just above the level of the inferior tibiofibular syndesmosis, about 4–7 cm proximal to the tip of the lateral malleolus (see Fig. 7.160). These fractures are transverse in orientation and occur predominantly in joggers ('runner's fracture'). An additional subgroup of fibular stress fractures occurs in middle-aged and elderly osteopaenic women about 3–4 cm above the tip of the lateral malleolus (Sherbondy and Sebastianelli 2006).

Distal tibial stress fractures

Distal tibial stress fractures are typically seen in runners and those involved in jumping sports (Shabat et al. 2002). In the skeletally mature athlete these fractures are typically sagittal in orientation, and occur at the junction between the medial malleolus and the tibial plafond (Shelbourne et al. 1988) (see Figs 7.161 and 7.162) and also in the distal tibial metaphysis (see Fig. 7.163). In the skeletally immature athlete these fractures may involve either the distal tibial metaphysis (see Fig. 7.164) or the distal tibial growth plate (see Fig. 7.165). Varus tilt of the plafond may predispose to distal tibial stress fracture (Okada et al. 1995).

Stress fractures of the talus

There are reports of stress fractures of the talus. Such stress fractures may involve the talar body (Bradshaw et al. 1996), the lateral process of the talus (Motto 1993; Black and Ehlert 1994) (see Figs 7.159 and 7.166) or the talar neck (Perry and O'Toole 1981) (see Fig. 7.167). As talar stress fractures are rare, the diagnosis may not be clinically suspected at first presentation. Stress fractures of the talar body are most common in long-distance runners (see Fig. 7.168), have a sagittal-oblique orientation and are often occult on plain films. MRI will usually demonstrate the fracture line and the extent of bone marrow oedema, while CT scanning helps to clarify the extent of the fracture line.

Fatigue and insufficiency fractures at the ankle

Subchondral fatigue or insufficiency fractures are a source of spontaneous onset of pain in the ankle. These injuries are most common in perimenopausal and postmenopausal women, but can also occur in amenorrhoeic younger women and patients who have severe osteoporosis for other reasons. Fatigue or insufficiency fractures at the ankle can involve the talar dome, distal fibula and distal tibia. Tibial and talar lesions typically parallel the subchondral plate, extend over less than 1 cm, are usually occult on plain x-ray, and can be relatively subtle on both MRI and CT. In the active phase, MRI will always show extensive surrounding marrow oedema (see Figs 7.169 and 7.170). In cases treated with a period of immobilisation, it is not uncommon for a new area of fracture to develop when the patient begins to mobilise again.

Tendon abnormalities at the ankle joint

Tibialis posterior tendon injuries

Sports-related posterior tibial tendon injuries tend to differ from those seen in the general population, with insertional changes that accompany a Type II os tibiale externum (syn. 'accessory naviscular') being more common in a sporting population and the overall severity of the process tending to be less pronounced. Karasick and Schweitzer (1993) found a 17% incidence rate of an associated os tibiale externum in patients with tibialis posterior tendon tears.

There is usually an insidious course of progressive tendon degeneration that ultimately leads to failure. The most frequent clinical presentation consists of peritendinitis and low-grade tendinopathy without a superimposed tear. Complete ruptures of the posterior tibial tendon do sometimes occur in athletes involved in jumping sports such as basketball, soccer and tennis. Infrequently, a tear of the flexor retinaculum attachment to the medial malleolus can result in posterior tibial tendon instability with anterior subluxation of the tendon (see Fig. 7.171).

Imaging of the tibialis posterior tendon

Tibialis posterior dysfunction produces alignment changes that are well demonstrated on a plain film foot series including AP and lateral views acquired with weightbearing. On the AP view there is mid-foot abduction with 'uncovering' of the medial aspect of the talar head, due to the unopposed action of the peroneus brevis, together with forefoot pronation, due to a loss of medial arch support (see Fig. 7.172). Bony irregularity and cystic change at the synchondrosis of a Type II os tibiale externum may indicate a chronic apophyseal stress reaction.

The plantar calcaneonavicular ligament cannot maintain the longitudinal arch of the foot by itself, and loss of tibialis posterior support results in midtarsal sagging.

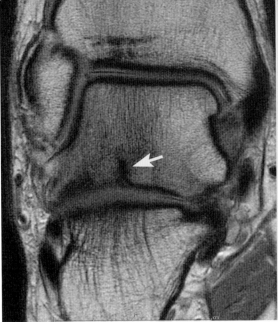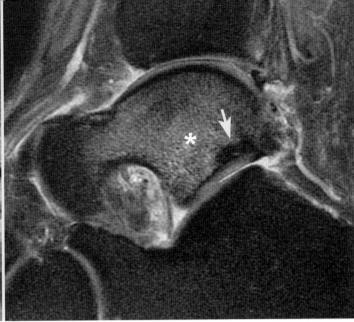

▲ **Fig. 7.159** Coronal PD and sagittal fat-suppressed PD-weighted MR images demonstrate an incomplete stress fracture of the body of the talus in a long-distance runner (arrows). Note the associated oedema shown as high signal in the talar body (asterisk).

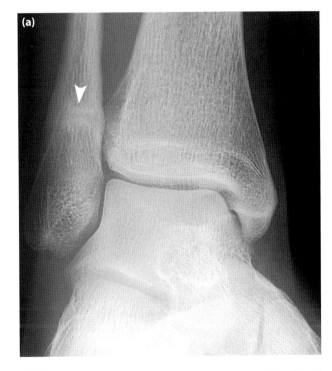

▶▼ **Fig. 7.160(a)** A stress fracture of the distal fibula always occurs above the level of the syndesmosis. In this case the fracture appears as a transverse band of sclerosis (arrowhead). No definite lucent fracture line can be seen.
(b) Coronal T1 and sagittal fat-suppressed PD-weighted MR images show a distal fibular stress fracture (white arrows). There is associated marrow oedema, partially mineralised periosteal reaction (white arrowheads) and intracortical hyperintensity (black arrow).

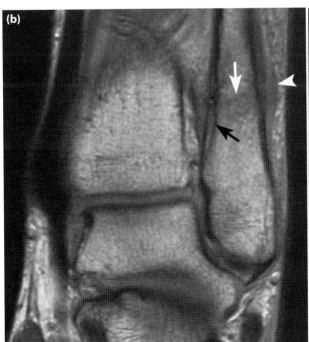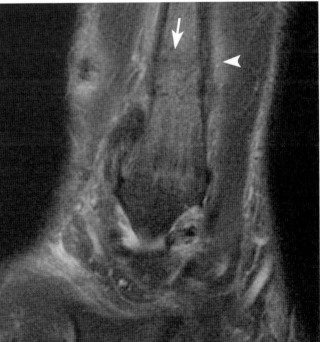

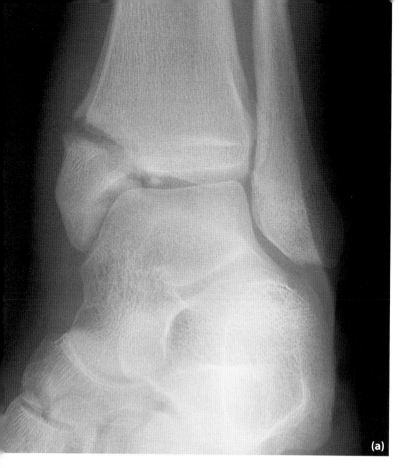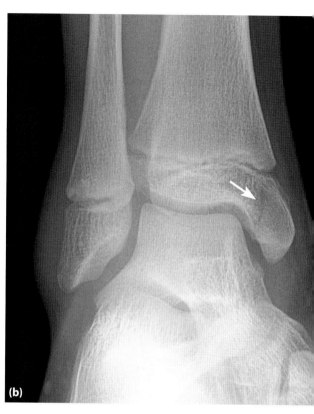

▲▼ **Fig. 7.161(a)** This stress fracture of the base of the medial malleolus occurred in a 17-year-old soccer player. The appearance is atypical, as medial malleolus stress fractures are usually vertical. There is established periosteal new bone present along the medial border of the distal tibial metaphysis and the appearance suggests that a stress reaction or partial fracture has converted to a complete fracture with an acute injury. **(b)** A junior soccer player shows an incomplete stress fracture in the medial malleolus of the distal tibial epiphysis (arrow). **(c)** A hockey player with medial ankle pain shows an incomplete stress fracture on plain films (left image) (arrow). A coronal STIR MR image (right image) shows considerable marrow oedema surrounding the fracture and confirms that the fracture is incomplete (arrow).

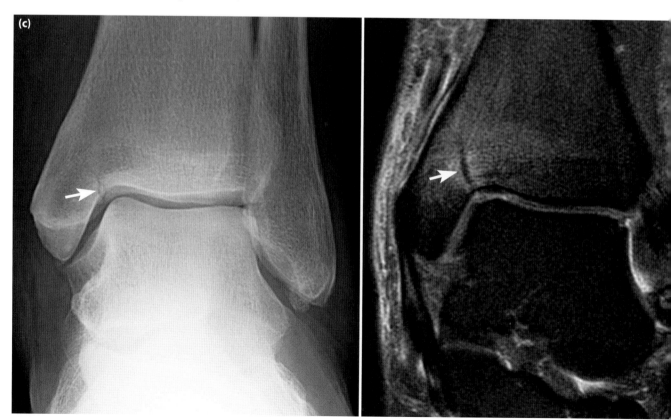

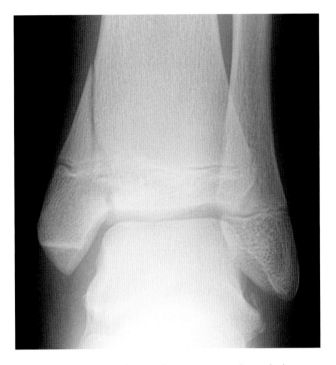

▲ **Fig. 7.162** A vertical stress fracture passes through the medial metaphysis and epiphysis of a skeletally immature soccer player. This appearance is characteristic of a medial malleolar stress fracture (see Fig. 7.50).

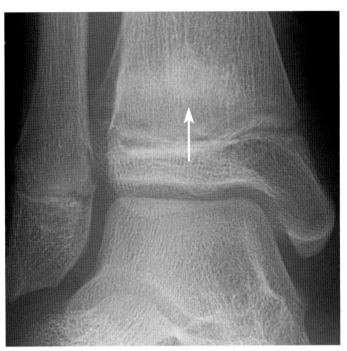

▲ **Fig. 7.164** A band of sclerosis traversing the distal tibial metaphysis in a school-aged cross-country runner indicates the presence of a stress fracture (arrow).

▼ **Fig. 7.163** Coronal PD and sagittal fat-suppressed T1-weighted MR images show a complex pattern of stress fractures at the distal end of the tibia that includes both vertical (arrowhead) and horizontal (white arrow) components. Note the associated marrow oedema (asterisk) and well-mineralised periosteal reaction on the dorsal surface of the distal tibia, with an ongoing hyperintense deep zone (black arrow). An ankle joint effusion is present.

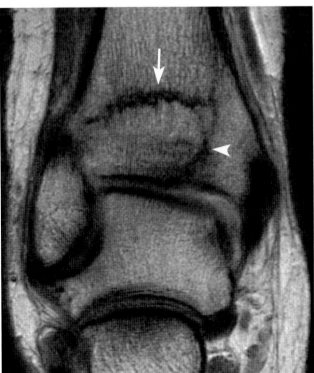

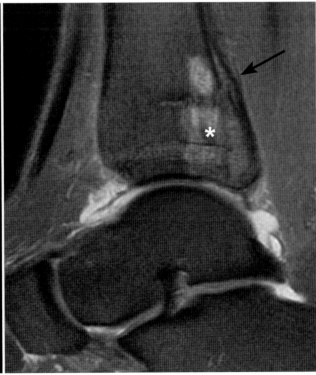

▶ **Figure 7.165** This is the typical appearance of a distal tibial growth plate stress fracture. The growth plate appears widened, with bony resorption mainly occurring on the metaphyseal side of the plate.

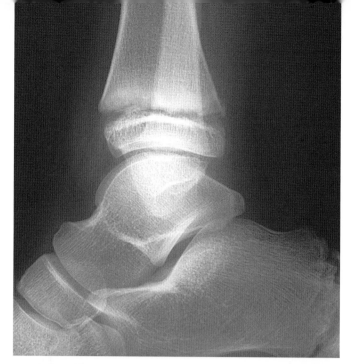

▼ **Fig. 7.166** Coronal and sagittal PD-weighted MR images demonstrate a chronic stress fracture extending across the base of the lateral process of the talus with non-union (arrows).

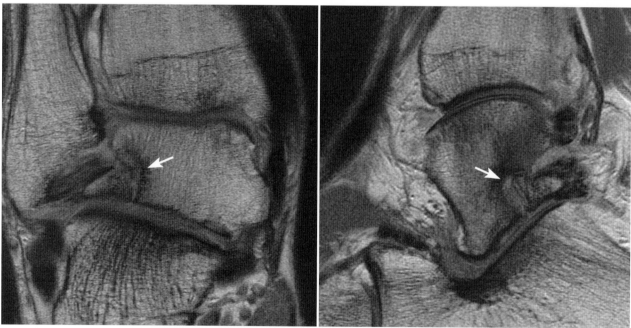

▼ **Fig. 7.167** A stress fracture involving the neck of the talus (arrowheads). No avascular changes can be seen on the fat-suppressed MR image.

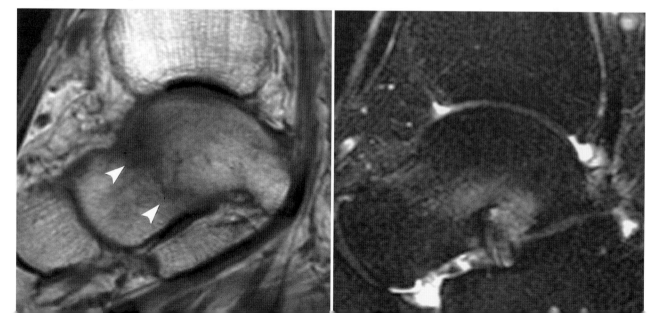

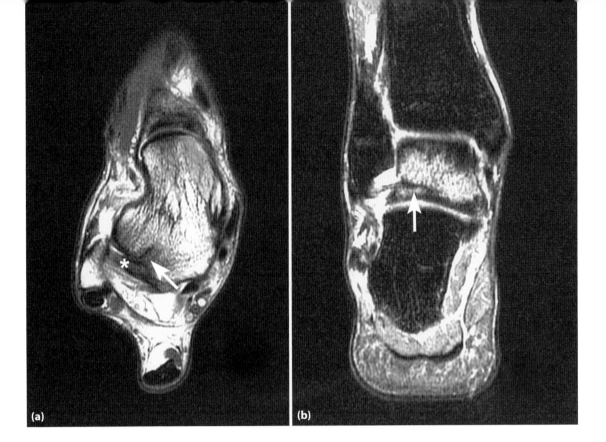

▲ **Fig. 7.168** A 400 m runner at the Sydney 2000 Olympics experienced sudden pain and disability soon after the start of the race, causing her to collapse.
(a) An axial PD-weighted MR image reveals a stress fracture of the posterior body of the talus (arrow) extending from the margin of attachment of the posterior talofibular ligament (asterisk).
(b) A coronal STIR image shows intense oedema throughout the talar body, and a fracture line extending roughly parallel to the subtalar joint (arrow).

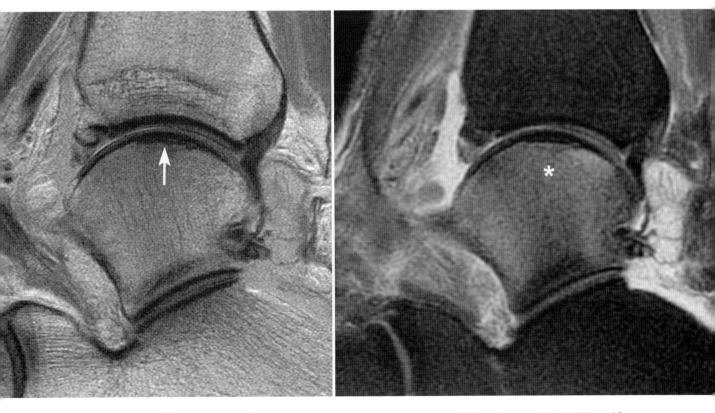

▲ **Fig. 7.169** A subchondral fatigue fracture of the talar dome has occurred in a 54-year-old female runner. Sagittal PD and fat-suppressed PD-weighted MR images show a subtle hypointense fracture line (arrow) with extensive surrounding marrow oedema (asterisk).

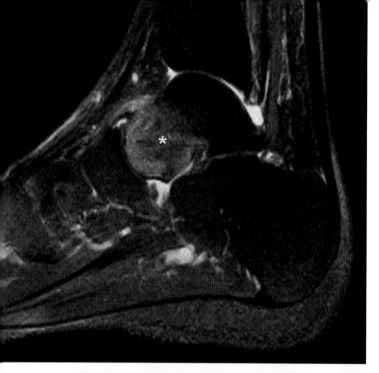

◀ **Fig. 7.170** An insufficiency fracture of the talar head and neck has developed in an athlete competing in the Masters Games. A sagittal fat-suppressed MR image shows marrow oedema associated with the fracture (asterisk).

▼ **Fig. 7.171** In this case there is stripping of the flexor retinaculum attachment to the medial malleolus, with associated anterior subluxation of the posterior tibial tendon. The patient was a soccer player with persistent medial ankle pain following an injury two years previously. Axial PD and fat-suppressed PD-weighted MR images show anterior subluxation of the posterior tibial tendon (asterisks) from the retromalleolar groove and periosteal stripping of a thickened and scarred flexor retinaculum away from its medial malleolus attachment (arrows). Medial malleolus = m.

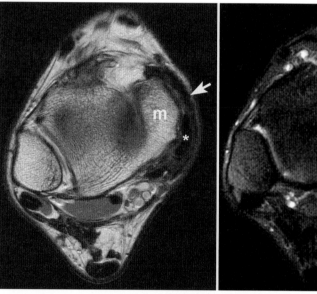

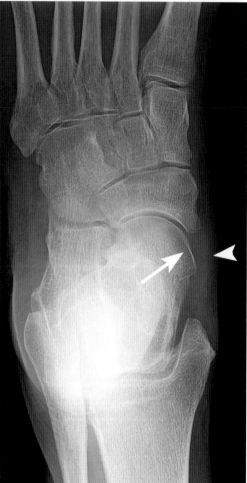

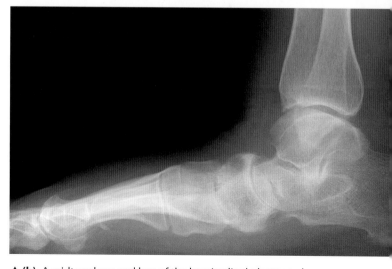

▲ **Fig. 7.172(a)** Tibialis posterior dysfunction produces midtarsal abduction, due to the unopposed traction of the peroneal muscles. There is uncovering of the medial articular surface of the talar head (arrow). Collapse of the medial column of the longitudinal arch of the foot causes forefoot pronation. Note the swollen distal tibialis posterior tendon (arrowhead).

▲ **(b)** A midtarsal sag and loss of the longitudinal plantar arch are common signs of tibialis posterior dysfunction. There is plantar rotation of the talus and loss of the normal talometatarsal alignment. The medial arch cannot be maintained without support of the tibialis posterior tendon.

This is seen on the weightbearing lateral view, where the long axis of the talus is no longer collinear with the long axis of the first metatarsal and there is a reduced lateral calcaneoplantar angle (which normally measures 15 to 30°). This deformity is accompanied by hind-foot valgus deformity.

The integrity of the posterior tibial tendon can be assessed using either ultrasound or MRI (see Fig. 7.173). Ultrasound has a number of advantages, including real-time clinical correlation, side-to-side comparison (useful for detecting subtle tendon swelling), and dynamic assessment of both tendon and synchondrosis stability. Ultrasound also has the ability to confirm a diagnosis of tendinopathy or peritendinitis using Power Doppler (see Figs 7.174 and 7.175). Ultrasound can occasionally struggle to differentiate a longitudinal split tear of tendon from a conspicuous hypoechoic connective tissue division between adjacent tendon fascicles. Real-time

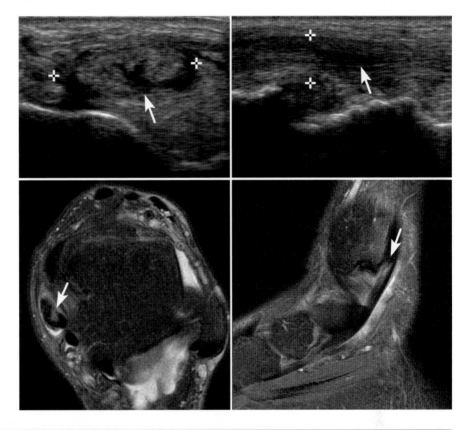

▶ **Fig. 7.173** An incomplete longitudinal split tear of the tibialis posterior tendon is demonstrated by ultrasound and MRI of the same case. The upper ultrasound images are transverse and long-axis views, while the lower images show the corresponding axial and sagittal fat-suppressed MR sections. Arrows indicate the incomplete longitudinal tear on a background of tendinopathy (callipers). Also note the associated tenosynovitis.

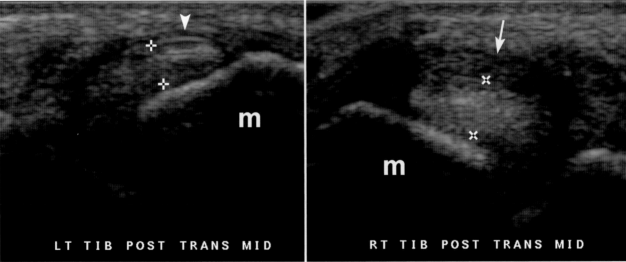

LT TIB POST TRANS MID   RT TIB POST TRANS MID

▲ **Fig. 7.174** Chronic right tibialis posterior tendinopathy and paratenonitis in a professional soccer player is demonstrated by ultrasound. Comparative transverse greyscale images of the tibialis posterior tendons of both ankles have been obtained at the level of the lower retromalleolar groove. The abnormal right tibialis posterior tendon (× callipers) is thickened by comparison with the left (+ callipers). There is an accompanying collar of marked peritendon thickening (arrow) but no associated tendon sheath effusion. At surgery, this corresponded with a chronically thickened paratenon without synovitis or thickening of the overlying flexor retinaculum. Medial malleolus = m. An arrowhead indicates the flexor retinaculum on the normal left side.

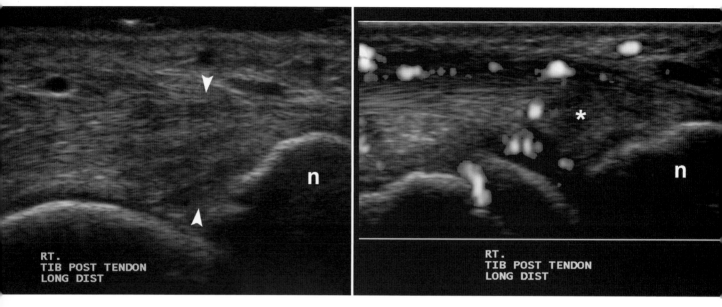

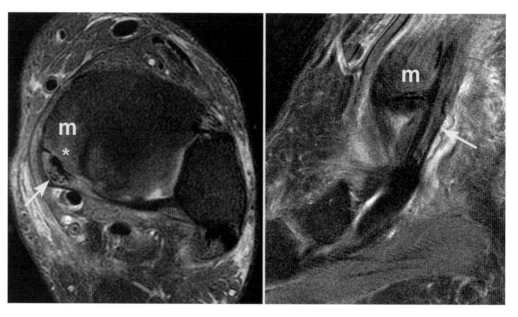

▲ **Fig. 7.175** Insertional tibialis posterior tendinopathy is demonstrated by long-axis greyscale and Power Doppler ultrasound images. The distal tendon segment shows heterogeneous hypoechoic echotexture indicative of tendinopathy (indicated by arrowheads on the greyscale image and asterisk on the Power Doppler image). There is both tendon and peritendon hyperaemia. Navicular = n.

▶ **Fig. 7.176** Posterior tibial tendinopathy with a complicating longitudinal tear is demonstrated by axial fat-suppressed T2 and sagittal fat-suppressed PD-weighted MR images. The torn segment is indicated by arrows. Note the reactive marrow oedema within the adjacent medial malleolus (asterisk). Subcutaneous oedema is noted. Medial malleolus = m.

features that favour a tear include lack of anisotropy (i.e. the hypoechoic division does not alter with transducer angulation) and the presence of differential motion between the fascicles on probing or with active use of the tendon.

MRI is effective at demonstrating tendon tears (see Fig. 7.176), flexor retinaculum avulsion and static posterior tibial tendon subluxations (Bencardino et al. 1997a). However, MRI can have difficulty demonstrating peritendinitis and mild degrees of tendinopathy, unless a fat-suppressed T1-weighted gradient echo sequence is included. A small amount of tendon sheath fluid is commonly seen in asymptomatic ankles and, as an isolated finding, should not be mistaken for tenosynovitis. Intravenous contrast is not routinely used but can help to confirm an MRI diagnosis of peritendinitis and also make tears more conspicuous. Occasionally, CT scanning is helpful in cases where the cause of tendinopathy or peritendinitis is an impinging bone spur arising from the margin of a previous medial malleolus fracture.

A painful os tibiale externum

An os tibiale externum is located on the posteromedial aspect of the tuberosity of the tarsal navicular. A Type I os tibiale externum is a small sesamoid contained within the insertional fibres of the posterior tibial tendon (see Fig. 7.177). The larger Type II os tibiale externum (8–12 mm in diameter) is joined to the navicular by a synchondrosis and serves as the dominant insertion of the posterior tibial tendon (see Fig. 7.178). A Type III os tibiale externum is a bony prominence continuous with the tuberosity of the navicular, with no separate ossicle

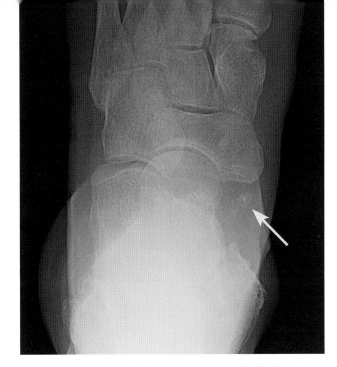

▲ **Fig. 7.177** This os tibiale externum is typical of a Type I accessory ossicle (arrow).

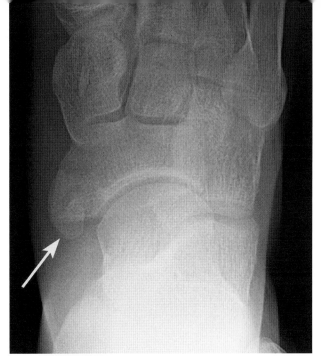

▲ **Fig. 7.178** A Type II os tibiale externum is 8–12 mm in diameter (arrow).

(see Fig. 7.179). In general, it is the Type II os tibiale externum that becomes symptomatic, most commonly occurring in adolescence or early adulthood. This typically presents with localised pain and tenderness arising from repetitive micro-trauma to the synchondrosis. There is rarely a history of significant trauma. Associated signs of tibialis posterior dysfunction may be present.

A routine plain film series of the foot is usually sufficient to demonstrate the os tibiale externum and any complicating bony irregularity or cystic change at the synchondrosis margins indicative of chronic apophysitis. An avulsion injury may be demonstrated by plain films (see Fig. 7.180). MRI may show marrow oedema within the os and thickening of the distal posterior tibial tendon (see Fig. 7.181). The presence of synchondrosis widening or fluid signal on MRI denotes disruption. Ultrasound can also dynamically assess the synchondrosis for disruption (Chen et al. 1997).

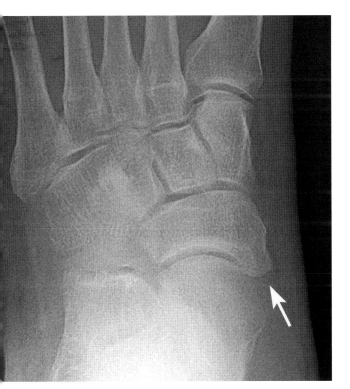

▲ **Fig. 7.179** A Type III os tibiale externum is fused with the navicular tuberosity and forms a bony prominence (arrow). No separate ossicle is present.

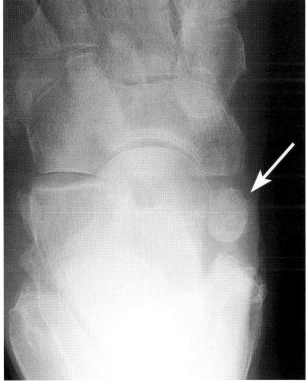

▲ **Fig. 7.180** Occasionally, tibialis posterior traction will cause avulsion of a Type II os tibiale externum (arrow).

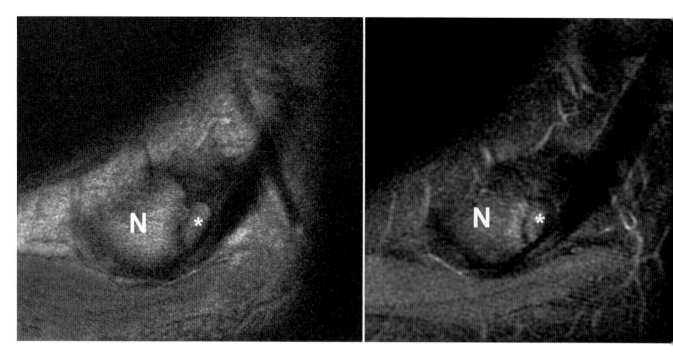

▲ **Fig. 7.181** Sagittal PD and fat-suppressed PD-weighted MR images demonstrate apophysitis associated with a Type II os tibiale externum. High marrow signal is present in the os tibiale externum and in the adjacent navicular. There is no separation at the synchondrosis. Tibialis posterior insertional tendinopathy is noted. The os tibiale externum is indicated by an asterisk. Navicular = N.

Flexor digitorum longus (FDL) tendinopathy

Injuries of the FDL tendon are rare. Imaging detects fluid within the proximal FDL tendon sheath in up to 25% of normal subjects (Schweitzer et al. 1994).

Flexor hallucis longus (FHL) tenosynovitis

FHL tenosynovitis produces posteromedial ankle pain with movement of the great toe, limited range of great toe motion, and tenderness over the fibro-osseous tunnel of the FHL on the posterior surface of the talus. A stenosing component is often present, and associated palpable crepitus or triggering can occur. Hamilton et al. (1996) found that 75% of dancers with FHL tenosynovitis also have symptoms of posterior ankle impingement. Although this process usually occurs at the level of the talar groove (see Fig. 7.182), a more distal form of FHL tenosynovitis can sometimes develop at the level of the great toe. Repetitive overload of the FHL tendon with secondary thickening of both the tendon and the retinaculum at the roof of the fibro-osseous tunnel is believed to be an important factor in dancers (Kolettis et al. 1996). The resulting stenosis limits tendon glide, produces tendon dysfunction

▼ **Fig. 7.182** FHL tendinopathy is demonstrated at the level of the sustentaculum tali by sagittal PD and oblique-axial fat-suppressed T2-weighted MR images. The FHL tendon shows a fusiform swelling and increased signal characteristic of tendinopathy (arrows). A partial tear is demonstrated at the tendon surface on the sagittal view.

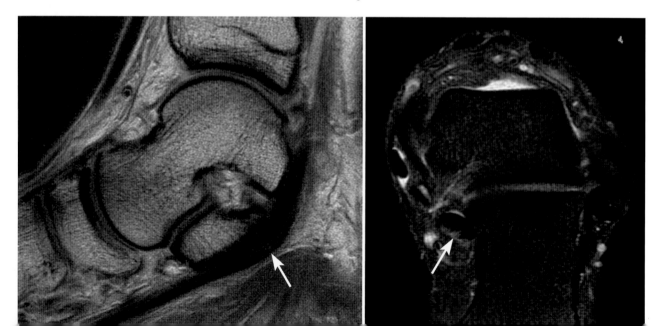

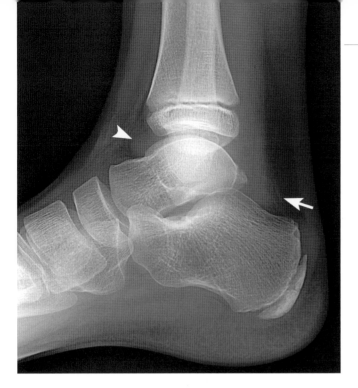

▲ Fig. 7.183 A lateral radiograph in a young athlete with FHL tenosynovitis demonstrates focal hazing of the pre-Achilles fat pad, immediately adjacent to the talar tunnel segment of the FHL tendon (arrow). Note the concurrent ankle joint effusion (arrowhead).

and results in tenosynovitis (see Fig. 7.183) (Hamilton 1982). The stenosis typically involves a relatively short 5 mm segment (Na et al. 2005). Contributing factors are thought to include poor en pointe technique, pronation of the foot and poor turn-out at the hips. Other impingement lesions can also be responsible. Operative findings can include thickening of the FHL tendon sheath, synovial hypertrophy, adhesions, localised FHL tendinopathy, a partial tear of the FHL tendon (see Fig. 7.184), and a tear of the distal FHL muscle (Kolettis et al. 1996).

MRI diagnosis of FHL tenosynovitis can be difficult, as fluid commonly distends the FHL sheath in asymptomatic ankles (Schweitzer et al. 1994). Additional MRI features are required to suggest a diagnosis of FHL tenosynovitis. These include tenosynovial thickening, retinacular thickening at the talar tunnel, FHL tendinopathy, and a prominent FHL sheath effusion in the absence of any explanatory ankle or posterior subtalar joint effusion. Tendon sheath enhancement after intravenous contrast injection is also relatively specific but not routinely performed.

Ultrasound has significant diagnostic advantages over MRI (see Fig. 7.185). These include better demonstration of subtle FHL tendinopathy, a more confident appreciation of synovitis and easy comparison of the thickness of the talar tunnel retinaculum with the asymptomatic side.

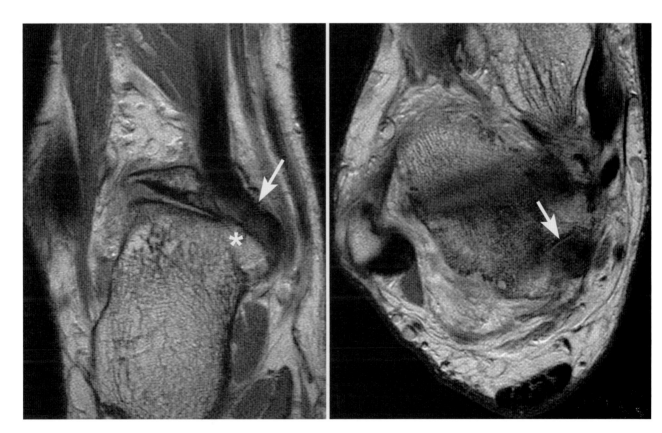

▲ Fig. 7.184 There is FHL tendinopathy and surface fraying secondary to impingement by osteophyte at the posterior margin of the subtalar joint. Coronal and axial PD-weighted MR images show a segment of FHL tendinopathy (arrows). Note that there is displacement and distortion of the FHL tendon by a broad but shallow osteophyte (asterisk) at the posterior margin of the subtalar joint. There is also subtle irregularity of the adjacent tendon surface due to fraying. The subtalar joint shows changes of osteoarthrosis.

▼ **Fig. 7.185** Ultrasound demonstrates FHL tenosynovitis in a 10-year-old netballer. Comparative transverse greyscale images of both FHL tendons have been obtained at the level of fibro-osseous talar tunnel. The abnormal right FHL tendon (asterisk) and overlying retinaculum (arrow) are both thickened by comparison with the left (arrowhead). Power Doppler imaging in this case shows peritendon hyperaemia. The corresponding plain film appearance is shown in Fig. 7.183. Tibialis posterior tendon = t. FDL tendon = f.

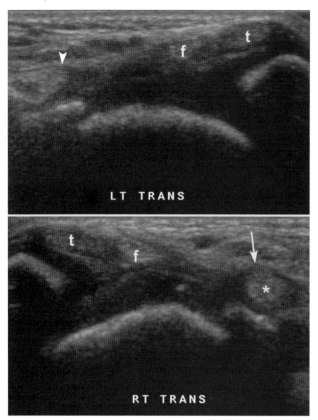

▼ **Fig. 7.186** A lateral plain film shows a collection of loose ossicles at the plantar aspect of the foot. The corresponding long-axis ultrasound image shows that these ossicles lie adjacent to the FHL tendon, within the tendon sheath (callipers). The ossicles produce echogenic foci with 'clean' posterior acoustic shadowing. The ossicles were asymptomatic.

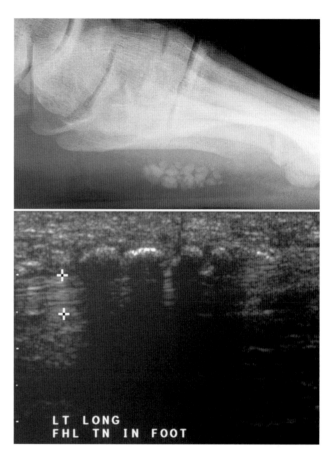

Dynamic ultrasound is helpful in assessment of FHL tendon glide, and accurate correlation of the site of clinical tenderness with the imaging appearance.

Other abnormalities that must be considered when evaluating the imaging appearance of the FHL tendon sheath include ganglion formation and loose bodies. The presence of internal septations or mass effect on the distal FHL muscle supports a diagnosis of a ganglion. Loose bodies may be asymptomatic (see Fig. 7.186).

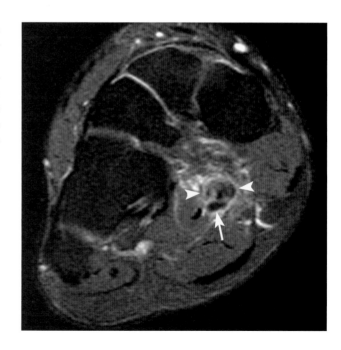

▶ **Fig. 7.187** A coronal fat-suppressed PD-weighted MR image at the level of the Knot of Henry shows an enlarged FHL tendon (arrowheads), with increased signal and an incomplete longitudinal split tear. Also note the associated peritendon hyperintensity. An arrow indicates the normal FDL tendon.

Therapeutic injection of the FHL tendon sheath is best performed under ultrasound guidance. Avoiding the posterior tibial neurovascular bundle requires either an oblique superior approach with the skin entry point just medial to the Achilles tendon, or a transverse approach at the level of the upper margin of the talar groove with the skin entry point lateral to the Achilles tendon.

Other rare types of FHL tendon pathology can occur. There are case reports of partial tears of the FHL tendon at the level of the Knot of Henry where a fibrous band connects the FHL and FDL tendons (see Fig. 7.187). The mechanism of injury in these cases is thought to relate to hyperextension of the great toe (Boruta and Beauperthuy 1997).

Peroneal tendinopathy and tears

The peroneal tendons evert the foot and are important dynamic stabilisers of the ankle. On the rare occurrence that both peroneal tendons are ruptured, the action of the tibialis posterior tendon is unopposed, producing a mid-foot malalignment in which there is medial subluxation at the talonavicular joint (see Fig. 7.188). A number of biomechanical factors are believed to predispose to peroneal tendon pathology. The peroneus longus and brevis tendons both course around the posteroinferior margin of the lateral malleolus, with the brevis at this level having a tighter arc of curvature and hence slightly higher mechanical loading. The peroneal tendons are also restrained by fascial planes at the level of the superior peroneal retinaculum, inferior peroneal retinaculum and cuboid tunnel. These are sites of relative constriction that predispose to peroneal peritendinitis (Burman 1953).

As the peroneus brevis tendon lies anterior to the peroneus longus tendon within the retromalleolar groove, it has been suggested that compression of the brevis against the malleolus by the longus may be a factor in the pathogenesis of peroneus brevis tendon longitudinal split tears (Sobel et al. 1992). Extension of the peroneus brevis musculotendinous junction into the retromalleolar groove and the presence of an accessory peroneus quartus have also been reported to predispose to peroneus brevis tendon tears.

The peroneus longus tendon curves around the calcaneum and beneath the cuboid, before coursing across the plantar aspect of the mid-foot, finally inserting at the base of the first metatarsal. Cavovarus hind-foot alignment creates a tighter arc of curvature, with increased loading of the longus tendon, and predisposes to longus pathology at both the cuboid tunnel and peroneal tubercle levels. Increased loading also explains why certain anatomical variants are more common in a cavovarus hind-foot, including:

- an os peroneum, which develops as a sesamoid, protecting the tendon against compressive stress as it turns around the lateral margin of the cuboid (see Fig. 7.189)
- hypertrophic spur formation at the peroneal tubercle of the calcaneum due to traction stress (see Fig. 7.190).

The longitudinal course of the peroneal tendons makes imaging assessment difficult. Several strategies can be used

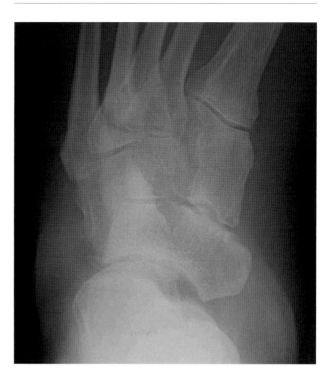

▲ **Fig. 7.188** In this case, both the peroneus longus and brevis tendons have ruptured leaving traction of the tibialis posterior unopposed. Medial subluxation of the midtarsal joint has occurred. Degenerative changes are noted in the navicular-medial cuneiform articulation.

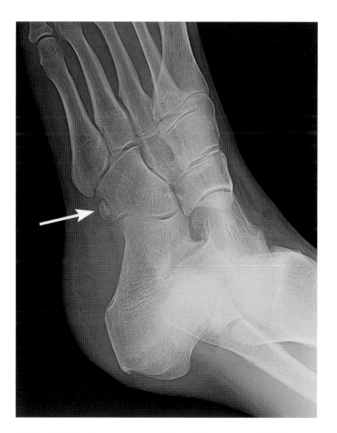

▲ **Fig. 7.189** An os peroneum (arrow) is a sesamoid that develops in the peroneus longus tendon, protecting the tendon as it turns around the edge of the cuboid (arrow).

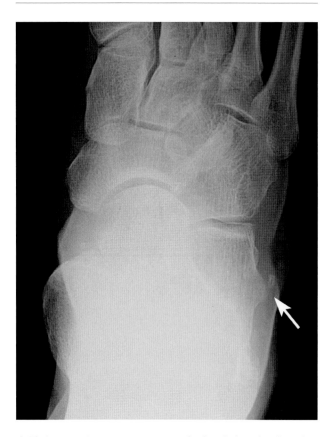

▲ Fig. 7.190 A prominent peroneal tubercle has developed on the lateral border of the calcaneum (arrow). Such a tubercle may cause abrasion to the peroneal tendons. A small ossicle adjacent to the tubercle may indicate an avulsion injury caused by retinacular traction.

to overcome this problem and provide improved diagnostic accuracy. Magic angle artefact on MRI can be minimised by using an axial pulse sequence with a TE above 60–70 msec. Also of help is an additional axial sequence acquired with the ankle in plantar flexion to produce a plane of section roughly perpendicular to the general arc of curvature of the peroneal tendons as they course around the lateral malleolus. As peroneus longus pathology may extend to the first metatarsal insertion, it is important that coronal and axial scans include this region.

Ultrasound can make it easier to appreciate subtle changes of peroneal tendinopathy and peritendinitis by allowing direct correlation between the site of clinical tenderness and the imaging appearance. Assessment of the peroneus longus by ultrasound at the cuboid tunnel level is difficult due to several factors, including the abruptly curving course of the tendon as it enters the tunnel, the thick overlying plantar skin, difficult transducer contact and anisotropy. Careful side-to-side comparison is helpful.

Peroneal peritendinitis (or tenosynovitis)

Peroneal peritendinitis is common in athletes after they undertake a marked increase in training intensity. This characteristically occurs early in the season (Sammarco 1994), with the athlete presenting with localised pain, swelling and tenderness. Peritendinitis reflects an increase in tensile and frictional loading associated with either acute or chronic overuse at sites of relative tendon sheath stenosis. These sites include the level of the superior peroneal retinaculum, inferior peroneal retinaculum and the cuboid tunnel. Synovitis can occasionally lead to tendon sheath adhesion. It should be noted that a small amount of peroneal tendon

▶ Fig. 7.191 MRI demonstrates a longitudinal tear of the peroneus brevis tendon with associated peroneal peritendinitis. These axial PD-weighted MR images show the peroneus brevis tendon (white arrows) separated into two halves by a zone of high signal. The adjacent peroneus longus tendon (arrowheads) is thickened and demonstrates intrasubstance tendinopathy. There is fluid within the FHL tendon sheath.

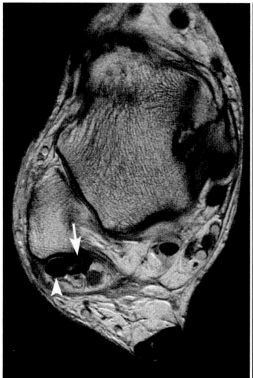
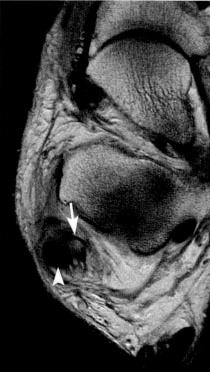

sheath fluid on imaging is a relatively non-specific finding, and is commonly seen in asymptomatic ankles. Kijowski et al. (2007) reported that the presence of circumferential fluid within the common peroneal sheath of more than 3 mm in maximal width is highly specific for peroneal tenosynovitis. Consequently, if there is only a small amount of fluid present, additional MRI signs must be used to diagnose peroneal peritendinitis. These can include tenosynovial thickening, oedema within the adjacent subcutaneous fat space, and peroneal tendinopathy (see Fig. 7.191). Additional help may be provided by MRI after intravenous contrast (looking for tendon sheath enhancement) or Doppler ultrasound (looking for tendon and/or peritendon hyperaemia).

Peroneus brevis tendinopathy and tendon tears

Tendinopathy of the peroneus brevis may be associated with chronic ankle instability, recurrent tendon subluxation and the presence of an accessory peroneus quartus (Jones 1993; Bonnin et al. 1997; Karlsson et al. 1998). Pathologic changes generally occur at or distal to the lateral malleolus. Peroneus brevis tendinopathy can occasionally result in central mucoid cystic degeneration without a surface tear, producing a 'pseudotumour' with consequent stenosing tenosynovitis at the level of the inferior peroneal retinaculum (Khoury et al. 1996) (see Fig. 7.192). More commonly, tendinopathy leads to surface tears that frequently extend over 2–5 cm (Jones 1993). Peroneus brevis tears characteristically progress from Grade 1 to Grade 4 (Sobel et al. 1992):

- **Grade 1:** Splayed-out tendon (sometimes difficult to differentiate from normal variation)
- **Grade 2:** Partial-thickness split
- **Grade 3:** Full-thickness split 1–2 cm in length
- **Grade 4:** Full-thickness split more than 2 cm in length.

Ultrasound has an overall high sensitivity and positive predictive value for peroneal tendon tears (Grant et al. 2005). Complete longitudinal tears are usually obvious (see Fig. 7.193), but incomplete tears can be quite subtle. The sonographic evaluation may be aided by a variety of techniques, including liberal use of stand-off gel, varying the angle of insonation and varying the degree of transducer pressure. Tendon examination is also improved by dynamic assessment during active foot circumduction, and occasionally by 'milking' any tendon sheath fluid to the level of the suspected tear. The significance of a splayed tendon with no discernible linear surface defect can be difficult to determine. While this has been reported to represent an incomplete tear (Grant et al. 2005), some surgeons describe the corresponding operative appearance as tendinopathy without a tear.

Peroneus longus tendinopathy and tendon tears

Tendinopathy and tears of the peroneus longus occur most commonly at the cuboid tunnel level in the cavovarus foot, but occasionally occur more proximally at the level of a prominent peroneal tubercle (see Fig. 7.194). There are isolated reports of a compartment syndrome complicating a peroneus longus tendon tear (Davies 1979; Arciero et al. 1984).

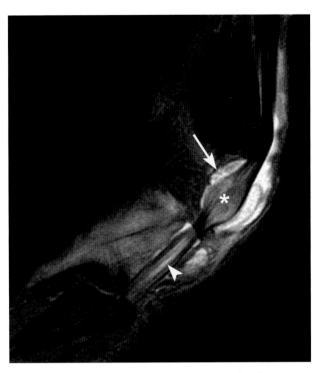

▲ **Fig. 7.192** A sagittal fat-suppressed PD-weighted MR image demonstrates myxoid degeneration of the mid-to-distal segments of the peroneus brevis tendon (asterisk). There is a superimposed longitudinal intrasubstance tear (arrowhead). Note the associated marked peroneal tendon sheath synovitis and effusion (arrow). The point of constriction between the mid and distal tendon segments is due to the overlying peroneal retinaculum.

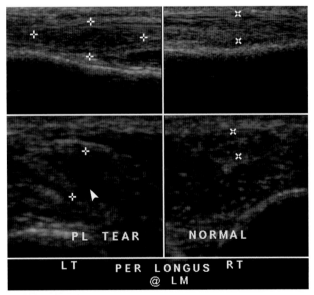

▲ **Fig. 7.193** A longitudinal tear of the left peroneus longus tendon is demonstrated by ultrasound. Comparison long-axis (top) and axial (bottom) ultrasound images have been obtained over the peroneus longus tendons at the submalleolar level. The left peroneus longus shows fusiform hypoechoic thickening due to tendinopathy (+ callipers) with a superimposed linear cleft of a longitudinal tear (arrowhead). The normal right peroneus longus is indicated by × callipers.

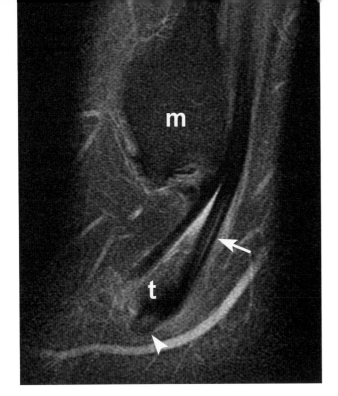

▲ Fig. 7.194 Peroneus longus tendinopathy and peritendinitis are demonstrated by a sagittal fat-suppressed PD-weighted MR image. There is increased tendon signal including a well-defined bright line of longitudinal tear along the submalleolar segment (arrow). The more distal pre-cuboid tunnel segment of the peroneus longus tendon also shows intrasubstance tendinopathy (arrowhead). Also note the accompanying peroneal tendon sheath effusion. Peroneal tubercle = t. Lateral malleolus = m.

Peroneal tendon subluxation and dislocation

The major stabiliser of the peroneal tendons at the lateral malleolus is the superior peroneal retinaculum. Retinacular incompetence resulting in peroneal tendon subluxation or dislocation can result from either an acute high-energy tear or an acquired laxity as a consequence of recurrent low-level interstitial trauma, as may occur with repeated inversion injuries (Jones 1993). A retromalleolar sulcus that is flat or posteriorly convex may also predispose to peroneal tendon subluxation, although this is of secondary importance to the status of the retinaculum (Trevino and Baumhauer 1992). Acute peroneal tendon dislocations are caused by forceful passive dorsiflexion and slight inversion at the ankle, which most commonly occurs in sports such as skiing, soccer, football, ice skating and basketball (Frey and Shereff 1988). The mechanism of injury in skiers involves catching the ski tip in the snow with the skier then falling forwards (Leach and Lower 1985). Although spontaneous reduction of the peroneal tendons can occur after an acute dislocation, the retinaculum is usually 'stripped' away from the malleolar attachment to create a pouch-like space that allows recurrent anterior tendon subluxation (Arrowsmith et al. 1983).

Plain films will occasionally show a cortical flake fracture at the posterolateral margin of the lateral malleolus due to avulsion by the superior peroneal retinaculum (see Fig. 7.195). Cavovarus hind-foot morphology and prominence of the peroneal tubercle may also be evident (Murr 1961). Although CT and MRI can each demonstrate static tendon subluxation or dislocation, ultrasound is the only imaging

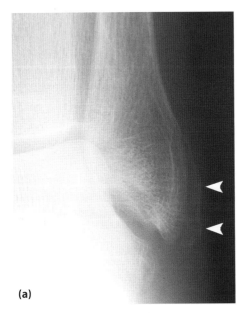

(a)

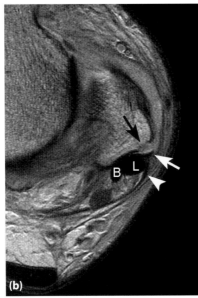

(b)

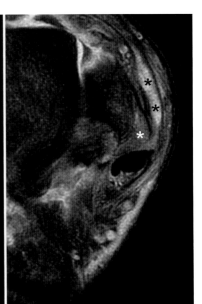

▲ Fig. 7.195(a) A linear fragment of cortical bone has been avulsed from the lateral malleolus by the superior peroneal retinaculum (arrowheads).

(b) An acute superior peroneal retinacular avulsion fracture is demonstrated by MRI. Axial PD and fat-suppressed T2-weighted MR images show a small avulsion bone flake (white arrow) with the attached superior peroneal retinaculum (arrowhead) separated and displaced away from the lateral malleolar fracture bed (black arrow). Note the corresponding marrow oedema within the lateral malleolus (white asterisk) and haemorrhage (black asterisks) extending along the lateral surface of the malleolus beneath a 'stripped' but intact deep fascial plane. Peroneus brevis tendon = B. Peroneus longus tendon = L.

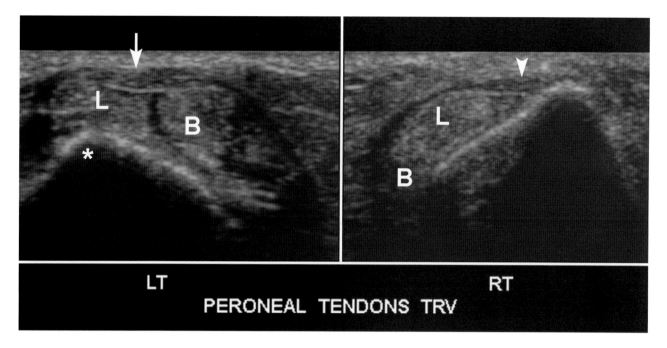

▲ **Fig. 7.196** Ultrasound demonstrates left peroneal tendon subluxation due to avulsion of the superior peroneal retinaculum. Comparison transverse ultrasound images have been obtained at the level of the retromalleolar groove. The left superior peroneal retinaculum (arrow) is thickened and has been avulsed away from its normal attachment at the posterolateral corner of the lateral malleolus (asterisk), and the left peroneus longus tendon shows slight anterior subluxation onto the lateral surface of the malleolus. Note the normal right superior peroneal retinaculum (arrowhead) and attachment. Peroneus brevis tendon = B. Peroneus longus tendon = L.

modality that provides a dynamic assessment of peroneal tendon stability. This is usually performed with the patient prone, the transducer transverse to the peroneal tendons at the retromalleolar groove level, and the tendons then observed during active ankle dorsiflexion-eversion. Additionally, the real-time examination should include peroneal tendon assessment during resisted contraction, most effectively achieved by examining the patient in a standing position during a heel-raise manoeuvre in which all weight is taken on the great toe. Peroneal tendon instability is demonstrated if ultrasound can show anterolateral tendon displacement beyond the corner of the retromalleolar groove and onto the lateral surface of the malleolus (see Fig. 7.196). Ultrasound should also evaluate the superior peroneal retinaculum itself both at rest and during each of these manoeuvres.

Another common cause of a posterolateral ankle click is the phenomenon of retrofibular intra-sheath peroneal tendon subluxation, which occurs as the peroneus brevis tendon suddenly shifts beneath the peroneus longus tendon within the retromalleolar groove. There is an associated popping and a palpable click but no subluxation anterior to the groove (Harper 1997). This phenomenon may or may not be associated with pain, and is readily demonstrated by dynamic ultrasound examination (Neustadter et al. 2004).

Painful os peroneum syndrome

Painful os peroneum syndrome (POPS) is a term that describes one or more of several conditions which may be associated with the presence of an os peroneum within the peroneus

longus tendon at the level of the cuboid tunnel (Sobel et al. 1994):

- acute os peroneum fracture (see Fig. 7.197), or diastasis of a multipartite os peroneum
- stenosing peroneus longus tenosynovitis secondary to callus formation after an os fracture or diastasis of a multipartite os
- attrition or partial rupture of the peroneus longus tendon proximal or distal to the os peroneum (see Fig. 7.198)
- frank rupture of the peroneus longus tendon at the proximal or distal margin of the os peroneum
- peroneus longus tendon and os peroneum entrapment secondary to a large peroneal tubercle on the lateral aspect of the calcaneum.

MRI and nuclear bone scans have identified an additional subgroup of patients with a painful and tender os peroneum who have corresponding bone marrow oedema but no fracture (see Fig. 7.199(a)). These patients also often show features of tendinopathy and peritendinitis within the adjacent peroneus longus tendon segments (see Fig. 7.199(b)). Differentiation of an os peroneum fracture from a multipartite os peroneum can be difficult. Acute fractures show no fracture margin sclerosis and the bone fragments typically fit together like pieces of a puzzle. Conversely, a finding of rounded, smooth sclerotic bone margins is consistent with a multipartite os peroneum. Fragment separation of 6 mm or more on plain film is associated with a full-thickness tear of the peroneus longus tendon (Brigido et al. 2005). The normal

(a)

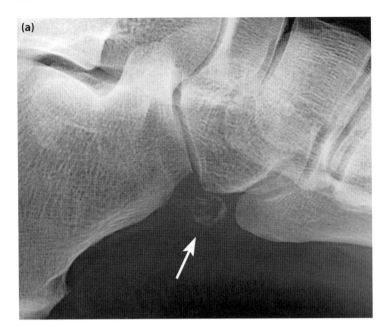

(b)

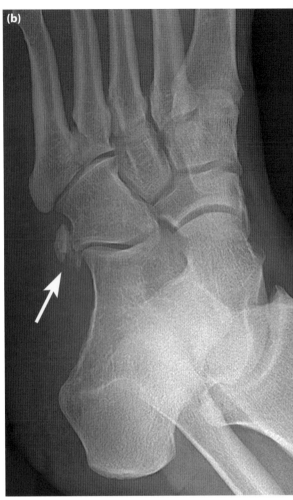

▲▶ **Fig. 7.197(a)** A fracture of the os peroneum produces localised tenderness and fragmentation of the os, which is seen on an oblique view of the foot (arrow). **(b)** A symptomatic os peroneum shows marked irregularity and fragmentation on plain films (arrow).

▼ **Fig. 7.198** A sagittal fat-suppressed PD-weighted MR image demonstrates an acute complete rupture of the peroneus longus, distal to the os peroneum (asterisk). The tendon proximal to the os shows diffuse high signal, swelling and mild retraction. There is high marrow signal within the os (arrow) and considerable surrounding oedema.

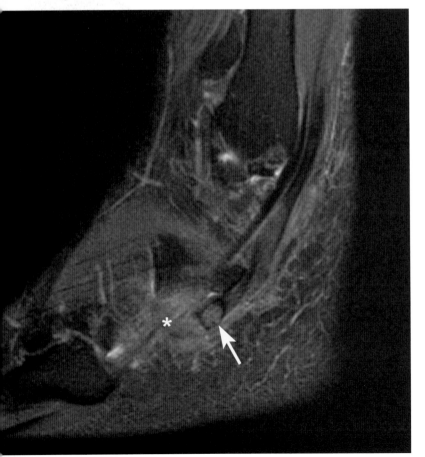

position of an os peroneum can be quite variable, but a location more than 2 cm proximal to the calcaneocuboid joint on an oblique plain film of the foot suggests a peroneus longus tear.

Symptomatic peroneus quartus

The peroneus quartus is a relatively common accessory muscle and tendon, with an incidence rate of 13–21%. This anomaly is usually asymptomatic. Originating from the distal fibula, intramuscular septum or peroneus longus, the tendon passes behind the retromalleolar groove of the fibula to insert at various sites, including the lateral border of the calcaneum (Sammarco and Brainard 1991), onto the peroneus longus or brevis tendons or at either the cuboid or the base of the fifth metatarsal. Because the peroneus quartus tendon accompanies the peroneus brevis, overcrowding may occur within the groove. This may contribute to peroneal tendinopathy, peritendinitis and dislocation (see Fig. 7.200). Best et al. (2005) reported a case of a symptomatic peroneus quartus, with resolution of symptoms following excision.

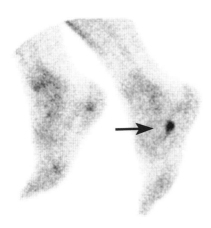

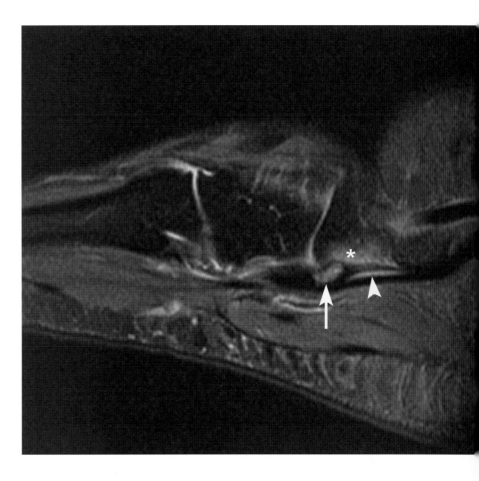

▲ **Fig. 7.199(a)** A nuclear bone scan shows increased uptake of isotope within an os peroneum following trauma (arrow). Bone injury has occurred, producing POPS.

▶ **(b)** Another example of POPS shows a longitudinal tear of the peroneus longus tendon proximal to the os (arrowhead). This sagittal fat-suppressed PD-weighted MR image shows associated marrow oedema within the os peroneum (arrow) and the adjacent margin of the calcaneum (asterisk).

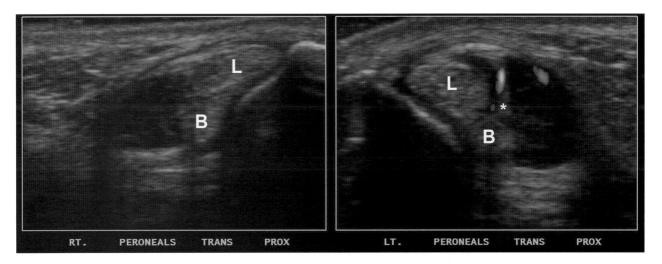

▲ **Fig. 7.200** Comparison transverse Power Doppler ultrasound images at the level of the retromalleolar groove demonstrate a symptomatic left peroneus quartus. Note the separate peroneus quartus tendon (asterisk), with associated muscle belly showing hyperaemia. There is a low-lying peroneus brevis muscle belly on the right. Peroneus longus = L. Peroneus brevis = B.

Miscellaneous conditions of the ankle

Thickened superior extensor retinaculum and ankle pseudotumours

Occasionally, focal thickening of the superior extensor retinaculum may develop at the level of the ankle joint. This is usually secondary to mechanical irritation associated with ill-fitting footwear, or is the result of an acute episode of blunt trauma.

A similar chronic injury, known as a shoe rim or shoe buckle pseudotumour, has been described in elite and professional ice skaters and snowboarders. These cases present as a painful supra-malleolar soft-tissue mass resulting from mechanical irritation of the subcutaneous fat over the fibula as it is compressed beneath the shoe rim. MRI shows a corresponding area of localised oedema in the subcutaneous fat (Anderson et al. 2004).

Malleolar bursopathy

Malleolar bursopathy is an adventitial bursopathy that has been described in figure skaters due to excessive compression and shear forces exerted on the malleolus by the boot. The medial malleolus is more commonly affected than the lateral malleolus. Symptom onset coincides with an increased level of training or the use of new boots. The MRI changes of adventitial bursopathy involve an initial oedematous stranding of subcutaneous fat and subsequent formation of a discrete fluid-filled bursa with a thick fibrotic wall (Brown et al. 2005).

Osteoid osteoma

An osteoid osteoma is a relatively common benign tumour of bone that is mostly seen in the 10–25 year age group with a 2:1 male preponderance. The clinical presentation usually includes night pain, which is characteristically relieved by aspirin. These lesions are typically small and can affect almost any bone, but are most frequent in the lower extremity. There is often a significant delay in the diagnosis of an osteoid osteoma in the ankle and foot, because the diagnosis is not considered. The subperiosteal region near the end of a long bone is most often affected, but less commonly osteoid osteomata may be intra-cortical or intra-medullary. Lesions that are intra-articular, subperiosteal or cancellous show much less surrounding sclerosis.

Plain radiographs are often normal or show extremely subtle changes. MRI usually shows a non-specific appearance of extensive surrounding bone marrow hyperintensity (see Fig. 7.201). The characteristic central nidus of an osteoid osteoma is usually obvious on CT scanning but is often occult on MRI (Davies et al. 2002). Ultrasound can occasionally demonstrate an intra-articular osteoid osteoma as a localised tender cortical irregularity with accompanying focal synovitis (Ebrahim et al. 2001). Many osteoid osteomata are amenable to CT-guided RF ablation.

Avascular necrosis of the talus

The talar dome and body are prone to avascular necrosis by virtue of a relatively tenuous blood supply associated with a large (60%) chondral surface area. AVN of the talus may be traumatic or atraumatic. Traumatic AVN is usually associated with fractures of the talar neck or body and has a higher incidence in cases of displaced fracture or a subtalar or ankle joint dislocation. Atraumatic AVN may be associated with many conditions, including corticosteroid therapy, alcoholism and systemic lupus erythematosus. AVN may be complicated by subchondral bone collapse and secondary degenerative osteoarthrosis.

On plain radiographs, talar AVN is usually manifest as a localised area of increased bone density. The development of osteopaenia in the talar body following trauma (Hawkins

▼ **Fig. 7.201** An intra-cortical osteoid osteoma of the talus is demonstrated by MRI and CT. A 26-year-old elite ballerina presented with persistent pain and anterior ankle impingement symptoms.
(a) A sagittal fat-suppressed PD-weighted MR image shows a non-specific appearance of a questionable shallow cortical erosion at the dorsal aspect of the talar neck (arrow), with associated marked subcortical marrow oedema and surrounding localised soft-tissue hyperintensity.
(b) A sagittal CT image demonstrates an intracortical nidus, which is diagnostic of an osteoid osteoma (arrowhead).

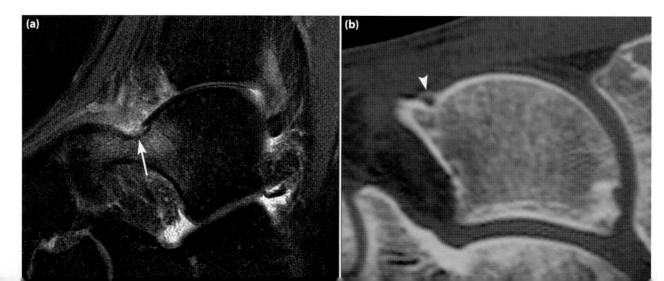

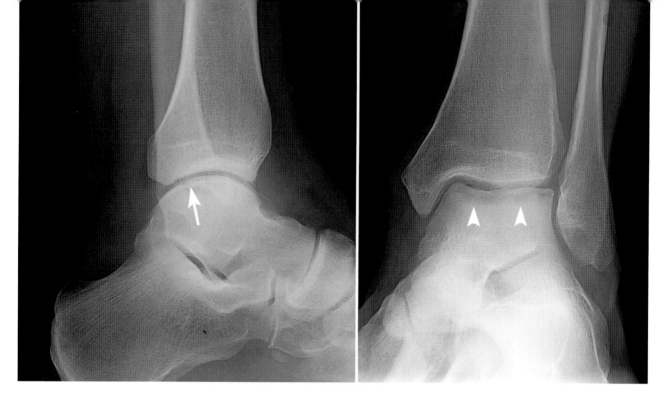

▲ **Fig. 7.202** Lateral and AP views of the ankle show changes of AVN involving the body of the talus. There is increased density of the body of the talus, and in the lateral view collapse of the articular surface of the talar dome is evident (arrow). A band of osteopaenia in the subchondral region of the dome on the mortise view indicates that some perfusion is occurring in this area (arrowheads). This is Hawkins sign, which suggests a favourable outcome.

sign) implies ongoing perfusion and is a good prognostic sign. Conversely, an absent Hawkins sign in the presence of osteopaenia, which typically affects the distal tibia and fibula 6–8 weeks after injury, indicates a high risk of AVN (Donnelly 1999) (see Fig. 7.202).

CT and MRI may show focal sclerosis with serpiginous margins, and are better than plain films at demonstrating any associated subchondral fracture and bone collapse. However,

MRI is more sensitive than CT for the diagnosis of talar AVN and is the preferred method of assessing progress. The typical MRI appearance consists of a geographic band of serpiginous marginating sclerosis (see Fig. 7.203). If the involved segment demonstrates marrow oedema-like signal on fat-suppressed PD or T2 sequences, then the marrow is likely to be viable. Conversely, if the marrow shows low signal on all sequences, then it is more likely to be non-viable.

▼ **Fig. 7.203** Spontaneous avascular necrosis of the talar dome is demonstrated in a 50-year-old male with a background history of old ankle trauma. Plain radiographs showed sclerosis, fragmentation and partial collapse of the talar dome. There was a corresponding marked isotope uptake at the talar dome on nuclear bone scan, and a large 'geographic' zone of well-marginated sclerosis and fragmentation are demonstrated by sagittal PD and fat-suppressed PD-weighted MR images.

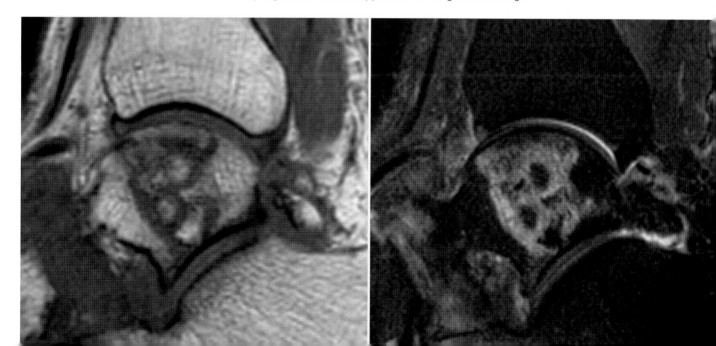

The foot

The foot functions as a platform of support and plays an important role in locomotion. To withstand and absorb the considerable loads and forces that occur with walking, running and jumping, the foot has longitudinal and transverse bony arches that are given static support by ligaments and dynamic support by muscles and tendons. Impact loading is largely cushioned by ligaments that support the sole.

Anatomically, the foot can be artificially divided into three sections and these divisions are used here. The talonavicular and calcaneocuboid articulations divide the hindfoot from the mid-foot and combine to form the transverse tarsal or Chopart joints. The hind-foot comprises the talus and calcaneum. The mid-foot consists of five tarsal bones, the cuboid, the navicular and three cuneiforms. Distally, the forefoot comprising the metatarsals and the phalanges is separated from the mid-foot by the tarsometatarsal (TMT) joints.

Biomechanically, these three sections interact, with the subtalar complex involved in hind- and mid-foot function, and the mid-foot and forefoot functioning together through a three-column structure. The first metatarsal and medial cuneiform form the medial column, with the middle column comprising the second and third metatarsals with the corresponding cuneiforms. The rigid lateral column is formed by the cuboid and fourth and fifth metacarpals and acts as the foot's shock absorber (Lawrence 2002).

Imaging the foot

Plain films are the first step in investigating sports-related conditions of the foot, with high-quality films required for the identification of the many subtle changes that should be noted. Correct positioning, high resolution and appropriate radiographic exposure are all required to image the soft tissues as well as the bony structures. Nuclear bone scans, CT, ultrasound and MRI may all contribute to the identification and characterisation of various conditions of the foot.

Plain films

Routine views of the foot

The routine views of the foot include AP, oblique and lateral views.

AP view

The AP view is obtained as a dorsiplantar projection with the primary beam centred at the base of the third metatarsal using a 5° cranial tube angle (see Fig. 7.204).

Oblique view

The oblique view is obtained by raising the lateral side 30° away from the cassette and directing the primary beam at the base of the fifth metatarsal (see Fig. 7.205). Together with the AP projection, this view is used to assess the toes, metatarsals and tarsal bones anterior to the ankle joint.

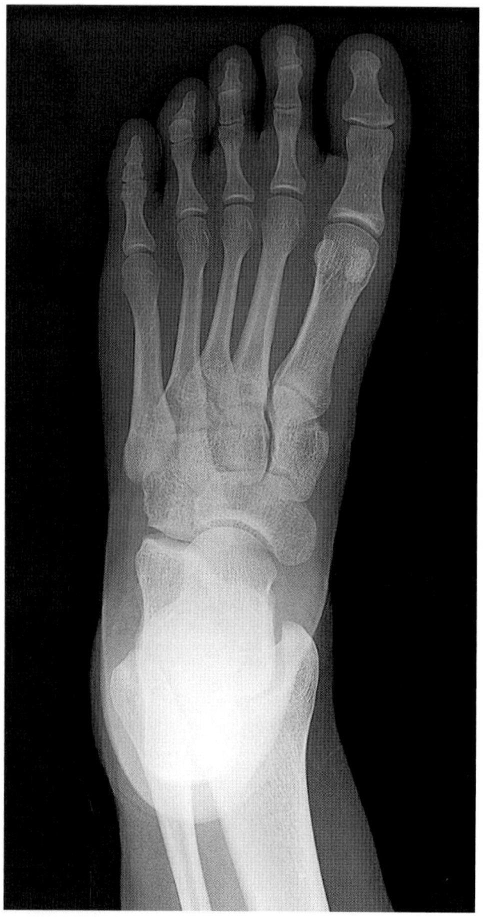

◀**Fig. 7.204** An AP view of the foot is an important routine view for the investigation of foot pathology. Using 5° of cranial tube angulation helps to display the joint spaces. The wedged shape of the foot means that the articular surfaces of the joint spaces are slightly oblique to a straight tube. The film is centred on the base of the third metatarsal and displays the foot from the tips of the toes to the mid hind-foot.

▶**Fig. 7.205** An oblique view complements the AP view, providing a further and different perspective of the toes, metatarsals and tarsal bones. Assessment of the lateral intertarsal joint spaces is improved and easily missed fractures of the base of the fifth metatarsal and anterior process of the calcaneum are usually well demonstrated. The foot is obliqued 30° by raising the lateral side of the foot and a straight tube is centred on the base of the third metatarsal.

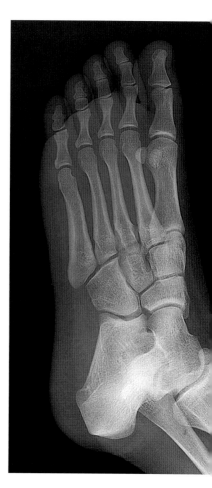

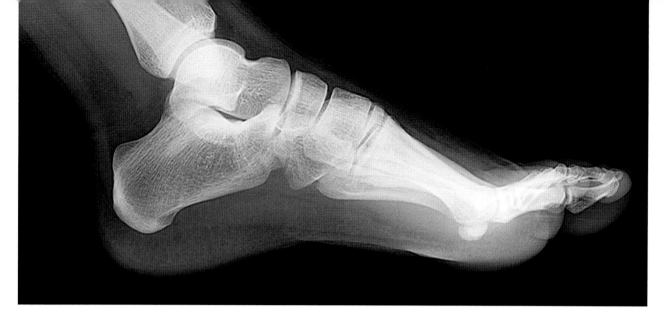

▲ **Fig. 7.206** Considerable information is available on a non-weightbearing lateral view and extremely important structures are displayed. As with a lateral view of the ankle, the malleoli should be superimposed, and in a true lateral projection bony structures and soft tissues from the heel to the toes are displayed. The exposure should allow assessment of the soft tissues of the Achilles and pre-Achilles fat pad, together with the sole and dorsum of the foot. Note the sclerotic bone island in the calcaneum.

Lateral view

Non-weightbearing lateral views are taken whenever possible with the medial side of the foot on the cassette, the malleoli superimposed and the primary beam centred over the metatarsal region (see Fig. 7.206). Occasionally, a marked hallux valgus deformity may prevent adequate positioning, in which case the lateral side of the foot should be placed on the cassette. When a foreign body is suspected in the plantar soft tissues, a weightbearing technique should not be used. Similarly, when soft-tissue swelling is to be identified, as in swelling of the plantar fascia, a weightbearing film is unsuitable.

Additional plain film views of the foot

Depending on the clinical presentation, the standard series may be complemented by extra views. These views often replace the need for more sophisticated tests, by supplying information that enables a diagnosis to be established.

Subtalar joint views

Specific views of the subtalar joint are used to demonstrate conditions of the subtalar joint such as degenerative changes, to assess the extent of a fracture of the lateral process of the talus or calcaneum, and to show a tarsal coalition. To demonstrate the posterior subtalar joint, there are two oblique views that should be added to the standard views.

The internal oblique view is obtained with 20° of internal rotation of the ankle. The beam is centred 3 cm below the lateral malleolus, with a 15° cranial tube angulation. In this view the posterior subtalar joint is imaged front-on (see Fig. 7.207).

The external oblique view produces a true lateral view of the posterior subtalar joint. The ankle is externally rotated 45° and, with a 15° cranial tube angle, the beam is centred 2.5 cm below the medial malleolus (see Fig. 7.208).

Harris-Beath view

This additional subtalar joint view has been previously discussed on page 538.

Axial view of the heel

When calcaneal injury is clinically suspected, an axial view is required for examination of the medial and lateral calcaneal tubercles. This view is similar to a Harris-Beath view, but uses a 40° tube angle (see Fig. 7.209).

▼ **Fig. 7.207** A true AP view of the posterior subtalar joint is obtained with internal rotation of the ankle and tube angulation, as described in the text.

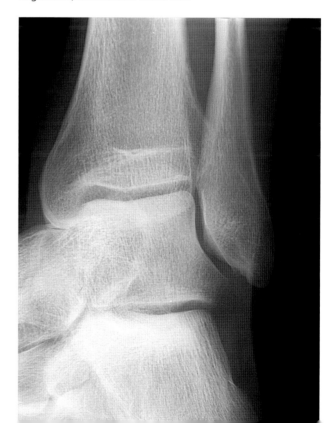

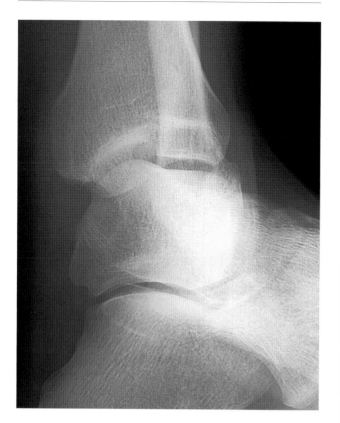

▲ **Fig. 7.208** Using 45° of external rotation of the ankle, the posterior subtalar view is imaged side-on.

Weightbearing AP and lateral views

These views are valuable for the assessment of changes in alignment, occurring in conditions such as hallux valgus deformity, tibialis posterior dysfunction and Lisfranc fracture-dislocation (see Figs 7.210, 7.211 and 7.212). A weightbearing lateral view will accentuate loss of the longitudinal plantar arch (see Fig. 7.213), together with joint space narrowing in the ankle and subtalar joints.

Navicular view

This view is used when a stress fracture of the navicular is suspected and is obtained by tilting the foot so that the primary beam demonstrates the proximal and distal

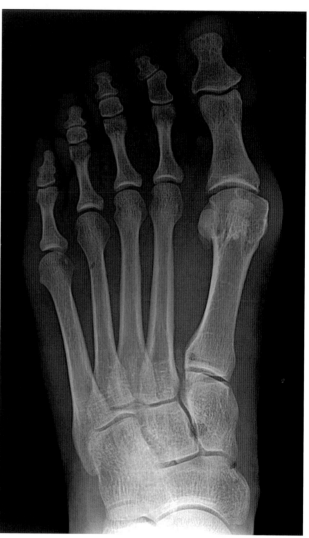

▲ **Fig. 7.210** A weightbearing view is valuable for demonstrating conditions that cause a change in foot alignment. Weightbearing tends to exaggerate the deformity. In this case a weightbearing AP view shows moderate hallux valgus deformity. There is lateral subluxation of the sesamoids and soft-tissue thickening is present over the medial aspect of the first metatarsophalangeal joint. Note the os intermetatarseum between the bases of the first and second metatarsals. This accessory ossicle is discussed later in the chapter.

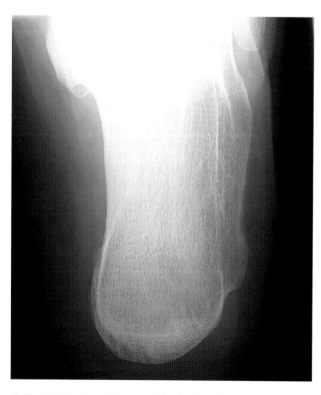

▲ **Fig. 7.209** The axial view of the heel is obtained in the supine position, with the foot held at 90° to the cassette. The patient holds their foot in this position by applying traction with a strap or bandage. Using 40° of cranial tube angulation, the beam is centred on the sole at the level of the fifth metatarsal.

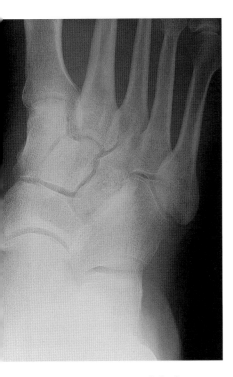

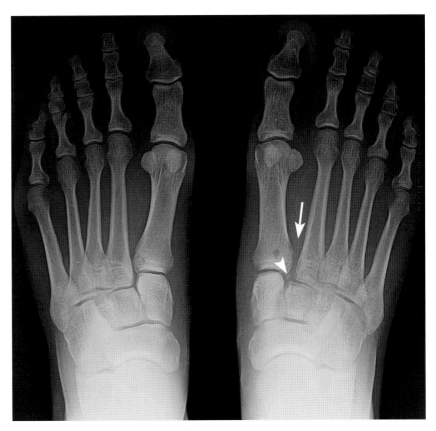

▲ Fig. 7.211 Changes of tibialis posterior dysfunction are well demonstrated with a weightbearing view. There is mid-foot abduction with uncovering of the medial aspect of the talar head and forefoot pronation.

▲ Fig. 7.212 Weightbearing helps demonstrate a Lisfranc fracture-dislocation on the right side by increasing the gap between the first and second metatarsal bases (arrow). This is a homolateral-type Lisfranc fracture-dislocation, involving the first, second and third TMT joints. A small fragment has been avulsed by the Lisfranc ligament (arrowhead).

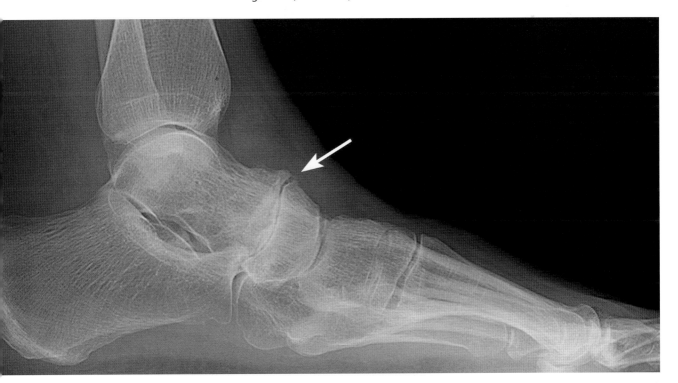

▲ Fig. 7.213 A weightbearing lateral view of the foot is sensitive to changes in alignment of the longitudinal arch. In this case there is moderate loss of the longitudinal plantar arch, due to mild midtarsal sag, raising the possibility of underlying tibialis posterior dysfunction. Marked degenerative changes are demonstrated at the talonavicular joint (arrow).

▶ **Fig. 7.214** Elevation of the forefoot using a 15° sponge will improve assessment of the proximal and distal articular surfaces of the navicular. In this case, there is a complete stress fracture of the navicular with deformity of its proximal articular surface. Wide separation of the fragments has occurred (arrowheads).

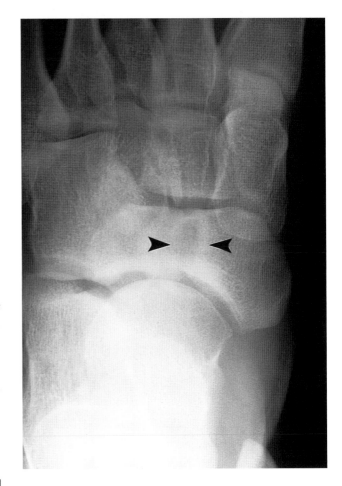

articular surfaces of the navicular and facilitates the identification of subtle stress fracture lines (see Fig. 7.214). A 15° wedge is placed under the forefoot to rotate the navicular into a vertical position.

Skyline view of the sesamoids

When there is clinical suspicion of a sesamoid fracture or sesamoiditis, a skyline view of the sesamoids should be obtained. The patient lies prone, with the toes held dorsiflexed by pressing the toes against the cassette. The medial border of the foot should be vertical. A 10° cranial tube angle is used to produce a tangential view of the sesamoids and the median ridge on the plantar aspect of the head of the first metatarsal (see Fig. 7.215). The medial sesamoid may be further imaged using an oblique AP view, by elevating the medial side of the foot (see Fig. 7.216).

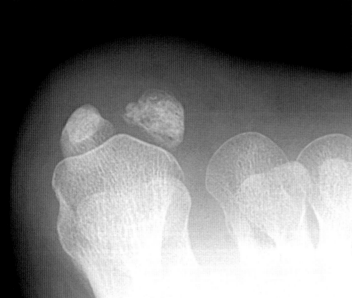

▲ **Fig. 7.215** A skyline view of the great toe sesamoids will demonstrate the sesamoids and the sesamoid articulations and profile the median ridge of the first metatarsal head. In this case, there is altered bony architecture in the lateral sesamoid, with fragmentation and compression. The appearance is that of lateral sesamoiditis.

▶ **Fig. 7.216** By elevating the medial border of the foot and centring on the sesamoid, the medial sesamoid is well demonstrated. In this case, no plain film change can be seen.

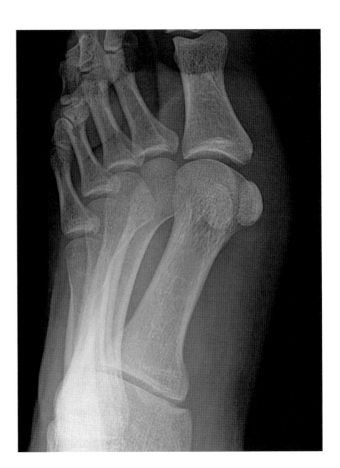

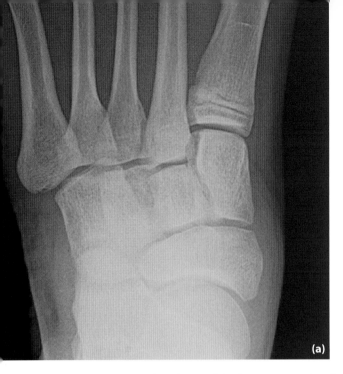

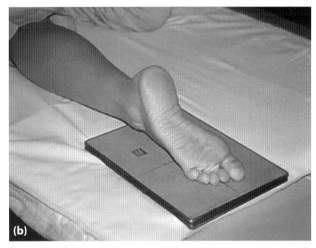

▲ **Fig. 7.217(a)** A plantodorsal view of the foot is extremely valuable for demonstrating the TMT joints.
(b) For a plantodorsal view of the mid-foot, the foot lies with its dorsal surface flat on the cassette, as shown in this photograph. A straight tube is used, centred on the TMT joints, which are identified by palpating the base of the fifth metatarsal.

Plantodorsal view of the mid-foot

One of the most valuable of all the extra foot views is the plantodorsal view. This is easy and quick to obtain and should be added to the basic series of images if there is clinical suspicion of TMT joint injury or a stress fracture of the base of the second metatarsal. It is difficult to assess the TMT joints on routine views due to the obliquity of the articular surfaces. This obliquity is overcome by rolling the patient prone and using a straight tube centred on the base of the second metatarsal (see Figs 7.217 and 7.218). The primary beam will then be parallel with the joint surfaces. Examples of the advantages of a plantodorsal mid-foot view are shown throughout the chapter in Figs 7.281, 7.299, 7.300 and 7.308.

Os tibiale externum view

The os tibiale externum is an accessory ossicle situated on the plantar aspect of the proximal surface of the navicular tuberosity. The tuberosity and os tibiale externum may produce a medial bony prominence. This ossicle may become symptomatic due to rubbing on footwear, by direct trauma or traction by the tibialis posterior tendon. To help with assessment of the ossicle and the adjacent tuberosity, an oblique view with a 30° elevation of the medial side of the foot should be acquired (see Fig. 7.219).

Views of the toes

Following a toe injury, plain films including AP, oblique and lateral views should be obtained (see Fig. 7.220). A 15° cranial tube angulation improves definition of the interphalangeal joints. Overall resolution is improved if the film is obtained PA rather than AP, allowing the toes to lie directly on the cassette. A wooden spatula is useful for separating the toes when obtaining a lateral view.

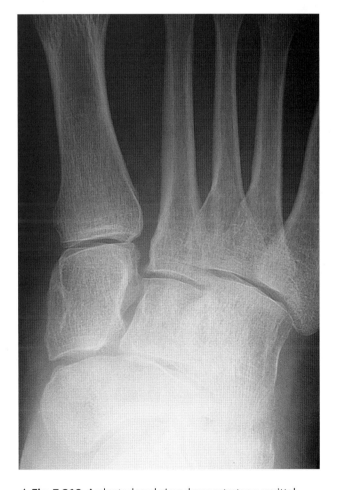

▲ **Fig. 7.218** A plantodorsal view demonstrates a sagittal diastasis, which extends between the middle and medial cuneiforms and then separates the navicular and the medial cuneiform. The TMT joints are all well demonstrated. Sagittal diastasis injuries are discussed later in the chapter.

▶ **Fig. 7.219** A special view to demonstrate an os tibiale externum requires a 30° elevation of the medial border of the foot. This obliquity brings both the os and the navicular tubercle into profile. In this case there is irregularity and cyst formation along the synchondrosis, suggesting a previous destabilisation.

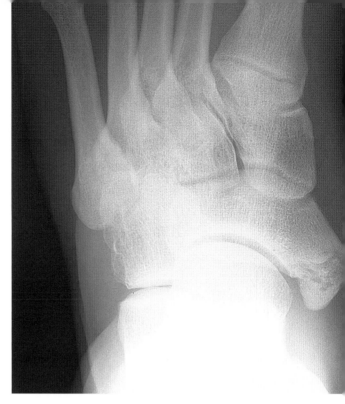

▼ **Fig. 7.220** An injury of the great toe is demonstrated on AP, oblique and lateral views, which constitute a normal toe series. A large bone fragment has been avulsed from the plantar aspect of the base and proximal shaft of the distal phalanx. This injury has presumably occurred as the result of forced extension against strong FHL contraction. The fragment appears to be hinged on the plantar plate.

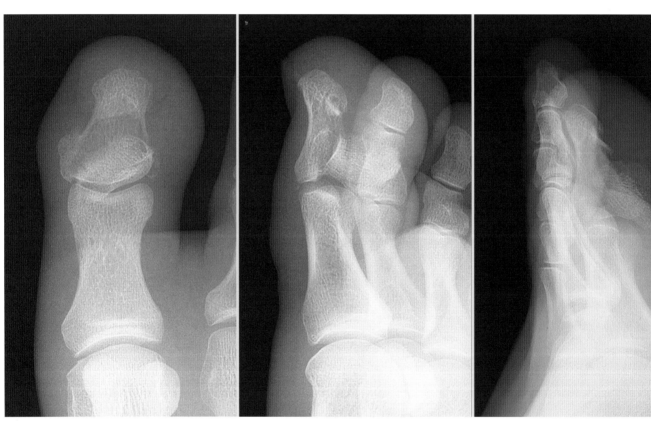

Tips on looking at plain films of the foot

As with the ankle, it is important to identify soft-tissue swelling as this will immediately guide the radiologist or clinician to likely sites of clinical interest. The swelling may be centred over a particular joint, as will often occur at the first or fifth metatarsophalangeal (MTP) joints (see Fig. 7.221) or, in the lateral view, dorsal soft-tissue swelling will often focus attention on the site of interest. Foreign bodies may require exclusion and consequently it is important to examine the sole of the foot carefully.

Next, the foot should be inspected for any loss of normal bone and joint alignment and configuration. This will be accentuated with weightbearing AP and lateral views.

▶ **Fig. 7.221(a)** Soft-tissue swelling is a handy marker of abnormalities. For example, in this case the experienced eye will be drawn to the first MTP joint and the base of the fifth metatarsal where soft-tissue swelling is present. These areas deserve careful inspection.

(b) In a 41-year-old male, soft-tissue swelling is centred over the lateral aspect of the fifth MTP joint and this should immediately attract attention. In the oblique view, a translucent area is demonstrated within this swelling. This is likely to be an abscess. The adjacent joint appears normal, but destruction of the articular surfaces of the fifth distal interphalangeal joint has the appearance of an old septic arthropathy. In addition, vascular calcification is seen between the first and second and the second and third metatarsals. This suggests that the patient may be diabetic, predisposing to the infection. Deformity of the head of the first proximal phalanx may have originated from a previous infection.

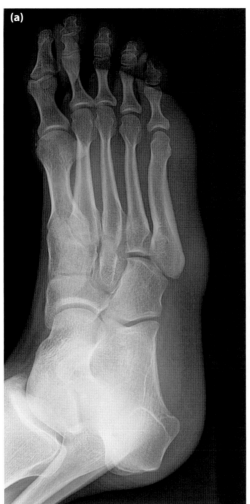
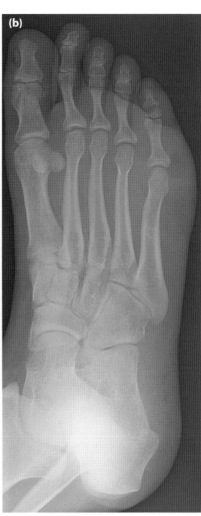

▶ **Fig. 7.222** This is a typical example of a bunionette. When there is lateral prominence of the head of the fifth metatarsal, rubbing on footwear may produce a tender lump known as a bunionette (arrow) overlying the metatarsal head.

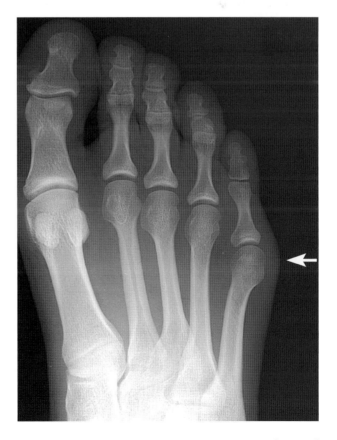

Alignment may be altered with conditions such as a hallux valgus, metatarsus primus varus deformity, a bunionette (see Fig. 7.222), Morton's foot (see Fig. 7.223), a prominent navicular tuberosity or os tibiale externum, tibialis posterior dysfunction and rupture of both peroneal tendons, and Lisfranc injury (see Fig. 7.224). Toe alignment should also be assessed. All these conditions will be discussed later in the chapter.

On the lateral view, talometatarsal alignment should be assessed to detect pes cavus (see Fig. 7.225) or pes planus deformities (see Fig. 7.226). The long axis of the talus should normally be collinear with the long axis of the first metatarsal.

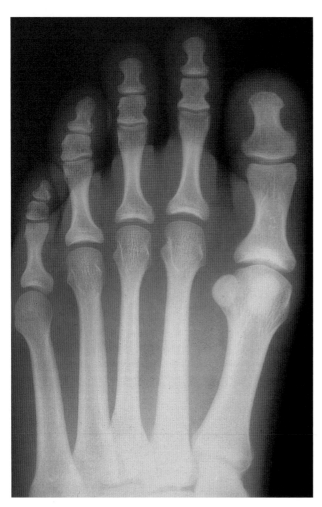

▲ **Fig. 7.223** A Morton's foot has a short first metatarsal. This is a particularly important anomaly in a ballerina, with the second ray exposed to excessive loading when in the en pointe position.

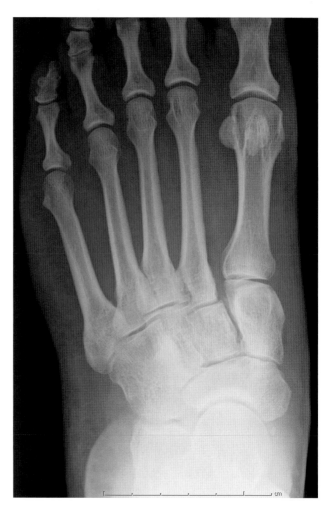

▲ **Fig. 7.224** There is a malalignment at the second TMT joint, due to a Lisfranc injury.

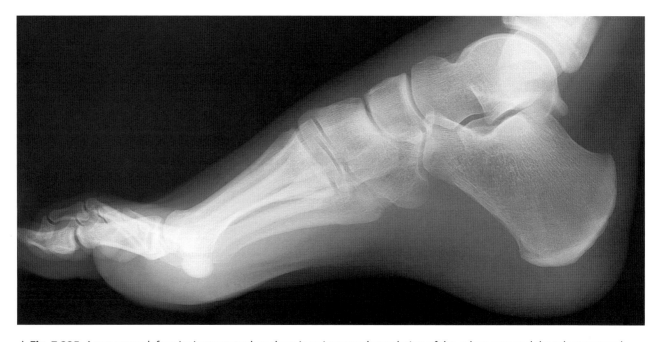

▲ **Fig. 7.225** A pes cavus deformity is present when there is an increased angulation of the calcaneum and the talometatarsal angle is positive. This is an important anomaly, and is discussed later in the chapter.

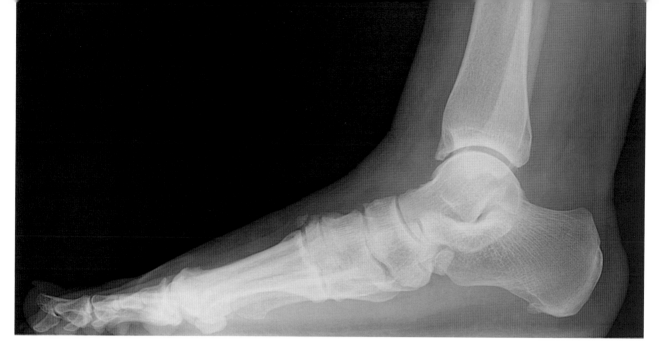

▲ **Fig. 7.226** In this case there is loss of the medial longitudinal plantar arch, due to tibialis posterior dysfunction. Other structures involved in arch support, including the spring ligament, plantar fascia and deltoid ligament, may also fail, leading to pes planus by allowing peritalar lateral subluxation.

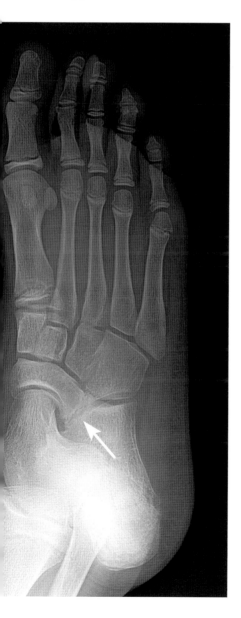

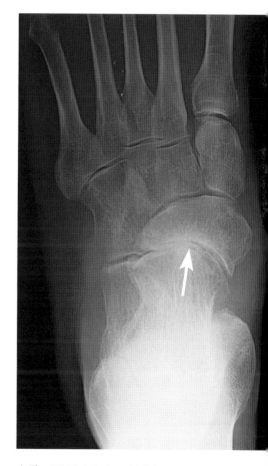

All intertarsal joint spaces should be of similar width and their articular surfaces congruent. Assessment of these spaces and alignments will enable the diagnosis of conditions such as coalition (see Fig. 7.227), osteoarthrosis (see Fig. 7.228) and subtle subluxations (see Fig. 7.229). Particular joint spaces, including the second and third MTP joint spaces, and the intercuneiform articulations are sometimes difficult to examine. However, examining the AP and oblique views together will usually allow adequate assessment.

Imaging the foot with nuclear bone scans

A nuclear bone scan is an economic alternative to MRI for imaging conditions such as bone stress (see Fig. 7.230), fractures (see Fig. 7.231), osteochondritis, enthesopathies (see Fig. 7.232) and impingements. However, further characterisation of the process is usually required by CT or MRI, as the uptake of isotope is generally non-specific.

◀ **Fig. 7.227** Intertarsal coalition will cause obliteration of the affected joint space if the coalition is bony, or narrowing if the coalition is fibrous or cartilaginous. In this case, there is a broad calcaneonavicular coalition, which appears to be of mixed cartilaginous and fibrous type (arrow).

▲ **Fig. 7.228** Intertarsal joint spaces will be narrowed or obliterated when osteoarthrosis is present. In this case, advanced degenerative changes involve the talonavicular joint, with joint space obliteration (arrow).

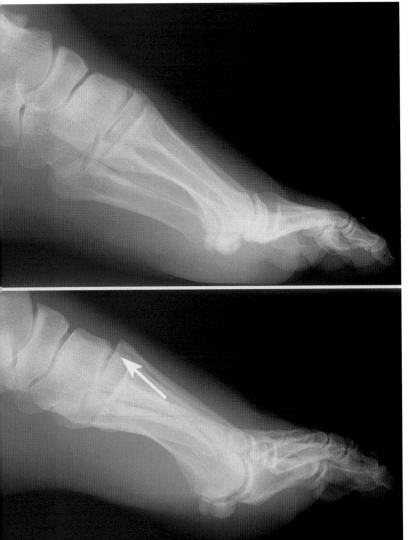

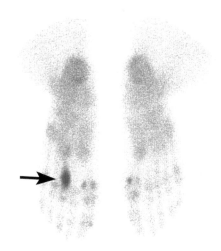

▲ **Fig. 7.230** A nuclear bone scan shows increased uptake of isotope in the shaft of the right third metatarsal (arrow). The appearance is typical of a stress fracture.

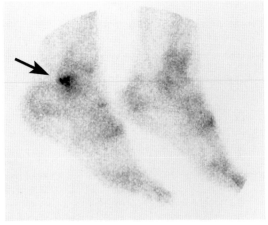

▲ **Fig. 7.229** In this case, a Lisfranc fracture-dislocation was suspected clinically, and a subtle first TMT joint subluxation was demonstrated by altering the angle of the lateral view (arrow).

▲ **Fig. 7.231** A fracture of the posterior process of the talus is demonstrated by a nuclear bone scan (arrow).

Imaging the foot with ultrasound

Soft-tissue changes such as tendinopathy (see Fig. 7.233), bursopathy, ganglion cysts, foreign bodies, a Morton's neuroma (see Fig. 7.234) and injury to the plantar fascia are well demonstrated by ultrasound (see Fig. 7.235). Ultrasound is also commonly used for imaging-guided injections and aspirations.

CT and MRI of the foot

In areas where complex bony anatomy is difficult to assess on plain films, MDCT may be extremely useful. The ability of this technology to produce high-resolution images in any plane is employed to demonstrate complex injuries of the foot such as a Lisfranc fracture-dislocation (see Fig. 7.236). Surface rendering and 3D reconstruction improve the understanding of complex foot injuries (see Fig. 7.237).

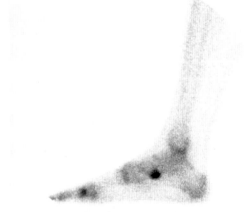

▲ **Fig. 7.232** A localised increase in uptake of isotope is present at the navicular tuberosity, due to enthesopathy at the insertion of the tibialis posterior tendon.

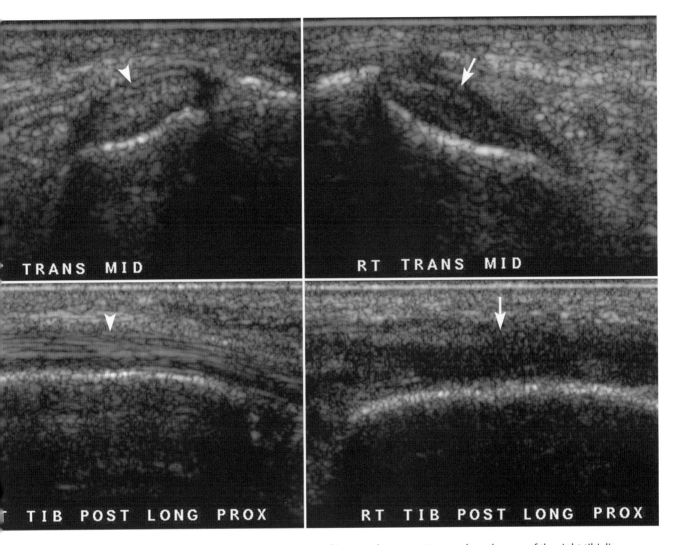

▲ **Fig. 7.233** Comparison transverse and long-axis ultrasound images demonstrate complete absence of the right tibialis posterior tendon with hypoechoic synovial thickening filling the otherwise empty sheath (arrows). A normal tendon is shown on the left (arrowheads).

▶ **Fig. 7.234** A long-axis ultrasound image obtained over the plantar aspect of the third metatarsal interspace in a patient with recurrent pain following a Morton's neurectomy shows a stump neuroma at the proximal neurectomy margin (callipers). The common digital nerve is indicated by arrowheads.

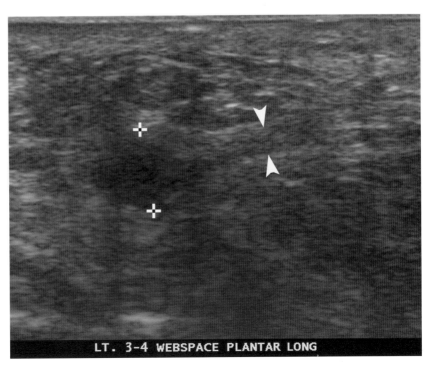

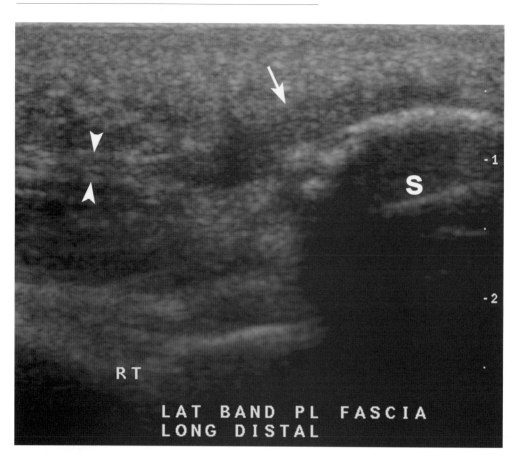

◀ Fig. 7.235 A long-axis ultrasound image has been obtained at the fifth metatarsal insertion of the lateral band of the plantar fascia. This shows localised hypoechoic fascial thickening and enthesial bone surface irregularity, which corresponded to the site of pain and tenderness reported by the patient and is a variant of plantar fasciitis (arrow). The normal fascial segment proximal to the insertion is indicated by arrowheads. Styloid process of the fifth metatarsal = S.

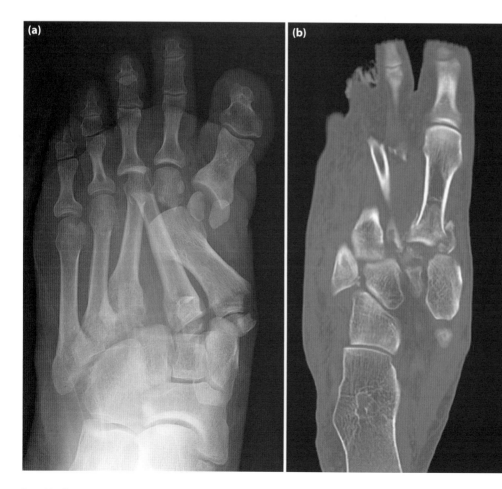

◀ Fig. 7.236(a) Gross foot deformity is demonstrated on plain films. There are fracture-dislocations of the TMT joints, a fracture of the neck of the second metatarsal, and dislocations of the third and first MTP joints. The extent and displacement of the injuries is difficult to visualise on plain films. **(b)** An axial CT image is also difficult to interpret.

▶ **Fig. 7.237** A 3D MDCT image helps in the preoperative assessment of the complex injuries shown in Fig. 7.236, allowing a better understanding of the deformities.

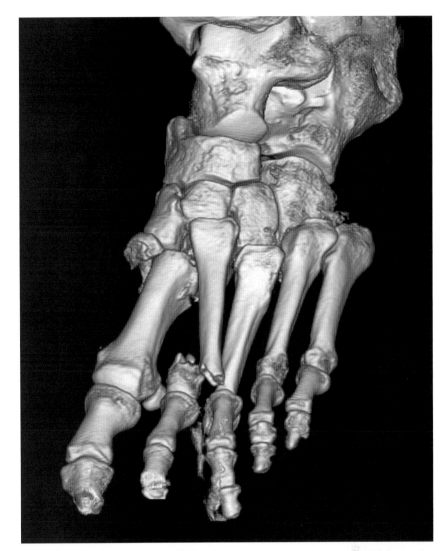

MRI provides a comprehensive demonstration of foot anatomy and the changes of many sports-related conditions. Appropriately tailored protocols using high-resolution scan techniques provide the best results. Common applications include bone stress reactions (see Fig. 7.238), plantar fasciitis (see Fig. 7.239), bursopathies (see Fig. 7.240), tendinopathies and ligament injuries.

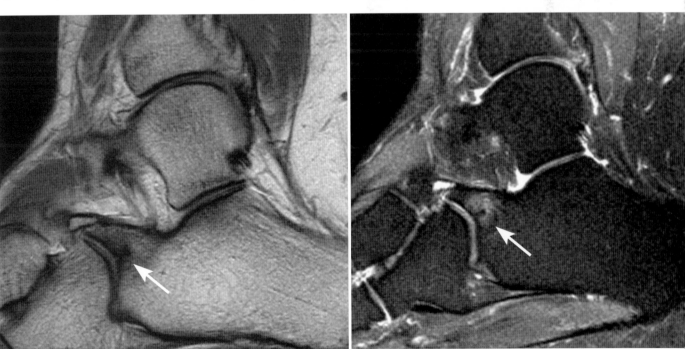

▲ **Fig. 7.238** MR images demonstrate a chronic stress fracture at the base of the anterior process of the calcaneum. Sagittal PD and fat-suppressed PD-weighted images show an incomplete hypointense fracture line with associated marrow oedema (arrows).

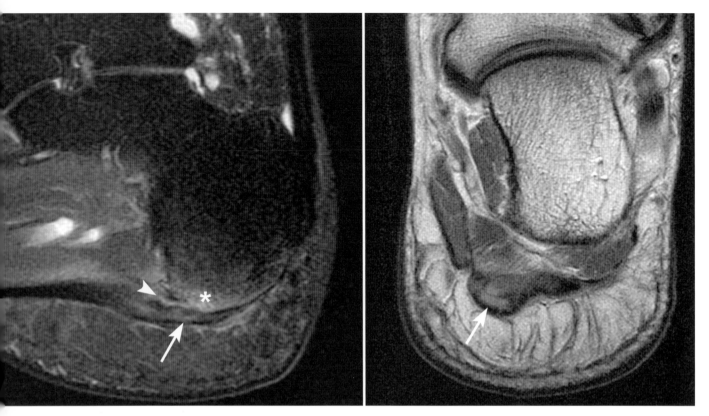

▲ **Fig. 7.239** MRI demonstrates typical changes of plantar fasciitis. Coronal PD and sagittal fat-suppressed PD-weighted MR images show oedema in the calcaneum (asterisk) and in adjacent soft tissues at the thickened fascial attachment to the calcaneum (arrows). A superimposed thin line of marked hyperintensity is consistent with a complicating intrasubstance tear (arrowhead). Also note perifascial oedema.

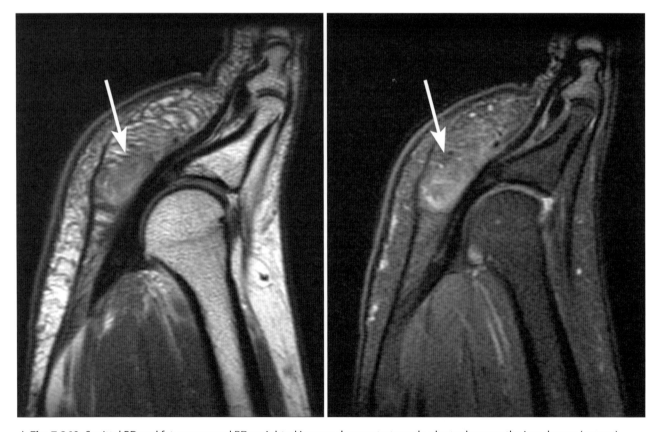

▲ **Fig. 7.240** Sagittal PD and fat-suppressed PD-weighted images demonstrate early plantar bursopathy in a dancer (arrows). Note the high signal of the bursal contents with fat-suppression.

Sports-related injuries of the forefoot

The forefoot lies distal to the TMT joints and includes the metatarsals, the MTP joints and the toes. Toe injuries result from their vulnerable position and digital fractures are the most common forefoot fracture. Metatarsals are susceptible to both acute and stress fractures and specific metatarsal fractures are of great importance to the athlete. These include any fracture of the first metatarsal, an acute or overuse fracture at the base of the second metatarsal, and the Jones fracture of the fifth metatarsal. Other overuse injuries that may disrupt an athlete's career include plantar plate rupture and sesamoiditis.

Conditions of the great toe: 'turf toe' (first MTP joint capsuloligamentous injury)

The term 'turf toe' arose from the observation that the likelihood of injuries to the capsule of the first MTP joint increased in athletes playing sports on artificial surfaces (Bowers and Martin 1976). The mechanism of injury is varied. Most commonly, a valgus mechanism causes disruption of the medial collateral ligament (MCL) complex at the metatarsal attachment, resulting in an acute hallux valgus deformity. Hyperextension mechanisms may be associated with disruption of the plantar plate and chondral injury occurs at the dorsal aspect of the joint. Less commonly, a varus mechanism may tear the lateral collateral ligament (LCL) and produce a hallux varus deformity.

Plain radiographs may detect capsular avulsion fractures (see Fig. 7.241), impaction fractures at the metatarsal head (see Fig. 7.242), sesamoid fractures (see Fig. 7.243) and sesamoid retraction. The AP view should be performed with weightbearing to assess alignment. Plain films are often normal and MRI is then the imaging method of choice to detect injury to ligaments, chondral surfaces and plantar plates (see Fig. 7.244). Immediately after injury, capsular disruption is usually obvious on MRI, with the tear defect seen as an area of fluid signal intensity. In late subacute and chronic cases, scar response may obscure the point of tear and make an accurate diagnosis more difficult. In cases of plantar plate tear, careful assessment of the relative positions of the sesamoids and correlation with plain radiographs is required to detect retraction (see Fig. 7.245). Chondral and osteochondral lesions can be identified on MRI if appropriate cartilage-sensitive PD and fat-suppressed PD sequences are utilised (Potter, Linklater et al. 1998). The identification of chondral flaps (see Fig. 7.246) is of particular relevance because these are a potential source of ongoing mechanical symptoms that may be amenable to arthroscopic debridement.

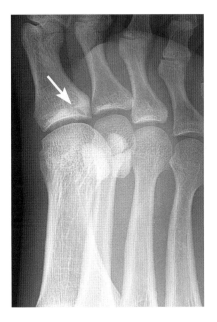

▲ **Fig. 7.241** In a case of ongoing symptoms at a site of previous hyperextension injury to the first MTP joint, an oblique plain film shows sclerotic changes around a focal lucency at the site of an old capsular injury (arrow).

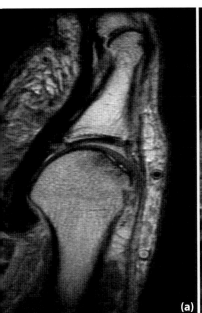
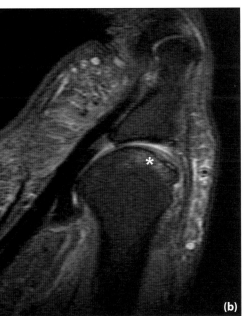

◄ **Fig. 7.242(a)** A sagittal PD-weighted image of the great toe shows a subchondral fracture of the head of the first metatarsal. There is compression of the cortex, and a fluid line and abnormal marrow signal are demonstrated. The overlying articular cartilage also shows an abnormal high signal.
(b) A sagittal fat-suppressed PD-weighted image shows oedema in the subchondral bone (asterisk) and in the articular cartilage. A joint effusion is noted.

(a)　　　　(b)

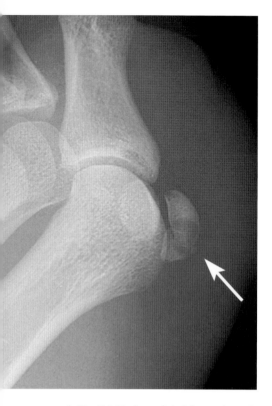

▲ **Fig. 7.243** A medial oblique view of the sesamoids shows an acute fracture of the medial sesamoid (arrow).

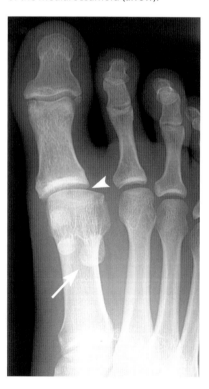

▲ **Fig. 7.245** A plain film shows retraction of both the lateral sesamoid and the proximal moiety of the medial sesamoid (arrow). There is medial subluxation of the first MTP joint, due to lateral collateral ligament rupture (arrowhead).

Conditions of the lesser toes: plantar plate rupture

The plantar plate is a thickened fibrocartilaginous portion of the MTP joint capsule that cushions the weightbearing plantar aspect of the metatarsal head and is integral to MTP joint stability. The plate must withstand tensile forces and compressive loads during walking and running. These forces are most pronounced at the second metatarsal head and are magnified by elongation of this metatarsal, hallux valgus deformity and high-heeled shoes with constricted toe boxes (Umans and Elsinger

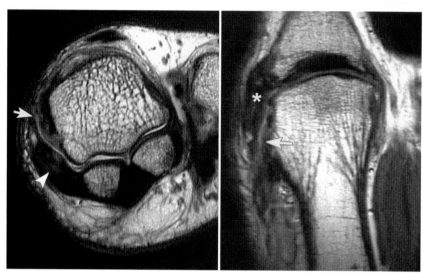

▲ **Fig. 7.244** 'Turf toe' is demonstrated in a 22-year-old rugby league player who sustained an injury six months prior to MRI. The PD-weighted images show a non-acute tear of the first metatarsal head insertion of the MCL (arrows) and medial sesamoid collateral ligament (arrowhead). There is hypertrophic scarring along the distal segment of the torn MCL (asterisk).

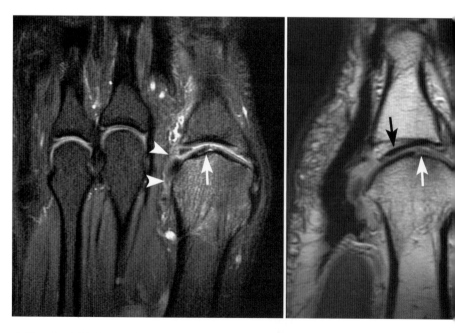

▲ **Fig. 7.246** 'Turf toe' is demonstrated by sagittal PD and axial fat-suppressed PD-weighted MR images. The images show hyperintensity indicative of capsular injury in the distribution of the LCL (arrowheads), marrow oedema within the metatarsal head, and a fluid line beneath the central articular cartilage of the metatarsal head due to basal chondral delamination (white arrow). There is also a full-thickness displaced chondral flap on the phalangeal side of the joint (black arrow).

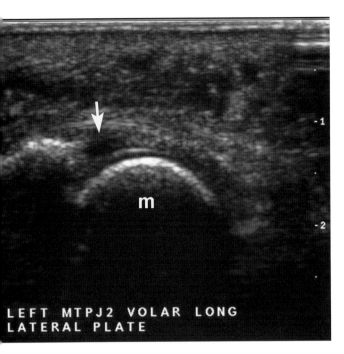

LEFT MTPJ2 VOLAR LONG
LATERAL PLATE

▲ **Fig. 7.247** Ultrasound demonstrates plantar plate rupture. A long-axis image obtained over the lateral side of the plantar plate of the second MTP joint shows an echo-free fluid gap indicative of a tear (arrow). Metatarsal head = m.

▶ **Fig. 7.248** A sagittal fat-suppressed PD image of the first MTP joint shows changes of chronic capsulosynovitis with rupture of the plantar plate. The plane of rupture is shown as a fluid line adjacent to the plantar margin of the base of the distal phalanx. An arrow indicates signal hyperintensity within the plantar plate and a joint effusion is noted.

2001). Chronic overload leads to plantar plate degeneration and attrition with eventual rupture and synovitis (see Figs 7.247 and 7.248). Ultrasound is useful for detecting plantar plate degeneration and associated capsulosynovitis, but is less reliable than MRI at directly visualising a rupture (see Fig. 7.249). Plantar plate injury may present clinically with metatarsalgia accompanied by capsular swelling and joint tenderness. At the second metatarsophalangeal joint, medial crossover deformity of the second toe is common. Rupture tends to occur at the lateral plantar plate insertion at the proximal phalanx, often in association with a tear of the phalangeal collateral ligament (Umans and Elsinger 2001).

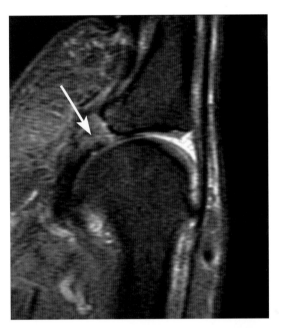

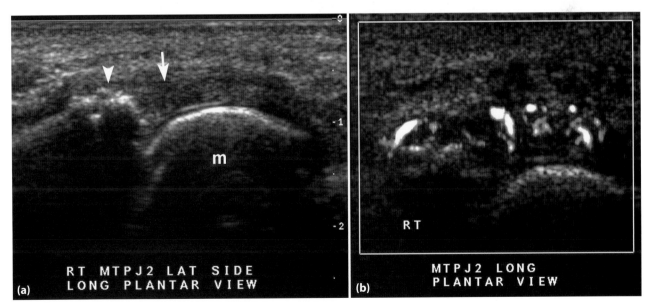

(a) RT MTPJ2 LAT SIDE LONG PLANTAR VIEW

(b) MTPJ2 LONG PLANTAR VIEW

▲ **Fig. 7.249** Plantar plate degeneration and MTP joint capsulosynovitis are demonstrated by ultrasound.
(a) A long-axis greyscale image obtained over the lateral side of the plantar plate of the second MTP joint shows mildly heterogeneous plantar plate echotexture (arrow) and degenerative enthesial bone surface irregularity at the adjacent phalangeal insertion (arrowhead). Metatarsal head = m.
(b) A corresponding Power Doppler image demonstrates florid plantar plate hyperaemia. With this pattern and degree of hyperaemia, an underlying tear of the plantar plate is likely, despite the lack of direct visualisation.

Toe deformities

'Hammer-toe', 'claw-toe' and medial crossover toe deformities are often associated with MTP joint plantar plate tears. 'Hammer-toe' deformity is a flexion deformity of the proximal interphalangeal (PIP) joint with dorsiflexion of the MTP joint and either neutral alignment or hyperextension at the distal interphalangeal (DIP) joint. This can involve multiple toes or it can be isolated to the second toe, when it is commonly associated with a hallux valgus deformity or a long second metatarsal (see Fig. 7.250).

'Claw-toe' deformity usually involves multiple toes and results from flexion contracture at the interphalangeal joints, the overall appearance being similar to 'hammer-toe' but involving a flexion deformity at the DIP joint. This can cause painful callosities over the dorsal aspect of the interphalangeal joints, MTP joint subluxations and metatarsal head overload (see Fig. 7.251).

Medial crossover deformity is characterised by hyperextension of the second toe with accompanying overlap of the great toe. This may be painful and is associated with second toe MTP joint capsular changes, which include LCL rupture, MCL shortening and medial displacement of both the plantar plate and accompanying flexor tendon. Imaging may demonstrate flexor tendinopathy or peritendinitis at the metatarsal head level (see Fig. 7.252).

The MTP joints

First MTP joint anatomy

The first MTP joint undergoes considerable loading with walking (0.4–0.6 × body weight), running (2–3 × body weight) and jumping (8 × body weight). The presence of a thick plantar capsule with fibrocartilaginous medial and lateral plantar plate and sesamoid bones all help to withstand these stresses. The sesamoids articulate with articular facets on the plantar surface of the first metatarsal head. They are linked by a thick intersesamoid ligament. The MCL complex helps withstand valgus loads and consists of the MCL proper and the medial sesamoid collateral ligament. The latter provides important stability to the medial sesamoid articulation during the toe-off phase of walking and running. The LCL complex provides stability during varus stress.

Imaging of the first MTP joint

A routine plain film series of the great toe should include AP, lateral and oblique views. In acute trauma, it can also be helpful to include both the left and right great toes on the AP view, as this can make proximal retraction of the sesamoids more conspicuous in cases of plantar plate disruption. If sesamoid pathology is suspected, an additional skyline view of the sesamoids should be obtained to enable assessment of their articulation with the first metatarsal head and their bony architecture (see Fig. 7.253).

MRI, using a small surface coil, is the imaging method of choice for examining the first MTP joint and assessing capsuloligamentous trauma, osteochondral pathology and sesamoid abnormalities (see Fig. 7.254). Accurate assessment of the capsuloligamentous complex and chondral surfaces requires high-resolution scan technique utilising an 8 cm field of view and a 2 mm slice thickness for both sagittal and axial (long-axis) images. As the orientation of the first MTP joint differs from that of the lesser MTP joints, these imaging planes must be plotted from a short-axis sequence that has first been acquired in the plane of the sesamoids.

CT is occasionally helpful in the assessment of sesamoid pathology and in the rare event of a suspected osteoid osteoma. Nuclear bone scanning can have a role in detecting sesamoiditis and marrow oedema, but lacks specificity compared to MRI (see Fig. 7.255).

Sesamoid bone stress, sesamoiditis and sesamoid fractures

Normal sesamoids vary considerably in appearance, and consequently abnormalities are often difficult to diagnose on plain film. Up to 30% of sesamoids in asymptomatic individuals are bi- or multipartite, separated by synchondroses (Biedert and

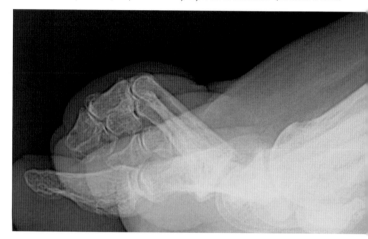

▲ **Fig. 7.250** This shows 'hammer-toe' deformity of the lesser toes.

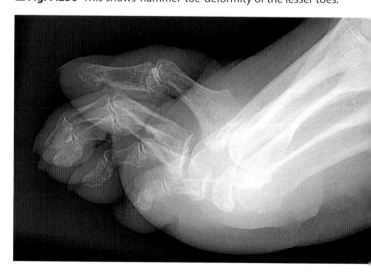

▲ **Fig. 7.251** 'Claw-toe' deformity occurs with flexion of both the proximal and distal interphalangeal joints. Callosities may develop over the dorsal aspect of the interphalangeal joints.

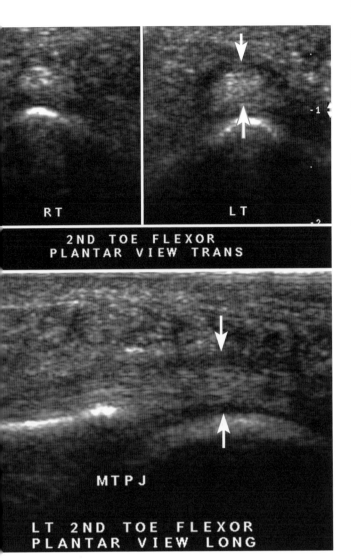

2ND TOE FLEXOR
PLANTAR VIEW TRANS

MTPJ

LT 2ND TOE FLEXOR
PLANTAR VIEW LONG

▲ **Fig. 7.252** Flexor tendinopathy of the second toe is demonstrated by ultrasound. Transverse and long-axis images obtained over the second toe flexor tendon at the MTP joint level show a segment of abnormal fusiform tendon thickening and hypoechoic peritendon thickening (arrows).

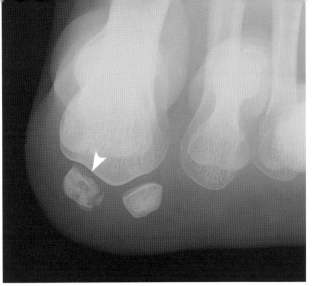

▲ **Fig. 7.253** A sesamoid view shows sesamoiditis of the medial sesamoid. There is sclerosis, fragmentation and compression of the sesamoid (arrowhead).

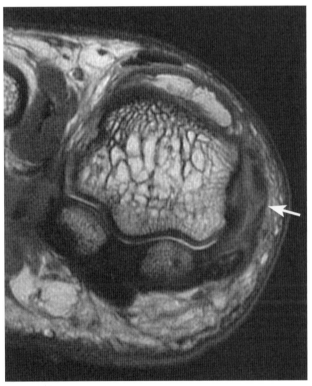

▲ **Fig. 7.254** A PD-weighted MR image demonstrates a subacute tear of the medial collateral ligament at the metatarsal head attachment (arrow).

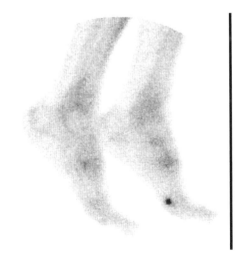
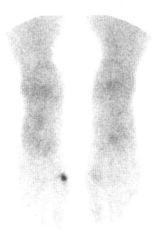

◀ **Fig. 7.255** A nuclear bone scan demonstrates increased uptake of isotope in the medial sesamoid, indicating either a fracture or sesamoiditis.

Hintermann 2003). The synchondrosis between two moieties of a bipartite sesamoid is usually about 1 mm wide and has smooth corticated margins. Nuclear bone scans, CT scanning and MRI can all play an important diagnostic role. Nuclear bone scans are non-specific and other imaging methods are required to differentiate acute fractures from stress fractures and sesamoiditis. A CT scan in the sagittal and axial planes will generally differentiate an acute fracture from a stress fracture, and MR imaging may be necessary to characterise the AVN process of sesamoiditis.

Sesamoiditis

Sesamoiditis is a post-traumatic avascular process, common in runners and dancers and particularly affecting those with a high plantar arch. Sesamoiditis presents as pain along the plantar aspect of the first MTP joint, which may be dull and is often likened to a stone bruise, although occasionally it is severe enough to interfere with walking. The pain is exacerbated by direct palpation, and tenderness is increased with dorsiflexion of the great toe. Either the medial or the lateral sesamoid can be affected, with the medial side being more often involved (Hulkko et al. 1985). The biomechanics of the injury appears to be dorsiflexion and abduction of the great toe with contraction of the flexor hallicus brevis, a movement pattern that occurs in activities such as dancing, rhythmic gymnastics and long jumping (Biedert and Hintermann 2003).

With continual loading the sesamoid undergoes an avascular evolution, with sclerosis, fragmentation and collapse eventually demonstrated on plain films and CT (see Fig. 7.256). Initially, plain films may be normal and a nuclear bone scan or MRI will help to establish the diagnosis in the early stages (see Fig. 7.257). On MRI, active bone stress of recent onset is manifest as marrow oedema on fat-suppressed sequences

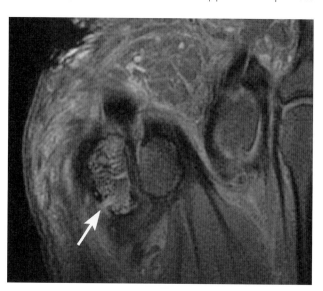

▲ **Fig. 7.257** The medial sesamoid is bifid. An axial PD-weighted MR image demonstrates a fracture in the proximal moiety (arrow).

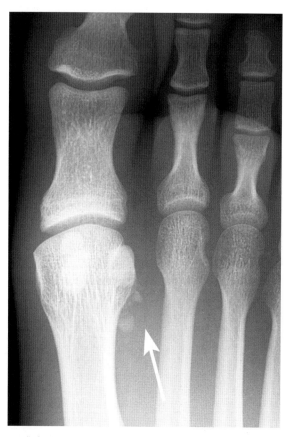

▲ **Fig. 7.256** Fragmentation of the lateral sesamoid in a cricketer (a fast bowler) results from a sesamoid stress fracture (arrow).

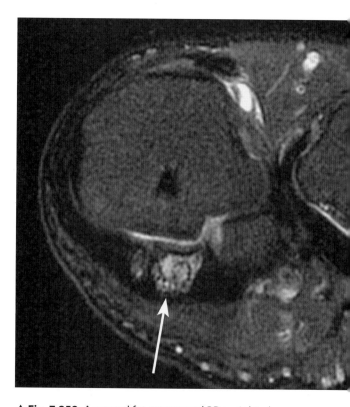

▲ **Fig. 7.258** A coronal fat-suppressed PD-weighted MR image shows marked oedema and fragmentation of the medial sesamoid (arrow). The appearance is that of sesamoiditis. The lateral sesamoid appears normal.

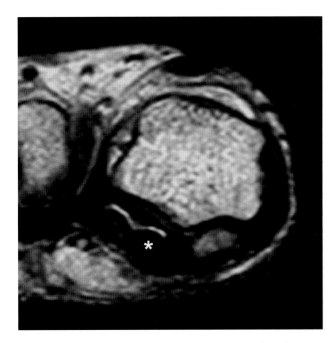

▲ **Fig. 7.259** A coronal PD-weighted MR image of the first metatarsal head shows that the lateral sesamoid is avascular, with no viable marrow fat signal demonstrated (asterisk). Fluid is noted in the joint space between the sesamoid and the metatarsal head.

(see Fig. 7.258). With chronicity and the development of sclerosis, MRI may show low signal intensity. AVN is likely when the marrow space is diffusely dark on all pulse sequences (see Fig. 7.259).

Acute sesamoid fractures

Acute sesamoid fractures are usually the result of direct trauma to the dorsum of the first MTP joint (see Fig. 7.260). Fracture lines can sometimes be difficult to distinguish from the synchondrosis of a bipartite sesamoid, and the composite size of the bipartite moieties is a helpful distinguishing feature in this situation. A nuclear bone scan followed by CT can be helpful in establishing the diagnosis of an acute fracture. Using MRI, an acutely disrupted synchondrosis shows fluid signal intensity, while intact synchondroses are only mildly hyperintense on sequences. A finding of cystic change at the margins of a synchondrosis is usually indicative of degeneration involving the synchondrosis.

Hallux valgus and metatarsus primus varus

Hallux valgus deformity is a common lesion of the first MTP joint with radiographic features including valgus angulation of the great toe, reactive overgrowth of bone at the medial aspect of the first metatarsal head with overlying soft-tissue thickening ('bunion') and degenerative osteoarthropathy at the first MTP joint. There is also lateral subluxation of the sesamoids due to erosion of the median ridge on the plantar aspect of the first metatarsal head, which normally separates the sesamoid articulations (Haines and McDougall 1954) (see Fig. 7.261).

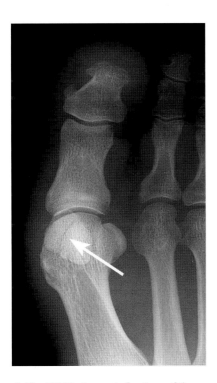

▲ **Fig. 7.260** An acute fracture of the medial sesamoid has resulted from a stomping injury to the dorsum of the first MTP joint (arrow).

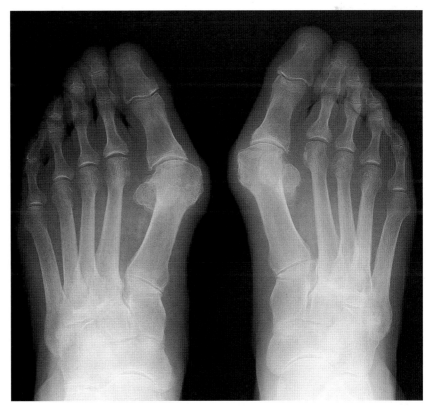

▲ **Fig. 7.261** Marked bilateral hallux valgus deformities are present.

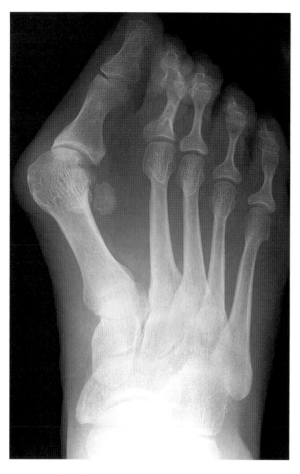

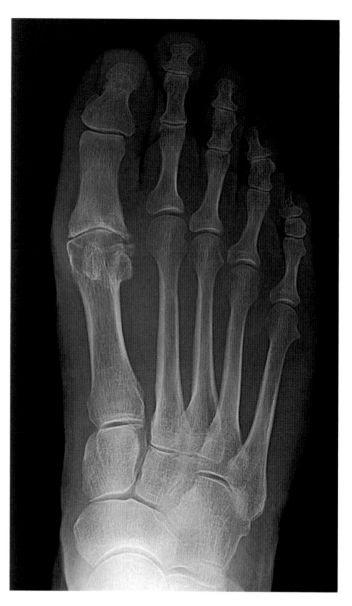

▲ **Fig. 7.262** Metatarsus primus varus deformity is present when the intermetatarsal angle between the first and second metatarsals exceeds 10°.

▶ **Fig. 7.263(a)** Hallux rigidus deformity is a painful degenerative process that involves the first TMT joint, with progressive joint space narrowing.

▼ **(b)** In addition to joint space narrowing, a characteristic of hallux rigidus deformity is the development of a spur from the dorsal aspect of the head of the first metatarsal (arrow). Clinically, dorsiflexion of the great toe is limited.

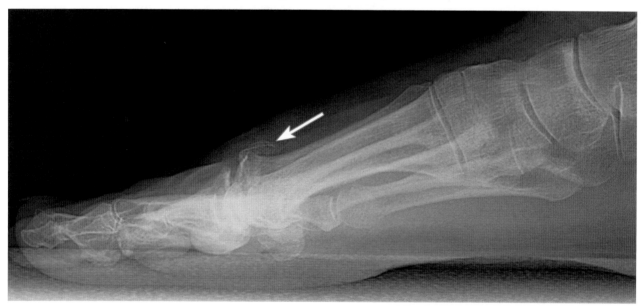

Metatarsus primus varus deformity is a developmental anomaly (splay foot) in which the first TMT joint is angled inferomedially to produce an increased gap between the first and second metatarsals (see Fig. 7.262). Hallux valgus deformity is invariably associated.

Weightbearing films should be obtained to properly assess hallux valgus and metatarsus primus varus deformities.

Hallux rigidus

Hallux rigidus is a premature degenerative condition of the great toe in which there is loss of the first MTP joint space and dorsal osteophyte formation at the metatarsal head and base of the proximal phalanx of the MTP joint of the great toe (see Fig. 7.263). Resulting impingement causes pain and limitation of dorsiflexion of the great toe.

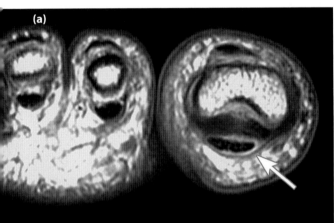

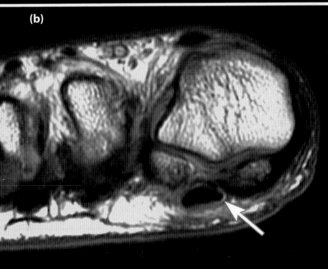

▲ **Fig. 7.264** Coronal PD-weighted images obtained at the level of the neck **(a)** and head **(b)** of the first metatarsal demonstrate changes of distal FHL tenosynovitis. Effusions surround the tendon at both levels (arrows).

Distal FHL tenosynovitis

Distal FHL tenosynovitis is a rare condition occurring at the level of the first metatarsal head in runners. The pathology involves the segment of FHL tendon that passes between the sesamoids, and is usually 'stenosing' in type with an associated restriction of great toe flexion (Gould 1981). The differential diagnosis includes an overlying plantar fat pad bursopathy (see Fig. 7.264).

Metatarsal fractures

Metatarsal fractures are a common sporting injury, frequently resulting from overuse and occasionally from acute trauma.

Acute fractures

The metatarsals are supported by intermetatarsal ligaments and intrinsic muscles, providing stabilisation that will, in most cases, reduce displacement of metatarsal shaft fractures, unless this inherent soft-tissue support is also compromised. Traction exerted by the flexor tendon tends to displace fractures of the metatarsal neck by rotating the metatarsal head in a plantar direction (see Fig. 7.265). This displacement may be important, as subsequent malunion can alter foot biomechanics and result in metatarsalgia or plantar keratosis (Asherman 2000).

Acute fractures may also involve the proximal shaft of the metatarsals, 1.5–3.0 cm from their base, often the result of jumping down onto a hard surface. These fractures are of particular interest, due to a tendency to delayed union (see Fig. 7.266). Fractures of the fifth metatarsal at this site characteristically present management problems due to either delayed union or non-union (see Fig. 7.267). These fractures were first described by Robert Jones in 1902 and are known as 'Jones' fractures. The mechanism of injury involves an adduction force applied to a grounded forefoot with the ankle in plantar flexion (Landorf 1999). The Jones fracture has a transverse orientation and is differentiated from a stress fracture by the absence of bony sclerosis at the fracture site. There is thought to be a relatively poor blood supply in this region and delayed union is common, often requiring bone grafting and internal fixation. It has been suggested that the relative avascularity of the proximal shaft of the fifth metatarsal is due to small-calibre vessels and that these are compressed during weightbearing (Acker and Drez 1986). Roca et al. (1980) also proposed that there is tensile stress occurring in the lateral aspect of the cortex in this area, produced by contraction of the peroneus brevis, and that this stress contributes to delayed healing.

Another fracture of the fifth metatarsal is of particular interest. A spiral fracture of the distal shaft and neck of the fifth metatarsal is known as a 'dancer's fracture' (O'Malley et al. 1996). Traditionally this is a ballet injury, occurring as an inversion injury as the dancer fell from a demi-pointe position. However, this fracture is also commonly seen in many other sporting activities (see Figs 7.268 and 7.269).

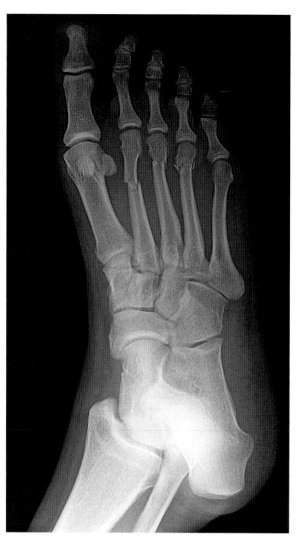

◀ **Fig. 7.265(a)** Fractures of the distal shaft of the second metatarsal and the necks of the third and fourth metatarsal have resulted from jumping onto a hard surface. The distal fragments are displaced or angled in a plantar direction by traction by the flexor tendon.

▼ **(b)** This shows fractures involving the heads of the second to fifth metatarsals. Involvement of the articular surface will predispose to early degenerative changes.

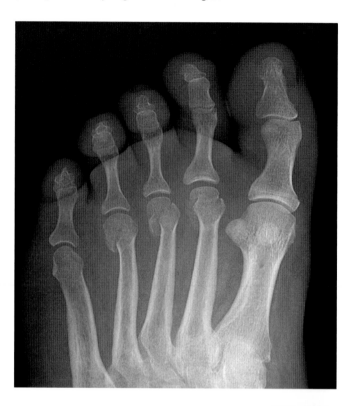

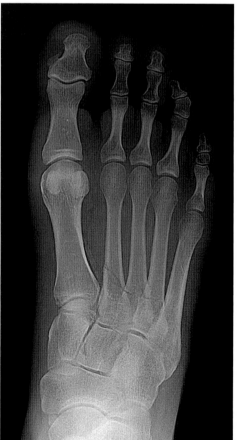

◀ **Fig. 7.266(a)** Fractures involving the proximal shafts of the second, third and fourth metatarsals were caused by jumping onto a hard surface. Fractures 1.5–3 cm from the metatarsal bases may have difficulty healing and signs of delayed or non-union can develop.

▶ **(b)** A fracture of the base of the fifth metatarsal has progressed to non-union. The fracture margins have developed well-defined cortical margins, with fragment separation.

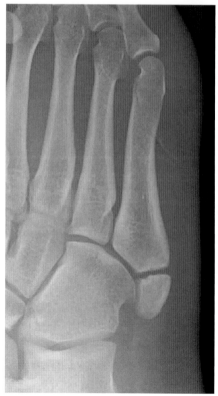

▶ **Fig. 7.267(a)** A Jones fracture is an acute transverse fracture of the proximal shaft of the fifth metatarsal in an area of poor blood supply.
(b) The same fracture imaged six weeks later shows delayed union, with bony resorption at the fracture margins. Cystic changes are also developing (arrow). Internal fixation is often required to help achieve a satisfactory outcome.

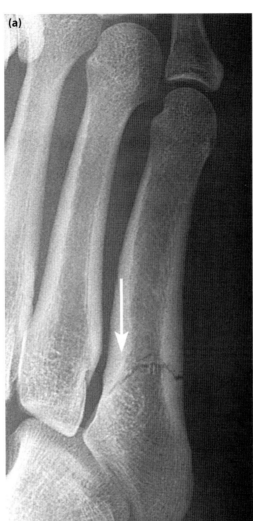

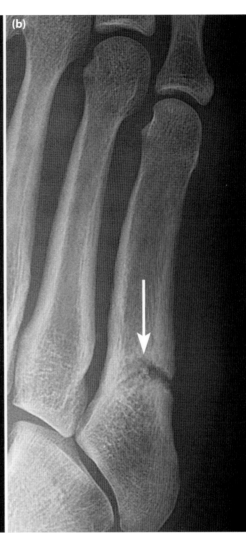

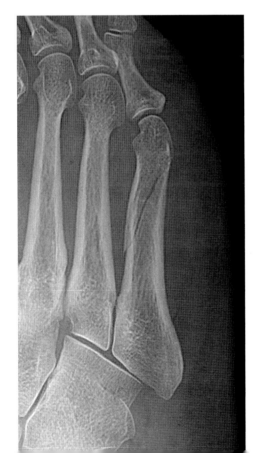

◀ **Fig. 7.268** A spiral fracture of the distal shaft of the fifth metatarsal is encountered in sport due to a twisting force to the foot. This fracture is known as a 'dancer's fracture' because it characteristically occurs in dancing. In this case, the fracture is undisplaced.

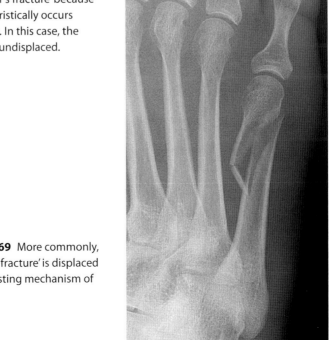

▶ **Fig. 7.269** More commonly, a 'dancer's fracture' is displaced by the twisting mechanism of the injury.

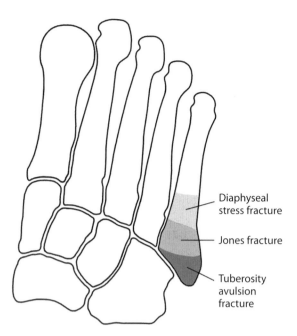

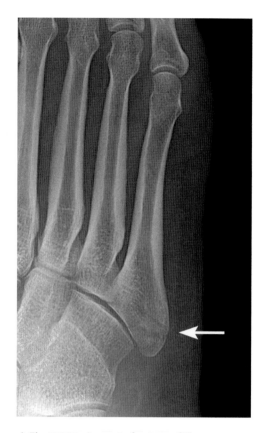

▲ **Fig. 7.270** This line drawing demonstrates the areas of the fifth metatarsal involved by a styloid process avulsion fracture, a Jones fracture and a fifth metatarsal stress fracture.

Fractures of the proximal fifth metatarsal

The most common injury of the fifth metatarsal is a transversely oriented avulsion fracture involving the styloid process at the base of the fifth metatarsal (see Fig. 7.270). These fractures extend across the styloid process and may involve the fifth TMT joint (see Fig. 7.271). An avulsion fracture of the styloid process should not be confused with a normal unfused apophysis, which has a longitudinal orientation and is located on the lateral aspect of the base of the fifth metatarsal (see Fig. 7.272). The peroneus brevis, peroneus tertius, adductor digiti minimi and the lateral band of the plantar aponeurosis all insert into the base of the fifth metatarsal.

An avulsion fracture at the base of the fifth metatarsal is a common injury caused by a sudden pull of the peroneus brevis tendon or plantar aponeurosis attachments during plantar flexion and inversion of the foot (Richli and Rosenthal 1984). The apophysis at the base of the fifth metatarsal can also occasionally be avulsed (see Fig. 7.273(a)) or fractured (see Fig. 7.273(b)).

Stress fractures

Metatarsal stress fractures are very common in athletes and account for 2–28% of all stress fractures (Johnson et al. 1999). At the Sydney 2000 Olympics, metatarsal stress fractures represented 23.3% of all bone stress imaged (Flahive and Anderson 2004). The proposed causes include muscle fatigue resulting in loss of ability to absorb shock, and repetitive bone stress due to muscular contraction producing osteoclastic activity that eventually overwhelms the new bone formation. Stress fractures can involve any of the metatarsals and the majority will heal without problems. The most common stress fractures involve the distal shaft or neck of the second and third metatarsals (see Fig. 7.274).

▶ **Fig. 7.272** A normal apophysis of the styloid process has a vertical orientation (arrowhead). There is also a fracture of the styloid process, which passes horizontally across the process (arrow).

▲ **Fig. 7.271** An acute fracture of the styloid process of the fifth metatarsal is characteristically caused by an inversion injury of the ankle and is a commonly missed fracture. The fracture passes transversely across the styloid process to involve the fifth TMT joint (arrow).

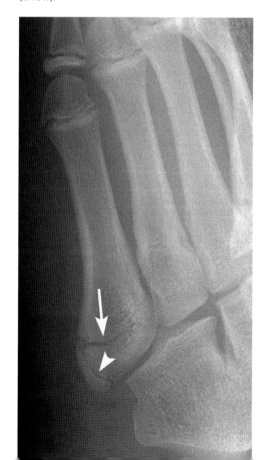

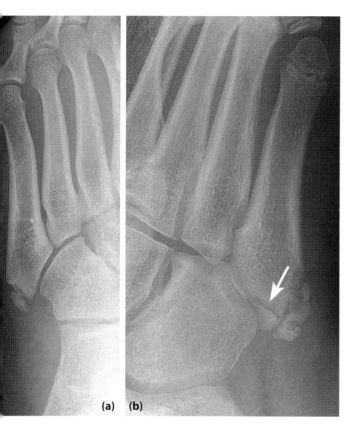

▲ **Fig. 7.273(a)** Avulsion of the apophysis occasionally occurs. **(b)** The apophysis may also be fractured. A styloid process fracture (arrow) passes horizontally across the process and through the apophysis.

Certain fractures are of special interest, because delayed union and non-union are common complications that can have a devastating outcome for an athlete. These fractures include stress fractures at the junction of the metaphysis and diaphysis of the third, fourth and fifth metatarsals, which are further discussed below. Stress fractures at the base of the second metatarsal are of particular interest, since these are prone to occur in ballerinas and are potentially a career-ending injury.

The diagnosis of metatarsal bone stress reactions and stress fractures is usually straightforward. A suspicion of bone stress is raised by the onset of exercise-induced pain, which is relieved by rest, and the development of localised bone tenderness. If the diagnosis is made before an actual fracture line has appeared, an early return to full activity can be anticipated. Early in the bone stress continuum, plain films are normal and either a nuclear bone scan or MRI scan is necessary to confirm the clinical diagnosis (see Fig. 7.275).

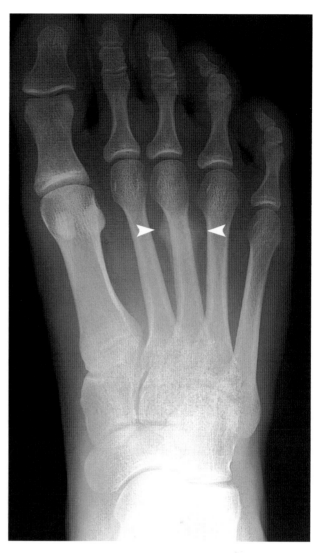

▲ **Fig. 7.274** A stress fracture of the distal shaft of the third metatarsal is a common metatarsal stress fracture. In this case there is considerable periosteal new bone (arrowheads).

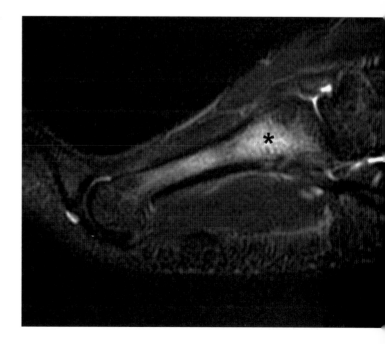

▶ **Fig. 7.275** An athlete competing at the Sydney 2000 Olympics presented with discomfort in the first MTP joint on push-off. A sagittal STIR MR image of the first metatarsal shows extensive high marrow signal (asterisk), indicative of bone stress. No fracture could be seen on a subsequent CT scan.

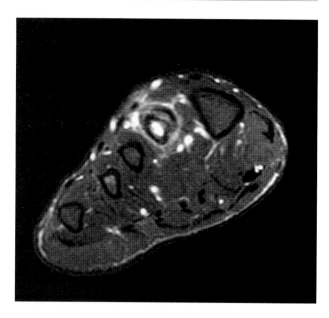

▲ **Fig. 7.276** A coronal STIR MR image of a track and field athlete competing at the Sydney 2000 Olympics shows an established stress fracture of the second metatarsal, involving the medial cortex with slight displacement. Note the surrounding high signal, indicating oedema in the periosteum and adjacent soft tissues.

Stress fractures occur less frequently in the first metatarsal than in the lesser metatarsals (Johnson et al. 1999). The second and third rays are most often affected (see Fig. 7.276). The second metatarsal accounts for just over 50% of metatarsal stress fractures, and the third metatarsal accounts for about 40%. Asymptomatic generalised cortical thickening along the shafts of the second and third metatarsals is a legacy of chronic bone stress and is extremely common in athletes (see Fig. 7.277).

Stress fractures of the second metatarsal

Stress fractures commonly involve the neck or shaft of the second metatarsal (see Figs. 7.278 and 7.279). In addition, there are two types of stress fractures that involve the base of the second metatarsal. The first type is a transverse fracture that occurs at the junction of the metaphysis and the diaphysis about 7 mm from the articular surface, without involving the second TMT joint (see Fig. 7.280). This stress fracture is similar to the Jones fracture of the fifth metatarsal and is extremely difficult to heal. The second type extends into the second TMT joint. This is an important stress fracture that is also resistant to healing. This fracture is oblique in orientation and occurs in a characteristic position (Harrington et al. 1993). The fracture plane is orientated at 90° to the direction of pull of the Lisfranc ligament, suggesting that stress applied by this ligament plays a role in the biomechanics of injury. These oblique stress fractures occur in classical ballet and jumping sports. In ballet, there is an association with the en pointe position, particularly if the ballerina has a short first

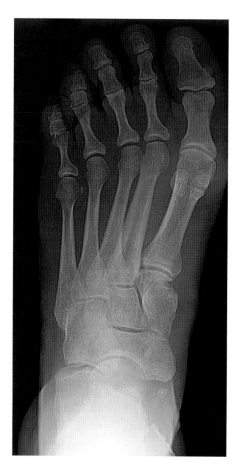

▲ **Fig. 7.277** Generalised cortical hypertrophy of the second metatarsal results from recurrent stress and is common in the sporting population.

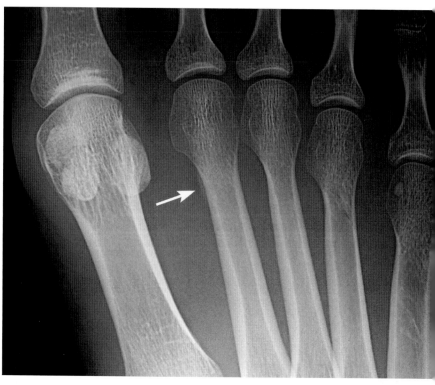

▲ **Fig. 7.278** A subtle periosteal reaction is the earliest plain film sign of a stress fracture of the neck of the second metatarsal (arrow). High-quality plain films are necessary to detect these subtleties.

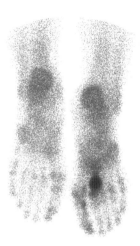

▲ **Fig. 7.279** A nuclear bone scan demonstrates a stress fracture of the mid-shaft of the second metatarsal.

metatarsal (Morton's foot). As previously noted, if this anomaly is present, the loading that occurs en pointe is transmitted along the second ray alone.

If a stress fracture is clinically suspected, a routine plain film foot series should include a plantodorsal projection of the TMT region. This additional view is helpful for demonstrating the base of the second metatarsal and the second TMT joint (see Fig. 7.281). If the plain films are normal, a nuclear bone scan or MRI is then required to confirm the presence of a fracture (see Fig. 7.282). A CT examination is able to show a frank fracture, but cannot detect the marrow changes that

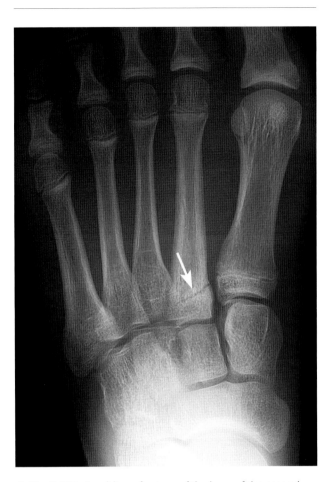

▲ **Fig. 7.281** An oblique fracture of the base of the second metatarsal is well demonstrated by a plantodorsal view of the tarsometatarsal region (arrow). The fracture extends to involve the articular surface at the base of the metatarsal.

▼ **Fig. 7.280** This shows a transverse stress fracture of the proximal shaft/base of the second metatarsal (arrowheads). There is also a stress fracture of the neck of the third metatarsal (arrow).

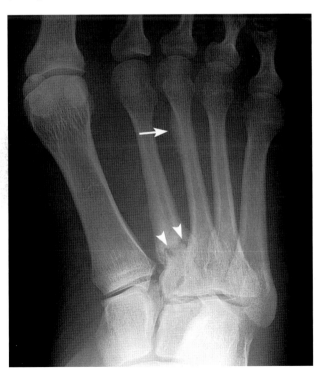

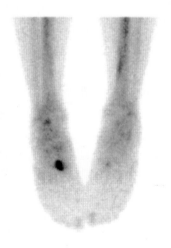

▲ **Fig. 7.282** A nuclear bone scan shows increased uptake of isotope at the second TMT joint. This may indicate a stress fracture, bone stress reaction or synovitis. An MRI examination is necessary to help characterise the change, as management differs for each condition.

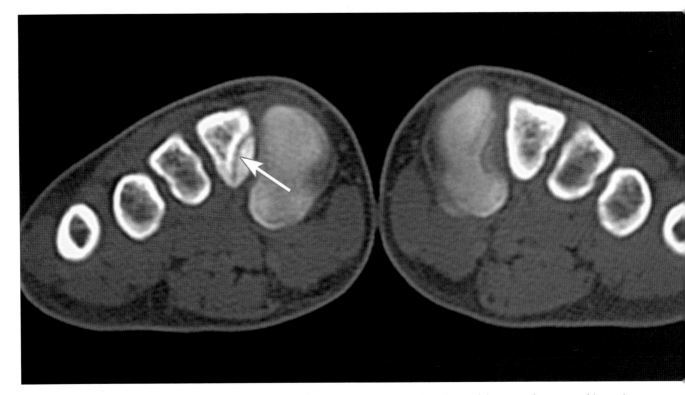

▲ **Fig. 7.283** A CT scan shows the characteristic configuration of a stress fracture of the base of the second metatarsal (arrow). The location and axis of the fracture correspond with the direction of traction exerted by the Lisfranc ligament and the fracture is presumably the result of repetitive stress applied by the ligament.

typify an early stress reaction (see Fig. 7.283). Consequently, MRI is the most useful imaging method for the differentiation of bone stress reaction from stress fracture and TMT joint synovitis (see Fig. 7.284). All three conditions will produce a positive nuclear bone scan of similar appearance.

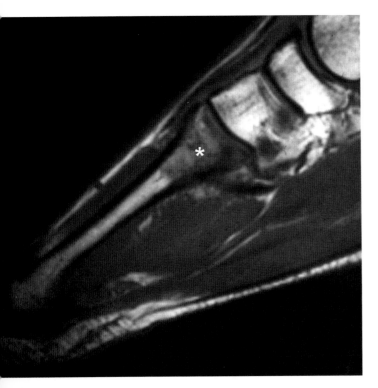

Stress fractures of the base of the fourth metatarsal

The clinical course of fractures involving the fourth metatarsal at the metaphyseal-diaphyseal junction is similar to that occurring with the Jones fracture of the fifth metatarsal. Saxena et al. (2001) reported five cases of this fracture and showed that all had prolonged healing. It was suggested that the anatomy of the metatarsal base contributed to the delayed healing. The long plantar ligament and a secondary slip of the tibialis posterior tendon both attach to the base of the fourth metatarsal, each exerting traction stress, predisposing to delay union. Theodorou et al. (1999) described an association between metatarsus adductus and stress fractures of the lateral metatarsals.

Stress fractures of the base of the fifth metatarsal

Stress fractures may also occur in the region of a Jones fracture, although it has been noted that stress fractures tend to occur slightly more distally than acute fractures and are often about 3 cm from the base (Landorf 1999). Stress fractures are most often seen in runners, are prone to delayed union or non-union (see Fig. 7.285) and may progress to complete fractures (see Fig. 7.286).

◀**Fig. 7.284** A sagittal T1-weighted MR image of the second metatarsal in a ballerina shows abnormal marrow signal in the base and proximal shaft (asterisk). No fracture line can be detected. The appearance is that of bone stress.

▶ **Fig. 7.285(a)** This is the typical appearance of a stress fracture of the fifth metatarsal, occurring in a middle-distance runner. There is cortical hypertrophy and a transverse fracture extending from the lateral margin (arrow). Such fractures have difficulty healing and may progress to a complete fracture. **(b)** A stress fracture in a track and field athlete appears to be progressing to a complete fracture and shows definite changes of delayed or possible non-union.

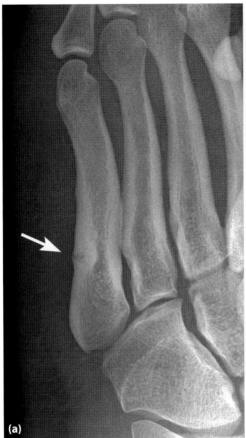
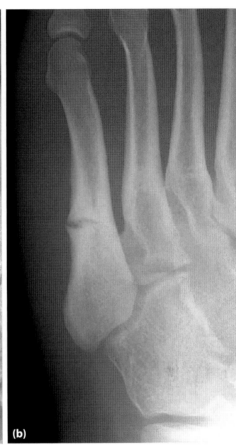

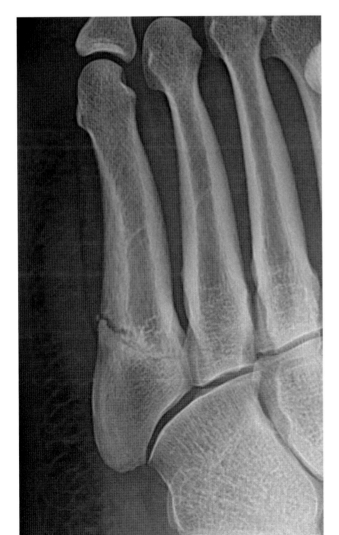

◀ **Fig. 7.286** This fifth metatarsal stress fracture has progressed to a complete fracture.

Other conditions of the forefoot

Freiberg's infraction

In the skeletally immature athlete, an osteochondritis may develop in the epiphysis of the head of the second, third or fourth metatarsals. There is a preponderance of this condition in females by a ratio of 5:1. The radiographic appearance is that of an avascular process with sclerosis, fragmentation and collapse occurring just before or as the epiphyses are closing (see Figs 7.287, 7.288 and 7.289).

It should be noted that although this condition is most common in adolescence, Freiberg's infraction may occur after the metatarsal epiphyses have closed (see Fig. 7.290).

Bunionette formation

A bunionette is a painful prominence at the lateral aspect of the fifth MTP joint that is a less pronounced mirror image of hallux valgus deformity (Karasick 1995). It is due to chronic adventitial bursopathy over a prominence produced by splaying of the forefoot, lateral bowing of the fifth metatarsal or an enlarged metatarsal head (see Fig. 7.291).

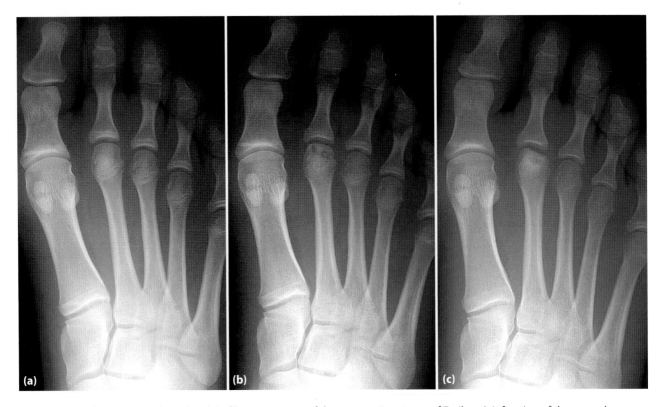

▲ **Fig. 7.287** These images show the plain film appearance of the progressive stages of Freiberg's infraction of the second metatarsal.

(a) There is increased density of the epiphysis of the second metatarsal head. This is typical of an avascular change. The appearance is otherwise normal.

(b) With progression of the avascular process, there is fragmentation and compression of the sclerotic epiphysis.

(c) Healing has now occurred and the deformity is permanent. The growth plate is closed.

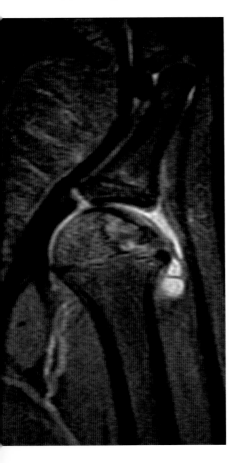

◀**Fig. 7.288** A sagittal fat-suppressed PD-weighted MR image shows a sharp sclerotic line of demarcation between the normal and avascular areas of the epiphysis. The articular surface over the abnormal area has become depressed and fragmentation is noted. An effusion is present.

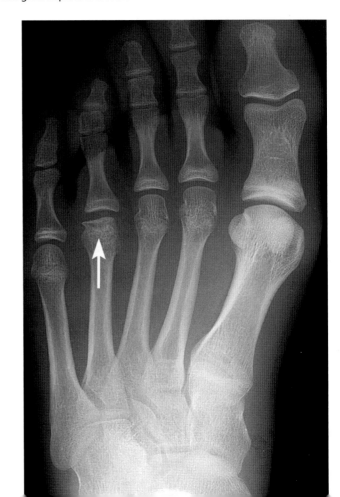

▶**Fig. 7.289** Any of the second to fifth metatarsals may be involved. Here the fourth metatarsal is involved (arrow).

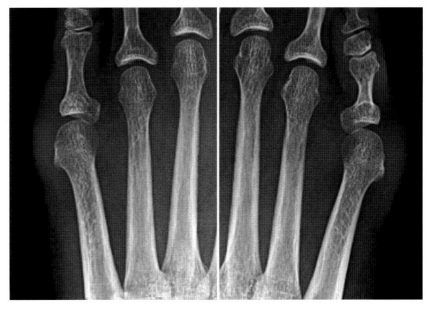

▲ **Fig. 7.291** Bilateral bunionettes are present, associated with lateral prominence of the fifth metatarsal heads. Note the lateral soft-tissue thickening over the lateral aspect of the metatarsal heads bilaterally.

Painful os intermetatarseum

The os intermetatarseum is an accessory ossicle that occurs at the dorsal margin of the interval between the bases of the first and second metatarsals (see Fig. 7.292). It has an incidence rate of approximately 3% and, rarely, may be symptomatic. Symptomatic cases may show increased uptake of isotope on a nuclear bone scan or bone marrow oedema on MRI. It should be noted that a branch of the deep peroneal nerve passes superficial to the os, and if the os protrudes dorsally as shown in Fig. 7.292(b), associated irritation from footwear may contribute to the symptoms.

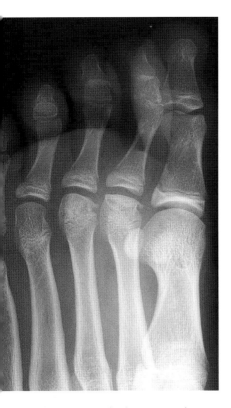

▲ **Fig. 7.290** Multiple metatarsal epiphyses may be involved. In this case, Freiberg's infraction involves the second and third metatarsal epiphyses.

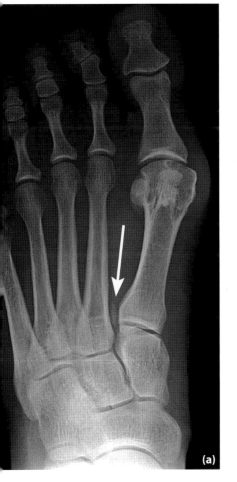

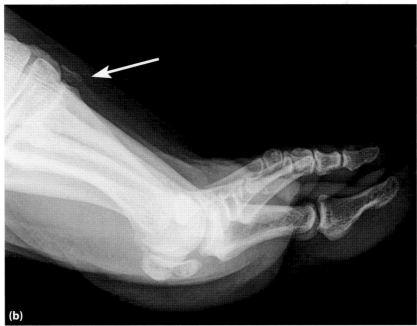

◄▲ **Fig. 7.292(a)** An os intermetatarseum is present on the dorsal aspect of the interspace between the first and second metatarsals (arrow).
(b) The os may protrude dorsally as shown in this lateral view (arrow).

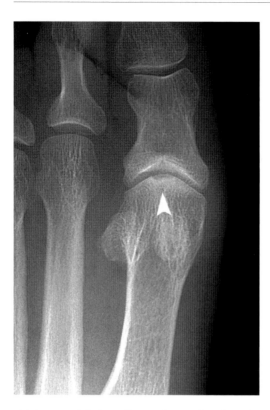

▲ Fig. 7.293(a) A small area of osteochondritis dissecans has developed in the articular surface of the first metatarsal head (arrowhead). The area is well demarcated and sclerotic changes are noted in the surrounding bone.

▼ (b) Osteochondritis dissecans is present in the medial aspect of the articular surface of the second metatarsal head (arrowhead).

Osteochondritis dissecans of the MTP joints

Changes of osteochondritis dissecans occasionally affect the heads and bases of the first and second metatarsals (see Figs 7.293 and 7.294).

Morton's neuroma

Morton's neuroma is a common cause of metatarsalgia. The underlying lesion is a degenerative thickening of the common digital nerve with accompanying endoneural fibrosis and mucoid degeneration in loosely adherent perineural fibroadipose tissue. The contiguous intermetatarsal bursa also shows increased ground substance in the subsynovial lining and areas of fibrinoid degeneration and necrosis in the bursal lining (Bossley and Cairney 1980). A small amount of watery fluid is often present within the bursa and can be appreciated on pre-operative imaging. This condition most often affects the third or second web spaces, and is regarded as an entrapment neuropathy caused by repetitive compression of the common digital nerve against the transverse metatarsal ligament. Females are more frequently affected than males, the highest incidence rate occurs in mid-life, and multiple web spaces of both feet are commonly involved. The diagnosis and localisation of a Morton's neuroma is usually clinical, but ultrasound or MRI can assist whenever the physical findings are atypical or localisation to a particular web space is difficult (Kaminsky et al. 1997; Read et al. 1999) (see Figs 7.295 and 7.296).

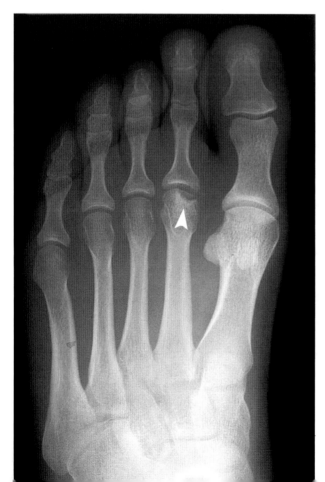

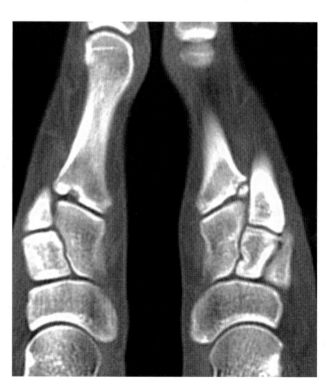

▲ Fig. 7.294 Small areas of osteochondritis dissecans have developed in the articular surface at the base of both first metatarsals.

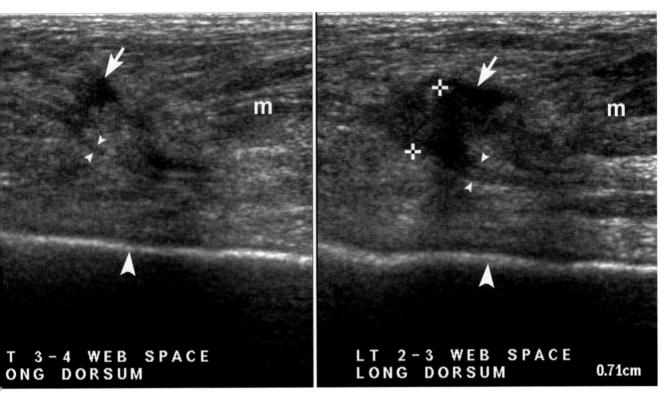

T 3-4 WEB SPACE
ONG DORSUM

LT 2-3 WEB SPACE
LONG DORSUM 0.71cm

▲ **Fig. 7.295(a)** A Morton's neuroma is demonstrated by ultrasound. Long-axis views have been obtained over the dorsal aspect of the second and third web spaces (respectively) of the left foot at the MTP joint level. An ovoid hypoechoic thickening of the common digital nerve is demonstrated within the second web space, measuring 7 mm in dorsiplantar diameter (indicated by + callipers). This appearance is consistent with a Morton's neuroma. The normal third web space is included for comparison. Long-axis imaging from the dorsal aspect of the foot provides an excellent global overview of web space anatomy in the orientation of the affected nerve, but can nevertheless occasionally be difficult due to beam-thickness artefact creating an area of acoustic shadowing in patients with a narrow interspace. Small arrowheads indicate the common digital nerves. Large arrowheads indicate the plantar skin surface. Arrows indicate the intermetatarsal bursae. Interosseous muscle = m.

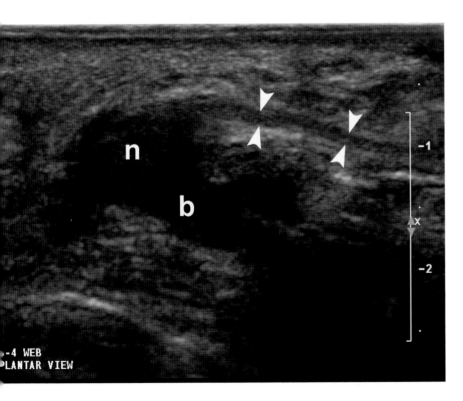

-4 WEB
PLANTAR VIEW

◀ **(b)** A further example of a Morton's neuroma is demonstrated by ultrasound. A long-axis view has been obtained over the plantar aspect of the third web space at the MTP joint level. An ovoid hypoechoic thickening (n) of the common digital nerve is demonstrated, and the appearance is consistent with a Morton's neuroma. Arrowheads indicate the normal segment of common digital nerve proximal to the neuroma. Fluid is seen within the adjacent intermetatarsal bursa (b). Imaging from the plantar aspect of the foot better demonstrates the digital nerve, and is essential when a narrow metatarsal interspace makes imaging from the dorsal aspect difficult. However, this approach offers a less effective understanding of overall web space anatomy.

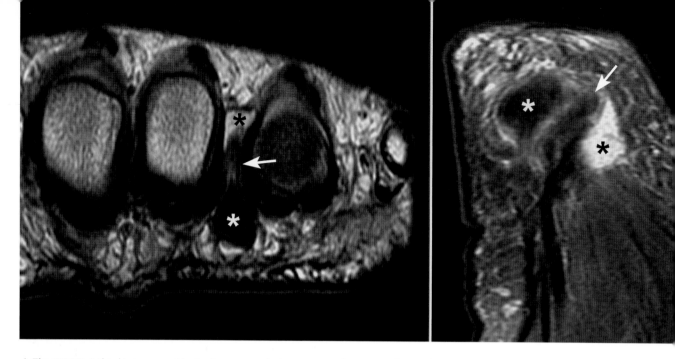

▲ **Fig. 7.296** A third interspace Morton's neuroma is demonstrated on coronal T2 and sagittal fat-suppressed PD-weighted MR images (white asterisks). Note the perineural mucoid degenerative thickening (arrows) and effusion within the adjacent intermetatarsal bursa (black asterisks).

Therapeutic injection of a Morton's neuroma under ultrasound control, coupled with an appropriate orthotic, allows successful conservative management in many patients. A study by Maja Markovic (personal communication, 2007) showed that 66% of patients had a positive outcome nine months after injection and did not require surgery. The method of injection under ultrasound control is discussed with images (see Fig. 7.297).

Plain films are usually normal, although they remain important for the exclusion of other potential causes of metatarsalgia, such as metatarsal stress fractures, or Freiberg's infraction. It must be appreciated that small neuromata can sometimes be missed by ultrasound and MRI, particularly by inexperienced operators. Consequently a negative scan will not exclude the diagnosis. Furthermore, a clinically obvious neuroma probably does not require imaging (Sharp, Wade

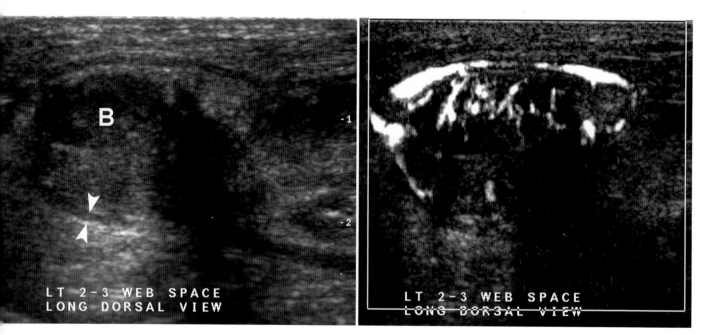

▲ **Fig. 7.297** Ultrasound demonstrates an inflammatory intermetatarsal bursopathy. A long-axis greyscale image obtained over the dorsal aspect of the second web space shows an ovoid hypoechoic soft-tissue thickening (B) that superficially simulates a Morton's neuroma in both position and appearance. A corresponding Power Doppler image demonstrates florid hyperaemia, which is atypical for Morton's neuroma and is more in keeping with intermetatarsal bursopathy. This case proved to be the initial presentation of psoriatic arthritis. Arrowheads indicate the common digital nerve, which remains normal in size and distinct from the adjacent bursal change. This is another important differentiating feature from a Morton's neuroma.

et al. 2003). Small neuromata may also be asymptomatic. An imaging size of 5 mm has been suggested as the threshold beyond which a neuroma is likely to cause symptoms (Redd et al. 1989). Mistaking an inflammatory intermetatarsal bursopathy as a neuroma is a potential pitfall in sonographic diagnosis and Power Doppler interrogation is an important aid in avoiding this error.

Acute sports-related injuries of the mid-foot

Mid-foot injuries are uncommon. When the injury is the result of high-energy trauma, the resultant disruption of integrity is usually easily recognised. Ligamentous, articular, bony and soft-tissue injury can occur alone or in combination. The injuries are rarely isolated and there is commonly an extension into neighbouring structures. It is important to remember to search for associated forefoot and hind-foot injuries, as the mechanics of the trauma will generally affect more than a single area. Mid-foot injuries include fractures of the navicular, cuboid and cuneiforms and injury to the transverse tarsal and TMT joints.

Lisfranc fracture-dislocations

Traumatic injuries of the TMT joint complex may not only include the TMT articulations, but also extend into the mid-foot to include the cuneiforms, cuboid and navicular with disruption of the intercuneiform, cuneiform-cuboid and naviculocuneiform joints (Myerson et al. 1986) (see Fig. 7.298). The stability of this complex requires both intact bony architecture and intact ligamentous supports. An important feature of the bony architecture is the transverse arch created by the alignment of the three cuneiforms and the cuboid, with a mortise formed by the recessed intermediate cuneiform, into which the base of the second metatarsal is locked by the Lisfranc ligament. This provides rigid stability to the junction of the mid-foot and forefoot and is the key to Lisfranc injury (Peicha et al. 2002). A shallow mortise predisposes to a Lisfranc fracture-dislocation. The TMT joints are supported by a vast network of dense plantar ligaments, interosseous ligaments and capsular structures. The Lisfranc ligament is the largest and strongest of the interosseous ligaments, coursing obliquely from the plantolateral aspect of the medial cuneiform to the plantomedial aspect of the second metatarsal base. Intermetatarsal ligaments pass between the bases of the second to fifth metatarsals providing important stability, but there is no intermetatarsal ligament between the bases of the first and second metatarsals.

A spectrum of injury to the Lisfranc ligament is possible, ranging from a stable sprain to laxity or fracture-dislocation. Sports-related trauma producing these injuries usually involves axial loading of the foot while in a position of extreme plantar flexion. Such an injury may occur in a fall where the plantar-flexed foot folds beneath the athlete, and is then compressed by the athlete's body weight or the weight of another athlete. This typically occurs in sports such as football, basketball and gymnastics (Faciszewski et al. 1990; Thompson

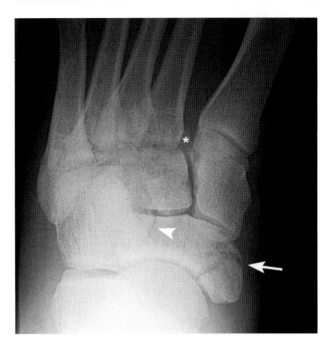

▲ **Fig. 7.298** A large bone fragment has been avulsed from the lateral border of the medial cuneiform (asterisk) by the Lisfranc ligament and there is lateral subluxation of the second TMT joint. This TMT joint complex injury extends into the mid-foot to involve the articulation between the medial and middle cuneiforms, and there is a fracture of the body (arrowhead) and tuberosity of the navicular (arrow). There is also disruption of the naviculocuneiform joints.

and Mormino 2003). Other less common mechanisms can include minimal twisting trauma and forceful forefoot abduction. Most sports-related Lisfranc injuries are low energy and the clinical and radiographic findings are subtle. The patient usually complains of forefoot pain, particularly with weightbearing. There may be swelling and ecchymosis at the plantar aspect of the mid-foot, tenderness over the TMT joints, and pain on passive abduction and pronation of the forefoot (Curtis et al. 1993). In high-energy injuries, the pattern of fracture-dislocation is highly variable but fractures are often multiple and comminuted.

Lisfranc fracture-dislocations have been classified as:

- homolateral, in which the TMT subluxations all occur in the same direction (see Fig. 7.299)
- divergent, in which the first TMT joint is displaced medially and separated from the other TMT joints, which are displaced laterally (see Fig. 7.300).

In Vouri and Aro's (1993) series of 66 cases, 95% had metatarsal fractures. The second metatarsal was the most frequently injured. This injury is more common than has been reported (Shapiro et al. 1994). In addition to a transverse disruption of the TMT joints, the disruption may occasionally be longitudinal, producing a deformity known as a 'sagittal diastasis', characterised by widening of the gap between the first and second metatarsal bases and the medial intercuneiform interval (Mantas and Burks 1994) (see Fig. 7.301). With both patterns of injury, extension can occur into neighbouring areas.

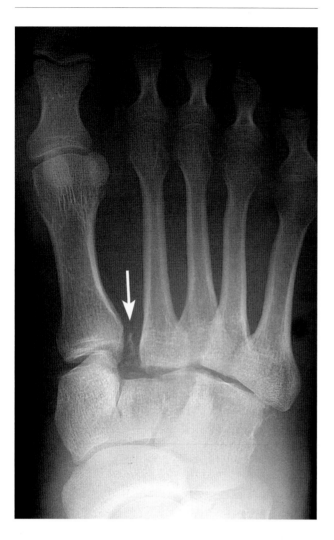

◀ **Fig. 7.299** A Judo player at the Sydney 2000 Olympics presented with a stomping injury to the foot. A homolateral Lisfranc fracture-dislocation is demonstrated, with lateral subluxation of all TMT joints. A number of bone fragments have been avulsed by the Lisfranc ligament (arrow). Note that the articulation between the middle and lateral cuneiforms is also disrupted, with deformity of the mortise for the base of the second metatarsal.

▼ **Fig. 7.300** A divergent Lisfranc fracture-dislocation of the TMT joints is well demonstrated using the plantodorsal technique. The base of the first metatarsal is displaced slightly medially, while the remaining TMT joints are subluxed laterally. Disruption of the articulation between the navicular and medial cuneiform is also present. Note the small avulsed ossicles (arrow).

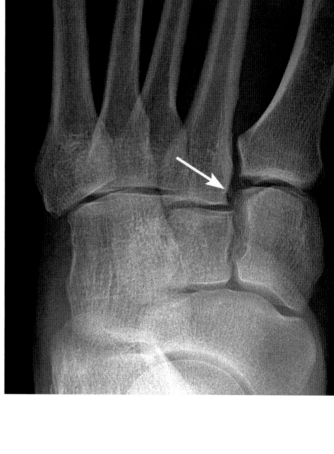

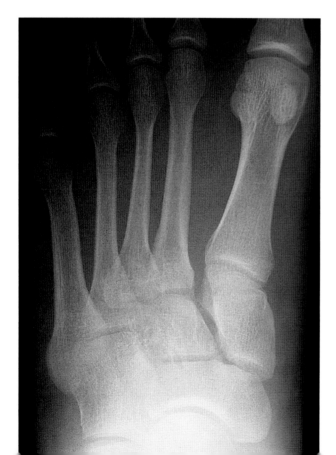

◀ **Fig. 7.301** A sagittal diastasis occurs when the force on the tarsometatarsal region is vertical, rather than transverse. There is widening of the space between the bases of the first and second metatarsals and this disruption characteristically continues proximally to widen the joint between the middle and medial cuneiforms. In this case, the force has continued and the articulation between the navicular and the medial cuneiform is also widened, with medial subluxation of the medial cuneiform.

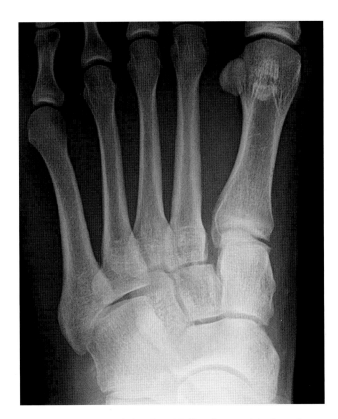

▲ **Fig. 7.302** A weightbearing AP film shows widening of the space between the first and second metatarsals and subluxation of the second, third, fourth and fifth MTP joints.

Imaging a Lisfranc injury

Plain films are an important initial step in imaging a Lisfranc injury and will more often than not provide the correct diagnosis if obtained with care. Cases may be missed on initial plain films due to the tendency of Lisfranc subluxations to spontaneously reduce at rest. It is essential that weightbearing views are obtained and, if doubt persists, an abduction stress view is extremely helpful (as described below).

Plain films in the AP and lateral projections are obtained with weightbearing (see Fig. 7.302). Oblique and lateral non-weightbearing views may also be helpful for identifying subtle subluxations (see Fig. 7.303).

A forefoot view with adduction stress may confirm the presence of TMT instability following a subtle Lisfranc injury. Interpretation is assisted by evaluating the 'medial column line' as reported by Coss (1998). A line is drawn from the medial aspect of the navicular to touch the medial border of the medial cuneiform and when continued should intersect the base of the first metatarsal (see Fig. 7.304). If the TMT

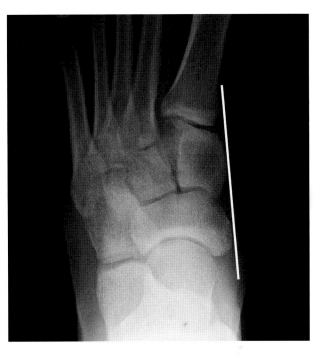

▲ **Fig. 7.304** Coss's line demonstrates lateral subluxation of the first TMT joint. Coss's line touches the medial border of the navicular and medial cuneiform and, in a normal study, should intersect the base of the first metatarsal.

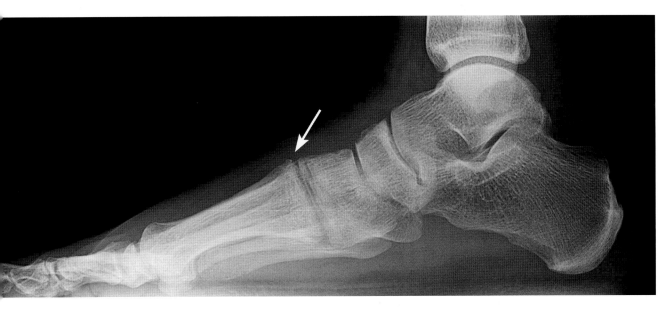

▲ **Fig. 7.303** A lateral weightbearing view shows subluxation at the first TMT joint (arrow).

complex is unstable, the line will not pass through the base of the first metatarsal when abduction stress is applied. This is a far more accurate test than measuring the space between the first and second metatarsals.

Early diagnosis of an unstable Lisfranc injury allows appropriate management and reduces the likelihood of a poor functional outcome. Unstable Lisfranc injuries carry a high risk of post-traumatic mid-foot osteoarthropathy.

Important radiographic criteria of normal alignment include congruence of the second metatarsal and intermediate cuneiform, congruence of the base of the first metatarsal with the medial cuneiform and congruence of the longitudinal arch on weightbearing lateral plain films (Faciszewski et al. 1990). The absolute distance between the bases of the first and second metatarsals should not exceed 3 mm. Transverse fractures at the base/shaft junction of the second metatarsal may occur just distal to the insertion of the Lisfranc ligament and, in this situation, the ligament itself usually remains intact.

Rarely, the tarsometatarsal disruption is gross (see Fig. 7.305), but more commonly when the injury results from a sporting activity the changes are subtle and a careful inspection is essential. An avulsed fragment can sometimes be seen on plain films and, if identified, is diagnostic of a Lisfranc injury. Such fragments are small and easily missed (see Figs 7.306 and 7.307). The initial series is incomplete without a plantodorsal image to help define details of the mortise at the base of the second metatarsal (see Fig. 7.308).

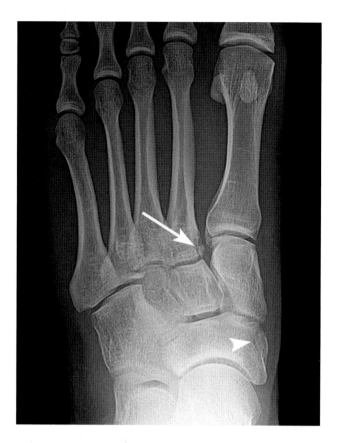

▲ **Fig. 7.306** A small fragment lies in the fracture bed on the medial aspect of the base of the second metatarsal (arrow). These small avulsed fragments are diagnostic of a Lisfranc injury and when there is a clinical suspicion of a Lisfranc injury, a search for these fragments is important. There is also an undisplaced fracture of the navicular tuberosity (arrowhead).

▼ **Fig. 7.305** A gross homolateral Lisfranc fracture-dislocation has resulted from a fall, disrupting all TMT joints. There is almost complete lateral dislocation of the first and second MTP joints. A fracture of the distal medial cuneiform is noted.

▼ **Fig. 7.307** A plantodorsal view improves the definition of the tarsometatarsal area. The articular surfaces of the joints can be assessed and subtle subluxations can be seen more easily. In this case a large fragment is demonstrated avulsed from the medial margin of the base of the second metatarsal by the Lisfranc ligament (arrow). Slight displacement has occurred.

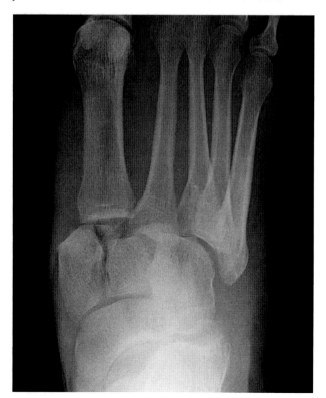

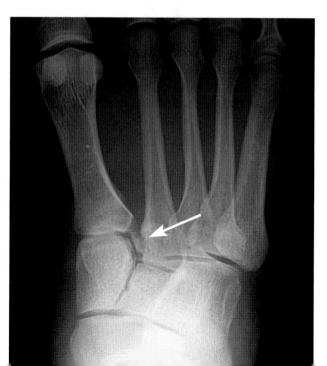

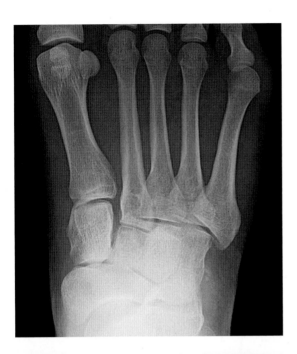

Often, plain films are not definitive and a nuclear bone scan may be used to confirm a fracture-dislocation, with increased uptake occurring in a characteristic pattern (see Fig. 7.309). CT and MRI can also help to confirm the diagnosis, with CT providing the best characterisation of fractures and the best assessment of non-weightbearing alignment (Preidler et al. 1999) (see Figs 7.310 and 7.311). However, high-resolution MRI allows the most comprehensive assessment of the TMT complex (Potter, Deland et al. 1998) (see Fig. 7.312).

◀**Fig. 7.308** A plantodorsal view shows subluxation of the first and fifth TMT joints. There is also loss of congruity at the articulation between the medial and middle cuneiforms.

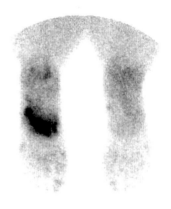

▲ **Fig. 7.309** A nuclear bone scan shows the characteristic uptake of isotope seen following a Lisfranc fracture-dislocation.

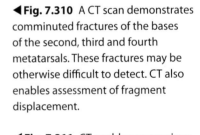

◀**Fig. 7.310** A CT scan demonstrates comminuted fractures of the bases of the second, third and fourth metatarsals. These fractures may be otherwise difficult to detect. CT also enables assessment of fragment displacement.

◀**Fig. 7.311** CT enables comparison with the asymptomatic side. There is a sagittal diastasis on the right side, and the increased gap between the right first and second metatarsal bases is easily appreciated (asterisk).

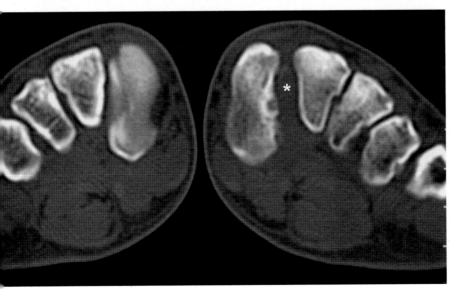

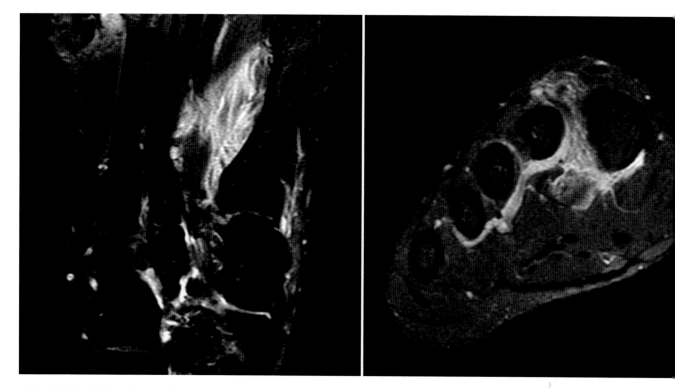

▲ **Fig. 7.312** Axial and coronal fat-suppressed PD MR images graphically demonstrate an injury to the Lisfranc ligament, separation of the bases of the first and second metatarsals, and widening of the joint between the medial and middle cuneiforms. Associated haemorrhage extends both longitudinally and transversely.

Acute navicular fractures

Acute navicular fractures are subdivided into three types:

1. capsular avulsion fractures
2. navicular tuberosity fractures
3. navicular body fractures.

Capsular avulsion fractures are common and result from traction by the dorsal talonavicular or tibionavicular ligaments (Goldman 1985) (see Fig. 7.313).

Fractures of the navicular tuberosity are generally secondary to a forced eversion injury. Tuberosity injuries may destabilise the transverse tarsal joint, with associated injuries to the spring ligament, deltoid ligament or posterior tibial tendon (Pinney and Sangeorzan 2001) (see Fig. 7.314). These fractures may also result from direct trauma, or contraction of the tibialis posterior due to an acute eversion or valgus injury of the foot. They may be associated with a subtalar subluxation injury (Bartz and Marymont 2001).

Navicular body fractures are often comminuted and produce articular disruption (see Fig. 7.315). These fractures have been classified into three types

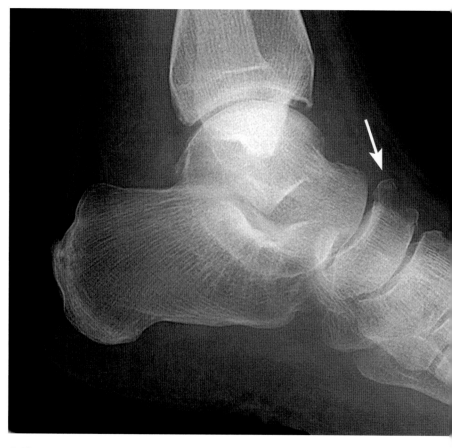

▲ **Fig. 7.313** Fragments have been separated from the dorsal margin of the navicular as a result of avulsion by the dorsal talonavicular, tibionavicular and dorsal naviculocuneiform ligaments (arrow).

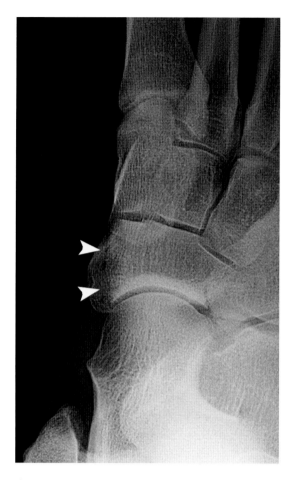

▲ Fig. 7.314 Fractures of the navicular tubercle may be avulsion fractures due to traction of the tibialis posterior tendon or the anterior fibres of the deltoid ligament (arrowheads). As shown in Figs 7.298 and 7.306, a fracture of the navicular tubercle may also occur as an extension of tarsometatarsal complex injuries.

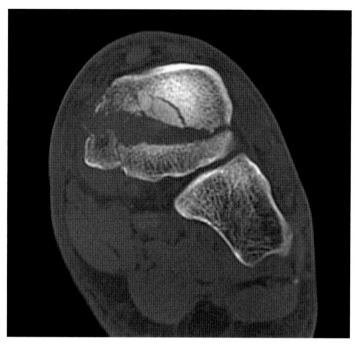

▲ Fig. 7.315 Acute fractures of the body of the navicular are usually the result of high-level trauma, such as may occur in motor sports or equestrian events. In this case, there is a horizontal fracture traversing the navicular body.

▼ Fig. 7.316 A plantodorsal view demonstrates a Lisfranc injury extending to involve the medial cuneiform. There are small avulsed ossicles in the area of the Lisfranc ligament with a fragment separated from the lateral margin of the medial cuneiform and base of the first metatarsal (arrow). The first TMT joint is disrupted with joint space widening, and a fracture involves the articular surface of the medial cuneiform and extends through the cuneiform to emerge medially (arrowhead).

with respect to the plane of the fracture. This classification is beyond the scope of this book. Navicular body fractures have a high incidence of avascular necrosis.

Cuneiform fractures

Acute fractures and dislocations of the cuneiforms are rare and, when they occur, are due to direct trauma or are secondary to a Lisfranc fracture-dislocation of the TMT joints (see Fig. 7.316), particularly when a sagittal diastasis extends between the middle and medial cuneiforms (see Fig. 7.317). Vouri and Aro (1993) reported 66 TMT injuries and found that 39% had fractures, dislocations or fracture-dislocations involving the navicular, cuboid or cuneiforms. There are reported cases of isolated fractures of the medial cuneiform. Rarely, an avulsion fracture can occur at the medial aspect of the medial cuneiform due to tibialis anterior tendon traction (see Fig. 7.318).

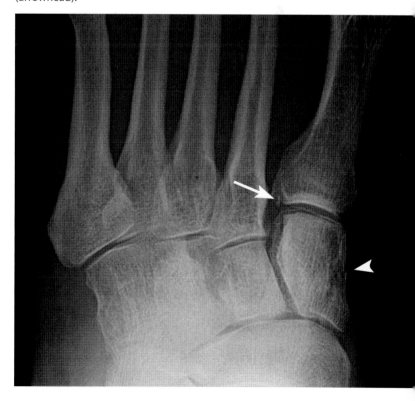

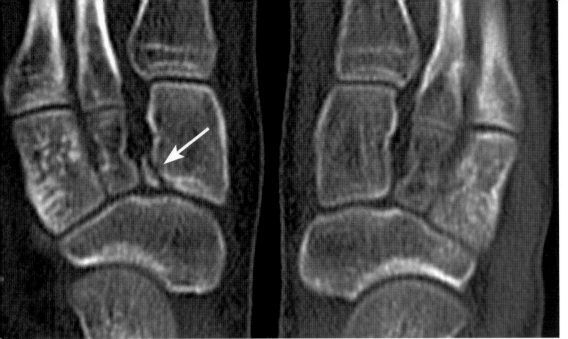

Cuboid fractures

There are four recognised acute fractures of the cuboid. These fractures are commonly associated with a Lisfranc fracture-dislocation. They usually involve the bases of the first to fourth metatarsals and the distal articular surface of the cuboid (see Fig. 7.319).

Small avulsion fractures of the lateral margin of the cuboid adjacent to the calcaneocuboid articulation are extremely common following an inversion injury and result from traction by the plantar calcaneocuboid ligament (see Fig. 7.320).

Compressive body (or 'nutcracker') fractures can arise when there is forced forefoot abduction on a fixed hind-foot, which crushes the cuboid between the bases of the lateral metatarsals and the anterior process of the

(a)

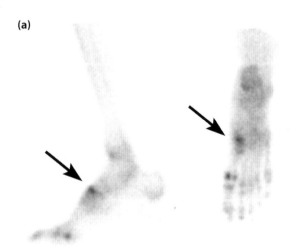

(b)

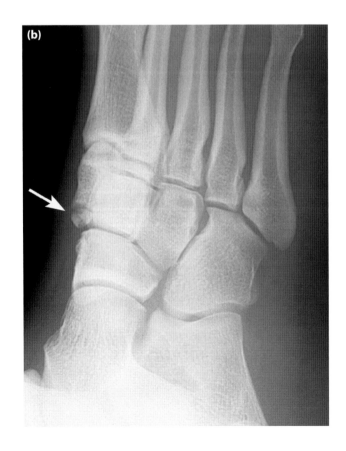

▲ **Fig. 7.318(a)** Following the sudden onset of pain and tenderness over the medial mid-foot, a nuclear bone scan demonstrates increased uptake of isotope in the proximal medial cuneiform (arrows).

▶ **(b)** The increased uptake of isotope on the nuclear bone scan was shown to be due to a small avulsion fracture at the dorsal corner of the proximal surface of the medial cuneiform. The history and clinical appearance suggest the cause to be traction by the tibialis anterior tendon.

calcaneum (see Fig. 7.321). With a severe abduction force, there will be shortening of the lateral column, with associated calcaneocuboid ligament rupture and subluxation at the midtarsal joint, or an avulsion fracture at the navicular tuberosity (Andermahr et al. 2000). Peroneus longus tendon dysfunction may occur if the fracture produces an irregular peroneal groove.

A fracture due to direct trauma may result in comminution of the cuboid. These fractures are uncommon as a result of sport.

Cuboid subluxation

Cuboid subluxation is a poorly recognised cause of lateral foot pain and is most commonly reported in ballet dancers. It is seen as a sudden injury in male dancers landing from a jump or as an overuse injury of gradual onset in female dancers performing repetitive pointe work (see Fig. 7.322). There is weakness in push-off, and the dancer may be unable to move from a flat foot to a demi-pointe or full pointe position. The cuboid is displaced in a plantar direction, due to either a rotational stress associated with forefoot inversion or eversion, or a medial rotation force exerted by reflex contraction of the peroneus

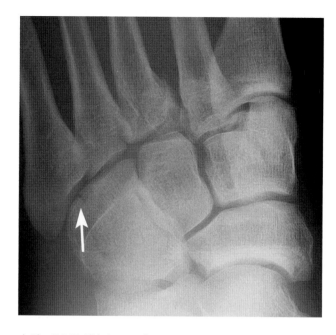

▲ **Fig. 7.319** This image demonstrates the usual pattern of fractures associated with a Lisfranc injury. There are commonly fractures of the bases of the second to fourth metatarsals and a fracture of the distal articular surface of the cuboid (arrow).

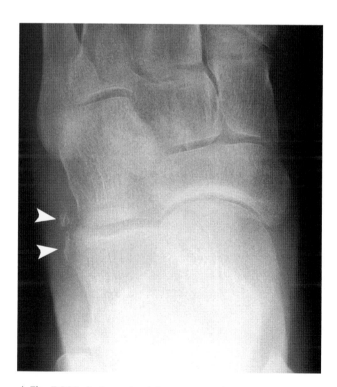

▲ **Fig. 7.320** An inversion injury commonly causes avulsion injuries at the lateral margin of the calcaneocuboid articulation, with separation of small bone fragments (arrowheads).

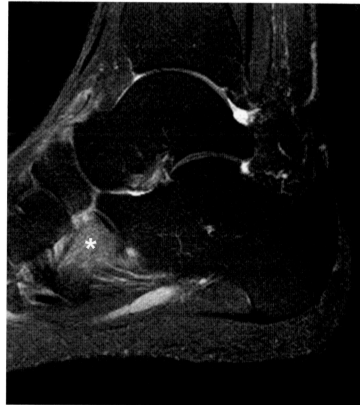

▲ **Fig. 7.321** Following an abduction force, there has been a compressive injury of the cuboid. A sagittal fat-suppressed PD-weighted MR image demonstrates marrow oedema in the body of the cuboid (asterisk).

longus after an ankle inversion injury. Pain is reproduced by direct pressure over the plantar aspect of the cuboid (Marshall and Hamilton 1992). The diagnosis is usually established from the history and physical examination. Imaging tests are often negative, but abnormal calcaneocuboid alignment is occasionally evident on the oblique and lateral plain film views of the foot (Ebraheim et al. 1999) (see Fig. 7.323). It has been suggested that a calcaneocuboid angle of 10° or more on varus stress radiographs and the presence and size of any associated avulsion fracture be used to guide treatment (Andermahr et al. 2000) (see Fig. 7.324).

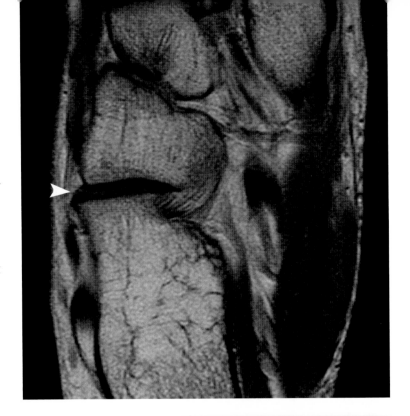

▶ **Fig. 7.322** Cuboid subluxation in a 14-year-old dancer is demonstrated by MRI. A coronal PD-weighted MR image of the symptomatic right calcaneocuboid joint shows mild calcaneocuboid subluxation (arrowhead). This can be a difficult assessment on both x-ray and MRI due to normal variation. However, congruent joint margin alignment should normally be seen on at least one image from any contiguous MRI series.

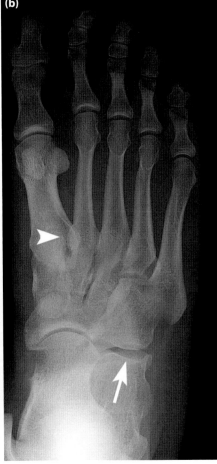

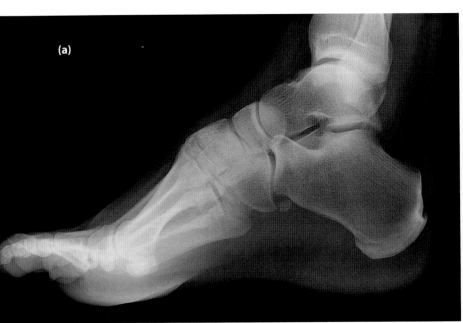

▲ **Fig. 7.323(a)** Subluxation of the cuboid has occurred due to a fall resulting in twisting of the foot. In the lateral view, subluxation of the cuboid is demonstrated, with loss of congruity at the calcaneocuboid articulation and disruption of the fourth and fifth TMT joints. The os peroneum has been displaced by the cuboid rotation.
(b) In the oblique view, a spiral fracture of the first metatarsal is a manifestation of the twisting mechanism of injury (arrowhead). Loss of calcaneocuboid congruity is again demonstrated (arrow), and a fracture of the distal articular surface of the cuboid is easily defined. This is difficult to see on the lateral view.

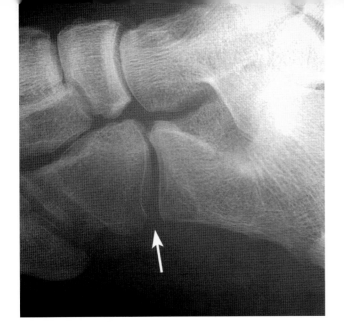

▲ **Fig. 7.324** Cuboid subluxation is demonstrated by a stress view. There is loss of congruity at the calcaneocuboid articulation, with widening of the joint space laterally (arrow). Instability extends across both midtarsal joints, with subluxation of the talonavicular joint also noted.

Overuse sports-related injuries of the mid-foot

Navicular stress fractures

Navicular stress fractures are relatively common and constitute up to 35% of all stress fractures. In the Sydney 2000 Olympics, bone stress was diagnosed in 67 athletes. Of these, 14.6% involved the navicular (Flahive and Anderson 2004). This fracture typically occurs in the sagittal plane and begins at the dorsal aspect of the proximal articular surface of the navicular at the junction of the middle and lateral thirds. Delayed diagnosis is common due to vague clinical presentation and negative plain film findings. The delay in diagnosis averages between four and seven months after the onset of symptoms (Torg et al. 1982; Khan et al. 1992). Navicular stress fractures are most common in sports requiring explosive push-off or change of direction, such as track events, football, rugby and basketball (Fitch et al. 1989; Khan et al. 1994).

Fitch et al. (1989) implicate shear forces transmitted through the second metatarsal and the intermediate cuneiform during foot strike as a likely mechanism. In support of this hypothesis is the anecdotal observation of an increased incidence of navicular stress fractures in athletes with a long second metatarsal or a relatively short plantar-flexed first metatarsal (Pavlov et al. 1983). Fitch et al. further suggested that metatarsus adductus and pronation during weightbearing and push-off increase the degree of shear stress. A varus or cavovarus hind-foot has also been reported as being relatively common in athletes with navicular stress fractures, as this tends to produce a stiffer foot which is less able to absorb and dissipate impact stress during the gait cycle (Lee and Anderson 2004). Additionally, the central third of the navicular is less vascular than the medial and lateral thirds (Golano et al. 2004).

Torg et al. (1982) described a tender area over the dorso-central aspect of the navicular, later referred to as the 'N spot' by Khan et al. (1994). Provocation of symptoms with percussion over the navicular and hopping on the plantar-flexed foot are described signs (Lee and Anderson 2004).

Imaging investigations should begin with plain films (see Fig. 7.325). The series should include a navicular view, which is an AP projection with a 15° wedge beneath the forefoot to

▼ **Fig. 7.325(a)** A pole vaulter at the Sydney 2000 Olympics presented with chronic mid-foot pain. Plain films demonstrate a well-established navicular stress fracture running across the navicular in the sagittal plane. This is the usual site of a fracture, but it is unusually well defined and easy to see (arrow). **(b)** This is the more typical appearance of a navicular stress fracture on plain films. The fracture line is usually subtle and any alteration of bony architecture should be viewed with suspicion. Traumatic deformity of the distal articular surface of the navicular is profiled using the navicular view (arrowhead).

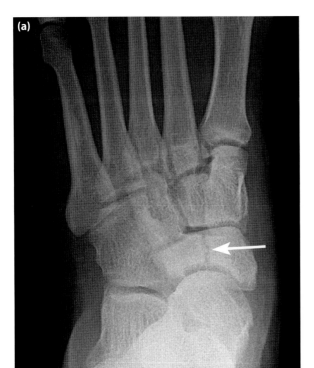

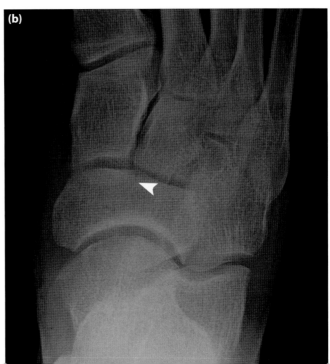

allow the primary x-ray beam to profile the articular surfaces (see Fig. 7.326). The normal variant of an unfused accessory centre of ossification (os supranaviculare) at the dorsal aspect of the proximal articular margin should not be confused with a stress fracture, although a CT may be required to help make this differentiation (see Fig. 7.327). Even a minor change in bony architecture on plain films can suggest a fracture. Nuclear bone scanning is sensitive in detecting both stress reactions and a stress fracture (see Fig. 7.328). However, when there is an abnormality demonstrated by an area of increased isotope uptake, further imaging with CT or MRI is necessary to help characterise the nature of the change (see Fig 7.329).

MRI should be optimised for the detection of fracture lines by using 2–3 mm thick slices that are oriented both along and perpendicular to the axis of the navicular. MRI findings may include bone marrow oedema, a fracture line, sclerosis and cystic change (see Fig. 7.330). CT best demonstrates the fracture line and is preferably performed using fine-collimation multi-detector technology to allow 0.5–2.0 mm thick multiplanar reformations providing high spatial detail (see Fig. 7.331). In addition, CT will detect associated fracture line sclerosis and cystic change, both of which are reported to carry a poorer prognosis.

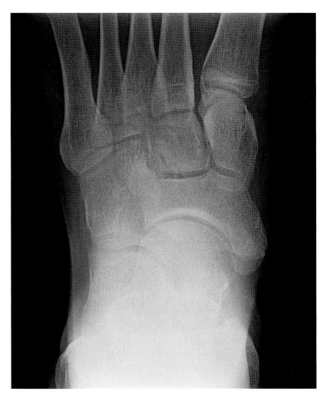

▲ **Fig. 7.326** Using 15° of elevation of the forefoot will improve assessment of the navicular, by bringing its articular surfaces into alignment with the primary x-ray beam.

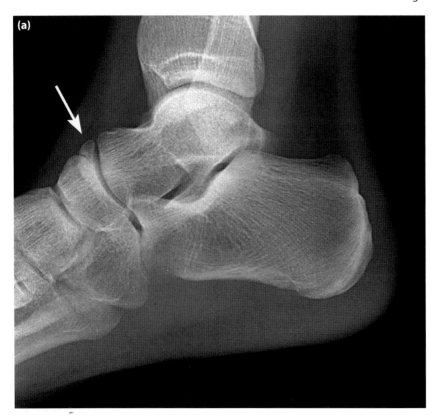

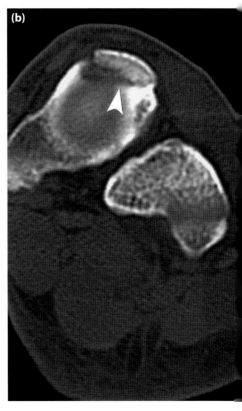

▲ **Fig. 7.327(a)** An ossicle at the dorsal aspect of the proximal articular surface of the navicular is a common accessory ossicle known as an os supranaviculare (arrow).
(b) Occasionally, an os naviculare and a small stress fracture may be difficult to differentiate on plain films and a CT is helpful. In this case CT demonstrates a stress fracture involving the superior margin of the proximal articular surface of the navicular (arrowhead).

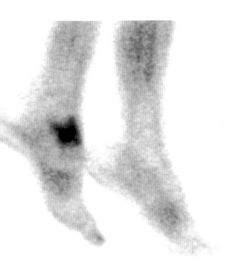

▲ Fig. 7.328 A nuclear bone scan shows uptake of isotope consistent with a navicular stress fracture.

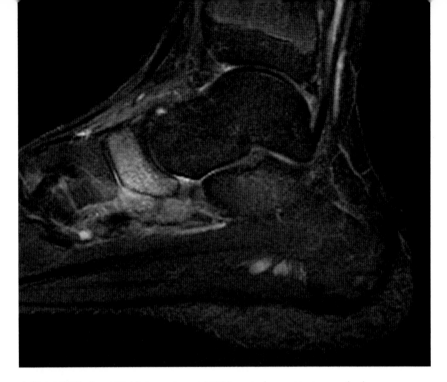

▲ Fig. 7.329 A sagittal fat-suppressed MR image demonstrates marked marrow oedema secondary to a navicular stress fracture.

▶ Fig. 7.330 An axial fat-suppressed MR image shows a navicular stress fracture in typical position (arrow). Extensive marrow oedema is present throughout the navicular.

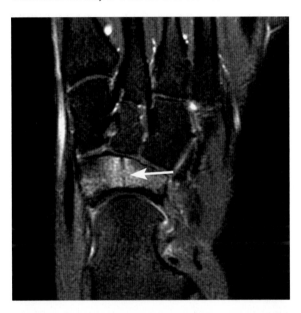

Assessment of stress fracture healing requires correlation with a previous imaging study, preferably using the same modality. The MRI criteria for healing include regression of bone marrow oedema and, if visible, a decrease in extent and definition of the fracture line. Kiss et al. (1993) described slight dorsal cortical bridging as the earliest CT sign of healing. This may be seen as early as six weeks after the commencement of treatment. Kiss et al. also reported a series in which frank non-union occurred in 39% of cases.

▶ Fig. 7.331(a) An axial CT image shows a typical stress fracture involving the right navicular in the sagittal plane (arrowhead). The fracture is incomplete. **(b)** An early incomplete stress fracture is demonstrated by CT (arrowhead). Stress fractures commence on the dorsal aspect of the proximal articular surface of the navicular.

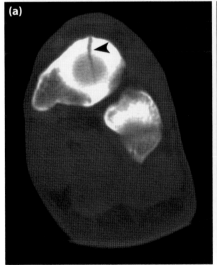
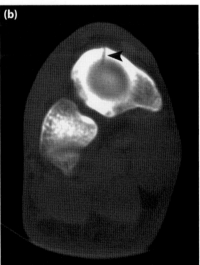

Cuboid stress fractures

Cuboid stress fractures in athletes are unusual (Beaman et al. 1993), but may be seen as a complication of plantar fascial rupture (Yu and Solmen 2001) and may mimic peroneal tendonitis (see Fig. 7.332).

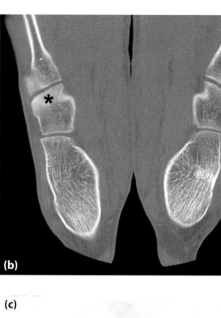

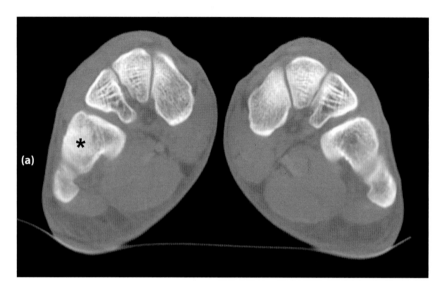

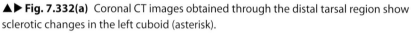

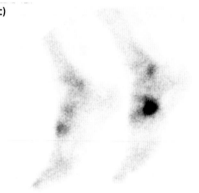

▲▶ **Fig. 7.332(a)** Coronal CT images obtained through the distal tarsal region show sclerotic changes in the left cuboid (asterisk).
(b) An axial CT image shows the sclerosis demonstrated in the coronal image to lie in the subchondral bone adjacent to the left fourth TMT joint (asterisk).
(c) A nuclear bone scan shows marked uptake of isotope in the left cuboid, typical of a stress reaction.

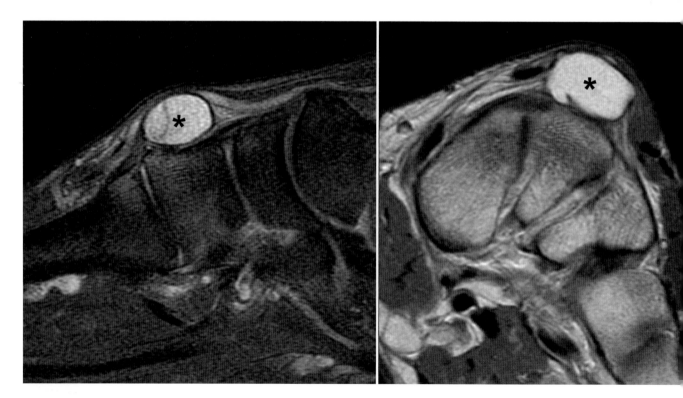

▲ **Fig. 7.333** MRI demonstrates a ganglion on the dorsum of the mid-foot, just proximal to the second TMT joint (asterisks). The ganglion caused deep peroneal nerve entrapment. The ganglion is shown as an encapsulated high signal mass on sagittal fat-suppressed and coronal PD-weighted images. The neck of origin of the ganglion cannot be identified.

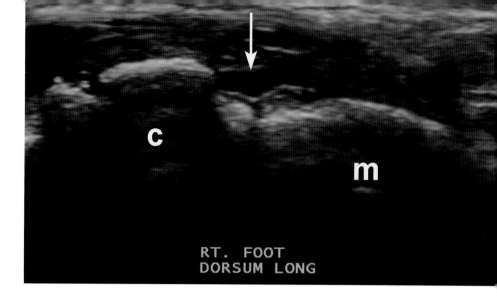

► Fig. 7.334 A long-axis ultrasound image obtained over the dorsal aspect of the third TMT joint shows a small ovoid ganglion cyst (arrow). Lateral cuneiform = c. Third metatarsal = m.

RT. FOOT
DORSUM LONG

Other mid-foot conditions

Mid-foot ganglia

Ganglion cysts in the mid-foot region are frequent incidental findings on MRI and ultrasound. These ganglia are often asymptomatic. The foot is the second most common site for ganglia after the hand and wrist. Although usually occurring adjacent to joints or tendon sleeves, communication with the synovial space is not always demonstrated. Lateral mid-foot ganglia most commonly arise from the dorsal capsule of the fourth TMT joint, often extending proximally with a thin neck that can sometimes be difficult to identify (see Fig. 7.333). On MRI, ganglia are slightly lower in signal intensity than muscle on T1-weighted images and homogeneously bright on T2-weighted images. They possess a thin fibrous capsule that may enhance with IV contrast. However, areas of nodular or irregular internal enhancement should not be seen, and if present, would raise the possibility of a neoplastic process. On ultrasound, most ganglia have either a simple rounded appearance or a lobulated septate appearance with a smooth thin wall, predominantly echo-free interior and posterior acoustic enhancement (see Fig. 7.334).

Insertional tibialis anterior tendinopathy

The tibialis anterior tendon inserts at the dorsomedial aspect of the medial cuneiform and at the base of the first metatarsal. Insertional tibialis anterior tendinopathy most commonly occurs in patients over 50 years of age. However, downhill runners, skiers and soccer players are predisposed to tibialis anterior tendinopathy secondary to tendon overload associated with forced plantar flexion of the foot (Bencardino et al. 2001). Plain radiographs may demonstrate soft-tissue swelling and a small bony spur on the medial cuneiform at the tendon insertion (see Fig. 7.335). In the early stages, MRI may demonstrate thickening of the peritendon space and a bursopathy deep to the tibialis anterior insertion. With chronicity, there may also be thickening and mild intra-tendon signal hyperintensity due to tendinopathy (see Fig. 7.336). A tear is indicated by frank fluid signal interrupting fibre continuity. Ultrasound provides equivalent information and has the advantage of easy comparison with the contralateral side. Power Doppler may also detect intra-tendon or peritendon hyperaemia.

▼ Fig. 7.335(a) A spur is present at the insertion of the tibialis anterior (arrow). **(b)** Soft-tissue calcification is seen adjacent to the spur at the insertion of the tibialis anterior (arrow). The appearance is almost certainly indicative of insertional calcific tendinopathy.

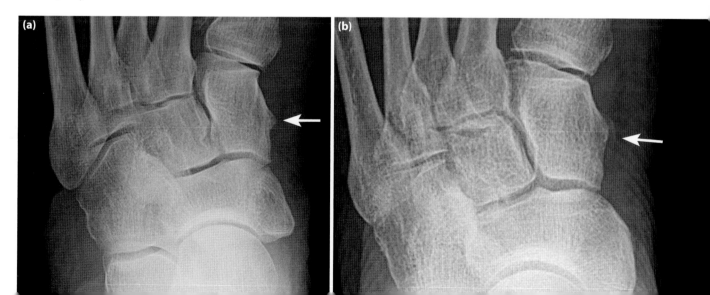

(a)

(b)

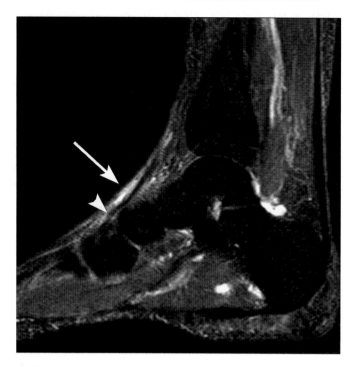

▲ Fig. 7.336 A sagittal STIR MR image shows changes of insertional tibialis anterior tendinopathy. There are high signal changes in the peritendon space (arrow) and high signal within the distal tendon segment just proximal to its insertion (arrowhead).

Osteochondritis of the navicular

Osteochondritis of the tarsal navicular (Kohler's disease) is a self-limiting condition that is characterised by sclerosis and collapse of the developing navicular. Most cases are unilateral, and the highest incidence occurs in males aged 3–7 years. Spontaneous radiographic resolution occurs over a period of two to four years. On plain films, the chondral surfaces are unaffected and the surrounding joint spaces are preserved throughout the process (see Fig. 7.337).

Meuller-Weiss syndrome: a comma-shaped navicular

In this condition, the navicular is compressed and fragmented laterally, often with medial and dorsal displacement of navicular fragments (see Fig. 7.338). The division between the fragments characteristically passes obliquely through the bone (see Fig. 7.339). The navicular assumes a comma-like shape. This syndrome is seen in otherwise healthy adults and is due to spontaneous osteonecrosis of the navicular (see Fig. 7.340).

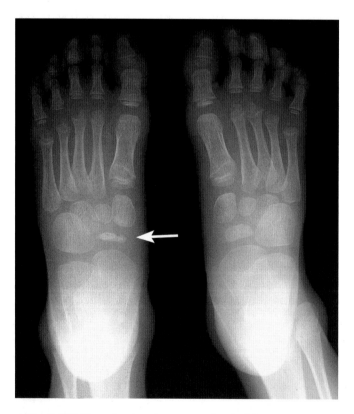

▲ Fig. 7.337 There is sclerosis, compression and fragmentation of the left navicular (arrow). Note that the distance from the surrounding tarsal bones is normally maintained, when compared to the right side, suggesting that the nucleus of ossification of the navicular is surrounded by additional cartilage. This is the typical appearance of Kohler's disease.

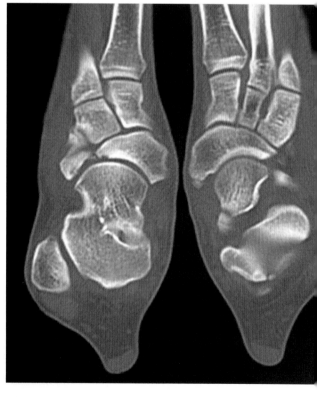

▲ Fig. 7.338(a) CT shows a comma-shaped navicular present bilaterally, with characteristic narrowing occurring laterally. There is fragmentation of the left navicular laterally. This condition is known as Meuller-Weiss syndrome. The patient is a 19-year-old male who was able to play soccer at a high standard despite this deformity.

▶ **Fig. 7.338(b)** Lateral views of the feet of the same patient show abnormal navicular configuration and dorsal protrusion, which is a constant characteristic of this condition.

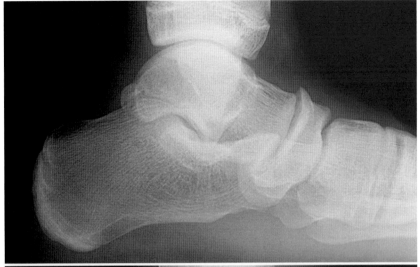

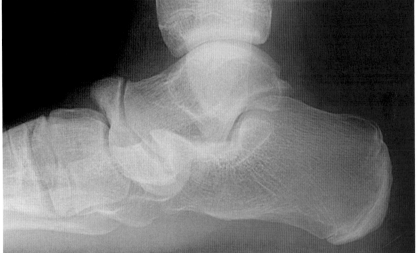

None of the reported cases of Meuller-Weiss syndrome have had abnormalities as children and the condition has no association with Kohler's disease (Sharp, Calder et al. 2003) (see Fig. 7.341). In the majority of cases, the cause of the spontaneous osteonecrosis remains uncertain and chronic stress has been suggested (Manter 1946; Sarrafian 1987). The condition is often bilateral but of different severity.

CT examination is required to accurately define the degree of fragment displacement. Haller et al. (1988) reported that MRI shows considerable decreased signal intensity throughout the navicular on T1-weighted images, with increased signal demonstrated in areas of active stress on T2-weighted images. In spite of Brailsford (1939) reporting that the disorder is characterised by a chronic clinical course of pain, disability and progressive deformity, in the authors' small series of five cases, two cases were playing sport at a high level.

A navicular deformity identical to that seen following spontaneous osteonecrosis in otherwise healthy individuals has also been reported in patients with rheumatoid arthritis, renal failure, lupus erythematosus and trauma (Haller et al. 1988). This indicates that the osteonecrosis is not always spontaneous.

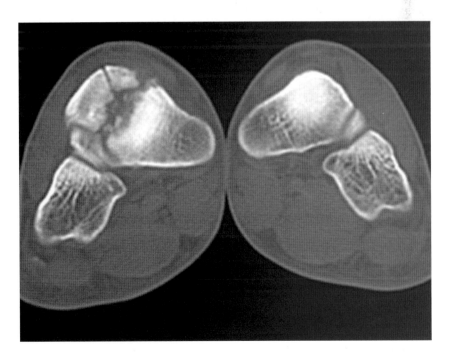

▲ **Fig. 7.339** Although the changes of Meuller-Weiss syndrome are bilateral, the changes are more marked on the left, where there is noticeable lateral fragmentation.

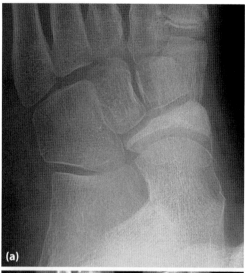
(a)

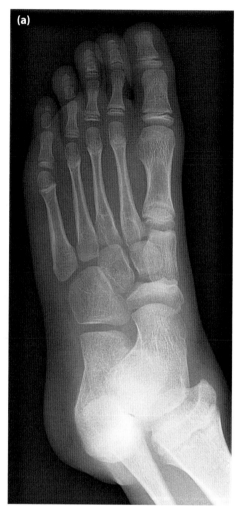
(a)

◀ **Fig. 7.340(a)**
A 14-year-old male shows the classic plain film changes of Meuller-Weiss syndrome. The navicular is wedged or comma-shaped and shows increased density, consistent with osteonecrosis.
(b) CT examination of the same case as in Fig. 7.341(a) shows compression and fragmentation of both naviculars laterally. Note that the fragmentation is oblique. There is increased density when compared with the surrounding tarsal bones.

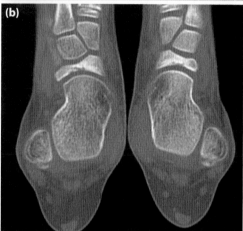
(b)

▶ **Fig. 7.341(a)** A 9-year-old boy is the youngest patient in the authors' series with Meuller-Weiss deformity of the navicular. There is narrowing and sclerosis of the lateral aspect of the navicular. This deformity was asymptomatic, with the patient presenting with forefoot trauma.

▼ **(b)** A lateral view of the same case shows an abnormal shape and bone density of the navicular. The navicular protrudes slightly on the dorsal profile of the foot. Fragmentation is noted.

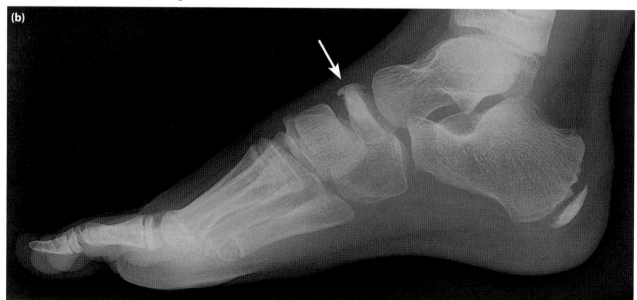
(b)

Osteochondritis dissecans of the navicular

Occasionally, changes of osteochondritis dissecans (OCD) may involve the proximal articular surface of the navicular (Haller et al. 1988) (see Figs 7.342 and 7.343).

Mid-foot arthropathy

Osteoarthrosis at the navicular-medial cuneiform articulation or first TMT joint can mimic insertional tibialis anterior tendon pathology. Sometimes this may remain occult to plain radiographic assessment. In these situations nuclear bone scans may localise the pathology, although MRI is the imaging method of choice because it enables simultaneous assessment of the tibialis anterior tendon.

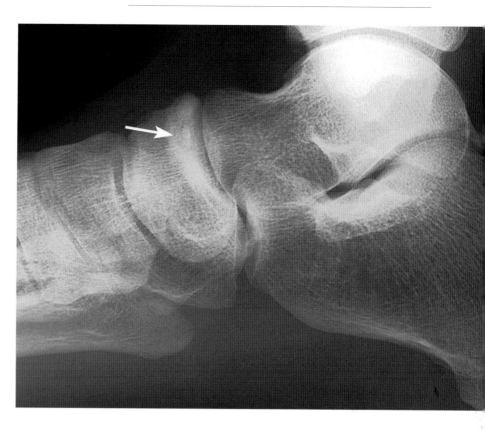

▲ **Fig. 7.342** An area of OCD is present superiorly on the proximal articular surface of the navicular. An ossicle is noted in a well-demarcated translucent area (arrow).

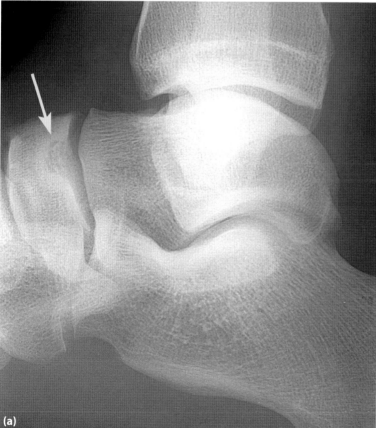

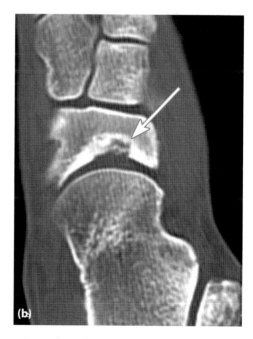

▲ **Fig. 7.343(a)** A well-demarcated bony deficiency is present on the proximal articular surface of the navicular (arrow). This area has a sclerotic margin and no contained ossicle can be seen. It is difficult to differentiate old OCD from a developmental ossification defect. A similar problem may be encountered on the tibial plafond and talar dome.
(b) A CT scan of the same case demonstrates the defect (arrow) and an unusual configuration of the proximal articular surface of the navicular. The appearance would favour a developmental ossification defect.

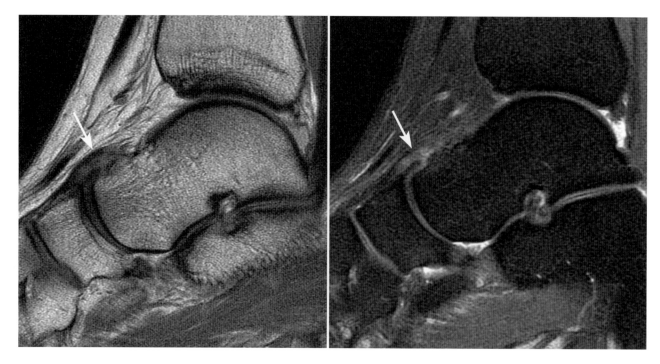

▲ **Fig. 7.344** MRI illustrates post-traumatic thickening of the dorsal talonavicular joint capsule in the acute or subacute phase, showing hyperintense changes on sagittal PD and fat-suppressed PD sequences (arrows).

Sports-related injuries of the hind-foot

Injuries of the talonavicular–middle subtalar joint complex

The talonavicular and middle subtalar joints are in communication and are referred to as the talonavicular–middle subtalar joint complex. They constitute the medial component of the transverse tarsal joint complex. The transverse tarsal joint acts synchronously with the subtalar and ankle joints during gait.

Injuries to the talonavicular–middle subtalar joint complex typically have a plantar flexion-inversion mechanism and are usually associated with a sprain or an avulsion of the dorsal talonavicular joint capsule. There is often an associated cortical flake avulsion fracture at the talar head insertion and a post-traumatic synovitis may develop at the dorsal recess of the talonavicular joint (see Fig. 7.344). On MRI the avulsion fracture fragment may be quite subtle (see Fig. 7.345). An associated injury at the plantar margin of the talar head is often present on MRI, with bone marrow oedema at the plantar aspect of the talar head, focal depression of the subchondral plate and an overlying chondral lesion.

Tarsal coalition

Tarsal coalition is an abnormal fusion between two or more bones of the hind-foot, attributed to a failure of segmentation and differentiation of primitive mesenchyme (Harris 1965). Coalitions are best classified as osseous, non-osseous (fibrous or cartilaginous) or partially osseous (Kulik and Clanton 1996). The clinical presentation is usually one of pain and restricted movement developing in the second or third decade of life. Associated rigidity of the hind-foot predisposes to chronic lateral ankle ligament complex instability (Sammarco and DiRaimondo 1988), and tarsal coalition is also an important cause of adolescent spastic flat foot. Multiple coalitions may be associated with syndromes such as fibular hemimelia and underlying genetic abnormalities.

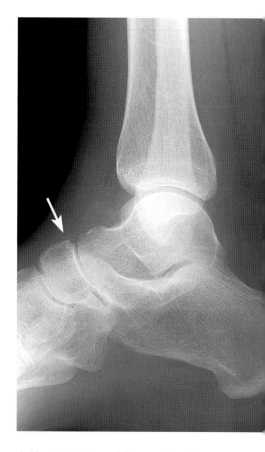

▲ **Fig. 7.345** A small fragment has been avulsed from the dorsal margin of the navicular adjacent to the talonavicular joint (arrow). As shown in this case, these fragments are often subtle. Note the bony calcaneonavicular coalition.

Calcaneonavicular coalition

Osseous calcaneonavicular coalitions appear radiographically between eight and 12 years of age. This condition is best demonstrated on an oblique plain film view of the foot (see Fig. 7.346). Non-osseous coalitions are more difficult to identify on plain films, but should be suspected whenever there is elongation and 'squaring' of the anterior process of the calcaneum with a narrowed calcaneonavicular interval and matching irregularity of the cortical margins (see Fig. 7.347). CT and MRI offer a more detailed assessment (see Fig. 7.348). CT has the advantage of examining both ankles simultaneously and demonstrates the full extent of an osseous coalition. In the authors' experience, a combination of MRI and weightbearing radiographs provides the most comprehensive assessment of non-osseous tarsal coalitions. MRI is particularly suited to the evaluation of

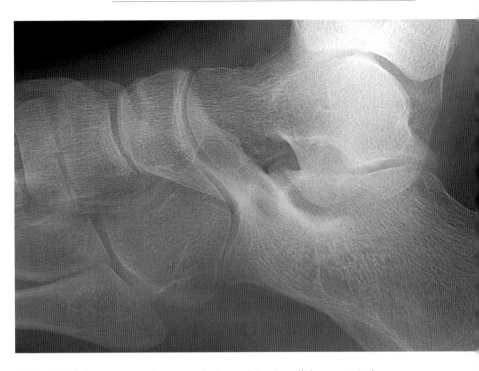

▲ **Fig. 7.346** An osseous calcaneonavicular coalition is well demonstrated on an oblique view of the foot.

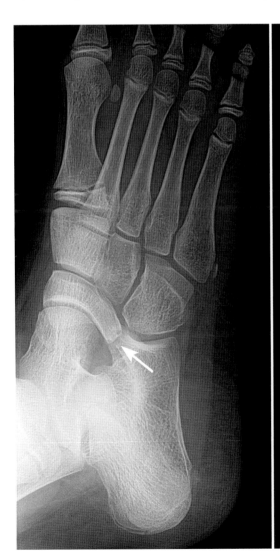
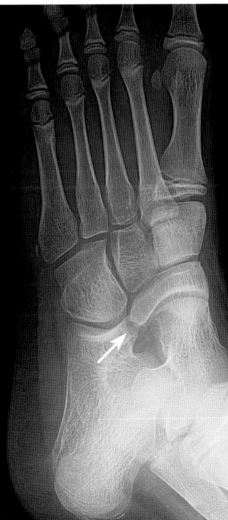

◀**Fig. 7.347** Bilateral fibrous or cartilaginous calcaneonavicular coalitions are demonstrated by oblique views (arrows). There is bony irregularity at the apposing margins of the coalitions. The nature of the bridging tissue cannot be characterised on plain films. An MRI examination would be necessary for further assessment.

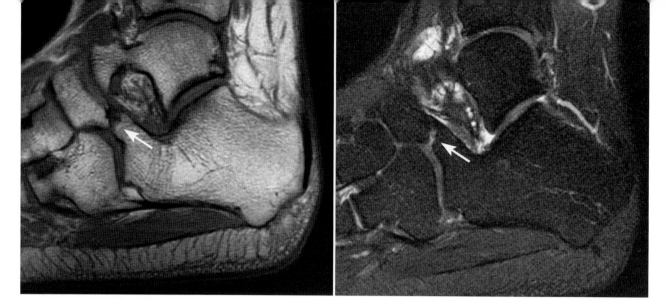

▲ **Fig. 7.348** Sagittal T1 and fat-suppressed PD-weighted MR images demonstrate a non-osseous calcaneonavicular coalition (arrows), with the bridging tissue showing mixed signal characteristics. Fibrotic and ganglionic changes are noted in the sinus tarsi and a ganglion is noted on the dorsal aspect of the head of the talus.

fibrous coalitions, although it is possible for the inexperienced to interpret the bifurcate ligament and plantar fibres of the spring ligament as a fibrous calcaneonavicular coalition. Calcaneonavicular coalition is best seen with a combination of sagittal and axial images. The addition of an oblique image in the plane of the calcaneonavicular interval is generally not required.

Talocalcaneal coalition

Although calcaneonavicular coalition is reported as the most common coalition, the authors suspect that this is because talocalcaneal coalition is frequently missed and the diagnosis is usually delayed.

Talocalcaneal coalition involves fusion across the middle subtalar joint at the level of the sustentaculum tali. Less commonly there may be a syndesmosis between the posterior margin of the sustentaculum and the antero-inferior margin of the medial tubercle of the posterior process of the talus (McNally 1999). An osseous talocalcaneal coalition is demonstrated on a true lateral plain film of the ankle as a continuous bony bridging of the middle subtalar joint (the 'C' sign) that is commonly accompanied by talar 'beaking', which develops as the result of altered

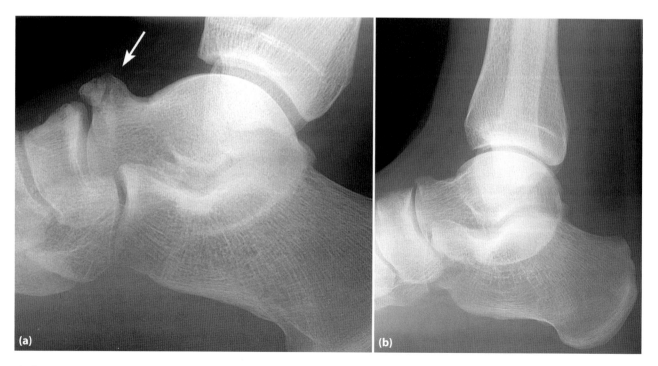

▲ **Fig. 7.349(a)** An osseous talocalcaneal coalition is present demonstrating a prominent associated talar 'beak' on the talar head (arrow). Having a bony bridge across the middle subtalar joint, a continuous cortical line runs unbroken from the talar dome to the undersurface of the sustentaculum tali. This produces a 'C' sign, which is well shown in this case.
(b) In this case of bony talocalcaneal coalition a 'C' sign is well shown, but only a small talar 'beak' is present.

subtalar joint biomechanics. The importance of obtaining a true lateral view must be stressed, as a false positive diagnosis will commonly occur with obliquity (Shaffer and Harrison 1980). Fusion of the middle subtalar joint produces a ball-and-socket movement in the sagittal plane at the talonavicular joint. This change in dynamics produces superior elongation of the talar articular surface with development of a talar 'beak' and flattening of the undersurface of the talar neck (see Fig. 7.349) (Conway and Cowell 1969). Talar beaking is more obvious than the 'C' sign and the experienced eye, having seen a 'beak', will immediately examine the posterior margin of the sustentaculum. Lateur et al. (1994) noted that the 'C' sign is non-specific, as it can also be caused by a planovalgus foot and is seen in calcaneocuboid coalition, as shown in Fig. 7.378. In addition, not all talocalcaneal coalitions have talar beaking.

If there is suspicion of a talocalcaneal coalition on the initial plain film series, a Harris-Beath view should be obtained (see Fig. 7.350). The method of obtaining this view is described on page 538.

Helical MDCT producing detailed multiplanar reformations will adequately demonstrate bony and osteocartilaginous coalitions, but will not detect a fibrous coalition (Kumar et al. 1992; Wechsler et al. 1994). The CT signs of a non-bony talocalcaneal coalition may be quite subtle and include bony irregularity, narrowing of the subtalar joint and mild adjacent sclerosis (see Fig. 7.351(a)). The extent of osseous coalition should be quantified, estimating the percentage area of the joint involved (see Fig. 7.351(b)).

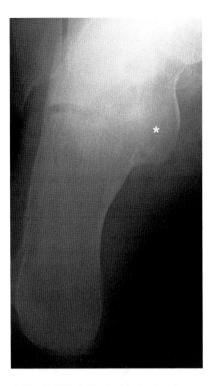

▲ **Fig. 7.350** A Harris-Beath view is an easy and efficient method of imaging a bony talonavicular coalition. The bony bridge across the middle subtalar joint is indicated by an asterisk.

(a)

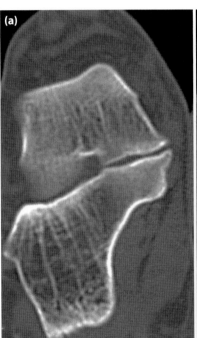
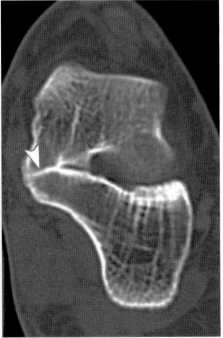

(b)

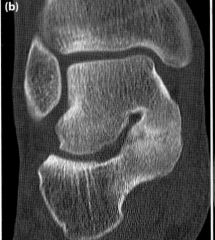
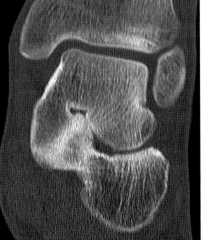

◀ **Fig. 7.351(a)** CT is useful for assessing coalitions. In this case, there is narrowing and irregularity of the middle subtalar joint on the left, which indicates a fibrous or cartilaginous coalition. The left coalition is mixed, with about 50% bony (arrowhead) and the remainder being fibrous or cartilaginous.

(b) There is an atypical bilateral medial talocalcaneal coalition. The coalition is largely osseous, with a minor fibrous or cartilaginous segment laterally on the right side. In this type of talocalcaneal coalition, there is an unusual medial process arising from the talus, and the sustentaculum tali is abnormally formed. There is no 'C' sign, and the talus has a characteristic lateral profile (see Figs 7.15 and 7.352).

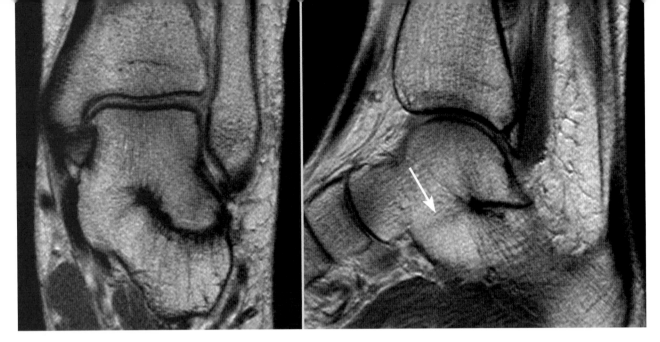

▲ **Fig. 7.352** A similar atypical talocalcaneal coalition is demonstrated by coronal and sagittal PD-weighted MR images. This is a medial coalition of an anomalous medial process of the talus across the middle subtalar joint (arrow). The sustentaculum tali cannot be identified. Note the absent 'C' sign on the sagittal image and the unusual hump on the posterior profile of the body of the talus. The coalition partly involves the posterior subtalar joint.

Osseous and fibrous coalitions are well assessed by MRI, and this test should be considered whenever there is a clinically suspected coalition but a negative CT scan (Wechsler et al. 1994; Harty and Hubbard 2001) (see Fig. 7.352). Standard ankle MRI protocols will demonstrate most talocalcaneal coalitions but can occasionally miss small fibrous extra-articular coalitions unless additional thin sagittal and mild reverse-tilt coronal images are included. Generally, fibrous coalitions are of low signal intensity and cartilaginous coalitions are of low-to-intermediate signal intensity. There may be cystic change and bone marrow oedema at the coalition margins.

If there is an associated ganglion or bony spurring arising from the medial margin of the coalition, then impingement on neurovascular structures in the adjacent tarsal tunnel should be considered.

Talonavicular coalitions and other rare coalitions

Talonavicular coalitions are unusual and are evident on plain films (see Fig. 7.353). There have also been reported cases of calcaneocuboid coalitions and, if osseous, these are also

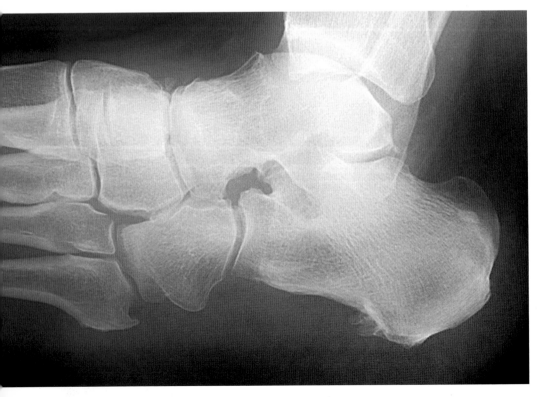

◀ **Fig. 7.353** This shows a bony talonavicular coalition. Note that the naviculocuneiform articulation has developed a rounded configuration, presumably enabling limited talonavicular-type joint function.

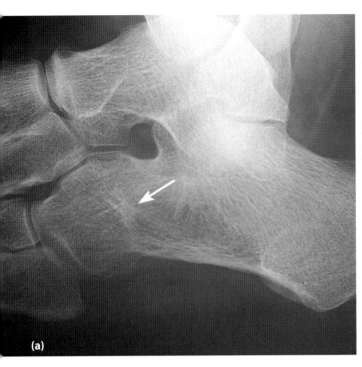
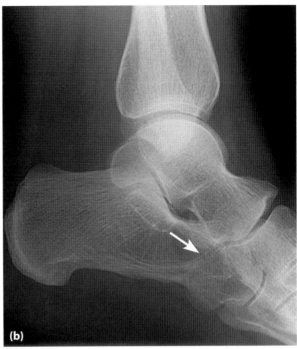

▲ **Fig. 7.354(a)** Multiple coalitions are present involving the talonavicular, calcaneocuboid and third TMT joints. As in Fig. 7.353, the naviculocuneiform coalition has developed a rounded configuration. **(b)** A calcaneocuboid coalition is present (arrow). Note the talar 'beaking', which has presumably developed as a manifestation of abnormal midtarsal movement.

obvious on plain films (see Fig. 7.354). This anomaly may be accompanied by peroneal spasm (Zeide et al. 1977). Coalition between the navicular and medial cuneiform occurs rarely (see Fig. 7.355(a)), and coalition may occur between the middle and medial cuneiform (see Fig. 7.355(b)).

There are reports of excision of symptomatic cuboid–navicular coalitions with resolution of patient symptoms (Johnson et al. 2005). First metatarsal–medial cuneiform coalitions have also been reported, with symptomatic cases having been non-osseous and incomplete (Tanaka et al. 2000).

▼ **Fig. 7.355(a)** There is a coalition between the navicular and medial cuneiform (arrow). This appears to be fibrous or cartilaginous, although MRI would be necessary for further characterisation. **(b)** A partial osseous coalition joins the middle and lateral cuneiforms (arrowheads).

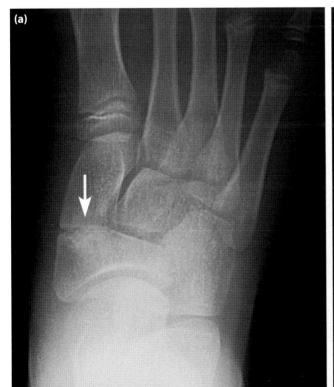
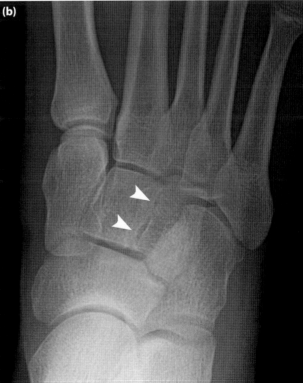

This disorder may be mistaken for a degenerative arthropathy on plain radiographs.

Os sustentaculi

An os sustentaculi represents a potentially painful variant of a talocalcaneal coalition, where the middle calcaneal articular facet is a separate ossicle and there is a fibrous coalition between the os and the talus and a fibrous or fibrocartilaginous linkage with the remainder of the calcaneum (Mellado et al. 2002) (see Fig. 7.356). The MRI appearance has been reported by Bencardino et al. (1997b).

The subtalar joint and sinus tarsi

The subtalar joint and the sinus tarsi are best regarded as a complex. The components of this complex are the anterior and posterior compartments of the subtalar joint and the contents of the sinus tarsi. The posterior compartment of the subtalar joint is the largest component and does not communicate with the anterior compartment. The anterior compartment includes both the middle subtalar joint and, when present, the anterior subtalar joint. The middle subtalar joint communicates with the talonavicular joint, and the anterior subtalar joint is only variably present and relatively small in size. The subtalar joint and ankle joint make up the functional unit of the hind-foot (Keefe and Haddad 2002).

The subtalar joint complex facilitates the conversion of the hinge movement of the ankle into intricate triaxial rotation and translation of the hind-foot (Perry 1983). The normal motion of the joint is approximately 25° of inversion-supination and 10° of eversion-pronation (Keefe and Haddad 2002). The primary ligamentous stabilisers of the subtalar joint are the CFL, the interosseous talocalcaneal ligament (ITCL) and the cervical ligament.

Because normal movement of the subtalar joint is required to provide transverse rotatory motion that occurs between the foot and the leg during walking and running, abnormal subtalar joint movement may stress the knee and hip. Subtalar instability may result from a severe hind-foot supination injury, and is in essence a continuation of the standard ankle inversion and plantar flexion sprain. It has also been speculated that isolated subtalar instability may alternatively develop after an inversion injury with the ankle in dorsiflexion.

Plain film views of the subtalar joint

Investigation of subtalar joint problems should commence with a routine plain film series of the ankle plus specific subtalar joint views. Supplementary projections include internal and external oblique views and a Harris-Beath view. The method of acquiring these views has already been discussed (see pages 538 and 621).

Because the anatomy of the subtalar joint is complex and superimposition often makes plain films difficult to interpret, additional imaging methods are usually required to diagnose conditions such as chondral lesions, early osteoarthropathy, fractures of the posterior or lateral processes of the talus, avascular necrosis and synovitis. Nuclear bone scans (see Fig. 7.357), CT and MRI can all be used to supplement the

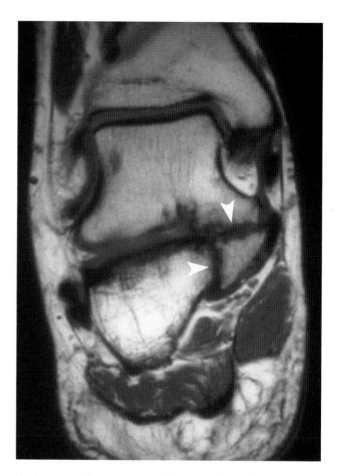

▲ **Fig. 7.356** A coronal T1-weighted MR image demonstrates fibrous or cartilaginous coalition between both the calcaneum and sustentaculum tali and articulation between the sustentaculum tali and the talus (arrowheads). The sustentaculum tali has developed as a separate ossicle.

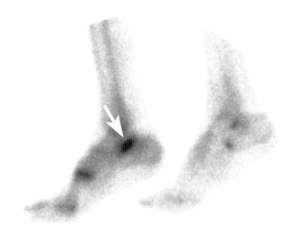

▲ **Fig. 7.357** There is increased uptake of isotope along the talar margin of the posterior subtalar joint of the right foot (arrow). Note the straight inferior edge of the uptake, indicating the joint line. In this case, the increased uptake was indicative of bone stress. Also note the uptake in the right first TMT joint.

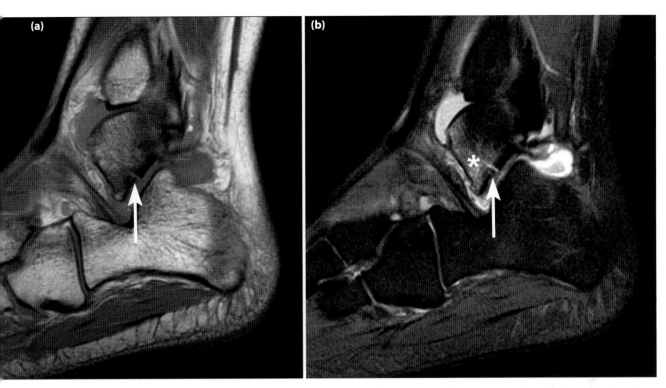

▲ **Fig. 7.358** Sagittal T1-weighted **(a)** and fat-suppressed PD-weighted **(b)** MR images demonstrate a fracture involving the talar articular surface of the posterior subtalar joint (arrows). This fracture involves the lateral process of the talus. Note the associated marrow oedema (asterisk) and accompanying ankle and subtalar joint effusions.

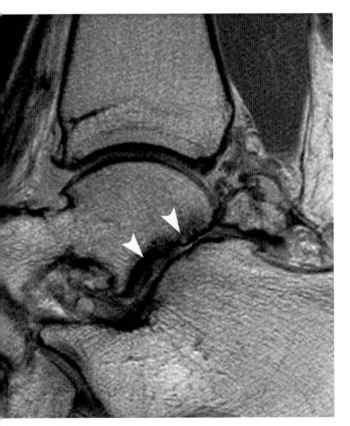

▲ **Fig. 7.359** A sagittal PD-weighted MR image demonstrates changes of osteoarthrosis involving the posterior subtalar joint (arrowheads). There has been destruction of articular cartilage with consequent joint space narrowing and subchondral sclerosis, more marked on the talar side of the joint.

assessment of bone and soft-tissue anatomy (see Figs 7.358 and 7.359).

Conditions of the subtalar joint and sinus tarsi

Focal chondral abnormalities and osteoarthropathy involving the posterior subtalar joint

The reliable detection of chondral lesions involving the posterior subtalar joint by MRI requires the use of high-resolution scans. The relevance of these changes has increased due to the development of arthroscopic techniques for the examination of the posterior subtalar joint.

Subtalar joint stress

Bone marrow oedema may be seen at the margins of the posterior subtalar joint in adolescents with peroneal spasm. This is sometimes quite extensive and usually reflects low-grade subchondral bone stress secondary to a spastic flat foot rather than underlying subtalar joint pathology. Similarly, in adults with advanced posterior tibial tendon dysfunction, marrow oedema may be seen at the anterolateral margin of the talar body and the adjacent base of the anterior process of the calcaneum, reflecting abutment arising from planovalgus deformity. This may sometimes be associated with localised lateral hind-foot pain (Malicky et al. 2002).

Sinus tarsi syndrome

The sinus tarsi is a cone-shaped cavity at the lateral aspect of the foot which is bounded superiorly by the neck of the talus and inferiorly by the dorsal margin of the anterior process of the calcaneum. The apex of the cone is directed medially and merges with the tarsal tunnel. The sinus tarsi contains several important stabilisers of the hind-foot, including the ITCL posteromedially, the cervical ligament anterolaterally and the insertion of the three roots of the inferior extensor retinaculum. Posteriorly the sinus tarsi is demarcated by the anterior capsule of the posterior subtalar joint.

Sinus tarsi syndrome consists of pain in the region of the sinus tarsi, which usually responds to injection and is associated with subjective hind-foot instability (Brown 1960). Frey et al. (1999) suggested that sinus tarsi syndrome is an inaccurate term, and should be replaced with a more specific diagnosis whenever possible. In a series of 14 patients with a pre-operative diagnosis of sinus tarsi syndrome, arthroscopy enabled a specific diagnosis in all cases. An ITCL tear was identified in 10 patients, arthrofibrosis in two patients and osteoarthritis in two patients. Plain radiographs, CT or MRI may demonstrate a bony spur or ossicle at the dorsal margin of the anterior process of the calcaneum as sequelae of a prior traction injury at the origin of the extensor digitorum brevis muscle. Infiltration of the sinus fat planes on MRI is a feature of sinus tarsi syndrome (see Fig. 7.360). However, a variety of conditions can produce infiltration including sinus tarsi ganglia, pigmented villonodular synovitis (PVNS), and abutment between the base of the anterior process of the calcaneum and the anterior margin of the lateral process of the talus. The signal characteristics of the infiltrate will therefore vary according to the type, severity and chronicity of the underlying pathology (see Fig. 7.361). In selected cases, ultrasound-guided injection of the sinus tarsi or aspiration of ganglia may be performed.

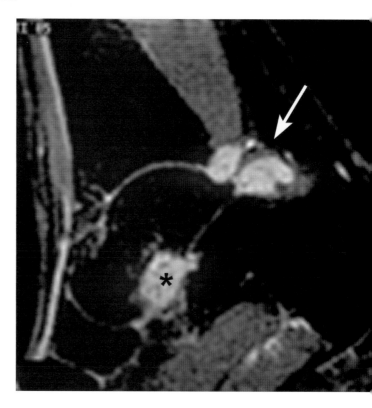

▲ **Fig. 7.361(a)** A sagittal STIR MR image shows replacement of the normal sinus tarsi fat by a ganglion (asterisk). Ganglia are also noted posterior to the ankle and subtalar joints (arrow).

▼ **(b)** A sagittal PD-weighted MR image shows fibrotic infiltrate in the sinus tarsi, replacing the normal sinus fat. This is shown as thickened hypointense bands of tissue replacing the normal bright fat signal (asterisk).

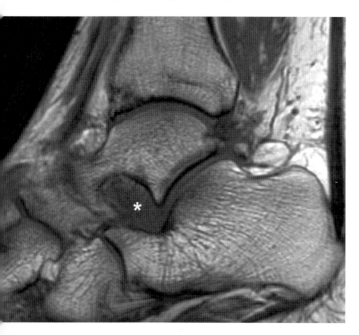

▲ **Fig. 7.360** This sagittal T1-weighted MR image shows infiltration of the sinus tarsi and loss of normal fat signal (asterisk). The fat in the sinus tarsi should have a similar signal to that seen in the pre-Achilles fat pad. There are many possible causes for this appearance.

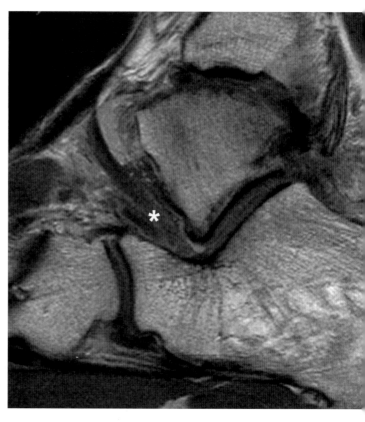

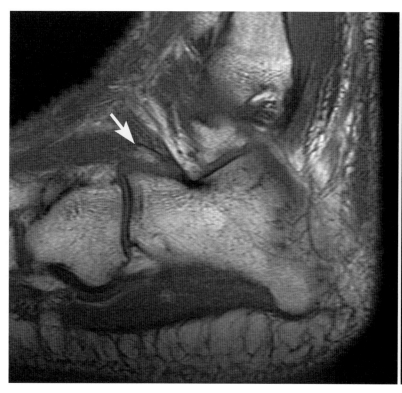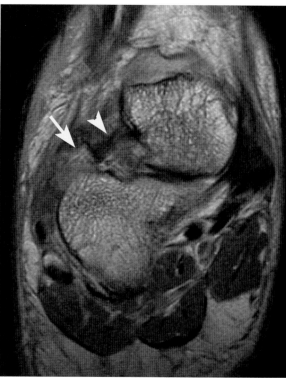

▲ **Fig. 7.362(a)** Sagittal and coronal PD-weighted MR images demonstrate an avulsion fracture at the calcaneal insertion of the cervical ligament. Note the avulsed bone fragment (arrows) and cervical ligament (arrowhead).

▼ **(b)** A PD-weighted coronal MR image demonstrates chronic scarring of the cervical ligament (arrow). The cervical ligament is thickened and hypointense.

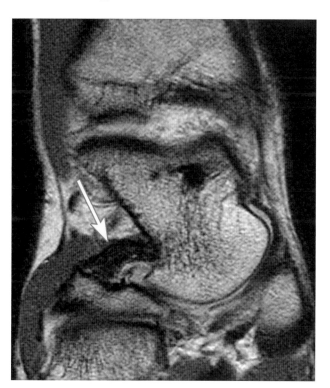

MRI provides assessment of the sinus tarsi ligaments, which may be injured in 43–60% of acute ankle sprains (Breitenseher et al. 1997) (see Fig. 7.362). Non-acute tears of the ITCL often manifest on MRI as focal ligamentous attenuation and signal hyperintensity.

Fractures of the anterior process of the calcaneum

An avulsion fracture of the anterior process of the calcaneum usually results from traction at the bifurcate ligament insertion or the extensor digitorum brevis (EDB) muscle origin. The mechanism of injury typically involves inversion of a plantar-flexed ankle. Alternatively, forced dorsiflexion and eversion may compress the anterior process between the cuboid and the talus, resulting in a shear fracture (Berkowitz and Kim 2005). These fractures commonly involve the dorsal margin of the calcaneocuboid joint. Small avulsion fractures that are entirely extra-articular can also occur. A variable fracture plane can make plain film detection difficult. The fracture line is usually seen on an oblique view of the foot, but occasionally several views must be obtained with differing obliquity to identify and confirm a fracture (see Fig. 7.363). Occasionally, an accessory ossicle (an os calcaneum secundarium) may simulate a fracture of the anterior process of the calcaneum. The absence of any associated bone marrow oedema on MRI can help to differentiate an accessory ossicle from a recent fracture (see Fig. 7.364). If the plain films are negative but clinical suspicion of an anterior process fracture remains high, the diagnosis can be made by nuclear bone scanning, CT or MRI (see Figs 7.365 and 7.366).

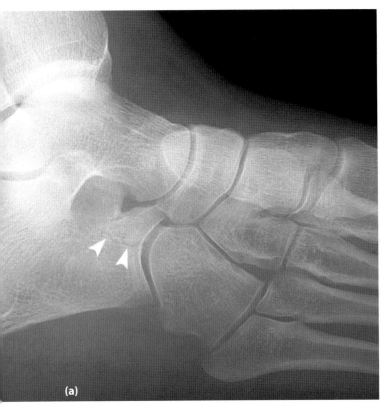

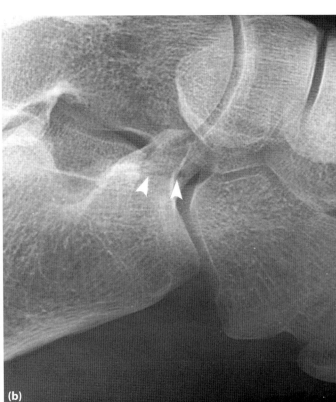

▲ **Fig. 7.363(a)** A fracture of the anterior process of the calcaneum can be difficult to display on plain films due to the varying plane of the fracture. In this case, a fracture is well displayed on an oblique view of the foot (arrowheads). **(b)** A fracture with a different fracture plane is well seen when the foot is more lateral (arrowheads).

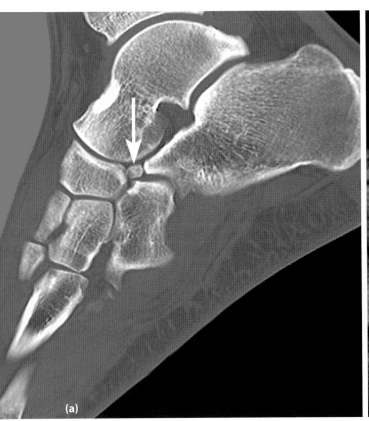

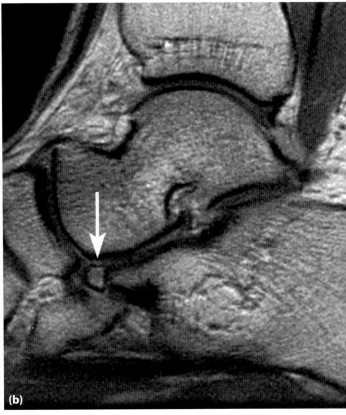

▲ **Fig. 7.364** An os calcaneum secundarium is a normally occurring accessory ossicle and should not be confused with a fracture. This accessory ossicle is demonstrated on CT **(a)** and MRI **(b)** (arrows). The ossicle has a well-defined cortical margin.

◀**Fig. 7.365** If the plain film changes are not clear, MDCT provides a high-resolution imaging method of confirming the presence of a fracture of the anterior process of the calcaneum (arrow).

▼**Fig. 7.366** A sagittal fat-suppressed MR image demonstrates an oblique fracture through the tip of the anterior process of the calcaneum (arrow). There is marrow oedema involving the affected process and an associated effusion.

Tarsal tunnel syndrome

Tarsal tunnel syndrome is caused by compression of the tibial nerve or one or more of its branches within the tarsal tunnel, as the nerve passes the medial malleolus. There are many possible causes of this syndrome, including space-occupying lesions such as a ganglion, lipoma, neuroma or an accessory FDL tendon. Other developmental anomalies that have been thought to predispose to this syndrome include a vertical talus and valgus hind-foot deformity.

Athletes usually present with intermittent sharp or burning pain that is triggered and accentuated by prolonged running and radiates along the foot to the toes. There may be accompanying numbness or paraesthesia. The symptoms most frequently occur in the dermatomal distribution of the medial plantar nerve and can sometimes be bilateral. Ultrasound and MRI can both have a role in the investigation of tarsal tunnel syndrome (see Figs 7.367 and 7.368).

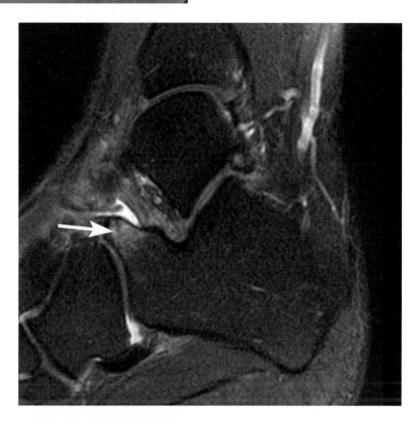

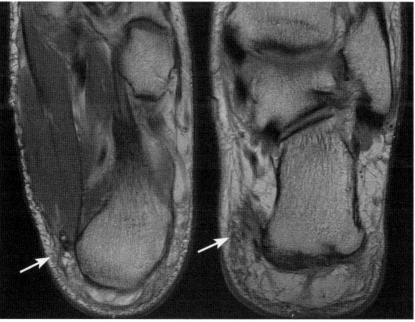

◀**Fig. 7.367** Axial and coronal PD-weighted MR images show a localised zone of irregular intermediate signal in the fat spaces surrounding the medial calcaneal neurovascular bundle secondary to post-traumatic scarring (arrows). Scar encasement of the medial calcaneal nerve was responsible for this patient's plantomedial heel pain.

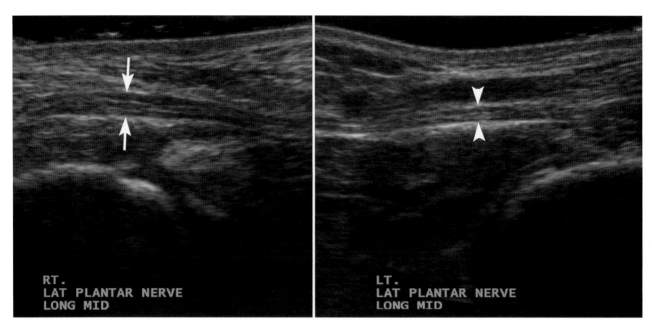

▲ **Fig. 7.368** Tarsal tunnel syndrome is demonstrated in a 22-year-old female dancer who underwent FHL tenosynovectomy that was initially successful. However, 10 months later posteromedial ankle pain occurred, radiating distally into the foot on lunge movements. Long-axis ultrasound images of the right and left lateral plantar nerves were obtained at the tarsal tunnel level. There is fusiform swelling of the right lateral plantar nerve (arrows) when compared with the normal left lateral plantar nerve (arrowheads).

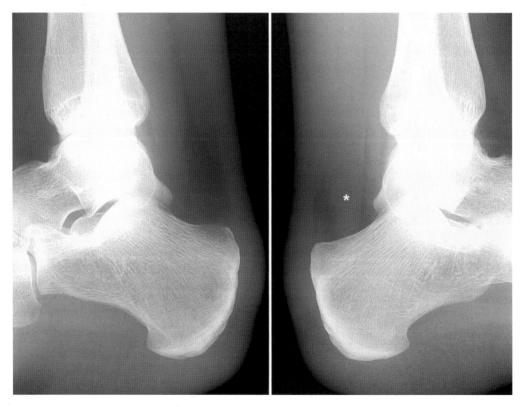

▲ **Fig. 7.369** An accessory soleus muscle on the right produces a soft-tissue density that traverses the pre-Achilles fat pad (asterisk). The left side is normal and is included for comparison.

Accessory muscles of the hind-foot

Accessory soleus muscle

Of particular importance in sports medicine is the recognition of an accessory soleus muscle. This is a normal variant with its own fascial sheath and a tenuous blood supply that can produce exercise-induced calf pain due to claudication or compartment syndrome (Mansberg and Van Niekerk 1991). The typical accessory soleus inserts on the calcaneum 1 cm anterior to the medial margin of the Achilles insertion, coursing superficial to the crural fascia. Lateral radiographs may demonstrate a soft-tissue stripe that traverses the pre-Achilles fat space (see Fig. 7.369). The diagnosis can be made by ultrasound but is often subtle and easily missed. MRI is definitive (see Fig. 7.370). It should be noted that a low-lying soleus muscle can also cause exertional calf pain (see Fig. 7.371).

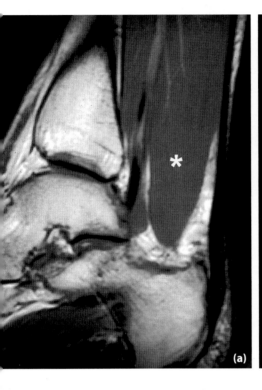

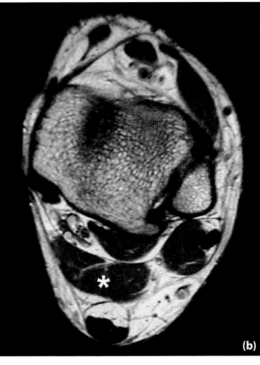

◀ **Fig. 7.370(a)** A large accessory soleus is demonstrated on a sagittal T1-weighted MR image (asterisk). The accessory soleus can vary greatly in size and a large example may completely obliterate the pre-Achilles fat pad.
(b) An axial PD-weighted MR image shows a moderate-sized accessory soleus muscle lying anterior to the Achilles tendon and posterior to the FHL (asterisk).

(a)

(b)

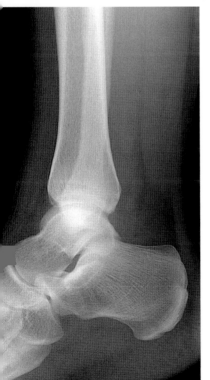

◀ **Fig. 7.371(a)** A low-lying soleus muscle–tendon junction is demonstrated by plain film. There is an unusually low extension of the soleus muscle, an anomaly that may be symptomatic.
▼ **(b)** Sagittal and axial T1-weighted MR images show a low distal myotendinous junction of the soleus muscle (S) (arrow). This was responsible for an exercise-induced compartment syndrome in an 18-year-old elite disabled athlete. The treatment involved partial excision.

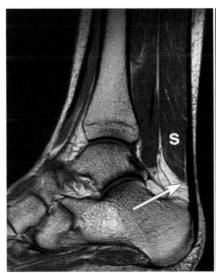

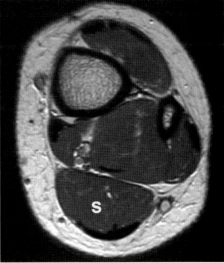

Accessory FDL muscle

This anomaly has a 6–8% incidence rate and becomes symptomatic when the tendon passes through the tarsal tunnel. The muscle originates from the FHL or the flexor retinaculum (see Fig. 7.372).

Behind the ankle joint, the muscle tracks posteromedial to the FHL and posterior tibial neurovascular bundle. The accessory FDL enters the tarsal tunnel medial and separate to the FHL and wedges between the FHL and the flexor retinaculum (see Fig. 7.373), passing posterolateral to the lateral plantar nerve. At the level of the sustentaculum tali, the muscle or tendon blends with the quadratus plantae.

Other accessory muscles

The peroneocalcaneus internus (PCI) has a 1% incidence rate, originates from the lower third of the fibula and descends immediately posterolateral to the FHL tendon with only a very thin intervening fat plane. The PCI enters the calcaneal groove lateral to the FHL before finally inserting at a small tubercle on the medial aspect of the calcaneum below the sustentaculum. Being separated from the neurovascular bundle by the intervening tendon of the FHL, the thin peroneocalcaneus internus tendon is unlikely to cause tarsal tunnel syndrome. If the accessory soleus passes deep to the crural fascia, it is known as tibiocalcaneus internus. The peroneus quartus is discussed elsewhere in this chapter.

The heel

Routine plain film views of the heel

A routine series of plain films of the heel includes lateral and axial views (see Fig. 7.374). The lateral view of the heel must be carefully positioned, with the ankle in a true lateral position and the malleoli superimposed. The axial view demonstrates the calcaneal tuberosity and is helpful in the assessment of subtle fractures. The method of obtaining this view is discussed on page 622.

On the lateral view, the pre-Achilles fat pad should be carefully examined. This should be of homogeneous fat density, apart from a few traversing

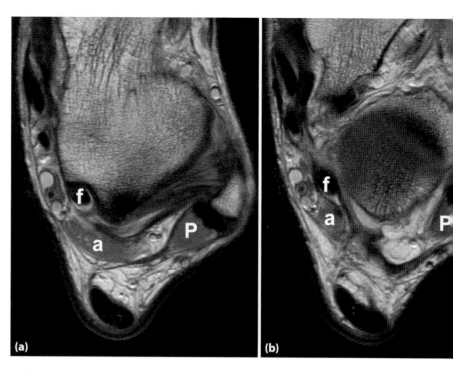

▲ **Fig. 7.372** Axial PD-weighted MR images have been obtained at the level of the talar groove **(a)** and at the level of the subtalar joint **(b)**. At the level of the talar groove, an accessory FDL muscle (a) is demonstrated originating from the flexor retinaculum and lying posterior to the FHL (f). At the level of the subtalar joint, the accessory FDL is seen within the tarsal tunnel posterior to the FHL (f). Peroneal muscle = P.

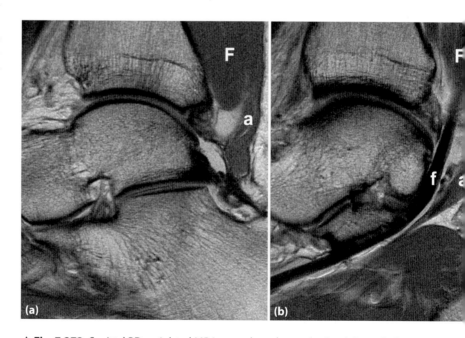

▲ **Fig. 7.373** Sagittal PD-weighted MR images have been obtained through the lateral tubercle of the posterior process of the talus **(a)** and at the level of the tarsal tunnel **(b)**. The midline image shows both the accessory FDL (a) and the FHL (f). At the level of the tarsal tunnel, the accessory FDL muscle and tendon (a) run posterior and medial to the FHL tendon (f). At the level of the sustentaculum tali, the tendon of the accessory FDL merges with the quadratus plantae.

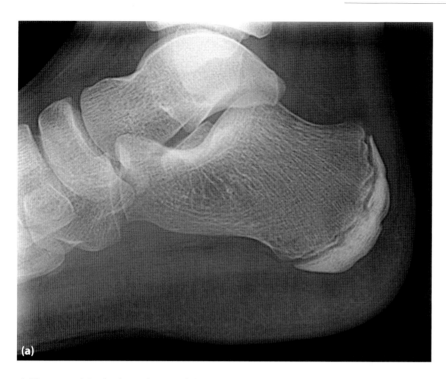
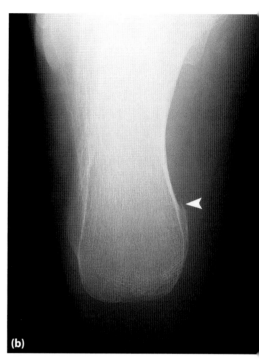

▲ **Fig. 7.374(a)** This lateral view of the heel in an immature athlete shows the normally dense calcaneal apophysis and considerable soft-tissue detail. In particular, the Achilles insertion and the plantar fascia should always be carefully examined. **(b)** The axial view is helpful in identifying fractures of the calcaneal tuberosity. In this case, a subtle fracture of the medial tuberosity is demonstrated (arrowhead).

vessels. The soleus muscle, Achilles tendon, plantar fascia, posterior ankle joint and FHL muscle should all be identified and examined. CT scanning may be necessary to confirm subtle calcaneal fractures or to determine the exact extent of joint involvement (see Fig. 7.375). Although plain films can provide an indication of soft-tissue abnormalities, these changes may be subtle and are better assessed by ultrasound or MRI.

Abnormalities of the Achilles tendon

Common conditions of the Achilles tendon are usually related to overuse and characteristically include tendinopathy and peritendinitis in males over 30 years of age, although anyone starting a sporting activity or significantly increasing the frequency or intensity of Achilles loading is at risk. Non-insertional Achilles tendinopathy and paratenonitis are the most frequent tendon problems in athletes (Brukner 1997).

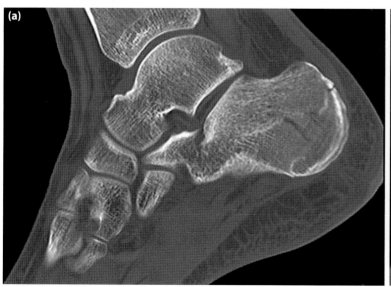
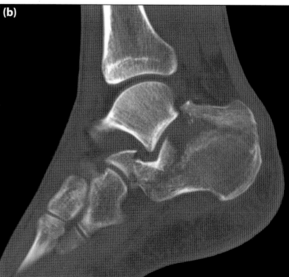

▲ **Fig. 7.375(a)** The high-resolution of MDCT demonstrates subtle calcaneal fractures that are difficult to see on plain films. **(b)** The complexities and displacement of fragments with more severe injuries are well displayed by MDCT.

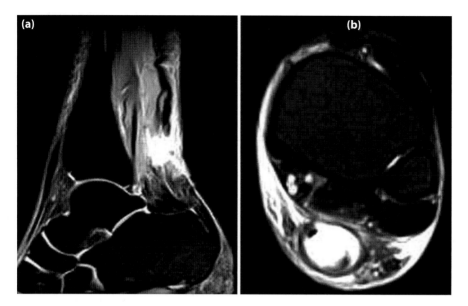

▲ **Fig. 7.376** Sagittal and axial STIR MR images dramatically demonstrate rupture of the Achilles tendon.
(a) The sagittal image shows a complete tear about 4–5 cm proximal to the Achilles insertion, with retraction of the proximal tendon. **(b)** Haematoma distends and is largely contained by the Achilles paratenon, which has become expanded.

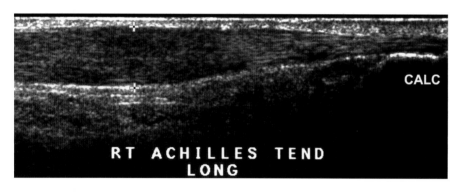

◀ **Fig. 7.377** Uncomplicated non-insertional Achilles tendinopathy is demonstrated by ultrasound. A long-axis ultrasound image of the Achilles tendon shows hypoechoic fusiform swelling of the proximal tendon segment (callipers) with fibrillar echotexture remaining discernible throughout. Calcaneum = CALC.

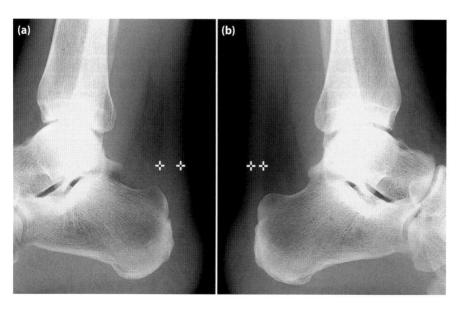

◀ **Fig. 7.378** Plain films show changes of distal Achilles tendinopathy. There is swelling of the abnormal right tendon **(a)** by comparison with the normal left side **(b)** (callipers). Also note the associated reaction within the pre-Achilles fat pad.

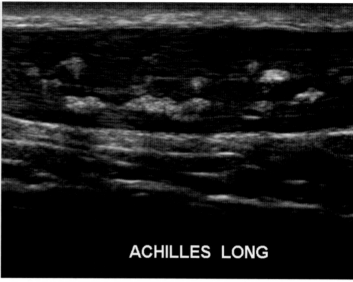

▲ **Fig. 7.379** Ultrasound demonstrates chronic Achilles tendinopathy with calcification. Transverse and long-axis greyscale ultrasound images show hypoechoic fusiform Achilles tendon thickening and multiple contained calcifications are shown as coarse echogenic foci casting posterior acoustic shadows.

Ultrasound and MRI are equally as effective at imaging Achilles tendon pathology, but surgeons faced with making a decision to operate often favour MRI for the more panoramic and less operator-dependent nature of this test. A fat-suppressed short TE (T2*-weighted) gradient-echo sequence should be routinely included in the MRI scan protocol, as this is the most sensitive sequence for tendinopathy. As many as 25% of intratendinous Achilles lesions may be missed by MRI if this technique is not used, although the high sensitivity of the gradient-echo sequence can sometimes lead to an over-estimation of lesion size (Karjalainen et al. 2000). Additional PD, fat-suppressed T2 or STIR sequences are also important (see Fig. 7.376).

Non-insertional Achilles tendinopathy is a degenerative process that results from either chronic repetitive loading or, less commonly, direct trauma. The clinical syndrome of tendon pain and thickening occurs in about 10% of runners, but can also be seen in other sporting activities such as dancing (Brukner 1997). Running produces forces up to eight times the body weight on the Achilles tendon, sometimes for prolonged periods (Soma and Mandelbaum 1994). Factors that may increase the load on the tendon and predispose to symptomatic tendinopathy include incorrect running technique, poorly fitted shoes, hyperpronation of the foot, contracture of the gastrocnemius-soleus complex, abnormal biomechanics and external pressure (Mazzone and McCue 2002). Although the tendinopathy process may occur at virtually any location within the tendon, the upper third is most often affected, probably due to its relative hypovascularity (see Fig. 7.377). There may be associated peritendon changes (see Fig. 7.378). Imaging is often used to confirm the clinical diagnosis and exclude complications such as an intra-tendon 'cyst' due to accumulated gel-like proteoglycans, calcification resulting from fibrocartilaginous metaplasia (see Fig. 7.379), and partial-thickness tear due to progressive tendon weakening (see Figs 7.380 and 7.381).

Insertional Achilles tendinopathy is usually insidious in onset and is associated with increased activity and pressure from shoes against the posterior heel in subjects with either Haglund deformity (discussed further below), or prominent spurring or intrasubstance calcification at the insertion of the Achilles tendon (see Fig. 7.382). Tenderness and swelling are localised to the calcaneal tendon insertion. Surgery may be required to excise calcifications or exostoses in recalcitrant cases. MRI or ultrasound will help to exclude a more proximal tendinopathy that would not benefit from such excision.

Achilles peritendinitis and paratenonitis are essentially synonymous terms that denote a clinical syndrome of pain and swelling due to inflammation of the peritendinous and perimysial structures associated with the proximal tendon and myotendinous junction. There are both acute and chronic forms of the condition, which is most common in runners. An acute inflammatory response may form within the loose areolar peritendon connective tissues and overlying paratenon after an episode of acute overuse or blunt trauma (see Fig. 7.383). Although the Achilles tendon lacks a true synovial sheath, it nevertheless moves or 'glides' within a thin fibrous membrane (the 'paratenon') that covers the dorsal, medial and lateral tendon surfaces and lies beneath the subcutaneous fascia cruris (Józsa and Kannus 1997). In acute paratenonitis, fibrinous exudate within this fibrous sheath may produce palpable crepitus on attempted movement of the Achilles tendon and eventual adhesions if the process persists (Kvist and Kvist 1980). Alternatively, chronic paratenonitis can develop as an overuse syndrome of gradual onset in which no prior acute episode can be elicited. In this condition there is tender fibroblastic thickening and adhesion of the paratenon (either diffuse or nodular) but no effusion or crepitus (see Fig. 7.384). The normal paratenon is quite thin but can still be appreciated on both ultrasound and high-resolution MRI as a distinct layer against the Achilles tendon.

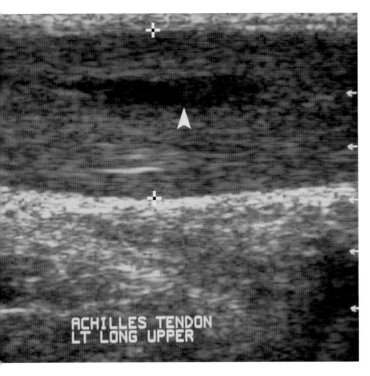

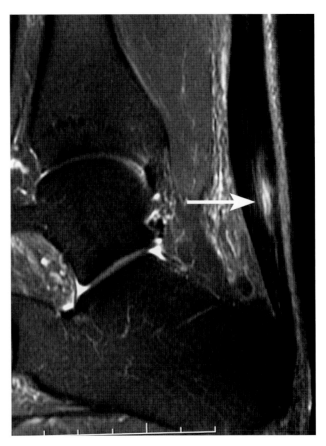

▲ **Fig. 7.380(a)** Complicated non-insertional Achilles tendinopathy is demonstrated by ultrasound. A detailed long-axis ultrasound image of the proximal Achilles tendon segment shows fusiform tendon thickening due to tendinopathy (callipers) and a superimposed central anechoic focus with loss of fibrillar echotexture (arrowhead), indicating either cystic degeneration or an intrasubstance tear. In practice, a careful consideration of the patient's history is often helpful in deciding which of these two possibilities is more likely.

▼ **(c)** Ultrasound demonstrates a longitudinal tear of the Achilles tendon (callipers). Long-axis and transverse images show a hypoechoic split in the Achilles tendon. Slight swelling of the tendon is noted.

▲ **(b)** A sagittal fat-suppressed MR image demonstrates linear high signal in a fusiform Achilles tendon, about 5 cm proximal to its insertion. The appearance is that of a longitudinal tear in an area of tendinopathy (arrow). Also note the high signal in the peritendon spaces.

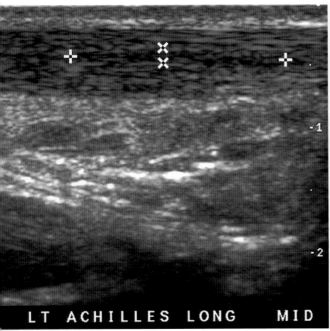

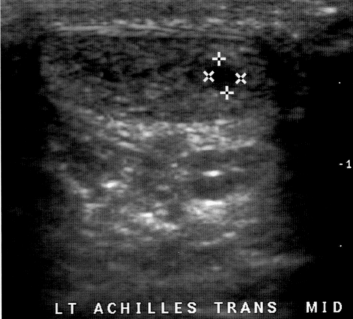

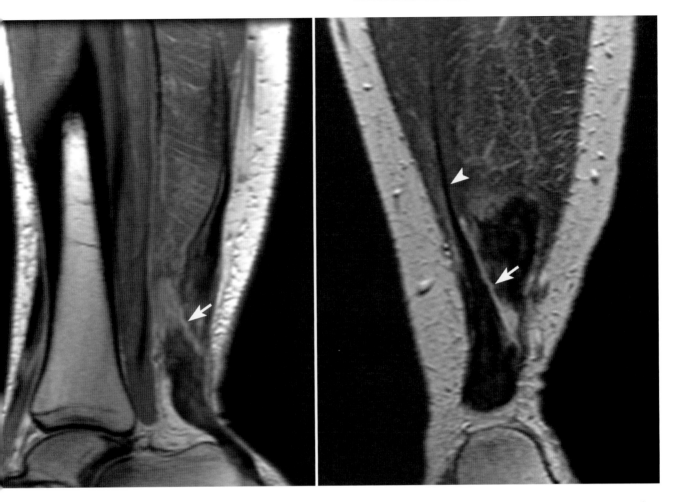

▲ **Fig. 7.381** Sagittal and coronal PD-weighted images show the high signal line of an oblique tear through the mid-portion of Achilles tendinopathy (arrows). Note the intact medial soleal tendon (arrowhead).

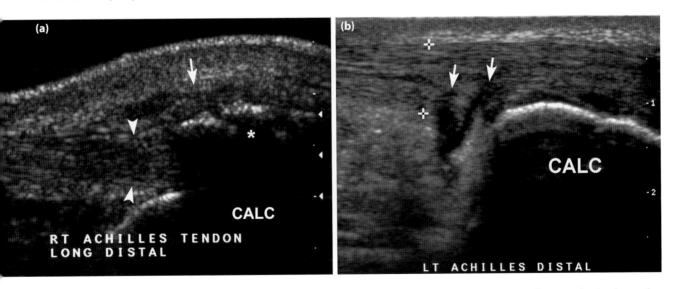

▲ **Fig. 7.382(a)** Insertional Achilles tendinopathy is demonstrated by ultrasound. A long-axis ultrasound image obtained over the calcaneal insertion of the Achilles tendon shows thickening of the distal tendon segment (arrowheads), prominent calcification and/or bone spurring at the calcaneal attachment (asterisk), and thickening of the overlying superficial calcaneal bursa (arrow). Calcaneal tuberosity = CALC.

(b) A partial-thickness tear of the Achilles tendon in its distal segment is shown by ultrasound. A long-axis ultrasound image demonstrates a ragged transverse hypoechoic defect in fibre continuity at the deep surface of the Achilles tendon just above the calcaneal tuberosity (arrows). The tendon at this level shows background changes of tendinopathy with thickening (callipers) and heterogeneous hypoechoic echotexture. Calcaneal tuberosity = CALC.

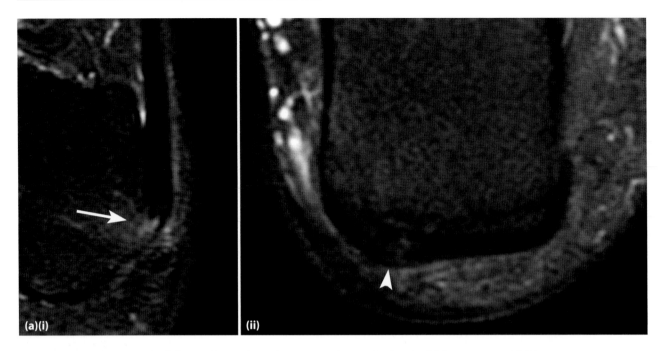

▲ **Fig. 7.383(a)** Insertional Achilles tendinopathy is demonstrated on sagittal and axial fat-suppressed MR images.
(i) The sagittal image shows irregular high signal in the Achilles tendon, with oedema extending into the adjacent calcaneum, indicative of both tendinopathy and enthesopathy (arrow).
(ii) The axial image shows localised swelling of the tendon and patchy high signal at the affected insertion (arrowhead).
▼ **(b)** Acute Achilles paratenonitis is demonstrated by transverse ultrasound images of the proximal Achilles tendon segment. The Achilles tendon (arrow) appears uniform in thickness and normal in echotexture, but there is marked hypoechoic thickening of the surrounding paratenon (arrowhead). The Power Doppler image (right) shows associated hyperaemia in the line of both the paratenon and the pre-Achilles fat pad.

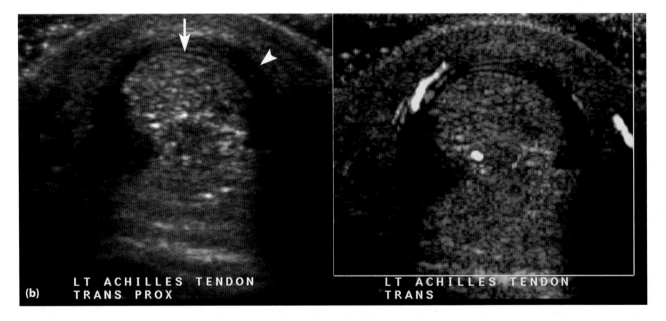

MRI findings in paratenonitis include thickening of the paratenon and high signal within the adjacent pre-Achilles fat pad on fat-suppressed T2 or STIR sequences. Ultrasound also shows thickening of the paratenon, increased fat pad echogenicity and variable peritendon hyperaemia. Small peritendon effusions are occasionally seen in acute cases. Although the clinical diagnosis is usually straightforward, imaging can help to exclude coexistent intra-tendinous lesions that may preclude a therapeutic steroid injection and

that also indicate a poorer prognosis (Karjalainen et al. 2000). Paratenonitis responds well to corticosteroid injections, which can be guided by ultrasound for the greatest accuracy.

Achilles tendon rupture can be spontaneous or traumatic, partial or complete, transverse (see Fig. 7.385(a)) or longitudinal (see Fig. 7.385(b)). Although a variety of pathological processes can potentially weaken a tendon and predispose it to rupture, the vast majority of Achilles ruptures (both spontaneous and traumatic) occur on a background of tendon degeneration or 'tendinopathy' (Kannus and Józsa 1991). Acute traumatic tears in young athletes are usually partial, while complete Achilles ruptures are more common in older athletes. Complete ruptures classically occur 2–6 cm above the calcaneal insertion within the zone of relative tendon hypovascularity (Lagergren and Lindholm 1959). Although the clinical diagnosis of a complete tear is usually obvious to an experienced physician, nevertheless a delayed or missed diagnosis of Achilles rupture occurs in

20–30% of cases (Inglis et al. 1976). The reasons for this can include haematoma obscuring the tendon defect, some retention of plantar-flexion power due to other flexors (including the plantaris) and a false-negative Thompson test, which can arise if the accessory ankle flexors are squeezed during the physical examination (Saltzman and Tearse 1998).

Although ultrasound can be highly accurate for the diagnosis of Achilles rupture, there are some important pitfalls for inexperienced operators. These include the missed diagnosis

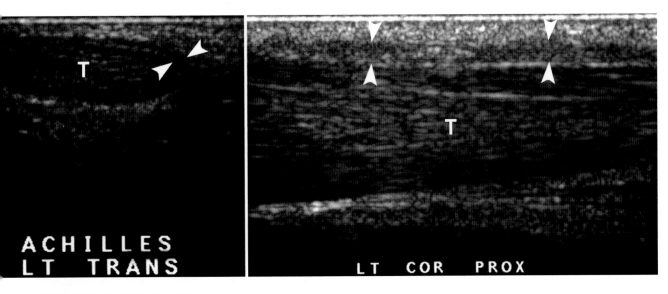

▲ Fig. 7.384 Ultrasound demonstrates chronic Achilles paratenonitis. Transverse and long-axis coronal ultrasound images of the proximal Achilles tendon segment are shown. The Achilles tendon (T) appears normal in size and texture, but there is localised hypoechoic thickening of the medial paratenon (arrowheads).

◄ Fig. 7.385(a) There is a complete mid-segment Achilles tendon rupture. A sagittal PD-weighted MR image shows complete interruption in tendon continuity, retraction of the proximal stump and the resulting gap filled largely by fat (arrow). There are changes of underlying tendinopathy at the separated proximal and distal tendon stumps (asterisks).

▼ (b) An Achilles tendon mid-segment partial-thickness tear is present. A long-axis ultrasound image demonstrates a hypoechoic longitudinal tear (callipers) within the central substance of the Achilles tendon. Arrowheads indicate the Achilles tendon surfaces. Calcaneal tuberosity = CALC.

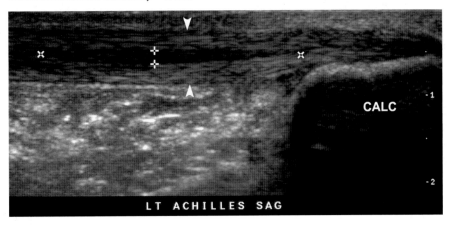

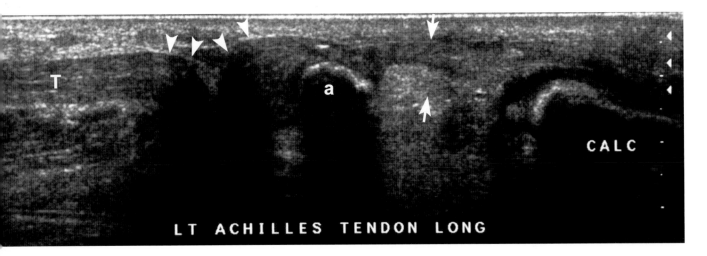

LT ACHILLES TENDON LONG

▲ **Fig. 7.386** Achilles tendon avulsion is demonstrated on a panoramic long-axis ultrasound image. The Achilles tendon (T) shows a complete avulsion of the calcaneal attachment, with retraction of the tendon stump and accompanying bone fragment (a) by approximately 3 cm. The retracted tendon segment has buckled (arrowheads), creating a hypoechoic zone due to anisotropy. The tendon gap (arrows) is not fluid-filled, but is instead echogenic due to contained organising haemorrhage and prolapse of the pre-Achilles fat pad. This complex sonographic pattern is a potential pitfall in the interpretation of ultrasound that leads to false negative examinations by inexperienced operators.

of a complete tear arising from failure to appreciate a tendon 'gap' that has filled with echogenic haematoma (see Fig. 7.386), and the falsely reassuring diagnosis of a 'partial tear' arising from failure to appreciate (and failure to alert the referring physician to) the significance of a high-grade lesion that is functionally equivalent to a complete tear and in need of surgical repair. Consequently, when reporting partial tears, the radiologist should always attempt to estimate the percentage of cross-sectional area of tendon involved and measure any gap resulting from fibre retraction. Chronic ruptures may result in tendon ossification (see Fig. 7.387).

Haglund's syndrome and heel bursopathy

The retrocalcaneal bursa lies in the sulcus between the Achilles tendon and the posterior surface of the calcaneum. This sulcus can be identified on a lateral plain film of the heel, and normally contains fatty tissue of similar density to the pre-Achilles fat pad. When retrocalcaneal bursopathy develops, the fatty tissue in the sulcus is replaced with water-equivalent density (see Fig. 7.388). An isolated retrocalcaneal bursopathy can develop with acute or repetitive trauma, or alternatively in association with arthropathies. On ultrasound, the retrocalcaneal bursa is distended if it measures more than 3 mm in thickness (see Fig. 7.389).

Haglund's syndrome is the most common condition of heel pain. This syndrome usually involves a combination of distal Achilles tendinopathy, tendo-Achilles bursopathy and retrocalcaneal bursopathy. The tendo-Achilles bursa lies in the subcutaneous soft tissues superficial to the Achilles tendon and the chronic bursopathy produces an enlargement known as a 'pump-bump' because it invariably results from repetitive friction from footwear (see Fig. 7.390). A bony prominence on the superior aspect of the posterior calcaneal margin may predispose an athlete to Haglund's syndrome. This is known as the bursal projection of the

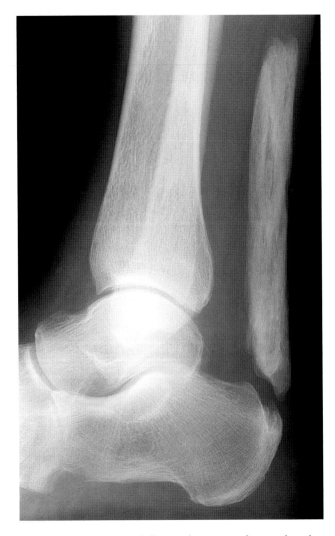

▲ **Fig. 7.387** Chronic Achilles tendon rupture has produced ossification. The only trauma that this patient could recall was caused by jumping into a lifeboat during World War II.

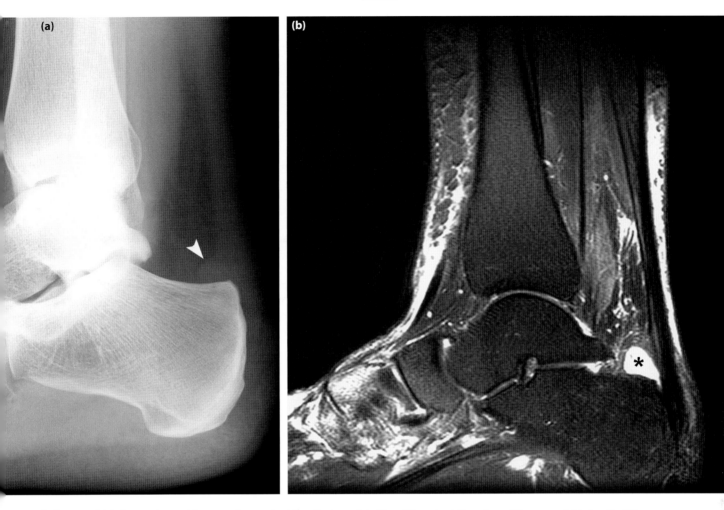

▲ **Fig. 7.388(a)** Retrocalcaneal bursopathy can be identified on plain films. There is obliteration of the normal fat density filling the sulcus between the lower Achilles tendon and the superoposterior margin of the calcaneal tuberosity. A distended bursa of water density has a rounded configuration (arrowhead). **(b)** A sagittal STIR MR image demonstrates the typical MRI appearance of a retrocalcaneal bursopathy (asterisk).

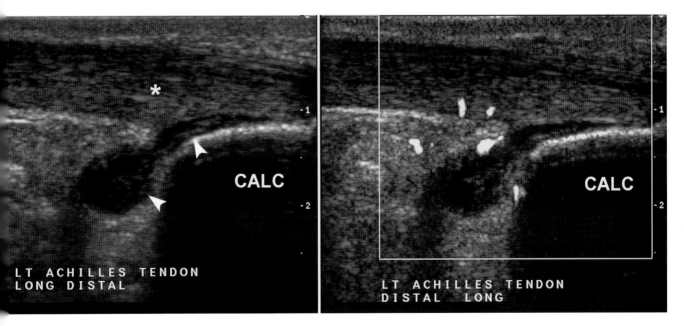

▲ **Fig. 7.389** Retrocalcaneal bursopathy is demonstrated by ultrasound. Long-axis greyscale and Power Doppler ultrasound images demonstrate synovial thickening, mild effusion and hyperaemia associated with a distended retrocalcaneal bursa (arrowheads). Also note the accompanying mild distal Achilles tendinopathy (asterisk). Calcaneum = CALC.

▲ **Fig. 7.390** Tendo-Achilles bursopathy is demonstrated by ultrasound. There is chronic adventitial bursal thickening with associated hyperaemia overlying the Achilles tendon insertion (arrowheads). The normal Achilles tendon is indicated by an arrow. Calcaneum = CALC.

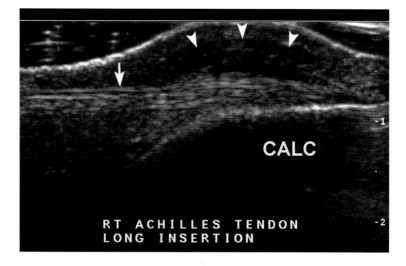

calcaneum (see Fig. 7.391). The presence of a prominent bursal projection is determined by drawing 'pitch lines' (see Fig. 7.392). Ultrasound or MRI will demonstrate the full extent of any associated Achilles tendinopathy and bursopathy.

Changes in the pre-Achilles fat pad

The normal pre-Achilles fat pad is triangular in shape with sharply defined margins and uniform fatty density. The borders of the fat pad are the FHL muscle anteriorly, the musculotendinous junction of the Achilles and Achilles tendon posteriorly, and the superior border of the calcaneum inferiorly. The fat pad should be routinely assessed on plain radiographs for any alterations in density, as these can be important clues to underlying pathology (see Fig. 7.393).

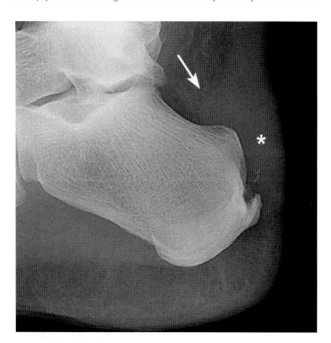

▲ **Fig. 7.391** Haglund's syndrome is readily recognised on plain film. There are four changes to be noted: (i) insertional Achilles tendinopathy, (ii) retrocalcaneal bursopathy, (iii) tendo-Achilles bursopathy and (iv) a bursal protrusion of the superoposterior angle of the calcaneum. In this case, Achilles tendinopathy is seen as swelling of the distal tendon, with calcification within the tendon adjacent to the insertion. Spur formation is also present at the Achilles insertion. The swelling of tendinopathy has merged with the 'pump bump', which is indicative of a superficial Achilles bursopathy (asterisk). A retrocalcaneal bursopathy is present, obliterating the retrocalcaneal sulcus (arrow). There is a prominent calcaneal bursal protrusion.

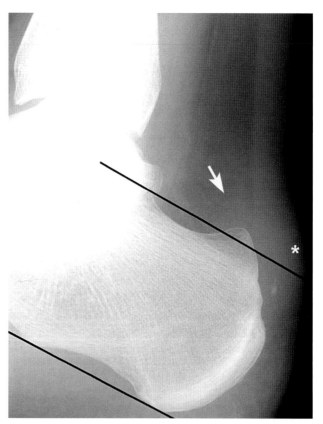

▲ **Fig. 7.392** 'Pitch lines' are a guide to the prominence of a bursal protrusion of the calcaneum. A line is drawn along the inferior margin of the calcaneum to guide the placement of a second parallel line tangential to the anterosuperior corner of the calcaneum. If any of the posterosuperior corner of the calcaneum lies above this line, this is considered abnormally prominent. Also note the other components of Haglund's syndrome in this case (arrow and asterisk).

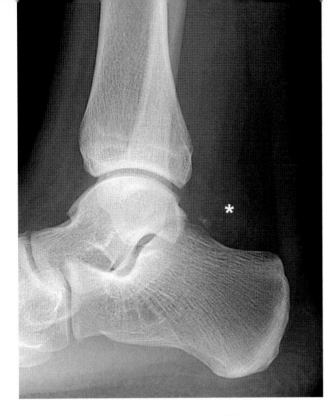

▲ Fig. 7.393 The pre-Achilles fat pad should be a homogeneous fat density; any other densities in this triangle are likely to indicate an abnormality. The fat pad should be carefully examined for altered densities. In this case, there is a rounded density protruding beyond the margin of the FHL (asterisk). This is most likely a large ganglion, and ultrasound or MRI would be necessary to further characterise this change.

Calcaneal fractures

Acute fractures of the calcaneum are usually related to impact from jumping or falling. The majority are comminuted compression injuries that involve the subtalar joint and depress the articular surface of the posterior facet. Plain films should include a lateral view of the hind-foot, AP and oblique views of the foot and an axial view of the heel, which can sometimes be difficult to obtain following an acute fracture. The degree of calcaneal deformity is quantified on the lateral view by measuring Böhler's angle (also known as the tuber-joint angle). This angle is normally 20 to 40° (see Fig. 7.394). The AP image of the foot should be assessed for fracture extension into the calcaneocuboid articulation, and the axial radiograph should be assessed for medial and lateral wall comminution or any increase in transverse dimension of the calcaneum. MDCT provides a more definitive assessment of calcaneal fractures (see Fig. 7.395).

Calcaneal stress fractures usually involve the posterior calcaneal tuberosity (see Fig. 7.396). The typical calcaneal stress fracture is oriented in an oblique coronal plane extending parallel to the line of the force transmitted between the Achilles tendon and plantar fascia, and identified on lateral radiographs as an ill-defined sclerotic band extending across the calcaneal tuberosity parallel to the posterior margin. Less commonly, the anterior process and anterior body may be involved (see Fig. 7.397).

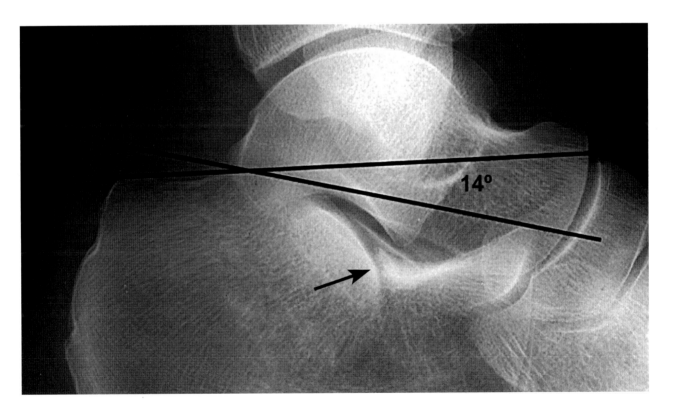

▲ Fig. 7.394 Böhler's angle is formed by the intersection of two lines, one drawn between the dorsal margin of the anterior process of the calcaneum and the posterior articular corner of the posterior calcaneal facet, and the other drawn between the far posterosuperior corner of the calcaneal tuberosity and the posterior articular corner of the posterior calcaneal facet. A normal angle is 20 to 40°. In this case, a fracture of the calcaneum extends into the subtalar joint, decreasing Böhler's angle.

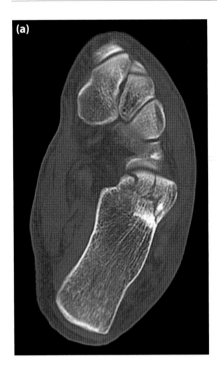

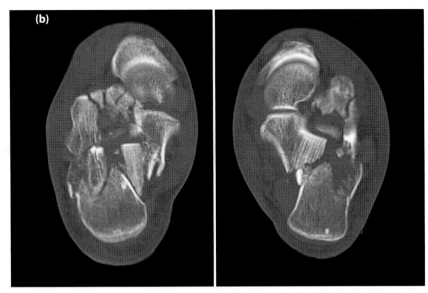

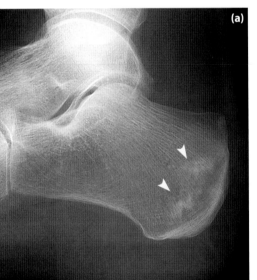

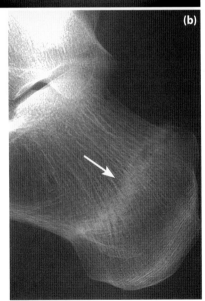

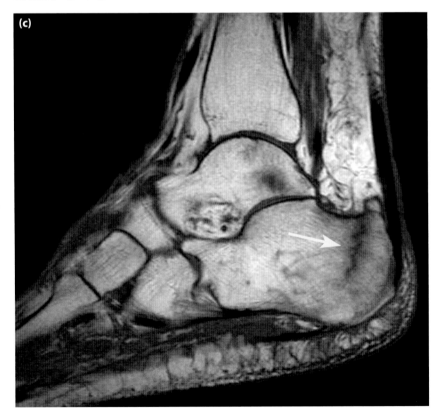

◀▲ Fig. 7.395(a) An axial MDCT image demonstrates a comminuted fracture of the anterior process of the calcaneum, with only minor displacement.
(b) A 29-year-old male in an intoxicated state decided to jump from a first-floor balcony. Axial MDCT images of both feet demonstrate gross bilateral hind-foot comminution.

◀▼ Fig. 7.396(a) This lateral plain film of the heel shows the typical appearance of calcaneal stress fractures. The fractures tend to run roughly parallel to the posterior margin of the calcaneal tuberosity (arrowheads). Occasionally, a fracture line is evident, but more often the bone stress appears as an indistinct sclerotic smudge.
(b) This is an insufficiency fracture extending across the calcaneum with a typical appearance and orientation (arrow). A discrete fracture line is developing at the superior aspect of the sclerotic band.
(c) A sagittal T1-weighted MR image demonstrates an insufficiency fracture of the calcaneum (arrow).

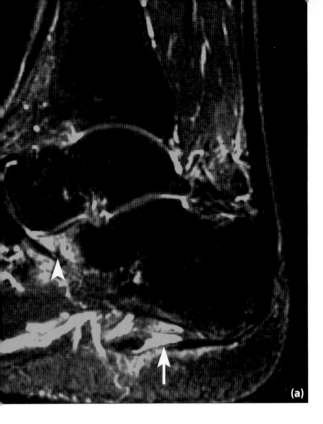

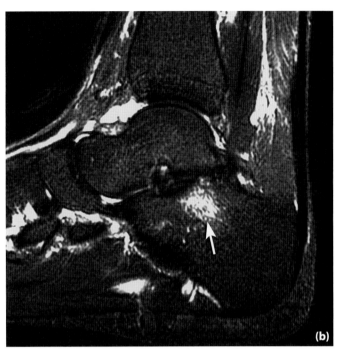

▲▼ **Fig. 7.397(a)** A middle-distance runner at the Sydney 2000 Olympics withdrew from his race with a rupture of the plantar fascia. The rupture is complete, with retraction of the distal stump. High signal of fresh haemorrhage fills the gap (arrow). This sagittal STIR MR image also demonstrates increased marrow signal in the anterior process of the calcaneum due to an underlying chronic stress fracture, seen as a hypointense line extending from the inferior margin of the base of the process (arrowhead).
(b) A sagittal STIR MR image shows a localised area of high signal in the subchondral bone beneath the calcaneal facet of the posterior subtalar joint (arrow). This change was clinically consistent with bone stress. No fracture line is evident. The patient was an Olympic female basketball player and the scattered small effusions and high signal noted in muscle are normal for an athlete performing at this level of competition.
(c) Axial PD and fat-suppressed PD-weighted images show a subchondral calcaneal stress fracture in the anterior process of the calcaneum at the calcaneocuboid articulation (arrow). Note the considerable associated marrow oedema (asterisk).

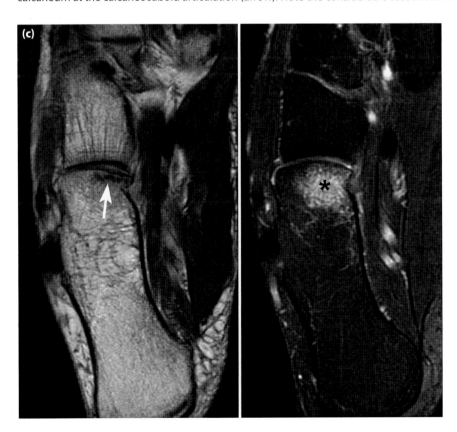

In the sporting population, these injuries are most commonly seen in runners (Eisele and Sammarco 1993). A reactive effusion is commonly present within the retrocalcaneal bursa, and calcaneal stress fractures can be mistaken both clinically and sonographically for retrocalcaneal bursitis if careful attention is not paid to the precise point of maximal tenderness. MRI or nuclear bone scans are usually diagnostic. An assessment of underlying bone density is also advisable, particularly in amenorrhoeic female athletes.

Rarely, the superior angle of the calcaneal tuberosity can be avulsed by the Achilles tendon. This is known as a 'beak' fracture (see Fig. 7.398(a)). Bone spurs at the Achilles insertion may also be avulsed (see Fig. 7.398(b)), and avulsion fractures may occur at the origin of the extensor digitorum brevis (see Fig. 7.399).

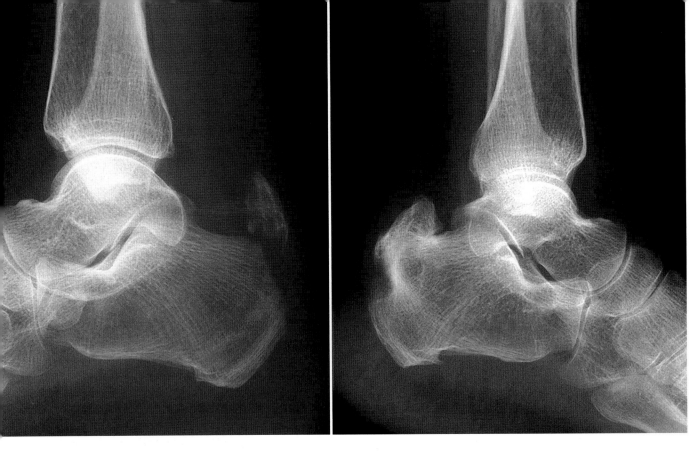

▲ **Fig. 7.398(a)** There has been an avulsion fracture of the posterosuperior corner of the left calcaneum caused by Achilles tendon traction. This is known as a 'beak' fracture. Retraction of the fragment has occurred. A similar fracture has previously occurred on the right side. Osteopaenia appears to be present.

▼ **(b)** A variation of the 'beak' fracture is the avulsion of a bony spur that has developed at the Achilles insertions. In this case, there are bilateral spurs and avulsion of the left spur has occurred, with retraction of the fragment.

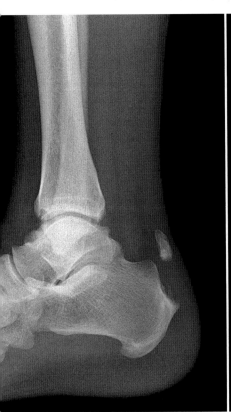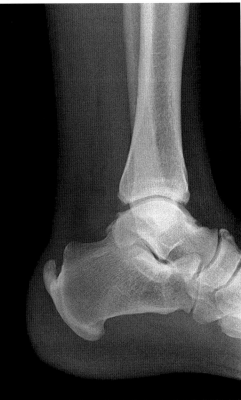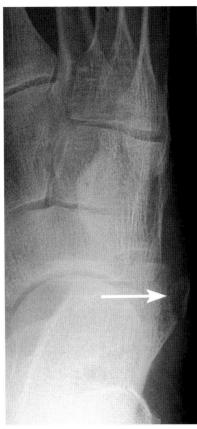

▲ **Fig. 7.399** A further calcaneal avulsion fracture may occur at the origin of the extensor digitorum brevis (arrow).

Sever's disease

Sever's disease is a para-apophyseal bone stress reaction of the calcaneal tuberosity in children, most common in boys between six and 10 years of age. The relevant MRI finding consists of marrow oedema within the metaphyseal region of the calcaneal tuberosity adjacent to the apophysis (Ogden et al. 2004) (see Fig. 7.400). It should be noted that oedema-like signal within the calcaneal apophysis itself can be a normal finding that persists after both heel pain and metaphyseal oedema resolve. Apophyseal fragmentation and sclerosis on plain radiographs are also normal findings that do not indicate Sever's disease.

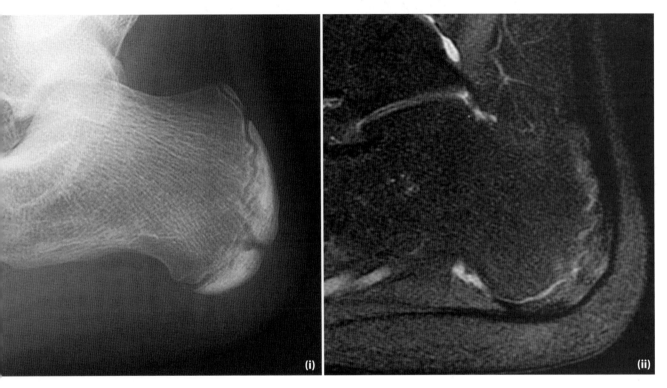

▲ **Fig. 7.400(a)** Sever's disease is demonstrated in an 11-year-old female athlete with persistent heel pain. **(i)** A plain film shows a sclerotic calcaneal apophysis, which is divided by a cleft. Both these findings are normal. **(ii)** A fat-suppressed PD image demonstrates high signal within the apophysis itself, which is also a normal finding. However, there is also abnormal subtle bone marrow oedema within the metaphyseal region of the calcaneal tuberosity adjacent to the apophysis.

▶ **(b)** An athletic 11-year-old boy presented with severe heel pain. Sagittal T1 and STIR MR images demonstrate a combination of Sever's disease and features of Haglund's syndrome. There is marrow oedema along the full length of the metaphyseal side of the calcaneal apophysis indicative of Sever's disease (arrowheads). Also note a prominent bursal projection of the calcaneum, with an effusion in the adjacent retrocalcaneal bursa (asterisk) and localised tendinopathy in the distal Achilles segment and the overall appearance is consistent with Haglund's syndrome (arrow).

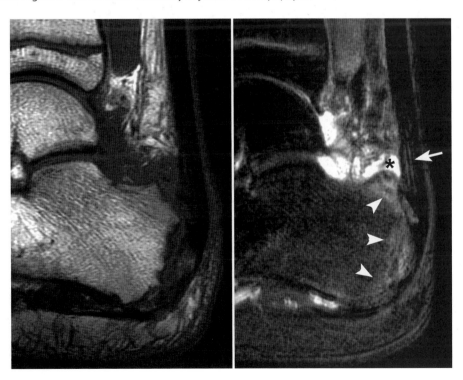

Plantar fascial pathology

The plantar fascia is a thickened fibrous aponeurosis along the inferior contour of the foot that originates primarily from the calcaneal tubercle but also receives a small contribution of fibres continuing on from the Achilles tendon, which pass around the heel. The medial band is the dominant and thickest portion of the fascia, originating from the medial process of the calcaneal tubercle and inserting distally into the transverse metatarsal ligaments, adjacent fibrous flexor sheaths and skin.

The lateral band is rudimentary or absent in 10% of the population (Lee et al. 1993), originates from the lateral process of the calcaneal tubercle and inserts distally into the base of the fifth metatarsal. The plantar fascia provides both static support for the longitudinal arch of the foot and dynamic shock absorption during foot strike while walking or running. When running, the plantar fascia effectively stores energy during the heel-off phase of gait due to elastic stretch, and then releases that energy by passive contraction during toe-off to assist foot acceleration (the 'windlass mechanism').

Plantar fasciitis is the most common cause of inferior heel pain. It may affect up to 10% of running athletes (Baxter 1994) and is among the five most common foot and ankle injuries observed in professional footballers, baseball players and basketball players (Moseley and Chimenti 1995). The term 'fasciitis' is misleading because the underlying pathology is degenerative rather than inflammatory, with repetitive micro-trauma resulting in micro-tears and incomplete repair. The calcaneal origin is the weakest point of the plantar fascia, and

pathological change is most frequent at the attachment of the medial band. Occasionally the non-insertional fibres may be involved about 1.5–3.0 cm from the calcaneal origin and, rarely, the insertion of lateral band plantar fascia at the fifth metatarsal base may be affected. Insertional plantar fasciitis produces pain and tenderness localised to the medial process of the calcaneal tubercle. The pain is typically most severe on taking the first step of the morning.

High-quality plain films are acquired primarily to exclude other bony pathology such as a calcaneal stress fracture or a foreign body in the sole of the foot. Plain films may show a characteristic pattern of fusiform fascial thickening with displacement of the overlying fat line (see Fig. 7.401). Fascial calcification can occur secondary to old fascial disruption (see Fig. 7.402). A plantar calcaneal bone spur is a finding of little significance, as there is no correlation between heel pain and an exostosis (Schuberth 1990). Either ultrasound or MRI can be used to confirm a clinical diagnosis of plantar fasciitis and, more importantly, to detect a complicating partial tear (see Figs 7.403 and 7.404). A finding of a partial tear discourages corticosteroid injection and instead favours more conservative management. The MRI findings in plantar fasciitis include fascial thickening, focally increased signal intensity on all pulse sequences, peri-fascial oedema, and bone marrow oedema at the calcaneal enthesis. There are characteristic changes on a nuclear bone scan and ultrasound (see Figs 7.405 and 7.406). Ultrasound findings in plantar fasciitis can include localised tenderness, fascial thickening greater than 4 mm (Cardinal et al.

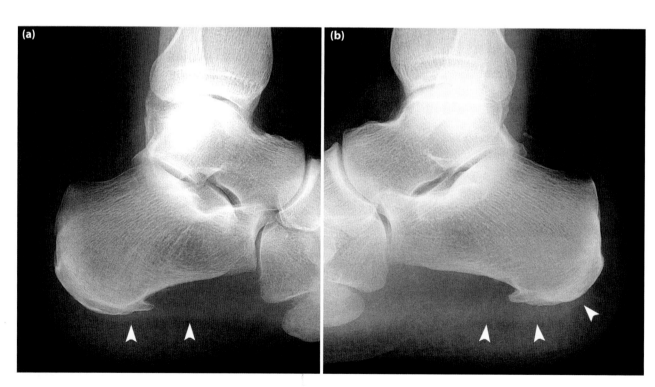

▲ Fig. 7.401 Plantar fasciitis is demonstrated on plain films.
(a) The contour of a normal plantar fascia is well demonstrated (arrowheads).
(b) Swelling of the plantar fascia occurs with plantar fasciitis and the rounded contour of this abnormality can be readily identified on plain films (arrowheads). Bilateral plantar spurs are present. These are of no clinical significance.

1996), hypoechogenicity and hyperaemia. Ultrasound-guided corticosteroid injection for plantar fasciitis is discussed further in Chapter 10.

Acute plantar fascial tears may be either spontaneous or traumatic. Spontaneous rupture can occur with or without a preceding clinical history of fasciitis (Leach et al. 1978). Traumatic ruptures are most commonly seen in jumping sports such as the long jump and triple jump. Fascial tears most often occur at or near the calcaneal insertion and may be partial or full thickness. They are readily diagnosed by either ultrasound (see Fig. 7.407) or MRI (see Figs 7.408 and 7.409).

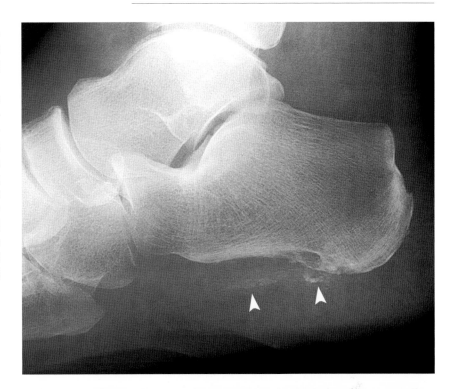

▶ **Fig. 7.402** Occasionally, plantar fascial calcification may occur in a patient with chronic plantar fasciitis complicated by a tear (arrowheads).

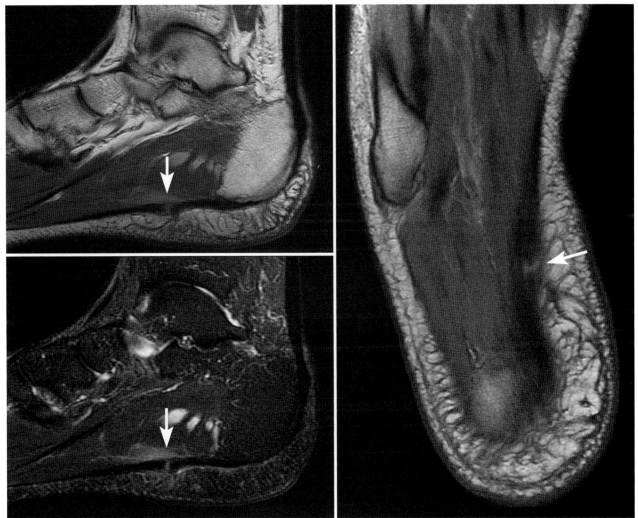

▲ **Fig. 7.403** Sagittal and axial PD-weighted and sagittal STIR MR images show a partial tear of the plantar fascia (arrows). Minor retraction has occurred and oedema is noted.

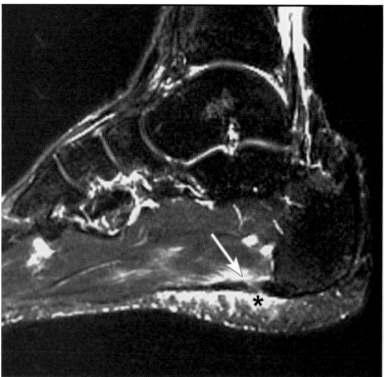

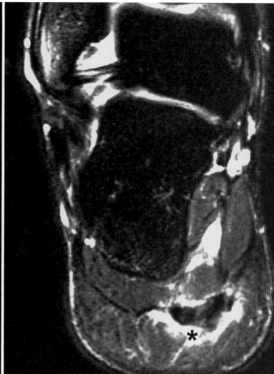

▲ Fig. 7.404 A pole vaulter at the Sydney 2000 Olympics was unable to compete due to a partial tear complicating plantar fasciitis (arrow). Considerable associated oedema or haemorrhage is shown on the sagittal and coronal STIR MR images (asterisks).

▶ Fig. 7.405 A nuclear bone scan shows increased uptake of isotope on the plantar border of the right calcaneum, indicating enthesopathy at the calcaneal attachment of the plantar fascia (arrow).

▼ Fig. 7.406 A long-axis ultrasound image demonstrates moderate swelling of the plantar fascia due to plantar fasciitis (callipers). A small non-acute complicating longitudinal intrasubstance tear is demonstrated at the calcaneal origin (arrowheads). Note that the configuration is similar to the plain film changes demonstrated in Fig. 7.401(b).

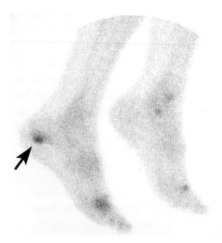

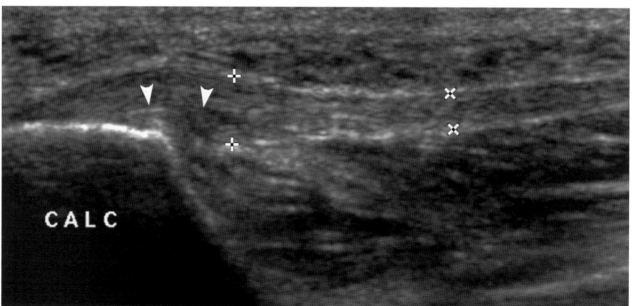

CALC

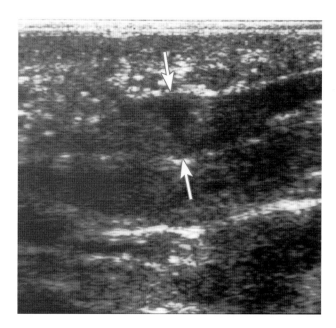

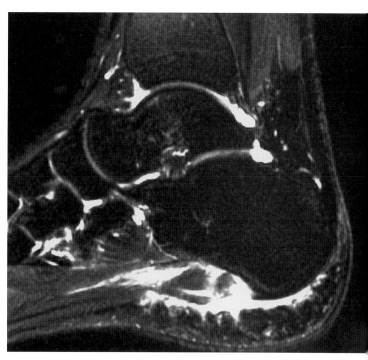

▲ **Fig. 7.407** Rupture of the mid-foot segment of the plantar fascia is demonstrated by ultrasound. A long-axis ultrasound image obtained over the proximal segment of the medial band of the plantar fascia about 3 cm distal to the calcaneal origin shows fusiform hypoechoic thickening of the fascia with a superimposed transverse hypoechoic cleft due to a tear (arrows).

▼ **Fig. 7.408** Sagittal and axial fat-suppressed PD-weighted MR images show an acute rupture of the medial band of the plantar fascia (arrows). There is retraction and laxity of the distal fascial segment with high signal in the surrounding tissues indicating associated haemorrhage.

▲ **Fig. 7.409** A triple-jump competitor at the Sydney 2000 Olympics ruptured his plantar fascia during take-off. There is fragmentation of the fascia and retraction of the distal segment. Considerable haemorrhage has occurred. Effusions in intertarsal, ankle and subtalar joints are a normal finding in an athlete competing at this level.

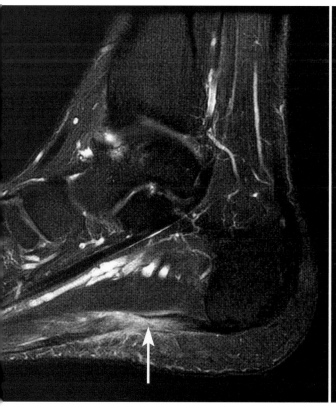

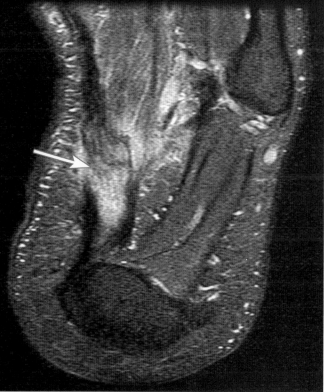

Plantar fibromatosis (Ledderhose disease)

Plantar fibromatosis is a condition characterised by a benign proliferation of fibrous tissue within the non-weightbearing portion of the plantar fascia. Patients present with one or more firm palpable nodules that may or may not have associated pain and tenderness. Lesions are multiple in one-third of cases, bilateral but often metachronous in 20–50% of cases, and have either concomitant or metachronous palmar involvement in about 50% of cases. Plantar fibromatosis can eventually extend to involve the skin or adjacent deep structures, but never metastasise. Plantar fibromata are usually well defined, but occasionally ill-defined fusiform hypoechoic nodules can be seen on ultrasound (see Fig. 7.410). They sometimes show marked vascularity on Power Doppler imaging. MRI typically shows a nodule of intermediate T1 and T2 signal intensity with a linear 'tail' of longitudinally oriented fascial extension (see Fig. 7.411) and hyperintensity on STIR images (see Fig. 7.412). Contrast enhancement is common. Plantar fibromatosis is more common in diabetics, epileptics and alcoholics with liver disease.

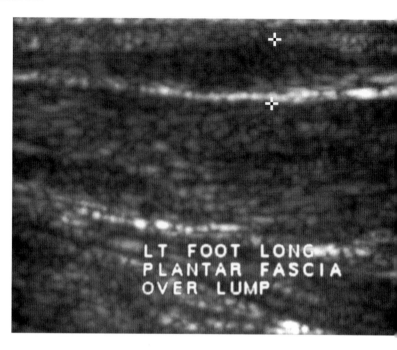

▲ **Fig. 7.410** A plantar fibroma is demonstrated by ultrasound. A long-axis ultrasound image of plantar fascia at the mid-foot level shows a focal fusiform intrasubstance hypoechoic thickening most pronounced along the line of the superficial fibres (callipers).

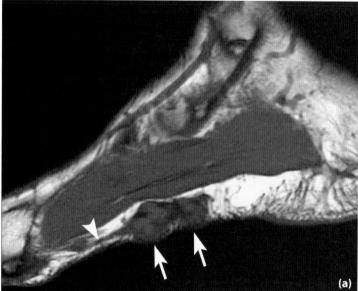
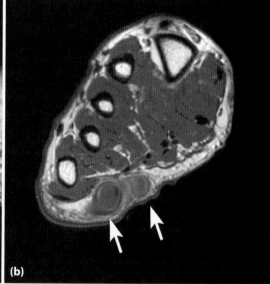

(a) (b)

▲ **Fig. 7.411** Sagittal and coronal PD-weighted MR images demonstrate nodular localised thickening of the plantar fascia in the mid-foot segment (arrows).
(a) In the sagittal image note the 'tail', which tapers distally in the line of the fascia (arrowhead).
(b) The coronal image shows the nodules to be discrete with well-defined margins.

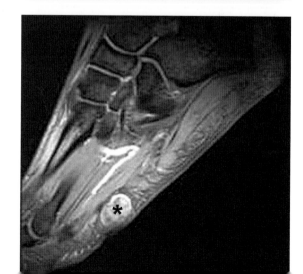

▶ **Fig. 7.412** This plantar fibroma is hyperintense on a sagittal T2*-weighted GRE MR image (asterisk).

References

Acker JH, Drez D, Jr. 'Nonoperative treatment of stress fractures of the proximal shaft of the fifth metatarsal (Jones fracture).' *Foot Ankle* 1986, 7(3): 152–5.

Alanen V, Taimela S, Kinnunen J, Koskinen SK, Karaharju E. 'Incidence and clinical significance of bone bruises after supination injury of the ankle. A double-blind, prospective study.' *J Bone Joint Surg (Br)* 1998, 80(3): 513–15.

Andermahr J, Helling HJ, Maintz D, Monig S, Koebke J, Rehm KE. 'The injury of the calcaneocuboid ligaments.' *Foot Ankle Int* 2000, 21(5): 379–84.

Anderson IF, Crichton KJ, Grattan-Smith T, Cooper RA, Brazier D. 'Osteochondral fractures of the dome of the talus.' *J Bone Joint Surg (Am)* 1989, 71(8): 1143–52.

Anderson J. *An Atlas of Radiography for Sports Injuries*. McGraw-Hill, Sydney, 2000.

Anderson SE, Weber M, Steinbach LS, Ballmer FT. 'Shoe rim and shoe buckle pseudotumor of the ankle in elite and professional figure skaters and snowboarders: MR imaging findings.' *Skeletal Radiol* 2004, 33(6): 325–9.

Anzilotti K Jr, Schweitzer ME, Hecht P, Wapner K, Kahn M, Ross M. 'Effect of foot and ankle MR imaging on clinical decision making.' *Radiology* 1996, 201(2): 515–17.

Arciero RA, Shishido NS, Parr TJ. 'Acute anterolateral compartment syndrome secondary to rupture of the peroneus longus muscle.' *Am J Sports Med* 1984, 12(5): 366–7.

Arrowsmith SR, Fleming LL, Allman FL. 'Traumatic dislocations of the peroneal tendons.' *Am J Sports Med* 1983, 11(3): 142–6.

Asherman DG. 'Injuries of the midfoot and forefoot.' *Current Opinion in Orthopedics* 2000, 11: 103–7.

Bagnolesi P, Carafoli D, Ortori S et al. 'Anterolateral fibrous impingement of the ankle: discrepancy between MRI findings and arthroscopy [Ab].' *Eur Radiol* 1998, 8: 1295.

Bartz RL, Marymont JV. 'Tarsal navicular fractures in major league baseball players at bat.' *Foot Ankle Int* 2001, 22(11): 908–10.

Bassett FH 3rd, Gates HS 3rd, Billys JB, Morris HB, Nikolaou PK. 'Talar impingement by the anteroinferior tibiofibular ligament. A cause of chronic pain in the ankle after inversion sprain.' *J Bone Joint Surg (Am)* 1990, 72(1): 55–9.

Baxter DE. 'The heel in sport.' *Clin Sports Med* 1994, 13(4): 683–93.

Beaman DN, Roeser WM, Holmes JR, Saltzman CL. 'Cuboid stress fractures: a report of two cases.' *Foot Ankle* 1993, 14(9): 525–8.

Bearcroft PWP et al. 'MRI of the ankle: effect of diagnostic confidence and patient management.' *Am J Roentgenol* 2006, 187: 1327–31.

Bencardino J, Rosenberg ZS, Beltran J, Broker M, Cheung Y, Rosemberg LA, Schweitzer M, Hamilton W. 'MR imaging of dislocation of the posterior tibial tendon.' *Am J Roentgenol* 1997a, 169(4): 1109–12.

Bencardino J, Rosenberg ZS, Beltran J, Sheskier S. 'Os sustentaculi: depiction on MR images.' *Skeletal Radiol* 1997b, 26(8): 505–6.

Bencardino JT, Rosenberg ZS, Serrano LF. 'MR imaging of tendon abnormalities of the foot and ankle.' *Magn Reson Imaging Clin N Am* 2001, 9(3): 475–92.

Berg EE. 'The symptomatic os subfibulare. Avulsion fracture of the fibula associated with recurrent instability of the ankle.' *J Bone Joint Surg (Am)* 1991, 73(8): 1251–4.

Berkowitz MJ, Kim DH. 'Process and tubercle fractures of the hind-foot.' *J Am Acad Orthop Surg* 2005, 13(8): 492–502.

Berndt AL, Harty M. 'Transchondral fractures (osteochondritis dissecans) of the talus.' *J Bone Joint Surg (Am)* 1959, 41A: 988–1020.

Best A, Giza E, Linklater J, Sullivan M. 'Posterior impingement of the ankle caused by anomalous muscles. A report of four cases.' *J Bone Joint Surg (Am)* 2005, 87(9): 2075–9.

Beumer A, van Hemert WL, Swierstra BA et al. 'A biomechanical evaluation of the tibiofibular and tibiotalar ligaments of the ankle.' *Foot Ankle Int* 2003, 24: 426–9.

Biedert R, Hintermann B. 'Stress fractures of the medial great toe sesamoid in athletes.' *Foot and Ankle Int* 2003, 24: 137–41.

Black KP, Ehlert KJ. 'A stress fracture of the lateral process of the talus in a runner. A case report.' *J Bone Joint Surg (Am)* 1994, 76(3): 441–3.

Bladin C, McCrory P. 'Snowboarding injuries. An overview.' *Sports Med* 1995, 19(5): 358–64.

Bonnin M, Tavernier T, Bouysset M. 'Split lesions of the peroneus brevis tendon in chronic ankle laxity.' *Am J Sports Med* 1997, 25(5): 699–703.

Boruta PM, Beauperthuy GD. 'Partial tear of the flexor hallucis longus at the knot of Henry: presentation of three cases.' *Foot Ankle Int* 1997, 18(4): 243–6.

Bossley CJ, Cairney PC. 'The intermetatarsophalangeal bursa—its significance in Morton's metatarsalgia.' *J Bone Joint Surg (Br)* 1980, 62B(2): 184–7.

Bowers KD Jr, Martin RB. 'Turf-toe: a shoe-surface related football injury.' *Med Sci Sports* 1976, 8(2): 81–3.

Bradshaw C, Khan K, Brukner P. 'Stress fracture of the body of the talus in athletes demonstrated with computer tomography.' *Clin J Sport Med* 1996, 6(1): 48–51.

Brailsford JF. 'Osteochondritis of the adult tarsal navicular.' *J Bone Joint Surg (Am)* 1939, 31: 111–20.

Breitenseher MJ, Haller J, Kukla C, Gaebler C, Kaider A, Fleischmann D, Helbich T, Trattnig S. 'MRI of the sinus tarsi in acute ankle sprain injuries.' *J Comput Assist Tomogr* 1997, 21(2): 274–9.

Brigido MK, Fessell DP, Jacobson JA, Widman DS, Craig JG, Jamadar DA, van Holsbeek MT. 'Radiography and US of os peroneum fractures and associated peroneal tendon injuries: initial experience.' *Radiology* 2005, 237(1): 235–41.

Brown JE. 'The sinus tarsi syndrome.' *Clin Orthop Relat Res* 1960, 18: 231–3.

Brown RR, Sadka Rosenberg Z, Schweitzer ME, Sheskier S, Astion D, Minkoff J. 'MRI of medial malleolar bursa.' *Am J Roentgenol* 2005, 184(3): 979–83.

Brukner P. 'Sports medicine. Pain in the Achilles region.' *Aust Fam Physician* 1997, 26(4): 463–5.

Burman M. 'Stenosing tendovaginitis of the foot and ankle, studies with special reference to the stenosing tendovaginitis of the peroneal tendons of the peroneal tubercle.' *AMA Arch Surg* 1953, 67(5): 686–98.

Burns J, Rosenbach B, Kahrs J. 'Etiopathogenetic aspects of medial osteochondritis dissecans tali.' *Sportverletz Sportsschaden* 1992, 6: 43–9.

Campbell DG, Menz A, Isaacs J. 'Dynamic ankle ultrasonography. A new imaging technique for acute ankle ligament injuries.' *Am J Sports Med* 1994, 22(6): 855–8.

Cardinal E, Chhem RK, Beauregard CG, Aubin B, Pelletier M. 'Plantar fasciitis: sonographic evaluation.' *Radiology* 1996, 201(1): 257–9.

Cardone BW, Erickson SJ, Den Hartog BD, Carrera GF. 'MRI of injury to the lateral collateral ligamentous complex of the ankle.' *J Comput Assist Tomogr* 1993, 17: 102–7.

Chen YJ, Hsu RW, Liang SC. 'Degeneration of the accessory navicular synchondrosis presenting as rupture of the posterior tibial tendon.' *J Bone Joint Surg (Am)* 1997, 79(12): 1791–8.

Clark TW, Janzen DL, Ho K, Grunfeld A, Connell DG. 'Detection of radiographically occult ankle fractures following acute trauma: positive predictive value of an ankle effusion.' *Am J Roentgenol* 1995, 164(5): 1185–9.

Conway JJ, Cowell HR. 'Tarsal coalition: clinical significance and roentgenographic demonstration.' *Radiology* 1969, 92(4): 799–811.

Cooper R, Allwright S, Anderson J. *Atlas of Nuclear Imaging in Sports Medicine.* McGraw-Hill, Sydney, 2003.

Coss S. 'Abductor stress and AP weightbearing radiography of purely ligamentous injury in the tarsometatarsal joint.' *Foot Ankle Int* 1998, 9: 537–41.

Curtis MJ, Myerson M, Szura B. 'Tarsometatarsal joint injuries in the athlete.' *Am J Sports Med* 1993, 21: 497–502.

Davies JA. 'Peroneal compartment syndrome secondary to rupture of the peroneus longus. A case report.' *J Bone Joint Surg (Am)* 1979, 61(5): 783–4.

Davies M, Cassar-Pullicino VN, Davies AM, McCall IW, Tyrrell PN. 'The diagnostic accuracy of MR imaging in osteoid osteoma.' *Skeletal Radiol* 2002, 31(10): 559–69.

DeAsla R, O'Malley M, Hamilton WG. 'Flexor hallucis tendonitis and posterior ankle impingement in the athlete.' *Techniques in Foot & Ankle Surgery* 2002, 1(2): 123–30.

De Simoni C, Wetz HH, Zanetti M, Hodler J, Jacob H, Zollinger H. 'Clinical examination and magnetic resonance imaging in the assessment of ankle sprains treated with an orthosis.' *Foot Ankle Int* 1996, 17(3): 177–82.

Donnelly EF. 'The Hawkins sign.' *Radiology* 1999, 210(1): 195–6.

Dhukaram V et al. 'Case report: Maisonneuve fracture in an adolescent.' *Foot and Ankle Surgery* 2003, 9: 241–4.

Ebraheim NA, Haman SP, Lu J, Padanilam TG. 'Radiographic evaluation of the calcaneocuboid joint: a cadaver study.' *Foot Ankle Int* 1999, 20(3): 178–81.

Ebraheim NA, Lu J, Yang H, Mekhail AO, Yeasting RA. 'Radiographic and CT evaluation of tibiofibular syndesmotic diastasis: a cadaver study.' *Foot Ankle Int* 1997, 18(11): 693–8.

Ebrahim FS, Jacobson JA, Lin J, Housner JA, Hayes CW, Resnick D. 'Intra-articular osteoid osteoma: sonographic findings in three patients with radiographic, CT, and MR imaging correlation.' *Am J Roentgenol* 2001, 177(6): 1391–5.

Egol KA, Parisien JS. 'Impingement syndrome of the ankle caused by a medial meniscoid lesion.' *Arthroscopy* 1997, 13(4): 522–5.

Eisele SA, Sammarco GJ. 'Fatigue fractures of the foot and ankle in the athlete.' *J Bone Joint Surg (Am)* 1993, 75(2): 290–8.

Enneking WF, Horowitz M. 'The intra-articular effects of immobilization on the human knee.' *J Bone Joint Surg (Am)* 1972, 54(5): 973–85.

Faciszewski T, Burks RT, Manaster BJ. 'Subtle injuries of the Lisfranc joint.' *J Bone Joint Surg (Am)* 1990, 72(10): 1519–22.

Feldman MD. 'Evaluation of intra-articular damage in displaced extra-articular ankle fractures.' Annual Meeting of the Eastern Orthopedic Association, Scottsdale, Arizona, 1997.

Fessell DP, van Holsbeek MT. 'Sonography of the foot and ankle.' In van Holsbeeck MT, Introcaso JH. *Musculoskeletal Ultrasound*, Mosby, St Louis, 2001, p. 610.

Fitch KD, Blackwell JB, Gilmour WN. 'Operation for non-union of stress fracture of the tarsal navicular.' *J Bone Joint Surg (Br)* 1989, 71(1): 105–10.

Flahive SR, Anderson IF. 'Bone stress in athletes at the Sydney 2000 Olympic Games.' *NZ J Sports Med* 2004, 32: 2–12.

Fortin PT, Guettler J, Manoli A 2nd. 'Idiopathic cavovarus and lateral ankle instability: recognition and treatment implications relating to ankle arthritis.' *Foot Ankle Int* 2002, 23(11): 1031–7.

Freiberger RH, Kaye JJ, Spiller J. *Arthrography*, Appleton-Century-Crofts, New York, 1979.

Frey C, Feder KS, DiGiovanni C. 'Arthroscopic evaluation of the subtalar joint: does sinus tarsi syndrome exist?' *Foot Ankle Int* 1999, 20(3): 185–91.

Frey CC, Shereff MJ. 'Tendon injuries about the ankle in athletes.' *Clin Sports Med* 1988, 7(1): 103–18.

Fritschy D. 'A rare injury of the ankle in competition skiers.' *Schweiz Z Med Traumatol* 1994(1): 13–16.

Funk JR, Srinivasan SC, Crandall JR. 'Snowboarder's talus fractures experimentally produced by eversion and dorsiflexion.' *Am J Sports Med* 2003, 31(6): 921–8.

Garrick JG. 'Epidemiologic perspective.' *Clin Sports Med* 1982, 1(1): 13–18.

Gerber JP, Williams GN, Scoville CR, Arciero RA, Taylor DC. 'Persistent disability associated with ankle sprains: a prospective examination of an athletic population.' *Foot Ankle Int* 1998, 19(10): 653–60.

Golano P, Farinas O, Saenz I. 'The anatomy of the navicular and periarticular structures.' *Foot Ankle Clin* 2004, 9(1): 1–23.

Goldman F. 'Fracture of the midfoot.' *Clinics in Podiatry* 1985, 2: 259–85.

Gould N. 'Stenosing tenosynovitis of the flexor hallucis longus tendon at the great toe.' *Foot Ankle* 1981, 2(1): 46–8.

Grant TH, Kelikian AS, Jereb SE, McCarthy RJ. 'Ultrasound diagnosis of peroneal tendon tears. A surgical correlation.' *J Bone Joint Surg (Am)* 2005, 87(8): 1788–94.

Haines RW, McDougall A. 'The anatomy of hallux valgus.' *J Bone Joint Surg (Br)* 1954, 36B(2): 272–93.

Haller J, Sartoris DJ, Resnick D, Pathria MN, Berthoty D, Howard B, Nordstrom D. 'Spontaneous osteonecrosis of the tarsal navicular in adults: imaging findings.' *Am J Roentgenol* 1988, 151(2): 355–8.

Hamilton WG. 'Stenosing tenosynovitis of the flexor hallucis longus tendon and posterior impingement upon the os trigonum in ballet dancers.' *Foot Ankle* 1982, 3(2): 74–80.

Hamilton WG, Geppert MJ, Thompson FM. 'Pain in the posterior aspect of the ankle in dancers. Differential diagnosis and operative treatment.' *J Bone Joint Surg (Am)* 1996, 78(10): 1491–500.

Harper MC. 'The deltoid ligament. An evaluation of need for surgical repair.' *Clin Orthop Relat Res* 1988, 226: 156–68.

Harper MC. 'Subluxation of the peroneal tendons within the peroneal groove: a report of two cases.' *Foot Ankle Int* 1997, 18(6): 369–70.

Harper MC. 'Delayed reduction and stabilization of the tibiofibular syndesmosis.' *Foot Ankle Int* 2001, 22(1): 15–8.

Harrington T, Crichton KJ, Anderson IF. 'Overuse ballet injury of the base of the second metatarsal. A diagnostic problem.' *Am J Sports Med* 1993, 21(4): 591–8.

Harris RI. 'Retrospect: peroneal spastic flat foot (rigid valgus foot).' *J Bone Joint Surg (Br)* 1965, 47A: 1657–67.

Harty MP, Hubbard AM. 'MR imaging of pediatric abnormalities in the ankle and foot.' *Magn Reson Imaging Clin N Am* 2001, 9(3): 579–602, xi.

Hauger O, Moinard M, Lasalarie JC, Chauveaux D, Diard F. 'Anterolateral compartment of the ankle in the lateral impingement syndrome: appearance on CT arthrography.' *Am J Roentgenol* 1999, 173(3): 685–90.

Hintermann B, Valderrabano V, Boss A, Trouillier HH, Dick W. 'Medial ankle instability: an exploratory, prospective study of fifty-two cases.' *Am J Sports Med* 2004, 32(1): 183–90.

Hopkinson WJ, St Pierre P, Ryan JB, Wheeler JH. 'Syndesmosis sprains of the ankle.' *Foot Ankle* 1990, 10(6): 325–30.

Hulkko A, Orava S, Pellinen P, Puranen J. 'Stress fractures of the sesamoid bones of the first metatarsophalangeal joint in athletes.' *Arch Orthop Trauma Surg* 1985, 104(2): 113–17.

Inglis AE, Scott WN, Sculco TP, Patterson AH. 'Ruptures of the tendo achillis. An objective assessment of surgical and non-surgical treatment.' *J Bone Joint Surg (Am)* 1976, 58(7): 990–3.

Johnson BA, Neylon T, Laroche R. 'Lesser metatarsal stress fractures.' *Clin Podiatr Med Surg* 1999, 16(4): 631–42.

Johnson TR, Mizel MS, Temple T. 'Cuboid-navicular tarsal coalition: presentation and treatment. A case report and review of the literature.' *Foot Ankle Int* 2005, 26(3): 264–6.

Jones DC. 'Tendon disorders of the foot and ankle.' *J Am Acad Orthop Surg* 1993, 1(2): 87–94.

Józsa L, Kannus P. *Human Tendons: Anatomy, Physiology and Pathology*, Human Kinetics, Champaign, IL, 1997.

Kaminsky S, Griffin L, Milsap J, Page D. 'Is ultrasonography a reliable way to confirm the diagnosis of Morton's neuroma?' *Orthopedics* 1997, 20(1): 37–9.

Kannus P, Józsa L. 'Histopathological changes preceding spontaneous rupture of a tendon. A controlled study of 891 patients.' *J Bone Joint Surg (Am)* 1991, 73(10): 1507–25.

Karasick D. 'Preoperative assessment of symptomatic bunionette deformity: radiologic findings.' *Am J Roentgenol* 1995, 164(1): 147–9.

Karasick D, Schweitzer ME. 'Tears of posterior tibial tendon causing asymmetric flatfoot: radiologic findings.' *Am J Roentgenol* 1993, 161: 1237–40.

Karjalainen PT, Soila K, Aronen HJ, Pihlajamaki HK, Tynninen O, Paavonen T, Tirman PF. 'MR imaging of overuse injuries of the Achilles tendon.' *Am J Roentgenol* 2000, 175(1): 251–60.

Karlsson J, Eriksson BI, Renstrom PA. 'Subtalar instability of the foot. A review and results after surgical treatment.' *Scand J Med Sci Sports* 1998, 8(4): 191–7.

Keefe DT, Haddad SL. 'Subtalar instability. Etiology, diagnosis, and management.' *Foot Ankle Clin* 2002, 7(3): 577–609.

Kennedy JG, Johnson SM, Collins AL, DalloVedova P, McManus WF, Hynes DM, Walsh MG, Stephens MM. 'An evaluation of the Weber classification of ankle fractures.' *Injury* 1998, 29(8): 577–80.

Kennedy MA, Sama AE, Sigman M. 'Tibiofibular syndesmosis and ossification. Case report: sequelae of ankle sprain in an adolescent football player.' *J Emerg Med* 2000, 18(2): 233–40.

Khan KM, Brukner PD, Kearney C, Fuller PJ, Bradshaw CJ, Kiss ZS. 'Tarsal navicular stress fracture in athletes.' *Sports Med* 1994, 17(1): 65–76.

Khan KM, Fuller PJ, Brukner PD, Kearney C, Burry HC. 'Outcome of conservative and surgical management of navicular stress fracture in athletes. Eighty-six cases proven with computerized tomography.' *Am J Sports Med* 1992, 20(6): 657–66.

Khoury NJ, el-Khoury GY, Saltzman CL, Kathol MH. 'Peroneus longus and brevis tendon tears: MR imaging evaluation.' *Radiology* 1996, 200(3): 833–41.

Kijowski R, De Smet A, Mukharjee R. 'Magnetic resonance imaging findings in patients with peroneal tendinopathy and peroneal tenosynovitis.' *Skeletal Radiol* 2007, 36: 105–14.

Kim DH, Berkowitz MJ, Pressman DN. 'Avulsion fractures of the medial tubercle of the posterior process of the talus.' *Foot Ankle Int* 2003, 24(2): 172–5.

Kiss ZS, Khan KM, Fuller PJ. 'Stress fractures of the tarsal navicular bone: CT findings in 55 cases.' *Am J Roentgenol* 1993, 160(1): 111–15.

Kolettis GJ, Micheli LJ, Klein JD. 'Release of the flexor hallucis longus tendon in ballet dancers.' *J Bone Joint Surg (Am)* 1996, 78(9): 1386–90.

Kulik SA Jr, Clanton TO. 'Tarsal coalition.' *Foot Ankle Int* 1996, 17(5): 286–96.

Kumar G et al. 'Superior tibiofibular joint disruption: as a variant of Masionneuve injury.' *Foot and Ankle Surg* 2004, 10: 41–3.

Kumar SJ, Guille JT, Lee MS, Couto JC. 'Osseous and non-osseous coalition of the middle facet of the talocalcaneal joint.' *J Bone Joint Surg (Am)* 1992, 74(4): 529–35.

Kvist H, Kvist M. 'The operative treatment of chronic calcaneal paratenonitis.' *J Bone Joint Surg (Br)* 1980, 62(3): 353–7.

Lagalla R, Iovane A, Midiri M, Lo Casto A, De Maria M. 'Comparison of echography and magnetic resonance in sprains of the external compartment of the ankle.' *Radiol Med (Torino)* 1994, 88(6): 742–8.

Lagergren C, Lindholm A. 'Vascular distribution in the Achilles tendon, an angiographic and microangiographic study.' *Acta Chir Scand* 1959, 116(5–6): 491–5.

Landorf KB. 'Clarifying proximal diaphyseal fifth metatarsal fractures. The acute fracture versus the stress fracture.' *J Am Podiatr Med Assoc* 1999, 89(8): 398–404.

Lateur LM, Van Hoe LR, Van Ghillewe KV, Gryspeerdt SS, Baert AL, Dereymaeker GE. 'Subtalar coalition: diagnosis with the C sign on lateral radiographs of the ankle.' *Radiology* 1994, 193(3): 847–51.

Lawrence SJ. 'Midfoot trauma, bony and ligamentous: evaluation and treatment.' *Current Opinion in Orthopedics* 2002, 13: 99–106.

Leach R, Jones R, Silva T. 'Rupture of the plantar fascia in athletes.' *J Bone Joint Surg (Am)* 1978, 60(4): 537–9.

Leach RE, Lower G. 'Ankle injuries in skiing.' *Clin Orthop Relat Res* 1985, (198): 127–33.

Lee S, Anderson RB. 'Stress fractures of the tarsal navicular.' *Foot Ankle Clin* 2004, 9(1): 85–104.

Lee TH, Wapner KL, Hecht PJ. 'Plantar fibromatosis.' *J Bone Joint Surg (Am)* 1993, 75(7): 1080–4.

Lindenfeld TN, Wojtys EM, Husain A. 'Surgical treatment of arthrofibrosis of the knee.' *Instr Course Lect* 2000, 49: 211–21.

Liu SH, Baker CL. 'Comparison of lateral ankle ligamentous reconstruction procedures.' *Am J Sports Med* 1994, 22: 313–17.

Liu SH, Mirzayan R. 'Posteromedial ankle impingement.' *Arthroscopy* 1993, 9(6): 709–11.

Loomer R, Fisher C, Lloyd-Smith R, Sisler J, Cooney T. 'Osteochondral lesions of the talus.' *Am J Sports Med* 1993, 21(1): 13–19.

Loren GJ, Ferkel RD. 'Arthroscopic assessment of occult intra-articular injury in acute ankle fractures.' *Arthroscopy* 2002, 18(4): 412–21.

Malicky ES, Crary JL, Houghton MJ, Agel J, Hansen ST Jr, Sangeorzan BJ. 'Talocalcaneal and subfibular impingement in symptomatic flatfoot in adults.' *J Bone Joint Surg (Am)* 2002, 84A(11): 2005–9.

Mangwani J. 'Chronic lateral ankle instability: review of anatomy, biomechanics, pathology and treatment.' *The Foot* 2001, 11: 76–84.

Mansberg VJ, Van Niekerk AL. 'The accessory soleus muscle: a case report and review of the literature.' *Australas Radiol* 1991, 35(3): 276–8.

Mantas JP, Burks RT. 'Lisfranc injuries in the athlete.' *Clin Sports Med* 1994, 13: 719–30.

Manter JT. 'Disruption of compressive forces in the joints of the human foot.' *Anat Rec* 1946, 96: 313–21.

Marshall P, Hamilton WG. 'Cuboid subluxation in ballet dancers.' *Am J Sports Med* 1992, 20(2): 169–75.

Mazur DW, Bartolozzi AR. *Ankle Soft Tissue Injuries in Sports Medicine 2* [Abstract], AAOS, 1999.

Mazzone MF, McCue T. 'Common conditions of the Achilles tendon.' *Am Fam Physician* 2002, 65(9): 1805–10.

McCrory P, Bladin C. 'Fractures of the lateral process of the talus: a clinical review. "Snowboarder's ankle."' *Clin J Sport Med* 1996, 6(2): 124–8.

McNally EG. 'Posteromedial subtalar coalition: imaging appearances in the three cases.' *Skeletal Radiol* 1999, 28: 691–5.

Mellado JM, Salvado E, Camins A, Ramos A, Sauri A. 'Painful os sustentaculi: imaging findings of another symptomatic skeletal variant.' *Skeletal Radiol* 2002, 31(1): 53–6.

Milz P, Milz S, Putz R, Reiser M. '13 MHz high-frequency sonography of the lateral ankle joint ligaments and the tibiofibular syndesmosis in anatomic specimens.' *J Ultrasound Med* 1996, 15(4): 277–84.

Milz P, Milz S, Steinborn M, Mittlmeier T, Reiser M. '13 MHz high-frequency ultrasound of the lateral ligaments of the ankle joint and the anterior tibia-fibular ligament. Comparison and results of MRI in 64 patients.' *Radiologe* 1999, 39(1): 34–40.

Milz P, Milz S, Steinborn M, et al. 'Lateral ankle ligaments and tibiofibular syndesmosis. 13 MHz high-frequency sonography and MRI compared in 20 patients.' *Acta Orthop Scand* 1998, 69: 51–5.

Moseley JB, Chimenti BT. 'Foot and ankle injuries in the professional athlete'. In *The Foot and Ankle in Sport*, Mosby, St. Louis, 1995, p. 321–8.

Mosier-La Clair SM, Monroe MT, Manoli A. 'Medial impingement syndrome of the anterior tibiotalar fascicle of the deltoid ligament on the talus.' *Foot Ankle Int* 2000, 21(5): 385–91.

Motto SG. 'Stress fracture of the lateral process of the talus: a case report.' *Br J Sports Med* 1993, 27(4): 275–6.

Muhle C, Frank LR, Rand T, Yeh L, Wong EC, Skaf A, Dantas RW, Haghighi P, Trudell D, Resnick D. 'Collateral ligaments of the ankle: high-resolution MR imaging with a local gradient coil and anatomic correlation in cadavers.' *Radiographics* 1999, 19(3): 673–83.

Murr S. 'Dislocation of the peroneal tendons with marginal fracture of the lateral malleolus.' *J Bone Joint Surg (Br)* 1961, 43: 563–5.

Myerson MS, Fisher RT, Burgess AR, Kenzora JE. 'Fracture dislocations of the tarsometatarsal joints: end results correlated with pathology and treatment.' *Foot Ankle* 1986, 6(5): 225–42.

Na JB, Bergman AG, Oloff LM, Beaulieu CF. 'The flexor hallucis longus: tenographic technique and correlation of imaging findings with surgery in 39 ankles.' *Radiology* 2005, 236(3): 974–82.

Neustadter J, Raikin SM, Nazarian LN. 'Dynamic sonographic evaluation of peroneal tendon subluxation.' *Am J Roentgenol* 2004, 183(4): 985–8.

Noyes FR, Barber-Westin SD. 'Reconstruction of the anterior and posterior cruciate ligaments after knee dislocation. Use of early protected postoperative motion to decrease arthrofibrosis.' *Am J Sports Med* 1997, 25(6): 769–78.

Nussbaum ED, Hosea TM, Sieler SD, Incremona BR, Kessler DE. 'Prospective evaluation of syndesmotic ankle sprains without diastasis.' *Am J Sports Med* 2001, 29(1): 31–5.

Ogden JA, Ganey TM, Hill JD, Jaakkola JI. 'Sever's injury: a stress fracture of the immature calcaneal metaphysis.' *J Pediatr Orthop* 2004, 24(5): 488–92.

Okada K, Senma S, Abe E, Sato K, Minato S. 'Stress fractures of the medial malleolus: a case report.' *Foot Ankle Int* 1995, 16(1): 49–52.

O'Malley MJ, Hamilton WG, Munyak J. 'Fractures of the distal shaft of the fifth metatarsal. "Dancer's fracture."' *Am J Sports Med* 1996, 24(2): 240–3.

Pankovich AM. 'Maisonneuve fracture of the fibula.' *J Bone Joint Surg (Am)* 1976, 58: 337–42.

Paterson RS, Brown JN. 'The posteromedial impingement lesion of the ankle. A series of six cases.' *Am J Sports Med* 2001, 29(5): 550–7.

Pavlov H, Torg JS, Freiberger RH. 'Tarsal navicular stress fractures: radiographic evaluation.' *Radiology* 1983, 148(3): 641–5.

Peicha G, Labovitz J, Seibert FJ, Grechenig W, Weiglein A, Preidler KW, Quehenberger F. 'The anatomy of the joint as a risk factor for Lisfranc dislocation and fracture-dislocation. An anatomical and radiological case control study.' *J Bone Joint Surg (Br)* 2002, 84(7): 981–5.

Perry DR, O'Toole ED. 'Stress fracture of the talar neck and distal calcaneus.' *J Am Podiatry Assoc* 1981, 71(11): 637–8.

Perry J. 'Anatomy and biomechanics of the hind-foot.' *Clin Orthop Relat Res* 1983, 177: 9–15.

Pinney SJ, Sangeorzan BJ. 'Fracture of the tarsal bones in the traumatized foot.' An AAOS monograph series, American Academy of Orthopaedic Surgeons, 2001, pp. 41–53.

Pneumaticos SG, Noble PC, Chatziioannou SN, Trevino SG. 'The effects of rotation on radiographic evaluation of the tibiofibular syndesmosis.' *Foot Ankle Int* 2002, 23(2): 107–11.

Potter HG, Deland JT, Gusmer PB, Carson E, Warren RF. 'Magnetic resonance imaging of the Lisfranc ligament of the foot.' *Foot Ankle Int* 1998, 19(7): 438–46.

Potter HG, Linklater JM, Allen AA, Hannafin JA, Haas SB. 'Magnetic resonance imaging of articular cartilage in the knee. An evaluation with use of fast-spin-echo imaging.' *J Bone Joint Surg (Am)* 1998, 80(9): 1276–84.

Preidler KW, Peicha G, Lajtai G, Seibert FJ, Fock C, Szolar DM, Raith H. 'Conventional radiography, CT, and MR imaging in patients with hyperflexion injuries of the foot: diagnostic accuracy in the detection of bony and ligamentous changes.' *Am J Roentgenol* 1999, 173(6): 1673–7.

Raatikainen T, Putkonen M, Puranen J. 'Arthrography, clinical examination, and stress radiograph in the diagnosis of acute injury to the lateral ligaments of the ankle.' *Am J Sports Med* 1992, 20(1): 2–6.

Read JW, Noakes JB, Kerr D, Crichton KJ, Slater HK, Bonar F. 'Morton's metatarsalgia: sonographic findings and correlated histopathology.' *Foot Ankle Int* 1999, 20(3): 153–61.

Redd RA, Peters VJ, Emery SF, Branch HM, Rifkin MD. 'Morton neuroma: sonographic evaluation.' *Radiology* 1989, 171(2): 415–17.

Richli WR, Rosenthal DI. 'Avulsion fracture of the fifth metatarsal: experimental study of pathomechanics.' *Am J Roentgenol* 1984, 143(4): 889–91.

Rijke AM, Vierhout PA. 'Graded stress radiography in acute injury to the lateral ligaments of the ankle.' *Acta Radiol* 1990, 31(2): 151–5.

Robinson P, White LM, Salonen DC, Daniels TR, Ogilvie-Harris D. 'Anterolateral ankle impingement: MR arthrographic assessment of the anterolateral recess.' *Radiology* 2001, 221(1): 186–90.

Roca J, Roure F, Fernandez Fairen M, Yunta A. 'Stress fractures of the fifth metatarsal.' *Acta Orthop Belg* 1980, 46(5): 630–6.

Rosenberg ZS, Cheung YY, Beltran J, Sheskier S, Leong M, Jahss M. 'Posterior intermalleolar ligament of the ankle: normal anatomy and MR imaging features.' *Am J Roentgenol* 1995, 165(2): 387–90.

Rubin DA, Tishkoff NW, Britton CA, Conti SF, Towers JD. 'Anterolateral soft-tissue impingement in the ankle: diagnosis using MR imaging.' *Am J Roentgenol* 1997, 169(3): 829–35.

Rubin G, Witten M. 'The talar-tilt angle and the fibular collateral ligaments.' *J Bone Joint Surg (Am)* 1960, 42a: 311–26.

Saltzman CL, Tearse DS. 'Achilles tendon injuries.' *J Am Acad Orthop Surg* 1998, 6(5): 316–25.

Sammarco GJ. 'Peroneal tendon injuries.' *Orthop Clin North Am* 1994, 25(1): 135–45.

Sammarco GJ, Brainard BJ. 'A symptomatic anomalous peroneus brevis in a high-jumper. A case report.' *J Bone Joint Surg (Am)* 1991, 73(1): 131–3.

Sammarco GJ, DiRaimondo CV. 'Surgical treatment of lateral ankle instability syndrome.' *Am J Sports Med* 1988, 16(5): 501–11.

Sarrafian SK. 'Functional characteristics of the foot and plantar aponeurosis under tibiotalar loading.' *Foot Ankle* 1987, 8: 4–18.

Saxena A, Krisdakumtorn T, Erickson S. 'Proximal fourth metatarsal injuries in athletes: similarity to proximal fifth metatarsal injury.' *Foot Ankle Int* 2001, 22(7): 603–8.

Schuberth JM. 'Trauma to the heel.' *Clin Podiatr Med Surg* 1990, 7(2): 289–306.

Schweitzer ME, van Leersum M, Ehrlich SS, Wapner K. 'Fluid in normal and abnormal ankle joints: amount and distribution as seen on MR images.' *Am J Roentgenol* 1994, 162(1): 111–14.

Shabat S, Sampson KB, Mann G, Gepstein R, Eliakim A, Shenkman Z, Nyska M. 'Stress fractures of the medial malleolus: review of the literature and report of a 15-year-old elite gymnast.' *Foot Ankle Int* 2002, 23(7): 647–50.

Shaffer HA Jr, Harrison RB. 'Tarsal pseudo-coalition: a positional artifact.' *J Can Assoc Radiol* 1980, 31(4): 236–7.

Shapiro MS, Wascher DC, Finerman GA. 'Rupture of Lisfranc's ligament in athletes.' *Am J Sports Med* 1994, 22(5): 687–91.

Sharp RJ, Calder JD, Saxby TS. 'Osteochondritis of the navicular: a case report.' *Foot Ankle Int* 2003, 24(6): 509–13.

Sharp RJ, Wade CM, Hennessy MS, Saxby TS. 'The role of MRI and ultrasound imaging in Morton's neuroma and the effect of size of lesion on symptoms.' *J Bone Joint Surg (Br)* 2003, 85(7): 999–1005.

Shelbourne KD, Fisher DA, Rettig AC, McCarroll JR. 'Stress fractures of the medial malleolus.' *Am J Sports Med* 1988, 16(1): 60–3.

Sherbondy PS, Sebastianelli WJ. 'Stress fractures of the medial malleolus and distal fibula.' *Clin Sports Med* 2006, 25(1): 129–37, x.

Siegler S, Block J, Schneck CD. 'The mechanical characteristics of the collateral ligaments of the human ankle joint.' *Foot Ankle* 1988, 8(5): 234–42.

Sijbrandij ES, van Gils AP, Louwerens JW, de Lange EE. 'Posttraumatic subchondral bone contusions and fractures of the talotibial joint: occurrence of "kissing" lesions.' *Am J Roentgenol* 2000, 175(6): 1707–10.

Sobel M, Geppert MJ, Olson EJ, Bohne WH, Arnoczky SP. 'The dynamics of peroneus brevis tendon splits: a proposed mechanism, technique of diagnosis, and classification of injury.' *Foot Ankle* 1992, 13(7): 413–22.

Sobel M, Pavlov H, Geppert MJ, Thompson FM, DiCarlo EF, Davis WH. 'Painful os peroneum syndrome: a spectrum of conditions responsible for plantar lateral foot pain.' *Foot Ankle Int* 1994, 15(3): 112–24.

Soma CA, Mandelbaum BR. 'Achilles tendon disorders.' *Clin Sports Med* 1994, 13(4): 811–23.

Sopov V, Liberson A, Groshar D. 'Bone scintigraphic findings of os trigonum: a prospective study of 100 soldiers on active duty.' *Foot Ankle Int* 2000, 21(10): 822–4.

Stiell IG, McKnight RD, Greenberg GH, McDowell I, Nair RC, Wells GA, Johns C, Worthington JR. 'Implementation of the Ottawa ankle rules.' *Jama* 1994, 271(11): 827–32.

Sugimoto K, Samoto N, Takakura Y, Tamai S. 'Varus tilt of the tibial plafond as a factor in chronic ligament instability of the ankle.' *Foot Ankle Int* 1997, 18(7): 402–5.

Takao M, Ochi M, Naito K, Iwata A, Kawasaki K, Tobita M, Miyamoto W, Oae K. 'Arthroscopic diagnosis of tibiofibular syndesmosis disruption.' *Arthroscopy* 2001, 17(8): 836–43.

Tanaka Y, Takakura Y, Sugimoto K, Kumai T. 'Non-osseous coalition of the medial cuneiform-first metatarsal joint: a case report.' *Foot Ankle Int* 2000, 21(12): 1043–6.

Theodorou DJ, Theodorou SJ, Boutin RD, Chung C, Fliszar E, Kakitsubata Y, Resnick D. 'Stress fractures of the lateral metatarsal bones in metatarsus adductus foot deformity: a previously unrecognized association.' *Skeletal Radiol* 1999, 28(12): 679–84.

Thompson MC, Mormino MA. 'Injury to the tarsometatarsal joint complex.' *J Am Acad Orthop Surg* 2003, 11(4): 260–7.

Torg JS, Pavlov H, Cooley LH, Bryant MH, Arnoczky SP, Bergfeld J, Hunter LY. 'Stress fractures of the tarsal navicular. A retrospective review of twenty-one cases.' *J Bone Joint Surg (Am)* 1982, 64(5): 700–12.

Trevino S, Baumhauer JF. 'Tendon injuries of the foot and ankle.' *Clin Sports Med* 1992, 11(4): 727–39.

Umans HR, Elsinger E. 'The plantar plate of the lesser metatarsophalangeal joints: potential for injury and role of MR imaging.' *Magn Reson Imaging Clin N Am* 2001, 9(3): 659–69, xii.

Usami N, Inokuchi S, Hiraishi E. *Pathophysiology and Treatment of Subtalar Instability*, Proceedings of AOFAS Annual Summer Meeting, Monterey, 1997.

Valderrabano V, Hintermann B, Horisberger M, Fung TS. 'Ligamentous posttraumatic ankle osteoarthritis.' *Am J Sports Med* 2006, 34(4): 612–20.

van Holsbeek MT, Powell A. 'Ankle and foot'. In Fornage BD. *Musculoskeletal Ultrasound*, Churchill Livingstone, New York, 1995, pp. 221–37.

Veltri DM, Pagnani MJ, O'Brien SJ, Warren RF, Ryan MD, Barnes RP. 'Symptomatic ossification of the tibiofibular syndesmosis in professional football players: a sequela of the syndesmotic ankle sprain.' *Foot Ankle Int* 1995, 16(5): 285–90.

Vouri J, Aro HT 'Lisfranc joint injuries: trauma mechanics and associated injuries.' *J Trauma* 1993, 72: 1519–22.

Wechsler RJ, Schweitzer ME, Deely DM, Horn BD, Pizzutillo PD. 'Tarsal coalition: depiction and characterization with CT and MR imaging.' *Radiology* 1994, 193(2): 447–52.

Wolin I, Glassman F, Sideman S, Levinthal DH. 'Internal derangement of the talofibular component of the ankle.' *Surg Gynecol Obstet* 1950, 91(2): 193–200.

Yu JS, Solmen J. 'Stress fractures associated with plantar fascia disruption: two case reports involving the cuboid.' *J Comput Assist Tomogr* 2001, 25(6): 971–4.

Zeide MS, Wiesel SW, Terry RL. 'Talonavicular coalition.' *Clin Orthop Relat Res* 1977, 126: 225–7.

Image acknowledgments

The authors wish to thank the following colleagues who kindly offered images for inclusion in this chapter:

- Dr Robert Cooper and Dr Stephen Allwright (Figs 7.33(a) and (b), 7.34 and 7.35, 7.57, 7.95, 7.96, 7.110, 7.119, 7.230, 7.231, 7.232, 7.255, 7.279, 7.282, 7.309, 7.318(a), 7.357 and 7.405)
- Dr Barry Figtree (Figs 7.148 and 7.149)
- Dr James Linklater (Figs 7.41, 7.53, 7.60, 7.66, 7.71, 7.72, 7.73, 7.75, 7.76, 7.79, 7.81, 7.83(a) and (b), 7.100, 7.101, 7.102, 7.103, 7.104, 7.105, 7.106, 7.120, 7.144, 7.145, 7.146, 7.147, 7.156, 7.157, 7.158, 7.165, 7.166, 7.169, 7.170, 7.171, 7.176, 7.186, 7.187, 7.191, 7.192, 7.194, 7.197(a), 7.198, 7.200, 7.238, 7.239, 7.240, 7.242, 7.244, 7.246, 7.248, 7.254, 7.258, 7.259, 7.288, 7.296, 7.321, 7.329, 7.330, 7.361(b), 7.362(b), 7.381, 7.399, 7.403 and 7.408)
- Dr Phil Lucas (Figs 7.43, 7.44, 7.52(a), 7.115, 7.121, 7.122, 7.125, 7.126, 7.127, 7.131, 7.137, 7.182, 7.187, 7.203, 7.264, 7.303, 7.336, 7.348, 7.356, 7.376, 7.380(c), 7.388(b), 7.396(c), 7.400(b), 7.411 and 7.412)
- Raouli Risti, Gosford Hospital (Figs 7.36, 7.37, 7.38, 7.58, 7.236(a) and (b), 7.237, 7.364(a) and (b), 7.365, 7.375(a) and (b), and 7.395(a) and (b))

These images have significantly added to the quality of the chapter.

The spine

**Jock Anderson and John Read
with Jennie Noakes and
Tony Peduto**

8

Serious spinal injuries are among the most feared injuries in sport. This is particularly so when the cervical region is involved. Fortunately, these injuries are uncommon. Most athletes and sports administrators involved in body-contact and high-speed sports are acutely aware of the catastrophic lifelong disability or death that can result from spinal trauma. Improved equipment, training supervision and rule changes have decreased the incidence of serious sports-related spinal injuries.

Even so, it is estimated that between 5% and 10% of the 10 000 cervical spine injuries seen annually in the United States have occurred as a result of involvement in sport (Maroon and Bailes 1998). In Australia, recreational and sporting injuries account for 15% of admissions to spinal cord injury units (Yeo et al. 1998), and a more recent study conducted in Germany found that on reviewing 1016 cases of traumatic spinal injury, 14.5% were caused by sport and recreational diving (Schmitt and Gerner 2001).

The overwhelming majority of spinal problems presenting to a sports medicine clinic do not involve fractures or dislocations, but are due to minor acute soft-tissue injuries such as paraspinal ligament sprain, muscle strains or chronic changes produced by the wear and tear of the repetitive stresses and strains placed on the spine by sport.

Most sports require the spine to move continuously. These movements occur at all spinal levels and between the spine and both the head and pelvis. To function normally, the spine must flex, extend, bend laterally and rotate. Each position must be counterbalanced by muscular and ligamentous forces so that different movements load the spine and intervertebral discs in a variety of ways. When these forces are coupled with the acute trauma of contact sport or the chronic cumulative trauma of activities such as gymnastics, it is no surprise that a wide range of spinal problems are encountered. Chronic back pain and disability are prevalent in athletes of all ages across a wide range of sports. Generally speaking, repetitive stress in the younger athlete may be associated with Scheuermann's disease and spondylolysis, whereas the middle-aged athlete is more prone to intervertebral disc rupture and the older athlete is more likely to suffer from degenerative spondylosis or spinal canal stenosis.

Imaging and the selection of the most appropriate imaging method play an important role in the management of these problems. The imaging specialist is very dependent on being supplied with pertinent history and relevant physical examination findings. An understanding of the mechanics and severity of the injury will enable the radiologist to plan the best imaging pathway. Plain films are the first step, occasionally followed by special additional views when indicated. In most cases this will be the only imaging required. Other imaging methods such as nuclear bone scans, CT and MRI may be required if important questions remain unanswered after plain films. When required, the imaging specialist can now offer a number of image-guided diagnostic and therapeutic interventional procedures for spinal conditions. These are discussed at length in Chapter 10.

Imaging the spine

Plain films

An appropriate plain film series and the method of acquiring these images will be discussed in detail for each anatomical area.

Nuclear bone scans

The role of nuclear bone scans is changing with the increased availability of MRI. In spite of this, nuclear medicine still plays a pivotal role in the diagnosis of spinal injuries. In the context of sporting injuries, bone scans are valuable for the identification of occult fractures in any area of the spine (see

Figs 8.1 and 8.2). Nuclear bone scans may play an important role in the demonstration of inflammatory processes such as discitis (see Fig. 8.3). Bone scans are also useful in helping to determine whether compression fractures or spondylolytic defects are recent or old, by assessing the intensity of isotope uptake (see Figs 8.4 and 8.5). Single photon emission computed tomography (SPECT) imaging is an axial tomographic technique that provides an accurate three-dimensional localisation of areas of increased isotope uptake (see Fig. 8.6). The lack of specificity may make the interpretation of areas of abnormal isotope uptake difficult, and other imaging methods are generally required to further characterise any detected abnormality.

CT

CT is the imaging method of choice for the demonstration of fine bone detail, such as is required for the detection and characterisation of fractures. CT may also be used for soft-tissue imaging but lacks the superior contrast resolution offered by MRI. In the cervical and thoracic regions, cord displacement by a bone fragment or haematoma can be assessed, although this role is being replaced by MRI as the technology becomes more widely available. In the lumbar region, CT is generally used for the demonstration of disc protrusions, (see Fig. 8.7) disc fragments and pars defects. CT is also used to demonstrate nerve roots and follow their

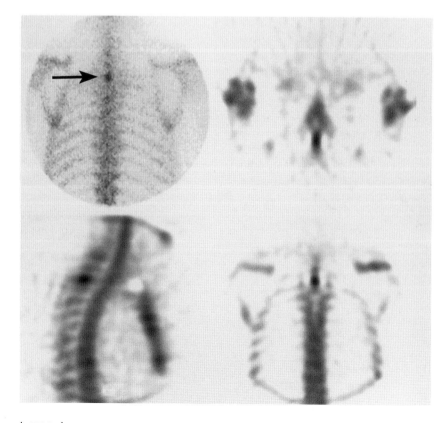

◀ **Fig. 8.1** Delayed planar and SPECT images demonstrate an occult fracture of the spinous process of the T2 vertebra (arrow). Following direct trauma, plain films had been negative.

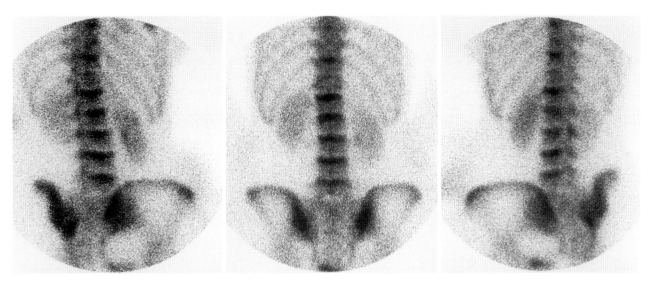

▲ **Fig. 8.2** A young skier experienced severe back pain following a skiing accident. Plain films were normal. A nuclear bone scan showed multiple occult compression fractures of endplates in the thoracic and lumbar regions. These fractures subsequently became evident on plain films.

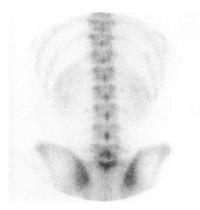

▲ **Fig. 8.3** Increased uptake of isotope is demonstrated at the margins of the L5/S1 disc. The appearance is consistent with discitis.

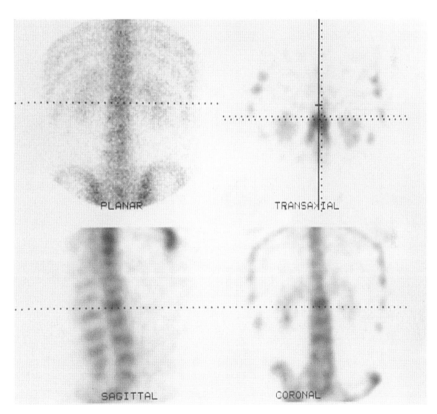

▲ **Fig. 8.4** Planar and SPECT images demonstrate a compression fracture of L1. This fracture is in the late phase of healing, as judged by the intensity of the isotope uptake.

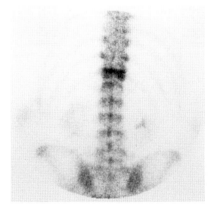

◀ **Fig. 8.5** A nuclear bone scan shows intense uptake of isotope, extending across the upper endplate of T12 and slightly into the body of the vertebra. The intensity of uptake suggests that this is a recent rather than an old fracture.

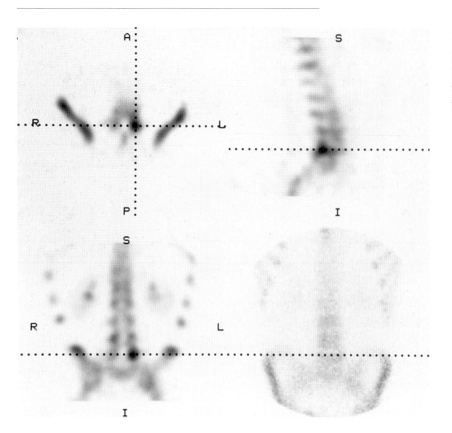

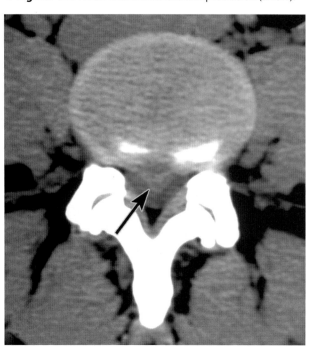

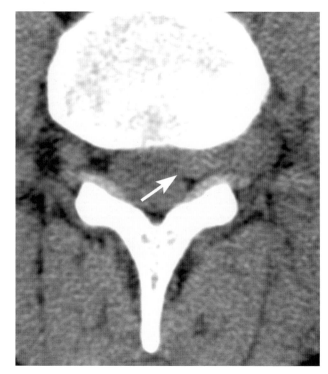

◄ Fig. 8.6 SPECT imaging allows a 3D localisation of an area of isotope uptake. In this case there are stress fractures of the left pars interarticularis of L5 and the right L4 pedicle.

pathways (see Fig. 8.8). Improvements in scanner hardware have led to the development of spiral and multislice CT techniques, allowing the acquisition of fine isotropic voxels and high-definition reformatted images in all planes (see Fig. 8.9). There is no longer difficulty detecting fracture lines that run along the same axial plane of scan acquisition. The use of computer workstations to view CT data enables comprehensive review and better 3D understanding of spinal injuries (see Fig. 8.10). CT myelography is no longer used routinely to demonstrate disc disease or spinal canal stenosis, having been replaced by MRI in most cases.

▼ Fig. 8.8 A sequestrated disc fragment lies in the left lateral spinal recess (arrow). There is considerable swelling of the nerve root on this side, which bulges laterally from the exit foramen. The right nerve root has passed through its exit foramen without complication.

▼ Fig. 8.7 A CT scan shows a central disc protrusion (arrow).

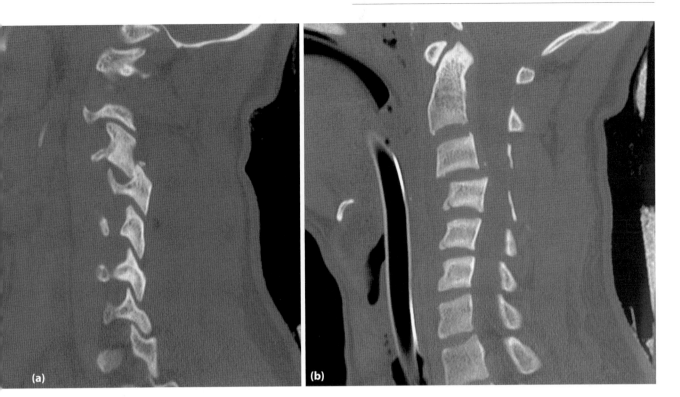

(a) (b)

▲ **Fig. 8.9** The development of multislice CT technology has made images such as these possible. Images can be reformatted in any plane. This is particularly helpful for the understanding of fracture dislocations of facet joints. This young surfer was found unconscious in the surf and was later shown to have a unilateral facet fracture/dislocation at the C3/4 level.
(a) A sagittal reformation through the facets shows a complete dislocation of the C3/4 facet joint, with the inferior C3 articular process having passed over the superior C4 articular process to become locked in the C3/4 exit foramen. Small fractures are also noted. **(b)** A further sagittal reformation through the vertebral bodies shows a C3/4 subluxation with 'teardrop'-type fractures involving the anteroinferior corners of the C4 and C5 vertebral bodies. Narrowing of the spinal canal is most marked at the C4 level.

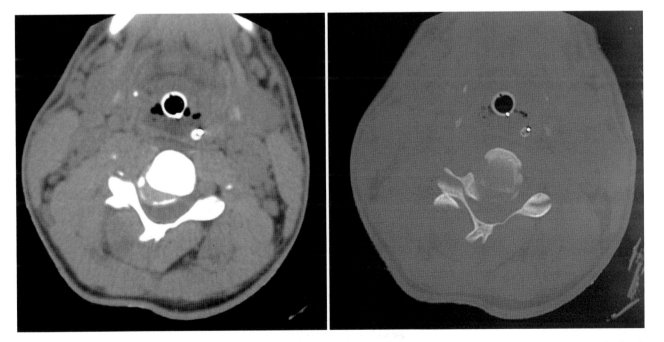

▲ **Fig. 8.10** To examine the relationship of the cord and the spinal canal in the case discussed in Fig. 8.9, axial CT scans at the level of the subluxation were obtained and then displayed after processing with bone and soft-tissue algorithms. The unilateral facet dislocation has caused rotation of the C3 vertebral body on C4, which is well demonstrated on these images. Compression of the cord is further demonstrated on the left image showing soft-tissue detail, while the bone image on the right shows the fracture dislocation at the right C3/4 facet. An endotracheal tube is noted.

MRI

MRI has become an important imaging method for the examination of spinal problems resulting from sport. MRI gives a panoramic view of the spine and has the ability to image in any plane with unsurpassed soft-tissue contrast. In acute injuries producing neurological signs and symptoms, MRI is used to exclude impingement upon neural elements (see Fig. 8.11). Trauma to the cord, including cord oedema, haematoma formation and transection are well demonstrated by MRI (see Figs 8.12 and 8.13). MRI does not easily detect subtle fractures and therefore complements rather than replaces CT. MRI may also be used to rapidly exclude significant ligamentous injuries in elite or professional athletes where a quick diagnosis and an assessment of prognosis are important considerations.

In chronic spinal conditions, the strength of MRI lies in the precise imaging of the spinal cord and its relationship to surrounding structures. Signal changes in discs can also be detected by MRI, reflecting biochemical alterations and disc dehydration (see Fig. 8.14). In addition, MR imaging is extremely sensitive to changes in the water content of bone marrow, which can indicate bone injury, stress reaction or discogenic marrow reaction at the vertebral endplates.

MRI scans have become significantly faster with the introduction of Fast (or Turbo) Spin-Echo (FSE) sequences, phased array coils and parallel imaging techniques. Now, the duration of most scan sequences is no longer than 2 to 3 minutes. Great care must be taken in moving and scanning the acutely injured spinal patient, with close monitoring by appropriate medical personnel and strict screening of patients and staff for metallic objects prior to entering the scan room.

Radiological evaluation of the cervical spine following trauma

Because of the potentially devastating consequences of an overlooked cervical spine injury, a radiograph of the cervical spine is routinely included in a general trauma series whenever there has been significant body trauma. The screening protocol consists of a cross-table lateral view of the cervical spine, taken with the patient supine, together with a supine chest image and an AP view of the pelvis. This cervical spine image is obtained with strict observation of spinal injury protocols whenever moving the patient. If the patient is wearing a hard collar, this is not removed (see Fig. 8.15).

The role of imaging the cervical spine at this initial stage of trauma management is to rule out clinically significant dislocations or fractures and to identify cervical spine instability patterns. Neurological symptoms and signs affect the extent of the initial plain film evaluation. For example, a patient with an acute neurological compromise or an abnormality on the initial lateral view would immediately proceed to cross-sectional imaging after the initial cross-table lateral view. Also, if the patient was experiencing 'burners' and 'stingers' suggestive of nerve root neuropraxia, or had transient quadriplegia indicative of cord neuropraxia, MRI would be indicated without further plain films. 'Burners' and 'stingers' describe a burning or stinging pain that radiates from the shoulder to the hand and may be associated with upper limb paraesthesia or weakness. This group of patients has been shown to have a high incidence of underlying spinal stenosis (Levitz et al. 1997).

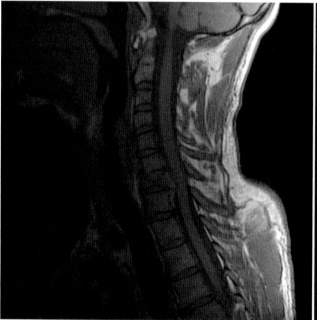
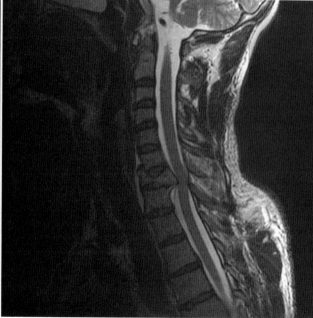

▲ **Fig. 8.11** Sagittal T1- and T2-weighted MR images demonstrate a burst fracture of the C7 vertebral body. A retropulsed fragment of bone compresses the cord against the posterior wall of the spinal canal. There has also been disruption of the posterior spinal elements at this level, consistent with a violent hyperflexion injury. Loss of spinolaminar alignment has occurred and there has been a fracture of the C6 spinous process with injury to the interspinous ligament.

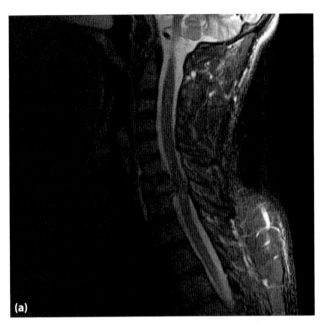
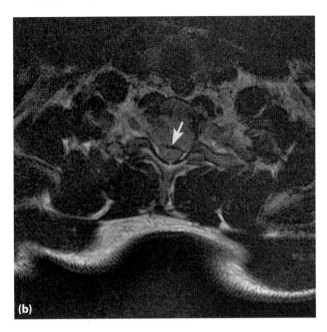

▲ **Fig. 8.12(a)** Further sequences used in the case shown in Fig. 8.11 provide more information. A sagittal GRE image shows high signal in the cord, indicating spinal cord oedema, and a small collection of blood is seen anterior to the vertebrae from C6 to T1. **(b)** A T2-weighted image shows the degree of cord compression and deformity (arrow) in the axial plane.

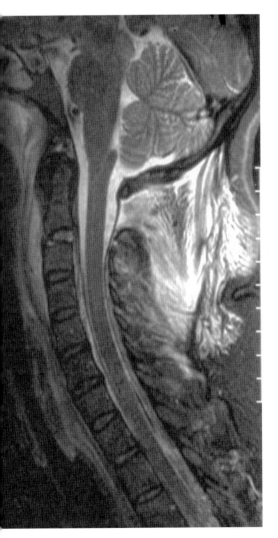

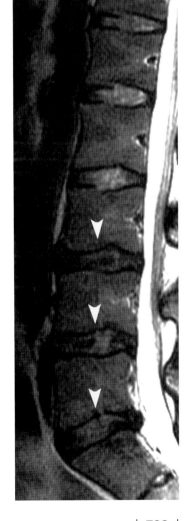

◀**Fig. 8.13** A sagittal fat-suppressed T2-weighted MR image shows a flexion injury at the C2/3 disc level, with rupture of the posterior longitudinal ligament and widening of the posterior disc space. There is a large haematoma anteriorly extending up to the base of the skull. A haematoma posteriorly indicates injury to the interspinous ligament and facet joints. There is altered signal in the C6 vertebral body and buckling of the anterior cortex, which is possibly pre-existing. No cord injury can be seen.

▶ **Fig. 8.14** A sagittal T2-weighted MR image shows loss of the normal high signal in the L3/4, L4/5 and L5/S1 discs (arrowheads). This change reflects decreased water content and is a sign of disc degeneration.

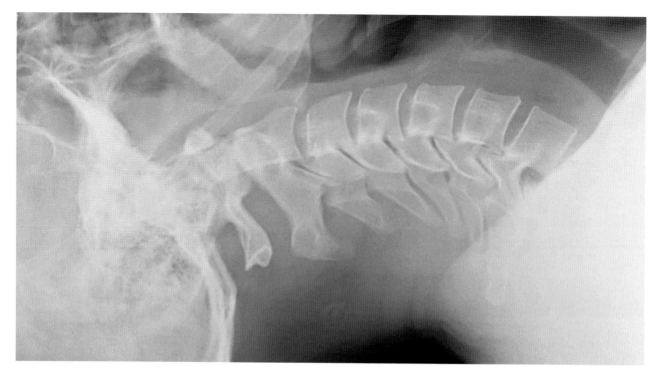

▲ **Fig. 8.15** A cross-table lateral image is generally of adequate standard to allow the exclusion of fractures, subluxations and soft-tissue swelling. The lower cervical region is often difficult to demonstrate and it should be remembered that a subluxation may only be seen on flexion and extension films obtained after the initial lateral view has been assessed and considered to be normal. In this case, apart from minor narrowing of the C5/6 disc space, no abnormality is evident.

If, after careful examination, the initial lateral image is considered to be technically satisfactory and shows no abnormality, the hard collar is removed and an 'open-mouth' AP view of the odontoid process and an AP cervical spine view are obtained. If these views are normal, the patient can be moved and a 'swimmer's' view may be obtained if visualisation of the lower cervical region has not been ideal on the initial lateral film. Also, if there is any persisting clinical suspicion of a subluxation, the hard collar is removed to obtain lateral flexion and extension views. In taking flexion and extension views, it is of great importance that the movement is performed unaided. The radiographer or assisting personnel should never hold the patient's head or force the cervical spine into flexion or extension. Unaided, the patient is protected from further injury by pain and muscle spasm. Subluxation may be demonstrated on these views that cannot be seen on the initial cross-table lateral image.

A routine non-traumatic cervical spine series

If a patient has symptoms related to the cervical spine without a history of acute trauma, a plain film series of the cervical spine is obtained. This series requires precise positioning and radiographic exposure to obtain adequate assessment of the bony structures and soft tissues. Jewellery and other radio-opaque artefacts should be removed prior to radiographic examination.

A routine cervical spine series consists of a neutral lateral view, lateral views in flexion and extension, an AP view of the cervical spine from C3 to T1, an 'open mouth' AP view of the atlantoaxial level and both oblique views.

The neutral lateral view

The neutral lateral view (see Fig. 8.16) is obtained with the patient erect, either standing or sitting. The patient's shoulder rests against the wall bucky to reduce movement. It is important to have the patient's head in a true lateral position as even a small amount of rotation makes the diagnosis of facet subluxation difficult. The angles of the mandible should be superimposed and the chin elevated to prevent superimposition of the mandible over the cervical spine. The beam is centred on the C4 vertebral body. To help assess the position of C4, remember that the C3 vertebral body is about 2 cm posterior to the angle of the mandible. Lowering of the shoulders is aided by expiration. Large muscle-bound athletes with broad shoulders, such as weightlifters and many footballers, are a radiographer's nightmare. Obtaining an adequate lateral view in athletes with this build is extremely difficult and visualisation of the lower cervical region usually depends on a 'swimmer's' view. In difficult patients, holding weights in both hands may help to depress the shoulders.

Flexion and extension views

The diagnosis of a facet subluxation often depends on flexion and extension views (see Fig. 8.17), which to some degree reproduce forces created by the dynamics of cervical spine movement.

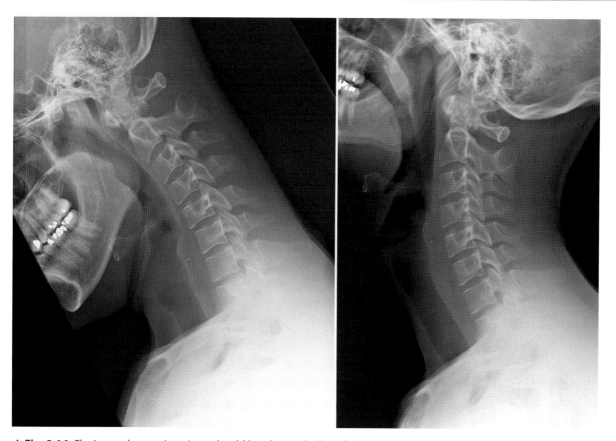

▲ **Fig. 8.16** Flexion and extension views should be obtained when there is a clinical suspicion of a subluxation or if restricted movement is noted.

▼ **Fig. 8.17** In the neutral view (right image) there is evidence of a flexion injury, with buckling of the anterior cortex of C6. With flexion (left image), subluxation is demonstrated at the C5/6 level.

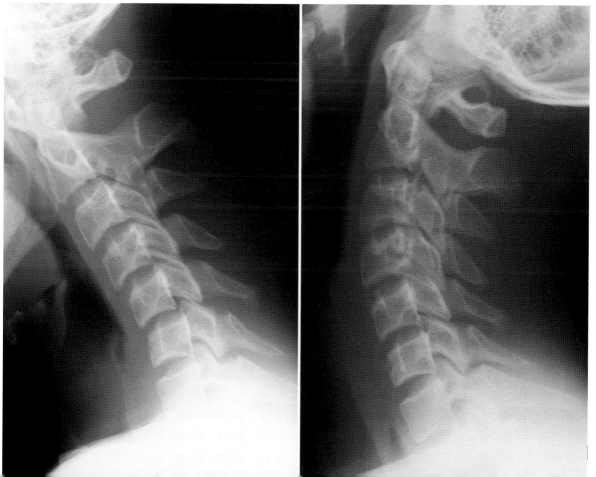

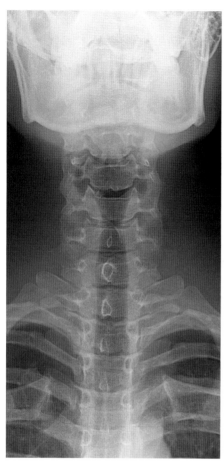

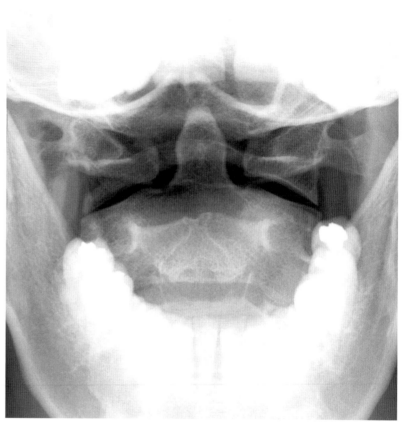

▲ **Fig. 8.18** An AP view displays the cervical spine from C3 to T1 and is valuable for the assessment of alignment of the spinous processes and identification of injury to the lateral masses. This example has been well positioned.

▲ **Fig. 8.19** A view of the atlantoaxial region is obtained through the open mouth and is an essential film in any cervical spine series. Fractures of the odontoid process, disruption of the atlantoaxial articulations and evidence of rotary C1/2 subluxation can be identified on this view.

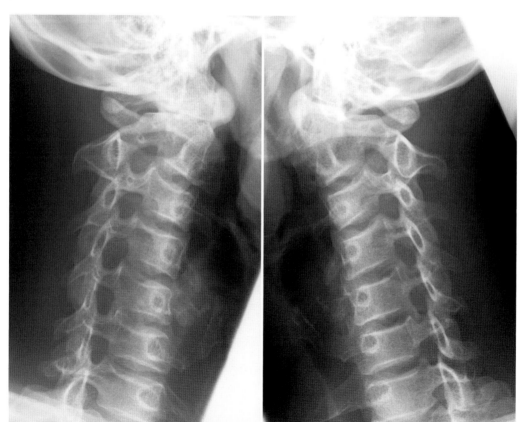

◀ **Fig. 8.20** Oblique views allow examination of the intervertebral foramina, aided by the use of cranial tube angulation. Alignment and integrity of the lateral masses and pedicles may also be assessed.

In addition to detecting evidence of subluxation, these views may identify spinal segments where there is less movement than normal. These 'functional' views are discussed in more detail later.

The AP view from C3 to T1

The AP view (C3 to T1) is taken with the patient standing against the wall bucky, the primary beam centred on the mid-thyroid cartilage, with 15° of cranial angulation. Care must be taken with positioning, and it is important that there is no lateral tilting (or rotation) of the head (see Fig. 8.18).

The AP view of the atlantoaxial region

An AP view of the atlantoaxial region (see Fig. 8.19) is obtained with the patient erect, through the open mouth and with a straight tube. The patient is positioned with a line from the lowest margin of the teeth to the tips of the mastoid processes, being perpendicular to the film. This often requires gentle neck extension. It is of great importance that the patient's head is straight. Slight head rotation makes the odontoid process appear off-centre relative to the lateral masses of the atlas, raising the possibility of rotary C1/2 subluxation.

AP oblique views

AP oblique views are obtained by rotating the entire patient 45° one way and then the other, obtaining images in each position. The chin is elevated, with the beam centred 2 cm above the thyroid cartilage, and 10 to 20° of cranial angulation is used to improve the display of the intervertebral foramina (see Fig. 8.20).

Tips on looking at plain films of the cervical spine

A routine checklist of assessment should be followed for each view of the cervical spine series. Although cervical vertebrae are anatomically complex, they should interlock like a jigsaw puzzle to create smooth arcs of alignment. The integrity of these arcs can be assessed on the lateral, AP and oblique views.

The lateral view

A suggested routine for the assessment of a lateral view of the cervical spine is as follows:

1. Count the vertebrae.
2. Check the alignment.
3. Assess the cervical lordosis.
4. Match the facet joint articular surfaces.
5. Inspect the disc spaces.
6. Examine the individual bony contours.
7. Assess the spinal canal diameter.
8. Examine the soft tissues.

9. Finally, go back and re-examine those areas where fractures commonly occur.

1. Count the vertebrae

In assessing the lateral view, the very first task is to count the vertebrae that have been demonstrated, making sure that the entire cervical spine has been adequately examined. Alignment at the C7/T1 level should be visible. As previously discussed, a 'swimmer's' view or possibly oblique views may be necessary to help examine the lower cervical region. Occasionally, CT scanning may be required if there is a high index of clinical suspicion and the additional views are still inadequate.

2. Check the alignment

Vertebral body alignments should then be assessed. Four unbroken smoothly curved lines must be present (see Fig. 8.21). The anterior and posterior margins of the vertebral bodies should form two curved parallel lines. The posterior margins of the articular masses (pillars) and the spinolaminar junctions should align as smooth arcs. The arc of posterior vertebral body alignment should be continuous with the clivus, and the spinolaminar line should be continuous with the posterior margin of the foramen magnum. Abrupt disruption of any of these lines is an indication of subluxation, dislocation, fracture or degeneration.

In children, there can be a physiological disruption of the vertebral alignment with a slight forward slip of one vertebra on the one below when the cervical spine is flexed. This occurs in the upper cervical region, most commonly at the C2/3 level (see Fig. 8.22), and results from ligamentous laxity ('pseudosubluxation'). To confirm that such alignment changes are physiological, a return to normal alignment should be seen with neck extension (see Fig. 8.23).

3. Assess the cervical lordosis

If the normal cervical lordosis is absent or there is a fixed flexion or extension deformity demonstrated with flexion and extension views, a particularly close review of the spine and correlation with clinical findings is required. However, loss of the normal cervical lordosis in the neutral position should not always be taken as a sign of injury or muscular spasm. Absence may also be due to the wearing of a hard collar or a chin-down position (also known as a Westpoint or Military position).

4. Match the facet joint articular surfaces

The facet joints and lateral masses should then be examined to confirm that the articular surfaces can be matched with their opposite number and that their posterior margins are aligned. Matching the articular surfaces of the vertebrae is an arduous task, but the evidence of a unilateral facet subluxation is often subtle and identification of this injury requires painstaking inspection of the film. If the film is a true lateral, a sudden change of facet alignment usually indicates subluxation (see Fig. 8.24).

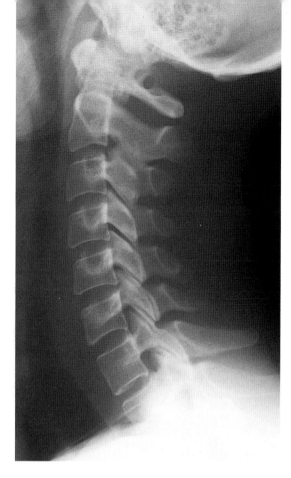

▲ Fig. 8.21(a) The first task is to count the vertebral bodies to confirm that the image adequately allows examination of the entire cervical spine. In this case the lower cervical spine is clearly seen and alignment can be assessed down to the mid-T1 vertebral body.

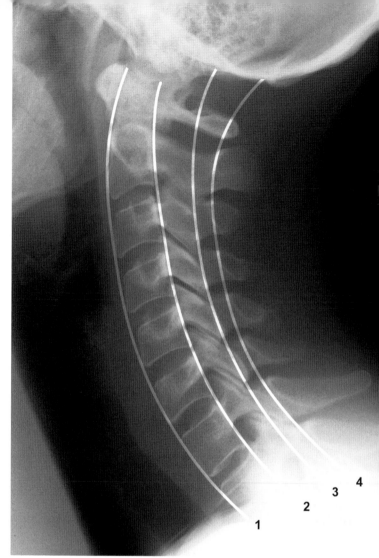

▲ (b) In a normal lateral view of the cervical spine, orderly alignment should be present. It is essential to be able to recognise four continuous smooth curves, as shown by the overlay. If these curves are unbroken, the cervical vertebrae have a normal anatomical relationship with each other.
The curves are:

1. the anterior borders of the vertebral bodies
2. the posterior borders of the vertebral bodies
3. the posterior margins of the lateral masses
4. the spinolaminar line.

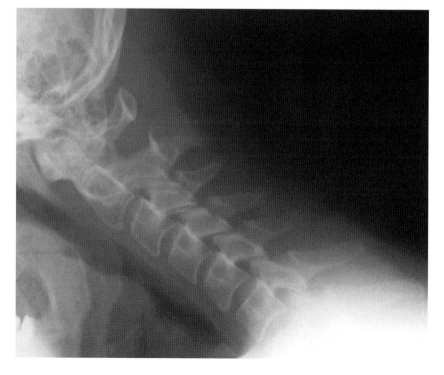

◀ Fig. 8.22 In children, physiological subluxations may occur in the upper cervical spine with flexion due to ligamentous laxity. This change is usually most marked at the C2 level. In this case minor pseudosubluxations are present at all levels from C2/3 to C5/6.

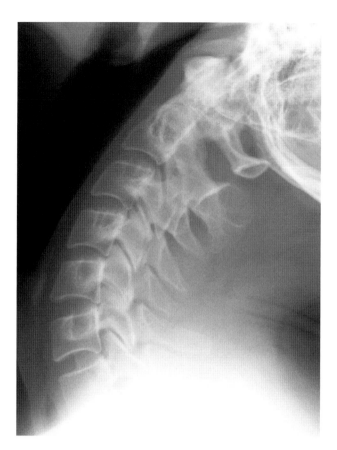

▲ **Fig. 8.23** When subluxations are seen in an immature cervical spine, a lateral view should be obtained in extension. If the alignment then returns to normal, as in this case, a diagnosis of physiological pseudosubluxation can be made.

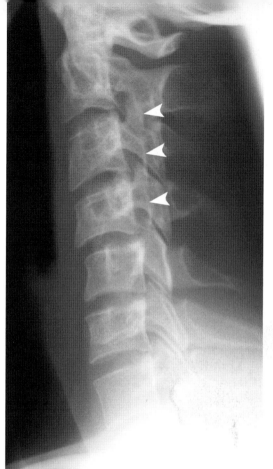

▲ **Fig. 8.24** Checking that the articular surfaces of each facet are neatly matched is an important task. In this case there is an abrupt change at the C4/5 level indicating the presence of a unilateral facet subluxation. Arrowheads indicate the posterior aspect of the lateral masses above the C4/5 level and these remain in constant alignment, indicating that the spine above the C4/5 level is rotated on the spine below this level.

If the film is not a true lateral because the whole body is turned, or if the head alone is turned, the task of matching the apophyseal articular surfaces is extremely difficult. Body and head rotation is easily assessed by looking at the angles of the mandible, which should be superimposed if the patient is in a true lateral position. It may then be possible to correlate the amount of offset of the facets with the degree of rotation of the mandible. If the offset is wholly the result of head rotation, the degree of offset will increase gradually the higher the level (see Fig. 8.25), whereas if the entire body is rotated, the degree of offset will remain constant throughout the cervical spine.

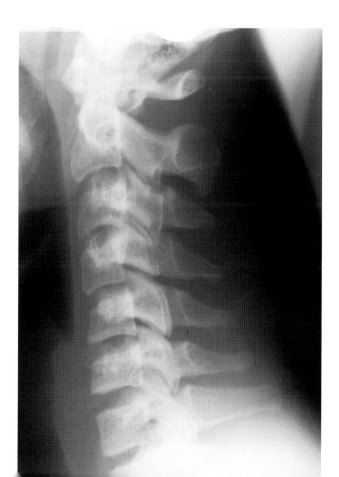

◀ **Fig. 8.25** In this example, the cervical facets above C5/6 are offset, and this appearance becomes increasingly prominent the higher the level. The degree of offset is gradual and progressive, and these changes are due to head rotation rather than subluxation, confirmed by noting the position of the angles of the mandible, which are considerably separated by rotation. Note the decreased vertical height of C6 compared to the vertebral bodies above and below. This is a common normal variant.

5. Inspect the disc spaces

The disc spaces in the cervical region are generally parallel and uniform. The endplates are examined for evidence of a compression injury. There is no definite increase in the width of the disc spaces with descending levels as there is in the lumbar region, but the spaces should not decrease when compared with those above. If there is a decrease in the width of a disc space, this will almost certainly indicate either disc degeneration or disc protrusion.

6. Examine the individual bony contours

Inspection of the individual bony contours is obviously an important step in the search for bone injury. Compression of a cervical vertebra may occur following an axial force, which, if combined with flexion, may cause a wedge deformity. This injury may occur alone or in conjunction with posterior ligament complex disruption. It is important to remember that an apparent slight relative reduction in height of C5 or C6 may be a normal variant. The vertical height of these vertebrae may be less than the vertebra above and below, as is shown in Fig. 8.66 on page 746.

The anterior cortical margin of each vertebra should be carefully examined for stepping or buckling that may follow a hyperflexion injury (see Fig. 8.26). It is also important to confirm that there is linear continuity of the anterior margin of C2 with the anterior margin of the odontoid process (see Fig. 8.27). Any deformity of the odontoid may require further investigation to exclude a fracture. The posterior arch of the atlas and the pars interarticularis of C2 may be injured by extension, and careful inspection of these structures is also advisable.

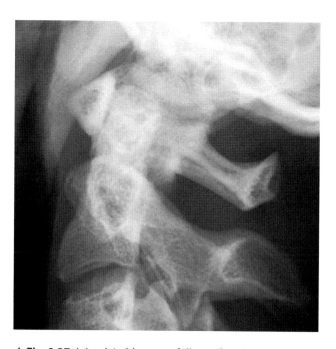

▲ **Fig. 8.27** It is advisable to carefully confirm that the normal smooth cortical continuity of the anterior margin of the body of the axis with the anterior margin of odontoid process has not been disrupted. A step or angulation may indicate an odontoid fracture. The odontoid process more generally should also be examined for evidence of injury. The posterior arch of the atlas and the pars interarticularis of the axis are common sites of injury due to extension forces and should become a part of the routine examination of the cervical spine. Remember that most fatal cervical spine injuries occur in the upper cervical region.

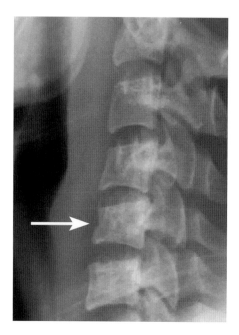

▲ **Fig. 8.26** There has been a compressive injury with cervical flexion producing buckling of the anterior margin of the C5 vertebral body (arrow). Note the soft-tissue swelling over the anterior aspect of the spine, due to a large haematoma associated with the flexion fracture.

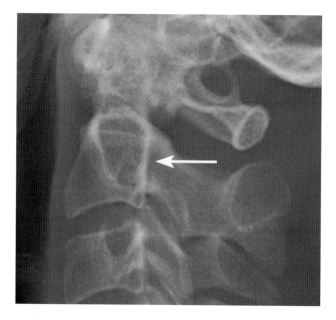

▲ **Fig. 8.28** A Harris ring is shown (arrow), although this example is larger than average. The ring is formed by end-on projection of the lateral mass of the cervical vertebral body. A ring is present at all levels, although the ring at C2 is always most prominent and any disruption at this level is more easily seen. When there is a fracture of the C2 body or lateral mass, the ring may appear fragmented and disrupted.

Oval or 'U'-shaped cortical outlines are superimposed on the vertebral bodies in the lateral view (see Fig. 8.28). These outlines are known as Harris or Axis rings (Mortelmans et al. 1999) and are created by the transverse processes and pedicles of the vertebrae. These should be carefully inspected for fragmentation or cortical irregularity, as evidence of a fracture of the lateral mass (see Figs 8.29 and 8.30). This is particularly important at the C2 level, where deformity of this superimposed outline may indicate a fracture of the base of dens or lateral mass of C2. Inspection of these superimposed contours offers an opportunity to diagnose fractures that are otherwise difficult to detect on a lateral view.

▶▼ **Fig. 8.29(a)** Following a surfing injury, a lateral plain film shows irregularity of the anterior margin of the Harris ring (arrow), and a fracture line can be seen projected over the base of the odontoid posteriorly, within the ring. These changes suggest an underlying injury at the atlantoaxial level. **(b)** A subsequent CT examination defines the fractures responsible for the deformity of the Harris ring. There are fractures of the lateral mass of the axis and the lateral mass and body of the atlas. **(c)** Reformatted CT images in the sagittal plane show the extent of the injury (arrows).

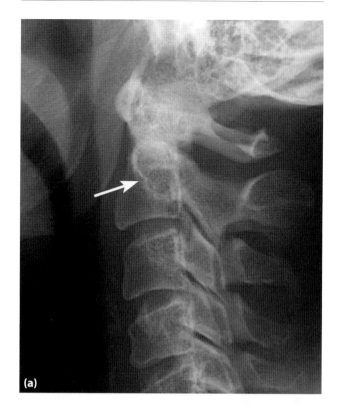
(a)

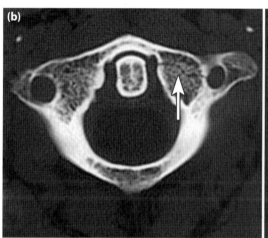
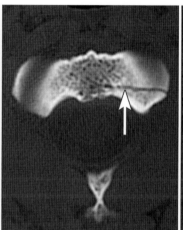
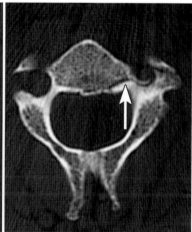
(b)

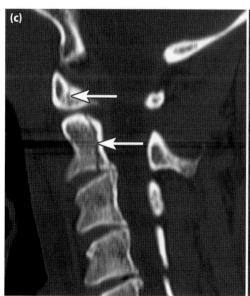
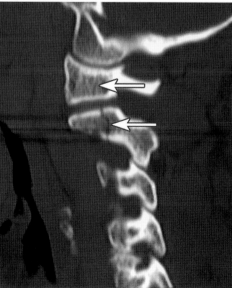
(c)

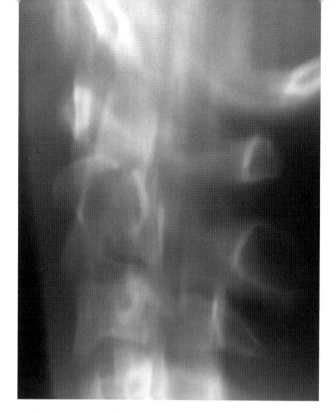

▲ **Fig. 8.30** In another case, a more obvious disruption of a Harris ring is demonstrated by conventional tomography.

Spinous processes may be injured in hyperflexion injuries. Consequently, the spinous processes and the interspinous spaces should be carefully assessed (see Fig. 8.31). The spaces between the spinous processes gradually increase at each level from C2 to C7, and will open and close with flexion and extension in a uniform fanlike manner. Following a hyperflexion injury, one space may become abnormally widened, indicating posterior ligament complex disruption. The shape of the spinous processes can be variable with dysplastic or bifid tips being quite common. The best location for inspection of the interspinous distance is between the bases of the spinous processes in the region of the spinolaminar line where there is less variability.

7. Assess the spinal canal diameter

In patients with episodic neurological symptoms such as 'stingers', assessment of the cervical spinal canal aperture is important. Direct AP diameter measurement or various ratios such as the Torg ratio may be used as a guide to congenital stenosis. This subject is discussed in more detail in the section on spinal canal stenosis (see page 758), where limitations of the Torg ratio are reviewed.

8. Examine the soft tissues

Any increase in thickness, anterior convexity or loss of definition of the anterior soft-tissue line can be a sign of haemorrhage resulting from cervical spine trauma (see Figs 8.32 and 8.33). An exception may be seen in children, when an apparent increase in prevertebral soft tissue can be due to poor pharyngeal aeration or, more superiorly, adenoidal hypertrophy.

The soft tissues anterior to the cervical spine are outlined against air in the adjacent pharynx. The soft-tissue thickness

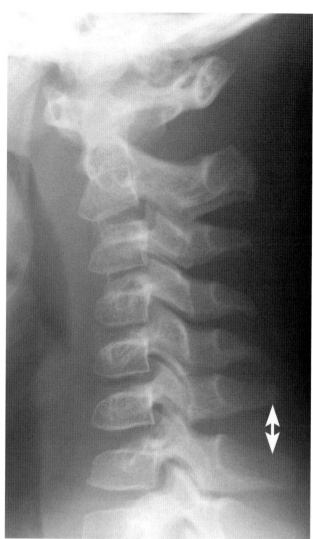

▲ **Fig. 8.31** The space between the C6 and C7 spinous processes is widened (arrows), when compared with the spaces above and below. This change has occurred as a consequence of subluxation at the C6/7 level due to a trampolining accident.

anterior to the mid-portion of the C2 vertebral body is normally up to 7 mm in adults, although on mobile films this distance may appear greater due to magnification (Harris and Yeakley 1989). The measurements at the C7 level should be less than 2 cm. This rule is easy to remember as '7 at 2 and 2 at 7'.

9. Re-examine the sites where fractures commonly occur

The final task in examining the lateral view is to re-examine the sites where fractures are likely to occur. These include the posterior arch of C1, the odontoid process, the posterior arch of C2 and the anterior margins of the vertebral bodies. In flexion, there may be widening of the anterior atlantoaxial joint indicating injury to the transverse ligament. On a lateral view, this joint space should remain less than 3 mm in an adult. In children, the joint space can be up to 4 mm wide due to the apparent space being partly composed of non-ossified cartilage (see Fig. 8.34) (Harris and Mirvis 1996).

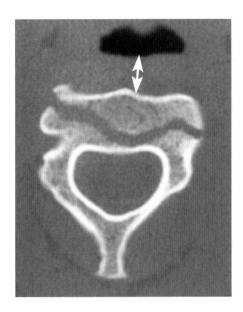

▲ **Fig. 8.32** A haematoma resulting from a fracture of the axis has produced anterior displacement of the pharynx (arrows). The upper limit of normal of the width of soft tissues at this level is 7 mm.

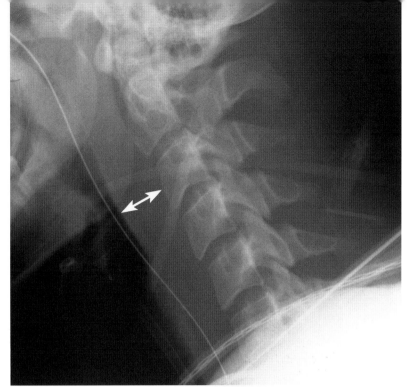

▲ **Fig. 8.33** Gross haemorrhage due to an atlanto-occipital fracture/dislocation has produced marked soft-tissue widening of the retropharyngeal space (arrows).

AP views

There are two AP views. The first is an AP view of the atlantoaxial joint. The atlantoaxial joint is examined in the frontal projection through an open mouth, with slight head extension to prevent the front teeth being superimposed over the odontoid. This position usually projects the posterior arch of the axis over the odontoid process and may produce an illusion of odontoid fracture due to a phenomenon of visual perception known as the 'Mach' effect (see Fig. 8.35).

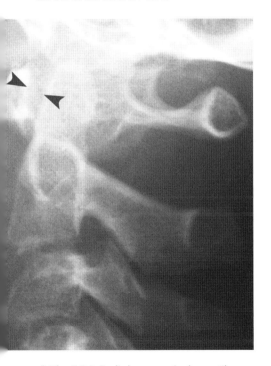

▲ **Fig. 8.34** Radiolucent articular cartilage and ligamentous laxity contribute to the width of the anterior atlantoaxial joint space in children (arrowheads). Consequently, the joint space may widen up to 4 mm in cervical flexion and still be considered normal.

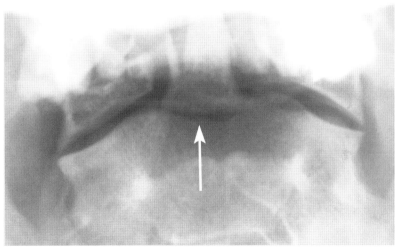

▲ **Fig. 8.35** The 'Mach' effect is an optical illusion appearing as a dark line, which is seen here crossing the base of the odontoid process (arrow). The dark line runs immediately adjacent to a white line caused by the posterior arch of the atlas. This dark line is a visual artefact that may sometimes be mistaken for a fracture.

There are three changes to search for on a view of the atlantoaxial joint:

1. A fracture of the odontoid process (or 'dens'), which is discussed further in the section on cervical spine injuries (see Fig. 8.36).
2. Divergent subluxation of the lateral masses of C1 at the atlantoaxial joints, which indicates a fracture of the atlas. On the AP view, the articular margins of the lateral masses of C1 and C2 should align, and even slight lateral subluxation of the lateral facets of the atlas may indicate a Jefferson fracture of the atlas (see Figs 8.37 and 8.38).
3. Rotary subluxation of C1 about the odontoid. The odontoid process should be centred between the lateral masses. Asymmetry is usually due to poor positioning and rotation of the head, but if the film is straight, a rotary subluxation may be present and CT scanning should be obtained to establish the diagnosis (see Fig. 8.39).

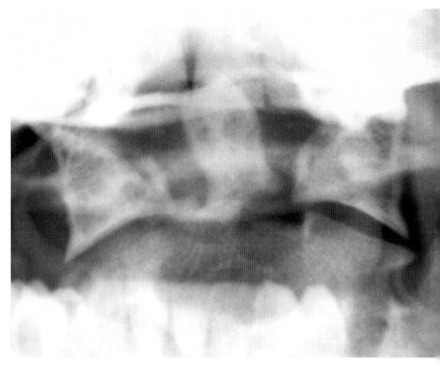

▲ **Fig. 8.36** A fracture involves the base of the odontoid with considerable displacement and lateral tilting of the process. Odontoid fractures can result from flexion or extension injuries, and lateral tilting of the head appears to have played a role in the mechanism of this fracture.

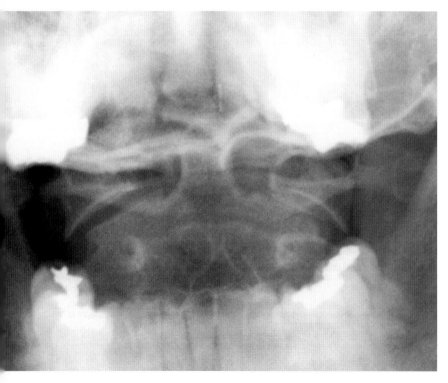

▲ **Fig. 8.37(a)** Lateral overhang of the facets of the atlas on an AP open-mouth view indicates slight C1 lateral mass subluxation at both lateral atlantoaxial joints. This is usually due to a Jefferson fracture of the atlas, which disrupts the bony ring both anteriorly and posteriorly allowing lateral separation of the fragments. When this sign is present, a CT scan of the atlas should be obtained.

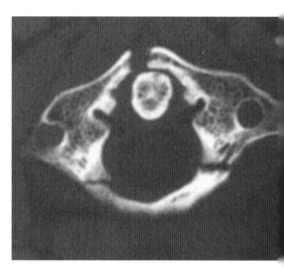

▲ **(b)** A CT scan of the atlas confirms the presence of a Jefferson fracture, demonstrating fractures of the anterior and posterior arches of the atlas with separation and lateral displacement of the lateral masses.

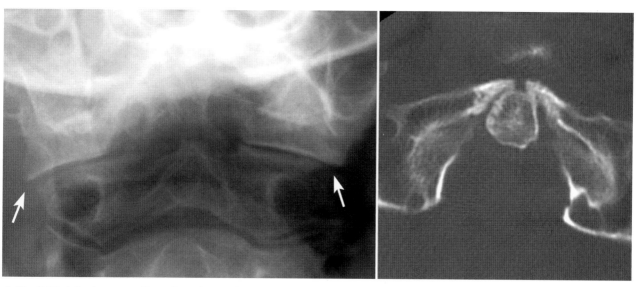

▲ **Fig. 8.38** A further case of lateral overhang of the facets of the atlas (arrows), due to a Jefferson fracture of the axis.

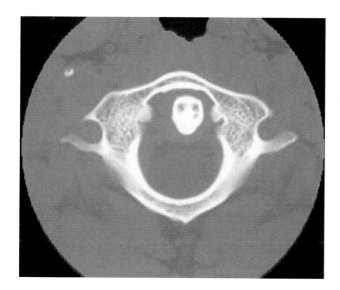

▲ **Fig. 8.39** A CT scan shows asymmetry and slight rotation of the axis relative to the odontoid. This suggests rotary subluxation, although review of the other CT images in this case would also be required to confirm the diagnosis.

▶ **Fig. 8.40** All spinous processes should align on the AP view. In this case there is an abrupt step in alignment at the C6/7 level, which reflects rotation of C6 on C7 due to a unilateral facet subluxation at the C6/7 level.

The second AP view shows the cervical spine from C3 to C7. There are three important features to assess on this view after trauma:

1. The spinous processes should align. If there is a sudden step in alignment, a unilateral facet subluxation is invariably present (see Fig. 8.40).

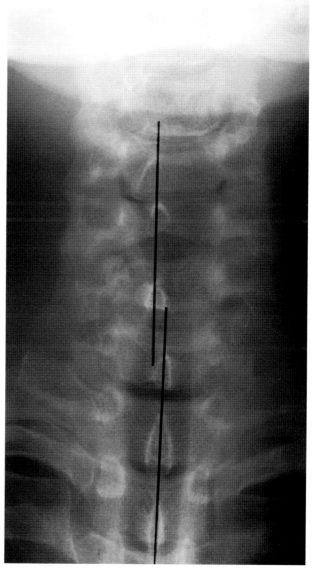

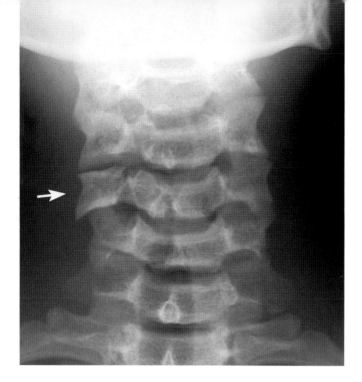

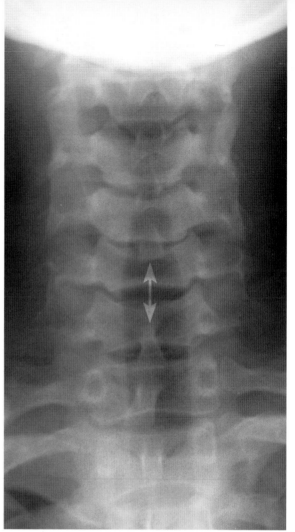

▲ Fig. 8.41 The usual smooth wavy contour created by the lateral margins of the cervical spine on the AP view is disrupted by a pillar fracture of C5 on the right (arrow).

▶ Fig. 8.42 A flexion injury may disrupt the posterior ligament complex. This complex includes the interspinous ligament, and injury to this ligament may manifest as a widened interspinous space that is out of step with the spaces above and below. In this case there is widening of the space between the C6 and C7 spinous processes due to a flexion injury at this level.

2. The lateral border of the lateral masses should describe a smooth wavy contour. This wavy contour is normally unbroken and irregularity of the profile may indicate a pillar fracture or facet subluxation (see Fig. 8.41). Fractures, particularly in the sagittal plane, can be detected with this view, although care must be taken not to confuse the laryngeal gas shadow with a fracture line.

3. The distance between the spinous processes should increase in a uniform progression from the proximal to the distal cervical spine. A widened interspinous space that is out of step with the spaces above and below may occur following a flexion injury which disrupts the posterior ligament complex (see Fig. 8.42).

Oblique views

Oblique views enable the intervertebral foramina to be examined. Consequently, oblique views are valuable in patients presenting with radicular pain. Osteophytes arising at the margins of the neurocentral joints as a result of disc degeneration may encroach on the intervertebral foramina and contribute to nerve root irritation (see Fig. 8.43). Oblique views are also valuable in confirming normal pedicle and facet alignment (see Fig. 8.44) and for the identification of pedicle fractures (see Fig. 8.45).

▶ Fig. 8.43 Osteophytes are demonstrated (arrow) at the C3/4 neurocentral joint encroaching on the intervertebral foramen.

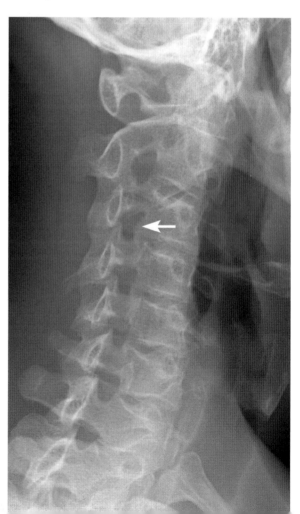

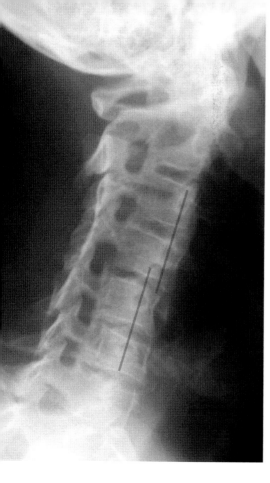

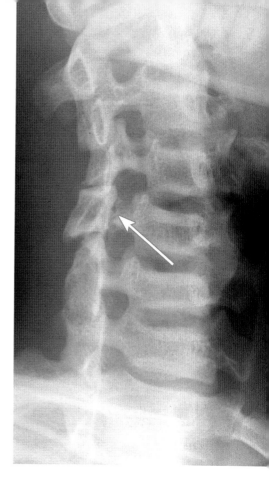

◄ **Fig. 8.44** Alignment of lateral masses and pedicles can be assessed on an oblique view. This case shows an abrupt loss of pedicle alignment due to rotation caused by a unilateral C4/5 facet subluxation.

▶ **Fig. 8.45** The pedicles and lateral masses are well seen in an oblique view. In this case, a fracture of the C5 pedicle at its junction with the lateral mass is demonstrated (arrow).

Additional radiographic views

The 'swimmer's' view

The most commonly used additional view is the 'swimmer's' view, so-called because it requires the patient to have one arm raised above their head and the other by their side, like a freestyle swimmer. In this position the shoulders are not super-imposed, enabling alignment at the cervicothoracic junction to be better imaged by reducing the overall thickness of tissue to be penetrated. This view is used whenever the cervicothoracic junction has not been adequately demonstrated on the routine lateral view (see Fig. 8.46(a)). The detail provided is invariably poor and vertebral alignment is usually the only dependable information available (see Fig. 8.46(b)). If doubt about the normality of alignment remains, a CT scan may be necessary to further assist with evaluation of this area.

▶ **Fig. 8.46(a)** A 'swimmer's' view is a valuable and much-used method of assessing the lower cervical spine and the cervicothoracic junction alignment. Note the narrowing of the C3/4 and C5/6 disc spaces.
(b) A swimmer's view shows a subluxation at the C6/7 level and a fracture of the C6 facet (arrow). As usual, the detail is poor, and other imaging methods can now be used for fracture characterisation.

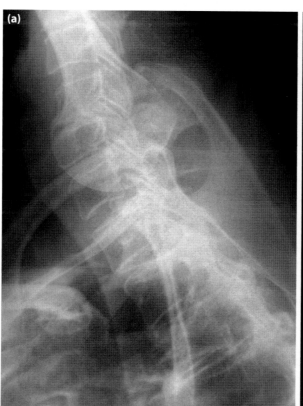

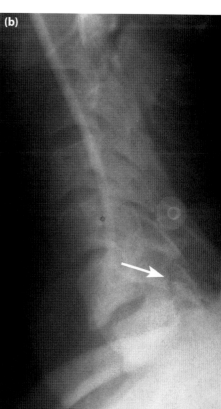

The pillar view

The pillar view is an AP view taken with 20 to 30° of caudal tube angulation, with a pad under the upper thoracic spine to elevate the shoulders and to allow extension of the cervical spine. The view is used to examine the facet joints and lateral masses to show pillar fractures and facet dislocations. Because there is hyperextension of the neck, the view should not be used if an unstable fracture or dislocation is suspected (see Fig. 8.47).

The moving jaw view

To acquire a moving jaw view, the patient continuously moves their jaw by saying 'mum-mum-mum' without moving their head. This blurs the mandible, and the entire cervical spine from the odontoid to T1 can be demonstrated on the one AP view (see Fig. 8.48).

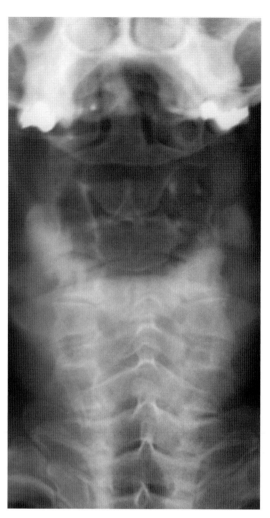

▲ **Fig. 8.48** An AP view taken with a moving jaw is a simple and efficient way of imaging the entire cervical spine from C2 to T1 with a single exposure. Movement produces blurring of the mandible.

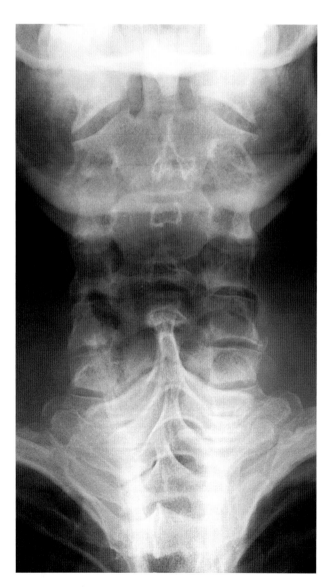

▲ **Fig. 8.47** The pillar view. This view should no longer be used as it requires neck extension, and far superior definition of the lateral masses and facet joints is obtained by CT scanning, without risking exacerbation of the injury.

Looking at MR images of the cervical spine

At a minimum, the typical protocol for spinal MR imaging should include a combination of axial and sagittal T1- and T2-weighted sequences:

- A sagittal T1-weighted FSE sequence will show anatomical detail of bone, cord and soft tissues. Alignments are well demonstrated (see Fig. 8.49).
- A sagittal T2-weighted FSE sequence is sensitive to the presence of water and consequently will demonstrate oedema or haematoma formation in the soft tissues as well as cord swelling or compression (see Fig. 8.50).
- Sagittal STIR or fat-suppressed T2-weighted FSE sequences can show subtle areas of high signal in the paraspinal soft tissues in cases of ligament injury, or marrow oedema due to fracture, contusion or stress reaction (see Fig. 8.51). Cord oedema associated with cord contusion may also be demonstrated.

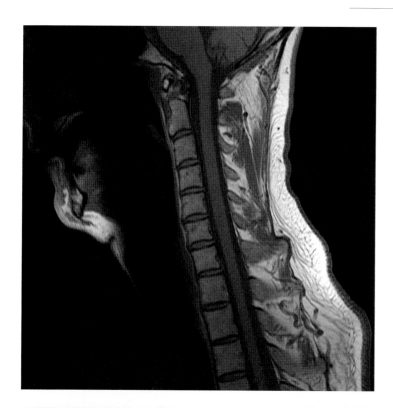

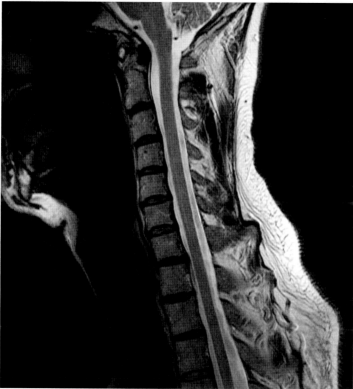

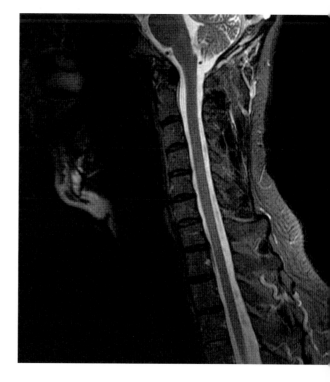

◀**Fig. 8.49** A sagittal T1-weighted image is the sequence best suited for the identification of many anatomical structures. Fat is bright and CSF relatively dark. The fat content of bone marrow means that bony structures are moderately bright. Ligaments and cortical bone are dark. Note the subtle increase in signal posterior to the C7/T1 disc. This represents a minor disc protrusion that is difficult to appreciate in the dark CSF background on this sequence.

◀**Fig. 8.50** A sagittal T2-weighted sequence is sensitive to water content and so is useful for the demonstration of oedema. The CSF is bright, providing a useful contrast to the cord, enabling easy identification of cord swelling and deformity. The small C7/T1 disc protrusion that was difficult to see on the T1 sequence is now more obvious due to the hypointense (dark) disc fragment and elevated overlying posterior longitudinal spinal ligament being silhouetted by bright CSF.

▶**Fig. 8.51** A sagittal STIR or fat-suppressed T2-weighted technique suppresses the high signal in fat and is sensitive to water content. As a consequence, such sequences may reveal areas of high signal due to localised oedema indicative of injury or other pathology within bone marrow, soft tissue or the spinal canal.

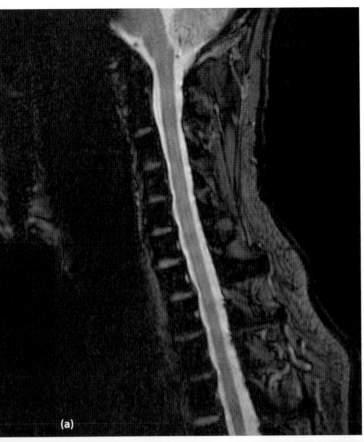

(a)

- Axial and sagittal T2*-weighted GRE sequences are sensitive to the presence of cord haematoma and disc disease (see Fig. 8.52).
- Axial T1- and T2-weighted images are essential to the assessment and localisation of injuries. They are a vital complement to the sagittal images and will often more clearly demonstrate findings such as migrated disc fragments, lateral recess pathology and foraminal changes. Cord signal changes that are appreciated only on the sagittal images and that are not confirmed on axial images are spurious (see Fig. 8.53).
- Coronal scanning with T1- or T2-weighting is sometimes used to assess alignment, lateral disc changes, paraspinal musculature and ligament injuries (see Fig. 8.54).
- T2-weighted oblique images have become increasingly popular for the examination of the nerve roots, exit foramina and the lateral masses (see Fig. 8.55).

Sagittal images must include the entirety of the lateral masses and ideally extend to the adjacent soft tissues. Slice thickness is 3–4 mm and a high-resolution matrix is used. Intravenous injection of gadolinium is sometimes necessary but not routine. Gadolinium may be helpful after spinal surgery in the differentiation of recurrent disc from scar formation, or in cases of suspected infection or tumour.

Figs 8.49–8.55 demonstrate the appearances of the different scan sequences on the same cervical spine. Different sequences extract different information.

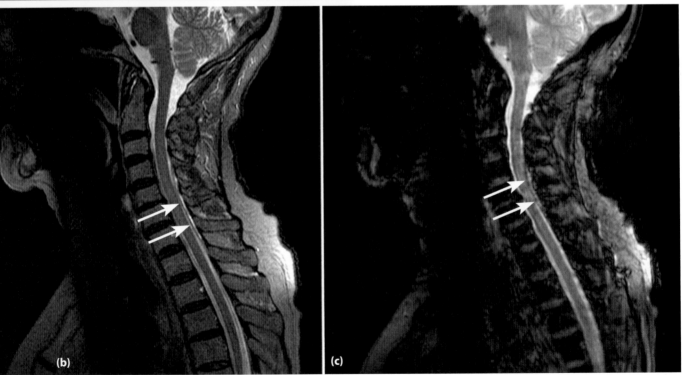

(b)

(c)

▲ **Fig. 8.52(a)** This image is an example of a sagittal T2*-weighted GRE sequence, which is sensitive to the presence of blood-breakdown products following haemorrhage. Also note the clear definition of the silhouette of the intervertebral discs.
(b) Another case demonstrates the value of a GRE sequence. A fat-suppressed T2-weighted FSE image shows an extradural collection of fluid (arrows).
(c) To differentiate between a CSF leak and blood, a T2*-weighted GRE image was obtained. The beaded hypointense appearance now seen at the margin of the collection on the GRE sequence represents 'blooming' due to the presence of blood breakdown products, indicating that this is a collection of blood (arrows).

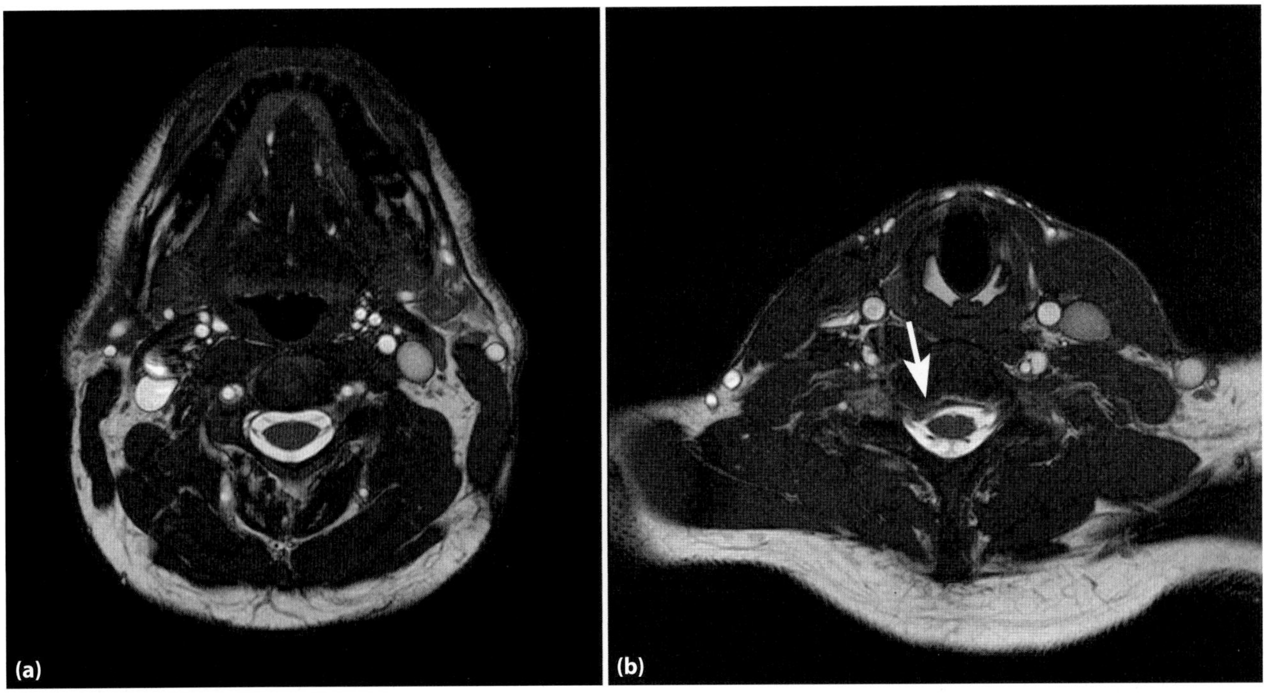

▲ **Fig. 8.53** Axial T2-weighted images from the case shown in Fig. 8.52 illustrate the complementary role to sagittal imaging. Axial images are sometimes more sensitive for the detection of pathology and they allow a more precise anatomical localisation and characterisation of abnormalities seen on sagittal images. The relationship of the cord to the spinal canal can be easily assessed, with bright CSF surrounding and highlighting this structure.

(a) An image from the upper cervical region shows a normal cord and spinal canal.

(b) An image, acquired at the C7/T1 level, shows a small disc protrusion (arrow) as previously noted on the sagittal images in Figs 8.49 and 8.50. The disc encroaches on the right lateral spinal recess, impinging on the ventral nerve root but not displacing the cord.

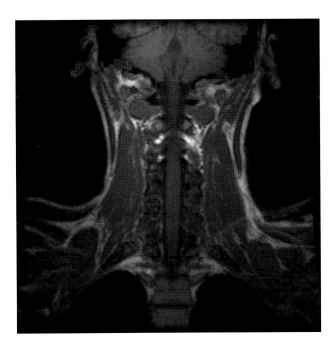

▲ **Fig. 8.54** Coronal scanning with T1-weighted or fat-suppressed T2-weighted images may be used to assess paraspinal musculature and ligament injuries. This example is a T1-weighted image.

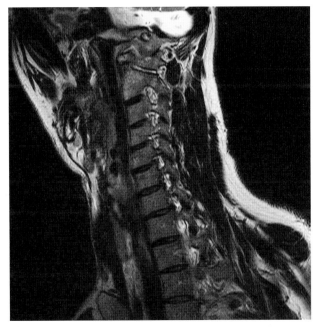

▲ **Fig. 8.55** An oblique sagittal T2-weighted image obtained with approximately 20° of obliquity clearly demonstrates the nerve roots in cross-section surrounded by perineural fat within the neural exit foramina. No foraminal compromise is present. Oblique images are also valuable for the examination of the exit foramina, pedicles and lateral masses.

Assessment of spinal structures for evidence of injury

As always, it is important to have a routine for film review so that care is taken to inspect each anatomical component in turn and no structure is overlooked. All images should be reviewed.

Interpretation of cervical spine injuries begins with assessment of the cord, looking for changes such as swelling (see Fig. 8.56), haemorrhage or compression (see Fig. 8.57). The epidural space is then examined to identify encroachment by bone, disc herniation (see Figs 8.58 and 8.59) or epidural haematoma (see Fig. 8.60). The ligamentous structures are examined to assess their integrity. Normal ligaments are hypointense structures, and the anterior and posterior longitudinal ligaments, the ligamentum flavum, and the interspinous and supraspinous ligaments should be examined in turn (see Fig. 8.61). Bony structures of the spinal column are assessed for vertebral body and posterior element fractures or subluxations and oedema related to contusion or overuse (see Fig. 8.62).

Vertebral artery occlusion may be associated with injuries that involve the lateral masses (see Figs 8.63 and 8.64) and cause vertebral artery dissection or tearing.

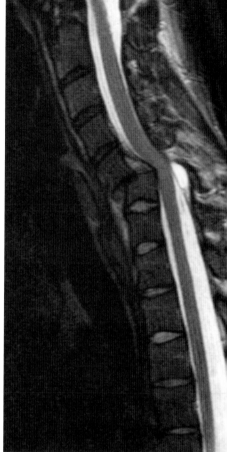

▲ **Fig. 8.57** A sagittal fat-suppressed T2-weighted MR image demonstrates gross injury to the cervical spine, following a violent hyperflexion force. There is a Grade II–III subluxation at the C5/6 level causing marked compression and distortion of the cord. Mild cord oedema is demonstrated on this sequence. High signal posteriorly indicates injury to the posterior ligament complex including injury to the ligamentum flavum. Haemorrhage extends along the anterior aspect of C2 to C4 and a collection is seen anterior to C6 and C7.

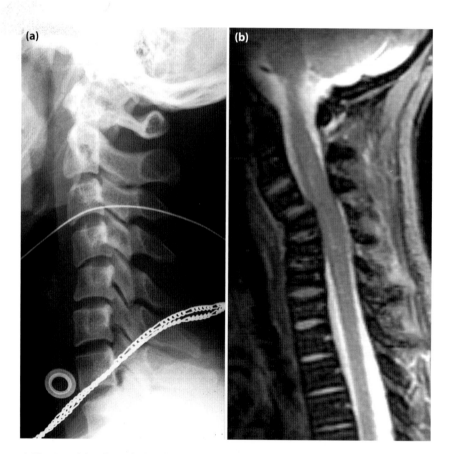

▲ **Fig. 8.56(a)** A lateral plain film demonstrates flexion deformity at the C4/5 level with widening of the disc space posteriorly and separation of the spinous processes, indicating disruption of the posterior ligament complex. **(b)** A sagittal STIR image of a different patient demonstrates changes of a hyperextension injury, with rupture of the posterior longitudinal ligament at the C3/4 level and a small step in the anterior margin of C4, which has resulted from a compression fracture. The cord is diffusely swollen and minor hyperintense signal in the cord at the C5/6 level indicates cord injury. The posterior ligamentous changes are not well demonstrated on this image.

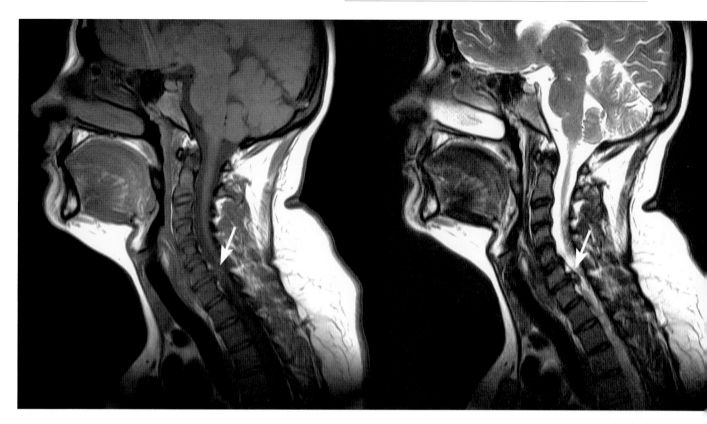

▲ **Fig. 8.58** Sagittal T1- and T2-weighted MR images demonstrate an acute disc herniation at the C6/7 level (arrows). Considerable elevation of the posterior longitudinal ligament is apparent, most obvious on the T2 image.

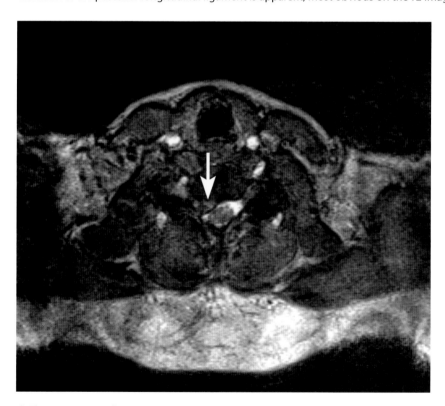

▲ **Fig. 8.59** An axial T2 image shows the disc protrusion of Fig. 8.58 producing right lateral spinal recess stenosis (arrow).

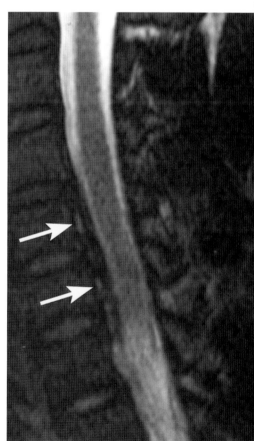

▶ **Fig. 8.60** With a T2* GRE sequence, blood-degradation products may produce hypointense signal. In this case an epidural haematoma is demonstrated, expanding the epidural space and compressing the cord (arrows).

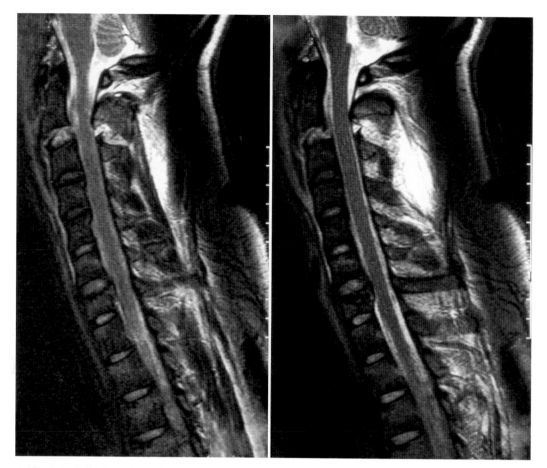

▲ **Fig. 8.61** Following a hyperflexion injury, sagittal fat-suppressed T2-weighted MR images demonstrate disruption of the C2/3 disc space, with rupture of the anterior and posterior longitudinal ligaments at this level. There is high signal posteriorly, indicating extensive injury to the posterior ligament complex and disruption of the ligamentum flavum at C2/3. No cord injury can be seen. Note the large haematoma anterior to the upper cervical spine, extending to the base of the skull. There has also been injury to the C7 vertebral body, with buckling of its anterior and posterior margins and abnormal signal in the vertebral body and neighbouring C6/7 disc.

▼ **Fig. 8.62(a)** This patient dived into shallow water, causing a flexion injury to the spine and a rotational component to the force, producing a unilateral facet joint fracture/dislocation. A sagittal T2-weighted MR image demonstrates buckling of the anterior margin of C5 secondary to compression and flexion, and there is slight compression of the inferior endplate of C6. There is rupture of the interspinous ligament in the upper cervical region. No cord injury can be seen. **(b)** The importance of examining the spine completely from one side to the other is illustrated here, in the same case as **(a)**. Another sagittal image, obtained through the right-sided facets, demonstrates a 'perched' dislocation of the C4/5 facet joint. The articular facet of C4 is indicated by the white arrowhead and the C5 articular surface by the black arrowhead. Obviously, the articular surfaces should appose.

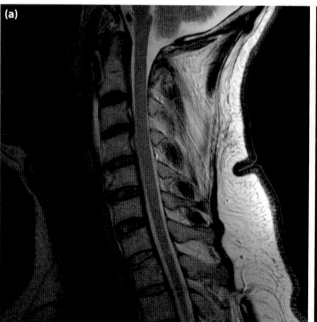

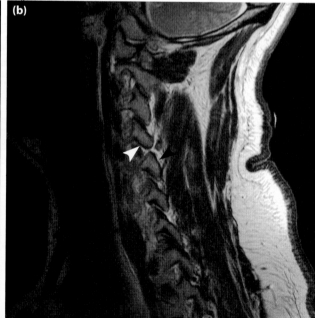

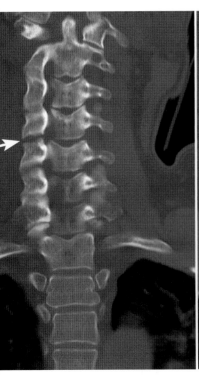
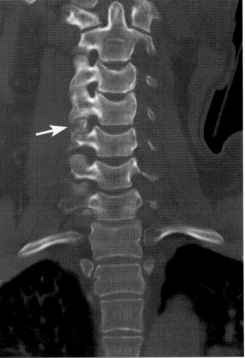
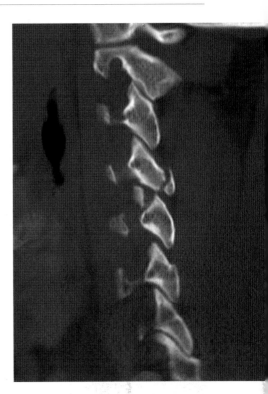

▲ **Fig. 8.63(a)** Further imaging from the case in Fig. 8.62(b) included CT to provide more precise bony detail of the facet injury. Multislice CT technology enables reformatted images of high quality in any plane and, in this case, reformatted coronal images clearly demonstrate the fracture/dislocation of the right C4/5 facet joint (arrows).

▲ **(b)** A reformatted sagittal CT image through the right-sided facet joints in the same case again demonstrates the 'perched' fracture/dislocation of the C4/5 facet.

▼ **Fig. 8.64** A magnetic resonance angiogram (MRA) acquired in the same case as Figs 8.62 and 8.63 demonstrates a complete occlusion of the right vertebral artery secondary to the C4/5 facet fracture/dislocation. A formal angiogram showed some retrograde filling into the upper end of the right vertebral artery from the basilar artery and it was noted that the right vertebral artery was considerably smaller than the left. Nevertheless, a small cerebellar infarct followed the occlusion of the vertebral artery. It remained uncertain whether there had been a dissection or extrinsic mechanical compression of the artery.

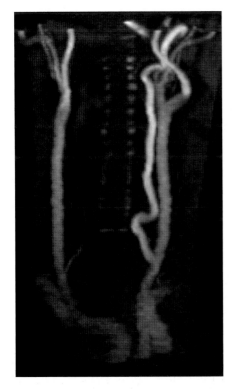

Cervical spine trauma

Sports-related injury to the cervical spine is usually the result of hyperflexion, hyperextension or axial compression. Injury biomechanics are rarely pure and the forces involved are usually a combination of the above with the addition of rotation. Torg et al. (1991) identified axial loading as the one element that was invariably common to all severe cervical spine injuries. The natural cervical lordosis helps to dissipate axial load in the cervical spine. If the spine is flexed, the ability of the spine to dissipate the energy of a sudden axial load is significantly reduced and a fracture may result. These fractures occur most often at the C4, C5 and C6 levels (Torg 1985). Factors that influence the severity and type of injury pattern include the direction and intensity of the force involved and the position of the neck at the time of injury.

Commonly missed fractures of the cervical spine are listed in Table 8.1.

Table 8.1 Easily missed fractures of the cervical spine

1. Wedge compression fractures
2. Clayshoveler's fractures
3. Teardrop fractures
4. Hangman's fractures
5. Odontoid process fractures

Cervical hyperflexion injuries

Cervical hyperflexion injuries with involvement of the posterior ligament complex and anterior subluxation

Cervical hyperflexion may injure the posterior ligament complex, which includes the interspinous ligament, facet joint capsules, ligamentum flavum and the posterior longitudinal ligament. These injuries may result in corresponding changes on plain films (see Figs 8.65 and 8.66), CT or MRI. These changes may include:

- injury to the posterior ligament complex, which allows anterior subluxation of the vertebra above and produces a step in posterior vertebral body alignment
- an angular kyphosis at the involved level with an abrupt alignment change due to widening of the posterior intervertebral disc space
- interruption of the spinolaminar line, due to anterior subluxation of the upper vertebra
- widening of the distance between the spinous processes at the level of injury
- loss of facet joint congruity, with partial or complete uncovering of the facet articular surface, in cases of facet subluxation (see Fig. 8.67).

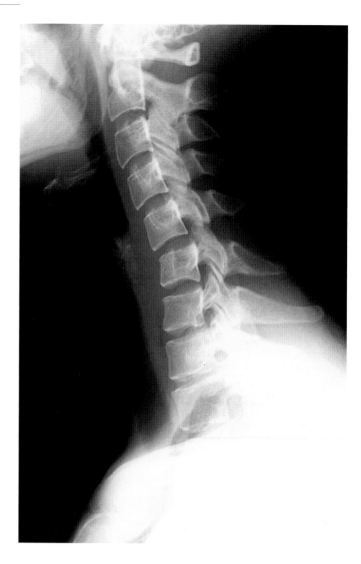

▶ **Fig. 8.65** A lateral plain film shows anterior movement of C5 on C6 with subluxation of the facets, moderate hyperkyphotic angulation and widening of both the interspinous distance and the posterior aspect of the C5/6 disc space.

▼ **Fig. 8.66** Widening of the interspinous space is a valuable plain film sign of subluxation (arrows). In this case, there is a subluxation at C7/T1.

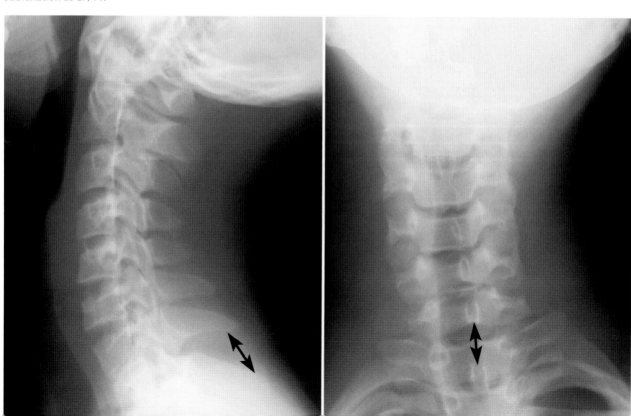

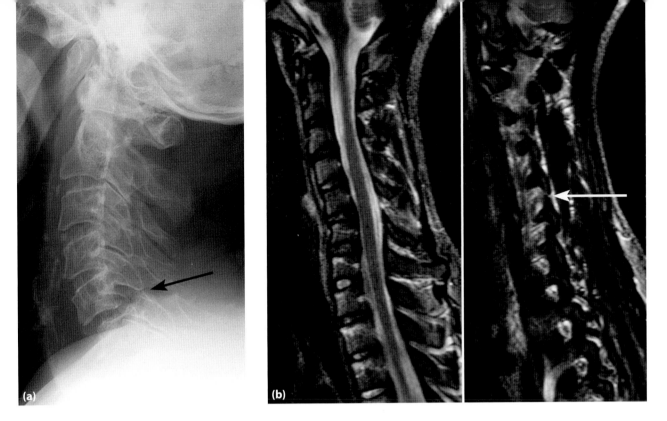

▲ **Fig. 8.67(a)** There is a unilateral facet dislocation at the C5/6 level with 'perched' facets (arrow). No fracture can be seen.
(b) Sagittal fat-suppressed T2-weighted MR images in the same patient as in **(a)** shows the C5/6 subluxation with perched facets (arrow). There is disruption of the ligamentum flavum, but an intact posterior longitudinal ligament. There is marrow oedema in several lower cervical and upper thoracic vertebral bodies consistent with bony contusions and/or occult incomplete fractures.

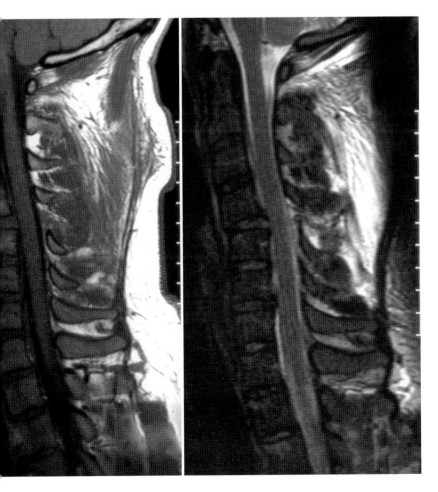

An angular kyphosis alone is non-specific, and may result from degenerative disease, patient positioning or muscle spasm. The essential diagnostic radiographic feature of this injury is facet joint subluxation. The probability of delayed instability resulting from this injury increases with the degree of ligamentous disruption, which is inferred by the degree of angular kyphosis and anterior vertebral body displacement. When the radiographic appearances on standard views are suspicious but not diagnostic, subluxation will usually be more definite on a flexion view. As previously stressed, this should only be performed under supervision, unaided and never beyond the limits of pain. MRI can also be helpful in showing disruption of the posterior ligaments in the acute injury setting (see Fig. 8.68).

◀ **Fig. 8.68** Sagittal T1- and fat-suppressed T2-weighted MR images demonstrate a typical flexion injury at the C4/5 level. A subluxation is present with slight forward shift of C4 on C5. There is rupture of the posterior longitudinal ligament and the ligamentum flavum. Widening of the space between the C4 and C5 spinous processes indicates injury to the facet joints at this level.

Vertebral body wedge compression fractures

Wedge compression fractures can occur with or without anterior subluxation (see Fig. 8.69). An isolated fracture of the vertebral body is stable. However, most hyperflexion injuries have associated posterior ligament complex disruption and instability may be present. This is especially so when a 'teardrop' fracture configuration is evident (see Fig. 8.70). The involved vertebral body shows loss of anterior height and a fracture step or angulation of cortex may be seen at the endplates or anterior cortical margin.

Clayshoveler's fractures

Clayshoveler's fracture is an avulsion fracture of a spinous process at the site of interspinous ligament insertion, and usually involves the lower cervical spine or T1 but with sparing of the spinal canal. This fracture may also result from forceful contraction of the trapezius or rhomboid muscles and has been reported in American football players (Nuber and Schafer 1987) and power lifters (Herrick 1981). The injury is stable when occurring in isolation (see Fig. 8.71).

Flexion teardrop fractures

Flexion injury may produce an oblique fracture through the anteroinferior vertebral body that results in a 'teardrop' fragment (see Fig. 8.72). This is a serious and unstable injury that is usually associated with spinal cord injury. The spine above the fracture level lies in flexion and previously described signs of posterior vertebral soft-tissue and ligament injury are present (see Fig. 8.73). Less commonly, it should also be noted that teardrop fractures can occur with either hyperextension or axial loading (Torg et al. 1991).

Bifacet dislocation

Bifacet dislocation is a severe hyperflexion injury with complete rupture of the posterior ligament complex, together with rupture of the intervertebral disc and anterior longitudinal ligament. The dislocation may be complete, with an anterior displacement of more than half the AP diameter of the vertebral body, or incomplete where anterior displacement is less than half the AP diameter of the vertebral body (see Fig. 8.74). The injury is unstable and is usually associated with spinal cord injury. The facets may become locked if they completely lose opposition and overlap. Perched facets occur when the apices of the upper and lower articular processes are directly opposed (see Figs 8.75 and 8.76). An MRI examination is mandatory before attempting reduction of a facet dislocation. If there is a haematoma associated with the dislocation, cord injury may result from the reduction.

▶ **Fig. 8.70** A lateral plain film shows a teardrop fracture of C6 and widening of the space between the C5 and C6 spinous processes indicates disruption of the posterior ligament complex.

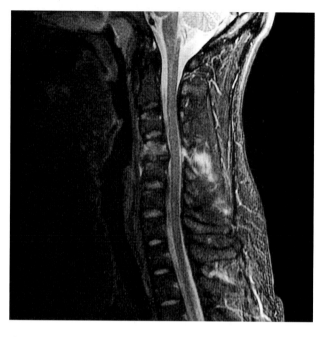

▲ **Fig. 8.69** An acute compression fracture of C4 is demonstrated on a fat-suppressed sagittal T2-weighted MR image, with marrow oedema throughout the vertebral body. Minor burst deformity is noted with slight retropulsion of the posteroinferior corner of the vertebral body. There is bulging of the anterior wall and a 'teardrop' fragment may be present, with involvement of the inferior endplate also noted. High signal posteriorly indicates disruption of the posterior ligament complex and rupture of the ligamentum flavum.

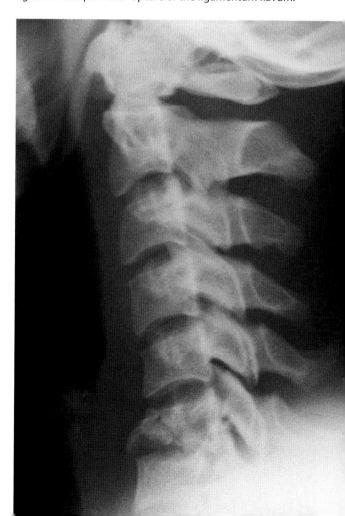

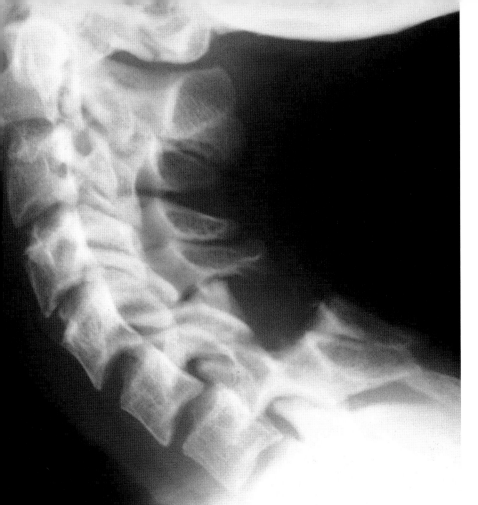

◀**Fig. 8.71** Clayshoveler's fracture is produced by traction of the interspinous ligament causing an avulsion fracture of a lower cervical spinous process. This fracture is stable, and the spinal canal is not involved.

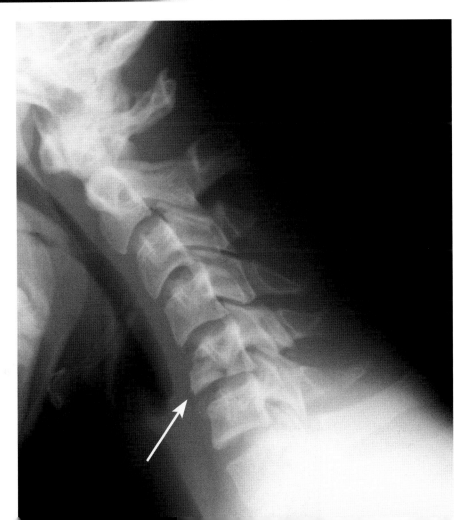

◀**Fig. 8.72** This is a typical plain film image of a flexion teardrop fracture. There is compression, wedge deformity and separation of an anteroinferior fragment (arrow). Disruption of the facet joints at this level is also noted.

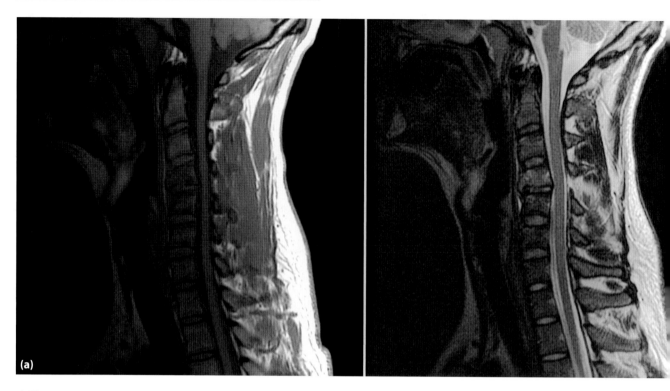

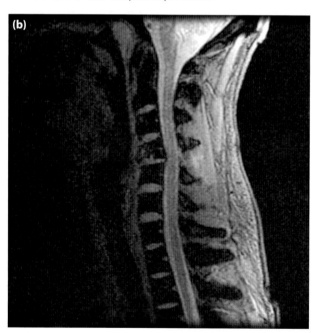

▲ **Fig. 8.73(a)** A teardrop fracture is an unstable fracture and is often associated with cord injury. T1- and T2-weighted MR images demonstrate wedge deformity of C4 with high signal in the vertebral body and 'teardrop' deformity at the anteroinferior corner. There are also fractures of the inferior endplates of C5 and C6. High signal posteriorly indicates trauma to the posterior ligament complex. No cord injury is evident.

▼**(b)** A T2*-weighted GRE image of the same case as **(a)** confirms the teardrop fracture of C4 and also shows a fracture of the C4 spinous process, with widening of the distance between the C4 and C5 spinous processes.

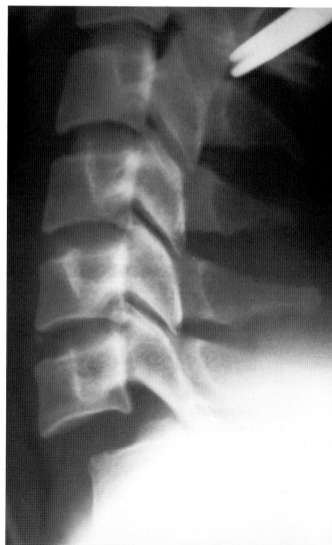

▶**Fig. 8.74** There is a complete dislocation at C6/7, with the facets of C6 having passed over the C7 facets into a 'locked' position.

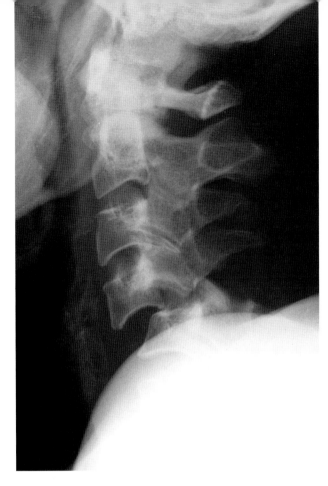

▲ **Fig. 8.75** A plain film shows bilateral facet dislocation at the C4/5 level. The facets are 'locked'.

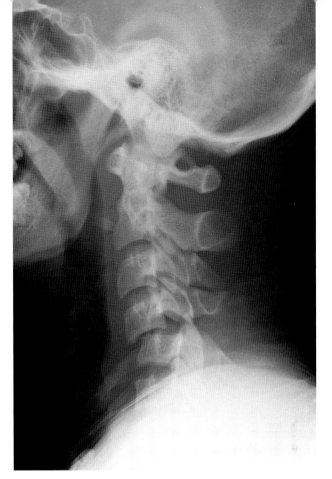

▲ **Fig. 8.76** 'Perched' facets are demonstrated at the C4/5 level with associated marked flexion deformity.

Unifacet dislocation

Unifacet dislocation results from a combination of hyper-flexion and rotation. This force causes the superior facet of the involved joint to pass anterior to the inferior facet while rotating towards the contralateral side. In a complete disloca-tion, there is locking of the superior facet of the joint within the exit foramen anterior to the inferior facet. The rotational component of this injury is a diagnostic feature. The spine below the level of injury is seen in a true lateral projection and the spine above will appear to lie in an oblique projection (see Fig. 8.77). The transition is abrupt and, unlike positional rotation, the bare facets of the dislocated joint can usually be seen. This injury is stable unless associated with a significant fracture. CT is helpful in confirming the diagnosis in uncer-tain cases and in detecting any associated fractures that are frequently occult on plain films.

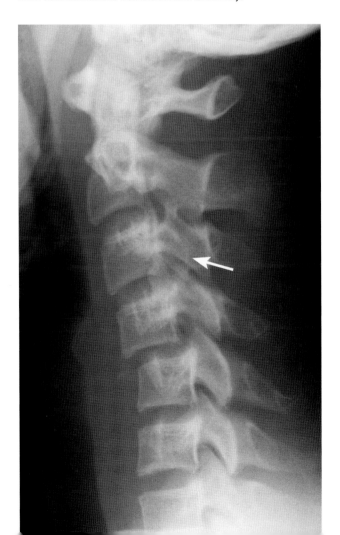

▶ **Fig. 8.77** There is unifacet subluxation at C4/5 with an angular kyphosis present at this level, together with a step in vertebral body alignment. At first glance the facets appear normally paired. However, above the C4/5 level, the facets on one side are stepped forward (arrow), indicating rotation of the spine above C4/5. In this case, the uncovered articular surfaces are obscured by superimposition. Note mild widening of the posterior interspinous space and a step in spinolaminar alignment at C4/5.

▶ **Fig. 8.78** A combination of axial and extension forces may produce a fracture of the posterior arch of the atlas (arrow), due to compression between the occiput and the usually sizable spinous process of the axis.

Cervical hyperextension injuries

Cervical hyperextension injuries are usually serious and commonly involve the upper cervical spine. They include fractures of the posterior arch of the atlas, extension sprain injuries, extension teardrop fractures, Hangman's fractures, odontoid process fractures and rotary atlantoaxial subluxation.

Fractures of the posterior arch of the atlas

When the head is hyperextended, the posterior arch of C1 is compressed between the occiput and the spinous process of C2, producing a fracture of the posterior arch of C1. The transverse ligament and the anterior arch are not involved, differentiating this fracture from a Jefferson fracture (see Fig. 8.78).

Extension sprain injuries

Extension injury to the cervical spine may result in soft-tissue injury only. An extension force may result in injury to the anterior longitudinal ligament without an avulsion teardrop-type fracture. Contusion injuries occur posteriorly (see Fig. 8.79).

Extension teardrop fractures

An extension teardrop fracture is an avulsion fracture, occurring when hyperextension of the cervical spine causes the anterior longitudinal ligament to avulse a fragment of bone from the anteroinferior corner of a vertebral body (see Fig. 8.80). This tends to occur in the lower cervical spine and associated buckling of the ligamentum flavum commonly causes cord injury.

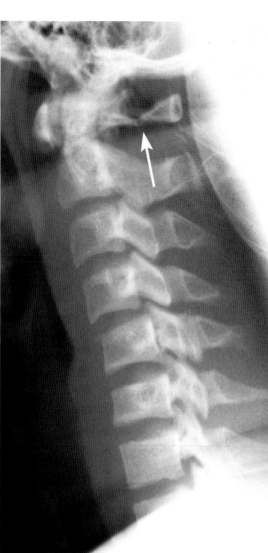

▶ **Fig. 8.79** Sagittal T1- and fat-suppressed T2-weighted MR images demonstrate an extension deformity at the C5/6 level. There has been rupture of the anterior longitudinal ligament at C5/6 and acute traumatic disc disruption with a posterior disc extrusion causing elevation of the posterior longitudinal ligament. The T2-weighted image shows buckling of the ligamentum flavum opposite the disc protrusion, adding considerable compression of the cord.

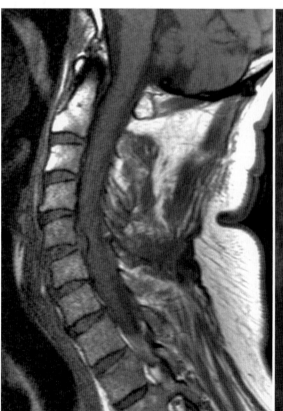

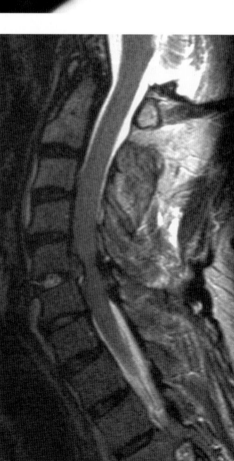

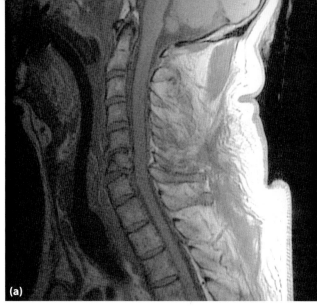
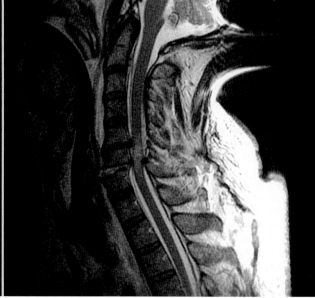

(a)

(b)

▲▶ **Fig. 8.80** An extension teardrop fracture is unstable and commonly associated with cord injury.

(a) T1- and T2-weighted MR images demonstrate an extension injury with a teardrop fracture fragment avulsed from the anteroinferior corner of the C6 vertebral body by the anterior longitudinal ligament. The anterior longitudinal ligament and the C6/7 disc have ruptured, with angular lordosis and retrolisthesis deforming the alignment. Mixed signal is present in the cord (Type III cord injury) and buckling of the ligamentum flavum would have probably contributed to cord damage. There is disruption of spinolaminar alignment and haemorrhage is present anteriorly.

(b) A corresponding STIR image shows a large soft-tissue haematoma posteriorly.

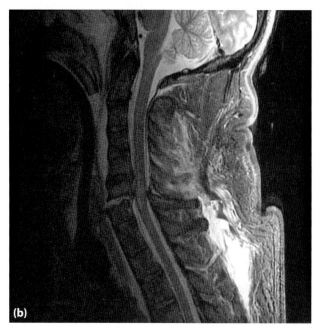

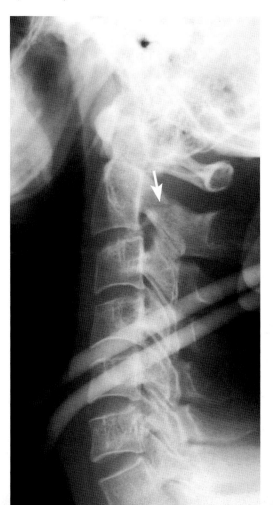

Hangman's fractures

Hangman's fracture results from an extension injury to the cervical spine, producing a traumatic spondylolisthesis of C2. Neurological injury does not usually occur unless there is involvement of the C2/3 facets. Effendi et al. (1981) described three types of injuries:

1. *Type I:* Hangman's fracture that involves the pars interarticularis of C2 and demonstrates less than 3 mm of displacement (see Fig. 8.81)
2. *Type II:* Hangman's fracture that demonstrates more than 3 mm of displacement and angulation; the fracture may involve the pars interarticularis, the pedicle or the body of C2 in the coronal plane (see Figs 8.82 and 8.83)
3. *Type III:* Hangman's fracture that involves the C2/3 facets, often with subluxation or bilateral dislocations (see Fig. 8.84).

◀ **Fig. 8.81** A Type I Hangman's fracture is an extension injury to the pars interarticularis of C2 (arrow).

▶ **Fig. 8.82** This is a displaced and angulated Type II Hangman's fracture, involving the junction of the vertebral body and pedicles of C2 (arrow).

Odontoid process fractures

Odontoid process fractures may result from either hyper-flexion or hyperextension injuries. Hyperflexion injuries cause the odontoid process to be displaced anteriorly. A hyperextension injury, such as a fall onto the forehead, may also cause an odontoid fracture in which the process is displaced posteriorly. Odontoid process fractures have recently been reclassified (Harris and Mirvis 1996) as either high or low:

- *High fractures* involve the dens (odontoid process) and were previously known as Type I and Type II fractures. They are almost invariably transverse or oblique disruptions through the base or lower portion of the dens with variable displacement (see Figs 8.85 and 8.86), and result in atlantoaxial instability until the fracture unites. The fracture may be very difficult to detect on a lateral film and careful attention to the dens and the anterior soft tissues is required. As previously discussed, the Mach effect may occasionally be mistaken for a fracture on plain films. An os odontoideum is now thought to be post-traumatic rather than developmental in origin (see Figs 8.87 and 8.88).

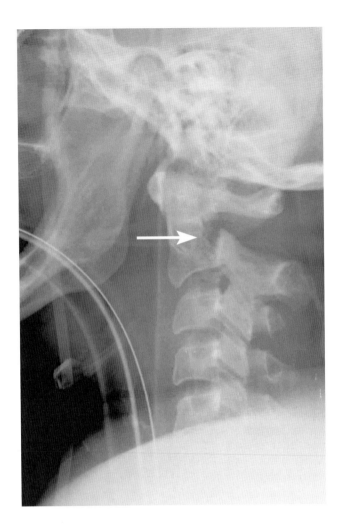

▼ **Fig. 8.83(a)** and **(b)** When there is angulation or 3 mm or more of displacement, the Hangman's fracture is classified as Type II (arrow).

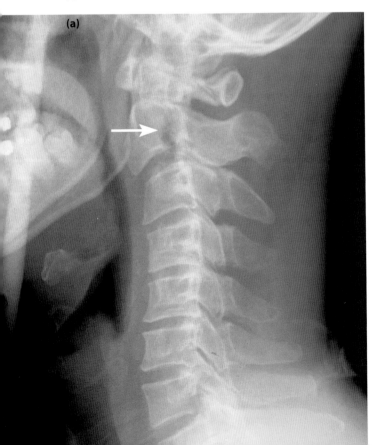

(a)

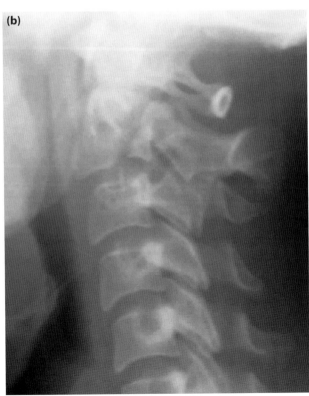

(b)

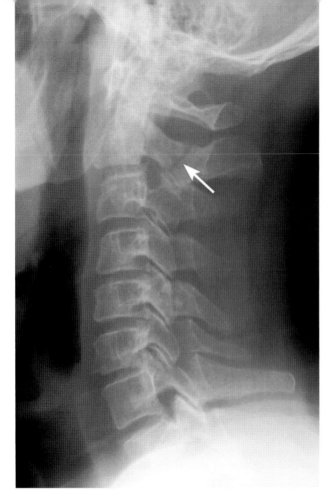

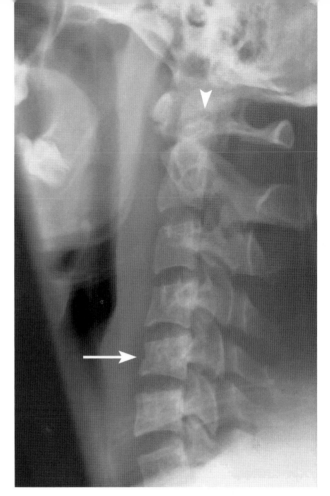

▲ **Fig. 8.84** This is a Type III Hangman's fracture where the C2/3 facet joints are involved (arrow). Although there is joint involvement, no subluxation or dislocation has occurred.

▲ **Fig. 8.85** There has been a fracture of the odontoid process (arrowhead) and the anterior arch of the atlas. The anterior atlanto-odontoid interval is widened, indicating injury to the transverse and alar ligaments. A large associated prevertebral haematoma is noted. There has also been a fracture of the C5 vertebral body with buckling of its anterior cortex (arrow).

- *Low fractures* involve the body of C2 and were previously known as Type III fractures. An example of a low fracture was shown in Fig. 8.29(b) and (c).

The distance between the posterior margin of the anterior arch of C1 and the anterior margin of the dens is normally 3 mm or less in adults (Harris and Mirvis 1996). This anterior atlantoaxial interval may be widened by either a dens fracture with posterior subluxation of the atlas or following an isolated rupture of the transverse ligament. The transverse ligament is generally ruptured with a low fracture but remains intact with a high fracture.

Rotary atlantoaxial subluxation

Rotary atlantoaxial subluxation is a common cause of torticollis in children and teenagers. It occurs when there is a fixed rotary subluxation of the atlas on the axis and rotary movement at this level becomes limited. The cause is unknown but an association with trauma and many other conditions, such as an upper respiratory infection or post head and neck surgery (Fielding and Hawkins 1977), is recognised.

▶ **Fig. 8.86** A fracture involves the base of the odontoid. There is posterior displacement of the odontoid and atlas together. The anterior atlantoaxial joint appears to be intact. It is likely that the fracture was the result of an extension injury.

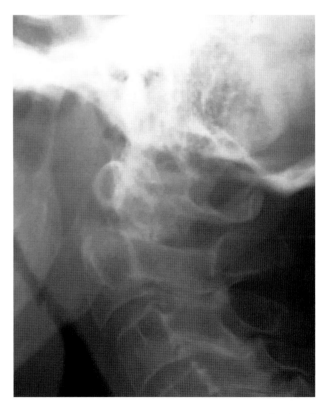

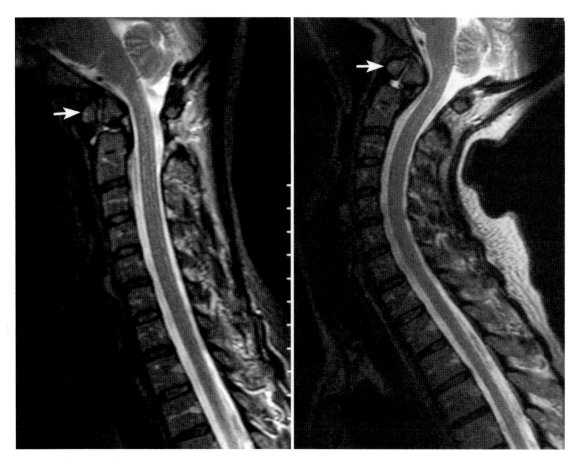

▲ **Fig. 8.87** Sagittal T2-weighted images have been acquired in flexion and extension. A non-acute non-united fracture of the odontoid is demonstrated (arrows). The odontoid fragment and atlas move dorsally together in extension, indicating disruption of the lateral atlantoaxial joints, but the anterior atlantoaxial joint appears intact.

▼ **Fig. 8.88** Flexion and extension views demonstrate instability at the atlantoaxial level due to a ununited fracture of the odontoid process. The atlas and odontoid fragment move together and displace dorsally with extension. This indicates that the anterior atlantoaxial joint is intact; subluxation of the lateral atlantoaxial joints occurs in extension.

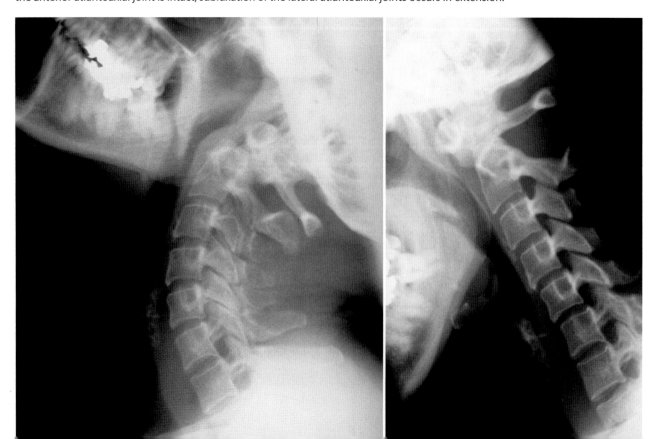

Plain films show asymmetry at the atlantoaxial joint with the odontoid sitting closer to one lateral mass than the other. Plain film diagnosis is technically difficult if a torticollis is present and the asymmetry is often produced by patient positioning.

CT examination is therefore necessary before a diagnosis can be made. Axial images are obtained with the head in maximal rotation, first one way and then the other, to demonstrate limitation in rotation. Rotation of C1 on C2 should be demonstrated before a diagnosis can be made (see Figs 8.89, 8.90 and 8.91).

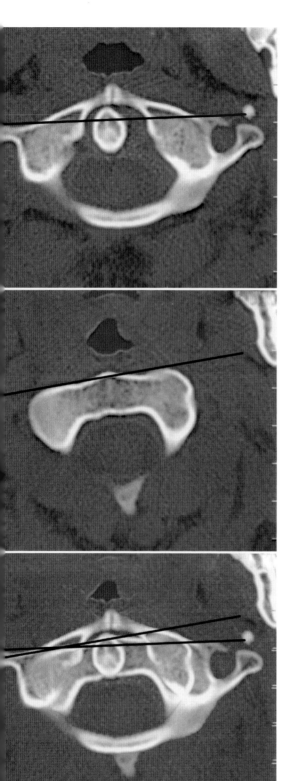

▲ **Fig. 8.89** An initial CT image of the atlas shows rotation and considerable asymmetry of the odontoid when compared with the lateral masses of the atlas (top image). An image through the body of the axis (centre image) has been superimposed on the top image to demonstrate more clearly the degree of rotation of the atlas on the axis (bottom image).

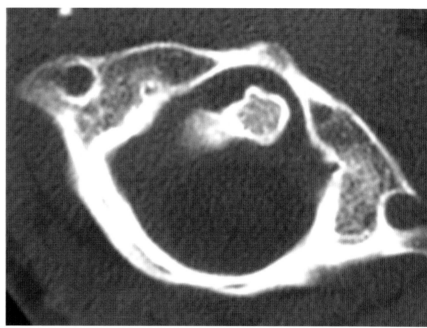

▲ **Fig. 8.90(a)** An axial CT image shows disruption of the normal atlanto-odontal relationship, with rotation and tilting of the atlas on the axis.

▼ **(b)** A reconstructed 3D image of the same case reveals an additional component of the lateral tilt to the atlas and helps to better understand the marked deformity present.

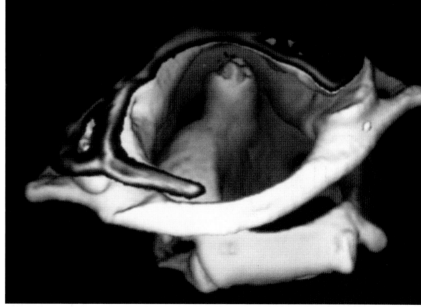

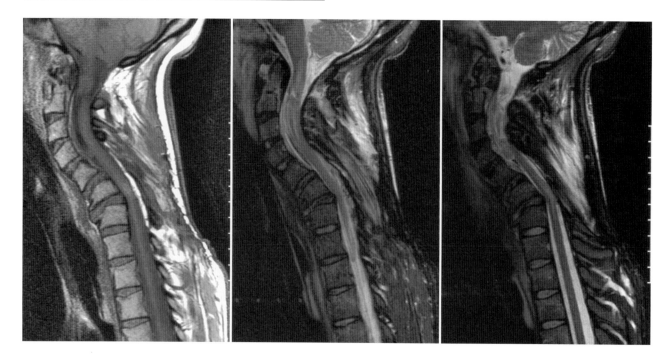

▲ **Fig. 8.91** A fracture of the odontoid process has produced a Kulkarni Type I spinal cord contusion injury and transection of the cord at the C2 level. Sagittal T1- and T2-weighted FSE images demonstrate a dens fracture with associated anterior and posterior soft-tissue swelling and haematoma. The cord shows patchy alteration of signal on the T1 image and central low signal with thick irregular surrounding high signal on the T2 image. There has been a previous teardrop-type compression fracture of C6 with subluxation, and C4, C5 and C6 cervical laminectomies are noted with kyphotic alignment of the spine at these levels. There is cord hyperintensity at the kyphotic C6/7 level.

Spinal cord injuries

Spinal cord injuries secondary to trauma are categorised as concussive, contusional or compressive (Benedetti 1996). Concussive injuries are transient and thought to be related to a brief deficiency of cord microcirculation (Dohrman et al. 1971). There are usually no abnormal imaging findings on MRI examination. Contusional injuries to the cord range from simple oedema to petechial haemorrhage and more severe haemorrhage that may result in liquefactive necrosis and cord disruption. Compressive injuries may occur due to a predisposing congenital stenosis, or in a normally developed spinal canal as the result of acute or chronic injury. Congenital and acquired spinal stenoses are discussed later in the chapter.

Kulkarni et al. (1987) described three MRI patterns of spinal cord injury that correlate to degrees of cord injury:

1. In a *Type I injury* (see Fig. 8.91), haemorrhage appears as inhomogeneous signal on a T1-weighted image and a central area of hypointensity on T2-weighting, with a thin rim of peripheral iso to hyperintensity.

2. The presence of oedema produces a *Type II injury*, which shows normal signal on T1-weighting and high signal on T2 in the area of injury (see Figs 8.92 and 8.93).

3. There is a mixture of blood and oedema in a *Type III injury*, which shows normal signal on a T1-weighted image and thick areas of mixed peripheral high signal and central low signal with T2-weighting (see Fig. 8.93).

Long-term follow-up studies performed on patients with these patterns revealed a better prognosis with a Type II pattern compared to patients with a Type I or mixed Type III pattern (Flanders et al. 1990).

Post-traumatic syrinx formation

A syrinx forms when CSF develops an expanded central cavity within the cord (see Fig. 8.94). A syrinx will form in 1–3% of patients after spinal injury (Williams 1979). Syrinx formation is twice as common in the thoracic spine as in the cervical spine. The syrinx can appear months or years after spinal trauma. Over time, a syrinx may elongate and destroy the centre of the cord (see Fig. 8.95).

Cervical spinal stenosis

The presence of spinal canal stenosis renders the athlete more vulnerable to neuropraxia of the cervical cord, producing a transient quadriplegia (Torg et al. 1986). Narrowing of the cervical canal may be developmental or acquired (Torg et al. 1996). A combination of a narrowed cervical canal and reduction of the normal cervical lordosis places the athlete at a significantly higher risk of cord injury. Torg et al. (1993) identified this sub-population from his review of the American National Football Head and Neck Injury Registry and termed this combination of radiographic findings as 'spear tackler's' spine (see Fig. 8.96).

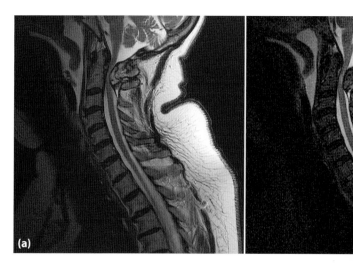

▲▶ **Fig. 8.92** A previous severe axial force had fractured the posterior arches of both atlas and axis. Healing produced hypertrophic bony callus, which progressively expanded and compressed the spinal cord at the level of the axis. The patient developed a progressive quadriparesis.
(a) Sagittal T2-weighted and STIR images demonstrate the cord compression caused by expanding new bone. Hyperintense signal in the cord is best demonstrated on the STIR sequence.
(b) An axial T2-weighted MR image demonstrates the extraordinary degree of cord compression (arrows), with accompanying signal changes.

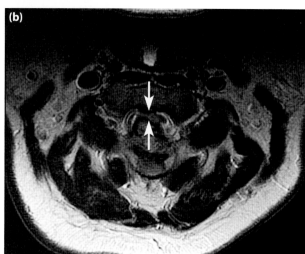

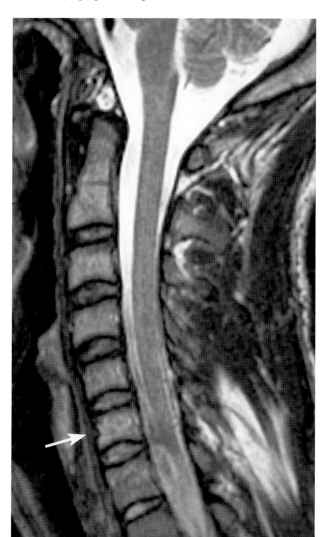

◀ **Fig. 8.93** A sagittal T2-weighted MR image shows that there has been a hyperflexion injury with compression of C6 producing buckling of its anterior margin (arrow). A subluxation has almost certainly occurred but has reduced. Alignment is now normal, but there is evidence of cord injury, with fusiform cord swelling and mixed signal abnormality. High signal posteriorly indicates that there is oedema associated with injury to the posterior structures at this level.

'Burners' and 'stingers' secondary to brachial plexus stretch or cervical nerve root neuropraxia are more prevalent in athletes with a narrowed cervical canal, whether developmental or acquired. In a study of 55 American football players with chronic burner syndrome, 53% had developmentally narrowed cervical canals and 93% had disc disease or narrowing of the intervertebral foramina (Levitz et al. 1997).

There are two types of canal stenosis: congenital canal stenosis and 'functional' or acquired canal stenosis.

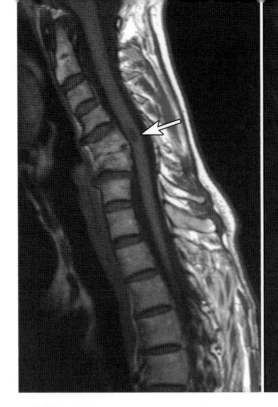

▶ **Fig. 8.94** Sagittal T1- and T2-weighted MR images show evidence of an old flexion injury at the C5/6 level. There has been fusion across the C5/6 disc space, with a kyphotic deformity persisting. Old fractures of C4 and C7 are also noted. Fluid is now present in the cord at the level of the previous C5 fracture and syrinx formation is occurring (arrow).

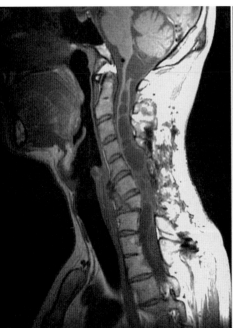
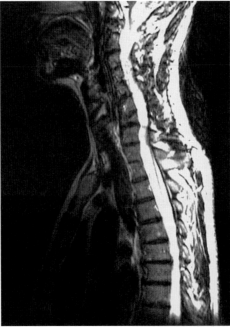

◀ **Fig. 8.95** Sagittal T1- and T2-weighted MR images demonstrate advanced post-traumatic syringomyelia with destruction of the centre of the cord in a Paralympian attending the 2000 Sydney Paralympics. An old flexion injury is noted at the T7/T1 level. Note the gross wasting of the neck muscles. Minimal cord tissue can be seen on the T2-weighted image.

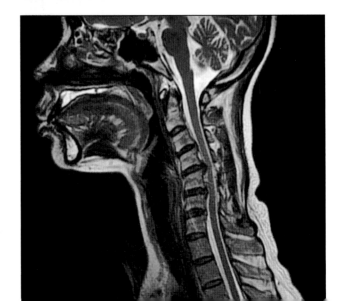

▶ **Fig. 8.96** This is an example of 'spear tackler's' spine. A sagittal T2-weighted image demonstrates reversal of the normal cervical lordosis. There are wedge deformities of C4, C5 and C6 due to previous injury and generalised disc dehydration. Disc protrusions at C4/5 and C5/6 cause further narrowing of a developmentally narrowed segment that extends from C3 to C7.

Congenital canal stenosis

Congenital canal stenosis is due to a narrowing of the AP diameter of the cervical spinal canal (see Fig. 8.97). The normal bony canal diameter on standard lateral films at the C4–C6 levels is approximately 18.5 mm. Severe stenosis is denoted by measurements of 13 mm or less (see Fig. 8.98). Torg et al. (1991) recommend that athletes with a canal measurement of 14 mm or less at any level (C3–C6) be advised against participating in contact sports. The ratio method of canal stenosis provides an assessment of canal stenosis that is unaffected by errors produced by magnification. The normal ratio of the canal diameter to the vertebral body diameter (at the same level) is approximately 1:1. A cut-off value of 0:82 was thought to be sensitive and specific in diagnosing congenital canal stenosis (Pavlov et al. 1987). The ratio, however, has a low positive predictive value, which precludes its use as a screening test (Torg et al. 1996).

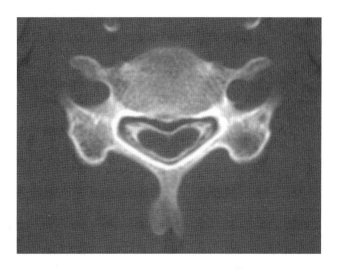

▲ **Fig. 8.97** An axial CT image shows underlying congenital canal stenosis with a reduced AP canal diameter.

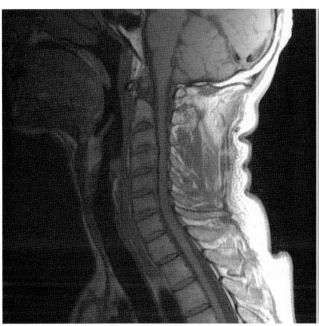

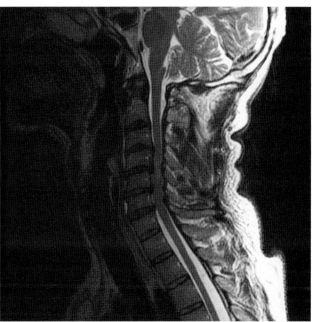

▲ **Fig. 8.98(a)** Sagittal T1- and T2-weighted MR images demonstrate a congenital canal stenosis from C2 to C6.
▶ **(b)** An axial T2-weighted MR image shows a corresponding reduction in the AP diameter of the spinal canal.

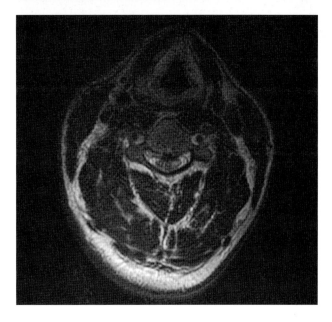

Herzog et al. (1991) showed that the Torg/Pavlov ratio produced a considerable number of false positive results. On reviewing CT scans of footballers, Herzog found that 70% had an abnormal ratio, although their cervical canals were of normal diameter. It was concluded that footballers often had large vertebral bodies and that there was no correlation between a Torg/Pavlov ratio of 0:8 and transient neuropraxia or permanent neurological deficit.

This method assesses bony narrowing only, and CT scanning or MRI is required to demonstrate the presence of a 'functional' stenosis, which assesses the available space in the CSF component of the spinal canal.

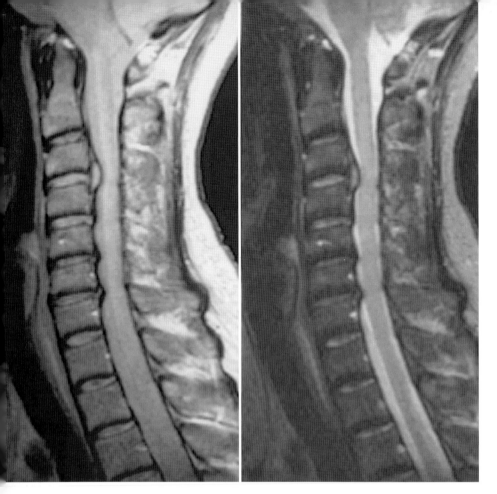

▲ **Fig. 8.99** 'Functional' stenosis is further complicated by a prominent C3/4 disc protrusion that has occurred on a background of congenital canal stenosis. Sagittal fat-suppressed T1- and T2-weighted MR images show a congenital stenosis extending from C3 to the C7 level, which is further complicated by small disc protrusions at C5/6 and C6/7. The recent C3/4 disc protrusion has produced additional cord displacement and compression.

'Functional' or acquired canal stenosis

In 1998, Cantu advocated the 'functional' definition of spinal stenosis. Functional spinal stenosis is present when the size of the canal is so small at any level that the CSF around the cord is obliterated, or the cord is deformed as shown by CT or MRI (see Fig. 8.99). Cantu suggests that any athlete with functional stenosis is at risk of quadriplegia and should not participate in contact sports. Functional canal stenosis is often produced by soft-tissue changes such as disc protrusions or buckling of ligaments. In these cases, the bony spinal canal may appear normal on plain films. Posterior protrusion of an intervertebral disc or osteophyte formation can cause significant canal narrowing, and impaction of the cord against these structures with hyperflexion can result in acute or chronic cord injury.

This does not minimise the need to look for evidence of congenital bony stenosis on plain films. On a background of congenital bony canal stenosis, even a small superimposed disc bulge may be sufficient to cause cord compression. Consequently, MRI is indicated in any case of neuropraxia or neurological deficit following injury.

Radicular symptoms following a cervical spine injury

Causes of radicular pain following cervical injury include:

- acute or chronic nerve root compression due to a focal disc protrusion (see Fig. 8.100)
- aggravation of a pre-existing degenerative foraminal stenosis
- spinal canal or foraminal stenosis
- brachial plexus neuropraxia (see Figs 8.101, 8.102 and 8.103)
- nerve root avulsion (see Fig. 8.104).

Generally, nerve root avulsion injuries are not amenable to surgical repair, while brachial plexus or peripheral nerve injuries can be repaired. Imaging of such injuries can be challenging, due to the high spatial resolution and large coverage usually required to image the nerves. High signal in the posterior paraspinal muscles due to denervation oedema on T2-weighted MR images and abnormal contrast enhancement of the affected muscles have been shown to be highly sensitive findings for cervical nerve root avulsion injury (Hayashi et al. 2002).

▲ **Fig. 8.100** A cervical disc protrusion, shown on non-contrast axial CT imaging, has produced lateral recess stenosis, with encroachment on the exit foramen and cord compression (arrow).

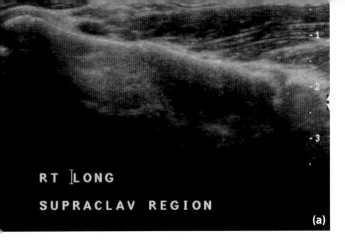

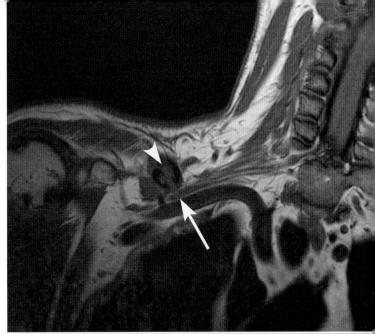

▲ Fig. 8.101 A footballer developed a right arm neuropraxia following a tackle and was subsequently noted to have a supraclavicular lump.
(a) The supraclavicular lump was imaged by ultrasound and a large right bony cervical rib with a distal pseudarthrosis was diagnosed.

▼ (b) Plain films confirmed this diagnosis, and showed a distal pseudarthrosis with an osteochondroma arising from the adjacent right first rib. A left bony cervical rib was also present.

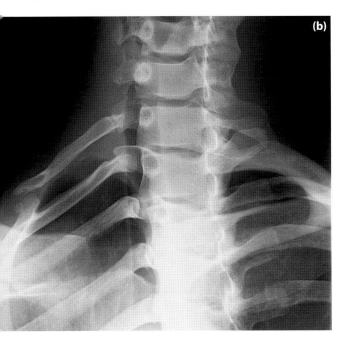

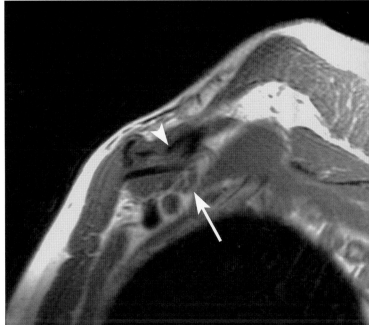

▲ Fig. 8.102 Coronal and sagittal T1-weighted images show a displaced bone fragment (arrowhead) originating from a comminuted mid-shaft clavicular fracture, pressing on the brachial plexus of an athlete and causing a C6 neuropathy (arrow).

▼ Fig. 8.103 An athlete fractured his clavicle prior to competing at the Sydney 2000 Olympics. To hasten recovery, he was injected with what was referred to as an 'osteoblastic factor', which produced a large soft-tissue mass that compressed the brachial plexus (arrows). He then presented with a C5 and C6 neuropathy.

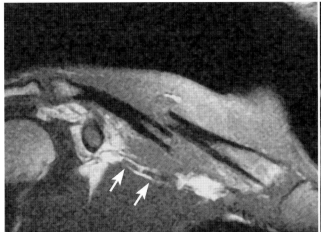

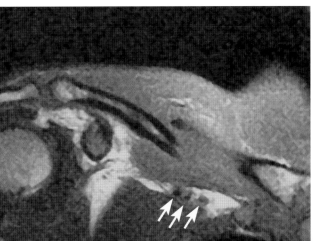

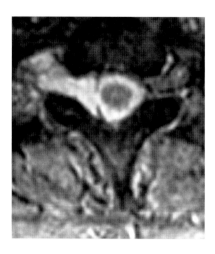

▲ **Fig. 8.104** An axial T2*-weighted GRE image shows a mid-cervical nerve root avulsion on the right side. This injury resulted from a traction force.

Imaging of the thoracic spine and lumbosacral spine

Routine views of the thoracic spine

The thoracic spine is not commonly injured as a result of sport. Hyperflexion injuries may occasionally cause a compression fracture or protrusion of a thoracic disc (see Fig. 8.105), but generally speaking the thoracic spine is not often the target of acute injury. Evidence of Scheuermann's disease is often seen in the thoracic spine of athletes, but is most often an incidental observation.

The plain film series of the thoracic spine includes an AP view and a lateral view:

- An AP view is obtained in the supine position, arms by the sides and shoulders at the same level. The knees are slightly flexed to reduce the dorsal kyphosis and, using a straight tube, the beam is centred 10 cm below the sternal notch (which is about the level of T7). Quiet breathing is allowed and this improves the image by blurring the lung markings (see Fig. 8.106(a)).

- A lateral view is best obtained erect, with the patient standing side-on to the upright bucky, with a shoulder touching the bucky for support. The arms are extended and the patient is steadied by holding a drip stand. The film is centred on T7 and again quiet breathing is allowed to blur unwanted information (see Fig. 8.106(b)).

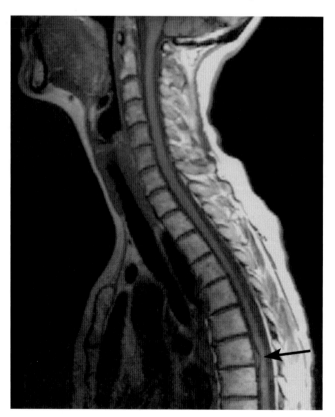

▲ **Fig. 8.105** There is protrusion of the T7/8 intervertebral disc, causing moderate cord compression (arrow).

▶ **Fig. 8.106(a)** and **(b)** AP and lateral views of the thoracic spine are generally the only imaging required for the investigation of thoracic spine symptoms. Nuclear bone scans may be necessary if plain films are normal but vertebral body compression is suspected clinically.

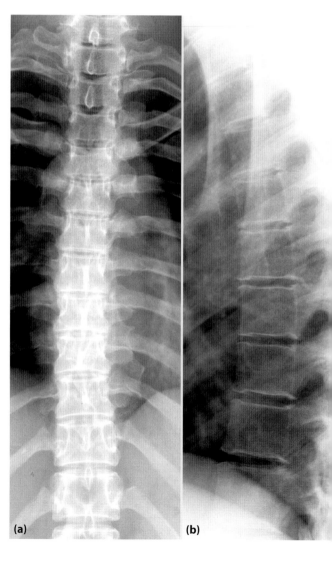

(a)   (b)

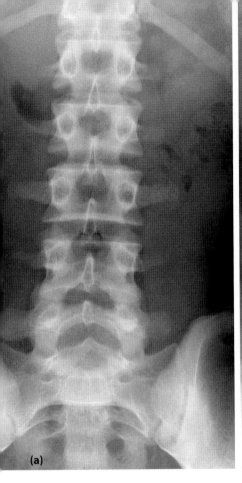
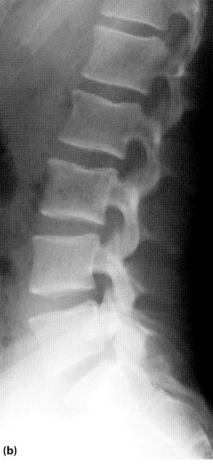

(a)   **(b)**

◄ **Fig. 8.107(a)** and **(b)** AP and lateral views of the lumbar spine are often the only views taken after acute trauma (see page 767). A cross-table lateral view is occasionally necessary. However, a full lumbar spine series is routine for all other problems of the lumbar region.

Additionally:

- If the patient is unable to stand, the image is obtained with the patient lying on their side on the table. Sponges are placed under the patient in an attempt to straighten the spine.
- Occasionally, an image centred on the thoracolumbar junction may be helpful for assessing compression fractures and determining the extent of Scheuermann's disease.
- When the patient's symptoms are located in the upper thoracic region, a 'swimmer's' view may be a helpful addition to the thoracic spine series.

Routine views of the lumbar spine

Unlike the thoracic spine, the lumbar spine is subjected to considerable wear and tear as a result of sport. The lumbar spine moves constantly and is subjected to considerable axial loading in many sports, resulting in overuse and acute injuries in all age groups.

A routine lumbar spine series includes an AP view, a lateral view, a coned lateral view of the lumbosacral junction and a coned angled view of the sacroiliac joints.

- An AP view is obtained with the patient supine and the knees flexed sufficiently to reduce the lumbar lordosis. The beam is centred at the level of the inferior costal cartilages, which corresponds to the level of L3. The film should be well coned to increase detail (see Fig. 8.107(a)).
- For a lateral view, the patient lies on their side, facing away so that the spine can be seen. The spine is straightened by placing a sponge under the lower thoracic spine. The knees are bent to provide support. The beam is centred 3 cm above the iliac crests and coning is important to help increase definition (see Fig. 8.107(b)).
- A coned lateral view of the L5/S1 level is an important view and care should be taken to ensure that the image is a true lateral. The patient is positioned as for the full lateral view and then the ankles and knees are separated by sponges, with support provided by sandbags. There is tight coning and the beam is centred 4 cm anterior to the L5 spinous process (see Fig. 8.108).

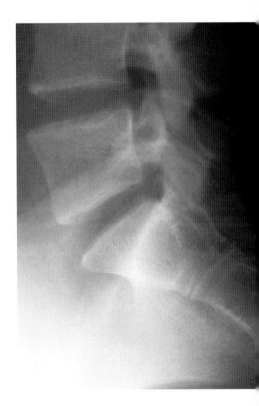

▲ **Fig. 8.108** A coned lateral view of the lumbosacral junction is a valuable component of a lumbar spine series, as this disc space is often difficult to assess on a full lateral view. The L5/S1 disc is frequently pathological but, being a transitional level, there can be considerable normal variation in the width of the disc space.

- Views of the sacroiliac joints may be obtained with the patient supine, using 30° of cranial tube angulation and with the tube centred 3 cm above the superior border of the symphysis pubis (see Fig. 8.109(a)). As discussed in Chapter 5, there is some support for the supine technique for plain films of the sacroiliac joints. This support is based on the joints being closer to the film in the supine position, increasing definition. Others prefer a prone technique, believing it to be superior because the joint orientation is such that the diverging beam in this position is better at demonstrating the joint space. If the prone position is used, the tube has 30° of caudal angulation and the beam is centred on the spinous process of L4.

Oblique views of the sacroiliac joints may be useful for better defining the joint margins. However, it must be remembered that views of the sacroiliac joints deliver a considerable dose of radiation to the pelvis and, if a CT examination is also being contemplated, oblique views should be omitted (see Fig. 8.109(b)).

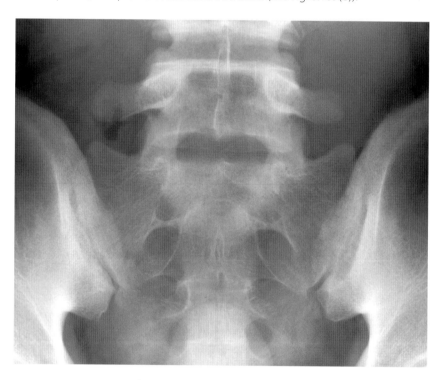

▶ **Fig. 8.109(a)** The sacroiliac joints can usually be adequately assessed on an angled AP or PA view. Rarely are oblique views or CT imaging necessary.

▼ **(b)** When appearances are equivocal for sclerosis or erosions on an AP or a PA view of the sacroiliac joints, oblique views may help to clarify the change. Oblique views are particularly valuable in confirming that the sclerosis of osteitis condensans ilii lies on the iliac side of the joint.

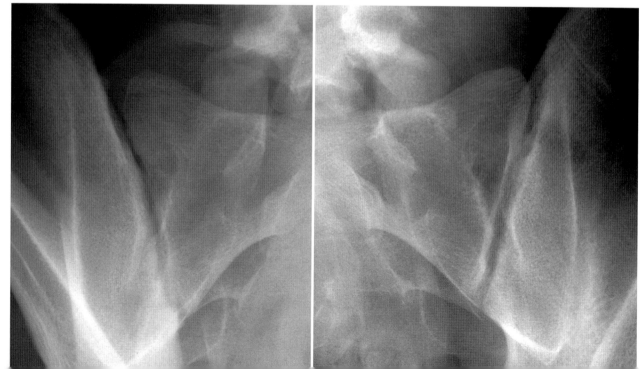

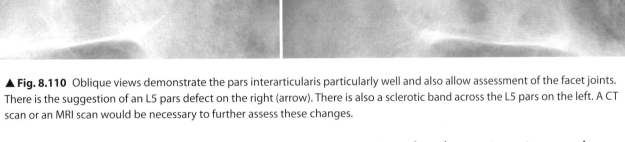

▲ **Fig. 8.110** Oblique views demonstrate the pars interarticularis particularly well and also allow assessment of the facet joints. There is the suggestion of an L5 pars defect on the right (arrow). There is also a sclerotic band across the L5 pars on the left. A CT scan or an MRI scan would be necessary to further assess these changes.

Oblique views of the lumbar spine are not obtained routinely, but may be helpful when a stress fracture of the pars interarticularis is suspected clinically. There may be wisdom in performing oblique views when investigating an athlete involved in a sport that involves repetitive hyperextension. These sports include diving, ballet, gymnastics and fast bowling in cricket. The facet joints are also well displayed on an oblique view (see Fig. 8.110).

Imaging the thoracic spine and lumbosacral spine following acute trauma

The initial radiographic assessment of acute injury to the thoracolumbar spine consists of AP and lateral views only. As the thoracolumbar junction is the most frequent site of injury,

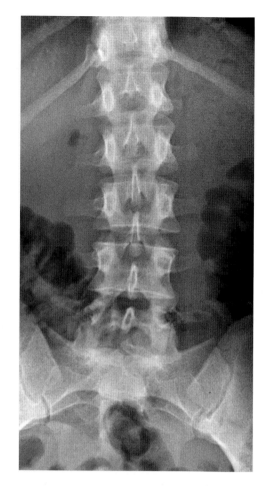

▶ **Fig. 8.111** Differentiating a postural curve from a true scoliosis can be difficult, and an erect film may solve the problem. In this case, lumbar curvature and pelvic tilt both disappeared on the erect film.

this region in particular must be well visualised. In the context of acute trauma, an initial shoot-through lateral image is acquired without moving the patient. Commonly missed fractures in the thoracic and lumbosacral spine are listed in Table 8.2.

Table 8.2 Easily missed fractures in the thoracolumbar spine

1. Fractures of the lumbar transverse process
2. Stress fractures of the pars interarticularis
3. Thoracolumbar burst fractures
4. Fractures of the rim apophysis

A useful approach to the evaluation of a lumbar spine series follows.

Alignment

On a lateral view, there is normally a continuous smooth alignment of the posterior vertebral margins (posterior cortical line), which should form a mild smooth kyphosis in the thoracic region and a mild lordosis in the lumbar region. There should be no abrupt step to indicate a spondylolisthesis or retrolisthesis. The thoracic kyphosis and the lumbar lordosis may show a generalised increase or reduction with flexion and extension. A common but non-specific finding is loss of the normal lumbar lordosis secondary to muscle spasm. This may also be produced by patient positioning.

On an AP view, the spine should be perfectly straight without a curvature to either side. Such curvature may be positional (see Fig. 8.111) or due to a pathological scoliosis. If a scoliosis is present, the vertebrae are rotated. Rotation is manifest by noting deviation of the spinous processes from the vertebral midline, and rotation also prevents superimposition of the posterolateral margins of the vertebral bodies in the lateral view (see Fig. 8.112). Other features of a scoliosis are discussed later.

Intervertebral disc height

Disc spaces are fairly uniform in the thoracic spine but in the lumbar spine they should increase slightly in width at each level from L1/2 to L4/5. The L5/S1 disc space height is extremely variable and can still be normal when significantly narrower than the L4/5 disc space height. Osteophytes or other signs of disc degeneration will indicate whether the disc space narrowing is at least in part degenerative.

Assessment of vertebral bodies

The number of lumbar vertebral bodies and the presence of transitional vertebrae should be noted. The diagnosis of six lumbar vertebrae can be made with certainty only when images of the thoracic spine are also available and counting down from T1 is possible. Normal variants are occasionally encountered in which there are ribs at L1 or no ribs at T12. Generally speaking, L3 has the longest transverse processes. The vertebral bodies should be assessed for any alteration in shape or contour, such as loss of height, osteophyte formation, endplate irregularity or cortical deficiency.

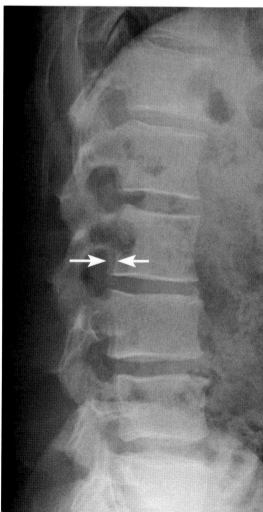

▶ **Fig. 8.112** A scoliosis is present when there is curvature of the spine and rotation of the vertebral bodies throughout the segment involved. On the lateral projection, rotation through the segment of curvature prevents superimposition of the posterolateral margins of the vertebral bodies (arrows). Note that the vertebrae in the lower lumbar region are in a true lateral position.

Spinal canal dimensions

The AP spinal canal dimension and the transverse interpedicular distance should remain constant throughout the lumbar spine. Measurements of the spinal canal are discussed in the section on lumbar spinal canal stenosis (see page 790).

Posterior elements

Each anatomical component of the posterior vertebral complex should be checked carefully. The pedicles are best seen on an AP view and should all be of similar density with a continuous well-defined cortical margin. The transverse processes are also best seen on an AP view. The pars interarticulares and the facet joints can be evaluated to some degree on an AP view, but are best demonstrated on an oblique view. A pars defect may be visible on a lateral view, but often requires an oblique film for confirmation. There is considerable overlap of the posterior elements on the lateral view, making assessment of all but the spinous processes difficult.

Soft-tissue signs

Soft-tissue signs are less helpful in the thoracic spine and lumbosacral spine than in the cervical spine. In the thoracic spine, a paravertebral soft-tissue swelling, seen as focal widening of the paraspinal soft tissues silhouetted by lung, may be a useful indicator of a haematoma associated with thoracic spine injury. In the lumbar region, the psoas shadows should be inspected for evidence of either widening due to a psoas haematoma or obliteration indicative of a retroperitoneal haematoma.

Fractures of the thoracolumbar spine

Thoracolumbar vertebral wedge compression fractures

Vertebral wedge compression fractures are the result of truncal flexion under axial load and are the most common bony injury encountered in the thoracolumbar spine. These injuries have been reported in waterski jumpers (Horne et al. 1987) and in athletes undertaking winter sports such as freestyle skiing, snow-boarding and snowmobiling (Keene 1987). The radiographic signs are best appreciated on a lateral view (see Fig. 8.113) and include:

- loss of anterior vertebral body height, resulting in wedging
- depression of the superior, or less commonly the inferior, vertebral endplate, causing linear sclerosis from trabecular impaction parallel to the depressed endplate
- preservation of the posterior cortical line of the vertebral body
- acute fracture changes at the anterior margin of the vertebral body, which may include a focal cortical break, an abrupt cortical step or cortical buckling.

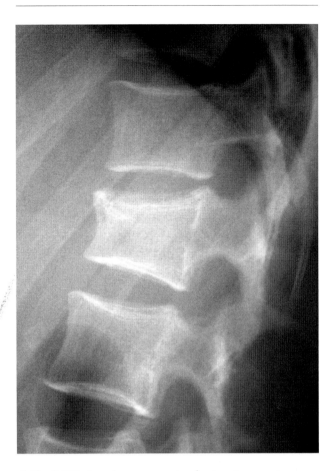

▲ **Fig. 8.113** A wedge compression fracture is present, resulting from combined axial and hyperflexion forces. There is no plain film evidence of any retropulsed bone fragment. This was confirmed by CT.

Marked loss of vertebral body height or significant fragmentation warrants further assessment with CT to define the extent of the injury and, in particular, to exclude a retropulsed bone fragment.

Burst fractures

A burst fracture is a vertebral compression injury that results in posterior displacement (retropulsion) of a vertebral body fragment into the spinal canal. Burst fractures are characteristically due to a hyperflexion injury, often caused by falling or jumping from a height. Burst fractures have been reported resulting from tobogganing accidents (Herkowitz and Samberg 1978) and bobsledding accidents (Oleson et al. 1995). Neurological deficit is present in approximately 50% of cases. It is therefore important to distinguish a burst fracture from a simple wedge compression fracture, and the key to this is to determine whether or not the fracture involves the posterior cortex of the vertebral body (see Fig. 8.114(a)). A retropulsed fragment is separated from the posterosuperior portion of the vertebral body and can usually be identified, although a CT scan is still advisable for confirmation (see Fig. 8.114(b)). Loss of definition of the posterior cortical line or loss of the normal concavity of the vertebra is highly suggestive of a burst fracture. On the AP view, the interpedicular distance

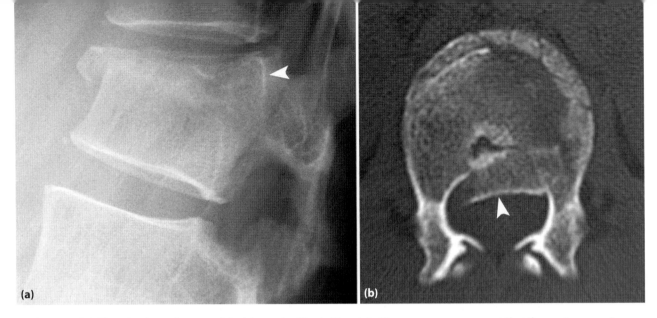

▲ **Fig. 8.114(a)** There is a burst fracture of the L1 vertebral body. The plain film appearances suggest that the posterosuperior corner of the vertebral body is displaced posteriorly (arrowhead), when compared with the posterior cortex of the vertebral body below. **(b)** A CT scan demonstrates a retropulsed bone fragment and the corresponding degree of encroachment on the vertebral canal (arrowhead).

may appear widened and a vertical component of the vertebral body fracture may be evident. A burst fracture has a variable degree of wedging and comminution. CT or MRI is indicated to confirm the diagnosis, determine the number and size of the retropulsed fragments, assess the degree of spinal canal compromise (see Figs 8.115 and 8.116) and define any associated injuries.

Transverse process fractures

A transverse process fracture (see Fig. 8.117) may be an avulsion injury at the site of the quadratus lumborum or psoas muscle attachment, or alternatively it may be the result of direct blunt trauma. The fracture line is vertical or oblique and frequently occurs at multiple levels. In the immature athlete, apophyses develop at the tips of the transverse processes and unfused apophyses can occasionally be avulsed (see Fig. 8.118). In contact

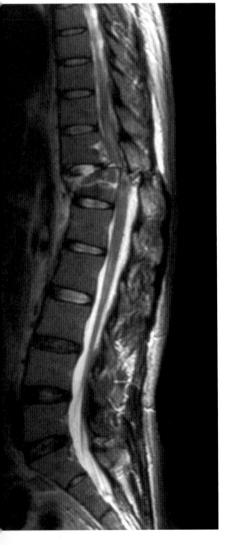

◀**Fig. 8.115(a)** A fat-suppressed T2-weighted MR image shows gross traumatic deformity at the thoracolumbar junction, resulting from a hyperflexion injury. There is a fracture of the T12 vertebral body, forward displacement of T11 on T12, and transection of the cord. The fracture passes horizontally through the spinous process of T11.

▼ **(b)** Axial MR images show substantial obliteration of the spinal canal at the T11/12 level by a bone fragment.

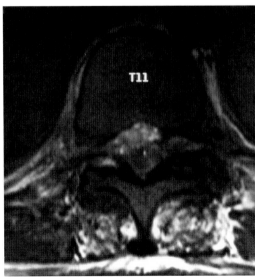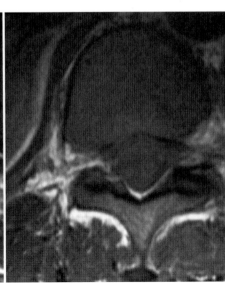

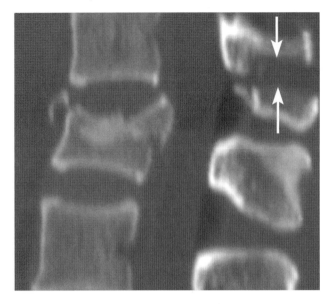

▲ **Fig. 8.116** A reformatted sagittal CT image of the case shown in Fig. 8.115 demonstrates compression of the T12 vertebral body with retropulsion of a posterosuperior fragment. A transverse fracture through the spinous process of T11 is also noted (arrows).

sports, transverse process fractures may be due to direct blunt trauma (see Fig. 8.119) and are less commonly associated with visceral injuries than transverse process fractures arising from motor vehicle trauma (Tewes et al. 1995). Stress fractures also occur in the transverse processes due to repetitive stress (see Fig. 8.120).

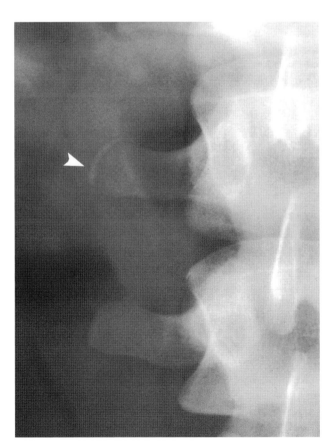

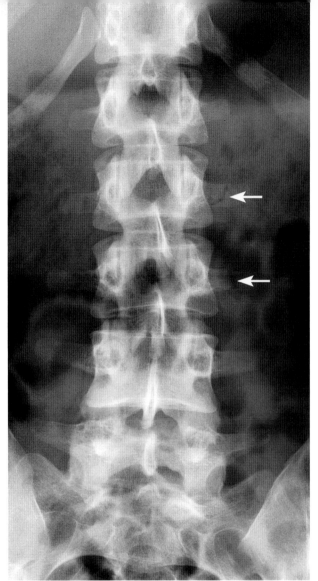

▲ **Fig. 8.117** Fractures of the transverse processes of L2 and L3 (arrows). No blunt trauma occurred and these fractures have resulted from an avulsion injury.

◄ **Fig. 8.118** A secondary ossification centre, which is normally present at the tips of the transverse processes in the immature athlete, has been avulsed and is slightly displaced (arrowhead).

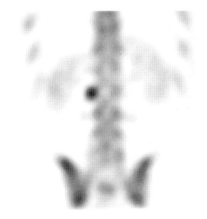

▲ **Fig. 8.119** During a rugby game, a knee to the back has fractured the right transverse process of L2. The fracture is demonstrated by a nuclear bone scan. The plain films were normal.

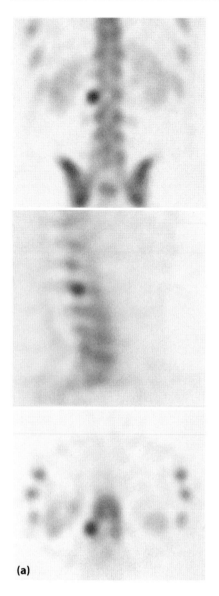

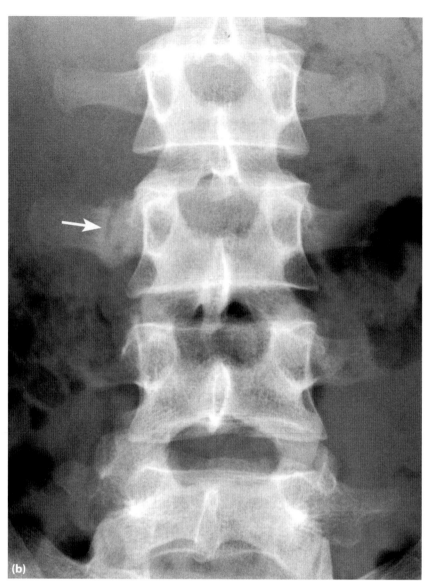

▲ **Fig. 8.120(a)** A nuclear bone scan demonstrates a stress fracture of the right transverse process of L3 in a professional dancer. **(b)** A plain film shows healing response at the stress fracture site (arrow), although the fracture line remains visible.

Other thoracolumbar spine conditions seen in athletes

Spondylolysis and spondylolisthesis

A defect of the pars interarticularis, or spondylolysis, is widely believed to be traumatic rather than developmental in origin (Resnick and Niwayama 1988). There is an incidence rate of approximately 6% in the general population, and a much higher incidence rate in sports that require lumbar hyperextension. The classic hyperextension sports associated with spondylolysis are diving, gymnastics, fast bowling in cricket and dancing. Other sports with a higher than normal incidence rate include throwing sports (such as javelin), weightlifting, rowing and football. Pars defects and associated spondylolisthesis are often asymptomatic (Beutler et al. 2003).

The vast majority of pars injuries are chronic stress fractures, although acute fractures can occur. The proposed mechanism is hyperextension with rotation, although torsion against resistance has also been proposed (Soler and Calderon 2000). The pars region acts as a bony fulcrum during spinal extension (see Fig. 8.121) and is therefore vulnerable to repetitive loading. Initially, a bone stress reaction is present, which may be demonstrated by SPECT bone scanning or fat-suppressed T2-weighted (or STIR) MR imaging (see Fig. 8.122). With ongoing stress and the development of increased reactive bony sclerosis, x-ray changes may become visible (see Fig. 8.123). A macroscopic lucent fracture line will form, initially partial but this may progress to complete fracture. The lucent fracture line first develops on the traction side of the bone strut, which is at the inferior bony cortex of the affected pars. Although stress fractures may heal with appropriate treatment, they may progress with continuing stress and result in complete defects (see Fig. 8.124), bony fragmentation and hypertrophic change. Spondylolisthesis may occur if the defects are bilateral (see Fig. 8.125).

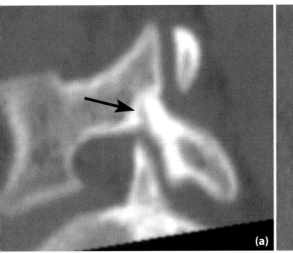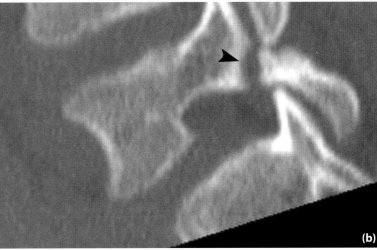

▲ **Fig. 8.121** These reformatted CT images clearly show the position of the pars interarticularis in relationship to the tip of the superior articular process of the lower vertebra. The articular process acts as a fulcrum under the pars. Both images show considerable bony sclerosis of the pars.
(a) An incomplete fracture has developed (arrow).
(b) At a more advanced stage, the fracture has progressed to become complete and a defect is present that demonstrates features of chronic non-union (arrowhead).

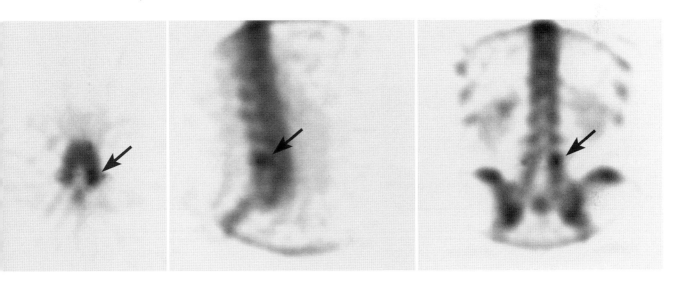

▲ **Fig. 8.122** A stress fracture involves the left pars interarticularis of L4. Increased uptake of isotope has been demonstrated and localised by SPECT imaging (arrows).

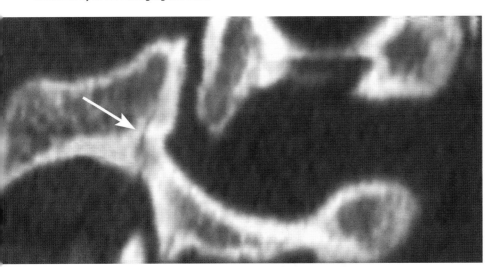

◀ **Fig. 8.123** A reformatted sagittal-oblique CT image demonstrates an incomplete fracture of the pars extending from the inferior margin (arrows).

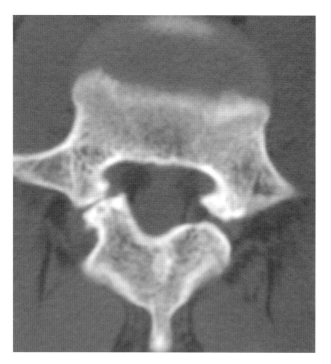

▲ **Fig. 8.124** Bilateral defects in the pars interarticularis have developed, with minor displacement. Changes of established non-union are present, with secondary degenerative features at the right-sided pseudarthrosis.

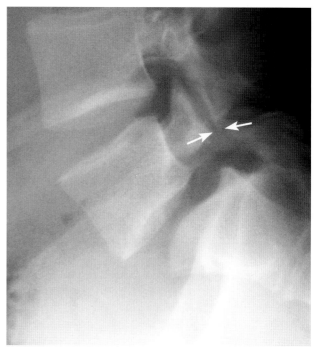

▲ **Fig. 8.125** Bilateral pars defects are present (arrows) and a Grade I–II spondylolisthesis has developed.

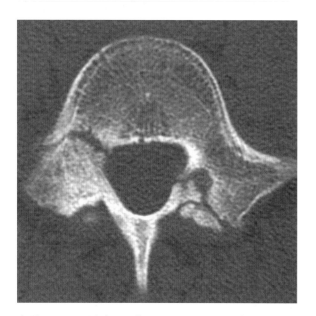

▲ **Fig. 8.126** A left pars fracture is present, with an accompanying contralateral pedicle fracture.

The presence of one pars fracture places the contralateral side at risk of a similar stress reaction and fracture, the degree of risk increasing with advancing spondylolysis. In a study of 13 young athletes with unilateral spondylolysis, 23% had a contralateral fracture or stress reaction (Sairyo et al. 2005). Contralateral fractures have been reported in the pars interarticularis, the pedicle and, less commonly, the lamina (Sairyo et al. 2005). Multiple contralateral fractures have been reported,

and bilateral pars fractures are also associated with other fractures of the posterior elements (Pascal-Moussallard et al. 2005) (see Fig. 8.126). In cricket fast bowlers, stress fractures occur on one side only, but involve a number of levels (see Fig. 8.127). These fractures occur on the contralateral side to the bowling action.

An early pars defect, defined as a negative x-ray and positive bone scan, has been shown to do well clinically with non-surgical management up to 11 years later. Unilateral defects, confirmed on CT, go on to union, but bilateral defects progress to non-union, pseudarthrosis, degeneration and slip. It is thought that the instability associated with bilateral defects hampers healing (Miller et al. 2004).

The degree of spondylolisthesis, or forward slip, is graded relative to the vertebral body AP diameter:

- *Grade I* is a forward slip of no more than 1/4 of the AP diameter of the vertebral body.
- *Grade II* is a forward slip of between 1/4 and 1/2 of the AP diameter of the vertebral body.
- *Grade III* is a forward slip between 1/2 and 3/4 of the AP diameter of the vertebral body.
- *Grade IV* is a forward slip greater than 3/4 of the AP diameter of the vertebral body.

Slip progression is more likely to occur before adulthood and appears to be related to disc degeneration.

Plain films are the first imaging investigation performed for lower back pain and are a useful screening test for many conditions. Contralateral pedicle hypertrophy and sclerosis may be visible. Chronic pars defects are often well seen on plain films (see Fig. 8.128).

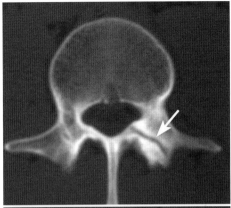

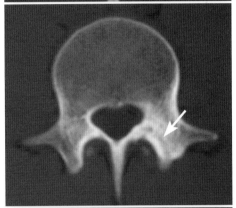

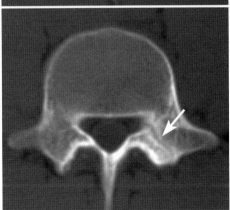

▲ **Fig. 8.127** A right-handed cricket fast bowler presented with back pain due to stress fractures of the L3, L4 and L5 vertebrae on the left (arrows). The bowling action caused pars stress fractures on the contralateral side to the bowling action.

In the absence of any strong clinical suspicion of chronic defects, oblique views are probably not warranted, given the high radiation dose that is used and the availability of other imaging methods. Oblique views may demonstrate defects or possibly sclerosis, but lack the resolution to identify all fractures. If there is strong clinical suspicion of chronic pars pathology in an athlete at high risk, oblique views may help to provide a quick diagnosis (see Fig. 8.129). Even if sclerosis of a stress reaction is seen on plain films, other imaging will still be required for further characterisation. Incomplete fractures are generally not shown on plain films. Consequently, it is debatable which imaging method should follow plain films for the investigation of suspected spondylolysis. SPECT imaging is sensitive for acute lesions and gives an indication of activity, but is insensitive to chronic healed defects, is non-specific and exposes the athlete to ionising radiation. SPECT scanning may also show asymptomatic areas of increased uptake in the spine of an athlete, creating further management problems.

Modern CT provides the highest resolution of bone detail and is excellent at showing the extent of fractures, but has the disadvantage of using ionising radiation and has a limited ability to screen for other conditions.

MRI is sensitive for acute and chronic lesions and has been shown to be positive in cases where SPECT imaging is negative, such as where contralateral stress is present. MRI also gives an indication of activity and screens for other abnormalities, but it can be difficult to discriminate between stress

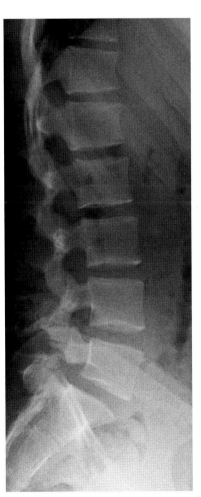

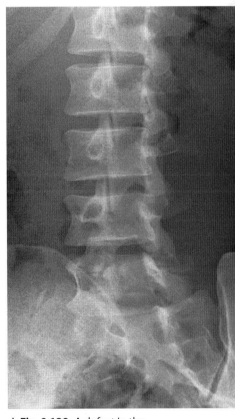

▲ **Fig. 8.129** A defect in the pars interarticularis of L5 is well demonstrated by an oblique plain film.

▲ **Fig. 8.128** A pars defect is often adequately seen on a lateral plain film.

reaction and an incomplete fracture. Therefore, an imaging protocol of MRI, followed by CT for acute or indeterminate cases, has been proposed (Campbell et al. 2005). It is probable that technical developments will further advance the role of MRI as a first-line investigation of spondylolysis.

Standard CT examinations of the lumbar spine are obtained in the axial plane of the intervertebral discs and do not resolve small pars defects well. Images are obtained in a plane relatively perpendicular to the pars interarticularis defect, either by the direct acquisition reverse gantry technique (see Fig. 8.130) or with modern multislice scanners by image reformations in the oblique sagittal plane (see Figs 8.131 and 8.132). The latter technique is sensitive for the detection of subtle fractures, and particularly for determining whether

a fracture is partial or complete. CT can help to assess the healing of acute stress fractures. Imaging signs of healing may take more than 12 weeks to appear.

Bone stress and active lesions are demonstrated as areas of bone marrow hyperintensity on fat-suppressed T2-weighted or STIR images (see Fig. 8.133). Thinner slices and a smaller field of view enable better visualisation of the pars. A normal pars interarticularis is best seen on sagittal T1 images as marrow continuity. Thickening of the anteroinferior cortex is a sign of an incomplete fracture and there may be sharp interruption of the cortical line with an acute defect (see Fig. 8.134). Complications such as spondylolisthesis and neural compression may also be assessed by MRI.

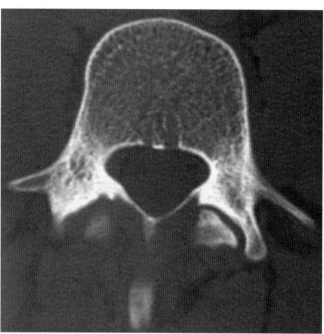
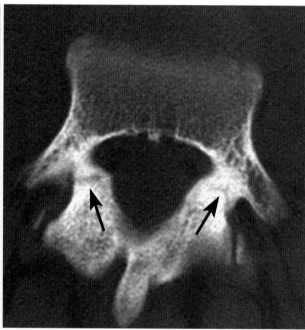

▲ **Fig. 8.130** A 19-year-old boxer presented with back pain and a stress fracture was suspected clinically. An initial CT series was normal. However, an angled reverse gantry tilt scan showed bilateral pars sclerosis and stress fractures (arrows).

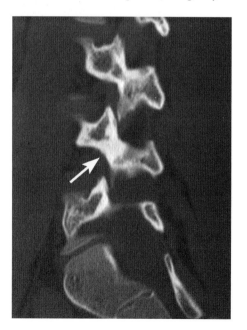
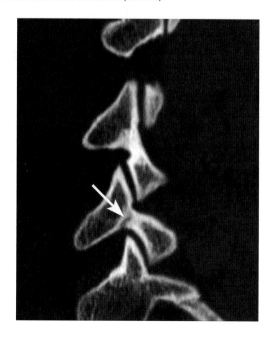

◀ **Fig. 8.131** A sagittal-oblique reformatted CT image shows sclerosis of the L4 pars without fracture (arrow).

▶ **Fig. 8.132** A sagittal-oblique reformatted CT image optimally displays the pars region and demonstrates an incomplete stress fracture of the L5 pars (arrow) and sclerotic changes at the L4 pars.

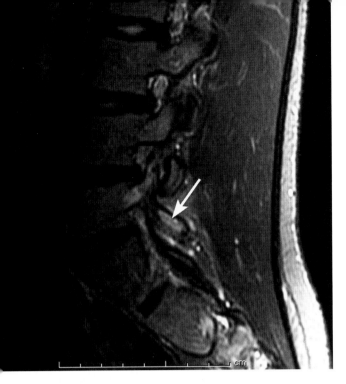

▲ Fig. 8.133 A sagittal STIR MR image shows high signal in the L5 pars interarticularis and pedicle regions (arrow) in this athlete with low back pain.

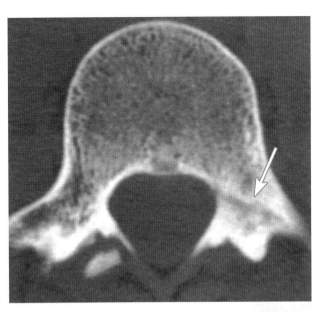

▲ Fig. 8.135 A 15-year-old cricketer presented with back pain and was found to have a stress fracture of a left-sided pedicle (arrow).

Other vertebral stress fractures

Although pars interarticularis fractures are the most common stress injury of the lumbar spine, other components of the posterior bony vertebral arch are also susceptible to stress, including the spinal lamina, the pedicles (see Fig. 8.135) and the spinous process (see Fig. 8.136). Stress fractures can also involve the transverse processes due to repetitive muscular traction (see Fig. 8.137). An example of this particular stress fracture has already been shown in Fig. 8.117.

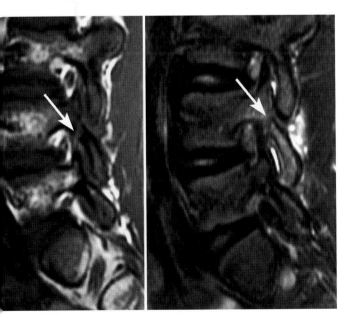

▲ Fig. 8.134 Sagittal T1-weighted and STIR images demonstrate an acute fracture of the pars interarticularis of L4 (arrows) in an 11-year-old athlete. The STIR image shows associated marrow oedema, facet joint effusion and soft-tissue oedema posteriorly.

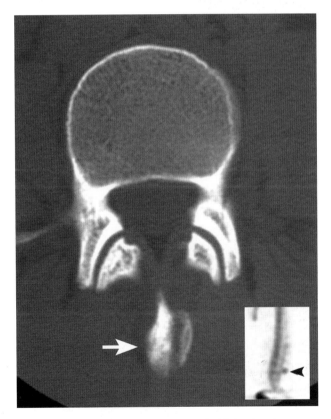

▲ Fig. 8.136 A ballet dancer presented with back pain after performing a season of *Swan Lake*, which required considerable flexion of the spine. A stress fracture of the spinous process of L4 was demonstrated by a CT scan (arrow), following a positive nuclear bone scan. The insert shows a SPECT image demonstrating increased uptake of isotope in the spinous process of L4 (arrowhead).

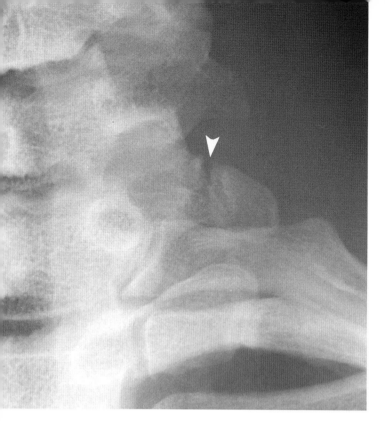

▲ Fig. 8.137 A stress fracture of the left transverse process of the C7 vertebral body has resulted from repetitive weightlifting activity in a body builder (arrowhead).

Stress fractures of the sacrum have been discussed in Chapter 5. These fractures present with low back or gluteal pain in runners and can be related to an increase in impact activity. Osteoporosis needs to be considered as a possible underlying factor in young female patients (Johnson et al. 2001).

Muscle injuries

Muscle strain is a common cause of lower back pain and imaging findings are usually negative. Uncommonly, an acute muscle tear may be demonstrated as a cause of back pain (see Fig. 8.138).

Interspinous bursopathy

Bursae may develop between the spinous processes as a result of repetitive spinal flexion and extension. They are more common in the mid- to lower lumbar spine and increase in prevalence with age. Interspinous bursopathy may develop, causing pain on extension. This condition has been described in basketball players and may be a precursor of Baastrup's syndrome where there is bony abutment of the spinous processes in extension (see Fig. 8.139).

Injury to the ring apophysis

The ring apophysis encircles the vertebral body endplates, fusing with the vertebral body by the age of 25 years. An avulsion fracture of a posterior apophyseal fragment is seen rarely in adolescents and young adults and usually involves the posteroinferior aspect of the L4 or L5 vertebral body (Laredo et al. 1986) (see Figs 8.140 and 8.141). There is always an associated disc herniation between the apophysis and the vertebral body. CT may be necessary to show the small avulsed fragment, which should be differentiated from an osteophyte, soft-tissue calcification within the posterior longitudinal spinal ligament or a chronic calcified herniated disc fragment.

Chronic injuries to the ring apophysis are thought to be the result of failure in tension shear at the attachment of

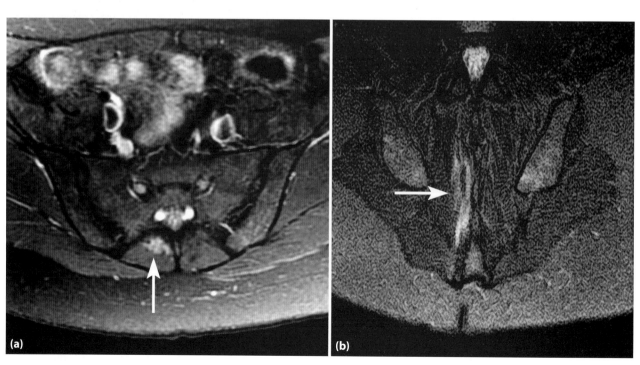

▲ Fig. 8.138 An acute injury to the right multifidus muscle is demonstrated by MRI as high signal within the muscle (arrows) on **(a)** axial and **(b)** coronal STIR images.

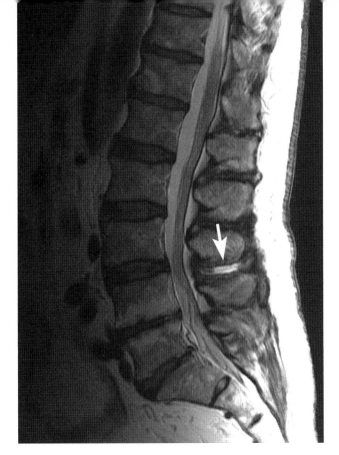

▲ **Fig. 8.139** A sagittal T2-weighted MR image demonstrates a linear area of high signal between the L3 and L4 spinous processes, typical of interspinous bursopathy (arrow). Disc degenerative changes are also present.

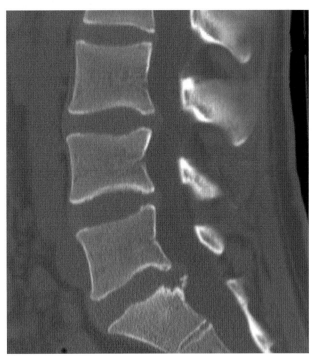

▲ **Fig. 8.140** A sagittal reformatted CT image of a young athlete shows a chronic injury to the posterior ring apophysis of S1, with mild posterior displacement of the apophysis and adjacent degenerate endplate change.

Sharpey's fibres to the apophysis, similar to other avulsion injuries in the immature skeleton. Hellstrom et al. (1990) described these vertebral ring apophyseal avulsions as occurring only in athletes.

Limbus vertebrae

A limbus vertebra is a normal variant and results from the lack of fusion of an ossification centre at either the anteroinferior aspect of a vertebral body in the cervical spine or the anterosuperior corner of a lumbar vertebral body (see Fig. 8.142). This should not be confused with a fracture. Both the unfused ossification centre and the adjacent vertebral body have well-corticated margins. In the lumbar region, a limbus vertebra can occur in association with Scheuermann's disease due to discal herniation beneath the apophyseal ring.

Schmorl's nodes and endplate injuries

Schmorl's nodes are common and are seen with similar frequency in both the young and old. The nodes represent changes at the discovertebral junction caused by small herniations of disc material through the vertebral body endplates, presumed to be due to compressive trauma or developmental defects in the endplates (see Fig. 8.143). Schmorl's nodes are incidental changes that are asymptomatic, although when they occur anteriorly they are often associated with Scheuermann's disease. Schmorl's nodes have also been reported in association

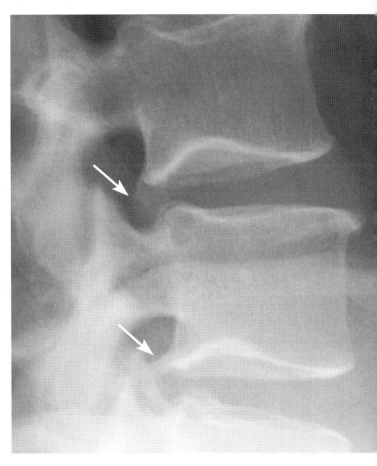

▲ **Fig. 8.141** There are non-acute fractures of the ring apophyses of L3 and L4 (arrows). Disc protrusions were found to be present at both levels.

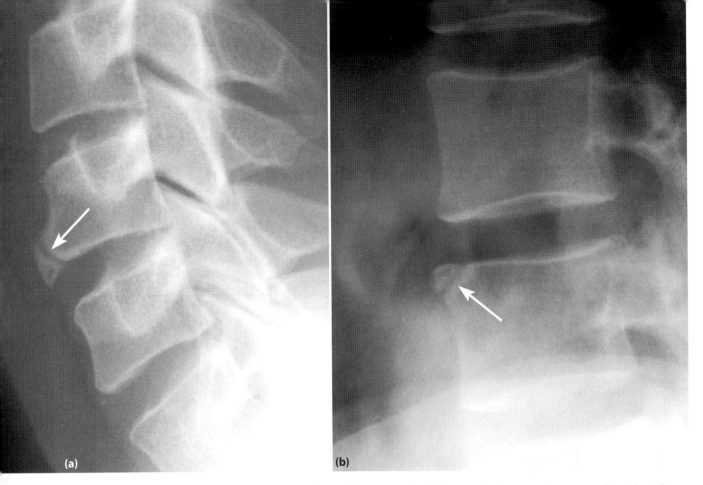

▲ Fig. 8.142 Limbus vertebrae are a normal variant, being due to an unfused ring apophysis appearing as a small ossicle at the corner of a vertebral body.

(a) In the cervical region, the ossicle is present at the anteroinferior corner of the vertebral body (arrow).

(b) The ossicle occurs at the anterosuperior corner of the vertebral body in the lumbar region (arrow).

The ossicles have a well-corticated margin, unlike a fracture.

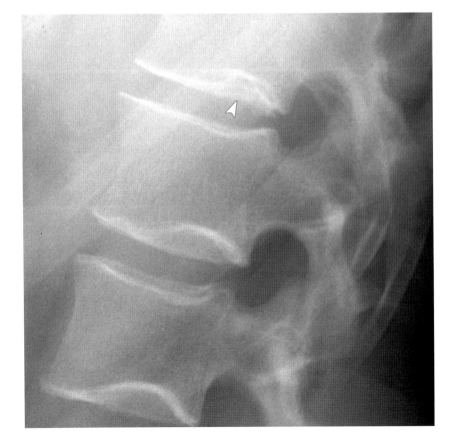

◄ Fig. 8.143 There are prominent posterior Schmorl's nodes present. The disc material lying in the upper node has calcified (arrowhead).

with moderate but not advanced disc degenerative changes. Hellstrom et al. (1990) demonstrated a higher rate of disc height reduction, Schmorl's nodes and abnormal vertebral configurations in athletes compared with the normal population. Excessive compressive loading of the spine affects normal growth at the apophyses and can result in wedging and uneven endplates. Anterior endplate lesions are strongly associated with excessive axial loading of the spine, particularly in the flexed position and during growth spurts.

Elite alpine skiers and ski jumpers have been shown to have a significantly higher rate of anterior endplate Schmorl's nodes than control subjects (Rachbauer et al. 2001) (see Fig. 8.144).

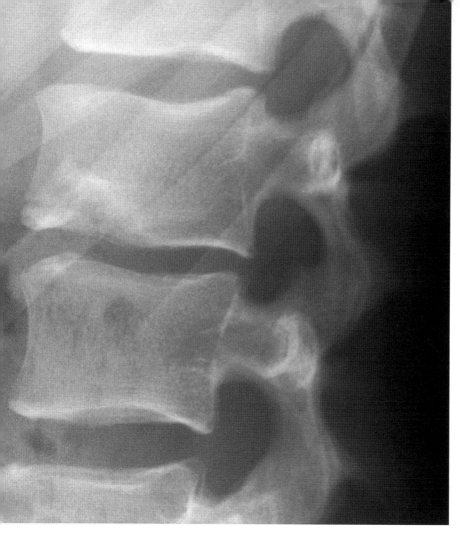

▲ **Fig. 8.144** A large anterior Schmorl's node is demonstrated. This defect clearly contains a large volume of disc material, resulting in reduction in the width of the disc space.

Increases in thoracic kyphosis and lumbar lordosis have been shown in adolescent athletes with greater cumulative training time, particularly in gymnasts (Wojtys et al. 2000).

Scheuermann's disease

Scheuermann's disease is a very common condition attributed to the protrusion of disc material through weakened vertebral endplates. The endplates may be thinner than normal and deformed by disc pressure, preventing normal ossification. The cartilaginous endplates may then degenerate and subsequent fissuring allows protrusion of disc material through the weakened endplates. These changes are thought to be due to mechanical stress on congenitally or traumatically weakened developing cartilaginous endplates (Resnick and Niwayama 1988).

Clinically, many patients are asymptomatic and no characteristic clinical presentation can be defined. Lumbar involvement is more likely to be painful than changes in the thoracic region. The condition settles with skeletal maturity, and old Scheuermann's disease of varying degrees is often noted as an incidental finding on spinal films obtained for other reasons in later life (see Fig. 8.145). Systematic disc degeneration eventually develops.

The radiographic appearances include undulating irregular endplates and Schmorl's nodes, which are characteristically anterior in position. This pattern of involvement is seen in the lumbar spine with less vertebral body wedging occurring when compared with the thoracic spine (see Figs 8.146 and 8.147). Schmorl's nodes have sclerotic margins and there is narrowing of the adjacent intervertebral disc space (see Fig. 8.148).

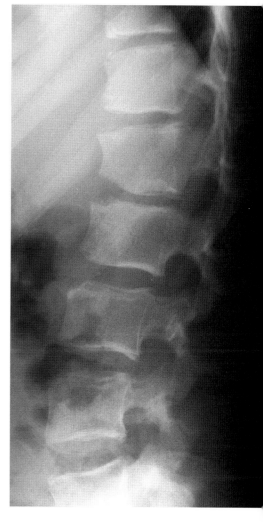

▲ **Fig. 8.145** A surprising number of skeletally mature elite athletes have evidence of old Scheuermann's disease, without ever having had back symptoms. Multiple vertebral bodies are deformed by large anterior Schmorl's nodes. No wedging is seen in the lumbar region, although there is wedging of T12 and narrowing of the T11/12 disc space. A kyphosis results at the thoracolumbar junction.

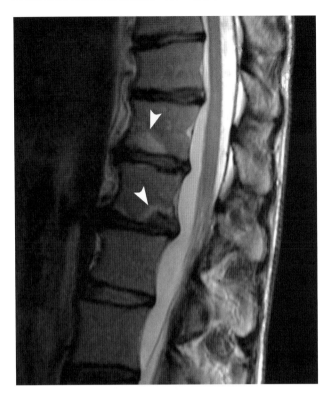

▲ **Fig. 8.146** A sagittal T2-weighted MR image demonstrates disc space narrowing, irregular endplates and increased marrow signal at the vertebral endplates (arrowheads).

▼ **Fig. 8.147** A plain film shows the typical lumbar changes of Scheuermann's disease. Findings include wavy endplates, disc space narrowing and anterior Schmorl's node formation. No wedging is present in the lumbar region but T12 is minimally wedged.

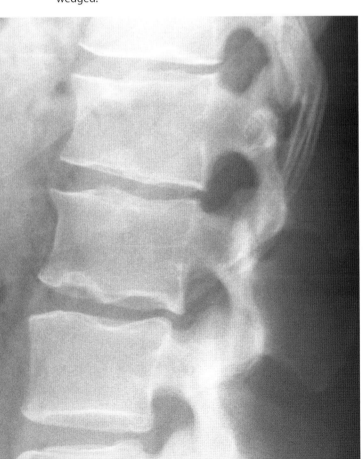

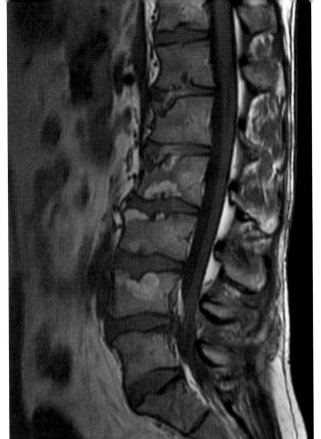

▲ **Fig. 8.148** Marked changes of Scheuermann's disease are present in the lumbar spine on a sagittal T1-weighted MR image. Note the reactive marrow changes at multiple endplates.

In the thoracic spine, where the changes are largely anterior, a kyphosis often develops due to anterior vertebral body wedging (see Fig. 8.149), and separated secondary ossification centres (limbus vertebrae) are noted.

The diagnostic criteria required to make a diagnosis of Scheuermann's disease are a matter of conjecture. Initially, it was considered necessary to have three vertebrae involved before a diagnosis could be made. It was then concluded that there could be one vertebra or five vertebrae involved. Sorenson (1964) introduced the criteria of three contiguous vertebrae, each with wedging of 5° or more. Wedging is absent when Scheuermann's disease involves the upper lumbar vertebrae and this form of the condition was excluded from such a definition by Alexander (1977).

Investigating lower back pain

The role and timing of imaging in patients presenting with lower back pain are currently being debated. Most patients will have a plain film series. While plain films do not often yield a specific diagnosis, they are useful in assessing weightbearing alignment, developmental variation and the background level of degenerative change. MRI provides more precise anatomical and pathological information than plain films without exposure to ionising irradiation, but whether this information alters patient outcome is disputed.

A recent study has shown MRI to be of no value in planning conservative treatment for lower back pain or radiculopathy and that patient knowledge of the imaging findings lessened their sense of wellbeing (Modic et al. 2005). Another study (Jarvik et al. 2003) has shown nearly identical outcomes comparing investigation with rapid MRI (an abbreviated examination) and a plain film series in patients with lower back pain. MRI was associated with a slight increase in the number of patients undergoing surgery. A third study (Gilbert et al. 2004) has shown that the early use of MRI or CT did not affect treatment overall, but did yield a small improvement in outcome. Imaging with MRI is thought to be desirable if lower back pain does not settle, helping to exclude unusual or unsuspected causes of back pain and to assess suitability for surgery.

Lumbar intervertebral disc degeneration

Intervertebral disc degeneration is common, and disc herniation is frequently implicated in back pain and radiculopathy. Loss of disc height results in excess axial load on the facet joints, which may in turn show degenerative changes and contribute to back pain (see Fig. 8.150).

The intervertebral disc is composed of a central nucleus pulposus and a surrounding annulus fibrosus. The annulus is composed of inner fibres that are connected to the cartilaginous endplates and outer Sharpey fibres that attach directly to the vertebral body. Disc degeneration is a result of mechanical stress and loss of hydration within the disc.

Increasing loss of disc hydration signal on T2-weighted MR images correlates with progressive degeneration. Lumbar intervertebral disc degeneration has been classified according to the MR appearances on T2-weighted images:

- *Grade 1:* Homogeneous hyperintense disc signal with clear distinction of the nucleus and annulus (see Fig. 8.151).

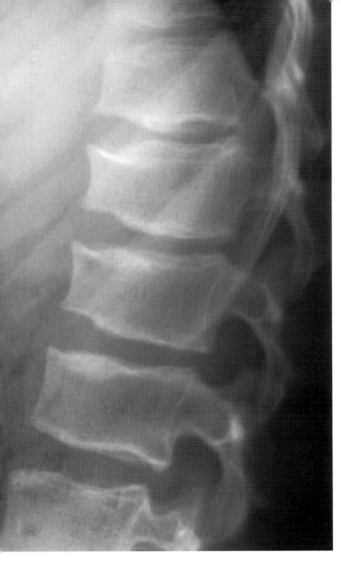

▲ **Fig. 8.149** Typical changes of thoracic Scheuermann's disease. There are anterior Schmorl's nodes and wedging is a feature, with a resultant kyphosis.

▼ **Fig. 8.150** Disc space narrowing may not cause pain per se. Narrowing increases loading of the facet joints, which in turn may produce degenerative joint changes.

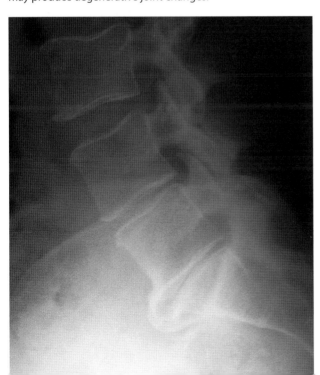

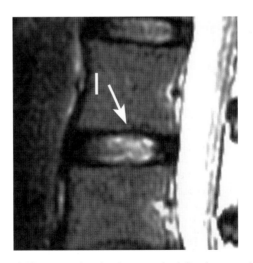

▲ **Fig. 8.151** Lumbar intervertebral disc degeneration is graded depending on the appearance of the disc, imaged by T2-weighted MRI. A Grade I disc shows a clear demarcation between the nucleus (high signal) and the annulus (low signal) (arrow).

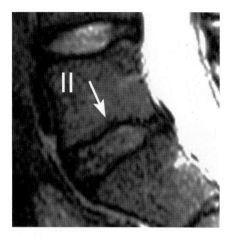

◀ **Fig. 8.152** In a Grade II disc degeneration, differentiation between the nucleus and the annulus is less apparent and hypointense horizontal lines are apparent through the nucleus (arrow).

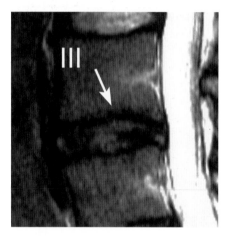

◀ **Fig. 8.153** In a Grade III disc degeneration, there is an inhomogeneous intermediate signal intensity throughout. Type 3 endplate changes are also present, with hypointense endplate bands seen on this T2 image (arrow).

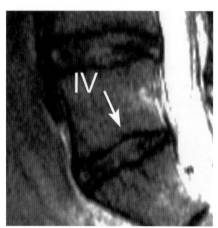

◀ **Fig. 8.154** In a Grade IV disc degeneration, there is no distinction between the nucleus and the annulus and moderate disc space narrowing. Type 3 endplate signal is again demonstrated (arrow).

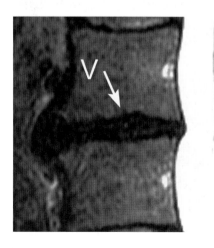

◀ **Fig. 8.155** In a Grade V disc degeneration, there is marked disc space narrowing and no distinction between the nucleus and annulus (arrow).

- *Grade II:* Inhomogeneous disc signal with or without horizontal bands (see Fig. 8.152).
- *Grade III:* Inhomogeneous intermediate signal intensity with unclear distinction between the nucleus and annulus (see Fig. 8.153).
- *Grade IV:* Intermediate to hypointense disc signal with a moderate decrease in height, with no distinction between the nucleus and annulus (see Fig. 8.154).
- *Grade V:* Hypointense collapsed disc space (see Fig. 8.155).

Plain film signs of disc degeneration appear relatively late and include disc space narrowing, a vacuum phenomenon and endplate sclerosis. Marginal vertebral body osteophytes develop in an attempt to contain the disc and osteophytes will often encroach on the neural exit foramina. Disc degeneration is common in asymptomatic people and is more common in athletes (Ong et al. 2003; Berge et al. 1999). Disc degeneration is most common at the L4/5 and L5/S1 levels and degenerative changes at one of these levels correlates with degenerative changes at the other (Martin et al. 2002). It is unlikely that disc degeneration itself is painful, but associated vertebral body endplate changes may well be a cause of painful symptoms (Weishaupt et al. 1998).

Modic et al. (1988) classified the changes in the MR appearance of endplates in degenerate discs as follows:

- *Type 1 endplate changes:* decreased signal intensity on T1, increased signal intensity on T2 (this change is seen in Fig. 8.146).
- *Type 2 endplate changes:* increased signal intensity on T1, mildly increased signal intensity on T2.
- *Type 3 endplate changes:* decreased signal intensity on both T1 and T2.

The histopathology of Type 1 changes shows disruption and fissuring of endplates with associated intra-osseous granulation tissue; Type 2 changes represent yellow fatty marrow replacement; and Type 3 changes correspond to endplate and marrow sclerosis.

The significance of endplate changes is controversial. There is evidence that Type 1 change is specific for discal pain and active segmental hypermobility (Toyone 1994). Another study has shown that moderate and severe Type 1 and Type 2 endplate abnormalities predict symptomatic painful discs. In the study by Weishaupt et al. (2001), a low prevalence of endplate abnormalities was shown in asymptomatic people. Progression from Type 1 to Type 2 changes has been shown to occur in patients over a period of a few years. Type 1 change seems to represent a more acute change, with Type 2 change being intermediate and Type 3 change chronic. Type 1 change has been demonstrated in association with instability and it may be that changes progress from Type 1 to Type 2 as the spine stabilises, with the converse occurring less frequently.

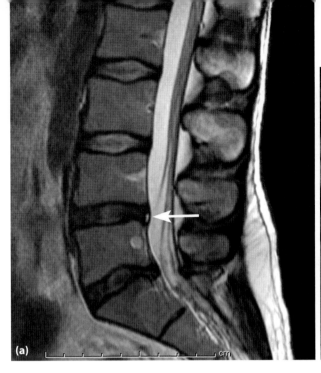

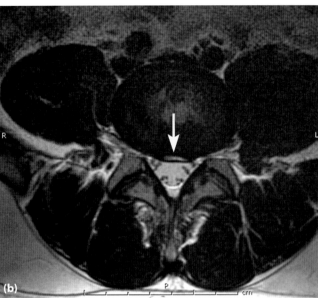

▲ **Fig. 8.156(a)** Sagittal and **(b)** axial T2-weighted MR images show a linear area of high signal in the peripheral posterior L4/5 intervertebral disc, indicating an annular tear (arrows).

Loss of disc height results in loss of tension of the surrounding ligaments, allowing hypermobility. Segmental motion has been shown to increase with the increasing severity of disc degeneration up to Grade IV, but to decrease when disc degeneration advances to Grade V. Presumably, at this latter stage osteophytes act to reduce movement. Facet joint osteoarthritis also has an effect on segmental motion (Fujiwara et al. 2000).

In a degenerate disc, small concentric tears form in the outer annular fibres and these may progress to radial tears. Hypointense degenerative discs on MRI have annular tears (see Fig. 8.156), and occasionally these can be visible as a linear area of hyperintensity on T2-weighted images described as a high-intensity zone (HIZ) (see Fig. 8.157). The high signal intensity is thought to represent neovascularity. There is ongoing debate as to whether a HIZ is a predictor of a painful disc. Hyperintensity and enhancement of an annular tear do not indicate activity of the tear (Munter et al. 2002).

The terminology for the altered morphology of a degenerate disc is as follows:

- *Annular bulge:* a generalised expansion of the disc concentrically beyond the vertebral body margin (see Fig. 8.158).

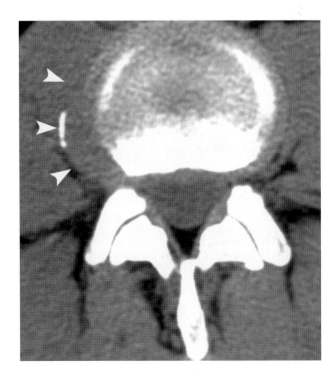

▲ **Fig. 8.157** Linear hyperintensity is noted in the annulus of this degenerative disc on a T2-weighted image (arrow). This is a high-intensity zone (HIZ) and it is debated whether this indicates a painful disc.

▲ **Fig. 8.158** An annular bulge is a generalised expansion of the disc beyond the vertebral body margin (arrowheads).

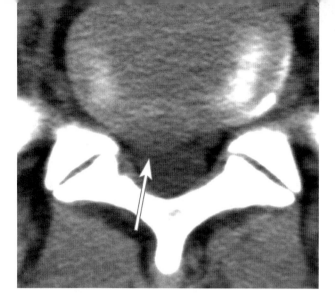

▲ **Fig. 8.159** A disc protrusion is a smooth focal or broad-based expansion of the intervertebral disc beyond its normal margin (arrow).

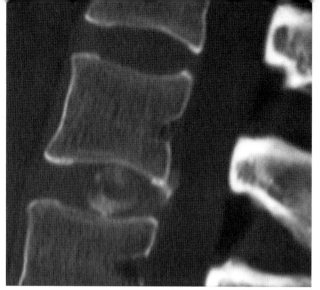

▲ **Fig. 8.160** A disc extrusion implies rupture of the annulus with a fragment of nucleus pulposis passing through the annular defect. This sagittal CT reconstruction shows the extrusion of calcified disc nuclear material with the fragment extending behind the vertebral body.

- *Disc protrusion:* a focal or broad-based smooth expansion of the annulus beyond the vertebral margin with an intact outer annulus (see Fig. 8.159).
- *Disc extrusion:* a disrupted outer annulus. The extruded fragment may migrate but remains beneath the posterior longitudinal ligament (PLL) (see Fig. 8.160).
- *Sequestrated disc:* a free disc fragment within the epidural space (see Fig. 8.161).
- *Herniation:* a general term encompassing abnormal morphology other than the annular bulge when precise characterisation is not possible.

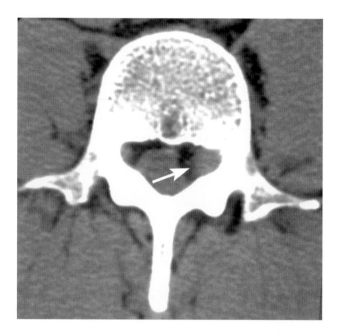

▶ **Fig. 8.161(a)** A sequestrated disc is a separated disc fragment that lies in the epidural space and moves often within this space to produce nerve compression (arrow).
▼ **(b)** T1- and T2-weighted MR images demonstrate a large L4/5 disc fragment almost completely obliterating the exit foramen at this level (arrows). Note the high endplate marrow signal at L5, which is brighter on the T2 image (Modic Type 1).

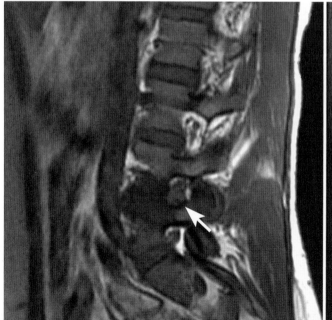

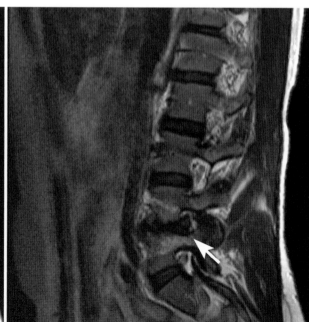

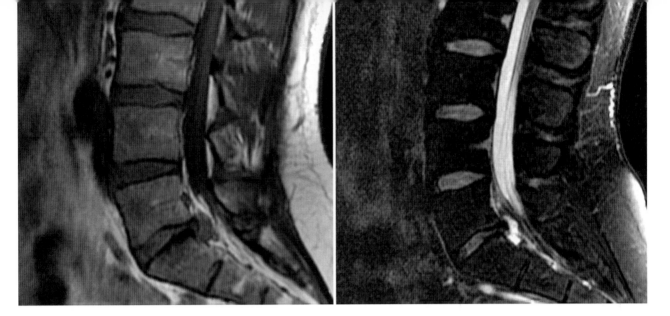

▲ **Fig. 8.162** Bleeding has occurred in conjunction with an L5/S1 disc protrusion. The haematoma is demonstrated on sagittal T1-weighted and STIR MR images.

People without back pain or radiculopathy can have abnormal MRI studies that show a disc protrusion. However, there is evidence that extrusions are more specific and are not usually found in asymptomatic populations (Weishaupt et al. 1998). An extruded disc fragment invokes a foreign body reaction and results in an inflammatory response that may cause pain. Granulation tissue may develop and further contribute to the mass effect. Disc extrusions with associated inflammation and granulation tissue have areas of high signal on T2-weighted MRI and have a better prognosis, being more likely to resorb and regress spontaneously. Hypointense disc extrusions are unlikely to resorb and carry a worse prognosis. A sequestrated fragment may have an associated haematoma that will regress (see Fig. 8.162).

There are two proposed mechanisms of disc herniation. The first is propulsion of material from the nucleus pulposus through a radial annular tear as a result of increased intradiscal pressure. The second is an endplate avulsion mechanism in which there is passage of disc material and osteochondral endplate fragments through a defect at the disc margin. The extruded portion of a disc contains material from the nucleus. Cartilage endplate material of presumed avulsive origin within the herniated disc has been shown experimentally to be associated with reduced inflammation and reduced neovascularisation, which may explain the poorer prognosis of some disc extrusions. Vertebral endplate abnormalities on MRI are associated with cartilaginous endplate fragments in the extruded material (Schmid et al. 2004).

Epidural fibrosis secondary to previous surgical intervention can be distinguished from recurrent disc extrusion on MRI with intravenous gadolinium. A disc fragment will show only rim enhancement (see Fig. 8.163), whereas a surgical scar

▼ **Fig. 8.163(a)** There is a large sequestrated disc fragment at L5/S1, demonstrated on a sagittal T2-weighted MR image (left image). Following intravenous gadolinium, there is corresponding rim enhancement on the T1-weighted image (arrows). **(b)** An axial image demonstrates the disc fragment (arrow).

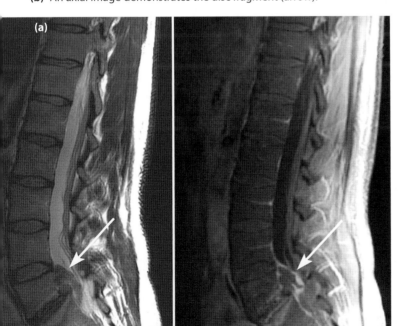
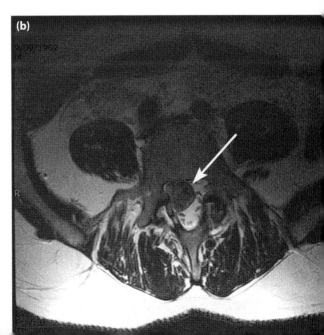

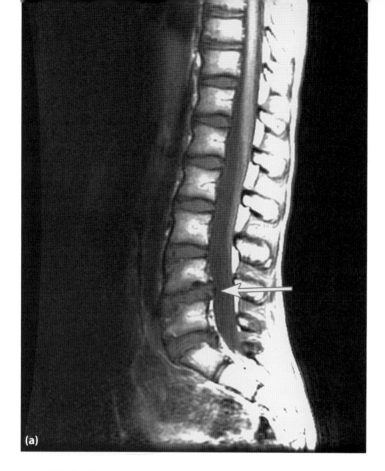

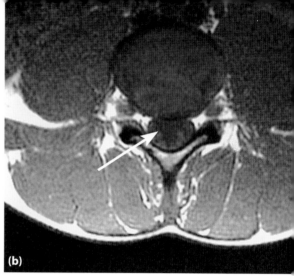

◀▲ **Fig. 8.164(a) and (b)** Sagittal and axial T1-weighted MR images demonstrate a focal central posterior L5/S1 disc protrusion (arrows).

will show diffuse enhancement. Thoracic intervertebral disc protrusions are commonly calcified and the vast majority of these will resolve without the need for surgery.

Nerve root compression

The effect of disc herniation depends on its location in relation to the nerves and its size in relation to the diameter of the spinal canal and exit foramina. Mechanical nerve root compression and nerve root irritation secondary to reactive inflammation around extruded nucleus material are both likely causes of sciatica. Simple contact of disc material with a nerve root is infrequently associated with symptoms. MRI can demonstrate disc contact with a nerve root,

◀▼ **Fig. 8.165(a) and (b)** Sagittal and axial T2-weighted MR images show a focal right posterolateral disc protrusion that encroaches significantly on the right lateral spinal recess (arrows). Note the high endplate marrow signal on the sagittal image.

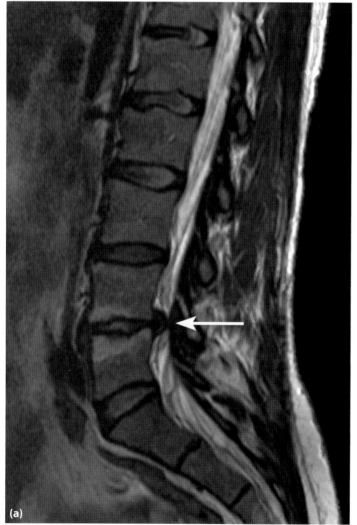

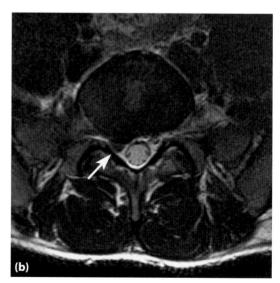

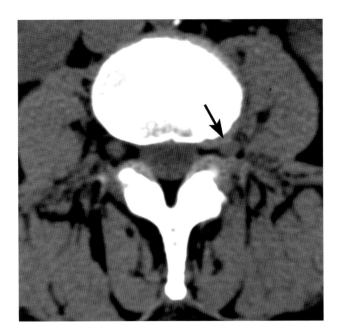

▲ **Fig. 8.166** A far lateral disc protrusion on the left side compresses and displaces the exiting nerve root beyond the neural foramen (arrow).

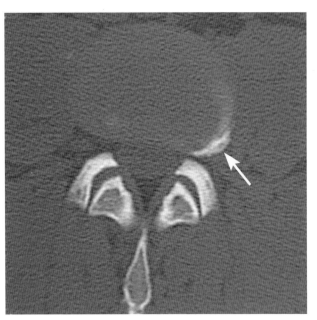

▲ **Fig. 8.167** Foraminal stenosis has been produced by a combination of osteophyte formation and a posterolateral disc protrusion (arrow).

nerve root displacement, nerve root compression and nerve root swelling immediately proximal or distal to the point of compression.

Nerve root compression with swelling is usually symptomatic (Weishaupt et al. 1998). A herniated central posterior (see Fig. 8.164) or posterolateral disc (see Fig. 8.165) may compress a nerve root within the spinal canal, lateral recess, neural exit foramen or beyond the foramen (far lateral protrusion) (see Fig. 8.166). Foraminal stenosis is usually due to disc margin osteophytes and associated annular bulging of the intervertebral disc (see Fig. 8.167). Facet joint hypertrophy can also narrow the neural exit foramen and contribute to nerve compression. Sequestrated or extruded fragments may cause compression almost anywhere (see Fig. 8.168).

Imaging patients in the seated position in both flexion and extension with an open 0.5T MR imager has more frequently demonstrated minor degrees of neural compression than conventional imaging. Positional pain differences appear related to position-dependent changes in foraminal size.

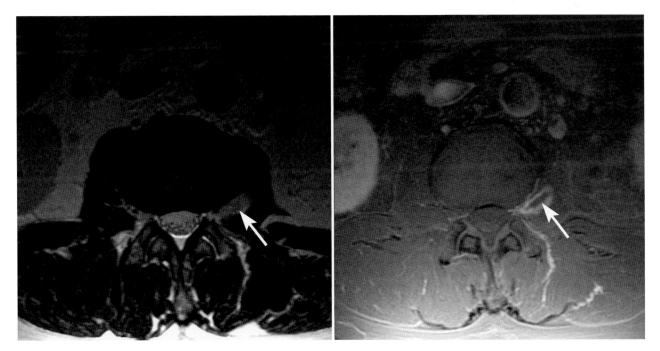

▲ **Fig. 8.168** A large far lateral left-sided disc extrusion is shown on axial T2 and fat-suppressed T1 post-intravenous gadolinium images. Note the rim enhancement following contrast, which confirms the disc fragment (arrows).

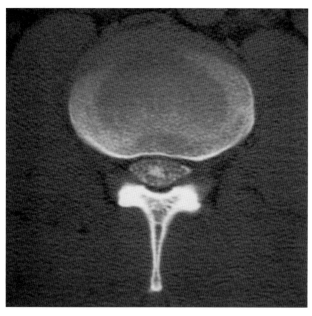

▲ **Fig. 8.169** An axial CT myelogram image demonstrates congenital spinal stenosis, with a reduction in all spinal canal dimensions.

Lumbar spinal canal stenosis

Central lumbar spinal canal stenosis may be developmental or acquired. Developmental canal stenosis is most commonly the result of short pedicles and may be asymptomatic, although such individuals are more susceptible to nerve root compression with mild degrees of superimposed acquired pathology. Spinal canal dimensions are substantially smaller in symptomatic patients than in asymptomatic controls (Pfirrmann et al. 2004) (see Figs 8.169, 8.170 and 8.171).

Acquired stenosis of the lumbar spinal canal is usually due to degenerative facet joint hypertrophy, with or without

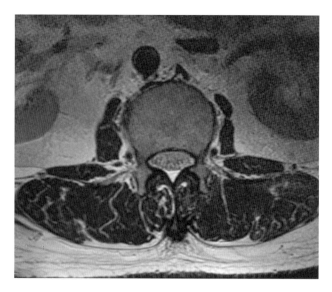

▲ **Fig. 8.170** An axial T2-weighted MR image demonstrates a developmental lumbar spinal stenosis due to short pedicles.

added spondylolisthesis and disc degeneration (see Fig. 8.172). Hypertrophy or buckling of the ligamentum flavum also often contributes to acquired stenosis (see Fig. 8.173).

Cross-sectional imaging measurements for central lumbar spinal canal stenosis are more accurate than plain film assessment. The published criteria include:

1. an AP diameter of less than 11.5 mm
2. an interpedicular distance (transverse diameter) of less than 16 mm
3. a canal cross-sectional area of less than 1.45 cm^2.

However, simple eyeball assessment of the images for thecal sac narrowing, obliteration of normal epidural fat planes and evidence of nerve root crowding and compression is usually sufficient and more meaningful.

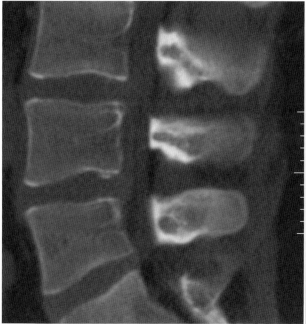
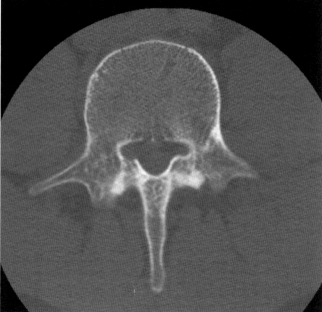

▲ **Fig. 8.171** Sagittal and axial CT images in this 23-year-old show marked developmental lumbar spinal canal stenosis.

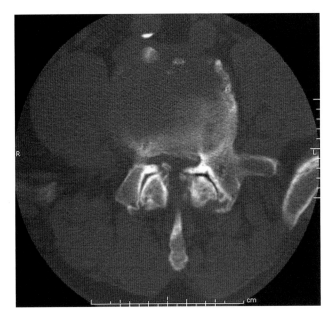

▲ **Fig. 8.172** An axial CT image shows the typical appearance of an acquired severe lumbar spine canal stenosis due to bilateral hypertrophic facet joint degeneration. Disc degeneration with marginal osteophyte formation is also present.

Facet joint degeneration

Facet joint osteoarthrosis may be primary or secondary. Primary osteoarthrosis can result from increased loading and abnormal movement which occurs in a facet joint that has an abnormal orientation (see Fig. 8.174). The most common cause of secondary osteoarthrosis is disc degeneration at the same level. The plain film changes of facet joint osteoarthrosis occur relatively late and include loss of articular

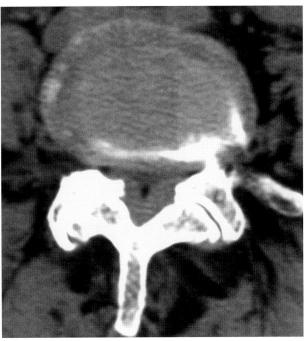

▲ **Fig. 8.173** A CT image demonstrates a severe central lumbar spinal canal stenosis due to the combined effects of marked hypertrophy of the ligamentum flavum, degenerative facet hypertrophy, a degenerative annulus bulge and developmentally short vertebral pedicles.

cartilage, subchondral sclerosis, subarticular cyst formation, bony hypertrophy with marginal osteophytic reaction and hypertrophy or buckling of the ligamentum flavum. Facet joint hypertrophic changes encroach on the subarticular gutter and result in lateral spinal recess stenosis

▼ **Fig. 8.174** Anomalous orientation of a facet joint predisposes the joint to the development of degenerative changes (arrows).

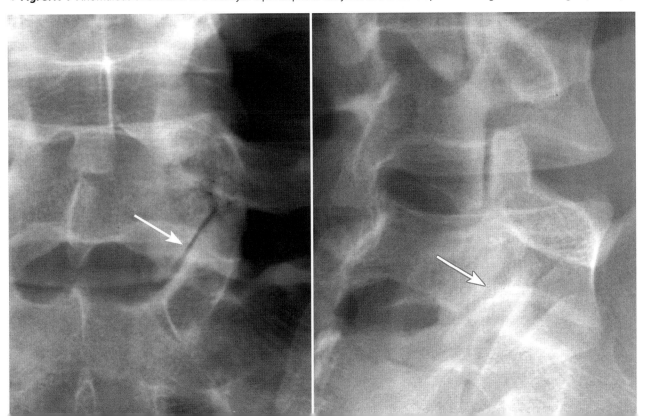

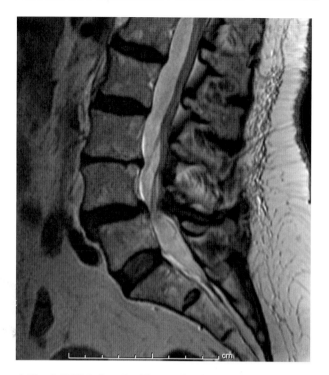

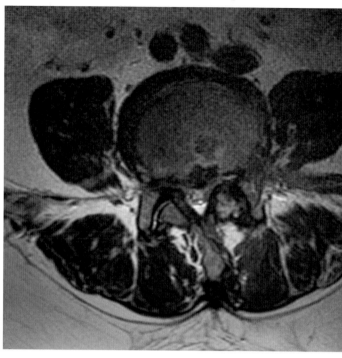

▲ **Fig. 8.175(a)** A sagittal T2-weighted MR image demonstrates diffuse degenerative changes at the lumbar discs and facet joints. The hypertrophic facet joints protrude into and cause narrowing of the spinal canal.

▲ **(b)** An axial T2-weighted image through the L5/S1 disc shows marked encroachment on the spinal canal by a combination of hypertrophic changes at the facet joints and degenerative disc disease, producing spinal canal stenosis.

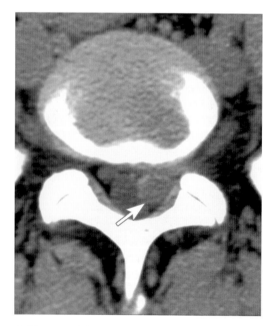

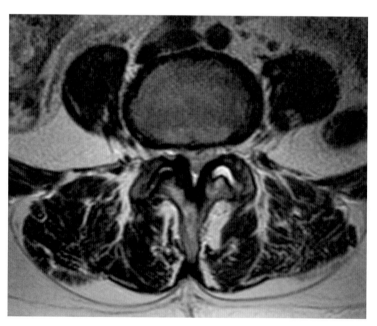

▲ **Fig. 8.176(a)** An axial CT image demonstrates a synovial cyst arising from a left-sided lumbar facet joint, encroaching on the left lateral spinal recess (arrow).

▲ **(b)** In another case, an axial T2-weighted MR image through the lower lumbar spine demonstrates peripheral calcification in a synovial cyst arising from the right-sided facet joint, resulting in right lateral recess stenosis.

(see Fig. 8.175). Facet joint subluxation, or degenerative spondylolisthesis, can result in central spinal canal stenosis and cause nerve compression. A facet joint synovial cyst may occasionally develop, causing posterolateral encroachment on the spinal canal, and is another potential source of nerve root compression. The cyst may be acutely painful if haemorrhagic, and may undergo rim calcification (see Fig. 8.176).

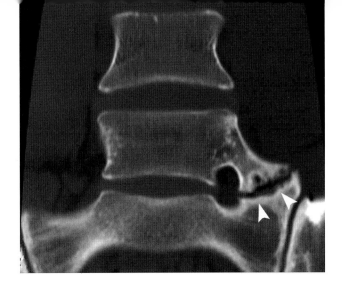

▲ **Fig. 8.177(a)** A coronal CT reformation demonstrates an elongated left L5 transverse process forming a pseudarthrosis with the left sacral wing. Degenerative changes have developed at the pseudarthrosis (arrowheads).

▼ **(b)** A nuclear bone scan demonstrates increased uptake of isotope at a pseudarthrosis on the left (arrow). The increased uptake of isotope is indicative of active degenerative changes.

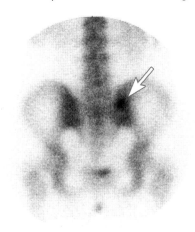

Lumbosacral pseudarthrosis

A developmentally enlarged transverse process of a transitional lumbosacral vertebra may articulate with the iliac wing or sacral ala and becomes painful if degenerative changes develop at the pseudarthrosis (see Fig. 8.177). Transitional vertebrae occur when there is sacralisation of L5 or lumbarisation of S1, and this anomaly may be unilateral (see Fig. 8.178(a)) or bilateral (see Fig. 8.178(b)). When the change is unilateral, there is often an associated lumbar scoliosis. The degenerative changes in a painful pseudarthrosis may respond to injection.

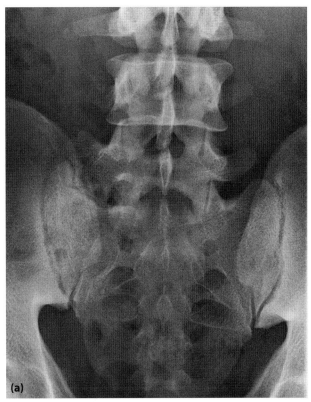

(a)

▲▼ **Fig. 8.178** Attempted sacralisation of L5 may be **(a)** unilateral or **(b)** bilateral (arrows).

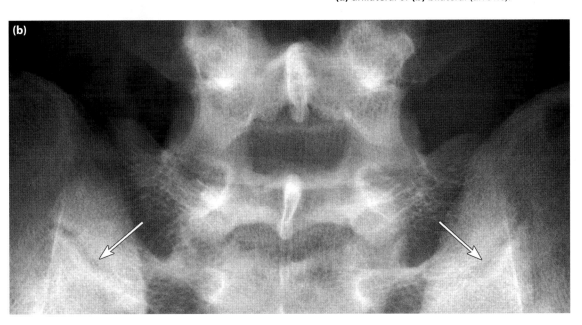

(b)

Idiopathic scoliosis

Idiopathic scoliosis most commonly occurs in female adolescents. There is deformity of the spine in three planes: coronal (lateral angulation), sagittal (straightening of the spine) and axial (rotation).

An erect AP x-ray of the thoracolumbar spine that includes the iliac crests is sufficient for an initial assessment. Curves are measured in the coronal plane using the Cobb angle. To measure this angle, the vertebrae with the greatest angulation at the upper and lower margins of the scoliosis are identified, and lines are drawn parallel to the upper and lower endplates, respectively, or to the pedicles if the endplates are not well seen. The perpendiculars to both these lines are drawn, and the angle between the intersecting perpendicular lines is the Cobb angle (see Fig. 8.179). Fusion of the iliac crest apophyses is an indication of skeletal maturity, at which time there is no further progression of scoliosis. The Risser sign grades the iliac crest apophyseal development from lateral to medial, with Grade 4 being when an apophysis is persisting medially and Grade 5 when fusion is complete. A leg-length discrepancy of more than 1 cm, based on a comparison of the heights of the iliac crests on a weightbearing pelvic x-ray, can be a correctable factor in scoliosis. A method of measuring leg-length discrepancy is shown in Chapter 5.

A structural curve is present if the Cobb angle is more than 10° and there is rotation. Idiopathic curves occur over a length of six to eight vertebrae, and the common idiopathic curve patterns are right thoracic, left lumbar, thoracolumbar and right thoracic with left lumbar. Other curve patterns require consideration of underlying developmental anomalies or other pathology. Lateral tilting (without rotation) on an erect film, which resolves on a supine film in an adolescent, is a sign of disc protrusion. A painful scoliosis always requires further investigation and may be due to an underlying tumour such as osteoid osteoma (Cummine et al. 2005).

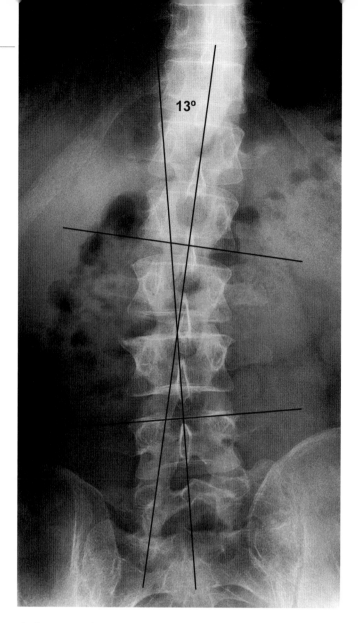

▲ **Fig. 8.179** There is a moderate lumbar scoliosis convex to the right. A pelvic tilt is noted to the right, raising the possibility of underlying leg-length discrepancy. The Cobb angle has been assessed.

Sacroiliac joints

The sacroiliac joints are strong inflexible joints due to their configuration and strong ligamentous supports. They are subjected to considerable stress in the young athlete. Imaging is generally unhelpful in sacroiliac joint strain and dysfunction, and the role of imaging is one of exclusion of other pathology such as inflammatory arthritis or infection.

The earliest plain film sign of seronegative inflammatory arthritis is subchondral bony erosion on the iliac side of the joint inferiorly. This causes loss of definition of the joint margins which is usually bilateral and symmetrical. Oblique views best demonstrate the joint spaces and joint margins. MRI is sensitive to changes of sacroiliitis, being able to demonstrate marrow oedema associated with early erosive change (see Fig. 8.180). The erosions are followed by bony sclerosis and ankylosis.

The radiographic grading of sacroiliitis changes in ankylosing spondylitis is as follows:

- *Grade 0:* Normal.
- *Grade 1:* Suspicious, with non-specific blurring of the joint margins.
- *Grade 2:* Minimal sclerosis, minor erosions.
- *Grade 3:* Severe erosions, widening of the joint space, definite sclerosis, some ankylosis.
- *Grade 4:* Complete ankylosis.

Osteitis condensans ilii is manifest as sclerosis on the iliac side of the joint. However, the joint margins remain well preserved, differentiating it from pathological conditions.

Septic arthritis at the sacroiliac joint is usually unilateral. Plain films are initially normal. CT can show early destructive changes and facilitate needle aspiration. MRI is sensitive to early and subtle sacroiliac joint and soft-tissue oedema and is the imaging test of choice.

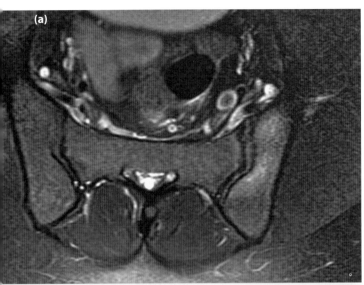

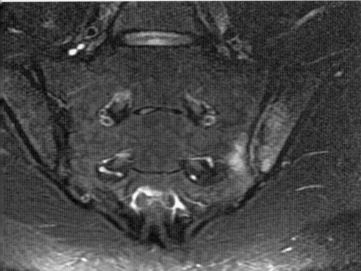

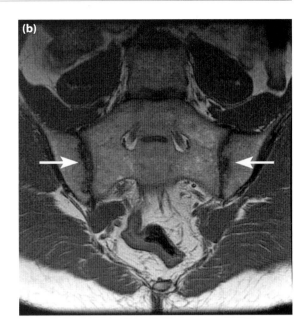

◀▲▼ **Fig. 8.180(a)** Axial and coronal STIR images are very sensitive to early bone marrow hyperintensity produced by sacroiliitis. The oedema precedes the erosive changes that may develop in the sacroiliac joints, shown in the lower image.
(b) This coronal T1-weighted MR image in a patient with enteropathic sacroiliitis shows bilateral asymmetrical sacroiliac joint erosions and sclerosis (arrows).
(c) Plain film changes appear late and include sclerosis with erosion of the joint margins.

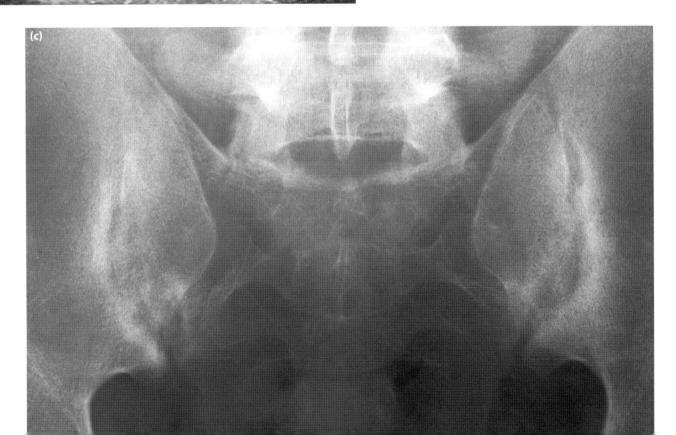

Mimics of traumatic disease

Discitis

Lumbar discitis occurs mostly in the second decade of life. Usually it is a primary infection of haematogenous origin caused by *staphylococcus aureus*. Frequently the clinical picture is one of non-specific back pain. The early imaging abnormalities are a single level increase in isotope uptake on nuclear bone scanning, and hyperintensity of both the disc and adjacent endplates on MRI. MR imaging findings with a high sensitivity for discitis include the presence of paraspinal or epidural inflammation, disc enhancement, hyperintensity of the disc on T2-weighted images, and erosion or destruction of at least one vertebral endplate. Plain film changes follow some weeks later with loss of intervertebral disc height and loss of definition of both adjacent vertebral endplates. With progression, there is increased lysis of the endplates followed by sclerosis as attempted healing occurs (see Fig. 8.181). Kyphosis and bony ankylosis may eventually result.

There are atypical manifestations of discitis where the classic findings may not be present, particularly if imaging is performed early in the course of the disease. For example, one or both endplates may appear normal, disc height may be normal or increased and there may be no enhancement following intravenous contrast. Serial MR imaging is helpful in these cases (Ledermann et al. 2003). Diffuse reactive bone marrow changes can be seen on MRI in the unaffected vertebrae of patients with infectious spondylitis (Stabler et al. 2000). Tuberculous discitis is characterised by calcification in the paraspinal soft-tissue inflammation, subligamentous spread and relatively late involvement of the disc compared to the bone (see Fig. 8.182).

Disc calcification in children

Disc calcification in children is a self-limiting condition, involving children 6–10 years old and manifests as acute pain and stiffness (see Fig. 8.183). The incidence between the sexes is equal and the cervical spine is the region most commonly involved. A disc protrusion may be associated. The condition resolves spontaneously over a few days or weeks with the disappearance of both the symptoms and the calcification. The cause is unknown (Resnick and Niwayama 1988).

▼ **Fig. 8.182** A coronal fat-suppressed T1-weighted image following intravenous gadolinium shows enhancement of tuberculous vertebral body osteomyelitis and a paravertebral abscess in the lower thoracic spine.

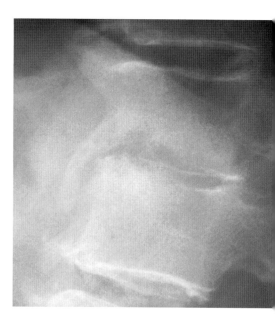

▲ **Fig. 8.181** There is destruction of neighbouring endplates at the T12/L1 level. Sclerosis and new bone formation indicate healing. The appearance is typical of discitis.

▼ **Fig. 8.183** Calcification is present in the C6/7 disc space, bulging anteriorly beneath the anterior longitudinal ligament (arrow). Pain and stiffness were present. The cause of this condition is unknown. Resolution was spontaneous.

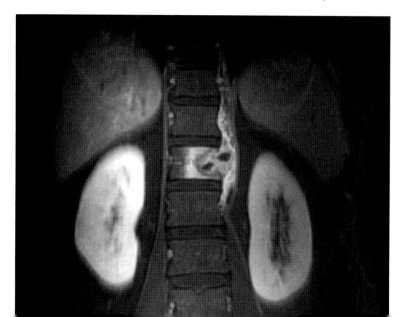

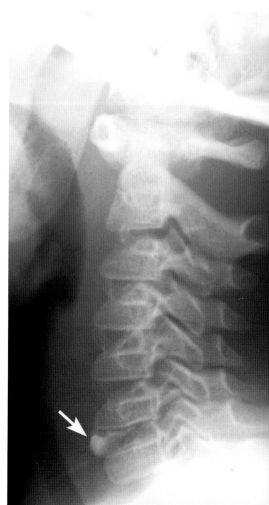

Spondyloarthropathy

Spondyloarthritis affects up to 2% of the population. Early diagnosis and treatment are important for improving the outcome. MRI detects the early oedematous stage of spondyloarthritis, characterised by high signal intensity on fluid-sensitive fat-suppressed sequences, while plain film changes of sclerosis are late and represent the post-inflammatory phase.

The early features of spondyloarthropathy are:

- anterior and posterior spondylitis (Romanus lesion), with inflammation at the site of attachment of the annulus fibrosis to the anterior and posterior vertebral body margins (an enthesitis)
- spondylodiscitis (Andersson lesion), with inflammatory involvement of the disc and endplates, progressing to endplate erosion (see Fig. 8.184)
- inflammatory arthritis of the facet, costotransverse or costovertebral joints
- enthesitis, typically at the interspinous ligament attachment to the spinous processes.

All of these manifestations can be detected in the early stage by MR imaging. Usually, these changes are accompanied by sacroiliitis, which can also be demonstrated early by MRI (Hermann et al. 2005).

Osteoid osteoma

In the spine, the classical although non-specific presentation of osteoid osteoma is a painful scoliosis. As elsewhere in the skeleton, the cardinal imaging feature is a focus of bony sclerosis with a contained lucent nidus. However, a prominent sclerotic reaction is not always present and the nidus is not always lucent. Plain film diagnosis in the spine is frequently difficult as there is considerable overlap of bony structures. A scoliosis is commonly present, and the osteoma is usually located at the apex

▲ **Fig. 8.184** This sagittal CT image shows the typical changes of spondylodiscitis, with endplate erosions and prominent vertebral body sclerosis on both sides of the disc. There is also anterior vertebral body new bone formation beneath the anterior longitudinal ligament of L5.

of the scoliosis on the concave side. An area of sclerosis may be evident, most often involving the posterior elements (see Fig. 8.185). Thin-section CT scanning targeted to the abnormal area is the test most likely to be diagnostic for osteoid osteoma, but SPECT or MR imaging may be necessary beforehand if the abnormality is difficult to localise (see Fig. 8.186). MRI is sensitive to marrow oedema associated with an osteoid osteoma, but frequently fails to show the nidus.

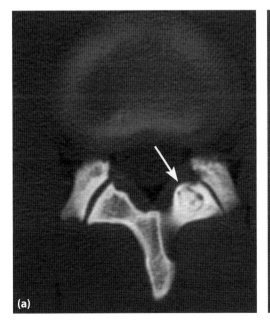

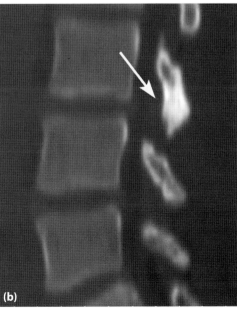

◀**Fig. 8.185** An Olympic athlete complaining of back pain was investigated by a lumbar CT examination, which disclosed a sclerotic expanded lamina containing a nidus within which was a sclerotic density (arrow). The clinical picture was consistent with an osteoid osteoma. The changes are demonstrated by **(a)** an axial CT scan (arrow) and **(b)** a reformatted sagittal image (arrow).

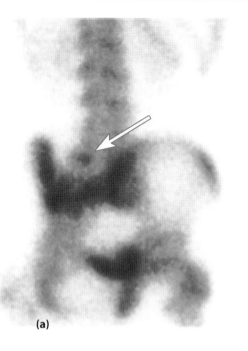
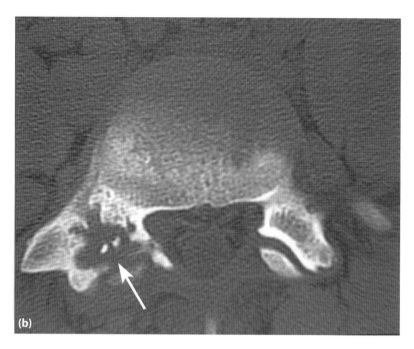

▲ Fig. 8.186(a) A nuclear bone scan demonstrates an area of increased uptake of isotope in the right side of the posterior arch of L5 (arrow). The appearances are non-specific and require characterisation by other imaging methods.
(b) A CT scan shows irregular destruction of the pedicle, extending into the facet articular surface (arrow). There is moderate sclerosis. Although atypical, this lesion proved to be an osteoid osteoma.

References

Alexander CJ. 'Scheuermann's disease. A traumatic spondylodystrophy?' *Skel Radiol* 1977, 1: 209.

Benedetti PF. 'MR imaging in emergency medicine.' *Radiographics* 1996, 16: 953–62.

Berge J, Marque B, Vital J-M, Senegas J, Caille J-M. 'Age-related changes in the cervical spine of front-line rugby players.' *Am J Sports Med* 1999, 27: 422–9.

Beutler W, Frederickson B, Murtland A et al. 'The natural history of spondylolysis and spondylolisthesis: 45-year follow-up evaluation.' *Spine* 2003, 28: 1027–35.

Campbell R, Grainger A, Hide I et al. 'Juvenile spondylolysis: a comparative analysis of CT, SPECT and MRI.' *Skeletal Radiol* 2005, 34: 63–73.

Cantu RC. 'The spinal stenosis controversy.' *Clin Sports Med* 1998, 17: 121–6.

Cummine JL, Stephen JPH, Taylor TKF. 'The role of the radiologist in the diagnosis of scoliosis: a new perspective.' www.spinecarefoundation.org (accessed 10 December 2005).

Dohrman GJ, Wagner FC, Buey PC. 'The microvasculature in transitory traumatic paraplegia: an electron microscopic study in the monkey.' *J Neurosurg* 1971, 35: 263–71.

Effendi B, Roy D, Cornish B, Dussault RG, Laurin CA. 'Fractures of the ring of the axis: a classification based on the analysis of 131 cases.' *J Bone Joint Surg* 1981, 63B: 319–27.

Fielding JW, Hawkins RJ. 'Atlantoaxial rotary subluxation.' *J Bone Joint Surg* 1977, 59: 37–44.

Flanders AE, Schaefer DM, Doan HT et al. 'Acute cervical spine trauma: correlation of MR imaging findings with degree of neurological deficit.' *Radiology* 1990, 177: 25–33.

Fujiwara A, Lim T-H, An HS, Tanaka N, J C-H, Andersson GBJ, Haughton VM. 'The effect of disc degeneration and facet joint osteoarthritis on the segmental flexibility of the lumbar spine.' *Spine* 2000, 25: 3036–44.

Gilbert FJ, Grant AM, Gillan MGC et al. 'Low back pain: influence of early MR imaging or CT on treatment and outcome: multicenter randomised trial.' *Radiology* 2004, 231: 343–51.

Harris JH Jr, Mirvis SE. *The Radiology of Acute Cervical Spine Trauma*, 3rd edn, Williams & Wilkins, 1996.

Harris JH Jr, Yeakley JS. 'Radiographically subtle soft tissue injuries of the cervical spine.' *Curr Probl Diagn Radiol* 1989, 18: 161–90.

Hayashi N, Masumoto T, Abe O et al. 'Accuracy of abnormal paraspinal muscle findings on contrast-enhanced MR images as indirect signs of unilateral cervical root-avulsion injury.' *Radiology* 2002, 223: 397–402.

Hellstrom M, Jacobsson B, Sward L et al. 'Radiologic abnormalities of the thoraco-lumbar spine in athletes.' *Acta Radiol* 1990, 31: 127–32.

Hermann K-GA, Althoff CE, Schneider U et al. 'Spinal changes in patients with spondyloarthritis: comparison of MR imaging and radiographic appearances.' *Radiographics* 2005, 25: 559–70.

Herkowitz HN, Samberg LC. 'Vertebral column injuries associated with tobogganing.' *J Trauma* 1978, 18: 806–10.

Herrick RT. 'Clay shoveler's fracture in power-lifting. A case report.' *Am J Sports Med* 1981, 9: 29–30.

Herzog RJ, Weins JJ, Dillingham MF. 'Normal cervical spine morphometry and cervical spine stenosis in asymptomatic professional football players. Plain film radiography, multiplaner computed tomography and magnetic resonance imaging.' *Spine* 1991, 16 (6 Suppl): 178–86.

Horne J, Cockshott WP, Shannon HS. 'Spinal column damage from water ski jumping.' *Skeletal Radiol* 1987, 8: 612–16.

Jarvik JG, Hollingworth W, Martin B et al. 'Rapid magnetic resonance imaging vs radiographs for patients with low back pain. A randomised controlled trial.' *J Am Med Assoc* 2003, 289: 2810–18.

Johnson AW, Weiss CB Jr, Stento K, Wheeler DL. 'Stress fractures of the sacrum.' *Am J Sports Med* 2001, 29: 498–508.

Keene JS. 'Thoracolumbar fractures in winter sports.' *Clin Orthop* 1987, 216: 39–49.

Kulkarni MV, McArdle CB, Kopanicky D et al. 'Acute spinal cord injury: MR imaging at 1.5T.' *Radiology* 1987, 164: 837–43.

Laredo JD, Bard M, Chretien J, Kahn MF. 'Lumbar posterior marginal intra-osseous cartilaginous node.' *Skeletal Radiol* 1986, 15: 201–8.

Ledermann HP, Schweitzer ME, MorrisonWB, Carrino JA. 'MR imaging findings in spinal infections: rules or myths?' *Radiology* 2003, 228: 506–14.

Levitz CL, Reilly PJ, Torg JS. 'The pathomechanics of chronic, recurrent cervical nerve root neuropraxia. The chronic burner syndrome.' *Am J Sports Med* 1997, 25: 73–6.

Maroon JC, Bailes JE. 'Athletes with cervical spine injury.' *Clin Sports Med* 1998, 17: 147–54.

Martin MD, Boxell CM, Malone DG. 'Pathophysiology of lumbar disc degeneration: a review of the literature.' *Neurosurg Focus* 2002, 13: 1–6.

Miller S, Congeni J, Swanson K. 'Long-term functional and anatomical follow-up of early detected spondylolysis in young athletes.' *Am J Sports Med* 2004, 32: 928–33.

Modic MT, Obuchowski NA, Ross LS et al. 'Acute low back pain and radiculopathy: MR imaging findings and their prognostic role and effect on outcome.' *Radiology* 2005, 237: 597–604.

Modic MT, Steinberg PM, Ross JS, Masaryk TJ, CarterJR. 'Degenerative disc disease: assessment of changes in vertebral body marrow with MR imaging.' *Radiology* 1988, 166: 193–9.

Mortelmans LJM, Geusens EAM et al. 'Harris or axis ring: an aid in diagnosing low (type 3) odontoid fractures.' *Europ J Surg* 1999, 165: 1138–41.

Munter FM, Wasserman BA, Wu H-M, Yousem DM. 'Serial MR imaging of annular tears in lumbar intervertebral discs.' *AJNR* 2002, 23: 1105–9.

Nuber GW, Schafer MF. 'Clay shoveler's injuries. A report of two injuries sustained from football.' *Am J Sports Med* 1987, 15: 182–3.

Oleson R, Nielson CS, Eiskjaer SP, Bunger CE. 'Spinal fractures in adults in bob-sled accidents.' *Ugeskr Laeger* 1995, 157: 1865–7.

Ong A, Anderson J, Roche J. 'A pilot study of the prevalence of lumbar disc degeneration in elite athletes with lower back pain at the Sydney 2000 Olympic Games.' *Br J Sports Med* 2003, 37: 263–6.

Pascal-Moussallard H, Broizat M, Cursolles J-C et al. 'Association of unilateral isthmic spondylolysis with lamina fracture in an athlete.' *Am J Sports Med* 2005, 33: 591–5.

Pavlov H, Torg JS, Robie B, Jahre C. 'Cervical spinal stenosis: determination with vertebral body ratio method.' *Radiology* 1987, 164: 771–5.

Pfirrmann CWA, Dora C, Schmid MR, Zanetti M, Hodler J, Boos N. 'MR image-based grading of lumbar nerve root compromise due to disc herniation: reliability study with surgical correlation.' *Radiology* 2004, 230: 583–8.

Rachbauer F, Sterzinger W, Eibl G. 'Radiographic abnormalities in the thoracolumbar spine of young elite skiers.' *Am J Sports Med* 2001, 29: 446–9.

Resnick D, Niwayama G. *Diagnosis of Bone and Joint Disorders*, 2nd edn, WB Saunders, Philadelphia, 1988.

Sairyo K, Katoh S, Sasa T et al. 'Athletes with unilateral spondylolysis are at risk of stress fracture at the contralateral pedicle and pars interarticularis.' *Am J Sports Med* 2005, 33: 583–90.

Schmid G, Witteler A, Willburger R, Kuhnen C, Jergas M, Koester O. 'Lumbar disk herniation: correlation of histologic findings with marrow signal intensity changes in vertebral endplates at MR imaging.' *Radiology* 2004, 23: 352–8.

Schmitt H, Gerner H. 'Paralysis from sport and diving accidents' *Clin J of Sports Med* 2001, 11: 17–22.

Soler T, Calderon C. 'The prevalence of spondylolysis in the Spanish athlete.' *Am J of Sports Med* 2000, 28: 57–62.

Sorenson KH. *Scheuermann's Juvenile Kyphosis*, Munksgaard, Copenhagen, 1964.

Stabler A, Doma AB, Baur A, Kruger A, Reiser MF. 'Reactive bone marrow changes in infectious spondylitis: quantitative assessment with MR imaging.' *Radiology* 2000, 217: 863–8.

Tewes DP, Fischer DA, Quick DC, Zamberletti F, Powell J. 'Lumbar transverse process fractures in professional football players.' *Am J Sports Med* 1995, 23: 507–9.

Torg JS. 'Epidemiology, pathomechanics and prevention of athletic injuries to the cervical spine.' *Med Sci Sports Exerc* 1985: 17: 295–303.

Torg JS, Naranja RJ Jr, Pavlov H, Galinat BJ, Warren R, Stine RA. 'The relationship of developmental narrowing of the cervical spinal canal to reversible and irreversible injury of the cervical spinal cord in football players.' *J Bone Joint Surg (Am)* 1996, 78: 1308–14.

Torg JS, Pavlov H, Genuario SE, Sennett B, Wisneski RJ, Robie BH, Jahre C. 'Neuropraxia of the cervical spinal cord with transient quadriplegia.' *J Bone Joint Surg (Am)* 1986, 68: 1354–70.

Torg JS, Sennett B, Pavlov H et al. 'Spear tackler's spine.' *Am J Sports Med* 1993, 21: 40–9.

Torg JS, Sennett B, Vegso JJ, Pavlov H. 'Axial loading to the middle cervical spine segment. An analysis and classification of twenty-five cases.' *Am J Sports Med* 1991, 19: 6–20.

Toyone T. 'Vertebral bone marrow changes in degenerative lumbar disc disease. An MR study of 74 patients with low back pain.' *J Bone Joint Surg (Br)* 1994, 76: 757–64.

Weishaupt D, Zanetti M, Hodler J, Boos N. 'MR imaging of the lumbar spine: prevalence of intervertebral disc extrusion and sequestration, nerve root compression, end plate abnormalities, and osteoarthritis of the facet joints in asymptomatic volunteers.' *Radiology* 1998, 209: 661–6.

Weishaupt D, Zanetti M, Hodler J, Min K, Fuchs B, Pfirrmann CWA, Boos N. 'Painful lumbar disk derangement: relevance of endplate abnormalities at MR imaging.' *Radiology* 2001, 218: 420–7.

Williams B. 'Orthopaedic features in the presentation of syringomyelia.' *J Bone Joint Surg* 1979, 61B: 314–23.

Wojtys EM, Ashton-Miller JA, Huston LJ, Moga PJ. 'The association between athletic training time and the sagittal curvature of the immature spine.' *Am J Sports Med* 2000, 28: 490–8.

Yeo JD, Walsh J, Rutkowski S et al. 'Mortality following spinal cord injury.' *Spinal Cord* 1998, 36: 329–36.

Image acknowledgments

The authors wish to thank the following colleagues who kindly offered images for inclusion in this chapter:

- Dr Jennie Noakes supplied 8.96, 8.101(a) and (b), 8.102, 8.134, 8.138, 8.139, 8.146, 8.148, 8.156(a) and (b), 8.160, 8.161(a) and (b), 8.162, 8.163(a), 8.165(a) and (b), 8.168, 8.169, 8.170, 8.171, 8.176(a) and (b), 8.177(a), 8.180(a), (b) and (c), 8.182, and 8.184.
- Dr Tony Peduto supplied images 8.13, 8.67(a) and (b), 8.87, 8.90, 8.91, 8.94, 8.115(a) and (b), and 8.116.
- Dr David Brazier and Sandy Huggett at the Royal North Shore MRI supplied figures 8.11, 8.12(a) and (b), 8.57, 8.58, 8.59, 8.69, 8.73(a) and (b), 8.79, 8.80(a) and (b), 8.98(a) and (b).
- Dr Raouli Risti, Adam Loveday and Adam Hill at the Gosford Hospital CT and MRI supplied figures 8.9, 8.10, 8.29(a), (b) and (c), 8.49, 8.50, 8.51, 8.52(a), (b) and (c), 8.53, 8.54, 8.55, 8.61, 8.62(a), 8.63(a) and (b), 8.64, 8.92(a) and (b).
- Dr Robert Cooper and Dr Stephen Allwright supplied images 8.1, 8.2, 8.3, 8.4, 8.5, 8.6, 8.119 and 8.122.
- Dr Jim Roche supplied figures 8.104 and 8.105.

These images have significantly added to the quality of the chapter.

The face, jaw and larynx
Jock Anderson and John Read

Sports-related facial trauma is a common injury and occurs in a great variety of different sporting activities. Facial soft-tissue trauma such as abrasions, cuts and bruises is extremely common, is generally unreported and rarely requires imaging unless an associated fracture or foreign bodies are suspected. So, when discussing facial injuries, the authors are almost always referring to facial fractures.

As might be anticipated, these injuries are most often seen in contact sports such as football, basketball, rugby, field hockey, martial arts and boxing, often caused by head clashes or contact with a knee or an elbow. Injuries may also occur from impact with sporting equipment, such as surfboards, skis, handlebars, hockey sticks, balls and bats (see Fig. 9.1). The more severe facial injuries are generally associated with high-velocity activities such as skiing, motor sports, cycling and equestrian pursuits. The frequency of facial injuries in particular sports has resulted in rule changes and the introduction of facial and mouth guards. In spite of these precautions, facial injuries can occur accidentally and unexpectedly in almost any sporting activity (see Fig. 9.2).

The incidence of facial fractures in sport: a literature review

In 2005, Romeo et al. published an article in the sports medicine literature reviewing facial trauma which stated that 10–42% of all such injuries occurred during a sporting activity. A finding common to many studies was that facial fractures occur predominantly in males aged less than 40, which is not surprising as this particular demographic is the most likely to be attracted to violent sports and to become involved in fights. The wide spectrum of sports producing facial injuries reflects the extensive variety of sports played in the countries in which the studies were performed. The following studies highlight the large variation in sports and associated injuries found in the literature.

A report from Cork in Ireland (Carroll et al. 1995) found that of all the facial injuries resulting from sport, 94.5% occurred in males and almost half of these injuries occurred playing Gaelic games. It is of no surprise that more than 50% of reported injuries were nasal fractures.

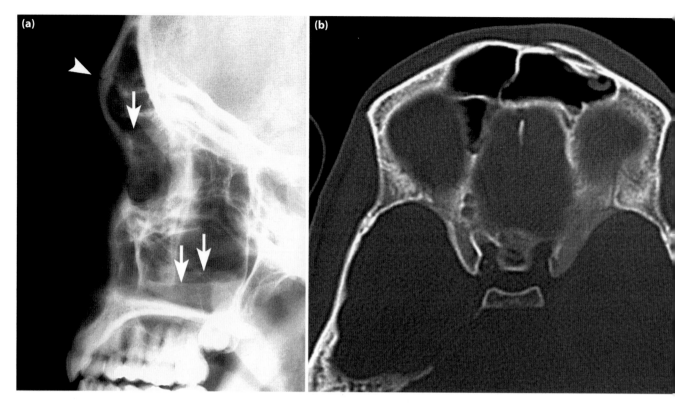

▲ **Fig. 9.1(a)** A surfer was struck on the forehead by a surfboard, causing a deep laceration. A subsequent plain film shows an associated fracture extending across the anterior wall of the frontal sinus (arrowhead). This lateral view has been acquired in the erect position and fluid levels are seen in the frontal sinus and in both maxillary antra (arrows). Fluid levels are commonly produced by haemorrhage associated with a fracture. **(b)** The bone injury is much easier to see on an axial CT image, which demonstrates comminution of the anterior wall of the frontal sinus with slightly depressed fragments.

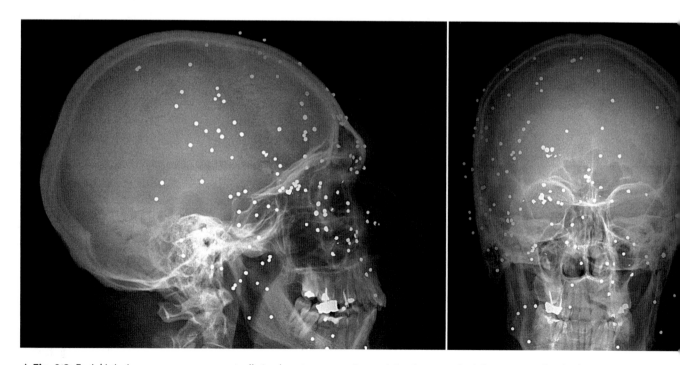

▲ **Fig. 9.2** Facial injuries may occur unexpectedly in almost any sporting activity. A young duck-hunter was shot by his companion when his movement in the undergrowth was mistaken for game. Bird-shot is scattered throughout the soft tissues of his face and unfortunately caused serious eye injuries.

Another report from The University Hospital in Bern (Switzerland) (Exadaktylos et al. 2004) found that of 750 patients with facial injuries, 90 (12%) suffered sports-related maxillofacial fractures. Of these, 27% were due to skiing and snowboarding. Soccer and ice hockey together accounted for 22% of injuries, and 21% were caused by cycling accidents. In addition, 68% of the cyclists, 50% of the ice hockey players and footballers and 48% of the skiers and snowboarders had isolated mid-face fractures.

Reporting from Innsbruck in Austria, Gassner et al. (1999) found that mountain bikers suffered a surprisingly high percentage of serious facial fractures. Cycling-related trauma represented 31% of all sports injuries and almost 50% of all traffic accidents. Of the 60 mountain bikers in this study, 55% had facial bone fractures, compared with 34.5% in street cyclists. Amazingly, 15.2% of the facial fractures in mountain bikers were LeFort type fractures, which are severe injuries causing gross disruption of the facial structure. These fractures are discussed later in the chapter.

In Australia, a review of 839 facial fractures from Adelaide, a stronghold of Australian Rules Football, found that 16.3% were sports-related (Lim et al. 1993). Males accounted for 93.4% of these cases, and 89% occurred in people less than 35 years. Australian Rules was associated with 52.6% of the injuries and cricket produced 14.6%. Horse-riding accidents produced the most severe injuries.

As interesting as these studies are, the great diversity of sports and conditions makes it difficult to extract information that can be helpful in dealing with facial trauma in other environments. Probably the most important advice to be gleaned is to avoid riding a bike in Austria and, in particular, to avoid mountain biking!

Imaging facial injuries

Following a facial injury, imaging is required whenever a fracture or foreign body is clinically suspected. Gradually, over the last decade, the use of plain films as the initial method of imaging facial trauma has decreased. This change has been driven by the continuous technological improvement and increased availability of CT, which is now the preferred initial imaging method. CT has been found to be more efficient, accurate, safe and cost-effective for the evaluation of facial injuries (Turner et al. 2004). Multi-detector CT (MDCT) has become the gold standard for imaging facial bones (see Fig. 9.3). The application of this technology to facial bone imaging is demonstrated and discussed later in the chapter.

In 2004, Turner et al. published findings of a study that examined the usage and cost of plain films and CT for facial bone injury in a level 1 trauma centre in 1992 and compared this with equivalent data from 2002. In the past, plain films were used as a screening test to help select those who might

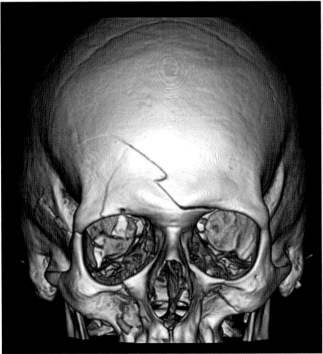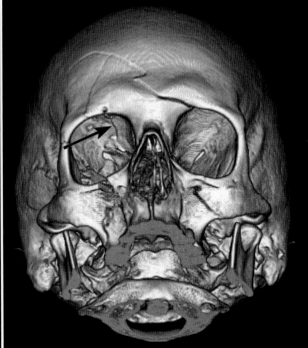

▲ **Fig. 9.3** Recent developments in CT technology have enabled the rapid acquisition of detailed volumetric scan data, which can then be post-processed to create reformatted 2D images in any plane or, as in this case, high-quality surface-rendered 3D images. These images greatly improve the surgical understanding of complex fractures. In the example shown here, a skydiving accident has produced highly complex fractures of the skull and facial bones. A fracture of the right frontal eminence extends posteroinferiorly into the temporal fossa and branches across the forehead to involve both superior orbital margins. The right supraorbital margin fracture extends posteriorly across the orbital roof (arrow) and lesser wing of the sphenoid, to involve the superior orbital fissure. Fractures also involve both inferior orbital margins and maxillae. There is a 'tripod' pattern of fracture on the right, with a depression of the zygomatic arch and rotation of the body of zygoma.

benefit from a CT scan. As a consequence, a significant number of patients had both tests. The plain film series for facial trauma is time-consuming and delivers significant exposure to radiation. The basic series includes Water's, Caldwell, lateral and basal views, with the additional possibility of nasal bone views. If there is also a mandibular series, AP mandible, reversed Towne's and oblique views of the mandible will be added. The radiation exposure is then further increased by having a CT scan, often including both axial and coronal acquisitions. Turner et al. found that in 1992 30% of patients had both plain films and single detector row CT. An interesting observation from this study was that the trend to increased use of CT and corresponding decreased use of radiography over a decade was not only cost-effective but also resulted in a lower overall radiation dose.

Although the skills needed for acquiring and examining plain films may not be called upon as much as in the past, these skills must be maintained for those occasions when CT is unavailable or not functioning. In remote areas in particular, plain films are still used for the diagnosis of facial injury and for the selection of patients who require transportation to a regional centre for CT. Consequently, it is still important to know which plain film views to request, how these views should be acquired and how they should be assessed.

Standard plain film views of the facial bones

If CT is unavailable, and plain films are to be acquired, multiple projections are necessary to assess the facial bone complex. In a patient who is able to sit or stand, a minimum series should include lateral, Caldwell, Water's and possibly basal views. An ideal series should include erect films for the detection of fluid levels and, if possible, the Water's and Caldwell views should be acquired posteroanterior, to increase detail resolution by reducing magnification. However, in practice, if the patient is seriously injured, supine and cross-table films may be all that are possible. Most likely, the patient will then be transported to the nearest regional centre with a CT service. For the badly injured patient, CT also provides an opportunity to examine the cervical spine and intracranial structures at the same time as the facial trauma. If a CT scan is inevitable on clinical grounds, plain films are totally unnecessary. A further important consideration is that hyperextension of the cervical spine is necessary for the Water's and basal plain film views, and movement may be unwise if any cervical spine injury is also suspected. With MDCT's ability to rapidly acquire a volume of data from which reformatted 2D images can be obtained in any plane, patient positioning need not be precise and the patient can remain comfortably immobilised.

Lateral view

To obtain a lateral view, the patient sits or stands with the side of their head against an upright bucky. The head is positioned with its sagittal plane parallel to the film and orbits at the same level. The orbitomeatal line is horizontal. The orbitomeatal line is the radiographic baseline of the skull and is a line drawn

from corner of the eye (outer canthus) to the external auditory meatus. For a lateral view, the tube is straight with the beam centred on the zygoma (see Fig. 9.4).

A true lateral view superimposes the orbits, maxillary antra and mandibular condyles. Consequently, anatomical detail may be difficult to identify. In spite of this, the view provides the best display of the sphenoidal sinus, the anterior and posterior walls of the frontal sinuses, and the anterior and posterior walls of the maxillary antra. The mandibular condyles may also be assessed (see Fig. 9.5). If the film has been taken erect, fluid levels may be seen. The presence of fluid levels increases the likelihood of a fracture.

Caldwell view

A Caldwell view is a valuable PA projection of the facial bones. The patient is positioned facing the bucky with their nose and forehead touching the bucky. The head is then positioned so that the orbitomeatal line is perpendicular to the bucky. The beam is centred to pass through the bridge of the nose

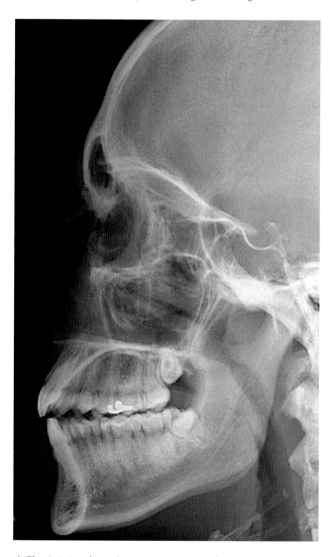

▲ **Fig. 9.4** In a lateral view, assessment of some anatomical structures is difficult due to superimposition. However, important information is nevertheless available, as will be discussed later.

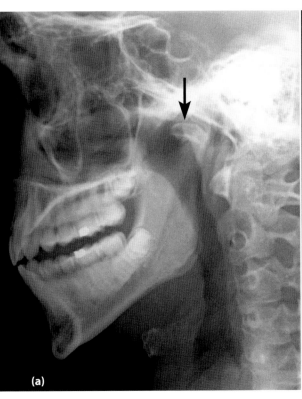
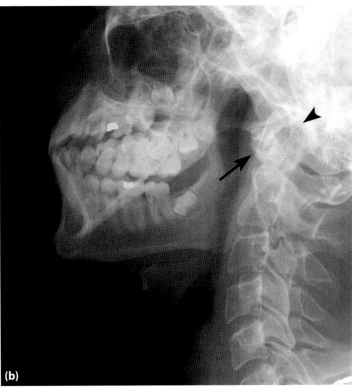

(a)
(b)

▲ **Fig. 9.5** In a correctly positioned lateral view of the facial bones, the mandibular rami, angles and bodies are superimposed. Deformity of the mandible may still be identified and, in particular, the condyles should be inspected to confirm that these lie in a normal position.

(a) In this case, there is fracture-dislocation of the right mandibular condyle. The displaced and dislocated right mandibular condyle can be identified (black arrow).

(b) The injury is confirmed on an oblique view, which shows the displaced condyle (black arrow) and an empty temporal articular fossa (arrowhead).

and with 15° caudal angulation to the orbitomeatal line. The margins of the upper half of the orbits, frontal sinuses and ethmoidal sinuses are all well displayed in this projection. However, the maxillary and sphenoidal sinuses are obscured by the superimposition of basal structures (see Fig. 9.6). As discussed later, by increasing the tube angle or by changing the centring position, the petrous ridge will be projected below the inferior orbital margin and the entire orbit may be demonstrated and assessed. This view is particularly useful for the examination of the medial wall of the orbit. Because the primary beam is at 15° to the horizontal plane, fluid levels will not be sharply defined.

▶ **Fig. 9.6** A Caldwell view is obtained with the tube angled 15° to the baseline of the skull. This projects the petrous ridge over the lower half of the orbits, obscuring the inferior orbital margins and other important structures. Nevertheless, this view is an important component of the facial bone series and is particularly valuable for assessment of the ethmoid air cells, the medial wall of the orbits, the superior orbital margin and the alveolar process of the maxilla, as shown later in Fig. 9.20.

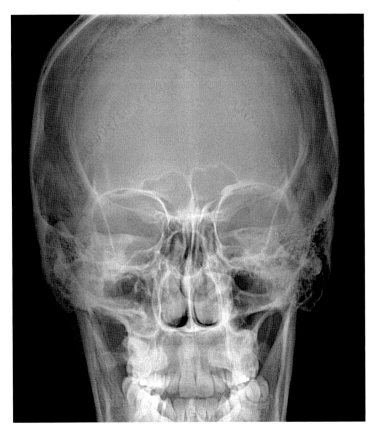

Water's view

A Water's view is an occipitomental projection. The patient is positioned with their chin resting on the surface of the upright bucky and their neck extended so that the baseline of the skull (the orbitomeatal line) is at 37 to 50° to the bucky. In this position, the tip of the nose will not be in contact with the bucky and is usually about 2 cm from the bucky's surface. A straight tube is used with the line of the primary beam passing through the corner of the eye.

Of all views, a Water's view is the most valuable as it demonstrates structures that are commonly injured and enables simple assessment of facial symmetry (see Fig. 9.7). The structures that are well demonstrated include the inferior orbital margins, the lateral walls of the maxillary antra, the zygomatic arches and the zygomaticofrontal sutures. Displacement of the nasal septum is best assessed on this view and, since a straight tube is used, fluid levels will be sharply defined.

▶ **Fig. 9.7** A Water's view presents facial bone symmetry more simply than seen in a Caldwell view. Important structures are presented without significant superimposition.

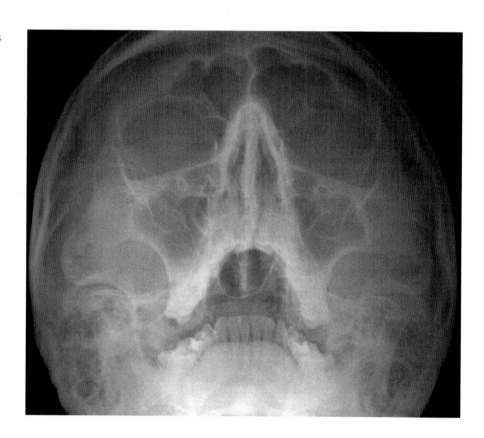

AP axial projection (reversed Towne's view)

A reversed Towne's view is specifically used to demonstrate the zygomatic arches and mandibular condyles (see Fig. 9.8). The patient rests the back of their head against the bucky and the baseline of the skull is at 90° to the bucky. There is a caudal tube angle of 30°, with the beam centred about 2–3 cm above the bridge of the nose. Coning to the area of interest improves definition of the image.

Basal view

A basal view is a submentovertical view, used to image the zygomatic arches and the lateral walls of the maxillary antra. If the view is obtained correctly, the arches will be demonstrated in profile (see Fig. 9.9). This view should not be attempted if there is possibility of cervical spine trauma, as the cervical spine has to be extended as much as the patient can manage, attempting to place the baseline of the skull as near as possible to a plane parallel to the bucky. The tube is angled to be at 90° to the arches, with the beam centred midway between the arches.

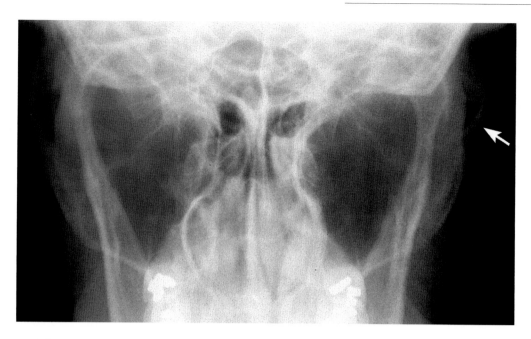

◀**Fig. 9.8(a)** A reversed Towne's view is valuable for demonstrating the zygomatic arches and the mandibular condyles. In this case, there is a depressed fracture of the left zygomatic arch (arrow).

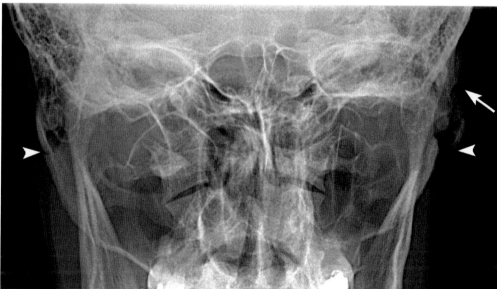

◀**(b)** The zygomatic arches and mandibular condyles are well demonstrated on a reversed Towne's view. This case shows fractures of both zygomatic arches (arrowheads). Considerable displacement has occurred on the left. There is also a second fracture of the left zygomatic arch, which is depressed (arrow).

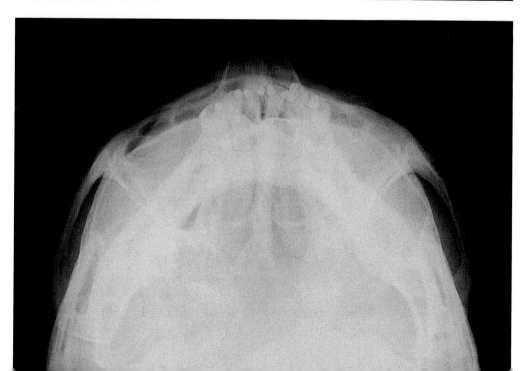

◀**Fig. 9.9** A normal basal view demonstrates the zygomatic arches in profile. This view allows identification of undisplaced zygomatic arch fractures with minor depression.

Nasal bone view

Injury to the nasal bones is common and there is an increasing tendency to diagnose and treat a broken nose on clinical grounds alone, without recourse to imaging. This means that nasal bone films are now requested less often. A complete radiographic series would traditionally include axial and both lateral projections. In practice, a single high-resolution coned lateral image is all that is necessary for assessment of the nasal bones and the anterior nasal spine of the maxilla (see Fig. 9.10). The nasal septum is usually well shown on a Water's view, but occasionally a CT is required to confirm a septal fracture (see Fig. 9.11). If associated ethmoidal or orbital involvement (nasoorbitalethmoid fracture) is suspected clinically, a CT scan is indicated (see Fig. 9.12).

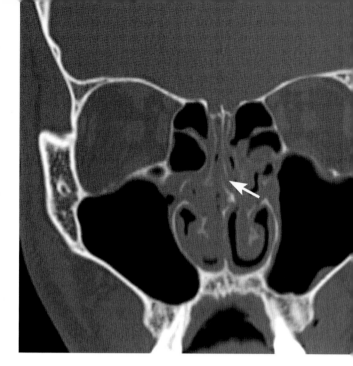

▲ **Fig. 9.11** Although the nasal septum is well demonstrated on a Water's view, a CT image is often necessary to definitely confirm the presence of a septal fracture (arrow).

▼ **Fig. 9.10** A nasal bone view demonstrates a minor fracture of the nasal bones with minimal depression of the distal tips. The anterior nasal spine appears normal (arrow). Note the groove of the nasociliary nerve running parallel to the profile of the nasal bones, and the nasomaxillary suture. The lines produced by the nasomaxillary and nasofrontal sutures are occasionally mistaken for fractures.

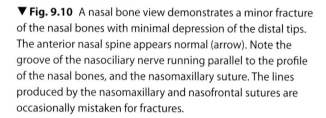

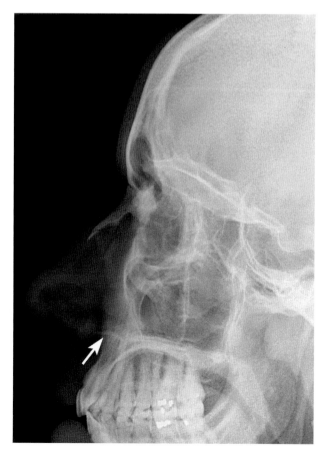

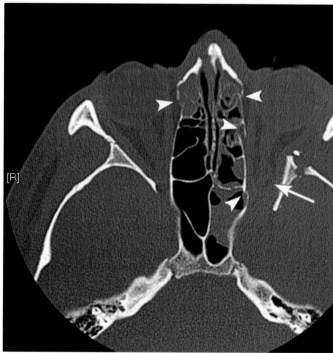

▲ **Fig. 9.12** An axial MDCT image demonstrates an extensive compressive injury to the middle third of the face. A nasoorbitalethmoid fracture has resulted. The fracture involves the right nasal bone with separation of the fragments and has extended posteriorly across the nasal septum into the ethmoid air cells. There is involvement of the medial walls of both orbits, particularly on the left where there are three fractures present (arrowheads). There is an undisplaced fracture of the lateral wall of the right orbit and comminution of the lateral wall of the left orbit. Note the widening of the left optic foramen, swelling of the adjacent extra-ocular muscle and subtle deformity of the related optic nerve segment. The possibility of an optic nerve injury is raised (arrow).

▶ **Fig. 9.13** Disturbances of bone and soft-tissue symmetry are often most easily appreciated on a Water's view. Note the minor mucosal thickening in both maxillary antra and the right nasal cavity in this case.

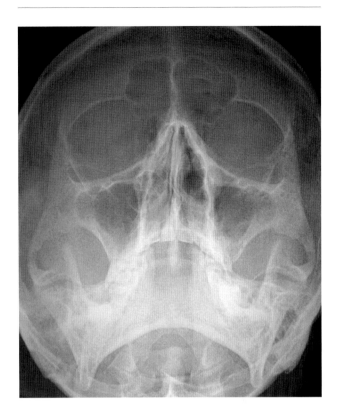

Tips on looking at plain films of the facial bones

There needs to be a disciplined approach to the assessment of a routine plain film series and it is important to know the radiographic anatomy demonstrated by the common views. The secret of identifying facial fractures is being able to recognise a loss of normal facial bone symmetry. It is a luxury for radiologists to have the normal side so readily available for comparison when unilateral injury has occurred (see Fig. 9.13). With the exception of air cell structures, symmetry is surprisingly precise. It is also important to know which structures are commonly injured by facial trauma, so that injury patterns can be recognised (see Fig. 9.14). The nasal bone, basal and Water's views are the easiest to examine. These views demonstrate structures that are commonly injured without being significantly obscured by radiographic superimposition. The Caldwell and lateral views are the most difficult to examine due to the anatomical complexity of the mid-face and inevitable superimposition.

The majority of facial fractures involve the orbits, so a disciplined and systematic examination of the orbits is always necessary. The orbital margins must be well displayed and carefully assessed, and the optic foramina and superior orbital fissures are important to inspect. Blowout fractures of the orbital floor are not uncommon and a search for this injury is an important part of the examination of the orbits (see Fig. 9.15). These fractures are discussed in detail later in the chapter. Fractures of the medial orbital wall may also be extremely subtle (see Fig. 9.16).

On reviewing each image, the first important assessment to make is whether the structures that should be displayed can be adequately assessed, and, if not, how an adjustment in radiographic positioning may improve the film.

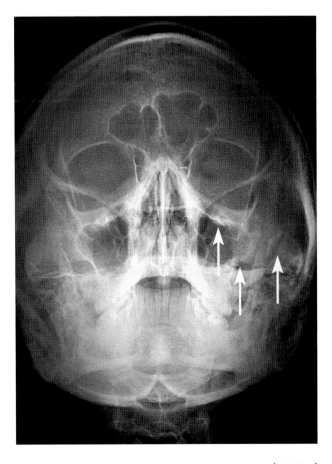

▶ **Fig. 9.14** Common injury patterns and disturbances of symmetry should be recognised. Fractures involve the left inferior orbital margin extending into the infraorbital foramen, the lateral wall of the antrum, and the junction of the body of the left zygoma and zygomatic arch (arrows). There is also minor displacement at the left zygomaticofrontal suture, with rotation of the zygoma. These fractures are not easily seen and could be overlooked. The diagnosis depends on noting the subtle loss of symmetry, which correlates with a common injury pattern known as a tripod fracture (discussed later in the chapter).

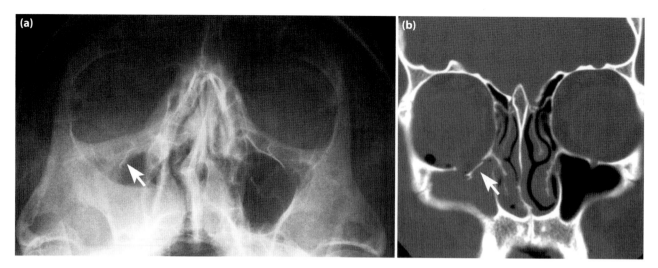

▲ **Fig. 9.15(a)** There is a large collection of fluid in the right maxillary antrum, which raises suspicion of an antral fracture. A linear bony fragment below the orbital floor (arrow) is abnormal because a similar structure cannot be seen on the left side. This raises the possibility of a blowout fracture of the right orbital floor. **(b)** A CT image of the same case shows opacification of the right antrum by fluid and confirms a blowout fracture of the orbital floor. The 'trapdoor' fragment is demonstrated (arrow), and there is associated orbital emphysema. The inferior rectus muscle lies just above the bony deficiency in the orbital floor, but no orbital contents can be seen to have passed into the antrum. This fracture is discussed in detail later in the chapter.

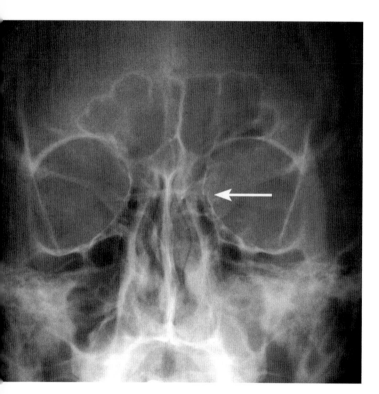

A Caldwell (PA) view is sensitive to small alterations of tube angulation. A true Caldwell view has 15° of caudal tube angulation to the baseline of the skull. With this angulation, the petrous ridge is projected through the centre of the orbit. Both the inferior orbital margin and orbital floor are partly obscured (see Fig. 9.17). If a straight tube is used, the petrous ridge is projected just below the superior orbital margin, with the majority of the orbit obliterated by this portion of the temporal bone. The zygomaticofrontal sutures and orbital structures such as the superior orbital fissure are difficult to see without angulation. The higher the centring point and/or

▲ **Fig. 9.16** A blowout fracture involves the medial wall of the left orbit, with clouding of the adjacent ethmoid air cells (arrow). This image has been obtained using a Caldwell view with 25° of caudal angulation to display the entire orbital margin. The use of a Caldwell view with varying angles is discussed below in the text.

▶ **Fig. 9.17** A true Caldwell view is obtained with the tube angled at 15° to the baseline of the skull and, with this projection, the petrous ridge projects across the centre of the orbits. This results in the inferior orbital margin and orbital floor being partly obscured.

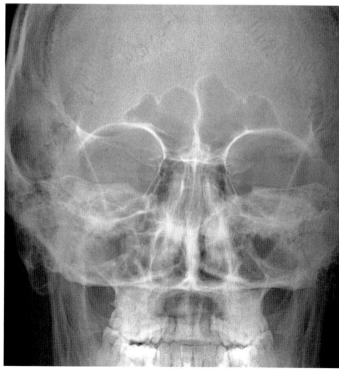

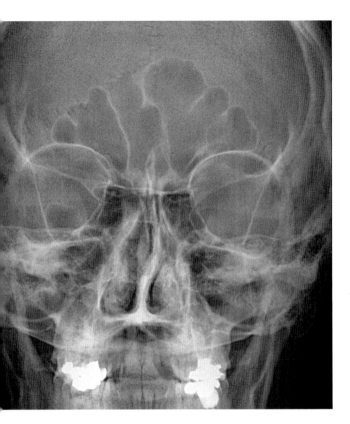

▲ **Fig. 9.18** The inferior orbital margin becomes clearly visible with about 20° of tube angulation.

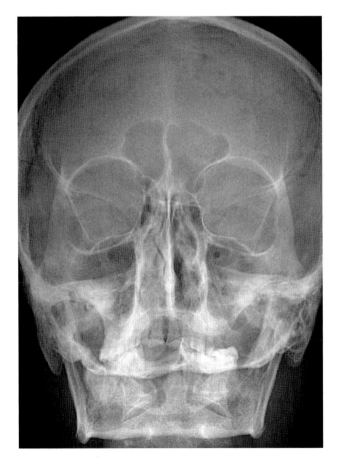

▲ **Fig. 9.19** A Caldwell view with 25° of tube angulation is the best plain film view for visualising the entire orbit.

the larger the tube angulation, the lower the petrous ridge and temporal bones will be projected in relation to the orbits. The inferior orbital margin and orbital floor are clearly seen at 20 to 25° angulation (see Figs 9.18 and 9.19). A Caldwell view shows many extremely important structures, the examination of which requires a disciplined routine (see Figs 9.20 and 9.21). As previously noted, fractures of the medial wall of the orbit may be extremely subtle and can be missed on a Water's view, as the medial wall is foreshortened in this view. A 25° Caldwell view demonstrates the orbital margins extremely well and in particular will show the medial wall, inferior orbital margin and orbital floor. These structures are usually partly obscured by soft tissues on a Water's view, particularly if the patient has a black eye (see Fig. 9.22).

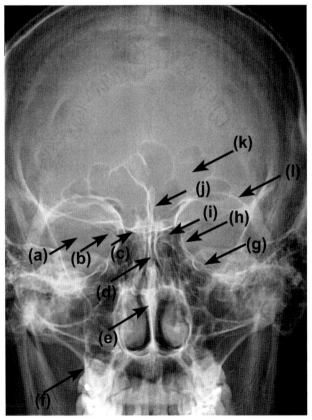

▲ **Fig. 9.20** The following structures are well demonstrated on a Caldwell view:
(a) greater wing of sphenoid
(b) lesser wing of sphenoid and superior orbital fissure
(c) cribriform plate
(d) perpendicular plate of ethmoid
(e) bony nasal septum
(f) alveolar process of the maxilla
(g) foramen rotundum
(h) medial wall of the orbit
(i) ethmoid air cells
(j) crista galli of ethmoid
(k) frontal sinus
(l) superior orbital margin

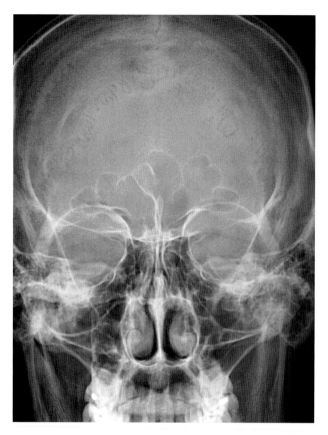

▲ Fig. 9.21 This is the same image as Fig. 9.20, without the labels.

A Water's view is the most valuable facial bone view. With increased angulation from extension of the head and neck, the petrous bones are projected below the inferior extent of the maxillary antra, enabling a clear assessment of the antral walls, body of zygoma, zygomatic arches, zygomaticofrontal sutures and orbits (see Fig. 9.23). Although the medial wall of the orbit is not ideally demonstrated, a Water's view demonstrates the orbital roof and will show extension of frontal sinus fractures into the orbital roof.

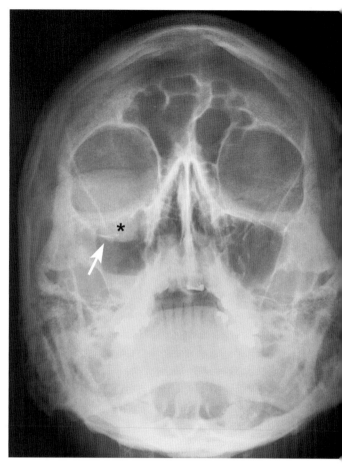

▲ Fig. 9.22 An athlete has a black eye on the right side, following an altercation with an opposition player. Obvious asymmetry is demonstrated on a Water's view. A fluid level is seen in the right antrum and there are characteristic changes of a blowout fracture of the right orbital floor. Diagnostic features include a soft-tissue opacity extending into the antrum from the orbital floor (asterisk), with an accompanying 'trapdoor' bone fragment (arrow). Note the generalised clouding of bone detail caused by the soft-tissue swelling associated with the black eye.

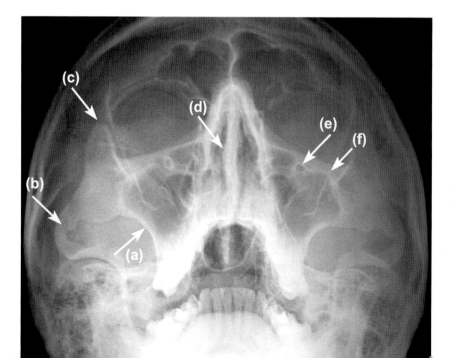

◀ Fig. 9.23 Particular structures are well demonstrated by a Water's view and these include: **(a)** the lateral walls of the maxillary antra, **(b)** zygomatic arches, **(c)** the zygomaticofrontal sutures, **(d)** the nasal septum, **(e)** the infraorbital foramen and **(f)** the inferior orbital margins. These structures are commonly injured by facial trauma, either individually (as in a blowout fracture) or in combination (as occurs in a tripod fracture).

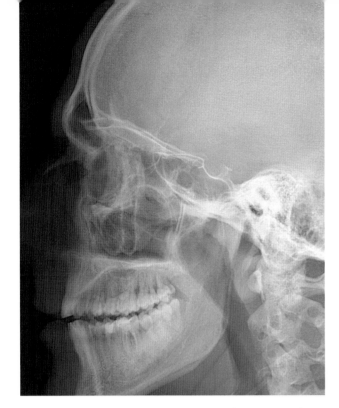

▲ Fig. 9.24 This image is a technically satisfactory normal lateral view. The assessment of the anatomical detail provided requires a disciplined search pattern. The important structures are labelled in Fig. 9.25.

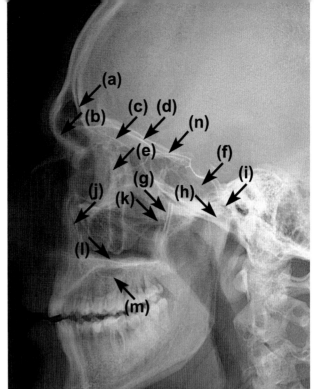

▲ Fig. 9.25 A normal lateral view demonstrates many important structures:
(a) posterior wall of the frontal sinus
(b) anterior wall of the frontal sinus
(c) medial orbital roof
(d) mid orbital roof
(e) lateral orbital margin
(f) sphenoid sinus
(g) pterygoid plates
(h) mandibular condyle
(i) temporomandibular joint
(j) anterior wall of the antrum
(k) posterior wall of the antrum
(l) hard palate
(m) antral floor
(n) cribriform plate

A lateral view demonstrates considerable anatomical detail but, as with a Caldwell view, suffers from superimposition, which makes the identification and assessment of individual structures laborious. Nevertheless, a lateral view provides important anatomical information (see Figs 9.24 and 9.25). As no tube tilt is used, fluid levels are well defined and usually indicative of fracture in a clinical setting of trauma (see Fig. 9.26).

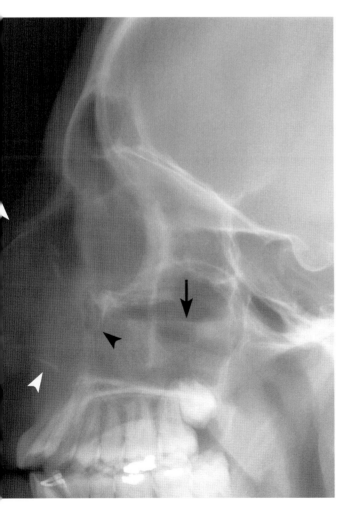

◄ Fig. 9.26 A lateral view shows multiple facial fractures. Fractures involve the nasal bones (white arrow) and the anterior nasal spine (white arrowhead). A fluid level (black arrow) demonstrated within the maxillary antrum calls for a careful inspection of the antral walls, and a fracture of the anterior antral wall can be seen below the anterior orbital margin (black arrowhead). It is not possible to determine the side of the injury from this view.

Although a nasal bone view would seem relatively simple to assess, fractures of the nasal bones are commonly missed and normal sutures are incorrectly called fractures. The normal nasofrontal and nasomaxillary sutures should be identified and should not be confused with fractures. Another normal line that may cause confusion is the groove for the nasociliary nerve, which runs parallel to the nasal profile (see Fig. 9.27). Any lucent line that is transversely oriented and located distal to the nasofrontal suture is likely to represent a fracture. However, the age of a nasal fracture is not always easy to determine on the basis of plain radiographs alone, as only 15% of old fractures heal by ossification and it is therefore not uncommon for old injuries to be mistaken for acute fractures. Remember to examine the anterior nasal spine of the maxilla, as a fracture of the spine may be associated with a nasal bone fracture (see Fig. 9.28).

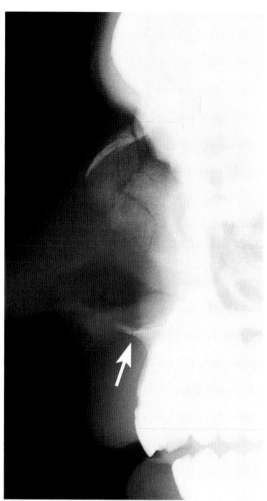

▲ **Fig. 9.28** A comminuted fracture of the nasal bones is demonstrated and the fracture is noted to extend across the nasomaxillary suture into the frontal process of the maxilla. Diastasis of the nasomaxillary suture has occurred. There is also a fracture of the anterior nasal spine with slight displacement (arrow).

CT examination of the facial bones

MDCT is now widely available for facial bone assessment and this technology offers rapid high-resolution imaging. The wide detector array of MDCT enables the acquisition of multiple-slice data from each revolution of the x-ray tube, with revolutions of less than 0.5 s possible. Such speed is helpful in successfully examining the badly injured or uncooperative patient. High spatial resolution is important for the identification of complex and subtle facial bone fractures, and MDCT has the ability to reformat data in any plane without loss of resolution. This is one of the most important features of this new technology (see Fig. 9.29). Using the same data, MDCT can also produce high-resolution surface-rendered 3D images, which assist in the interpretation and understanding of soft tissue as well as bony injury (see Figs 9.30 and 9.31). This realistic surface rendering and 3D appearance is created by illuminating the area with a virtual light and then displaying the intensity of the light that would be scattered back.

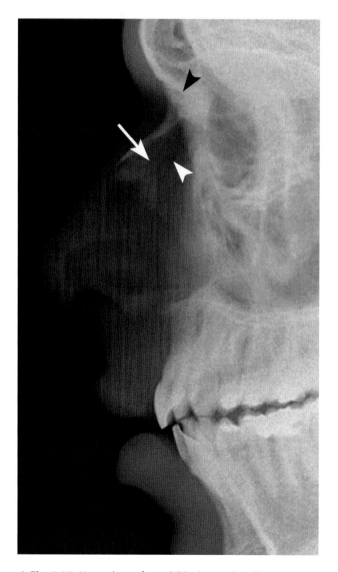

▲ **Fig. 9.27** Normal nasofrontal (black arrowhead) and nasomaxillary sutures (white arrowhead) should be identified and should not be confused with fractures. Diastasis of these sutures occasionally occurs. The groove for the nasociliary nerve may be mistaken for a fracture (white arrow).

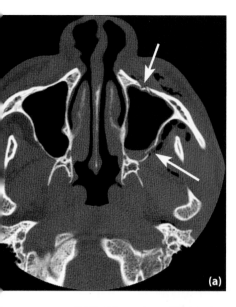

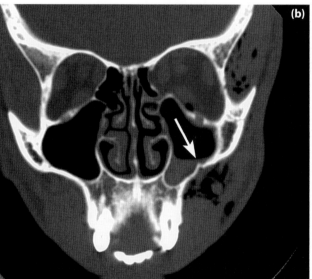

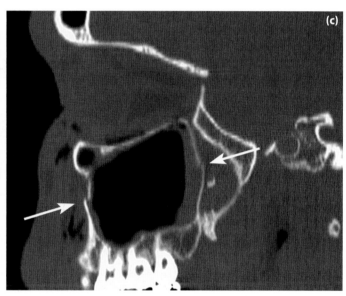

◀▼ **Fig. 9.29** A boxer competing at the Sydney 2000 Olympics presented with bruising and swelling below the left eye. Surgical emphysema was noted clinically. An MDCT examination was performed and reformatted images were then obtained in the axial, coronal and sagittal planes.

(a) An axial reformation shows fractures of the anterior and lateral walls of the left maxillary antrum (arrows). A small collection of fluid is present in the antrum. No other recent bone injury is seen in this plane. Soft-tissue swelling and surgical emphysema are present anteriorly and surgical emphysema is also noted deep to the zygoma, extending along the lateral aspect of the lateral antral wall. The nose shows features typical of a fighter.

(b) A coronal reformation shows surgical emphysema in the cheek, temporal fossa and orbit. Diastasis of the zygomaticofrontal suture is suspected. Slight displacement of a fracture through the lateral wall of the maxillary antrum is again demonstrated (arrow).

(c) A sagittal reformation shows fractures of the anterior and posterior walls of the maxillary antrum (arrows), and a fracture at the posterior aspect of the orbital floor. Surgical emphysema is noted in the orbit and cheek.

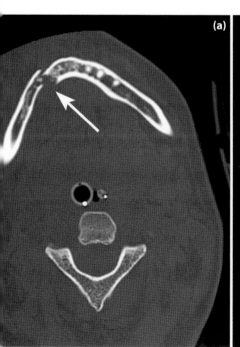

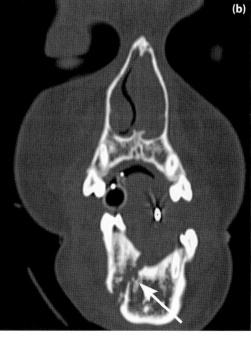

◀**Fig. 9.30** Following facial trauma, a series of high-resolution axial and coronal MDCT images were obtained, demonstrating a fracture of the right body of the mandible. An endotracheal tube is present. **(a)** is a representative axial reformation and **(b)** is a representative coronal reformation demonstrating the fracture (arrows). However, the overall fracture configuration and degree of resulting dental deformity are difficult to conceptualise from 2D images alone, and an improved understanding can be obtained from a 3D presentation of the same data.

▶ **Fig. 9.31** A surface-shaded 3D display of the same data set used to produce the 2D images in Fig. 9.30 gives the surgeon a better understanding of the mandibular fracture position and associated dental deformity. There is an oblique comminuted fracture of the right body of the mandible between the mental foramen and the symphysis. Deformity of the alveolar margin has resulted and the upper front teeth are missing. A search for the missing teeth would include a chest x-ray to exclude inhalation. The patient has been intubated.

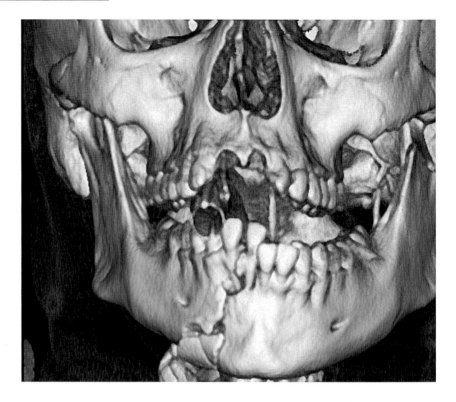

A potential downside of this technology is the radiation dose to the patient. This problem has been recognised, addressed and partly overcome through refinements of multi-detector technology and careful attention to optimal radiographic technique. The temptation to improve quality and produce pretty images by increasing x-ray tube output must be resisted. Instead, it is possible to employ low-dose techniques that still provide diagnostic information and are appropriately tailored to the specific area of clinical interest (see Fig. 9.32).

The use of other imaging methods

MRI is used for imaging of the articular disc of the temporomandibular joints (TMJs). This will be discussed in detail later in the chapter. No other application for MRI is recognised and neither nuclear bone scans nor ultrasound have a routine role in imaging the facial bones and mandible.

▶ **Fig. 9.32** Reducing the patient's exposure to radiation must always be considered when devising any CT imaging protocol. In this case the data acquisition was restricted to the area of clinical interest between the supraorbital ridge and alveolar margin.

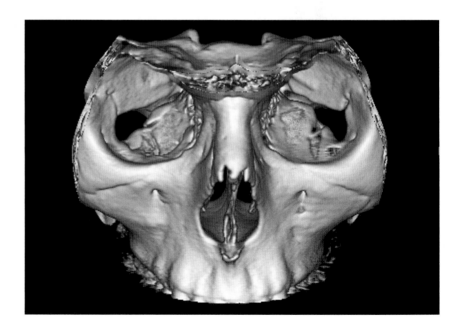

Facial fractures

On plain film views, facial fractures can be diagnosed by the identification of a lucent fracture line, diastasis of a suture or overlapping bone edges. Indirect signs include anatomical asymmetry, soft-tissue swelling, paranasal sinus opacification with or without an air-fluid level, soft-tissue emphysema and malocclusion. Frequently missed fractures of the facial region are listed in Table 9.1. CT displays normal symmetry particularly well (see Fig. 9.33) and abnormalities are easily detected (see Fig. 9.34). Fractures of the face may be classified as shown in Table 9.2

Table 9.1 Commonly missed fractures of the facial region

1. The second of bilateral mandibular fractures
2. Symphyseal fracture of the mandible
3. Isolated zygomatic arch fracture
4. Orbital wall fractures, particularly medial and lateral
5. Fractures of the frontal sinus and orbital roof
6. Medial maxillary-orbital fractures

Source: Johnson et al. (1984).

Table 9.2 Classification of facial fractures

Orbital fractures	Orbital rim fracture
	Blowout fracture
	Blow-in fracture
Zygomaticomaxillary fractures	Isolated zygomatic arch fracture
	Tripod fracture
Maxillary fractures	Isolated antral fracture
	Alveolar ridge fracture

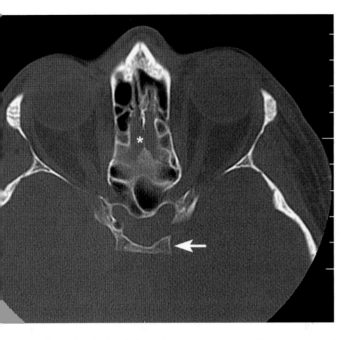

▲ **Fig. 9.33** Using CT imaging, symmetry is well demonstrated and subtle fractures can be identified easily. Although the air cells of the paranasal sinuses are characteristically asymmetrical, the symmetry of bony structures is otherwise normally precise. This axial image demonstrates normal and symmetrical orbits, and illustrates the ease with which the lateral and medial orbital walls may be assessed. At this level, the posterior cribriform plate (asterisk) and dorsum sellae (arrow) are demonstrated.

Orbital fractures

Orbital rim fractures

Orbital rim fractures usually occur from direct trauma caused by a head clash or the impact of a sporting implement. These fractures may be seen on plain films (see Fig. 9.35) but are best identified by CT (see Fig. 9.36). Inferior orbital rim fractures are common and are often a component of a more extensive fracture pattern, such as a tripod or zygomaticomaxillary fracture complex (see Fig. 9.37). Superior orbital rim fractures often extend into the roof of the orbit and frontal sinus (see Fig. 9.38). Lateral orbital rim fractures are characteristically associated with more complex tripod and LeFort fractures of the mid-face (see Fig. 9.39).

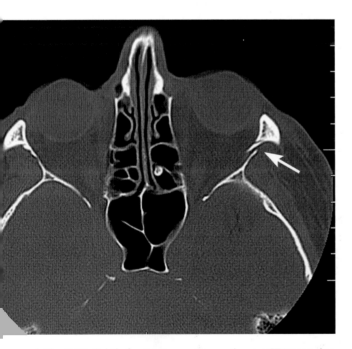

▲ **Fig. 9.34** Subtle fractures are seen easily on a CT image due to loss of symmetry. In this case there is a fracture of the lateral wall of the left orbit (arrow).

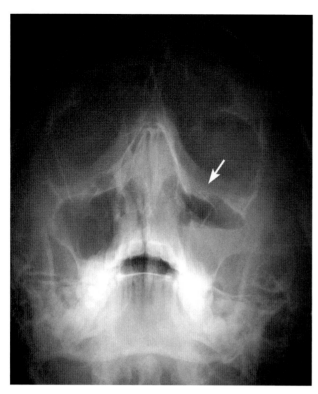

▲ **Fig. 9.35** A Water's view demonstrates an isolated fracture of the left inferior orbital rim, involving the infra-orbital foramen (arrow). The zygomatic arch and the lateral wall of the maxillary antrum are intact. A large collection of fluid is present within the antrum. A CT examination would be necessary for the assessment of the orbital floor, which is likely to be involved.

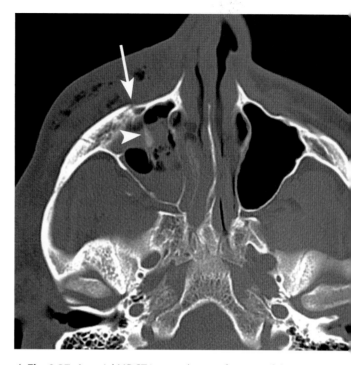

▲ **Fig. 9.37** An axial MDCT image shows a fracture of the right inferior orbital rim that extends across the orbital floor (arrow). There is marked swelling and surgical emphysema in the cheek, and fluid and air are present in the right antrum. An orbital floor bone fragment is noted (arrowhead).

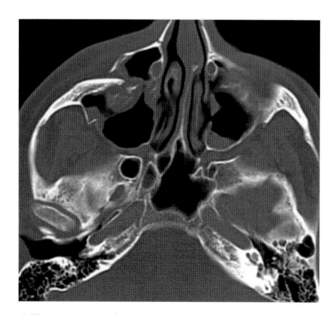

▲ **Fig. 9.36** An axial MDCT image demonstrates a depressed fracture of the right inferior orbital rim with buckling of the lateral antral wall. The zygomatic arch appears intact. This injury was the result of a head clash during a football game.

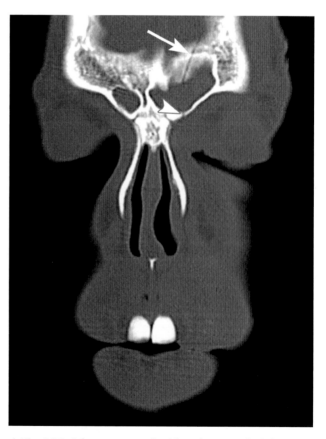

▲ **Fig. 9.38** A fracture extends obliquely across the left supra-orbital ridge (arrow) and involves the left frontal sinus and left orbital roof (arrowhead).

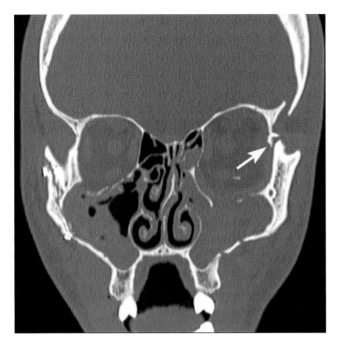

▲ **Fig. 9.39** A severe LeFort Type II–III mid-face fracture has resulted from anterior compression of the middle third of the face with the fracture line extending into the wall of the anterior cranial fossa on the left. There is also a fracture of the lateral orbital rim (arrow), a blowout fracture of the left orbital floor and medial wall, and fractures through the lateral wall of the maxillary antrum. There is also a blowout fracture of the right orbital floor and a fracture of the right zygoma. The maxillary antra are opacified by haemorrhage. A fracture of the nasal septum is noted.

Blowout fractures

A blowout fracture of the orbit is usually the result of a direct blow by an object of a similar size to the orbit. Blowout fractures most commonly involve the floor of the orbit, but can also involve the medial wall, the roof or the lateral wall, alone or in combination (see Figs 9.40, 9.41 and 9.42). It is postulated that raised intra-orbital pressure at the time of impact results in failure of the thinnest portion of the orbital wall. Buckling of the orbital floor may also result from a direct blow to the inferior orbital rim. A blowout fracture of the orbital floor acts like a trapdoor, allowing herniation of intraorbital fat with or without the inferior rectus muscle into the maxillary antrum (see Fig. 9.43). Enopthalmos, exophthalmos and diplopia on upward gaze may result. Infra-orbital nerve injuries are also common with resultant anaesthesia or hypoaesthesia in the distribution of the nerve. Figure 9.15 showed an example of the plain film changes of a blowout fracture of the orbital floor. These changes may include the presence of an air-fluid level in the maxillary antrum, a polypoid soft-tissue opacity projecting into the antrum from its roof, a subtle displaced bony fragment of orbital floor on the lateral or Water's view, and orbital emphysema. With MDCT, images reformatted in the axial, coronal and sagittal planes combine so that the most subtle fractures are easily seen. CT also provides assessment of the orbital contents, which can be injured in up to 30% of these cases (Hammerschlag et al. 1982; Tonami et al. 1987) (see Fig. 9.44).

Blow-in fractures

Blow-in fractures occur when fragments are displaced into the orbit, producing a decreased orbital volume (see Fig. 9.45).

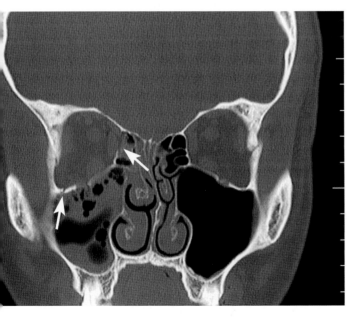

▲ **Fig. 9.40** A coronal CT image demonstrates fractures of the floor and medial wall of the right orbit (arrows). A mixture of haemorrhage and admixed air bubbles is noted in the maxillary antrum.

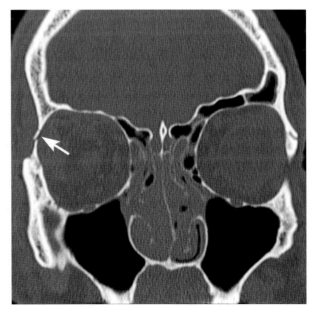

▲ **Fig. 9.41** A subtle fracture of the lateral wall of the right orbit is easily seen with high-resolution CT imaging (arrow). Unusually wide pneumatisation of the roof of the left orbit is present.

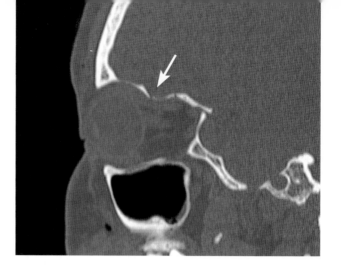

▶ **Fig. 9.42** A sagittally reformatted MDCT image demonstrates a blowout fracture of the orbital roof (arrow).

▼ **Fig. 9.43(a)** A blowout fracture involves both the floor and the medial wall of the right orbit, following trauma to the right eye (arrows). Fragments have been displaced outwards, consistent with transient increased intra-orbital pressure. A large deficit in the orbital floor has resulted and partial herniation of the inferior rectus muscle (asterisk) has occurred through the bony deficiency. Orbital fat has also herniated into the right maxillary antrum. Fluid opacifies the right ethmoid air cells and the right maxillary antrum. **(b)** A severe blowout fracture involves the floor and the medial wall of the right orbit (arrowhead). Substantial herniation of the inferior rectus muscle has occurred through the large defect in the orbital floor (asterisk). A small bone fragment has been displaced from the orbital floor into the centre of the antrum (arrow).

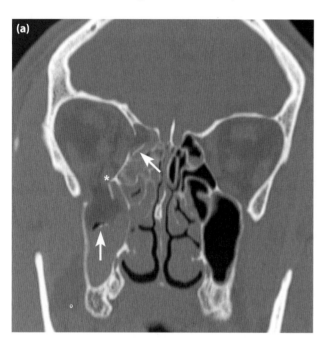

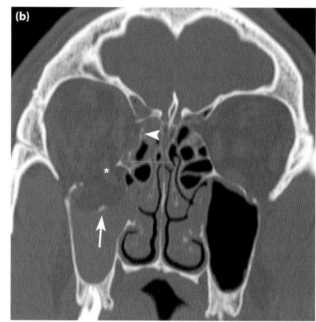

▼ **Fig. 9.44(a)** A violent punch has caused a blowout fracture of the right orbit, with extensive damage to the floor and the medial wall demonstrated on a coronal CT image. There are also fractures of the ethmoid air cells. Fluid fills the majority of the ethmoid air cells and the right maxillary antrum. There is swelling and surgical emphysema in the right cheek. Considerable air is present within the orbit and the eye is not evident in this plane, despite being demonstrated on the left. This is due to traumatic exophthalmos. **(b)** The traumatic exophthalmos is well seen on an axial CT image, with considerable protrusion of the right eye. Air is shown in the tissues around the eye and between the medial surface of the optic nerve and the medial rectus muscle.

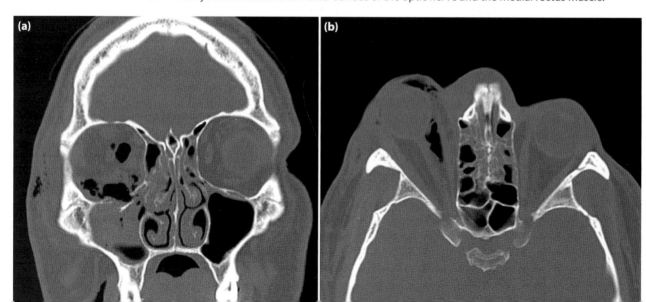

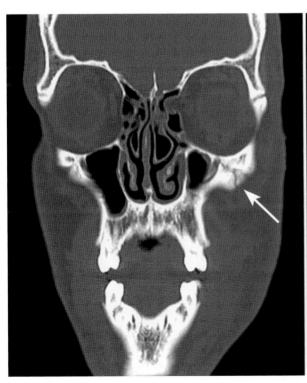

▲ **Fig. 9.45** A blow-in fracture of the superomedial wall of the left orbit follows an injury to the eye (arrow). Note the associated haematoma (asterisk) causing lateral displacement of the globe and optic nerve.

▶ **Fig. 9.46** An isolated zygomatic arch fracture is demonstrated by a Water's view (arrow).

Zygomaticomaxillary fractures

Isolated fractures of the zygoma and zygomatic arch

An isolated fracture of the zygomatic arch generally occurs from a direct blow to the side of the face (see Fig. 9.46). The fracture is usually in three parts with a depressed V-shaped central fragment. It is best appreciated on basal views and is often overlooked on other views (Dolan and Jacoby 1978). An isolated fracture of the body of the zygoma is unusual and occurs following direct trauma (see Fig. 9.47).

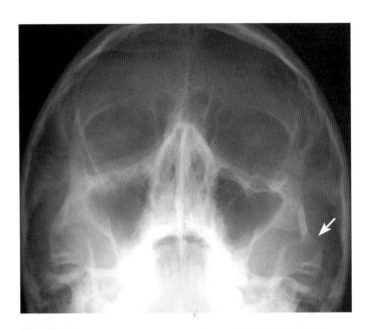

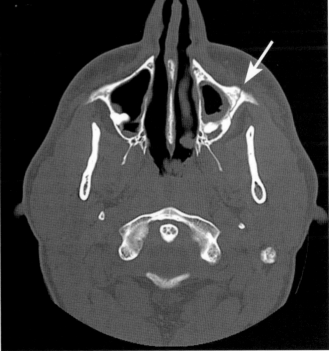

▲ **Fig. 9.47** A comminuted fracture of the body of the zygoma is demonstrated by coronal and axial MDCT images (arrows). This injury resulted from direct trauma.

Tripod fractures

Tripod fractures also result from a direct blow to the cheek and are characterised by a disruption of all three bony processes of the zygoma. There is disruption with diastasis of the zygomaticofrontal suture, a fracture of the zygomatic arch and a fracture of the inferior orbital margin in the region of the zygomaticomaxillary suture extending across the maxillary antrum to involve the lateral antral wall. This is one of the most common facial bone fractures and is well demonstrated using reformatted images and the 3D capabilities of MDCT (see Figs 9.48 and 9.49). There is often an air-fluid level in the maxillary antrum. Associated injury of the infra-orbital nerve is common. Displacement and rotation of the body of the zygoma occurs and this can be appreciated on CT (Rogers 1992).

Maxillary fractures

Isolated antral fractures

An isolated antral fracture is a rare injury and is difficult to assess on plain films. Most antral fractures occur in combination with other complex fracture patterns. CT clearly defines the diagnostic features of an isolated fracture of the maxillary antrum (see Figs 9.50, 9.51 and 9.52).

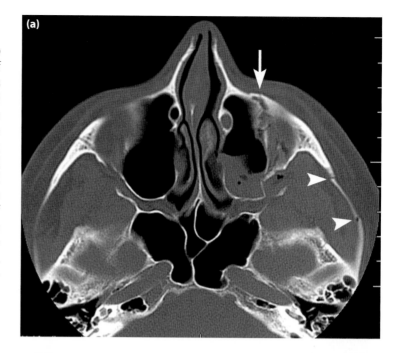

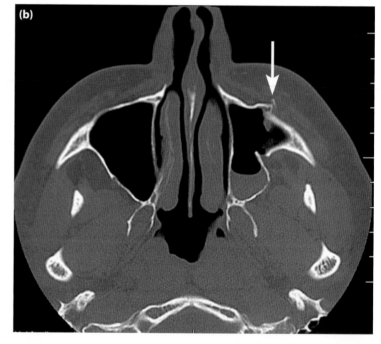

▶ **Fig. 9.48(a)** The tripod injury is a pattern of fractures so-called because the three processes of the zygoma are involved. An axial reformatted MDCT image shows fractures of typical tripod pattern. There are fractures of the left inferior orbital margin extending into the orbital floor (arrow), the lateral wall of the left antrum and the left zygomatic arch (arrowheads).
(b) An axial image acquired at a lower level shows fractures of the anterior wall of the left maxillary antrum (arrow) and considerable depression of the lateral wall. Isolation and rotation of the body of the zygoma can be appreciated. Fluid is present in the left antrum.
(c) Using the same volumetric MDCT scan data, coronal images were also generated. This image from the coronal series is useful for demonstrating marked depression of the lateral wall of the left maxillary antrum and depression of the lateral aspect of the orbital floor (arrow). There is also a fracture at the junction of the lateral antral wall and the alveolar process of the maxilla (arrowhead).

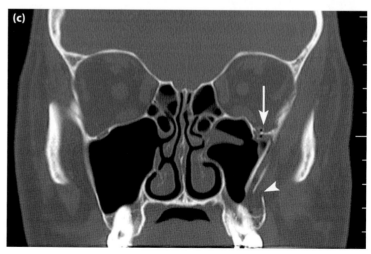

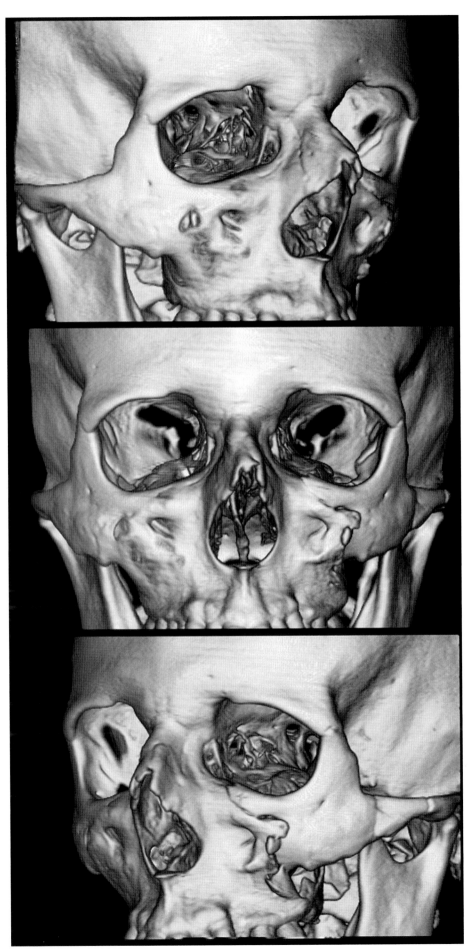

◀**Fig. 9.49** The MDCT scan data used in Fig. 9.48 was also processed to generate surface-shaded 3D images to improve the understanding of the cosmetic deformity caused by depression of the left zygoma. This 3D view of the facial bones can be rotated and viewed from any position.

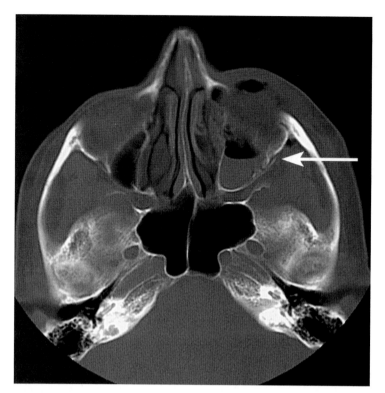

▲ **Fig. 9.50** An axial MDCT image shows periorbital soft-tissue swelling and surgical emphysema on the left. The swelling extends over the left cheek and there is a fracture of the lateral wall of the maxillary antrum (arrow), with surgical emphysema noted posterior to the zygoma. Fluid is noted in the maxillary antrum.

Alveolar ridge fractures

An alveolar ridge fracture is usually bilateral and on plain films there is displacement and malalignment of the teeth. An orthopantomogram (OPG) provides an ideal panoramic overview of dental alignment and CT is useful for the assessment of displacement and associated fractures. If teeth are missing, a chest x-ray should be obtained to exclude inhalation and avoid subsequent complications.

Bilateral mid-face fractures

LeFort fractures are usually serious high-energy impact injuries. They are generally associated with high-velocity sports such as skiing, cycling and motor sports or are the result of a fall from a height. LeFort fractures may be associated with both cervical spine and intracranial trauma. They are classified according to the pattern of disruption that occurs along lines of relative bony weakness (LeFort 1901). There is characteristically either partial or complete separation of the maxilla from the remainder of the facial skeleton or skull (see Fig. 9.53). There is often depression of the mid-face (see Figs 9.54 and 9.55). The ability of MDCT to generate reformations is a great help in the assessment of these complex and serious injuries.

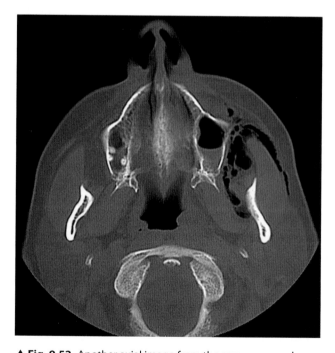

▲ **Fig. 9.51** A further axial image obtained at a lower level in the same patient as Fig. 9.50 shows increased surgical emphysema lying between the left lateral wall of the antrum and the masseter muscle. Air is also noted over the superficial surface of the masseter. Fluid within the left antrum and a fracture of the lateral antral wall are again noted (arrow).

▲ **Fig. 9.52** Another axial image from the same case as shown in Figs 9.50 and 9.51 at the level of the hard palate shows a spectacular pattern of surgical emphysema that has tracked down the cheek and surrounds the anterior two-thirds of the masseter, the medial margin of the temporalis and the lateral margin of the lateral pterygoid muscles.

▶ **Fig. 9.53** Mid-face fractures are usually bilateral. This is a typical case, demonstrated on an axial CT image. An anterior force has produced fractures that extend through the maxillary antra as well as causing depression of the middle third of the face (arrows). There are fractures involving the right zygoma and the zygomatic arch, and compression of the nasal septum is another common feature.

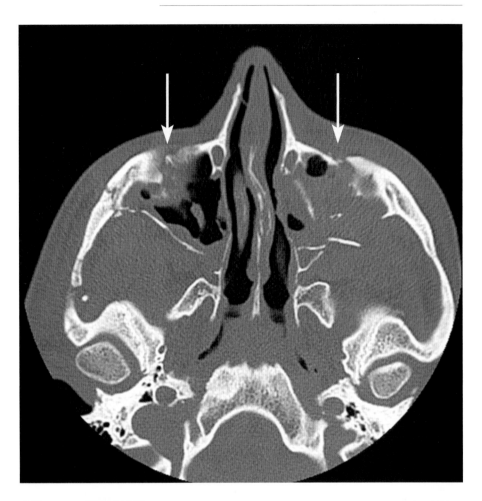

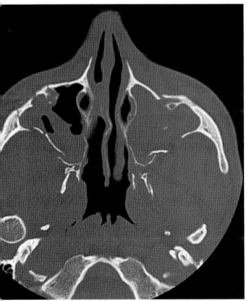

▲ **Fig. 9.54** A similar mid-face fracture image from a different case shows extensive fracturing of the maxillary antra. The bone injury extends posteriorly to disrupt the pterygopalatine fossae and pterygoid plates. Compression of the nasal septum is noted.

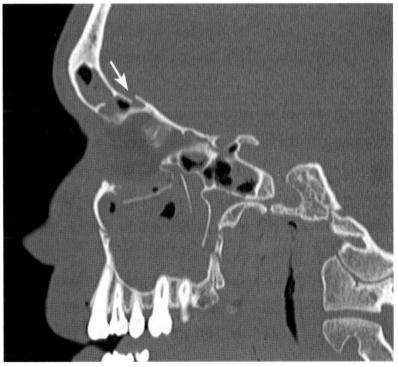

▲ **Fig. 9.55** Depression of the middle third of the face is best appreciated on images reformatted in the sagittal plane. In this case, fractures can be seen through the anterior and posterior antral walls, the pterygoid plate, orbital floor and base of the frontal sinus (arrow). Displacement at the latter fracture site demonstrates the degree of depression of the central face.

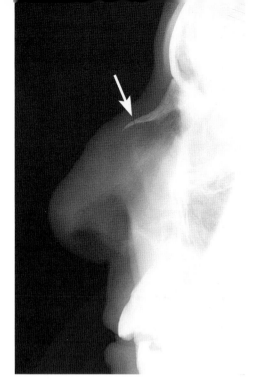

▲ **Fig. 9.56** A plain film demonstrates an undisplaced fracture of the tip of the nasal bones (arrow).

Nasal fractures

Nasal bone fractures

The medical literature indicates that a fractured nose is the most common of all facial fractures, although the incidence is difficult to determine as a large number of these injuries are unreported (Costello et al. 2005).

The nose is a prominent facial feature and this would undoubtedly contribute to the high frequency of nasal bone fractures. A simple fracture of the nasal bone invariably results from a direct blow to the nose. Soft-tissue swelling and deformity are usually obvious and the diagnosis is generally established clinically (Logan et al. 1994). As previously discussed, the value and accuracy of nasal bone radiographs is controversial, but a good lateral view can give a reasonable idea of the extent of a fracture and the degree of depression. For this reason, if imaging is to be performed at all, plain radiography remains the initial imaging method of choice (see Fig. 9.56). Nevertheless, MDCT is accurate in the diagnosis of nasal fracture and plays an important role in the diagnosis of complications (see Figs 9.57 and 9.58).

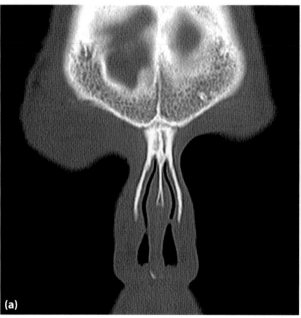

(a)

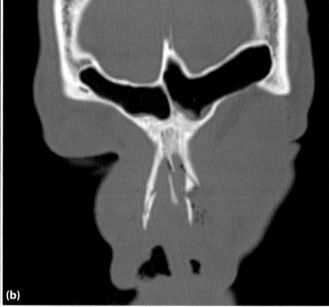

(b)

▲ **Fig. 9.57(a)** A coronal CT image demonstrates normal nasal bones and a normal nasal septum.
(b) In a different case, fractures of the nasal bones and nasal septum are well demonstrated by a coronal CT image. Surgical emphysema is also noted.

▶ **Fig. 9.58** An axial MDCT image is useful for demonstrating the nasal bones and nasal septum. The orbits, ethmoid air cells and perpendicular plate of the ethmoid are important structures to assess in the more extensive nasal injuries. The perpendicular plate of the ethmoid should be a direct continuation of the nasal septum and should merge with the rostrum of the sphenoid.

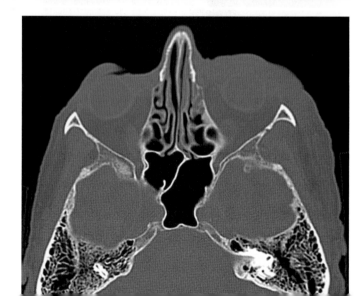

▼ **Fig. 9.59(a)** An axial image shows comminution of the nasal bones due to a compressive injury and there is a fracture of the nasal septum. Note the surgical emphysema in the soft tissues adjacent to the nasal bone fractures. **(b)** An axial image in a severe LeFort type injury demonstrates fracturing and compression of the nasal septum (arrow). Antral fractures are also noted.

Fractures of the nasal septum

Direct force to the nose may produce compression and fracture of the nasal septum. This may be suspected on a Water's view, although deviation of the nasal septum is a common normal variant and CT is usually required to differentiate a fracture from normal anatomical variation (see Figs 9.59, 9.60 and 9.61).

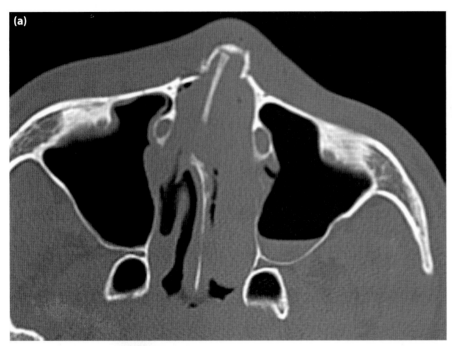

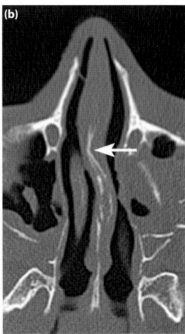

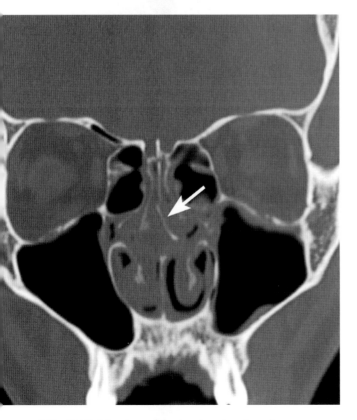

▲ **Fig. 9.60** A fracture of the nasal septum is well demonstrated on a reformatted coronal MDCT image (arrow).

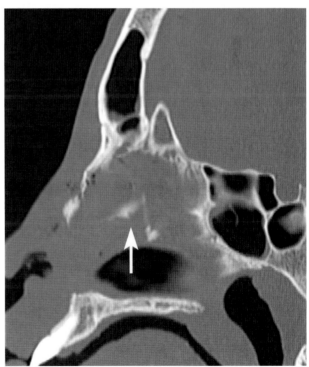

▲ **Fig. 9.61** In the same case as Fig. 9.59(a), a reformatted sagittal MDCT image graphically demonstrates a gross degree of nasal compression and buckling of the nasal septum (arrow). Surgical emphysema is again noted.

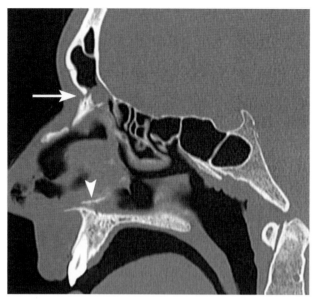

▲ **Fig. 9.62** A sagittal MDCT image shows a depressed fracture of the nasal bones, diastasis of the nasofrontal suture (arrow) and a fragment avulsed from the anterior nasal spine (arrowhead).

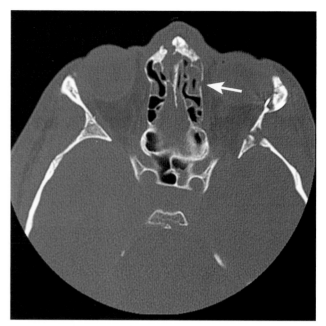

▲ **Fig. 9.63** An axial MDCT image demonstrates a nasoorbitalethmoid injury. The fracture involves the nasal bones and the force has been transmitted posteriorly as further fracturing along the nasal septum, ethmoid air cells, and medial and lateral walls of the left orbit (arrow).

Fractures of the anterior nasal spine of the maxilla

A fracture of the anterior nasal spine is a relatively uncommon injury that may either be associated with avulsion of the cartilaginous nasal septum or result from direct trauma. The fracture may occur in isolation or in conjunction with a nasal bone fracture, and is best visualised on sagittal MDCT images (see Fig. 9.62).

Nasoorbitalethmoidal fractures

A nasoorbitalethmoidal fracture is a more serious nasal injury, usually bilateral, and is caused by direct high-velocity trauma to the nasion. There is comminution and compaction of the thin nasal bones, ethmoid air cells, frontal sinuses and medial orbital walls (see Figs 9.63 and 9.64). Associated fractures of the cribriform plate (see Fig. 9.65) may be associated with CSF leak, and significant cerebral trauma is frequently present. Although these injuries may be suspected on plain films, MDCT provides the best assessment of fracture extent and displacement.

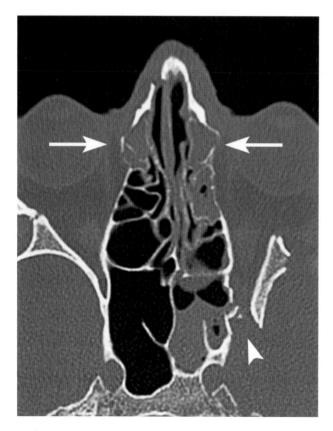

▲ **Fig. 9.64** An axial MDCT image demonstrates an example of nasoorbitalethmoid fracture resulting from a facial compression injury. The fracture involves the right nasal bone and compressive forces have produced buckling of the anterior ethmoid air cells with resulting fractures of the medial walls of both orbits (arrows). Fluid opacifies a number of air cells affected by this injury. The fracture also involves the left lateral wall of the sphenoid sinus, with opacification of the adjacent sinus. There is widening of the inferior orbital fissure on the left (arrowhead) and disruption of the lateral wall of the left orbit.

▶ **Fig. 9.65** Compression of the middle third of the face has produced marked nasal bone compression and fractures of the cribriform plate (arrows). Fluid is noted in the sphenoid sinus. These changes are well demonstrated on a reformatted sagittal MDCT image.

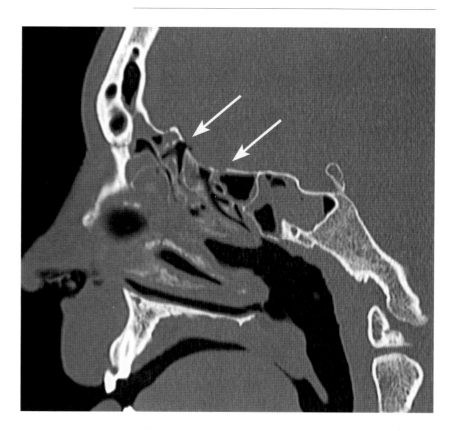

Mid-face fractures

The causes of mid-face fractures are similar worldwide. Motor vehicle accidents are the most common cause (the incidence ranges from 31% to 90%) with assaults being the next common (the incidence ranges from 3% to 33%). Fortunately, LeFort fractures resulting from sporting activities are uncommon.

There are many classification systems for mid-face fractures. None are ideal. The LeFort system is the most widely used classification, in spite of its shortcomings. The major fault with the LeFort system is that most mid-face fractures characteristically have features of more than one LeFort type, and most LeFort fractures have comminutions and displacements that do not comply with the other features of any specific type.

LeFort Type I fractures

A LeFort Type I fracture is a low transverse fracture that separates the maxillary alveolar process and palate from the maxilla. Fractures of the anterior and posterior maxillary walls and pterygoid plates are present (see Figs 9.66, 9.67 and 9.68).

LeFort Type II fractures

In a LeFort Type II fracture, a transverse/oblique fracture extends across the nasal bones and crosses the orbital rim. A LeFort Type II fracture characteristically involves the ethmoid air cells, medial and inferior orbital walls, maxillary antra and pterygoid plates (see Fig. 9.69). This results in a large pyramidal fragment, which can displace posteriorly.

LeFort Type III fractures

In a LeFort Type III fracture, a transverse fracture extends across the nasofrontal region, ethmoid air cells, inferior orbital

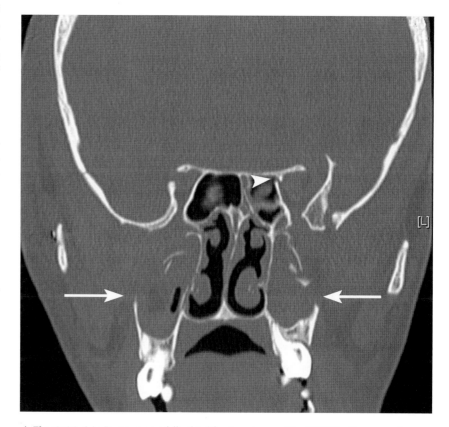

▲ **Fig. 9.66** A LeFort type middle third fracture imaged by MDCT in the coronal plane shows comminution of the maxillary antra with separation of the hard palate and alveolar process of the maxilla (arrows). These are features of a Type I fracture. There is also a fracture extending into the left middle cranial fossa and a fracture through the left half of the sphenoidal sinus that involves the medial wall of the optic canal (arrowhead).

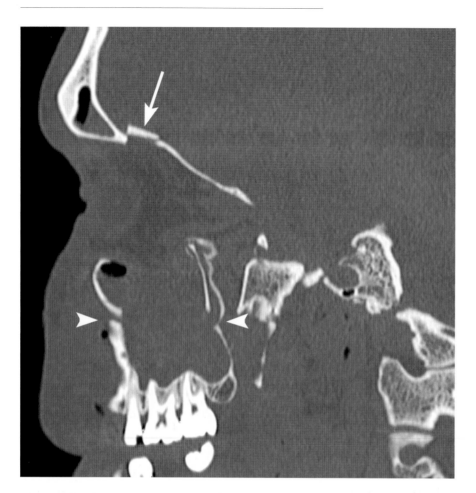

◄Fig. 9.67 A reformatted sagittal MDCT image shows fractures through the anterior and posterior walls of the maxillary antra (arrowheads) and a blowout fracture of the orbital floor with the hinged fragment lying against the posterior wall of the antrum. There is also a blowout fracture of the orbital roof (arrow).

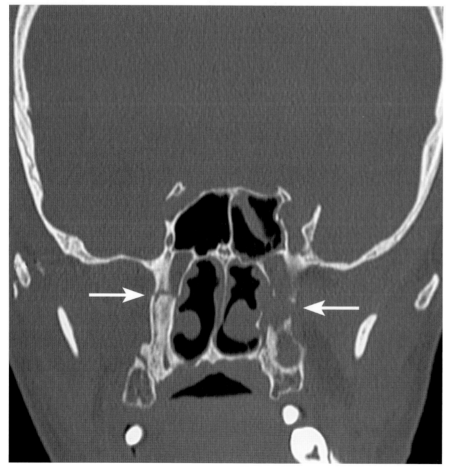

◄Fig. 9.68 A reformatted coronal MDCT image shows transverse fractures through the pterygoid plates (arrows), a feature of a LeFort Type I facial injury. There are also fractures of the base of the left orbit and the sphenoid on the left.

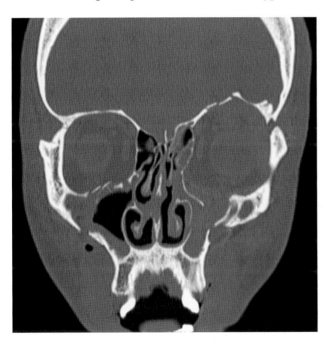

▲ Fig. 9.69 A severe facial trauma has produced injuries with LeFort Type II features. There has been a compressive injury to the middle third of the face, with changes more marked on the left. There are injuries to the nasal fossae, with buckling of the nasal septum and comminution of the walls of the left orbit, inferior orbital fissure and pterygopalatine fossa. Fractures enter the middle cranial fossa on the left. There are also fractures involving the right lateral orbital wall and zygoma.

▲ Fig. 9.70 Elongation of the orbit on the left side is characteristic of a LeFort Type III fracture. Fractures involve both maxillary antra, the floor of the right orbit, the left ethmoid air cells, and the medial and lateral walls, roof and floor of the left orbit. There is considerable intra-orbital but extra-ocular haematoma present, and inferolateral displacement of the lateral orbital margin and zygoma increases the apparent orbital size. There is separation of the hard palate and the alveolar process of the maxilla.

fissures, lateral orbital walls, zygomatic arches and pterygoid plates. This results in complete separation of the facial skeleton from the skull base. There is a characteristic elongation of the orbits on frontal views (see Fig. 9.70). In imaging these more severe injuries it is always important to remember that facial fractures may be associated with intracranial injury and trauma to the cervical spine (Costello et al. 2005).

Mandibular fractures

Fractures of the mandible are the result of a direct blow, commonly produced by a fist or a ball travelling at high speed. Fractures are often multiple due to the ring shape of the bone, and commonly there is a fracture on each side of the mandible. So if one mandibular fracture is seen a careful search should be made for a second fracture, which is commonly subcondylar or condylar.

Fractures of the body and angle of the mandible

The majority of mandibular fractures (50–70%) involve the body and angle of the mandible. The most common pattern is a fracture through the angle of the mandible on one side and a concomitant fracture through the body of the mandible on the opposite side. An angle fracture commonly involves the third molar tooth and the presence of third molars doubles the chance of an angle fracture (Dodson 2004). The fact that a fracture involves a tooth socket should be recognised and any missing teeth noted. When an angle fracture is present, the action of the masseter, temporalis and medial pterygoid may cause displacement by distraction of the proximal fragment.

Symphyseal and parasymphyseal fractures

Symphyseal and parasymphyseal fractures are unusual (accounting for 7–15 % of all mandibular fractures) and mostly occur following a direct blow to the chin, commonly due to a fall. Symphyseal fractures are often associated with bilateral fractures of the mandibular condyles. Although the symphysis usually fuses by one year of age, it can occasionally remain open until close to puberty and this variant should not be mistaken for a fracture.

Condylar fractures

Fractures of the condyles of the mandible usually occur at their bases and may be seen on plain films with a Towne's view or OPG. There is often dislocation of the TMJ and care should be taken to inspect the condyle and its relationship to the articular fossa. In children, fractures through the growth plate of the condyle can lead to growth arrest and underdevelopment of the mandible. MDCT is the examination of choice, and images are easy to acquire and interpret (see Fig. 9.71).

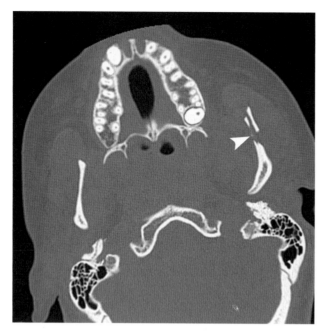

▲ **Fig. 9.71** An axial MDCT image shows a mandibular condyle fracture on the left (arrowhead). Further images of this case are shown in Figs 9.77 and 9.78.

Fractures of the ramus and coronoid process of the mandible

Fractures of the ramus and coronoid process of the mandible together make up 5% of mandibular fractures, are difficult to image on plain films and invariably require MDCT for diagnosis and delineation of fracture detail.

Imaging of the mandibular fractures

Although most fractures of the mandible can be demonstrated by plain films, some fractures are subtle and easily overlooked. For this reason, MDCT is now the imaging method of choice, as discussed below.

The standard plain film views of the mandible

PA view

The PA view is important for assessment of the integrity and symmetry of the mandibular bodies, angles and rami. It is also important to examine the symphysis and dental occlusion in this view (see Fig. 9.72).

Oblique view

An oblique view of each side of the mandible will demonstrate the body, angle, ramus and condylar regions without the superimposition of structures seen in the lateral view (see Fig. 9.73).

▶ **Fig. 9.72** A normal PA view of the mandible. Important features to examine include bony symmetry and dental occlusion, confirming that the spaces between the upper and lower front teeth are in alignment. The condyles are not well seen. Symphyseal fractures are notoriously difficult to identify and are commonly missed.

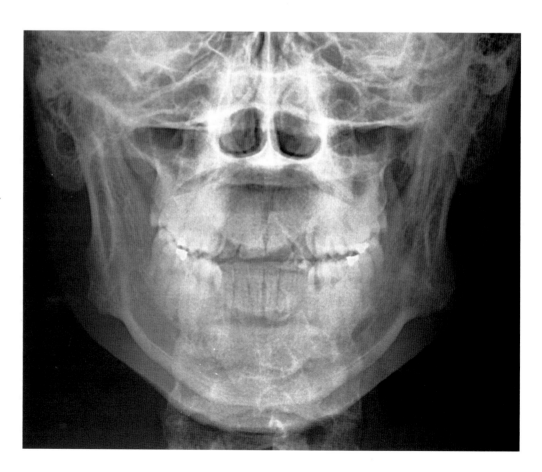

Lateral view

Although the lateral view shows superimposition of the mandibular structures, it nevertheless provides another view of the body and rami as well as helping to assess alignment (see Fig. 9.74).

Reversed Towne's view

A reversed Towne's view provides good visualisation of the mandibular condyles (see Fig. 9.75).

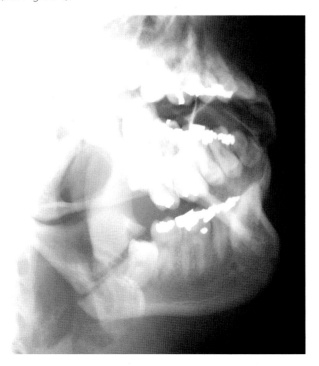

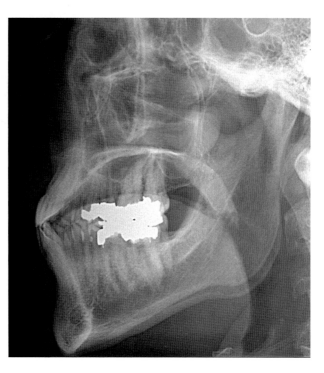

▲ **Fig. 9.73** An oblique view of the mandible is particularly valuable, allowing examination of the body, angle and ramus of the mandible. In this case, there is a fracture of the angle of the mandible extending into the socket of the unerupted third molar tooth. Moderate displacement has occurred.

▲ **Fig. 9.74** A lateral view of the mandible allows assessment of the body, angles, rami and condyles, although other views or CT are necessary to assess fracture detail and to determine the side of the injury.

▼ **Fig. 9.75** A reversed Towne's view is helpful for displaying the mandibular condyles in the AP projection.

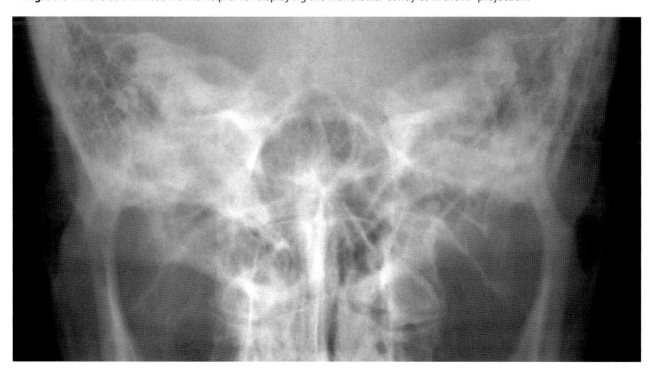

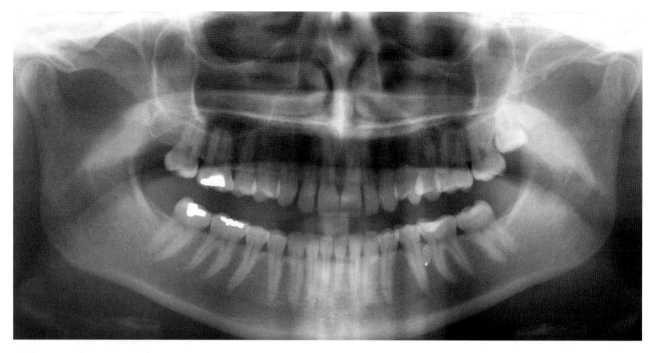

▲ **Fig. 9.76** This is a normal OPG. No mandibular abnormality is demonstrated. Dental detail is displayed.

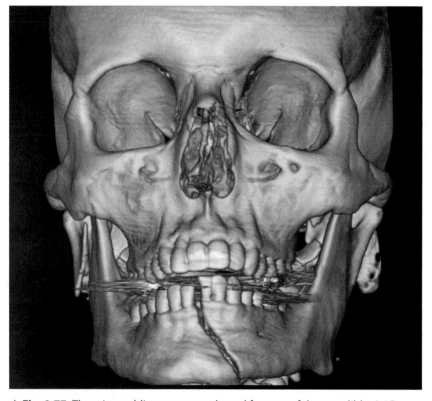

▲ **Fig. 9.77** There is an oblique parasymphyseal fracture of the mandible. A 3D surface-rendered display aids understanding of the degree of displacement and resulting dental malalignment. There is also a fracture through the base of the right mandibular condyle, which is difficult to see. Using the same scan data, the mandible can be disarticulated to enable improved understanding of such injuries.

Imaging with OPG

When available, the panoramic views provided by an OPG can be of great benefit in assessing fractures of the mandible and to a lesser extent the maxilla (Charlton et al. 1981) (see Fig. 9.76).

The use of MDCT for the imaging of mandibular fractures

The ability to obtain high-quality multiplanar reformations with MDCT is extremely helpful for the interpretation of mandibular fractures. In addition, surface-rendered 3D displays play an important role in the understanding of complex fractures, particularly when fracture displacement is to be surgically corrected (see Figs 9.77 and 9.78).

▼ **Fig. 9.78(a)** Disarticulation of the TMJs with rotation of the mandible enables a thorough examination of the fracture displacement from all angles. **(b)** Having a virtual eye behind the mandible, the fractures can even be examined at any angle from behind.

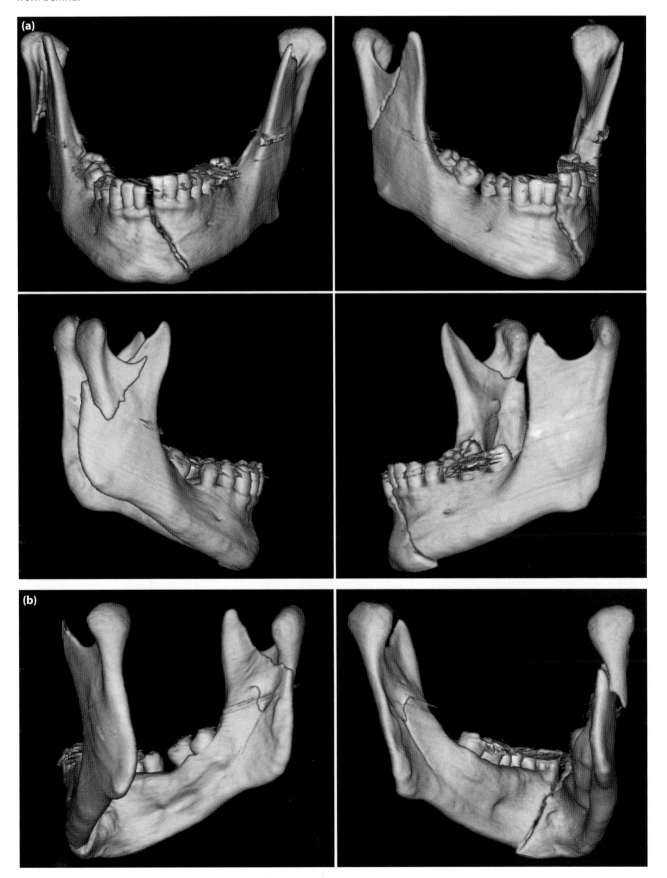

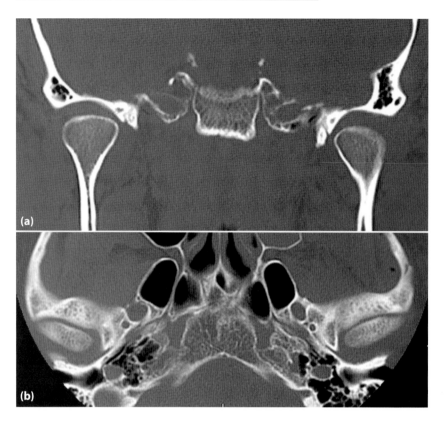

◀ **Fig. 9.79** Normal TMJs are well demonstrated in both the coronal and axial planes by MDCT. **(a)** The joints do not lie in the true coronal plane, as can be seen in **(b)**. As a consequence, coronal-oblique views are helpful if a fracture is present and displacement is to be carefully assessed.

The head of the mandible is elongated transversely. The upper, posterior and a negligible area on the anterior surface are covered by articular cartilage. An articular disc of fibrocartilage separates the articular surfaces of the mandible and temporal bone. The circumference of the disc is attached to the capsular ligament of the joint, dividing the joint into an upper and a lower compartment. With the TMJ at rest and the mouth closed, the mandibular head is in contact with the articular disc below the articular fossa. The head and the disc travel downwards and anteriorly as the mouth opens until they are positioned below the temporal eminence.

TMJ injuries

A direct blow to the mandible may transmit forces to the TMJs and cause a fracture or dislocation. Acute and repetitive trauma may result in disc displacement or degeneration, capsular adhesions, synovitis, osteochondritis dissecans, avascular necrosis or degenerative arthritis (Schellhas 1989).

Radiographic anatomy of the TMJs

The TMJ is a gliding joint, formed by the condyle of the mandible and the glenoid cavity of the temporal bone. The articular surface of the temporal bone consists of a concave articular fossa, which lies posterior to the temporal eminence.

Imaging of the TMJs

Plain films have a limited application in imaging of the TMJs, although as shown in Fig. 9.5, fractures of the mandibular condyles may be evident if displacement has occurred. Traditionally, plain films were acquired with the mouth open and closed to help assess bone injury and abnormal movement of the TMJ. Towne's and reversed Towne's views have also been used to image the mandibular condyles. These views were radiographically difficult to obtain and equally difficult to interpret due to bony superimposition. MDCT is the imaging method of choice for display of the bony structures of the TMJs (see Fig. 9.79). The joints lie in a plane that is slightly oblique to the coronal plane and the ability to reformat MDCT images in any plane is therefore a great advantage (see Figs 9.80 and 9.81).

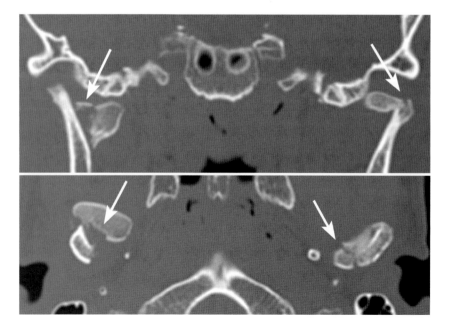

◀ **Fig. 9.80** Bilateral fractures of the mandibular condyles are demonstrated in coronal and axial planes (arrows). Both TMJs are dislocated. These injuries followed a fall, with a force to the tip of the mandible.

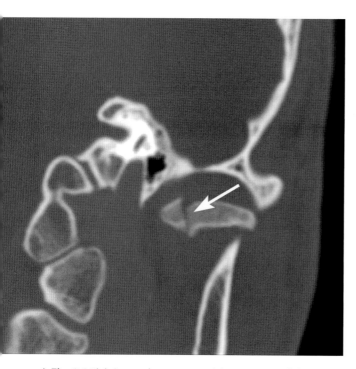

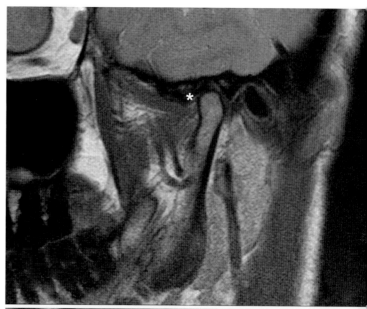

MRI is the diagnostic imaging procedure of choice for imaging the fibrocartilagenous disc of the TMJ (see Figs 9.82, 9.83, 9.84 and 9.85). Arthrography can also be used, and is especially helpful in cases of capsular adhesion or perforated disc (Schellhas et al. 1988).

If there has been internal derangement of the TMJs, the cartilaginous meniscus is best assessed with MRI or MR arthrography.

▲ **Fig. 9.81(a)** In another case, an oblique image of the left mandibular condyle shows a fracture of the condyle. Displacement at the condylar fracture site is well shown (arrow). The condyle lies in the articular fossa. A fracture of the neck of the condyle is also confirmed.

▼ **(b)** An oblique view of the right TMJ shows that the condyle lies in the articular fossa and demonstrates a fracture of the condylar neck (arrow).

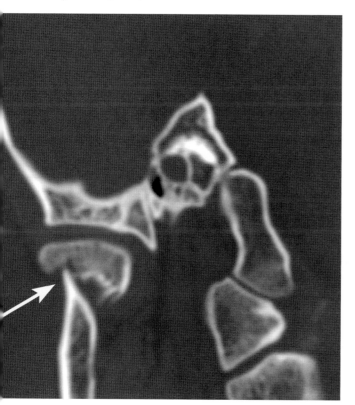

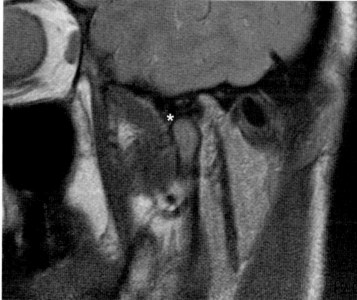

▲ **Fig. 9.82** A normal TMJ is demonstrated in mouth closed (upper image) and mouth open (lower image) positions by sagittal-oblique PD-weighted MR images. With the mouth closed, the articular disc (asterisk) lies in a normal position between the condyle and the articular fossa. On opening, excursion of the mandibular condyle is normal, reaching the apex of the temporal eminence and in this position the disc lies between the condyle and the temporal eminence (asterisk).

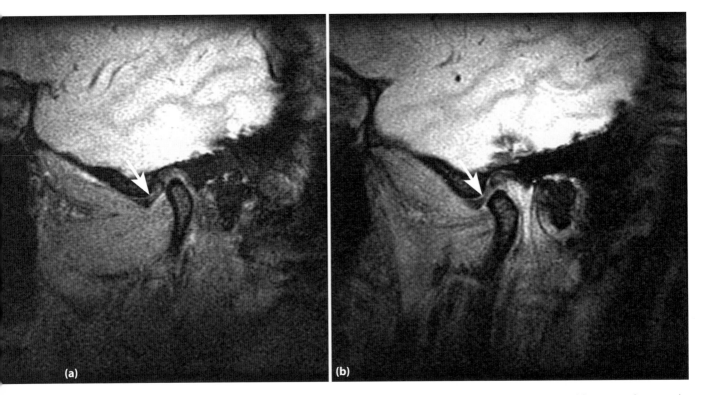

▲ **Fig. 9.83** A judo player at the Sydney 2000 Olympics was kicked in the jaw, following which she was unable to open her mouth normally. T2*-weighted GRE MR images were obtained in the sagittal plane with the mouth closed and with attempted mouth opening.
(a) There is anterior subluxation of the disc with the mouth closed. The disc has a characteristic bow-tie configuration and is indicated by an arrow.
(b) On opening, the disc does not move and blocks the normal anterior movement of the condyle (arrow). When partially open, the condyle recaptures the disc on the posterior aspect of the eminence and further movement is blocked.

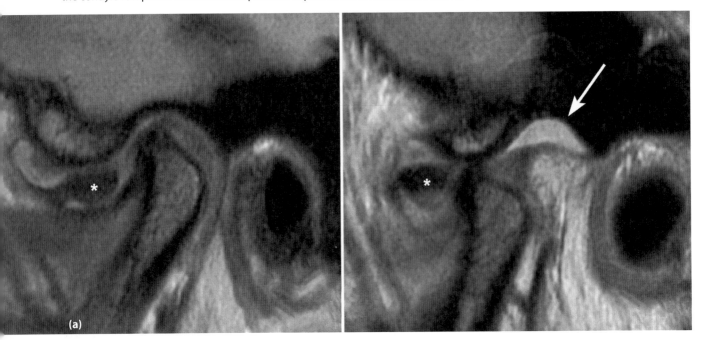

▲ **Fig. 9.84** Dislocation of the articular disc is demonstrated on sagittal PD-weighted MR images obtained with the mouth both closed and open.
(a) With the mouth closed, the disc (asterisk) lies below the apex of the temporal eminence instead of between the mandibular condyle and the articular fossa.
(b) On opening, the condyle reaches the apex of the temporal eminence, displacing the dislocated disc further anteriorly. An effusion is noted (arrow).

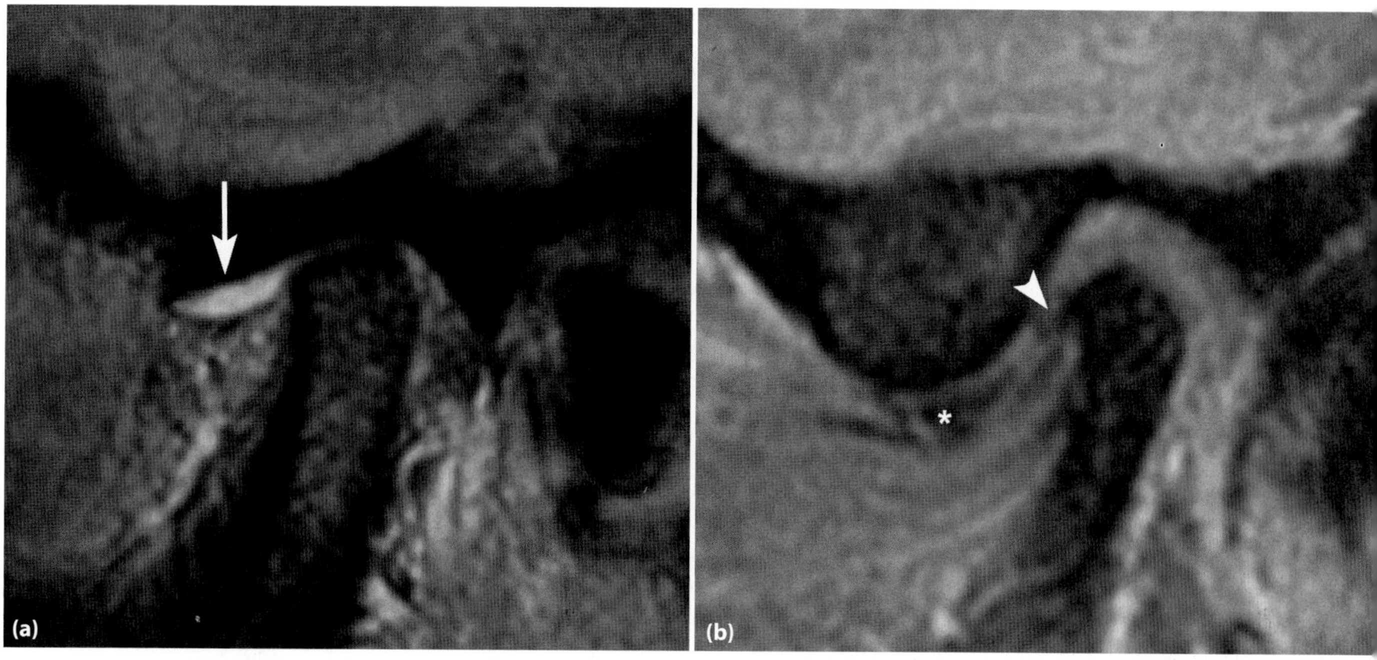

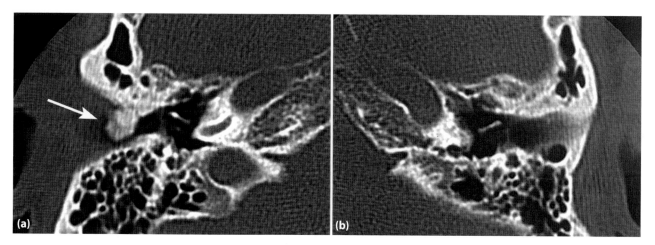

▲ **Fig. 9.85** Degenerative changes involve both TMJs on sagittal T2*-weighted GRE MR images obtained with the mouth closed.
(a) On the right side advanced degenerative changes are present with flattening of the articular surface of both the mandibular condyle and the temporal eminence. An effusion is present (arrow). The articular disc is not evident.
(b) On the left, the joint space is widened with the mouth closed, and the articular disc is dislocated (asterisk). An osteophyte is shown arising from the anterior aspect of the articular surface of the mandibular condyle.

A stress reaction secondary to sport: 'surfer's ear'

An exostosis may develop on the wall of the external auditory canal in response to repetitive stress caused by regular surfing in cold water. Over a number of years of surfing, these bony growths may completely obstruct the canal, causing deafness (Timofeev et al. 2004). In areas of Australia where the surfing culture is strong, the keen surfers can be recognised because they have blond hair and are deaf in one ear. This is because surfers routinely turn their head in the same direction when they pass through a wave, meaning that waves persistently break onto the same ear. The exostosis will then develop as a defence against this trauma (see Fig. 9.86).

▲ **Fig. 9.86** A CT scan demonstrates 'surfer's ear'.
(a) A large exostosis has developed at the entry of the right external auditory canal (arrow) in a dedicated surfer who has always turned his head to the right as he passes under a wave when paddling out through the surf. The exostosis has developed as a response to the repetitive stress caused by waves breaking on the right side of his head.
(b) Because the head is always turned the same way, the left ear is normal.

Fractures of the larynx

A laryngeal fracture is invariably due to a direct force to the neck and may constitute a medical emergency. Fortunately, this is an unusual sporting injury. Most laryngeal fractures are due to motor vehicle accidents, assaults, hanging and strangulation. Laryngeal injuries occur when a violent force compresses the larynx against the cervical spine. This force may result in devastating injuries including fractures, dislocations and mucosal tears.

The cervical spine and the mandible protect the larynx. In children, elasticity of the larynx offers additional protection against injury, but with advancing age and cartilaginous calcification, comminuted fractures of the larynx may occur. Males have a higher percentage of traumatic laryngeal injuries (Jewett et al. 1999) most likely due to a greater participation in violent sports and fighting.

Imaging of laryngeal injuries

MDCT is the imaging method of choice for laryngeal injuries. The rapid scan times and the ability to reformat in any imaging plane require only limited breath holding while still providing a detailed display of complex laryngeal anatomy (see Fig. 9.87). The 3D images may contribute to optimal imaging results (Lupetin et al. 1998) and may be especially useful when conventional CT, MRI and fibroscopy have failed to reveal laryngeal trauma (Kobayashi et al. 2004). MRI has not become popular for use in laryngeal imaging.

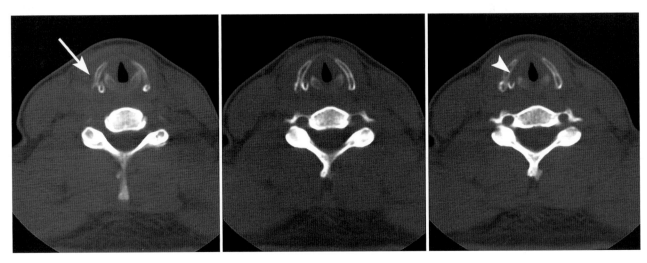

▲ **Fig. 9.87** A female basketball player at the Sydney 2000 Olympics was struck across the neck by an opponent and experienced pain over the larynx and difficulty in speaking. The airway was not obstructed. Axial CT images demonstrate a fracture of the right posterior horn of the thyroid cartilage (arrow). The separated fragment has become lodged in the adjacent cricothyroid joint. There is resultant widening of the joint (arrowhead).

References

Carroll SM, Jawad MA, West M, O'Connor TP. 'One hundred and ten sports related facial fractures.' *Br J Sports Med* 1995, 29: 194–5.

Charlton OP, Daffner RD, Gehweiler JA et al. 'Panoramic zonography of fractures of the facial skeleton.' *Am J Roentgenol* 1981, 137: 109–12.

Costello BJ, Papadopoulos H, Ruis R. 'Pediatric craniomaxillofacial trauma.' *Clin Pediatr Emerg Med* 2005, 6: 32–40.

Dodson TB. 'Third molars may double the risk of an angle fracture of the mandible. *Evid Based Dent* 2004, 5: 78.

Dolan DD, Jacoby CG. 'Facial fractures.' *Semin Roentgenol* 1978, 13: 37–51.

Exadaktylos AK, Eggensperger NH, Eggi S, Smolka KM et al. 'Sports related maxillofacial injuries: the first maxillofacial trauma database in Switzerland.' *Br J Sports Med* 2004, 38: 750–3.

Gassner R, Tarkin T et al. 'Mountainbiking, a dangerous sport: comparison with bicycling on oral and maxillofacial trauma.' *Int J Maxillofac Surg* 1999, 28: 188.

Hammerschlag SB, Hughes S, O'Reilly GV, Weber AL. 'Another look at blowout fractures of the orbit.' *Am J Roentgenol* 1982, 3: 331–5.

Jewett BS, Shockley WW, Rutledge R. 'External laryngeal trauma analysis of 392 patients.' *Arch Otolaryngol Head Neck Surg* 1999, 125: 877–80.

Johnson DH Jr, Colman M, Larsson S, Garner OP Jr, Hanafee W. 'Computed tomography in medial maxilla-orbital fractures.' *J Comput Assist Tomogr* 1984, 8: 416–19.

Kobayashi M, Seto A, Nomura T. '3D-CT highly useful in diagnosing foreign bodies in the paraesophageal orifice.' *Nippon Jibiinkoka Gakkai Kaiho* 2004, 107: 800–3.

LeFort R. 'Etude/experimentiale sur les fractures de la machoine superieure.' *Rev Chir* 1901, 23: 208–11.

Lim LH, Moore MH et al. 'Sports-related facial fracture: a review of 137 patients.' *Aust NZ J Surg* 1993, 63: 784–9.

Logan M, O'Driscoll K, Masterson J. 'The utility of nasal bone radiographs in nasal trauma.' *Clin Radiol* 1994, 49(3): 192–4.

Lupetin AR, Hollander M, Rao VM. 'Evaluation of laryngotracheal trauma.' *Semin Musculoskelet Radiol* 1998, 2: 105–16.

Rogers LF. *Radiology of Skeletal Trauma*, 2nd edn, Churchill-Livingstone, New York, 1992, pp. 365–437.

Romeo SJ, Hawley CJ, Romeo MW et al. 'Facial injuries in sport: a team physician's guide to diagnosis and treatment.' *The Physician and Sportsmedicine* 2005, 33(4): 45–53.

Schellhas KP. 'Internal derangement of the temporomandibular joint: radiologic staging with clinical, surgical, and pathological correlation.' *Magn Reson Imaging* 1989, 7: 495–515.

Schellhas KP, Wilkes CH, Omlie MR, Peterson CM, Jonnson SD, Keck RJ, Block JC, Fritts HM, Heithoff KB. 'The diagnosis of temporomandibular joint disease: two compartment arthrography and MR.' *Am J Roentgenol* 1988, 151: 341–50.

Timofeev I, Notkima N, Smith IM. 'Exostoses of external auditory canal: a long-term follow-up of surgical treatment.' *Otolaryngol* 2004, 29: 588–94.

Tonami H, Nakagawa T, Ohguchi M et al. 'Surface coil MR images of orbital blow out fractures: a comparison with reformatted CT.' *Am J Roentgenol* 1987, 8: 445–9.

Turner BG, Rhea JT, Thrall JH et al. 'Trends in the use of CT and radiography in the evaluation of facial trauma, 1992–2002: implications for current costs.' *Am J Roentgenol* 2004, 183: 751–4.

Image acknowledgments

The authors wish to thank the following colleagues who kindly offered images for inclusion in this chapter:

- Dr Raouli Risti, Gosford Hospital (Figs 9.3, 9.29(a), (b) and (c), 9.30(a) and (b), 9.31, 9.32, 9.45, 9.47, 9.48(a) and (b), 9.49, 9.77 and 9.78)
- Janeen Gibbs, The Royal North Shore Hospital (Figs. 9.12, 9.36, 9.37, 9.39, 9.40, 9.41, 9.42, 9.43, 9.44(a) and (b), 9.50, 9.51, 9.53, 9.54, 9.55, 9.58, 9.59(a) and (b), 9.60, 9.61, 9.62, 9.63, 9.64, 9.65, 9.66, 9.67, 9.68, 9.69, 9.70, 9.79, 9.80, 9.81 and 9.82)
- Lavier Gomes (Figs. 9.82, 9.84 and 9.85)
- Dr Peter Briscoe (Fig. 9.86)
- Dr Sharron Flahive (Fig. 9.1(a) and (b))

These images have significantly added to the quality of the chapter.

10

Intervention

Jock Anderson and John Read
with Gus Ferguson

The role of the radiologist within the team of specialists managing sports injuries continues to change and expand. Now, in addition to a diagnostic role, there is an expanding requirement for the radiologist to be directly involved in the management of injuries, by using imaging for the precise placement of needles for percutaneous injections and aspirations.

Some injections may be quite satisfactorily performed by the sports physician in their consulting rooms. Others, however, will require a more accurate and controlled procedure if complications are to be avoided and the best results achieved. The radiologist is uniquely placed to perform these more demanding interventions by using a variety of imaging tools such as fluoroscopy, CT and ultrasound. Because of the increased safety and improved results achieved by image guidance (Eustace et al. 1995), over the last decade there has been a constant growth in the demand for this service. The range of procedures and the sophistication of the requests have also increased. Such is the demand that 'intervention' has become a subspecialty within radiology and image-guided procedures are now a highly valued component of the therapeutic armamentarium of the sports clinician.

'Intervention' has become an additional chapter in this second edition in recognition of the importance of this subspecialty. This chapter offers an opportunity to review the literature and to identify and confront ethical dilemmas that arise from time to time in this subspecialty.

Ethical considerations and the position of the radiologist

Ethical issues abound in sports medicine, particularly in the area of masking of pain and in the use of particular drugs. The radiologist's involvement begins when they are asked to perform an interventional procedure. Although the radiologist is not the primary decision maker, and is in essence the technician carrying out the procedures requested by the sports medicine team, ethically and medicolegally the radiologist must take responsibility for the immediate and ongoing effects of the procedure on the health of the athlete. The radiologist must be aware of the ethical and/or legal considerations before deciding to proceed. Most of these issues will be confined to the professional relationship between the athlete and their immediate medical personnel, but some problems may flow over to the radiologist and it is likely that radiological encounters with these issues will increase.

The majority of these considerations can be dealt with on the sidelines or in the change rooms and the radiologist is rarely, if ever, called on for an opinion or to help with an injection. However, with the appearance of mobile image intensifiers, ultrasound machines in suitcases and the installation of imaging facilities in the new generation of change rooms, it is only a matter of time before the radiologist will be positioning needles for nerve root blocks and masking the pain of a fracture. Radiological involvement already occurs at the Olympic Games and the Commonwealth Games and as a part of World Cup meetings in all sports. Consequently, it is essential for the sports medicine radiologist to have a clear understanding of the position of intervention in each sport.

A radiologist may also become caught up in conflicts of interest. Conflicts of interest may exist between the short- and long-term health of the athlete, their commercial interests, their career ambitions and the commercial or sporting interests of a team or club. At times, the pressures of team responsibilities or even the academic research interests of a sports physician may influence management decisions.

It is advisable for a radiologist to consider the following:

- how they would handle a request for an injection of local anaesthetic to mask pain, enabling an athlete to train and compete with an injury
- how to handle a request for the injection of a drug such as corticosteroids that is on the restricted list.

Masking pain

Pain is the body's major defence against injury, so logic would suggest that to remove this defence is to invite progression of an injury already present, or to allow new injuries to occur to the anaesthetised area. There is considerable anecdotal evidence to suggest that the use of pain-killing local anaesthetic injections in professional sports is widespread (Nelson 2002). The authors certainly have had first-hand experience of this phenomenon at the Sydney 2000 Olympics, where there was an extraordinary demand for interventional procedures to be performed at the Imaging Service within the Village Polyclinic.

In professional football, this practice probably began in the United States in the 1960s and in Australia in the 1970s (Orchard 2002). Based upon a documented case series of injuries encountered as a team physician in the professional Australian Football League and National Rugby League codes over a six-year period, John Orchard (2001) challenged physicians to either ban this particular use of local anaesthetic injections or produce guidelines for its rational use.

The Australian College of Sports Physicians (ACSP) recognised that the practice of using local anaesthetic in sport was almost exclusively confined to sports medicine practitioners and, on behalf of the ACSP, Locke (2002) offered the following position statement:

The ACSP:

- *acknowledges that there is a place for the use of local anaesthetic agents in professional sport;*
- *recognises that the use of local anaesthetic agents in the professional sporting environment is principally a matter between doctors and their patients;*
- *recognises that the use of local anaesthetic agents in professional sport requires discussion between doctors and their patients and informed formal consent of the patient given in an appropriate environment prior to the planned intervention;*
- *acknowledges the lack of scientific information regarding the use of local anaesthetic agents in the sporting environment and recommends that research be undertaken to increase the body of scientific knowledge;*
- *recommends that education and training of medical practitioners in the use of local anaesthetic agents in sport is appropriate;*
- *does not endorse the use of local anaesthetic injections in the sporting environment for children under 16 years of age.*

The National Collegiate Athletic Association (NCAA) in the United States has issued non-specific advice that the final decision is at the discretion of the individual treating physician, while the policy of the International Federation of Sports Medicine (FIMS) states that the physician may not in any way mask pain in order to enable the athlete's return to sport if there is any risk of aggravating the injury. Orchard (2004) emphasises that the financial benefits of remaining on the playing field will often blur judgement in relation to both the short- and longer-term risks of injury. These include tendon and ligament rupture, accelerated joint degeneration, fracture, pneumothorax, dislocation and even inadvertent nerve block causing short-term loss of strength and coordination, which may occur following femoral, obturator or sciatic nerve blocks (Orchard 2004). Injections around the ankle, thumb and wrist should not be undertaken lightly, with preliminary imaging being advisable to exclude tendon injury and minimise any subsequent risk of complete rupture requiring surgery. From a workers compensation perspective, the direct relevance of local anaesthetic injections to long-term disability is extraordinarily difficult to define. There is often no single incident in time that can be identified as the specific cause for degenerative joint disease and there are also many other factors that may play a part in its development. Imaging-guided and aseptically controlled injections off-field are likely to be safer than those performed clinically during a game.

The use of corticosteroids

Corticosteroids are not 'anabolic' agents, but have nevertheless been included on the banned list of the World Anti-Doping Agency (WADA). Corticosteroid injections are permitted out of competition, but are only allowable in competition *if the national sporting federation is notified*. If their use is contemplated, then an abbreviated Therapeutic Use Exemption (TUE) form must be completed and forwarded to the national sporting body.

The subject of doping in sport is beyond the scope of this text. A wealth of information is available on the Internet and the full list of banned substances is available from WADA. WADA was established following the Lausanne World Conference on Doping in Sport in 1999, and its mission is to promote and coordinate the fight against doping in sport, in all its forms, at an international level. It combines the resources of governments and sporting bodies to enhance and supplement existing efforts to educate athletes about the harms of doping and to promote fair play. The World Anti-Doping Code was accepted at the Copenhagen World Conference on Doping in Sport in 2003 by major sports federations, key stakeholders and governments. The Australian Sports Commission together with the National Sporting Organisations (NSO) enforces anti-doping policies and programs. The NSO works with the Australian Sports Drug Agency (ASDA) to ensure that Australia maintains its respected anti-doping program.

The side effects of corticosteroid preparations

The most frequently encountered side effect is a 'post-injection flare', which is transient pain thought to be due to a crystal-induced synovitis arising from the steroid suspension. This occurs in about 5% of cases, usually in the first six to 36 hours and runs a self-limiting two- to three-day course. Management includes non-steroidal anti-inflammatory drugs (NSAIDs) and icing. Other adverse effects occur infrequently and may include a vasovagal reaction and a transient hyperglycaemia in poorly controlled diabetics. Subcutaneous fat and skin atrophy with depigmentation may result from either direct infiltration of subcutaneous fat or overdistension of the joint,

▼ **Fig. 10.1** Pericapsular calcification at the bases of the second and third proximal phalanges has followed a corticosteroid injection, performed 12 months previously, for a 2–3 web space Morton's neuroma.

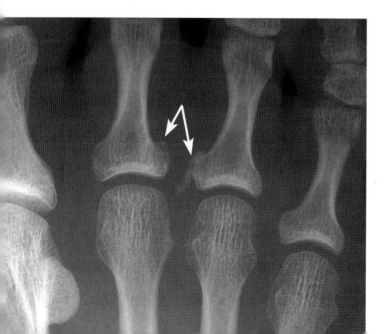

producing reflux of corticosteroid back along the needle tract. Facial flushing has also been observed, and needle trauma may occur to structures such as muscle, nerves and articular cartilage. Asymptomatic pericapsular calcification may also result from a corticosteroid injection (see Fig. 10.1).

Infection is rare, with an incidence rate of 1 in 15 000, but it is a serious complication that requires prompt and aggressive management. Despite anecdotal reports, there is no convincing evidence that an intra-articular corticosteroid injection causes either an avascular necrosis of bone or a neuropathic joint (Newberg 1998). Nevertheless, injections into large weightbearing joints for osteoarthritis are probably best performed only as a late-stage temporising measure for those patients with severe pain who are inevitably proceeding to joint replacement surgery. No more than three injections of the same joint should be performed within a 12-month period, spaced at minimum intervals of four months.

Absolute contraindications to corticosteroid injection include infection, an allergic diathesis or a history of a previous anaphylactic reaction to an injected pharmaceutical. As the injection of multiple joints at the same time has the potential to transiently suppress the hypothalamic-pituitary-adrenal axis for two to seven days, high-dose injections are probably best restricted to one large joint at a time. Additionally, the interval between such injections should preferably be more than six weeks (Gray and Gottlieb 1983; Fadale and Wiggins 1994).

Table 10.1 lists reported complications and side effects of corticosteroid injection for athletic injuries.

Table 10.1 Reported complications and side effects of corticosteroid injection for athletic injuries

Reported complications and side effects	Incidence
Post-injection pain	9.7%
Skin atrophy	2.4%
Skin depigmentation	0.8%
Localised erythema/warmth	0.7%
Facial flushing	0.6%
Tendon rupture	Unknown
Fascial rupture	Unknown
Subcutaneous atrophy	Unknown
Axillary nerve injury	Unknown
Mycobacterium infection	Unknown

Source: Nichols (2005).

Non-spinal intervention in sports medicine

Joint injections

Joint injections can have both a diagnostic and therapeutic value. Many joints cannot be consistently injected by palpation alone, even though the clinician may be confident that the drug has been accurately delivered. Jones et al. (1993) showed that, surprisingly, only 10% of palpation-guided joint injections were actually intra-articular, and Eustace et al. (1995) showed that only 42% of palpation-guided glenohumeral joint injections actually reached their intra-articular target. Obviously, having a skilled imaging-guided injection under fluoroscopic (see Fig. 10.2), CT or ultrasound guidance (see Fig. 10.3) must have a significant influence on the outcome of a therapeutic injection, with the drug reaching the planned target. When intra-articular injections are used for diagnostic purposes, a false negative or positive result is likely each time the injection misses the joint.

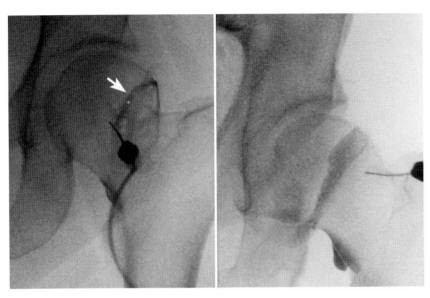

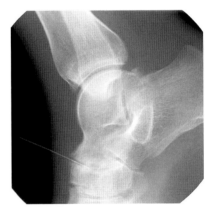

▲ **Fig. 10.2(a)** Fluoroscopic images of the hip show a needle well positioned in the joint space. With injection, the contrast runs freely away from the needle tip (arrow) and in the right-hand image is seen to pool in the dependent part of the joint.

▲ **(b)** Fluoroscopic guidance enables a needle to be precisely placed in a narrowed, arthritic joint.

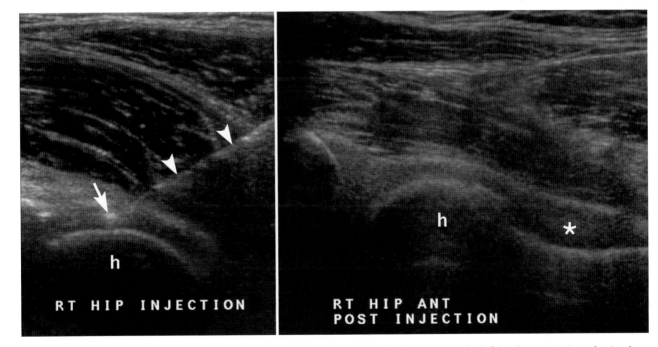

▲ **Fig. 10.3** An ultrasound-guided injection of the hip joint is demonstrated. The image on the left is a long-axis view obtained over the anterior aspect of the hip joint with the needle (arrowheads) in situ. The needle tip (arrow) is located immediately deep to the anterior joint capsule over the mid anterior convexity of the femoral head (h). Injection was performed without resistance and without focal accumulation or blebbing at the needle tip. The image on the right is a panoramic long-axis view of the femoral head and neck obtained following injection to confirm distension of the anteroinferior joint recess by the injectate (*).

As a variety of techniques can be used to inject joints, only general concepts are included in this discussion.

Preparation for the procedure

- A signed consent form should be obtained.

- Strict asepsis must be observed.

- Needle calibre and length should be selected according to the size and depth of the joint to be injected. Larger calibre needles, up to 18 gauge, may allow easier and more effective joint aspiration. This is of importance when a tense effusion requires decompression for pain relief, or when a specimen of joint fluid is to be obtained for analysis. Large needles can also make the injection of large joints easier by minimising the potential for complete burial of the needle tip within relatively thick articular cartilage.

- The chosen needle approach depends to some extent upon the imaging method chosen for guidance, but is preferably the shortest and least painful pathway that offers the lowest risk of complication.

Imaging of the procedure

Each interventional procedure requires adequate documentation by means of the acquisition of images. The space injected should be recorded, otherwise the procedure may lack diagnostic specificity. This is particularly important where the targeted joint may communicate with other articulations, bursae or tendon sleeves, and it is important to outline the injected compartments with a small amount of contrast agent (see Figs 10.4 and 10.5). The image becomes an important part of the patient's records from both a clinical and medicolegal viewpoint. Pre-operative fluoroscopically guided injections of the foot and ankle give the surgeon a greater level of confidence (Lucas et al. 1997). As an alternative to fluoroscopy, ultrasound-guided injections can be used with a small amount of contrast agent mixed with the injectate and an immediate post-injection plain film image obtained.

Choice of drugs to be injected

A mixture of corticosteroid and bupivacaine 0.5% is typically injected. The total volume of injectate should not exceed the capacity of the targeted joint, as capsular overdistension is painful and, as previously noted, can have adverse consequences if reflux occurs along the needle tract. The patient should carefully note any degree of pain relief provided by the bupivacaine over a period of three to four hours following the injection, as this is important diagnostic information. The joint should be rested for several days to minimise the risk of post-injection steroid 'flare'. Some practitioners also include a 48-hour course of NSAIDs and intermittent icing as an added precaution. The effectiveness of the injected corticosteroid is assessed after two weeks, the usual period of clinical follow-up.

There are a variety of commercially available corticosteroid preparations. These vary considerably with regard to solubility, potency, speed of onset and duration of effect. The

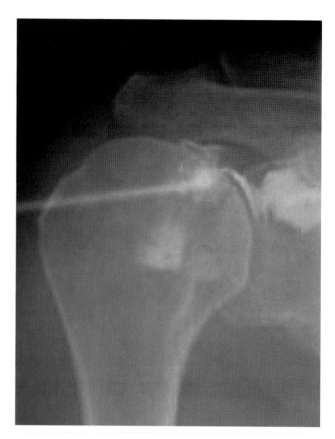

▲ **Fig. 10.4** Fluoroscopic images are often of poor quality, but are usually sufficient to help assess needle position. In this case, the needle is well positioned, with contrast outlining the joint space and running down the bicipital groove around the tendon of the long head of the biceps.

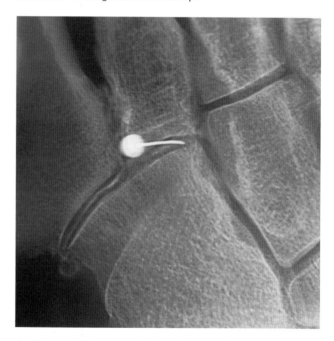

▲ **Fig. 10.5** A fluoroscopically guided needle placement has enabled accurate placement of the needle tip in the medial aspect of the fourth tarsometatarsal articulation. With injection of contrast, correct needle placement is confirmed and a common cavity is demonstrated between the fourth and fifth tarsometatarsal joints.

more soluble agents have a faster onset, shorter duration of therapeutic effect and a lower propensity for post-injection flare and subcutaneous fat atrophy. For joint injections, most physicians favour agents that contain both rapid and long-acting components. Betamethasone sodium phosphate is soluble and rapid acting, while betamethasone sodium acetate is less soluble but longer acting. Therapeutically, the role of joint injection with corticosteroid is for either pain relief or the management of an erosive arthritis. It is important to recognise that a steroid injection is not a treatment in itself. When properly considered, an intra-articular corticosteroid injection is merely an adjunct to the overall treatment plan and has variable success on patient outcome.

Conditions that may benefit from percutaneous intervention

Frozen shoulder

The term 'frozen shoulder' has been used since 1934 to describe a common syndrome of shoulder pain character-ised by generalised restriction of both passive and active glenohumeral joint movement. Plain films are typically normal, although demineralisation of the humeral head and neck occurs with prolonged inactivity. Later in 1945, Neviaser introduced the term 'adhesive capsulitis' to describe the same clinical entity based upon arthrographic findings. This term is misleading because there are no intracapsular or extracapsular adhesions (Bunker 1985). The aetiology of 'frozen shoulder' is unknown, but an association with diabetes is recognised in about 10% of cases.

Despite an excellent prognosis in the vast majority of cases, 'frozen shoulder' may take an average of two years to resolve. A minority of cases have long-term disability and pain (Binder et al. 1984; Shaffer et al. 1992). A variety of treatments have been advocated, some of which require intervention. These procedures include a suprascapular nerve block, an intra-articular injection of corticosteroid and glenohumeral joint hydrodilatation with capsular rupture, either alone or with an intra-articular injection of corticosteroid.

A joint injection can be a painful procedure, requiring either fluoroscopic or ultrasound guidance (see Figs 10.6 and 10.7). Jacobs et al. (1991) demonstrated pain relief but no more than 5° improvement in movement with corticosteroid injected alone or in combination with mild joint distension using a local anaesthetic volume of no more than 10 cc. The authors' experience with this procedure is that most patients report 80–90% pain relief and subsequently show slow resolution over many months, provided that the condition is not aggravated by ongoing provocative shoulder activities. Full-blown hydrodilatation procedures that combine intra-articular corticosteroid and saline with intentional rupture of the joint capsule can be extremely painful. Usually 10–55 cc of normal saline is used, but occasionally as much as 100 cc may be used and the subsequent pain may be such as to require parenteral narcotic analgesia. Bell et al. (2003) found that substantial pain relief occurred in 89% of cases and there was 20–39° improvement in range of motion at two months

post-hydrodilatation. Bell et al. (2003) also found that diabetic patients have more pain at presentation and less reliable relief of pain after hydrodilatation.

Osteitis pubis

The value of corticosteroid injection in the management of osteitis pubis remains unproven. In 1995, Holt et al. reported the use of clinically guided injection of the pubic symphysis that provided an overall good result in a small group of intercollegiate athletes. However, the consistency of injections performed by palpation alone is questionable. The potential exists for the local anaesthetic and corticosteroid to leak into the periarticular tissues and to confuse the diagnostic assessment, by fortuitously acting to reduce pain arising from adjacent soft-tissue pathology.

Imaging-guided injection of the symphyseal cleft can be performed under fluoroscopic, ultrasound or CT control (see Fig. 10.8). O'Connell et al. (2002) reported a technique of symphyseal injection under fluoroscopic guidance in 16 elite athletes with suspected osteitis pubis. Puncture of the interpubic disc alone caused groin pain prior to the injection of contrast medium in 10 patients, and the provocative instil-lation of 1.0 ml of non-ionic contrast produced groin pain in the remaining six. This was followed by the therapeutic injection of 20 mg of prednisolone acetate and 1 ml of 0.5% bupivacaine. Fourteen (87.5%) of the 16 patients experienced immediate but subtotal relief of groin pain and were able to resume sporting activities 48 hours after the procedure; ten (62.5%) reported substantial but incomplete pain relief two weeks after the procedure; and five (31.2%) were completely symptom-free at six months. The study concluded that in athletes, symphyseal cleft injection can produce an objective diagnosis and short-term symptom relief allowing involve-ment in sporting events.

Ganglia

Ganglia are cysts that contain a transparent clear or straw-coloured mucinous fluid and have a fibrous wall without any recognisable epithelial lining. Ganglia arise either as a synovial herniation that may communicate with a joint, bursa or ten-don sleeve or as a focus of advanced mucoid degeneration within dense connective tissues.

For practical purposes, the terms 'ganglion cyst' and 'syn-ovial cyst' are interchangeable. The latter term is often used to describe cystification of a normally occurring synovial recess, such as a Baker's cyst. Mixed terminology or interchangeable usage is often encountered in radiology reports.

If contrast medium is injected into a joint adjacent to a wrist ganglion, a communication with the ganglia is often demonstrated. However, injection of the ganglion itself usually fails to show any communication with the joint, suggesting the presence of a 'one-way valve' mechanism (Jayson and Dixon 1970; Andren and Eiken 1971; Dalinka et al. 1981).

Ganglion cysts are most common in the extremities, but can occur within connective tissue at any site that is subjected to trauma or repeated mechanical loading. They occur at all ages and carry no malignant potential. A

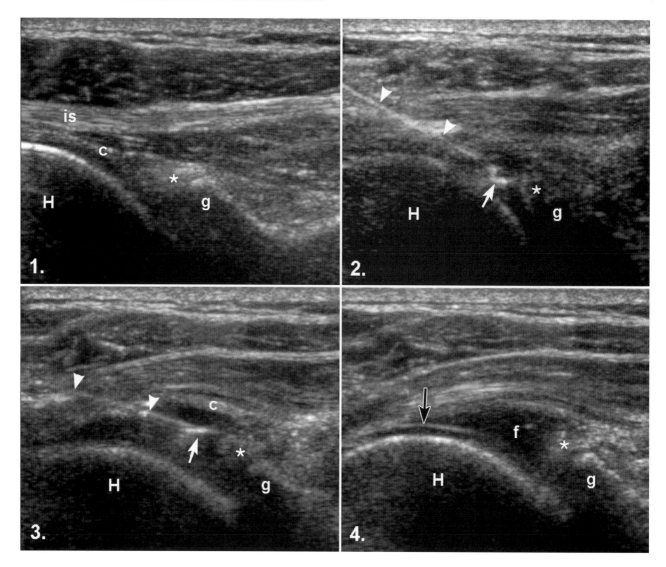

▲ **Fig. 10.6** Ultrasound guidance is used for a glenohumeral joint injection.

1. A pre-injection long-axis image is obtained of the infraspinatus tendon (is) at the posterior aspect of the glenohumeral joint showing the recognisable anatomic landmarks of the humeral head (H), posterior glenoid rim (g), posterior glenoid labrum (*) and the posterior glenohumeral capsule (c).

2. The needle (arrowheads) is positioned with the tip (arrow) preferably between the free margin of the posterior glenoid labrum and the hypoechoic articular cartilage of the humeral head. Note the bevel of the needle is facing upwards, as this orientation has an advantage of avoiding needle-tip deflection during passage through the overlying infraspinatus tendon.

3. For intra-articular injection, the needle tip (arrow) often requires initial rotation through 90° or 180° to find an intracapsular position that will allow resistance-free injection. Note the bevel in this case is now facing downwards. Injected sonolucent fluid has displaced the posterior joint capsule (c) away from the humeral head, confirming the intra-articular placement of the injectate.

4. A post-injection image following withdrawal of the needle shows sonolucent fluid (f) distending the posterior glenohumeral joint recess, revealing the reflective acoustic interface of the articular cartilage (black arrow) at the posterior surface of the humeral head.

Source: Modified from Zwar et al. (2004), with permission.

careful analysis is advisable to avoid confusion with other solid mass lesions that can sometimes have a similar MRI appearance (see Fig. 10.9). Other cystic lesions may have a similar appearance on ultrasound. These include an aneurysm, abscess, oil cyst, haematoma, seroma or a neoplasm with a cystic component. On ultrasound, most ganglia have a simple rounded appearance with a smooth thin wall, although they may be lobulated or septated. Normally, the interior of the ganglion is predominantly echo-free and the ganglion wall is thin and smooth. There is posterior acoustic enhancement. A progressively tapering 'neck' pointing to the probable site of origin is present in many cases. Ganglia arising from joints may show intra-osseous extension and in some cases demonstrate an adjacent zone of reactive synovitis with accompanying hyperaemia on Doppler ultrasound. Leaking cysts may show localised

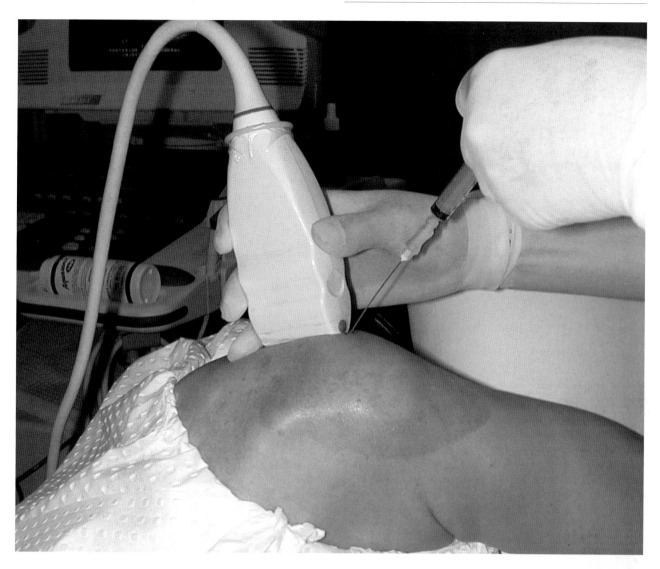

▲ **Fig. 10.7** Transducer positioning and needle alignment for a glenohumeral injection are demonstrated. Passing the needle along the imaging plane of the ultrasound transducer enables real-time visualisation. In this example, a glenohumeral joint injection is performed using a posterior approach. *Source*: From Zwar et al. (2004), with permission.

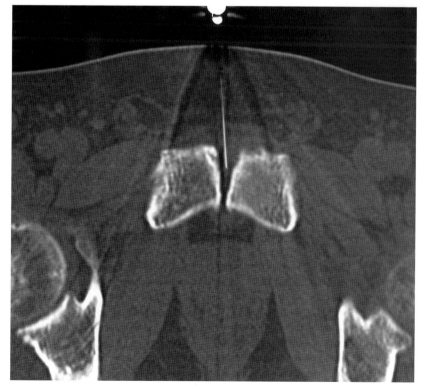

▶ **Fig. 10.8** Using CT guidance, the needle is satisfactorily positioned in the symphysis pubis.

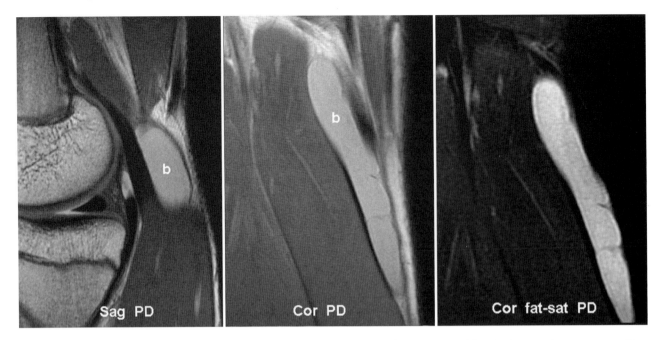

▲ **Fig. 10.9(a)** A semimembranosis-gastrocnemius bursopathy has developed in a 14-year-old patient, secondary to overuse. The imaging appearances superficially mimic a Baker's cyst on MRI and synovial chondromatosis on ultrasound. Note the subtle but diffuse 'cobblestone' pattern of internal signal on both PD and fat-suppressed PD-weighted MR imaging. This appearance could easily be mistaken for fluid with poor greyscale windowing.

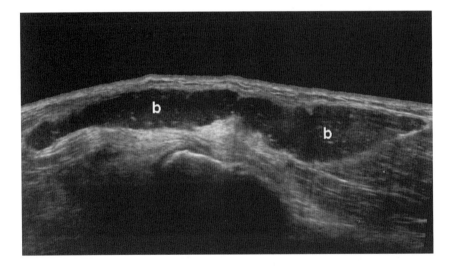

◄ **(b)** Corresponding long-axis ultrasound images show a bursa distended predominantly by weakly reflective tissue rather than fluid, and additional scattered foci of bright reflectivity casting acoustic shadows and thus simulating chondromatosis. Histopathology showed fibrofatty tissue containing a cystic space comprised of fibrous tissue lined by a synovial layer with hyperplasia and nodular areas of focal wall infolding. Increased mucoid ground substance and fibrinoid degeneration of collagen typical of overuse were noted in the surrounding fibrofatty spaces. There were no inflammatory cells. Semimembranosis-gastrocnemius bursa = b.

wall thickening and irregularity at the leak point. Chronic or previously ruptured cysts with inflammatory changes may contain low-level internal echoes on ultrasound (Fornage and Rifkin 1988).

Ganglia are harmless and may be left untreated. Spontaneous resolution is common, with 33–45% of untreated patients 'ganglion-free' at six years and 51–63% 'ganglion-free' at ten years (Burke et al. 2003). Children have been reported to show a rate of 63–79% spontaneous resolution (Rosson and Walker 1989; MacCollum 1977). If active treatment is planned, options may include intervention. The ganglia may be simply aspirated, or there can be needle aspiration and a corticosteroid injection:

- *Needle aspiration alone* Wide bore needle aspiration alone has a recurrence rate of 60–70% at 12 months, whether or not there have been multiple wall punctures (Nield and Evans 1986; Richman et al. 1987; Burke et al. 2003). Improved results of 85–88% resolution have been reported after several repeated aspirations (Zubowicz and Ishii 1987; Oni 1992). Because aspiration reassures patients that no malignancy is present, this procedure decreases the frequency of surgical excision (Stephen et al. 1999).

- *Needle aspiration and a corticosteroid injection* Varying results have been reported when needle aspiration is supplemented with an injection of corticosteroid. Some authors report no difference in recurrence rate (Varley et al. 1997; Wright et al. 1994), whereas others report lower recurrence rates in the 40–50% range (Holm and Pandey 1973; Burke et al. 2003). The rationale for steroid use is unclear, as most ganglia have no associated inflammatory component. The catabolic properties of corticosteroids theoretically delay the healing of the puncture site and possibly help to maintain a 'leaky' or weakened lesion, which is then more susceptible to spontaneous decompression.

- *Injection of hyaluronidase* Mixed results have also been reported if hyaluronidase (up to 150 units in 1 ml) is instilled into a ganglion 24 hours prior to needle aspiration and corticosteroid steroid injection (Otu 1992; Paul and Sochart 1997). A cure rate of 89–95% was found if hyaluronidase is included, but Seki and Bell (1997) reported only about a 50% cure rate after three treatments regardless of the injection type.

Methods of ganglion aspiration

Needle aspiration procedures are best performed under real-time ultrasound control, as this provides direct visualisation of the needle tip and allows accurate and effective cyst evacuation (see Figs 10.10 and 10.11). Depending upon the size and depth of the ganglion and the viscosity of the mucinous fluid content, needle or sheath-needle sizes ranging up to 14 gauge may be necessary, with smaller calibres being tried first. In addition to aspiration, the authors also routinely 'fenestrate' the lesion using multiple needle passes through different portions of the ganglion wall before injecting a small amount of betamethasone (usually 5.7 mg), partly into the lumen of the emptied lesion and partly into the periganglionic space.

It should be noted that recurrence can occur even after surgical excision. Reported surgical recurrence rates vary from 1 to 28% (Angelides 1988; Clay and Clement 1988; Faithfull

▼ **Fig. 10.10** Ultrasound images demonstrate aspiration of a Baker's cyst under ultrasound control. A panoramic long-axis image on the left shows the Baker's cyst (b) in overview prior to needle aspiration. The lower left image shows visualisation of the needle (arrow) within the lumen of the cyst immediately prior to aspiration. The lower right image shows collapse of the cyst walls (arrowheads) at the conclusion of the aspiration procedure. The use of manual compression at the skin surface by an assistant during the aspiration process can help to 'milk' the cyst contents towards the needle tip and assist with its complete emptying.

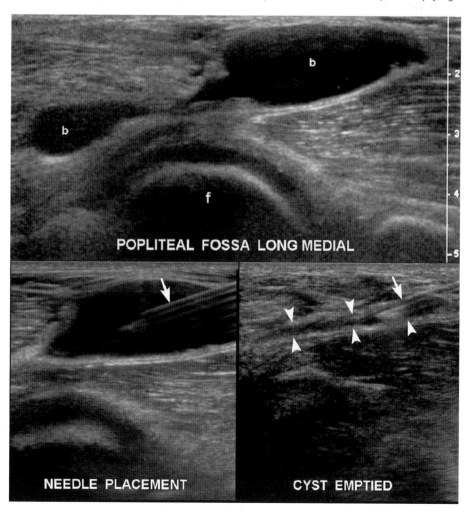

POPLITEAL FOSSA LONG MEDIAL

NEEDLE PLACEMENT

CYST EMPTIED

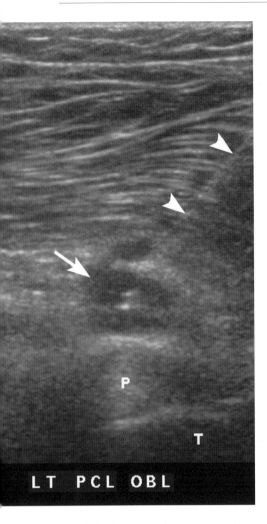

▲ Fig. 10.11 Aspiration of a posterior cruciate ligament (PCL) ganglion is performed under ultrasound control. Even though small in size or deep in location, ganglion cysts can be aspirated and injected under ultrasound control if they can be clearly visualised on preliminary real-time scanning. In this case, the echogenic bevel of the aspirating needle can be clearly seen on a long-axis ultrasound image within the central lumen of a small and relatively deep ganglion cyst lying immediately posterior to the lower end of the PCL in the midline of the popliteal fossa. The arrow indicates the ganglion. Arrowheads indicate the shaft of the needle. PCL = P. Tibia = T.

and Seeto 2000; Dias and Buch 2003; Burke et al. 2003). Post-surgical problems can include persistent scar tenderness, sensitivity, pain and numbness (Dias and Buch 2003; Jacobs and Govaers 1990).

Bursal injections

Bursopathy occurring in sport is usually caused by trauma, from either direct contusion or frictional overload or as the result of an impingement. The use of local anaesthetic and corticosteroid injections for the relief of pain is a well-accepted and generally effective clinical procedure. An injection of local anaesthetic alone is sometimes performed as a purely diagnostic procedure. For example, injection of the subacromial-subdeltoid bursa in the shoulder is performed as an 'impingement test'. Although bursal injections are often performed in the sports physician's office as a clinically guided procedure, imaging-guided injections are more accurate. Eustace et al. (1995) showed that only 29% of clinically guided injections for subacromial bursopathy actually reached the intended target. Imaging-guided bursal injections are generally best performed under real-time ultrasound control (see Figs 10.12 and 10.13).

The patient is preferably placed supine in order to minimise any risk of vasovagal collapse. The most distended portion of the bursa is targeted. The needle tip is introduced into the bursal space under sterile conditions and real-time control in the imaging plane of the transducer. Needle calibre and length are selected as appropriate for the depth of the particular bursa and pathology involved. 25-gauge needles are adequate if nothing more than simple injection is required, but 18-gauge needles (or larger) may be required if preliminary aspiration is indicated to decompress a painfully distended bursa or to obtain material for pathological

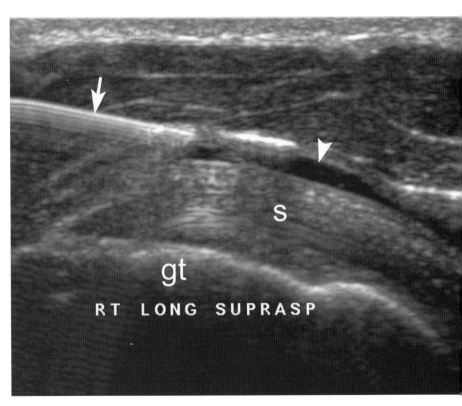

▲ Fig. 10.12 This long-axis ultrasound image demonstrates an ultrasound-guided injection of the subacromial-subdeltoid bursa. A long-axis view of the supraspinatus tendon (s) shows the needle (arrow) positioned within the subacromial-subdeltoid bursa. The injectate has not blebbed at the needle tip, but instead flows freely along the bursal space (arrowhead) above the supraspinatus tendon. Greater humeral tuberosity = gt.

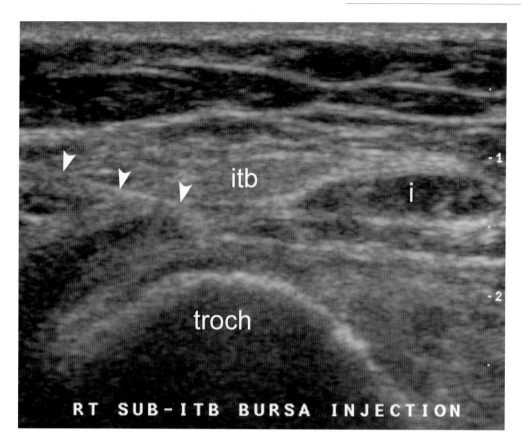

◀ **Fig. 10.13**
An ultrasound-guided injection of a trochanteric bursa. A transverse image obtained over the greater trochanter (troch) shows the needle (arrowheads) positioned with its tip immediately deep to the iliotibial band (itb). The injectate has not blebbed at the needle tip, but instead flows freely along the bursal space to spill into the rounded anterior recess of the sub-ITB or 'trochanteric' bursa (i).

assessment. Either local anaesthetic alone or a mixture of local anaesthetic and corticosteroid may then be injected in a volume that is appropriate for the capacity of the targeted bursa. Importantly, if the clinical setting is one of possible infection, steroid should not be injected until sepsis has first been ruled out.

Tendon intervention

Sports-related tendon disorders that commonly cause pain include tendinopathy and paratenonitis. The histopathology observed within the tendon in these conditions is predominantly that of collagen breakdown, mucoid degeneration and microvascular proliferation, with inflammatory cells and granulation tissue only observed if a healing partial tear is present. Some authors also report the presence of an inflammatory infiltrate within the paratenon (Puddu et al. 1976; Clancy et al. 1976; Harms et al. 1977; Kvist et al. 1985; Williams 1986), while other authorities state that this is rare in actual clinical practice (Brukner and Khan 2001). Paratenonitis can occur alone, where for example there is tendon impingement by bone spur, or in conjunction with tendinopathy, such as occurs in association with Achilles tendinopathy.

Acute paratenonitis is associated with swelling, hyperaemia, a scattered mild mononuclear infiltrate and a variable degree of fibrinous exudate that may cause palpable crepitus. Chronic paratenonitis is associated with mucoid degeneration in the areolar tissue (Brukner and Khan 2001), perivascular lymphocytic infiltration (Kvist et al. 1992) and a myofibroblastic reaction that thickens the peritendon and produces adhesions (Jarvinen et al. 1997). Tendinopathy may be a precursor of tenosynovitis, the term relating to inflammation of the synovial lining of the tendon sheath. This in turn may become thickened and swollen and may be accompanied by an effusion.

At the most basic level, the treatment of any sports-related tendinopathy requires facilitation of the normal process of tissue repair, promoting the healing of damaged or degenerate tendons by new healthy tendon tissue as efficiently as possible. Tendons have a slow metabolic rate and as a consequence heal slowly, with the recovery period often long and frustrating.

Peritendon injections

The injection of synthetic corticosteroid agents for rheumatologic conditions was possibly first introduced by Hollander (1953), and usage subsequently became widespread in sports medicine during the 1960s. Corticosteroid injections are now very commonly used for sports-related tendinopathy and provide effective pain relief, although this may be transient. The mechanism of corticosteroid pain relief remains unclear but is possibly related to inhibited prostaglandin release. Corticosteroids do not assist tissue repair and should be used as an adjunct to a wider treatment plan for tendinopathy rather than in isolation. Although injections may be performed by the sports physician in their clinical office by the use of 'feel' and surface anatomy, increasingly the procedure is performed by an off-site radiologist with the assistance of some form of real-time imaging guidance for greater accuracy.

Some physicians prefer to perform peritendon injections using non-steroidal agents. The options include:

(a) the use of techniques or substances that aim to stimulate a healing response by causing either a local tissue irritation (prolotherapy) or a proliferative pharmacological effect, such as 'dry needling', aprotinin, low dose heparin, calcium gluconate, saline, dextrose or autologous blood

(b) the use of sclerosants, such as polidocanol, which obliterate neovessels and have an anaesthetic effect.

All of these techniques are characterised by limited objective scientific evidence of benefit but enjoy very similar and largely uncontrolled clinical reports of a positive outcome in about 70% of cases. This leads the cynical observer to ask whether the type of agent injected actually matters (Orchard 2003). Alternative agents may possibly have a role in clinical situations where the risk of tendon rupture precludes or discourages the use of corticosteroid.

Techniques for peritendon injections

Imaging-guided peritendon injections are generally best performed under ultrasound control, although fluoroscopic or CT guidance may be useful alternatives for some deep tendons, such as the iliopsoas insertion and the origin of the hamstrings.

A variety of ultrasound techniques can be used, each being tailored to the clinical setting. The transducer may be held by either the interventionist or the sonographer. Each technique requires continuous observation of sterile 'no-touch' precautions. Some interventionists use a longitudinal approach with the needle advancing in the longitudinal plane of the tendon, and this is appropriate in many cases (see Fig. 10.14). However, the authors often prefer an approach that is transverse to the long axis of the tendon with the needle directed in the imaging plane of the transducer, especially when the tendon being targeted is curved. This allows direct visualisation of both the advancing needle tip and the dispersing injectate. The needle tip is first directed into the immediate peritendon space (see Figs 10.15, 10.16 and 10.17).

Before injecting, gentle negative pressure on the syringe will help to avoid inadvertent injection into a non-visualised blood vessel. Injection should then always be performed slowly and gently to avoid potential problems that can be associated with accidental intravasation, retrograde spill along the needle track into the subcutaneous space and injection of an incorrect peritendon space. In cases where the targeted injection space is a synovial sheath, focal accumulation or blebbing of injectate at the needle tip generally indicates an extra-synovial location and the need to re-position the needle before proceeding. Injection should never be made against a firm resistance, as this usually indicates that the needle tip is located within the substance of the tendon and that re-positioning is required.

Whenever corticosteroid is used, the volume chosen to be injected should always be appropriate to the targeted compartment, as overdistension may cause both pain and reflux of the injectate. The authors occasionally elect to follow the peritendon injection with a limited 'dry needling' procedure in which the abnormal tendon segment is peppered by several dry needle passes. This is easily performed while the needle is still in situ and the procedure may have an additional therapeutic value in its own right.

Complications of peritendon injections

Tendon or fascial rupture is the most feared complication of peritendon injections with corticosteroid, supported in the literature by isolated case reports (Blazina et al. 1973; Alexeeff 1986; Kerlan and Glousman 1989; Stannard and Bucknell 1993). However, uncontrolled case studies do not provide reliable evidence that corticosteroids damage human tendons when the underlying disease process itself could equally be responsible (Paavola et al. 2002). Moreover, a recent comprehensive review of the medical literature (Nichols 2005) has shown a relatively low overall reported complication rate for steroid injections when used to treat athletic injuries (see Table 10.1).

Nevertheless, a variety of precautions may be used to minimise the risk and medicolegal hazard of tendon rupture:

- using betamethasone rather than triamcinolone (Nichols 2005)
- resting the affected tendon for at least 10 to 14 days following injection
- not injecting around any tendon if either the history or imaging suggests a possible recent partial tear (within the previous three months)
- never directly injecting into the tendon itself, as hydraulic distension alone could cause a tear. Subsequent necrosis has also been reported in animal studies.
- not injecting around tendons that are routinely exposed to very high loads, such as the adductor longus, or those that are prime movers without agonists, such as the Achilles tendon
- obtaining a written informed consent.

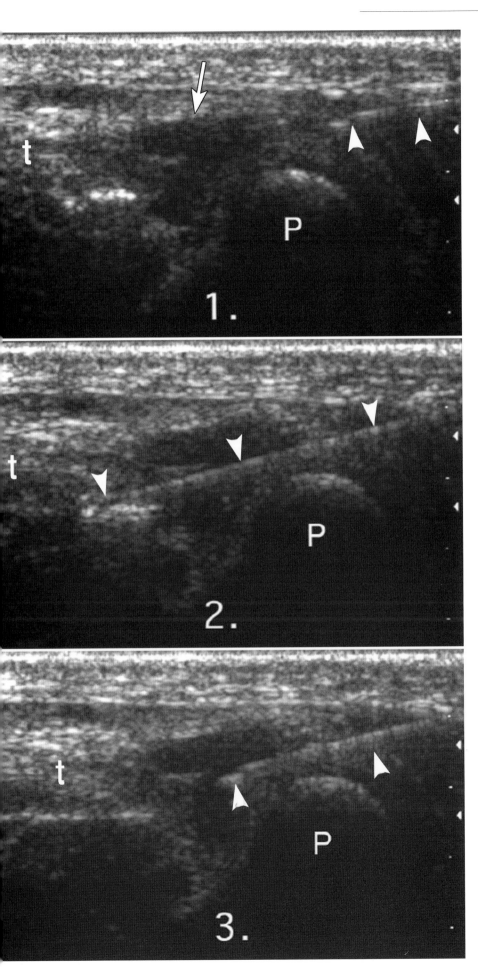

◄**Fig. 10.14** An ultrasound-guided injection of the adductor longus peritendon. Scans have been obtained in the long axis of the tendon with the patient's feet to the left of the images. The arrow indicates a zone of hypoechoic tendinopathy, with thickening and a small superimposed central echogenic band of a complicating chronic longitudinal intrasubstance tear at the origin of the adductor longus. Arrowheads indicate the needle.

1. For the initial injection, the needle tip is placed at the anterior surface of the conjoint tendon. Note the bevel is directed anteriorly.
2. For injection over the deep surface of the adductor longus tendon, the needle tip is advanced through the adductor longus tendon.
3. The 'dry' needle is subsequently passed back and forth through the abnormal tendon segment several times. Adductor longus tendon = t. Pubic crest = P.

Source: Modified from Read and Peduto (2000) with permission.

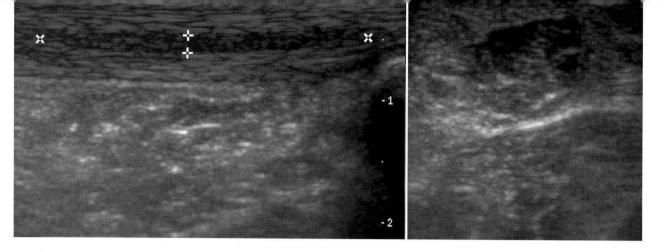

▲ **Fig. 10.15** A hurdler presented with considerable pain and disability due to an Achilles tendon tear (callipers). Local anaesthetic alone was injected into the paratenon anterior to the Achilles tendon, using a transverse approach. The pain was relieved and the athlete was advised to rest to prevent extension of the tear. The long-axis image on the left shows the injectate in the paratenon anterior to the tendon and the right image was obtained to assess the needle position in the axial plane.

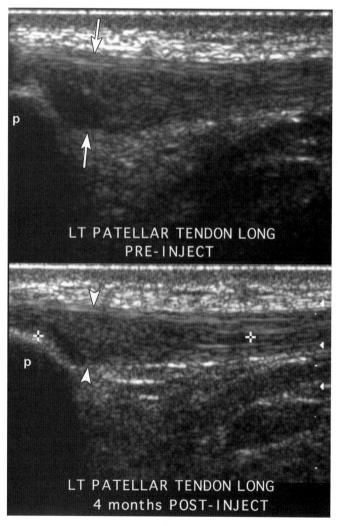

LT PATELLAR TENDON LONG
PRE-INJECT

LT PATELLAR TENDON LONG
4 months POST-INJECT

◄**Fig. 10.16** Progress long-axis ultrasound examinations show the result of peritendon injection for 'jumper's knee'. Peritendon injection was performed for a patient with symptomatic proximal patellar tendinopathy of the left knee. Corticosteroid was infiltrated along the deep peritendon space at the level of maximal tendinopathy (arrows), just below the inferior pole of patella. The needle approaches transversely from the medial side and passes beneath the tendon. This was followed by 'dry needling' of the deeper fibres of the involved segment. At four months post-injection, and following a treatment program that included eccentric strengthening, the patient was asymptomatic. Progress ultrasound examination showed a significant decrease in tendon swelling (arrowheads). Inferior pole of patella = p.

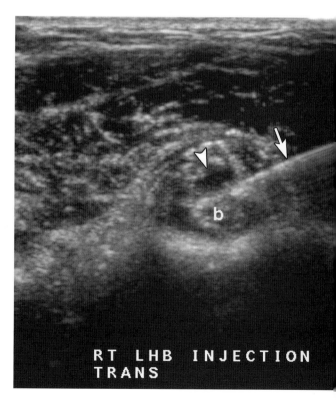

RT LHB INJECTION TRANS

▶ **Fig. 10.17** A transverse ultrasound image shows an ultrasound-guided injection of the tendon sheath of the long head of the biceps. Using a transverse approach under real-time control, the needle (arrow) is directed to the surface of the long head of the biceps tendon (b) at the level of the intertubercular humeral sulcus. The injected mixture of corticosteroid and bupivacaine flows without resistance or localised blebbing to outline the tendon with a uniformly hypoechoic collar of fluid (arrowhead). This confirms correct placement of the injectate within the tendon sheath.

Aspirations

Percutaneous imaging-guided needle aspirations can be used for diagnosis (when fluid is required for analysis) and for the treatment of conditions such as a cyst (ganglion), haematoma or calcific deposit. The method of aspiration of ganglia has already been described in the discussion on ganglia (see pages 847–52).

Aspiration of haematomata

Large muscle haematomata are painful due to the pressure effect created by distension of a relatively constrained and non-compliant fascial compartment. Needle aspiration can help to reduce pain, re-approximate torn muscle edges and reduce overall healing time (van Holsbeek and Introcaso 1992). It is unclear whether the risk of subsequent post-traumatic myositis ossificans might also be reduced. The aspiration is best performed in the earliest stages of clot evolution, which is when active bleeding has ceased but before significant clotting has taken place. As the haematoma ages and organises, ultrasound may show irregular walls, septation and increasing internal echogenicity. Muscle injuries studied in the rabbit model show that regenerating muscle fibres appear within the fibrin clot after four weeks and become more prominent after six weeks (Kim et al. 2002). Dystrophic calcifications can appear as early as two weeks on ultrasound and four weeks on plain films. After the first month, most haematomata will gradually resolve with anechoic spaces seen on ultrasound. Rarely, these may persist as muscle cysts.

It is important to remember that uniform semi-liquid or gelatinous consistency can occur during both the early and late stages of clot evolution, and may produce areas of hypoechoic or anechoic echotexture that can be easily mistaken for fluid consistency. Thus, percutaneous drainage can be unsuccessful, even in old echo-free collections (Wicks et al. 1978). For all of these reasons, attempted drainages are generally performed only for particularly large and painful haematomata, usually under real-time ultrasound guidance (see Fig. 10.18). Strict sterile procedure should be observed to minimise the risk of infection. Large-bore cannulas are more likely to be successful than fine needles. Complete evacuation may be impossible, but partial decompression can provide significant pain relief.

Aspiration of calcific tendinopathy

Calcium hydroxyapatite crystal deposition disease affecting tendons is a common idiopathic condition that can either be asymptomatic or cause severe pain and restriction. Needle aspiration under fluoroscopic or ultrasound guidance may play a role in the management of calcific tendinopathy. Aspiration is mostly used for calcific tendinopathy at the shoulder, although other sites may also be suitable if large calcific deposits are present.

Farin et al. (1995) described an ultrasound-guided aspiration technique utilising two separate but simultaneously placed 18–19-gauge needles. In this method, initial disruption of the calcific deposit with multiple needle passes is followed

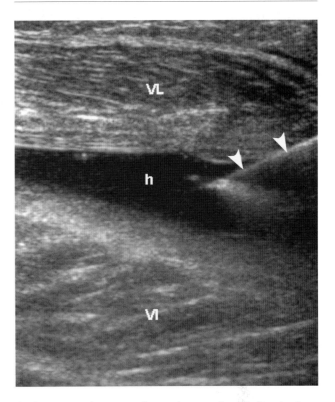

▲ **Fig. 10.18** This image shows ultrasound-guided aspiration of a thigh haematoma. A long-axis ultrasound image obtained over the anterolateral aspect of the thigh shows a needle in situ (arrowheads) with its tip positioned centrally within a largely anechoic haematoma (h). Vastus lateralis = VL. Vastus intermedius = VI.

by aspiration through one needle while lavaging with saline through the other. Finally, corticosteroid is injected into the overlying subacromial-subdeltoid bursa. This procedure has a reported clinical success rate of 60–74% (Farin et al 1995; Normandin et al. 1988; Pfister and Gerber 1997).

A simpler and less aggressive method of ultrasound-guided aspiration that also provides satisfactory results was subsequently reported by Aina et al. (2001). In this method, a single 22-gauge (or larger if desired) needle is positioned in the centre of the calcific deposit (see Fig. 10.19), and the needle tip is then rotated to cause fragmentation before lavaging with a 5–10 ml syringe filled with lignocaine 1%. The technique of lavage is to use the plunger of the syringe to repeatedly flush and aspirate, while at the same time monitoring the needle-tip position with ultrasound. Extracted calcium is identified as a white cloud of material mixing with the lignocaine and depositing in the dependent portion of the syringe (see Fig. 10.20). A combination of corticosteroid and 1–2 ml bupivacaine 0.5% is then injected into the overlying subacromial-subdeltoid bursa. The success of aspiration varies with the consistency of the calcification. Often the deposit is non-liquid and chalk-like, allowing only a small amount of material to be extracted. Much less commonly, the material is paste-like in consistency and dramatic decompression can be achieved rapidly. Even if the amount of calcific material removed is only small, mechanical fragmentation of the calcific deposit is thought to accelerate the usual process of spontaneous resorption.

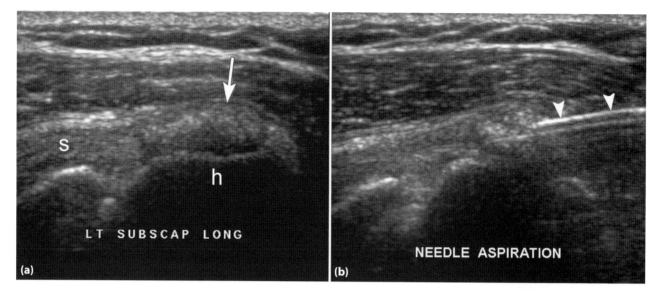

▲ **Fig. 10.19** These images demonstrate ultrasound-guided aspiration of an acute calcific subscapularis tendinopathy. A preliminary long-axis ultrasound image **(a)** of an acutely symptomatic subscapularis tendon shows a poorly marginated zone of echogenic tendon thickening due to non-shadowing calcium deposition (arrow). Similar image **(b)** obtained during aspiration shows an 18-gauge needle in situ (arrowheads). Note the needle tip is located centrally within the zone of calcification. Rotation of the bevel then assists with the fragmentation and aspiration of the deposit. Subscapularis tendon = s. Lesser humeral tuberosity = h.

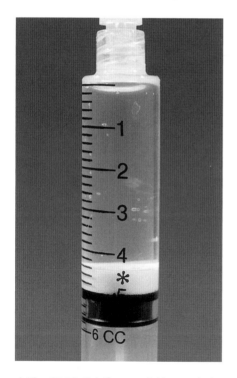

▲ **Fig. 10.20** Calcific material has settled to the base of the barrel of the syringe, following a lavage of calcific tendinopathy. A syringe filled with lignocaine 1% is used to repeatedly flush and aspirate with re-adjustment of the needle-tip position. Fragmentation of the calcific deposit is achieved by rotation of the bevel. Extracted calcium appears as a white cloud of material mixing with the lignocaine and settles dependently in the syringe.
Source: Aina (2001), used with permission.

Perineural injections of peripheral nerves

Perineural injection of corticosteroid and/or local anaesthetic can aid in both the diagnosis and treatment of certain nerve entrapment syndromes.

Diagnostic injections

Diagnostic injections of local anaesthetic will provide transient relief of pain and can help to:

- confirm a provisional diagnosis, such as median nerve compression at the carpal tunnel
- confirm the clinical relevance of an apparent imaging abnormality, such as posterior interosseous nerve entrapment at the elbow
- confirm the symptomatic sites when multiple imaging abnormalities have been demonstrated, such as Morton's neuromata within multiple web spaces.

Therapeutic injections

Therapeutic corticosteroid injections can have a role in the management of some forms of nerve entrapment. As many tunnel syndromes lack any true inflammatory infiltrate, the mechanism of beneficial corticosteroid effect is often unclear. Nevertheless, benefit has been verified by randomised, controlled double-blind trial for carpal tunnel syndrome (Gerritsen et al. 2002; Marshall et al. 2002). Other conditions of peripheral nerve entrapment for which perineural corticosteroid injection may be therapeutic include Morton's neuroma (see Fig. 10.21), posterior interosseous nerve entrapment at the elbow, meralgia paraesthetica, piriformis syndrome, tarsal tunnel syndrome and pudendal nerve entrapment.

Ultrasound is the imaging guidance most often used, and this offers accurate placement and minimises complications. Injection of the pudendal nerve is best performed under CT guidance (Hough et al. 2003). With all perineural injections, the nerve itself should be avoided. An intrafascicular injection of the median nerve may cause dysaesthesias that persist for months (Hunt and Osterman 1994). One exception to this rule, which offers an alternative strategy to corticosteroid for the injection treatment of Morton's neuroma, is chemical

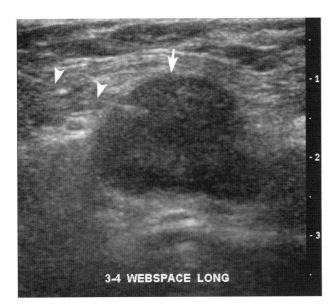

▲ **Fig. 10.21** A long-axis ultrasound image shows an ultrasound-guided perineural injection for Morton's neuroma. A distal interdigital approach has been taken, with the ultrasound transducer placed along the sole of the foot and oriented in a longitudinal plane between the third and fourth metatarsals. The needle (arrowheads) can be seen to enter an ovoid zone of hypoechoic soft-tissue thickening typical of Morton's neuroma (arrow). The thickened zone comprises both neural and perineural degenerative changes that cannot be clearly differentiated on imaging.

neurolysis of the common digital nerve using 4% ethyl alcohol solution (Dockery 1999).

Pudendal nerve entrapment is a condition that may arise in cyclists and equestrians. The entrapment presents with chronic perineal pain that is made worse with pressure or sitting and is relieved by standing. The perineal symptoms may present as penile, scrotal or labial pain or symptoms suggestive of chronic non-bacterial prostatitis or chronic pelvic pain syndrome in the male. The nerve becomes trapped between the sacrotuberous and sacrospinous ligaments or it may be compressed by the falciform process of the sacrotuberous ligament in the pudendal canal. Hough et al. (2003) described a technique of treating perineal nerve entrapment under CT guidance. Their technique is to inject with the needle tip adjacent to the pudendal nerve at the ischial spine, in the interligamentous space or at the pudendal canal.

Injections of the plantar fascia

Plantar fasciitis is a common condition that can occur at any age but is most frequently seen in overweight middle-aged women and is particularly prevalent in elite track and field athletes. Bilateral fasciitis carries a poorer prognosis and occurs in 20–30% of patients (this has an association with HLA B27 spondyloarthropathies, including psoriatic and reactive arthritis).

A wide variety of treatments exist, with relatively few randomised controlled trials providing good assessment of the management choices. In about 90% of cases, plantar fasciitis

is self-limiting and resolves with conservative treatment over a period of six to 18 months (Young et al. 2001). Imaging, which includes plain x-ray and either ultrasound or MRI, may be useful in ruling out differential diagnostic considerations such as a fascial tear, a stress or insufficiency fracture of the calcaneum, a contused heel pad or a foreign body.

Corticosteroid injections are usually reserved for resistant cases of plantar fasciitis and have a reported success rate of about 70% (Furey 1975; Kane et al. 1998). They provide only a short-term benefit, with decreased pain at one month and no difference at three to six months (Crawford et al. 1999). The injection itself is painful. Potential risks include fascial rupture and heel fat pad atrophy. Rupture of the plantar fascia after injection has been reported in almost 10% of patients (Acevedo and Beskin 1998) and has long-term sequelae in approximately 50% of these. Longitudinal arch strain is the most common ongoing effect, representing 50% of sequelae (Sellman 1994; Acevedo and Beskin 1998).

Accordingly, written informed consent should first be obtained. The injection approach is through the skin at the medial aspect of the foot rather than the thick specialised skin of the sole, as the latter is more prone to infection (see Fig. 10.22). A mixture of corticosteroid and local anaesthetic is infiltrated along the peritendon space associated with the deep surface of the fascia close to the bony insertion, avoiding injection of both the fascia itself and the overlying heel fat pad. The patient should rest the foot for 24 hours after the procedure, and repeat injections are probably best avoided.

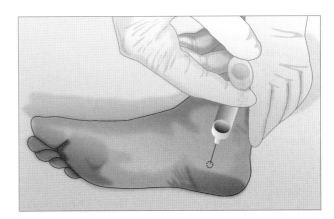

▲ **Fig. 10.22** A line drawing shows the medial approach used for injection of the plantar fascia.

Spinal intervention in sports medicine

Not all back pain needs investigation or treatment. Back pain is a common complaint in all age groups, often resulting from muscle soreness, and most acute-onset low back pain will resolve spontaneously.

The investigation and treatment of spinal pain using interventional procedures is a specialty in itself and requires patience, care and a thorough knowledge of spinal anatomy. It also demands an understanding of the potential hazards, particularly in the cervical spine. Many radiologists avoid intervention in the cervical region but it is hoped that this account will be helpful in encouraging a greater interest in this region. By following a few simple guidelines, most potential complications can be avoided.

Tips on injection technique

Precise needle placement is a critical skill that is developed from the art of thinking in a three-dimensional manner while directly watching the needle on real-time imaging. With experience, needle placement is also helped by an acquired 'feel', which is facilitated by good technique.

Control of the needle is most precise when:

- there is a clear understanding of the required anatomical pathway to be travelled by the needle to the target—this is best determined by reviewing previous imaging tests
- the forearm muscles of the operator are relaxed
- the needle tip is slowly and steadily advanced with gentle pressure, with one hand used to hold and orientate the needle while the other hand, at the same time, is used to advance the needle tip and sense the degree of tissue resistance (see Fig. 10.23).

Gentle hands can feel the needle tip progressing. They should recognise the pulsation of arteries and the differing densities of muscle, fascia, ligament and tendon, readily allowing an immediate easing-off of pressure when required. Force should never be an option, and using both hands gives the confidence required for both precision and the avoidance of complications.

Lumbar discography

Properly performed and correctly interpreted, lumbar discography can provide valuable and precise diagnostic information that cannot be provided by any other imaging technique. Although MRI may demonstrate a high intensity focus in the annulus as presumptive evidence of an annular tear, many of these assumed annular tears are asymptomatic. Discography is an imaging test designed to stimulate the intervertebral disc to determine whether it is the source of the patient's pain. The value of this procedure has repeatedly fallen into disrepute, largely due to two factors: first, the discographer's technique has been inconsistent and occasionally flawed; and second, the interpretation of the findings has been deficient, thereby not producing enough useful information.

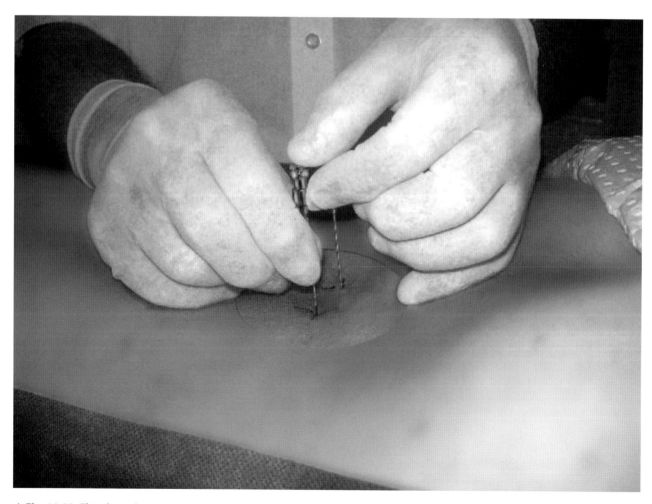

▲ **Fig. 10.23** This shows how needles can be progressively guided by the use of both hands. The wrist of the right hand rests on the patient while the fifth finger of each hand lies flat on the drape surface. This provides for a balanced position for both hands. The index finger and thumb of both hands are used to provide a controlled yet gentle progression of the needle tip.

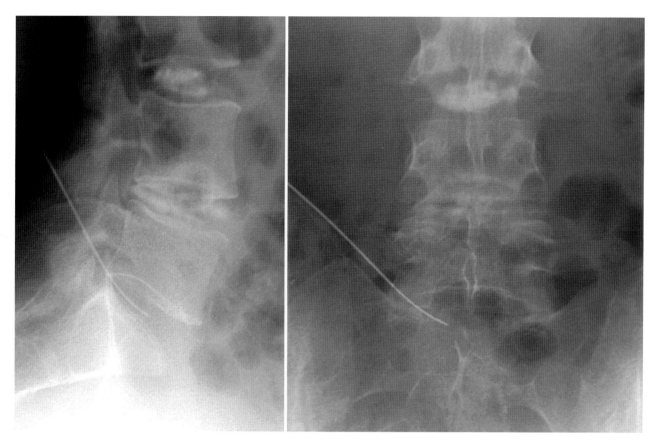

▲ **Fig. 10.24** Needle placement for an L5/S1 discogram has been achieved using fluoroscopic guidance. Note the significant preformed curve of the inner of the two concentric needles. The inner needle assumes the curve after leaving the outer needle (double-needle technique) helping to negotiate the difficult angle of approach. It is helpful to aim the needle at the angle between the iliac crest and the outer inferior angle of L5 on the AP view while intermittently checking the approach on the lateral projection. The ski-tip is bounced off the superior margin of S1.

The value of the procedure has often been controversial and an interesting debate was published by Bogduk and Modic (1996), each giving opinions from opposite perspectives. Bogduk emphasised that while CT and MRI have value in the investigation of radicular pain, they 'offer little in the investigation of back pain and somatic referred pain'. He notes that it is 'here that neuroradiologists and discographers part company'. On the other hand, Modic is of the opinion 'that discography has led to inappropriate surgery and that the potential for abuse or misuse is the responsibility of the proponents of discography'.

The procedure is of diagnostic value in patients:

- who have persistent pain for which no cause has been established by non-invasive imaging
- where the information provided by imaging with MRI or CT does not correlate with the clinical presentation
- in whom fusion is being considered and the spinal surgeon requires confirmation that the discs above and below the proposed fusion segment are pain free and that the disc at the proposed fusion level is responsible for the presenting symptoms.

Guyer and Ohnmeiss (1995) also made the point that limiting one's view purely to the clinical usefulness of the procedure for treatment, particularly surgery, may overlook the value of understanding the disease process for the peace of mind of the patient, their family and the physician. Understanding the source of the symptoms may be an important part of rehabilitation.

The technique of discography

A full and precise description of the technique of discography is beyond the scope of this text, but it will suffice to say that the technique is probably best learned from an experienced discographer. The abbreviated description that follows is an account of the procedure in the prone position. The authors believe that the prone position for discography is the most comfortable for the patient, is the position in which the radiologist can best understand the three-dimensional concept of anatomy, and is also a position allowing ease of patient management. However, for various technical and personal reasons, many differing techniques are used.

The procedure is best performed under fluoroscopic control (see Fig. 10.24), although thoracic discograms are safer under CT guidance (see Fig. 10.25). Schellhas et al. (1994) described a fluoroscopic technique in the thoracic region, which they found safe when performed by experienced operators. The authors believe that all discs, especially narrow discs, are easier to enter under fluoroscopic guidance than with CT.

Preparation for discography

First, informed consent should be obtained, witnessed and documented.

Light hypnotic sedation with a drug such as Diazopam (hypnovel) is an important and sensible preliminary for a smooth procedure and shows empathy with the patient. Often the procedure is uncomfortable. The dose should reflect the patient's anxiety and body weight. In addition, some patients will have been taking analgesia for some time and may exhibit drug tolerance and require a higher dose.

The disc level to be investigated is established under fluoroscopy. The skin and deeper tissues along the line of approach, especially the muscle fascia, are anaesthetised some 8 cm or so from the midline and more in larger patients. Note is made of the degree of the lordosis at the desired level in order to conceptualise its influence on any obliquity required. The influence of the lordosis is greatest at L5/S1. At this level, circumnavigation of the iliac crest also influences the angle of approach and the degree of obliquity required.

A double-needle technique is recommended (Fraser et al. 1987). At all levels, the prior shaping of the outer of the two concentric needles to form a 'ski-tip' will aid in the entry to the disc by providing a manoeuvrable tip that can bounce off the edge of the bony margin of the disc space. This is particularly important at the L5/S1 level where the angle is often steep. The prior shaping of the needle tip to form a steep curve will aid in negotiating awkward angles, allowing rotation of the curved tip and helping with its passage through the annulus and into the disc space.

The tip of the needle must lie in the nucleus prior to injection, since annular injections are useless. If the tip is in the annulus, the pressure of injection is generally high and should alert the discographer to the incorrect position. Even in normal discs, the annulus is sensitive and the passage through the annulus can be quite painful. If the injection is annular, the procedure will need to be repeated.

Cervical discograms

It is the considered opinion of the authors that cervical discography rarely provides useful information. It calls for a significantly different technique. A frontal approach is used for a single-needle technique, with the needle passing medial to the carotid artery and lateral to the larynx or trachea. While the technique is simple and much quicker than lumbar discograms, almost all cervical discs are sensitive and painful during injection and it is difficult for the patient to determine the offending disc from the adjacent levels.

Documentation

Documentation of the procedure should be accurate and reliable. The discographer should record observations in a consistent format. One such format that has stood the test of time is the DDD classification (Dallas discogram description) (Sachs et al. 1987). This has a reproducible reporting format and classifies the information. It relates to five different categories of information:

- *Category one* describes the percentage of annular filling with contrast and reflects general degeneration.
- *Category two* provides for a description of the degree and location of annular disruption. This is shown graphically in Fig. 10.26, illustrating how contrast escapes between the concentric layers of the annulus.
- *Category three* provides a reproducible format for reporting the clinical information produced by provoking pain. The patient's pain response is recorded on a visual analogue scale (VAS) together with its location and similarity to the clinical symptoms.
- *Category four* requires the contrast volume to be noted and whether the volume is related to the degree of pain provoked.
- *Category five* allows for comments and other information specific to the case.

Discography is followed by a post-discogram CT scan, which records visual information on disc morphology, annular disruption and disc protrusions, as seen in Figs 10.25 and 10.27.

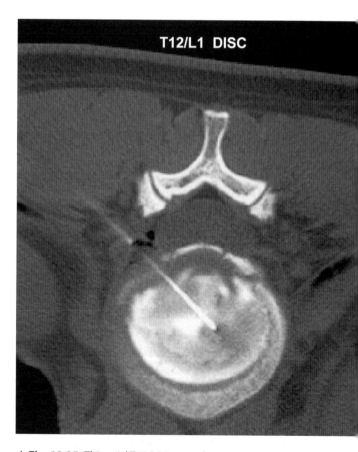

T12/L1 DISC

▲ **Fig. 10.25** This axial T12/L1 image demonstrates a discogram with contrast lying beneath the outer layer of the annulus. Note that the procedure has been performed under CT guidance at this level. The proximity of the lung is a concern and a pneumothorax must be avoided. Note the position of the needle tip in the centre of the annulus and the track of the needle lying just posterior to the exiting T12 nerve root. The DDD grading is 3 (see Fig. 10.26), with contrast extending to the outer layer of the annulus posteriorly.

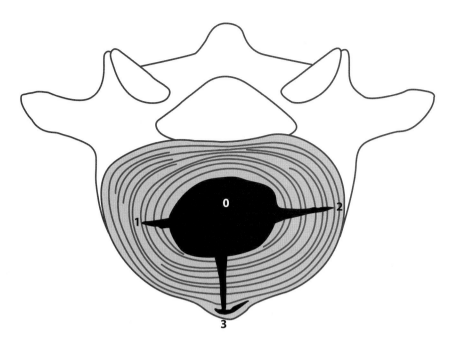

▲ **Fig. 10.26** This line drawing depicts the circumferential areas of the annulus and the grading of annular disruptions ranging from 0 to 3. The grading can be extended to include a complete disruption with contrast entering the epidural space.

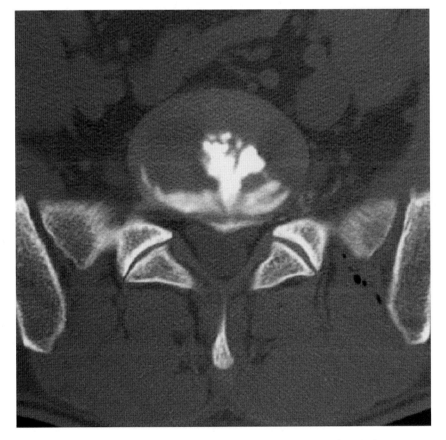

▲ **Fig. 10.27** This is the classic appearance of a contrast-enhanced L5/S1 discogram with a Grade 3 annular disruption associated with a prominent bulge of the annulus. Note also that the contrast has been correctly introduced into the centre of the nucleus. The injection exactly reproduced the patient's clinical presentation.

Complications

The prevention of infection and subsequent discitis is of paramount importance and the procedure calls for careful sterile conditions, a double-needle technique (Fraser et al. 1987) and the use of an antibiotic mixed with water-soluble non-ionic contrast for the injectate. While discitis is rare, it is devastating when it does occur. Awareness of this potential and the prophylactic use of antibiotics will significantly diminish the likelihood of this complication. An excellent publication on the experimental role of antibiotics in the prevention of discitis in sheep by Osti et al. (1990) illustrates the value of this precaution. The same article describes how an intravenous injection is of less value due partly to the half-life of the antibiotic, its peak serum level and the limited penetration of many antibiotics through the annulus. Therefore, for injection into the disc, the authors recommend a broad-spectrum antibiotic such as Cephazolin, mixed one part antibiotic to three parts of contrast.

Facet (zygopophyseal) joint intervention

At the outset, a word of caution about the radiological interpretation of facet joints is appropriate. Advanced degenerative arthropathy is often symptom free and, conversely, symptomatic joints may look pristine on imaging. If facet joint pain is suspected and the athlete has not responded to conservative measures, a diagnostic pain-blocking procedure may help to clarify the clinical picture.

Two imaging-guided procedures are used to block pain originating from a facet joint. Blocking can be achieved by either:

• injecting local anaesthetic into the joint or
• performing a medial branch block, which blocks the nerve supply to the joint.

The most reliable method of anaesthetising a facet is to block the nerve supply to the facet by performing a medial branch block. If the pain is

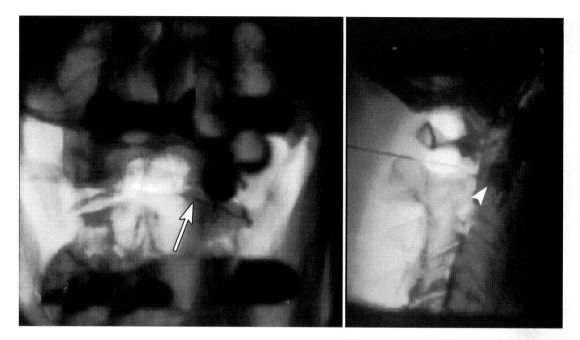

▲ **Fig. 10.28** A C1/2 intra-articular injection has been performed under fluoroscopic guidance. A posterior approach has been used with the needle passing between the thecal sac medially and the vertebral artery laterally. Note the contrast in the joint (arrow) and in the lateral recess (arrowhead) confirming that the needle is precisely placed in the narrow target.

eliminated following the block, then this is good evidence that the pain source has been found. If the pain is not alleviated, then it is likely that its origin lies elsewhere. If positive, medial branch blocks can be followed by a per-cutaneous radiofrequency neurotomy, a procedure that will be discussed later (see page 869).

Injection into facet joints: cervical

In the cervical spine, with the exception of the C0/C1 and C1/C2 synovial joints, intra-articular blocks have been superseded by medial branch blocks, which are easier and safer to perform (Lord et al. 1994). Intra-articular blocks are technically more difficult to perform and produce a generally less reliable result.

The C0/1 and C1/2 joints have a complex nerve supply and cannot be blocked other than by intra-articular injections. The medial branch of C2, the greater occipital nerve has been implicated in cervical-related headaches, although this remains controversial. It is also thought that branches from this nerve pass to the vertebral and superficial temporal arteries, in addition to supplying innervation to the lateral atlantoaxial joints. Potentially hazardous structures in this region make the procedure of intra-articular blocks at these levels unpopular with interventionists. However, the lateral atlantoaxial joints can be injected with anaesthetic and cortisone using a lateral or posterior approach under fluoroscopy or CT guidance. A small injection of contrast will confirm the intra-articular placement of the needle (see Fig. 10.28).

Injection into facet joints: lumbar

In the lumbar spine, intra-articular blocks are generally not long-lasting and are quite non-specific in their action. The inner wall of the joint cavity is essentially made up of the

ligamentum flavum. The joint cavity is of small capacity and, although the needle may be in the joint, the injected sub-stance may extravasate into the peri-articular tissues and very often rupture through the medial joint wall into the epidural space (see Fig. 10.29).

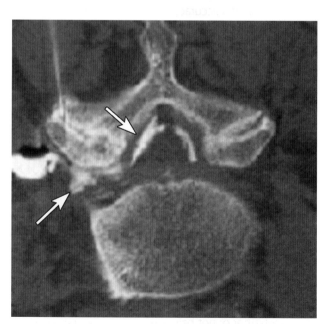

▲ **Fig. 10.29** An intra-articular injection has been performed under CT guidance, with 1.5 cc of injectate mixed with contrast. Note how little of the contrast is in the joint space and how much ends up outside the joint and in the epidural space (arrows). The clinical results achieved may be due to the epidural component and not to any effect in the joint itself. If the patient achieves pain relief, then the procedure has been of value, but the benefit is usually short-lived.

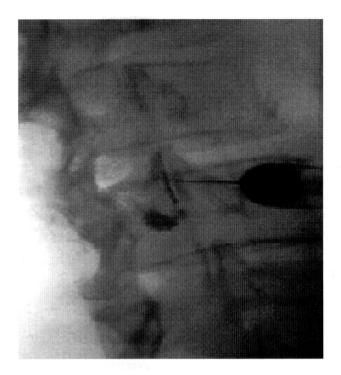

▲ **Fig. 10.30** Fluoroscopically guided intra-articular injections require a contrast injection on most occasions to ensure that the needle is in the joint. Note the extravasation of contrast from the upper and lower recesses.

Intra-articular blocks can be performed with either fluoroscopic (see Fig. 10.30) or CT guidance. CT has the advantage of allowing greater accuracy, especially in arthritic joints and particularly at the L5/S1 level where the obliquity of the joints can provide a problem. If CT is unavailable, fluoroscopy may be used, although needle placement guided by this imaging method is more difficult. An injection of contrast medium is invariably required for reassurance that the needle is in the joint. CT guidance allows an immediate correction of the angle of approach.

Having established that the needle is accurately placed, about 1 cc of long-acting local anaesthetic is injected. If appropriate, steroid will be added. The patient is then asked to document their response and a record is kept of the degree and length of pain relief. Occasionally, the response is prolonged and full recovery will occur. On other occasions, the response will be short-lived. If the clinical diagnosis is incorrect, there will be no improvement at all.

Medial branch blocks

Medial branch blocks are the most precise method of determining whether or not pain is emanating from a particular joint. The procedure has not only diagnostic value, but also potential therapeutic value, because a reproducible positive pain-relieving response from a medial branch block is an indication that the patient is likely to respond to more definitive treatment such as percutaneous radiofrequency neurotomy. In order to perform these blocks, a thorough knowledge of the anatomy of the spine is essential. The anatomy differs in the three regions of the spine.

Cervical spine medial branch blocks

In general terms, the nerve supply of the facet joints is from the medial branch of the posterior primary ramus at each segmental level, with each joint being supplied by the medial branch above and below the joint. The medial branch is specific in its action and has no cutaneous distribution with the exception of the third occipital nerve, which innervates skin in the suboccipital region.

C2/3 facet joint and third occipital nerve blocks

The third occipital nerve has been implicated in cervical-related headaches (Bogduk and Marsland 1986; Lord et al. 1994; Bogduk 1982). These often severe and persistent headaches tend to begin in the upper cervical region and radiate upwards behind the ear and over the vertex, occasionally reaching the frontal region. They have been shown to have a particular relationship to whiplash-type injuries (Bogduk 1982).

The nerve supply of the C2/3 joint is from the third occipital nerve, which is the dorsal ramus of C3. In 2001, Bogduk et al. published findings of dissections of the spinal nerves, noting that the third occipital nerve has a consistent pathway across the C2/3 joint. Afferent supply to the joint arises from either the third occipital nerve or its communication with the dorsal ramus of C2 (see Fig. 10.31).

Third occipital blocks are achieved by injecting small amounts (0.5 cc) of bupivacaine 2–3 mm apart along the joint line that passes obliquely downwards and backwards. The placement of electrodes for radiofrequency neurotomy mimics these positions.

C3–C7 facet joints

The C3–C7 facet joints have a predictable nerve supply from the medial branch above and below each joint. The target point from C3–C6 is the centre of the diamond-shaped articular pillar at each level (see Fig. 10.32). The C7 medial branch differs slightly in position and is best targeted at the anterior tip of the articular facet of C7.

The technique of cervical medial branch blocks

Bogduk et al. (2001) described in detail the procedure involved in performing medial branch blocks in the cervical region, with guidance by either fluoroscopy or CT. The authors prefer the use of CT, particularly in the cervical region, where minor degrees of rotation of the neck may give significant inaccuracy when viewed in the lateral projection (see Fig. 10.33)

The patient can be placed in either the prone or supine position. Either position allows a direct lateral approach directly onto the articular pillar. The authors prefer the supine position. Mostly the patient is more comfortable in the supine position, but in thick-necked athletes the lower cervical medial branch blocks are easier to approach in the prone position with a posterior approach. The skin is anaesthetised, avoiding deeper infiltration of muscle fascia and ligaments. This avoids any possible confusing removal of a pain source other than the joint. Each medial branch block requires no more than 1 cc of bupivacaine on the target nerve.

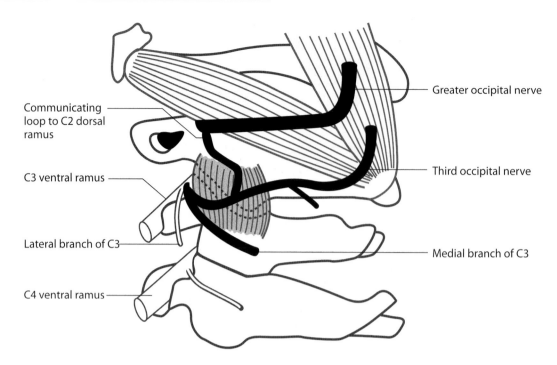

▲ Fig. 10.31 The posterolateral aspect of the left third occipital nerve crosses the lateral aspect and then the dorsal aspect of the lower half of the C2/C3 joint (dotted line). A branch to the semispinalis eventually passes dorsally to enter the skin over an area in the sub-occipital area. Articular branches to the joint arise from the third occipital nerve or the communicating loop to the C2 dorsal ramus, the greater occipital nerve. The lateral branch is shown as well as the deep medial branch of the C3 dorsal ramus crossing the C3 articular pillar forming the medial branch of C3.
Source: Modified from Bogduk and Marsland (1986).

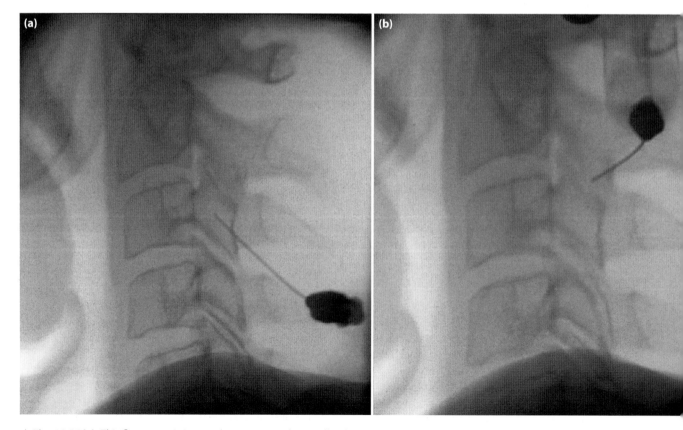

▲ Fig. 10.32(a) This fluoroscopic image demonstrates the needle placement required to block the deep medial branch of C3 over the articular pillar of C3. **(b)** The needle tip lies along part of the pathway of the third occipital nerve overlying the C2/3 joint.

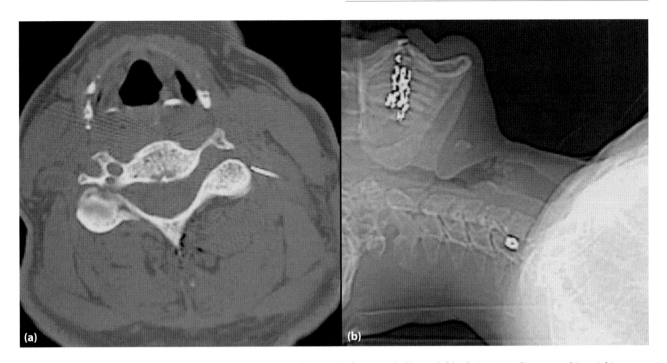

▲ **Fig. 10.33(a)** There has been a CT-guided placement of a needle for a medial branch block. Its tip is shown on this axial image over the articular pillar at C5. Note how the patient's neck has become slightly rotated to the right. This rotation can cause difficulty and perhaps incorrect placement under fluoroscopic guidance if not recognised.
(b) The lateral scout view shows the apparent position of the same needle, suggesting that it lies well anterior to the articular pillar. This illusion is created by the rotation of the neck.

Thoracic spine medial branch blocks

The thoracic medial branches describe a different course and are best targeted at the upper and outer tip of the transverse process at each level (Chua and Bogduk 1995). While these blocks can be performed under fluoroscopic guidance, the accuracy of CT in the thoracic region helps to avoid the potential complication of pneumothorax (see Fig. 10.34). According to Chua and Bogduk, the mid-thoracic medial branches are sometimes in the inter-transverse space a little above the tip of the transverse process, and are easier to target with CT.

Thoracic medial branch blocks are best performed in the prone position. The clinically diagnosed level is established and documented with imaging. A direct vertical approach onto the upper and outer tip of the transverse process is performed. A 22-gauge, 5 cm spinal needle is recommended, keeping in mind that the only significant procedural complication is caused by inserting the needle too deeply, thereby producing a pneumothorax. No more than 1 cc of bupivacaine is used to produce a block.

Lumbar spine medial branch blocks

The lumbar medial branches lie in a groove between the transverse process and the superior articular facet. Strictly speaking, each medial branch courses downward from the segment above, resulting in the L4 medial branch being below the L4/5 joint and the L5 medial branch passing through a groove just below and adjacent to the L5/S1 joint on the ala of the sacrum. While this is the strict anatomical

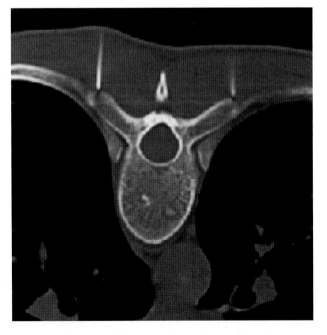

▲ **Fig. 10.34** An axial CT image shows the position of the needle tips for bilateral medial branch blocks and for radiofrequency neurotomy electrodes. In the thoracic region the needle tips are positioned at the upper and outer tip of the transverse process. The medial branches in the mid-thoracic region may lie in the inter-transverse space (Chua and Bogduk 1995).

nomenclature at each lumbar level, the target point is the most important practical point. For example, the L5/S1 joint is blocked by targeting the groove between the transverse process and the superior articular facet of L5 and the groove on the ala of the sacrum (see Fig. 10.35). Similarly, the L4/L5 joint is blocked by targeting the grooves between the transverse process and the superior articular facet above and below the joint (see Figs 10.36 and 10.37).

▶ **Fig. 10.35** The needle position for blocking the L5/S1 joint, with the needle tip between the superior facet of L5 and the groove in the ala of the sacrum.

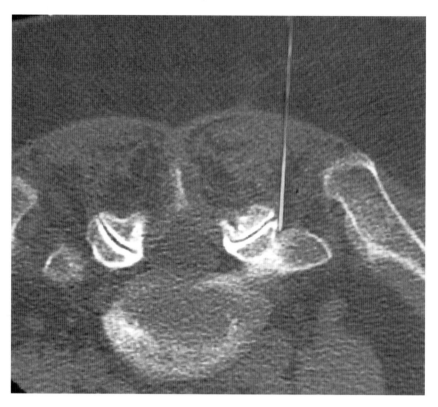

▼ **Fig. 10.36(a)** An axial CT image showing the needle position for a medial branch block at L4 on the right side. Note the position of the needle in the groove between the transverse process and the superior articular facet. It is of interest to note that there is a healing fracture of the transverse process on the left side (arrow). No more than 1 cc of bupivacaine is injected, with the needle tip seated on the periosteum during the injection. **(b)** Using CT guidance, needles are in the correct position for bilateral medial branch blocks at L4.

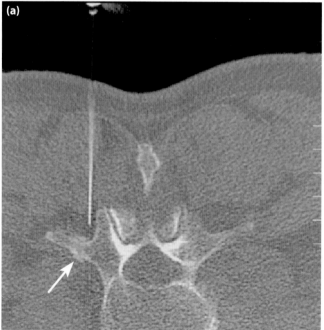

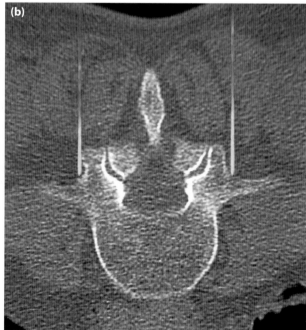

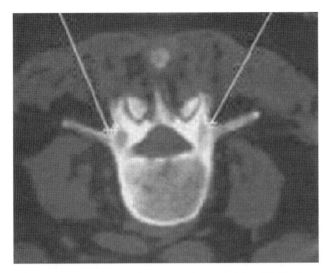

▲ **Fig. 10.37** The vertical approach for medial branch blocks can be modified if anatomy dictates. In this case, an oblique approach was chosen to position the needle tips for bilateral simultaneous injections.

After giving afferent supply to the joint, each medial branch continues to give segmental efferent supply to multifidus.

Lumbar medial branch blocks are performed under fluoroscopic or CT guidance. With either method, the procedure is performed in the prone position. With CT guidance, the target level and a line of approach are quickly established and documented. As in other areas, only the skin is anaesthetised to prevent loss of specificity, keeping in mind that muscle fascia can be a pain source. A direct vertical approach is the quickest and easiest method, although occasionally an oblique approach will be necessary when there is a steep angle between the transverse process and the vertebral body. No more than 1 cc of bupivacaine is injected.

Following the medial branch block procedure, the patient is asked to perform whatever activity normally produces their pain, and their degree of pain relief is documented hourly on a visual analogue scale.

The procedure is repeated after an appropriate interval, which can be as short as one day. The repeat procedure is to eliminate the 27% or so of patients who have a false positive or placebo reaction to the first medial branch block (Barnsley et al. 1993). The result of this second medial branch block is again documented. Some authors (for example, Barnsley et al. 1993) advocate using anaesthetic agents with a different length of action in a random manner to increase the specificity, although this is not always practical in a clinical setting. The ideal response is 100% pain relief in the topographically targeted region (Barnsley et al. 1993). In this case, the diagnosis of facet-related pain can be assumed to be correct with a fair degree of certainty.

It is important to realise that there are many causes of spinal-related pain and that medial branch blocks may not eliminate all of the patient's pain. It is the elimination of the targeted topographic pain that is the object of the exercise and it is imperative that this is kept in mind when interrogating the patient. Many patients will insist that they still have pain after the procedure, but careful questioning will reveal that the persisting pain is of a different character or in a differing region from that which was targeted. Not infrequently, following the relief produced by the medial branch block, pain of a different character is unmasked by the procedure and the interpretation of this phenomenon requires considerable experience on the part of the operator.

If the medial branch block response is deemed positive on two occasions, the decision can be made regarding whether or not it is appropriate to proceed to percutaneous radiofrequency neurotomy.

Percutaneous radiofrequency neurotomy

Although medial branch blocks can be utilised as a purely diagnostic procedure, their true value is to establish those patients who would benefit from percutaneous radiofrequency neurotomy (PRFN). This assumes the availability of a PRFN machine and a trained interventionist.

The procedure and technique closely follow that described for medial branch blocks, with a curved-tip electrode replacing the needle. The nerve is coagulated with radiofrequency with the nerve sheath remaining intact. There is a variable length of response depending on the patient's age and the length of the nerve segment coagulated. Some patients achieve up to two years of good pain relief. It is important to appreciate that not all patients are suitable for this procedure and the decision to proceed incorporates a number of factors, including the patient's age, athletic status and degree of disability. It is more appropriate for the mature skeleton as opposed to, for example, an adolescent with spinal pain.

Epidural injections

Epidural injections can be very effective in neural compression syndromes such as small disc protrusions in the cervical and lumbar spine, and especially in spinal stenosis. Anaesthetists are well experienced in performing this procedure blind for anaesthesia during surgery and childbirth. Their technique relies upon 'feel'. The ligamentum flavum is a tough membrane and protects the underlying epidural fat. The needle has a curved tip and is advanced into the ligamentum flavum. A syringe containing air is then attached to the needle and intermittent pressure is applied to the plunger as the needle is advanced through the ligamentum flavum. The air will remain compressed as long as the needle is within the ligament and the plunger will rebound when released. As soon as the needle tip 'pops' into the epidural space, the plunger will no longer be under pressure and the air will release easily into the epidural space.

Radiologists have the advantage of imaging to assist in needle placement and this advantage should be utilised. A quick and easy modification of the anaesthetists' technique is the interlaminar approach. After selecting the level, the ideal angle of approach is chosen and a 22-gauge spinal needle is advanced to the level of the ligamentum flavum. At this point, the air-containing syringe is attached and the process proceeds as described above with intermittent pressure on the plunger. As the needle 'pops' into the epidural space, the air will no longer be under pressure and will easily expel into the epidural fat. The great advantage of imaging is that an axial image at this stage will show the air in the epidural space and confirm that the needle is not inadvertently in the subarachnoid space or outside the central vertebral canal altogether. Even very tight canals can be entered using this technique and maximum concentration of corticosteroid can be delivered where it is most needed. A caudal approach via the sacral canal can also be employed.

Nerve root sleeve blocks

Nerve root sleeve blocks (NRSB) are variously called periradicular blocks and nerve sheath blocks. The clinical indication for this procedure in the athlete is the presence of performance-limiting radicular pain with or without confirmation of neural compression on CT or MRI. The procedure can be utilised for diagnostic as well as therapeutic purposes. The elimination of the patient's pain with an injection of bupivacaine will confirm the clinical diagnosis and the segmental level. The concomitant injection of cortisone is most often appropriate to prolong the effect.

Cervical spine NRSBs: technique and anatomy

In the cervical region, nerve root sleeve blocks can be performed relatively safely under CT guidance from C3 to C8. The anatomy is such that C3 exits via the C2/3 intervertebral foramen, C4 exits via the intervertebral foramen at C4/5 and so on, with C8 exiting at C7/T1.

The procedure can be performed in either the prone or supine position, but the supine position is more comfortable for the patient. In addition, the interventionist and nurse can monitor the reactions of the patient more easily in this position. CT guidance is used to follow the progress of the procedure. After establishing the entry point, an element of confidence can be achieved utilising a gentle two-handed needle approach, taking images as required to confirm the correct pathway of the needle. On aiming for the facet joint and after feeling the needle tip engaging bone, an image is obtained to confirm the position of the needle. The needle tip is then gently manoeuvred over the joint and into the intervertebral foramen, making sure that the needle remains posterior to the vertebral artery. It is likely that the nerve root will be touched or the perineural sheath penetrated, at which time the dermatome distribution of the root can be confirmed (see Fig. 10.38).

After confirming the position of the needle and that there is no sign of blood on gentle aspiration, a moderately firm injection of 1–3 cc of bupivacaine is made, followed by 1 or 2 cc of celestone chronodose, if this is appropriate. It is important that the patient understands that they may feel some pain but that they must remain perfectly still during the injection. A small prior injection of contrast can provide assurance that the needle is not intravascular. If the contrast outlines the nerve sheath then the needle is correctly placed and extravascular (see Fig. 10.39). This will also show the extent to which you may expect to achieve infiltration of the epidural space in the central vertebral canal. If the needle tip is intravascular, the contrast will dissipate and will not be seen on the CT image that follows. In the neck, the use of a 22-gauge, 5 cm, non-cutting, short-bevel spinal needle gives a significantly less likelihood of vascular (especially arterial) penetration than may occur using a 25-gauge cutting needle.

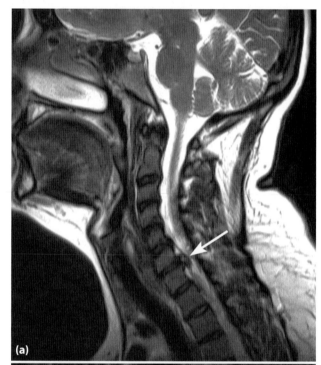

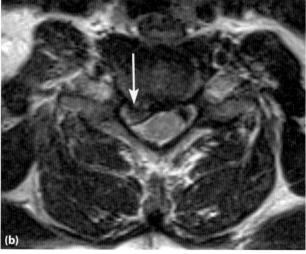

▲ **Fig. 10.38(a)** A sagittal MR image demonstrating an acute disc protrusion at the C6/7 level (arrow).

(b) An axial image of the same case showing the large disc fragment filling the right lateral recess at the C6/7 level (arrow), rotating and displacing the spinal cord.

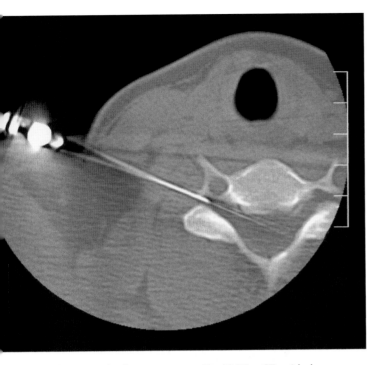

▲ **Fig. 10.39** In the same case as Fig. 10.38, a CT-guided interventional nerve root sleeve block has been performed for pain relief. The nerve was successfully blocked with 3 cc of bupivacaine followed by 2 cc of celestone chronodose for prolonged relief. Note the angle of approach with a 22-gauge, 5 cm needle, with its tip within the intervertebral foramen posterior to the vertebral artery. The carotid and jugular lie well anterior to the line of approach at this level, but become progressively more posteriorly placed as these vessels progress up the cervical region. They often lie parallel to the vertebral artery at C3/4, making the procedure technically more difficult at this level.

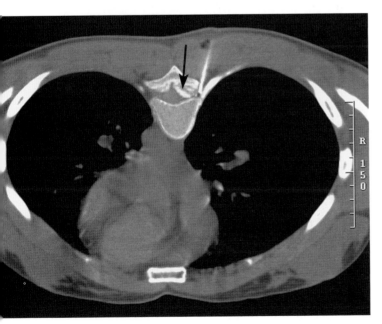

▲ **Fig. 10.40** Compression of an exiting mid-thoracic nerve root caused by a calcified and hypertrophied ligamentum flavum (arrow) in an elite javelin thrower. The needle is well positioned, with its tip lying adjacent to the exiting nerve root. Pain relief was achieved by an injection of bupivacaine.

The use of a 9 cm needle should be avoided in the neck. It is seldom necessary, even with athletes with a thick neck. Most nerve roots can be reached with a 5 cm needle and most often, except for very thin patients, the central canal is less likely to be inadvertently reached.

Complications

There have been reports of a number of complications from this procedure in the neck and a few in the lumbar region. Most of the complications have been assumed to have occurred as a result of vascular injury or penetration (Furman et al. 2003). In the neck, most, if not all, of these complications have occurred when the injections have been made blind, without imaging guidance, or have been performed with fluoroscopic guidance. Using CT for guidance with or without CT fluoroscopy gives a significantly increased level of confidence for needle placement and a reduced likelihood of complications. Axial images demonstrate the anatomy and identify the position of the vertebral and carotid arteries even without contrast, providing increased safety.

The most devastating complications occur when the cord or brain is involved from dissection of the vertebral artery or from what is presumed to be an inadvertent intra-arterial injection, either into the vertebral artery or into the tiny radicular artery that accompanies the nerve root in the intervertebral foramen. To some extent the prior injection of contrast will give the operator reassurance if the procedure is being performed under fluoroscopy, but this does not entirely eliminate the possibility. As previously noted, the use of a short, bevelled 22-gauge needle rather than a fine 25-gauge cutting needle reduces the likelihood of arterial penetration.

Thoracic spine NRSBs: technique and anatomy

Radicular pain due to neural compression is less common in the thoracic region but is nonetheless performance-limiting if the nerve root is being compromised. The compression is rarely due to a disc protrusion and is more likely to occur within the intervertebral foramen due to osteophytes or compression from the ligamentum flavum (see Fig. 10.40). This structure is often seen to calcify or ossify in older patients but may also calcify following trauma in younger patients and in athletes undertaking sports such as the shot-put, hammer throw and javelin, which are associated with extreme axial torsion.

For the procedure the patient is placed in the prone position. The symptomatic level is established clinically and the anatomical level is determined with imaging. By far the best method is to introduce the needle under CT guidance. A pneumothorax is much easier to avoid using this method. Following simple guidelines avoids problems. Having established the ideal angle of approach with CT and measured the depth to the target, the skin is anaesthetised. Gradual introduction of the needle, monitored with intermittent images to confirm the angle of approach, allows the interventionist to safely enter the target adjacent to the exiting nerve root. A contrast injection can be performed if required and this will show contrast entering the epineural space and often the epidural space. The nerve is blocked with 1 or 1.5 cc of bupivacaine. Celestone chronodose can be injected as well, if appropriate for the athlete.

Complications

Vascular penetration is much less likely in the thoracic region but is still a possibility and the same precautions need to be taken as in the cervical region. Infection is unlikely with aseptic precautions. Avoiding a pneumothorax needs to be a consideration.

Lumbar NRSBs: technique and anatomy

The clinical distinction between true sciatica (lumbar radicular pain) and referred pain from facet or discogenic pain can be difficult. Diagnostic lumbar nerve root blocks can be helpful in confirming the clinical impression of neural compression. The simultaneous injection of celestone chronodose can also be therapeutic by producing a more prolonged period of pain relief. In the lumbar region, CT guidance gives a confident approach and these blocks have a significantly lower morbidity than their cervical counterparts. The neural compression may be due to a disc protrusion, central spinal stenosis, foraminal stenosis or occasionally to a synovial cyst. Synovial cysts may sometimes be ablated by needle aspiration and corticosteroid injections (see Fig. 10.41).

Lumbar nerve root sleeve blocks can be performed under fluoroscopic (see Fig. 10.42) or CT guidance (see Fig. 10.43).

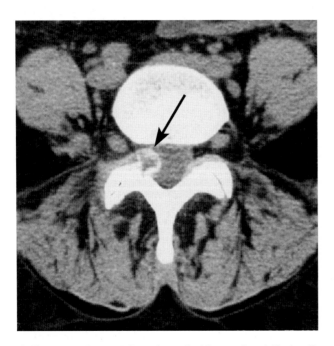

▲ **Fig. 10.41** A synovial cyst (arrow) with a partly calcified wall arising from an arthritic lumbar facet joint (arrow). Aspiration of these cysts can be achieved by using a pre-curved needle tip.

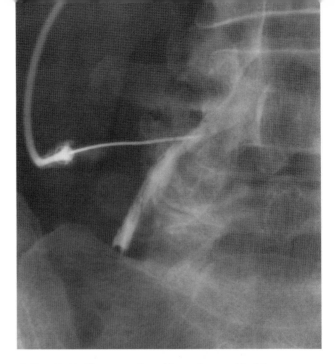

▲ **Fig. 10.42** Fluoroscopic guidance has enabled the placement of the needle tip into the perineural sheath, which is subsequently outlined by contrast.

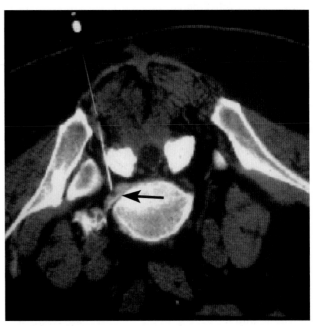

▲ **Fig. 10.43** An axial CT study shows contrast medium outlining the L5 perineural sheath at L5/S1 on the right (arrow). Occasionally, when the lumbar lordosis is marked, an angled gantry approach may be helpful.

The symptomatic level is established clinically, often with confirmatory imaging of nerve root compression. The patient is placed in the prone position and a needle is introduced obliquely from the flank to reach and penetrate the nerve sheath. This will confirm the dermatome distribution of the targeted root. This is followed by an injection of up to 3 cc of bupivacaine. This injection can be quite painful for a few seconds. After the effect of the anaesthetic is established, an injection of celestone chronodose can be performed to try to achieve a more prolonged period of pain relief. The downside of these injections in the athlete is that there is a period of motor disturbance for about eight hours, during which time motor weakness can be quite pronounced.

Complications

Apart from the previously noted transient pain on injection, possible motor disturbance and transient weakness, complications are unusual. There is also possibility of a haematoma and a theoretical chance of infection.

Unlike the cervical region, there are very few potential complications when performing lumbar and sacral NRSBs whether they are performed under CT guidance (preferred) or fluoroscopy.

Lumbar NRSBs do not share the potential vascular invasion complications associated with cervical injections. However, it should be recognised that the injection into the nerve sheath or into the perineural or periradicular tissues will often result in a degree of infiltration of injectate into the adjacent epidural space. This can easily be shown if contrast is simultaneously injected. The clinically evident complications associated with this spread are generally transient and of little consequence. Rarely, a patient experiences transient bilateral leg weakness due to transepidural spread of the anaesthetic agent. Conjecturally, some of the therapeutic effects of the steroid may be due to this epidural component of the injectate. Occasionally a patient will experience transient accentuation of their symptoms, usually settling in 24 to 48 hours.

Inadvertent injection into the subarachnoid space is rare but, in this regard, the presence of subarachnoid or Tarlov cysts should be recognised and represent a contraindication for this procedure in the sacral canal. Inadvertent injection of steroid into the subarachnoid space should be avoided to circumvent the implication that the subsequent development of adhesive arachnoiditis and aseptic meningitis may have been caused by the procedure. Additionally, a puncture of the subarachnoid space has the potential to produce a CSF leak, resulting in a low-pressure headache possibly requiring a blood patch (see below).

Infection is extremely rare when an appropriate aseptic technique has been used, although the potential for discitis should be kept in mind if the needle enters the annulus.

As with an injection of steroid elsewhere, occasional transient headaches, nausea or facial and sometimes widespread skin flushing may occur, settling within 24–48 hours and requiring no more than patient reassurance.

Spontaneous cerebrospinal fluid leaks

Spontaneous cerebrospinal fluid (CSF) leaks are most often spontaneous but occasionally are thought to be secondary to bony spurs in the cervical spine and possibly caused by a sharp calcified ligamentum flavum in the thoracic region. The exact aetiology in any one case is generally difficult to determine (Eross et al. 2002). The syndrome of low-pressure headaches is well recognised after lumbar puncture and

sometimes after spinal surgery. A spontaneous CSF leak can be difficult to treat. While not a common problem, it is assumed that the dura is torn or punctured and possibly precipitated by excessive spinal flexion. The syndrome of low-pressure headaches needs to be kept in mind for patients of all ages presenting with headaches that are present only in the erect posture and completely disappear when lying flat.

The condition can be diagnosed with CT myelography (see Fig. 10.44) or MRI where the CSF leak is seen into the epidural space. MRI may also show cerebral meningeal enhancement and a subdural collection. Radionuclide cisternography may aid in diagnosing this condition, but this method is more difficult to interpret precisely.

Initial treatment is conservative and includes horizontal bed rest and adequate hydration with intravenous infusion. If conservative measures fail, an epidural blood patch is worth considering (Dillo et al. 2002) (see Fig. 10.45). In the authors' experience of three cases, there was rapid and permanent relief following a CT-guided blood patch intervention. The authors' method utilises CT for guidance with spiral acquisition. The level and angle of approach are selected and documented at a site as close as practical to the level of the leak. A 22-gauge spinal needle is obliquely advanced into the epidural space and its position is confirmed with the

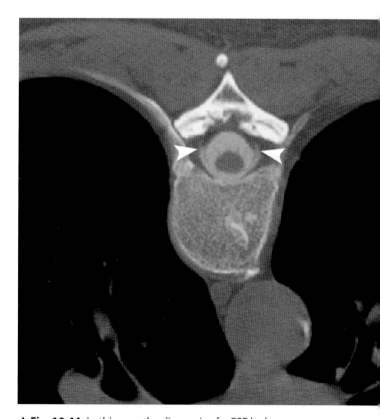

▲ **Fig. 10.44** In this case the diagnosis of a CSF leak was confirmed by injecting contrast into the lumbar subarachnoid space, which was then gravitated into the mid-thoracic region, where this axial CT image clearly shows the contrast leaking into the epidural space. Note the contrast spreading around the epidural space from anterior to posterior (arrowheads).

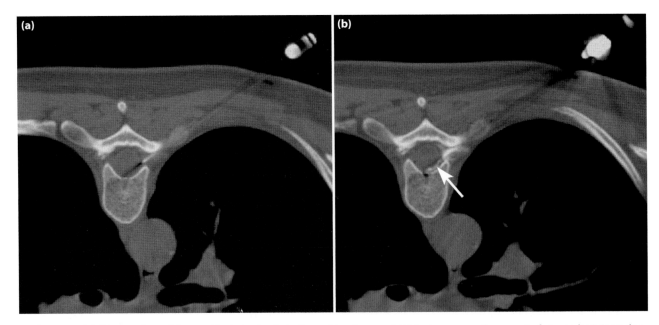

▲ **Fig. 10.45(a)** The artefact of the needle tip is clearly in the epidural space. At this stage a small amount of air can be injected to confirm that the needle is in the correct space. **(b)** The contrast-enhanced blood of the patient is injected into the epidural space (arrow). This patient had been incapacitated for several months with undiagnosed postural headache. Her symptoms resolved in less than one hour and she has remained completely symptom-free.

injection of a small volume of air or contrast. Next, 10–20 cc of the patient's own blood is drawn from an appropriate vein and mixed with 1 or 2 cc of contrast. This mixture is injected slowly into the epidural space while continually monitoring the progress of the contrast-enhanced blood with spiral acquisition to establish a good volume spreading upwards and downwards from the injection site. The volume injected may be limited if the patient experiences pain. The volume does not seem to be a major factor in achieving a positive result, which can be expected in less than an hour.

References

Acevedo JI, Beskin JL. 'Complications of plantar fascia rupture associated with corticosteroid injection.' *Foot Ankle Int* 1998, 19(2): 91–7.

Aina R, Cardinal E, Bureau NJ, Aubin B, Brassard P. 'Calcific shoulder tendinitis: treatment with modified US-guided fine-needle technique.' *Radiology* 2001, 221(2): 455–61.

Alexeeff M. 'Ligamentum patellae rupture following local steroid injection.' *Aust NZ J Surg* 1986, 56(9): 681–3.

Andren L, Eiken O. 'Arthrographic studies of wrist ganglions.' *J Bone Joint Surg (Am)* 1971, 53(2): 299–302.

Angelides AC. 'Ganglions of the hand and wrist.' In Green DP (ed.), *Operative Hand Surgery*, 2nd edn, Churchill Livingstone, New York, 1988. pp. 2281–99.

Barnsley L, Lord S, Bogduk N. 'Comparative local anaesthetic blocks in the diagnosis of cervical zygapophyseal joint pain.' *Pain* 1993, 55(1): 99–106.

Bell S, Coghlan J, Richardson M. 'Hydrodilatation in the management of shoulder capsulitis.' *Ausral Radiol* 2003, 47(3): 247–51.

Binder AI, Bulgen DY, Hazleman BL, Roberts S. 'Frozen shoulder: a long-term prospective study.' *Ann Rheum Dis* 1984, 43(3): 361–4.

Blazina ME, Kerlan RK, Jobe FW, Carter VS, Carlson GJ. 'Jumper's knee.' *Orthop Clin North Am* 1973, 4(3): 665–78.

Bogduk N. 'The clinical anatomy of the cervical dorsal rami.' *Spine* 1982, 7(4): 319–30.

Bogduk N. et al. 'Practice Standards & Protocols. Cervical medial branch blocks.' *Australian Musculoskeletal Medicine* 2001 (available at www.musmed.com/, accessed 16 October 2005).

Bogduk N, Marsland A. 'On the concept of third occipital headache.' *J Neurol Neurosurg Psychiatry* 1986, 49(7): 775–80.

Bogduk N, Modic MT. 'Lumbar discography.' *Spine* 1996, 21(3): 402–4.

Brukner PD, Khan K (eds), *Clinical Sports Medicine*, 2nd edn, McGraw-Hill, Sydney, 2001.

Bunker TD. 'Time for a new name for "frozen shoulder".' *Br Med J (Clin Res Ed)* 1985, 290: 1233–4.

Burke FD, Melikyan EY, Bradley MJ, Dias JJ. 'Primary care referral protocol for wrist ganglia.' *Postgrad Med J* 2003, 79(932): 329–31.

Chua WH, Bogduk N. 'The surgical anatomy of thoracic facet denervation.' *Acta Neurochir (Wien)* 1995, 136(3–4): 140–4.

Clancy WG Jr, Neidhart D, Brand RL. 'Achilles tendonitis in runners: a report of five cases.' *Am J Sports Med* 1976, 4(2): 46–57.

Clay NR, Clement DA. 'The treatment of dorsal wrist ganglia by radical excision.' *J Hand Surg (Br)* 1988, 13(2): 187–91.

Crawford F, Atkins D, Young P, Edwards J. 'Steroid injection for heel pain: evidence of short-term effectiveness. A randomized controlled trial.' *Rheumatology (Oxford)* 1999, 38(10): 974–7.

Dalinka MK, Turner ML, Osterman AL, Batra P. 'Wrist arthrography.' *Radiol Clin North Am* 1981, 19(2): 217–26.

Dias J, Buch K. 'Palmar wrist ganglion: does intervention improve outcome? A prospective study of the natural history and patient-reported treatment outcomes.' *J Hand Surg (Br)* 2003, 28(2): 172–6.

Dillo W, Hollenhorst J, Brassel F, von Hof-Strobach K, Heidenreich F, Johannes S. 'Successful treatment of a spontaneous cervical cerebrospinal fluid leak with a CT guided epidural blood patch.' *J Neurol* 2002, 249(2): 224–5.

Dockery GL. 'The treatment of intermetatarsal neuromas with 4% alcohol sclerosing injections.' *J Foot Ankle Surg* 1999, 38(6): 403–8.

Eross EJ, Dodick DW, Nelson KD, Bosch P, Lyons M. 'Orthostatic headache syndrome with CSF leak secondary to bony pathology of the cervical spine.' *Cephalalgia* 2002, 22(6): 439–43.

Eustace JA, Brophy DP, Gibney RP, Bresnihan B, FitzGerald O. 'Comparison of the accuracy of steroid placement with clinical outcome in patients with shoulder symptoms.' *Ann Rheum Dis* 1995, 38: 59–63.

Fadale PD, Wiggins ME. 'Corticosteroid injections: their use and abuse.' *J Am Acad Orthop Surg* 1994, 2(3): 133–40.

Faithfull DK, Seeto BG. 'The simple wrist ganglion: more than a minor surgical procedure?' *Hand Surg* 2000, 5(2): 139–43.

Farin PU, Jaroma H, Soimakallio S. 'Rotator cuff calcifications: treatment with US-guided technique.' *Radiology* 1995, 195(3): 841–3.

Fornage BD, Rifkin MD. 'Ultrasound examination of the hand and foot.' *Radiol Clin North Am* 1988, 26(1): 109–29.

Fraser RD, Osti OL, Vernon-Roberts B. 'Discitis after discography.' *J Bone Joint Surg (Br)* 1987, 69(1): 26–35.

Furman MB, Giovanniello MT, O'Brien EM. 'Incidence of intravascular penetration in transforaminal cervical epidural steroid injections.' *Spine* 2003, 28(1): 21–5.

Furey JG. 'Plantar fasciitis. The painful heel syndrome.' *J Bone Joint Surg (Am)* 1975, 57(5): 672–3.

Gerritsen AA, de Krom MC, Struijs MA, Scholten RJ, de Vet HC, Bouter LM. 'Conservative treatment options for carpal tunnel syndrome: a systematic review of randomised controlled trials.' *J Neurol* 2002, 249(3): 272–80.

Gray RG, Gottlieb NL. 'Intra-articular corticosteroids. An updated assessment.' *Clin Orthop Relat Res* 1983, 177: 235–63.

Guyer RD, Ohnmeiss DD. 'Lumbar discography. Position statement from the North American Spine Society Diagnostic and Therapeutic Committee.' *Spine* 1995, 20(18): 2048–59.

Harms J, Biehl G, von Hohbach G. 'Pathology of paratenonitis achilleae in athletes' (in German). *Arch Orthop Unfallchir* 1977, 88(1): 65–74.

Hollander JL. 'Intra-articular hydrocortisone in arthritis and allied conditions, a summary of two years' clinical experience.' *J Bone Joint Surg (Am)* 1953, 35–A(4): 983–90.

Holm PC, Pandey SD. 'Treatment of ganglia of the hand and wrist with aspiration and injection of hydrocortisone.' *Hand* 1973, 5(1): 63–8.

Holt MA, Keene JS, Graf BK, Helwig DC. 'Treatment of osteitis pubis in athletes. Results of corticosteroid injections.' *Am J Sports Med* 1995, 23(5): 601–6.

Hough DM, Wittenberg KH, Pawlina W, Maus TP, King BF, Vrtiska TJ, Farrell MA, Antolak SJ Jr. 'Chronic perineal pain caused by pudendal nerve entrapment: anatomy and CT-guided perineural injection technique.' *Am J Roentgenol* 2003, 181(2): 561–7.

Hunt TR, Osterman AL. 'Complications of the treatment of carpal tunnel syndrome.' *Hand Clin* 1994, 10(1): 63–71.

Jacobs LG, Barton MA, Wallace WA, Ferrousis J, Dunn NA, Bossingham DH. 'Intra-articular distension and steroids in the management of capsulitis of the shoulder.' *BMJ* 1991, 302: 1498–501.

Jacobs LG, Govaers KJ. 'The volar wrist ganglion: just a simple cyst?' *J Hand Surg (Br)* 1990, 15(3): 342–6.

Jarvinen M, Jozsa L, Kannus P, Jarvinen TL, Kvist M, Leadbetter W. 'Histopathological findings in chronic tendon disorders.' *Scand J Med Sci Sports* 1997, 7(2): 86–95.

Jayson MI, Dixon AS. 'Valvular mechanisms in juxta-articular cysts.' *Ann Rheum Dis* 1970, 29(4): 415–20.

Jones A, Regan M, Ledingham J, Pattrick M, Manhire A, Doherty M. 'Importance of placement of intra-articular steroid injections.' *BMJ* 1993, 307: 1329–30.

Kane D, Greaney T, Bresnihan B, Gibney R, Fitzgerald O. 'Ultrasound-guided injection of recalcitrant plantar fasciitis.' *Ann Rheum Dis* 1998, 57(6): 383–4.

Kerlan RK, Glousman RE. 'Injections and techniques in athletic medicine.' *Clin Sports Med* 1989, 8(3): 541–60.

Kim HJ, Ryu KN, Sung DW, Park YK. 'Correlation between sonographic and pathologic findings in muscle injury: experimental study in the rabbit.' *J Ultrasound Med* 2002, 21(10): 1113–19.

Kvist M, Jozsa L, Jarvinen M. 'Vascular changes in the ruptured Achilles tendon and paratenon.' *Int Orthop* 1992, 16(4): 377–82.

Kvist M, Jozsa L, Jarvinen M, Kvist H. 'Fine structural alterations in chronic Achilles paratenonitis in athletes.' *Pathol Res Pract* 1985, 180(4): 416–23.

Locke S. 'Local anaesthetic use in sport.' Australian College of Sports Physicians Position Statement, Cabal, 10–11 May 2002 (available at www.injuryupdate.com.au/images/research/Cabal02localdraft.pdf, accessed 2 November 2005).

Lord SM, Barnsley L, Wallis BJ, Bogduk N. 'Third occipital nerve headache: a prevalence study.' *J Neurol Neurosurg Psychiatry* 1994, 57(10): 1187–90.

Lucas PE, Hurwitz SR, Kaplan PA, Dussault RG, Maurer EJ. 'Fluoroscopically guided injections into the foot and ankle: localization of the source of pain as a guide to treatment—prospective study.' *Radiology* 1997, 204(2): 411–15.

MacCollum MS. 'Dorsal wrist ganglions in children.' *J Hand Surg (Am)* 1977, 2(4): 325.

Marshall S, Tardif G, Ashworth N. 'Local corticosteroid injection for carpal tunnel syndrome.' *The Cochrane Database of Systematic Reviews* 2002, 4. (Art. No. CD001554. DOI: 10.1002/14651858.CD001554.)

Nelson C. 'Anaesthetic injections in football: a case series helps to fill the information void.' *Sports Med Digest* 2002, 17: 53–5.

Neviaser J. 'Adhesive capsulitis of the shoulder: a study of pathologic findings in periarthritis of the shoulder.' *J Bone Joint Surg (Am)* 1945, 27: 211–22.

Newberg AH. 'Anaesthetic and corticosteroid joint injections: a primer.' *Semin Musculoskelet Radiol* 1998, 2(4): 415–20.

Nichols AW. 'Complications associated with the use of corticosteroids in the treatment of athletic injuries.' *Clin J Sports Med* 2005, 15(5): 370–5.

Nield DV, Evans DM. 'Aspiration of ganglia.' *J Hand Surg (Br)* 1986, 11(2): 264.

Normandin C, Seban E, Laredo JD, N'Guyen D, Kuntz D, Bard M. 'Aspiration of tendinous calcific deposits.' In Bard M, Laredo JD (eds), *Interventional Radiology in Bone and Joint*, Springer-Verlag, New York, 1988. pp. 258–70.

O'Connell MJ, Powell T, McCaffrey NM, O'Connell D, Eustace SJ. 'Symphyseal cleft injection in the diagnosis and treatment of osteitis pubis in athletes.' *Am J Roentgenol* 2002, 179(4): 955–9.

Oni JA. 'Treatment of ganglia by aspiration alone.' *J Hand Surg (Br)* 1992, 17(6): 660.

Orchard J. 'Is it safe to use local anaesthetic painkilling injections in professional football?' *Sports Med* 2004, 34(4): 209–19.

Orchard J. 'Tendon injections: does it matter what you use?' *Sport Health* 2003, 21(3): 25–7 (available at www.sma.org. au/publications/sporthealth/, accessed 12 October 2005).

Orchard J. 'Benefit and risks of using local anaesthetic for pain relief to allow early return to play in professional football.' *Br J Sports Med* 2002, 36: 209–13.

Orchard J. 'The use of local anaesthetic injections in professional football.' *Br J Sports Med* 2001, 35(4): 212–13.

Osti OL, Fraser RD, Vernon-Roberts B. 'Discitis after discography. The role of prophylactic antibiotics.' *J Bone Joint Surg (Br)* 1990, 72(2): 271–4.

Otu AA. 'Wrist and hand ganglion treatment with hyaluronidase injection and fine needle aspiration: a tropical African perspective.' *J Roy Coll Surg Edinb* 1992, 37(6): 405–7.

Paavola M, Kannus P, Jarvinen TA, Jarvinen TL, Jozsa L, Jarvinen M. 'Treatment of tendon disorders. Is there a role for corticosteroid injection?' *Foot Ankle Clin* 2002, 7(3): 501–13.

Paul AS, Sochart DH. 'Improving the results of ganglion aspiration by the use of hyaluronidase.' *J Hand Surg (Br)* 1997, 22(2): 219–21.

Pfister J, Gerber H. 'Chronic calcifying tendinitis of the shoulder—therapy by percutaneous needle aspiration and lavage: a prospective open study of 62 shoulders.' *Clin Rheumatol* 1997, 16(3): 269–74.

Puddu G, Ippolito E, Postacchini F. 'A classification of Achilles tendon disease.' *Am J Sports Med* 1976, 4(4): 145–50.

Read JW, Peduto AJ. 'Tendon imaging.' *Sports Medicine and Arthroscopy Review* 2000, 8: 32–55.

Richman JA, Gelberman RH, Engber WD, Salamon PB, Bean DJ. 'Ganglions of the wrist and digits: results of treatment by aspiration and cyst wall puncture.' *J Hand Surg (Am)* 1987, 12(6): 1041–3.

Rosson JW, Walker G. 'The natural history of ganglia in children.' *J Bone Joint Surg (Br)* 1989, 71(4): 707–8.

Sachs BL, Vanharanta H, Spivey MA, Guyer RD, Videman T, Rashbaum RF, Johnson RG, Hochschuler SH, Mooney V. 'Dallas discogram description. A new classification of CT/ discography in low-back disorders.' *Spine* 1987, 12(3): 287–94.

Schellhas KP, Pollei SR, Dorwart RH. 'Thoracic discography. A safe and reliable technique.' *Spine* 1994, 19(18): 2103–9.

Seki JT, Bell MSG. 'Treatment of carpal and digital ganglions by simple aspiration or aspiration and injection of corticosteroid and/or hyaluronidase.' *Canadian J Plastic Surg* 1997, 5(4): 233–7.

Sellman JR. 'Plantar fascia rupture associated with corticosteroid injection.' *Foot Ankle Int* 1994, 15(7): 376–81.

Shaffer B, Tibone JE, Kerlan RK. 'Frozen shoulder. A long-term follow–up.' *J Bone Joint Surg (Am)* 1992, 74(5): 738–46.

Stannard JP, Bucknell AL. 'Rupture of the triceps tendon associated with steroid injections.' *Am J Sports Med* 1993, 21(3): 482–5.

Stephen AB, Lyons AR, Davis TR. 'A prospective study of two conservative treatments for ganglia of the wrist.' *J Hand Surg (Br)* 1999, 24(1): 104–5.

Van Holsbeek M, Introcaso JH. 'Musculoskeletal ultrasonography.' *Radiol Clin North Am* 1992, 30(5): 907–25.

Varley GW, Needoff M, Davis TR, Clay NR. 'Conservative management of wrist ganglion. Aspiration versus steroid infiltration.' *J Hand Surg (Br)* 1997, 22(5): 636–7.

Wicks JD, Silver TM, Bree RL. 'Gray scale features of hematomas: an ultrasonic spectrum.' *Am J Roentgenol* 1978, 131(6): 977–80.

Williams JG. 'Achilles tendon lesions in sport.' *Sports Med* 1986, 3(2): 114–35.

Wright TW, Cooney WP, Ilstrup DM. 'Anterior wrist ganglion.' *J Hand Surg (Am)* 1994, 19(6): 954–8.

Young CC, Rutherford DS, Niedfeldt MW. 'Treatment of plantar fasciitis.' *Am Fam Physician* 2001, 63(3): 467–78.

Zubowicz VN, Ishii CH. 'Management of ganglion cysts of the hand by simple aspiration.' *J Hand Surg (Am)* 1987, 12(4): 618–20.

Zwar RB, Read JW, Noakes JB. 'Sonographically guided glenohumeral joint injection.' *Am J Roentgenol* 2004, 183(1): 48–50.

Image acknowledgments

The authors wish to thank the following colleagues who kindly offered images for inclusion in this chapter:

- Dr David Lisle, QDI (Figs 10.2(a) and 10.5)
- Dr Phil Lucas (Fig. 10.42)

These images have significantly added to the quality of the chapter.

Index